MW01640050

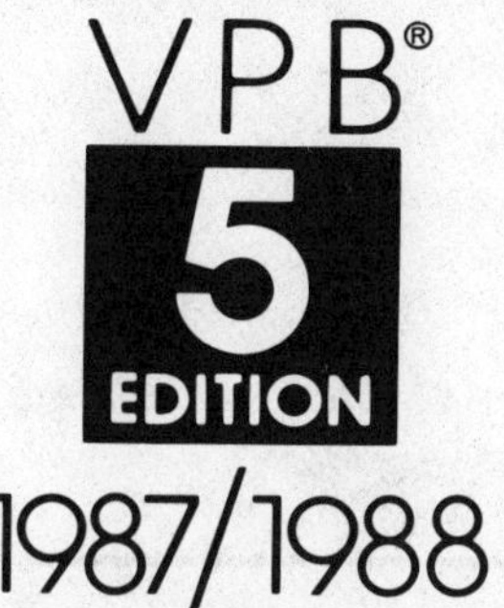

1987/1988

VETERINARY PHARMACEUTICALS AND BIOLOGICALS®

Andrew J. Weber
President/Publisher

Sandra Grey
Book Manager

Kim Townsend, DVM
Technical Editor

Margaret Rampey
Assistant Editor

Rosa Lee Metzler
Editorial Assistant

Scott Johnson
Director
Corporate Communications

Library of Congress Catalog Number LC85-647677
0-87489-843-9

Foreward to the Fifth Edition

This edition of VETERINARY PHARMACEUTICALS AND BIOLOGICALS includes the latest available information on pharmaceuticals and biologicals used in veterinary medicine. We have updated the appendixes, revised the indexes to better meet the practitioner's needs, and expanded the Product Information section with the addition of several new companies.

VPB is published biennially by Veterinary Medicine Publishing Company, Inc. in collaboration with the manufacturers whose products appear in the book. We wish to acknowledge the excellent cooperation we have received from the pharmaceutical industry in the preparation of this reference.

ANDREW J. WEBER
Publisher

DISCLAIMER: The information presented in this book has been supplied by the manufacturers in all cases. It must be pointed out that the information is presented as a reference and it remains the responsibility of the veterinarian to familiarize himself/herself with the information contained on the package insert accompanying each product. No reference to any name is intended as a suggestion to violate any trademarks or patents.

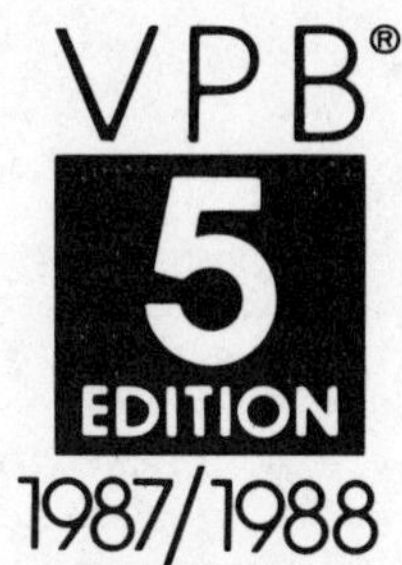

Contents

SECTION 1

Alphabetical List of Manufacturers

Manufacturers are presented alphabetically in this section. Following each manufacturer's name is a complete listing of products included in this edition. Where the symbol ♦ appears, the product can be visually identified by referring to Section 5, the Product Identification section.

PAGE

ADAMS VETERINARY RESEARCH LABS., INC. 502, 922
P.O. Box 971039
Miami, FL 33197
Anti-Crawl Residual Insecticide
Anti-Crawl Room Fogger
Anti-Sept
Caniderm Mist
Feliderm Mist
Feli-Tinic
Flea Off Dip
Flea Off Dust II
Flea Off Ear Mite Lotion
Flea Off Mist
Flea Off Residual Mist
Flea Off Shampoo
Klean Shampoo
Liquid Ear Dessicant
Lotion Of Sulfur
Nutri-Tinic
Pan-Otic
Pan-San
Skin Conditioner and Softener
Sulfur Shampoo
Sulfur Tar Shampoo
Surface Spray

AMERICAN HOECHST CORPORATION
See HOECHST-ROUSSEL AGRI-VET COMPANY

ANTHONY PRODUCTS COMPANY 505
5600 Peck Road
Arcadia, CA 91006
Dexameth-A-Vet Injection
Dex-A-Vet Injection
Diuride
Fura-Septin
Oxytocin Injection
Phen-Buta-Vet Injection & Tablets

BARRY LABORATORIES, INC. 509, 958
Veterinary Division
461 N.E. 27th St.
Pompano Beach, FL 33064
Allergenic Extract
Allergenic Extract, Flea Antigen
Allergenic Extract, Flea Antigen for Intradermal Testing
Allergenic Extract, Intradermal Test Kit
Allergenic Extract, Prescription Product

BEECHAM LABORATORIES 401, 509, 922
501 Fifth St.
Bristol, TN 37620
Amoxi-Drop
Amoxi-Inject for Cattle
Amoxi-Inject for Cats & Dogs
Amoxi-Sol/Amoxi-Bol
♦Amoxi-Tabs
Amp-Equine
Atrobac-P
Atrobac-R
Benza-Pen
Clavamox Drops
♦Clavamox Tablets
Coli-Bovis
Coli-Suis
Dariclox
Farrowgen
Granulex-V
IBR/BVD/PI_3
IBR/PI_3/Somubac
Imathal Equine
Leptomune-5
Leptopar
Lixotinic
Mycodex Aqua-Spray
Mycodex Creme HC
Mycodex Flea & Tick Spray
Mycodex Mini-Fog
Mycodex Pearlescent Grooming Shampoo
Mycodex Pet Shampoo with Pyrethrins
Mycodex Pet Shampoo with Allethrin
Mycodex Pet Shampoo with Carbaryl
Mycodex Pet Shampoo with 3X Pyrethrins
Mycodex Powder Plus
Mycodex Room and Carpet Accu-Spray
Mycodex Room Fogger
Mycodex Tar & Sulfur Pet Shampoo
Nasamune-IP
Orbenin-DC
Oti-Clens
Panacine RC
Panavac
Panavac RC
Penicillin G Procaine
♦Pet-Cal
♦Pet-Dec
Pet-Derm, III
Pet-F.A. Liquid
Pet-Tabs
♦Pet-Tabs/F. A. Granules
♦Pet-Tabs Feline
♦Pet-Tabs Jr.
Pet-Tabs Plus
Pet-Tinic
Pneumosuis II
Porci-Rab
Rabcine
Rabmune-3
Re-Sorb
Ripercol Piperazine
Salmonella Bacterin

(♦ Shown in Product Identification Section)

(◆ Shown in Product Identification Section)

(◆ Shown in Product Identification Section)

GLENWOOD INC. 937
83 N. Summit St.
Tenafly, NJ 07670
Calphosan Solution
Calphosan Suspension

GRANITE DIVISION, ENVIRONMENTAL DIAGNOSTICS, INC. 962
P.O. Box 908
2990 Anthony Road
Burlington, NC 27215
EZ-Screen: Aflatoxin
EZ-Screen: Chloramphenicol
EZ-Screen: Gentamicin
EZ-Screen: Neomycin
EZ-Screen: Penicillin
EZ-Screen: Sulfadimethoxine
EZ-Screen: Sulfamethazine
EZ-Screen Test System
EZ-Screen: Tylosin

HAVER 661, 937, 964
Mobay Corporation
Animal Health Division
Shawnee, KS 66201
Alobac-2
Baymix Crumbles
Caricide
Clostri-Bac 4
Clostri-Bac 7
Clostri-Bac 8
Clostri-Bac C&D
Clostri-Bac CS
Clostri-Bac CSN
Clostri-Bac CSP
Combot Liquid
Combot Paste
Combotel Paste
Co-Ral Animal Insecticide
Co-Ral Emulsifiable Livestock Insecticide
Co-Ral Livestock Duster
Co-Ral Pour-On
Co-Ral 25% Wettable Powder
Dexabiotic Aqueous Suspension
D.N.P.
Droncit Injectable
Droncit Tablets
Electrofin Powder
Electrofin Tabsules
Eltradd-4000
Encevac with Havlogen
Encevac-T with Havlogen
Encevac TC-4 with Havlogen
Ene-Pet Solution
Equicine II
Equicine–T
Equimate
Estrumate
Flea Antigen
Fleatol Shampoo
Foalchek
Hava-Cide Liquid
Hava-Span
Havidote
Havolac Food Supplement
Havo-Lep-5
Heifex Prostaglandin
H-L Bi-Pen
H-L Dex
Hy-Guard with Havlogen
Hypodermin Injection
Intranasal Bovine Rhinotracheitis
Kit-Tonne Laxative
KRS Spray Foam
Leg Tone Equine
Lysoff Insecticide
Neguvon Pour-On
Novin Injection
Novin Tablets
Odor-Ban Deodorant
Odor-Trol Tablets
Ovine-Ecthyma Vaccine
Para Ban-S
Paraboceptol–Bovine
Parabocine Bovine Rhinotracheitis-Parainfluenza 3
Para Mist Water Base
Para-M-1
Para Powder
Para-Premise
Para Pyrethrin Mist
Para S–1 Aerosol
Parguard
Proban
Pro-Kill Insecticide
Pro-Powder
Pro-Spot
Redwol with Spur
Rintal Paste
Rintal Suspension
Rompun 20
Rompun 100
Sendran Cat Collar
Sendran Flea and Tick Spray
Sendran Insecticide Shampoo
Sendran Liquid Tick & Flea Dip
Sendran Tick and Flea Collar
Spotton 20% Solution
Strepguard with Havlogen
Styquin
Styrid Caricide
Super-Tet
Tetanus Antitoxin
Thraxol–2
Tiguvon Pour-On (Cattle)
Tiguvon Pour-On (Swine)
Veltrim
Vercom Paste
Vibrio-Bac
Vibrio-Bac-H-L5
Vibrio-Bac-L
Vibrio-Bac-L5
Wart Vaccine

HILL'S PET PRODUCTS, INC. 937
P.O. Box 148
Topeka, KS 66601
Control Diet HRH
Prescription Diet Canine c/d
Prescription Diet Canine d/d
Prescription Diet Canine g/d
Prescription Diet Canine h/d
Prescription Diet Canine i/d
Prescription Diet Canine k/d
Prescription Diet Canine p/d
Prescription Diet Canine r/d
Prescription Diet Canine s/d
Prescription Diet Canine u/d
Prescription Diet Feline c/d
Prescription Diet Feline h/d
Prescription Diet Feline k/d
Prescription Diet Feline p/d
Prescription Diet Feline r/d
Prescription Diet Feline s/d
Science Diet Canine Growth
Science Diet Canine Maintenance
Science Diet Canine Performance
Science Diet Canine Senior
Science Diet Feline Growth
Science Diet Feline Maintenance
Science Diet Mixit

HOECHST-ROUSSEL AGRI-VET COMPANY 403, 682
Somerville, NJ 08876
Enzygnost Progesterone Test Kit
◆Lasix
Panacur (Horses)
Panacur Granules (Dogs)
Panacur Paste (Cattle)
Panacur Suspension (Cattle)
Regu–Mate
T–61 Euthanasia Solution

INTERNATIONAL MINERALS AND CHEMICAL CORP. 687
Animal Health & Nutrition Division
P.O. Box 207
Terre Haute, IN 47808
Ralgro

INTERNATIONAL MULTIFOODS
See OSBORN

LUITPOLD PHARMACEUTICALS, INC. 687
Animal Health Division
One Luitpold Drive
Shirley, NY 11967
Adequan

MOLECULAR GENETICS INC. 688, 965
10320 Bren Road East
Minnetonka, MN 55343
Coli-Tect 99
Genecol 99

MSD AGVET 403, 688
Division of Merck & Co., Inc.
P.O. Box 2000
Rahway, NJ 07065
Corid 9.6% Solution
Corid 1.25% Crumbles
Corid 20% Soluble Powder
◆Diuril Boluses & Tablets
Equizole A Liquid
Equizole Suspension
Eqvalan
Hydrozide Injection
Ivomec
Nalline Hydrochloride
Tresaderm

NORDEN LABORATORIES, INC. 693, 945, 965
601 W. Cornhusker
P.O. Box 80809
Lincoln, NE 68521
Anthelcide EQ Paste
Anthelcide EQ Suspension
Apralan
BovEye
BRSV
Calf-Guard
CalfSpan
Carmilax Bolets
Carmilax Powder
ClinEase-FeLV
Clostrin 7
CoughGuard-B
CoughGuard-BP
Cytobin Tablets
Darbazine Injection
Darbazine Spansule Capsules
E Coli Bac
Endurall-K
Endurall-R
ER Bac
ER Bac/Leptoferm-5
EVA
EVA/Leptoferm-5
Felobits
Felocell CVR
Felocine
Felomune CVR
Filaribits
Filaribits Plus
FirstDose CPV
Flea And Tick Powder for Cats & Dogs
Flea, Tick, and Mite Spray for Dogs, Cats, and Birds
Fleavol
Furacin Dressing
Furacin Soluble Powder
Furacin Water Mix
Furoxone Suspension
Geribits
Heathcliff's Flea And Tick Collar for Cats
Heathcliff's Flea And Tick Spray for Cats
Heathcliff's Flea, Tick, and Lice Dip for Cats
Leptoferm-P
Leptoferm-5
Leukocell
Life-Guard
Litterguard
Litterguard LT
Marmaduke Automatic Room Fogger
Marmaduke Flea & Tick Collar for Dogs
Marmaduke Flea And Tick Dip
Marmaduke Flea And Tick Spray for Dogs
Mitox Liquid
Neo-Darbazine
Norcalciphos
Nutriderm
Parvo-Vac
Parvo-Vac/Leptoferm-5
Pleuroguard
Pleuroguard 3
Pleuroguard 4
Pneumo-Guard H
Pragmatar*
Preg-Guard 9

(◆ Shown in Product Identification Section)

Pr–Vac
Pr–Vac—Killed
PR–VAC/Leptoferm-5
Rabguard-TC
Resbo BVD
Resbo IBL5
Resbo IBR
Resbo IBR-BVD
Resbo IBR-BVD-LP
Resbo IBR–LP
Resbo IBR-PI 3
Resbo 3
Resbo 4
Resbo 8
Rhinobac
Rhinobac-ER
Rhinobac-P
Rhinobac 3
Rhinomune
Rota-Vac TGE
Scourguard 3
Spanbolet II Tablets
Sulkamycin-S Bolettes
Sulkamycin-S Powder
Super Spray/Repellent for Dogs, Cats, and Horses
Temaril-P
Temaril-P Tablets
TGE Vaccine
Therabloat
Topazone
Tri-Sulfa-G
TSV-2
Vanguard CPV
Vanguard CPV (ML)
Vanguard DA_2L
Vanguard DA_2MP
Vanguard DA_2P
Vanguard DA_2P+CPV
Vanguard DA_2PL
Vanguard DA_2PL+CPV
Vanguard D–M
Vanguard DMP
Vibrin
Vibrio/Leptoferm-P
Vibrio/Leptoferm-5
Vi-Sorbin
Vi-Sorbits
Weanguard

OSBORN **403, 737, 946**
An Essar Corporation
P.O. Box 1590
Fort Dodge, IA 50501
Amcon
Beta-Con
◆Bovo-Cox Boluses
◆Bovo-Cox Calf Boluses
Bovo-Cox Powder
Bovo-Lyte Concentrate
Bovo-Lyte Powder
Butatron Oral Gel
◆Cal-Phos Palatabs
◆Carbam Palatabs
◆Carbam Tablets
Celulase
Conval
Dexamethasone Tablets
DXT–500
◆Dyrea–Aid Palatabs
Elpak–360
◆Endomagma Boluses
Endomagma Powder
Equi-Lyte Concentrate
Equi-Lyte Solution
◆Geriatric Vitamin Palatabs
Hema-Glo
IVS-1830
Kalamino
Kal-K-Dex
Ketoban
LBA Bolus
LBA-Gel
LBA Powder
Magnadex
Med-A-Sul
Mer-A-Lite
◆Methapyrin Boluses
Methionine Palatabs
Nitrozone Ointment
NRG–Plus
Plexamino Bolus
Plexamino II

SG–Seven
◆Sustain III
◆Sustain III Calf Bolus
Triple Sulfa-699
TS-543
◆Viceton Tablets
Vita-Glo
◆Vita-Min Palatabs

PFIZER, INC. **744, 947**
Agricultural Division
235 E. 42nd St.
New York, NY 10017
Combiotic
Liquamast
Liquamycin Injectable 50 mg/ml
Liquamycin 100 mg/ml
Liquamycin La–200
Nemex
Nemex Tabs
Nemex–2
Paratect
Pen BP-48
Procaine Penicillin G
Strongid Paste
Strongid-T
Terra–Cortril Spray
Terramycin Ophthalmic Ointment
Vitamin A & D Injectable

PHARMADERM **753**
A Division of Altana Inc.
60 Baylis Road
Melville, NY 11747
Cat Lax

PIONEER BRAND MICROBIAL PRODUCTS **754**
Pioneer Hi-Bred Intl., Inc.
P.O. Box 258
Johnston, IA 50131
BRSV Vac
BRSV Vac 2
BRSV Vac 3
BRSV Vac 4
BRSV Vac 9
Horizon I
Neo-Vac 7
Probiocin
Probiocin Brand Bolus
Probiocin Brand Dispersible
Probiocin Brand Equine One Gel
Probiocin Brand Granules
Probiocin Brand Pet Gel
Probiocin Brand Ruminant Gel
Probiocin Brand Swine Gel
TGE/Ecoli-Vac 4-C
TGE/Neo-Vac 7
TGE-Vac

PITMAN-MOORE, INC. **405, 761, 947, 966**
P.O. Box 344
Washington Crossing, NJ 08560
Bactassay*
Bactrovet*
Bactrovet Tablets
Bordegen*
Canex* Solution
Cerbinol* Solution
Conofite* Cream, 2%
Conofite* Lotion, 1%
Dermassay
Diryl*
Disposaject*
D-Tec CB
D-Tec DF
D–Tec* Foal IgG
D–Tec* MP
Ectoral
Entromycin* Powder
Equine Infectious Anemia
Filarassay*F
Fungassay*
FVR*–C–P
FVR*–C–P (MLV)
Imrab
Imrab–1
Inflogen
Inflogen–T
Innovar–Vet Injection
Kat–A–Lax*
K.F.L.*
Leukassay-B
Leukassay* F
Levasole* Cattle Wormer Boluses
Levasole* Gel
Levasole* Injectable Solution
Levasole* Sheep Wormer Boluses
Levasole* Soluble Drench Powder for Cattle & Sheep
Levasole* Soluble Drench Powder for Sheep
Levasole* Soluble Pig Wormer
Lubrivet* Concentrate
Metofane*
Ovassay*
Paladin*
Pellitol* Ointment
Pestisol*–R
P/M* Naloxone HCl
Porcimune*
Porcimune* B
Progestassay
Pseudovax*
Quantum*
Quantum* 4
Quantum* 6
Rhivin*
Rhusigen
Sirlene
Sprecto* Cat Insecticide Collar
Sprecto CCR
Sprecto*–CF Insecticide Fogger
Sprecto* Dog Insecticide Collar
Sprecto*–D Triple Action Dip
Sprecto*–F Total Release Fogger
Sprecto* with Repellent
Stiglyn* 1:500
Stresnil* Injection
Swivax* 6
Swivax* 6 & PVR
Swivax* 8
Telmin
Telmin* B
Telmin* Suspension
Telmin* Syringe Formula
Telmintic* Powder
Tetnogen
Tissuvax* 5
Tissuvax* 6
Titan*3
Toxoplasma Gondii Antibody Test
Triple-E
Triple-E FT
Triple-E T
◆Vermiplex* Capsules
Vetrachloracin
Vetropolycin* HC
Vetropolycin* Ophthalmic Ointment
Vitamycin*
V–Tergent* 8X
Weladol* Antiseptic Shampoo
Weladol* Disinfectant

THE PURDUE FREDERICK COMPANY **784**
100 Connecticut Ave.
Norwalk, CT 06856
Betadine Aerosol Spray
Betadine Ointment
Betadine Solution
Betadine Surgical Scrub

RHONE-POULENC INC. **785**
Feed Additives Division
500 Northridge Road
Suite 620
Atlanta, GA 30338
Deccox

A.H. ROBINS COMPANY **405, 786**
1407 Cummings Drive
Richmond, VA 23220
Bovicon-PM
Carpet Control
Dopram-V Injectable
Elanone–V
Guailaxin
Precon–PH
◆Robamox–V Tablets
Robamox–V Veterinary Oral Suspension
◆Robaxin-V Injectable & Tablets
Robinul-V Injectable
◆Viokase—V
◆Z–Bec

(◆ Shown in Product Identification Section)

ROCHE ANIMAL HEALTH AND NUTRITION, HOFFMANN-LA ROCHE INC. 405, 793
340 Kingsland St.
Nutley, NJ 07110
(201) 235-5000
◆Albon Boluses
◆Albon Injection-40%
Albon Soluble Powder
◆Albon-S.R. Bolus
◆Albon Tablets & Oral Suspension 5%
Albon 12.5% Drinking Water Solution
Alfavet
Injacom
Injacom 100
Injacom 100 +B-Complex
Ipropran

SOLVAY VETERINARY, INC. 406, 801
P.O. Box 7348
Princeton, NJ 08540
Crystiben
Crysticillin 300/AS
◆Dirocide Tablets & Syrup
Distrycillin– A.S.
Eclipse 1
Eclipse 1 KP
Eclipse 3
Eclipse 3 KP
Eclipse 3 KP-R
Eclipse 4
Eclipse 4 KP
Eclipse 4 KP-R
Equipoise
Flea Collar For Cats
Flea Collar For Dogs
Follutein
Fromm D
Galaxy DA_2L
Galaxy DA_2PL
Galaxy 6 MHP
Galaxy 6 MHP-L
Galaxy 6 MP-L
Panodry
Panolog Cream Veterinary
Panolog Ointment Veterinary
Parvoid 2
◆Princillin Boluses
◆Princillin 125, 250 & 500 Capsules
Princillin Soluble Powder
Psittacoid
Rabvac 1
Rabvac 3
Re-Covr Injection
◆Task
◆Task Tabs
Vetalog Cream
Vetalog Oral Powder
Vetalog Parenteral
◆Vetalog Tablets
◆Vetisulid Bolus, Injection, Oral Suspension & Powder
Xenodine
Xenodine Spray

SPECIALTY PET PRODUCTS, INC. 947
P.O. Box 58
Nashville, TN 37202
ANF Puppy Food
ANF 30
Tamiami Cat Food

E.R. SQUIBB & SONS
See SOLVAY VETERINARY, INC.

SYNTEX ANIMAL HEALTH, INC. 407, 820, 949
4800 Westown Parkway, Suite 200
West Des Moines, IA 50265
Subsidiary of Syntex Agribusiness, Inc.
Palo Alto, CA
Amcal Bolus
Anaprime
Benzelmin Equine Anthelmintic Paste
Benzelmin Equine Anthelmintic Suspension
Benzelmin Pellets
Benzelmin Plus
Benzelmin Powder
◆Bovilene
Dia–Glo L.A.
Dia–Glo S.A.
Diamino 4X
◆Di-Trim Tablets
Di-Trim 24% Injection
Di-Trim 48% Injection
Di-Trim 400 Oral Paste
Domoso Gel
Domoso Solution
Equine Proleen 775
Equiproxen
Flucort Solution
◆Flucort Tablets
Neo-Synalar Cream
Optiprime
Proleen T20
Repose
Spectinomycin Oral
Synalar Cream
Synotic Otic Solution
◆Synovex C
◆Synovex H
◆Synovex S
◆Tranvet Chewable Tablets

TECHAMERICA GROUP, INC. 846, 976
15th & Oak
P.O. Box 338
Elwood, KS 66024
Acepromazine Maleate Injection
Acepromazine Maleate Tablets
Adenomune-7
Adenomune 7-L
Aminoplex–C
Aminoplex Solution
Anestatal
Borditech-P
Borditech P-E
Bova Creme
Bronchicine
Calcium Gluconate
Cal–Phos
C.C.S.N.S.
Clostridial-7-Way
CMPK
Combiplex-B
Controller Flea & Tick Collar
Controller Flea-Kill Mist
Controller House & Carpet Spray
Deltox C & D
Dermaquel Pet Shampoo (w/Complex Iodine)
Dermaquel Pet Shampoo (Neutral concentrate)
Dermaquel (w/Sulfa-Tar)
Dexamycin
Dexasone
Dextrose Solution, 50%
Diasystems-Canine Parvo
Diasystems-FeLV
DiaSystems-Ovucare Cowside
DiaSystems-Ovucare 96 Well Plasma
Disal Injection
Disal Tablets
Dizan Tablets
Dual-Pen
Electro Solution
Erocon
Gentamicin Sulfate Injection
Herd-Vac 10
IBR-BVD PI 3
IBR-BVD-PI 3-Lepto 5
IBR-BVD-PI 3-Pasteurella
IBR-BVD-PI 3-SomnuTech
IBR-BVD-P13-VIBRIO-Lepto
IBR-PI 3
Iodo-Cam
Iron Dextran Complex Injection
Lepto 5
Medamycin
Medamycin-100
Methylprednisolone Acetate Injectable
Methylprednisolone Tablets
Multi–B Super
Nemacide –C
Nemacide Chewable Tablets
Nemacide Oral Syrup
Nemacide Tablets
Neo–Sul Jr.
Neo–Sul Sr.
Neurosyn
Nitrofurazone Dressing 0.2%
Nitrofurazone Soluble Powder
Nitrofurazone Solution 0.2%
Omnivac PRV
Oxytocin
Paramune-5
Parvocine
Parvocine-MLV
Parvotech-Lepto 5
Pen-Aqueous
Pen–Strep
Premier
Premier-IB
Premier IBL-5
Premier IBL-SomnuTech
Premier IBP
Premier IBPL5
Respomune-CP
Revive
Rhinopan-MLV
Somnutech
Tanisol
Tylosin Injection
Vibrio–Lepto 5
Vitamin A-D Injectable
Vitamino 4X

3M/ANIMAL CARE PRODUCTS 869
225-1N 3M Center
St. Paul, MN 55144
Duratrol #1488 Household Flea Spray
Duratrol #1489 Yard and Kennel Concentrate–Flea Spray
Sectrol Concentrate
Sectrol #1495 Pet and Household Flea Spray
Sectrol Two-Way Flea Foam
Sectrol Two-Way Pet Spray

THE UPJOHN COMPANY 407, 872, 951
7000 Portage Road
Kalamazoo, MI 49001
◆Albaplex Tablets
Bio-Delta
Biolyte
Biosol–Aquadrops
◆Biosol Bolus
Biosol Liquid
◆Biosol Tablets
Biosol 325
Brytin
Cheque Drops
◆Cortaba
◆Delta Albaplex
Depo–Medrol
DEPO-Penicillin
Drygard
ECP
Forte–Topical
◆Lincocin for Intramuscular, Intravenous, & Oral Use
Lincocin Soluble Powder
Lincocin Sterile Solution
Lutalyse
◆Medrol
Mitaban Liquid Concentrate
Mycitracin Sterile Ointment
Neo–Delta–Cortef
Neo–Predef
Neo–Predef with Tetracaine
Panmycin Aquadrops
◆Panmycin Hydrochloride
Petdrops
Predef 2X
Prostin F2 Alpha
Quartermaster* Suspension
Solu–Delta–Cortef
Special Formula 17900–Forte
Tritop Topical Ointment
Unilact Liquid or Powder
◆Unipet–C Tablets
◆Unipet Senior
◆Unipet Tablets

VET-A-MIX, INC. 408, 900, 952
604 W. Thomas Ave.
Shenandoah, IA 51601
Add-Plex
Ade-Sol
Aqua-Lite
Avi-Con
Bio-Meth
Bio-Tin 100
Bloat-Pac
Bovi-Form K
Diet-Derm
◆Diro-Form

(◆ Shown in Product Identification Section)

VPB®
5
EDITION
1987/1988

SECTION 2

Product Name Index

Products in this section are arranged alphabetically. The product name is followed by the name of the manufacturer and page number where full information is provided. Where the symbol ◆ appears, the product can also be visually identified by referring to Section 5, the Product Identification section.

(◆ Shown in Product Identification Section)   (Products without page numbers are not described)

(◆ Shown in Product Identification Section) (Products without page numbers are not described)

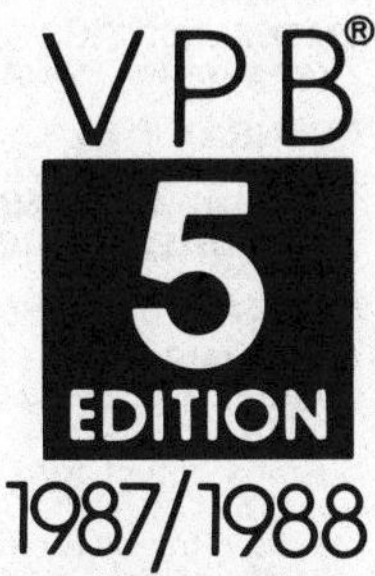

SECTION 3

Product Category Index

Products described in the Product Information, Diets and Nutritional Supplements, or Diagnostic Aids and Supplies sections are listed according to their classifications. The headings and sub-headings have been determined by the Publisher with the cooperation of the individual manufacturers. In cases where there were differences of opinion, or where the manufacturer had no opinion, the Publisher has made the final decision.

P

PANCREATITIS

PARASITICIDES, HOME USE

PARASITICIDES, LARGE ANIMALS EXTERNAL

PARASITICIDES, LARGE ANIMALS INTERNAL

PARASITICIDES, SMALL ANIMALS EXTERNAL

W

WARTS
(see under BOVINE VACCINES)

WATER

Injectable

WOODEN TONGUE
(see under ACTINOBACILLOSIS/ACTINOMYCOSIS)

WOUNDS

Z

ZINC

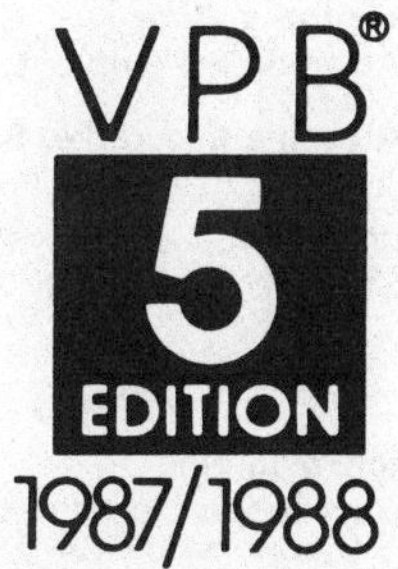

SECTION 4

Active Ingredients Index

In this section, the products described in the Product Information, Diets and Nutritional Supplements, and Diagnostic Aids and Supplies sections are listed under generic and chemical name headings according to the principal ingredient(s). The headings under which products are listed have been determined by the Publisher with the cooperation of the individual manufacturers.

R

S

T

Memorandum

Memorandum

VPB
5
EDITION
1987/1988

SECTION 5

Product Identification

Designed to help you identify products, this section contains full-color reproductions selected for inclusion by participating manufacturers.

Because tablets and capsules, for the most part, are shown here, you should not infer that these are the only dosage forms. Other dosage forms may be available. Refer to the product's description in the Product Information section or check directly with the manufacturer.

While every effort has been made to reproduce products faithfully, this section should be considered only as a quick reference identification aid.

LIST OF MANUFACTURERS

ALPHABETICAL BY PRODUCT

BEECHAM

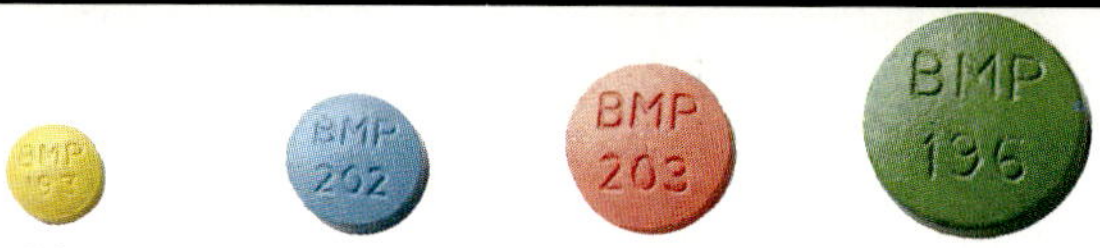

50 mg. 100 mg. 200 mg. 400 mg.

Amoxi-Tabs™ (Amoxicillin)

Beecham

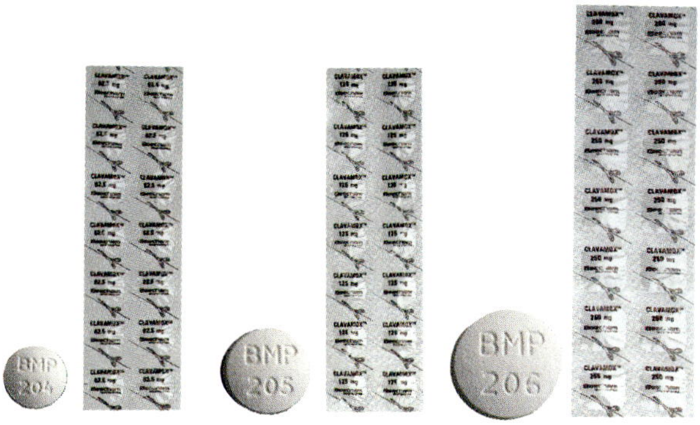

62.5 mg. 125 mg. 250 mg.

Clavamox® Tablets
(Amoxicillin Trihydrate/Clavulante Potassium)

Beecham

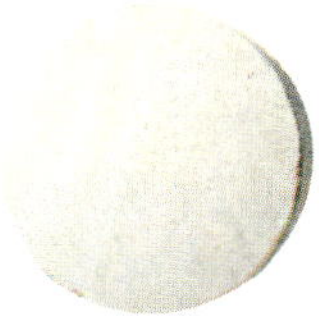

Pet-Cal™
(Calcium PO_4, Calcium CO_3, Vitamin D_3)

Beecham

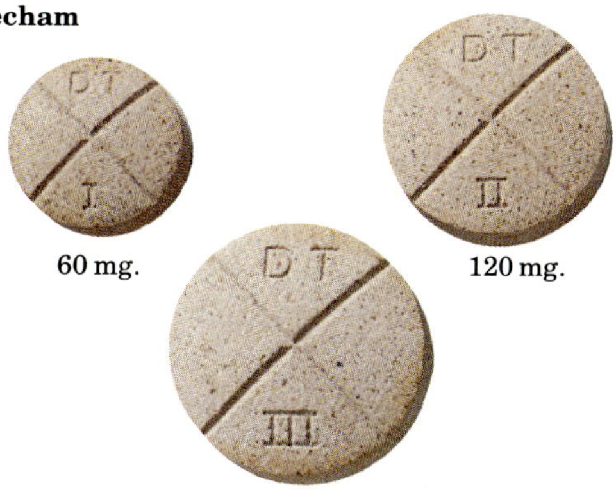

60 mg. 120 mg. 180 mg.

Pet-Dec®
(Chewable Diethylcarbamazine Citrate)

Beecham

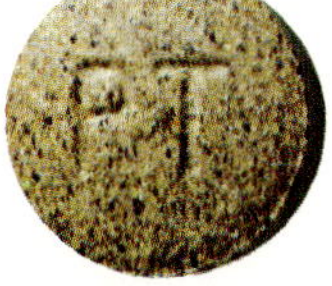

Pet-Tabs®
(Multi-Vitamin-Mineral Combination)

Beecham

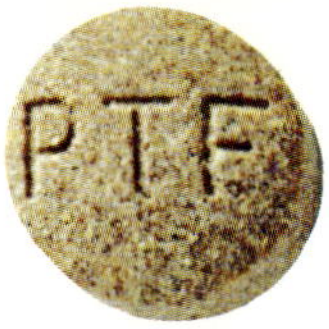

Pet-Tabs® Feline
(Vitamin, Mineral Supplement)

Beecham

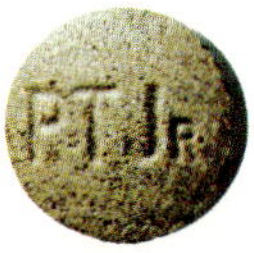

Pet-Tabs® Jr.
(Multi-Vitamin-Mineral Combination)

BRISTOL

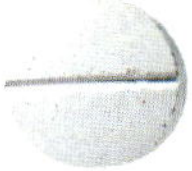

Amforal® Tablets
(Kanamycin SO4, Aminopentamide hydrogen sulfate, Pectin, Bismuth subcarbonate, Activated Attapulgite)

Bristol

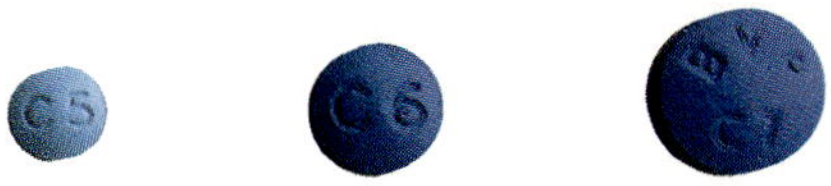

50 mg. 100 mg. 200 mg.

Cefa-Tabs
(Cefadoxil)

Bristol

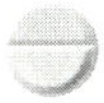

Centrine® Tablets
(Aminopentamide hydrogen sulfate)

Bristol

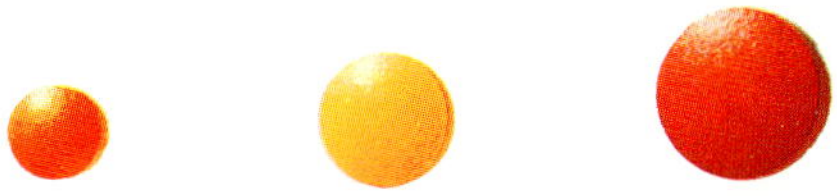

50 mg. 100 mg. 200 mg.

Hetacin®-K Tablets
(Hetacillin)

Bristol

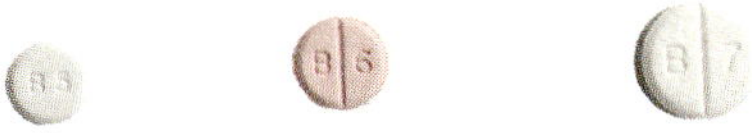

1 mg. 5 mg. 10 mg.

Torbutrol
(Butorphanol tartrate)

COOPERS

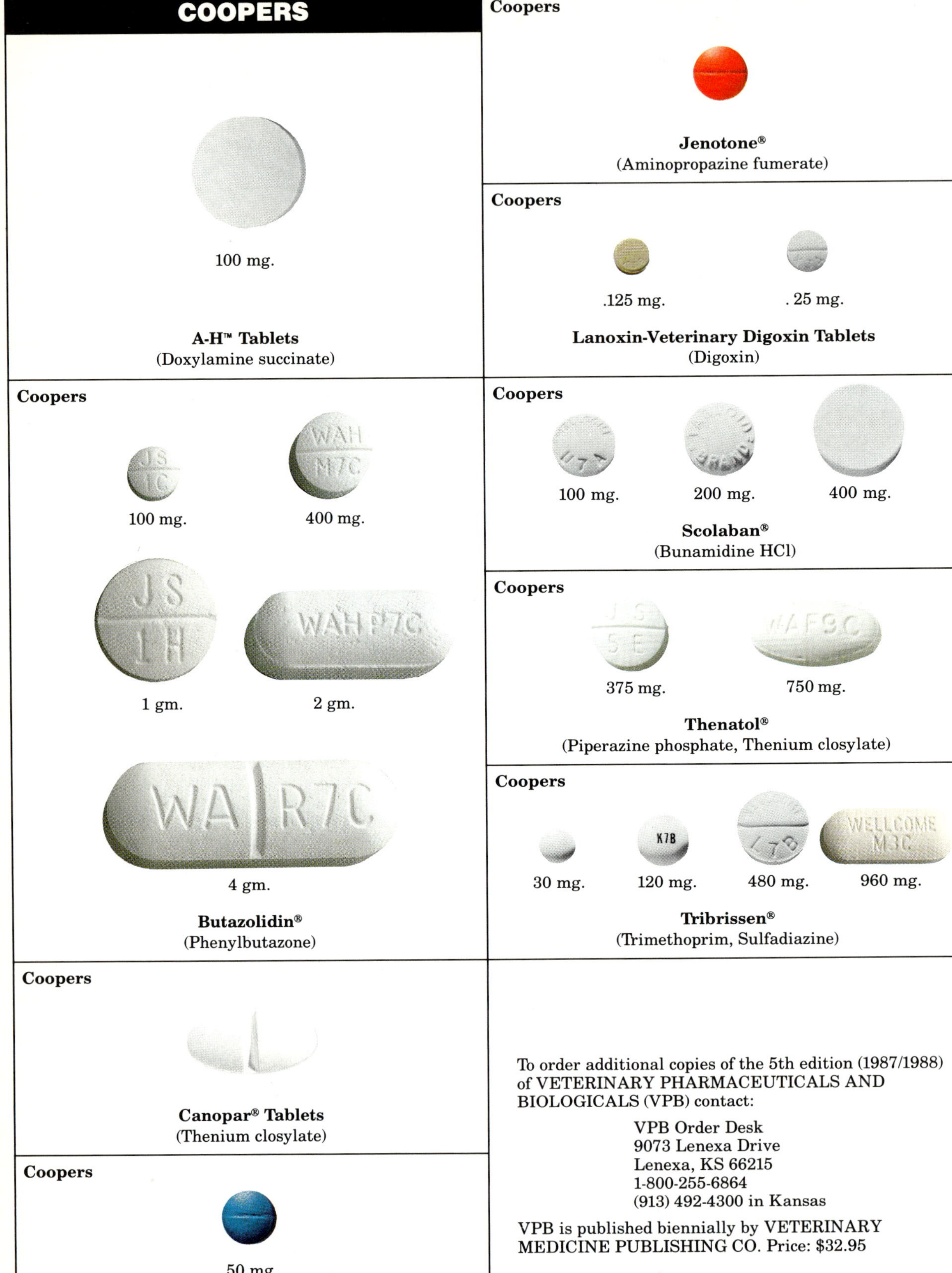

100 mg.

A-H™ Tablets
(Doxylamine succinate)

Coopers

.125 mg. . 25 mg.

Lanoxin-Veterinary Digoxin Tablets
(Digoxin)

Coopers

100 mg. 400 mg.

1 gm. 2 gm.

4 gm.

Butazolidin®
(Phenylbutazone)

Coopers

Canopar® Tablets
(Thenium closylate)

Coopers

50 mg.

Diquel®
(Ethylisobutrazine HCl)

Coopers

Jenotone®
(Aminopropazine fumerate)

Coopers

100 mg. 200 mg. 400 mg.

Scolaban®
(Bunamidine HCl)

Coopers

375 mg. 750 mg.

Thenatol®
(Piperazine phosphate, Thenium closylate)

Coopers

30 mg. 120 mg. 480 mg. 960 mg.

Tribrissen®
(Trimethoprim, Sulfadiazine)

DANIELS

425 mg.

Pancrezyme™
(Pancreatin)

Daniels

0.1 mg. 0.2 mg. 0.3 mg. 0.4 mg.
0.5 mg. 0.6 mg. 0.7 mg. 0.8 mg.

Soloxine®
(Levothyroxine Sodium)

Daniels

400 mg.

Uroeze™/Uroeze™ Chewable
(Ammonium Chloride)

EVSCO

50 mg. 100 mg.
200 mg. 300 mg. 400 mg.

Difil® Tabs
(Diethylcarbamazine citrate)

FORT DODGE

250 mg.

Mylepsin
(Primidone)

Fort Dodge

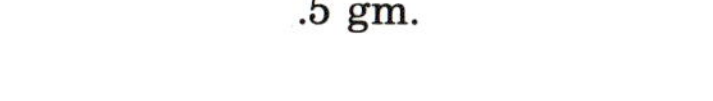

.5 gm. .25 gm.

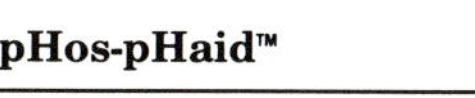

pHos-pHaid™

Fort Dodge

5 mg. 10 mg. 25 mg.

PromAce
(Acepromazine Maleate)

HOECHST-ROUSSEL

12.5 mg. 50 mg.

Lasix®
(Furosemide)

Hoechst-Roussel

2 g.

Lasix Bol-O-Tabs (Furosemide)

MSD AGVET

Diuril Tablet
(Chlorothiazide)

Diuril Bolus
(Chlorothiazide)

OSBORN—AN ESSAR CORPORATION

Bovo-Cox® Calf Bolus (Sulfaquinoxaline)

Osborn Line

Bovo-Cox® Bolus (Sulfaquinoxaline)

Osborn Line

(Calcium, Phosphorus, Vitamin D)

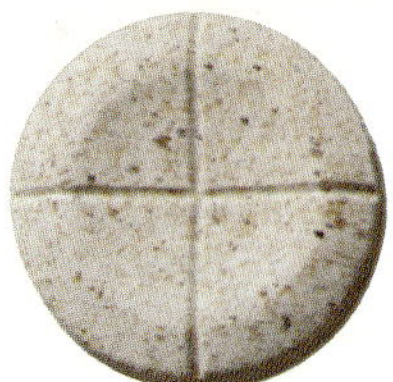

Cal-Phos Palatabs®

Osborn Line

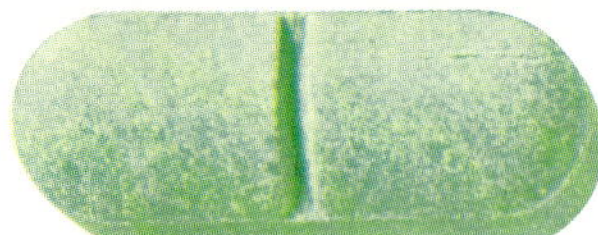

Methapyrin® Bolus
(Sulfamethazine, Neomycin base, Pyrilamine maleate, Methylatropine nitrate)

Osborn Line

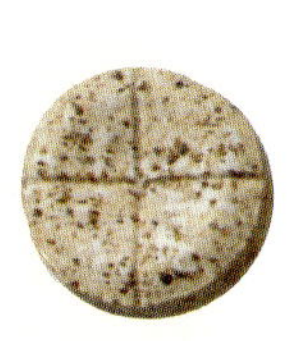

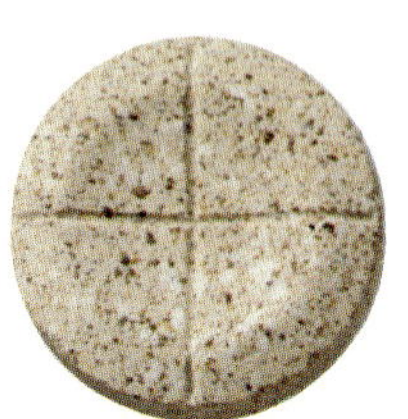

60 mg. 120 mg. 180 mg.
Palatabs

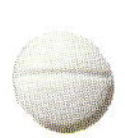

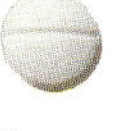

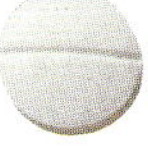

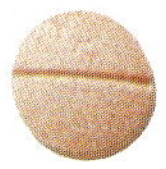

50 mg. 100 mg. 200 mg.

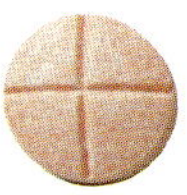

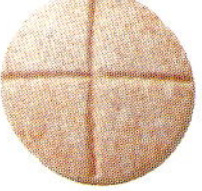

300 mg. 400 mg.
Tablets

Carbam®
(Diethylcarbamazine citrate)

Osborn Line

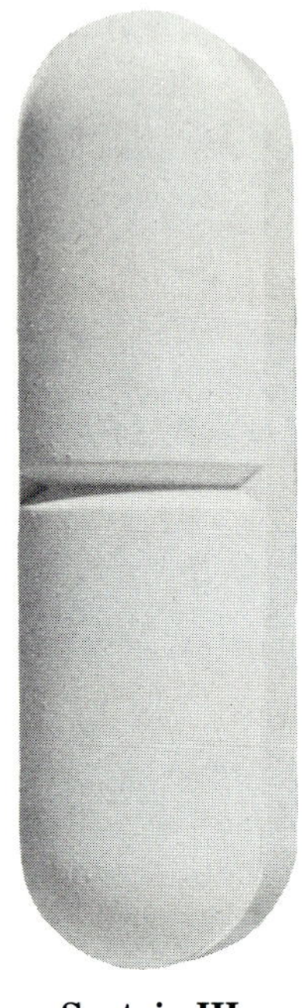

Sustain III **Sustain III Calf Bolus**
(Sulfamethazine Sustained Release)

Osborn Line

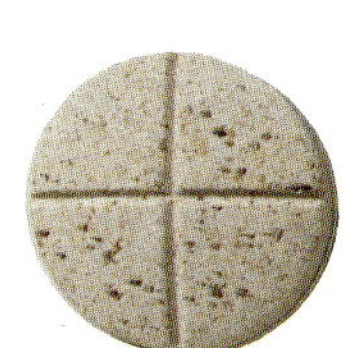

Dyrea-Aid Palatabs® **Geriatric Palatabs®**

(Colloidal Aluminum Silicate, Kaolin, Pectin, Methyl Atropine Nitrate)

Osborn Line

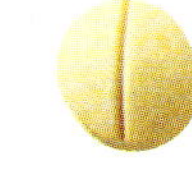

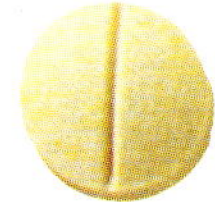

100 mg. 250 mg. 500 mg.
Viceton Tablets™
(Chloramphenicol Tablets)

Osborn Line

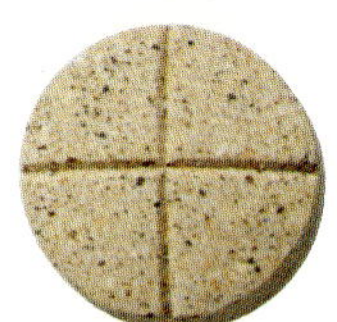

Vita-Min Palatabs®
(Vitamins, Minerals)

Osborn Line

(Attapulgite, Carob pulp, Citrus pectin, Magnesium trisilicate, Aluminum silicate)

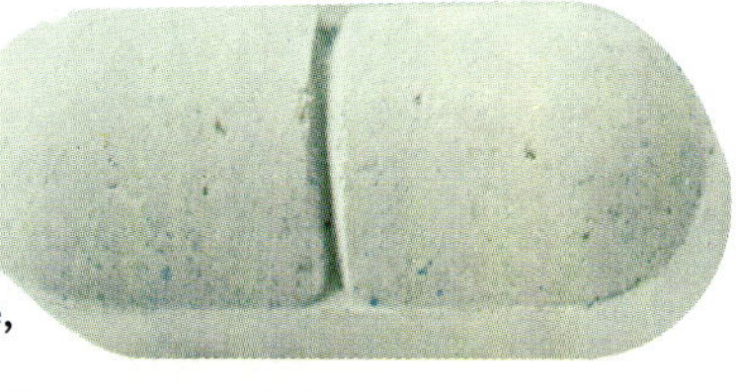

Endomagma™ Bolus

Designed to help you identify drugs, this section contains color reproductions of products selected for inclusion by participating manufacturers.

PITMAN-MOORE

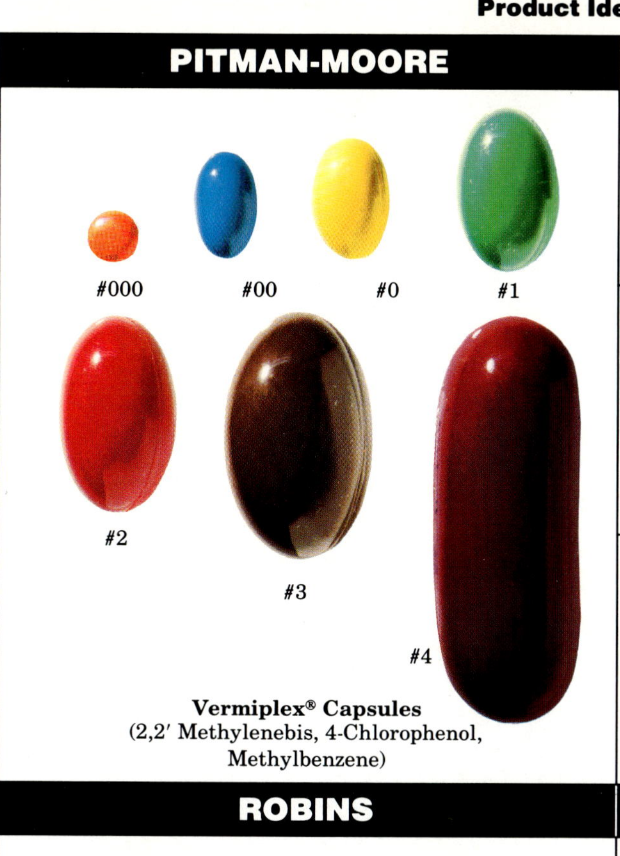

#000 #00 #0 #1

#2 #3 #4

Vermiplex® Capsules
(2,2′ Methylenebis, 4-Chlorophenol, Methylbenzene)

Robins

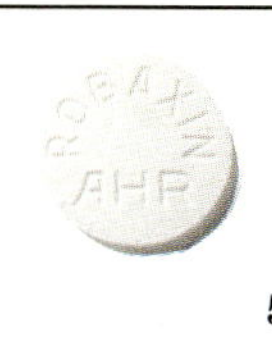

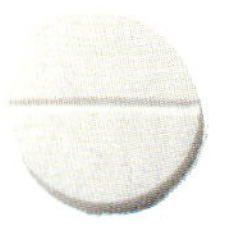

500 mg.

Robaxin®-V
(Methocarbamol)

Robins

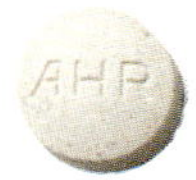

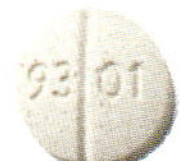

425 mg.

Viokase®-V Tablets
(Pancreatic Enzymes)

Robins

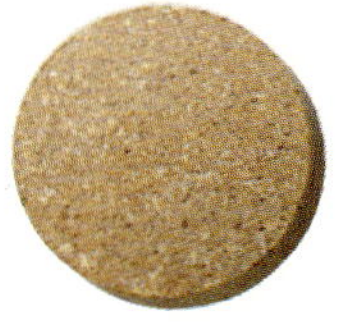

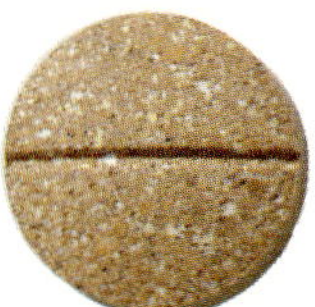

Z-BEC® Veterinary
(Zinc/Vitamin Supplement)

ROBINS

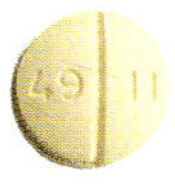

10 mg.

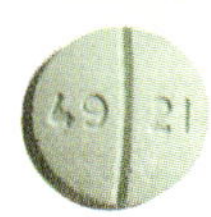

25 mg.

Elanone® V Tablets
(Lenperone Hydrochloride)

Robins

50 mg.

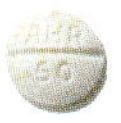

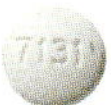

100 mg.

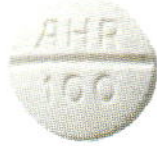

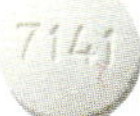

200 mg.

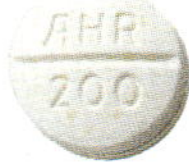

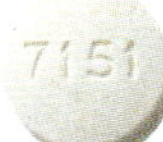

400 mg.

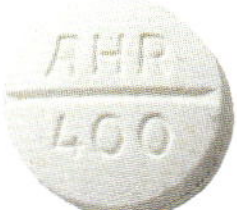

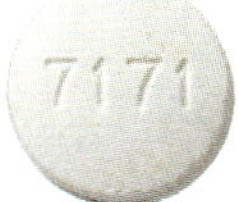

Robamox®-V Tablets
(Amoxicillin Trihydrate)

ROCHE

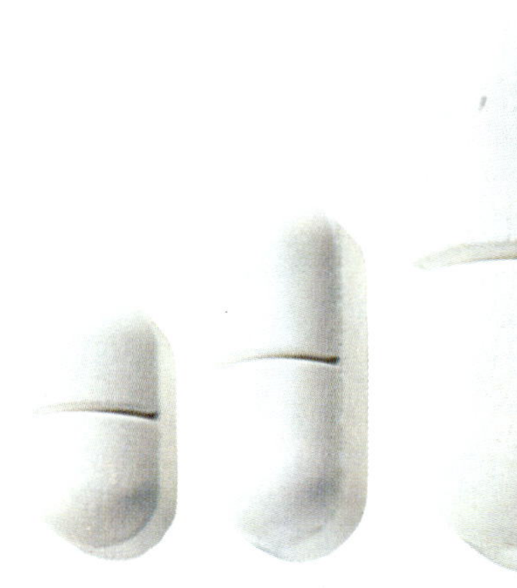

2.5 g. 5 g. 15 g.

Albon® Boluses
(Sulfadimethoxine)

Roche

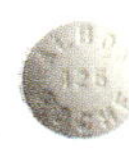

125 mg.

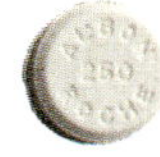

250 mg.

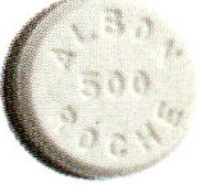

500 mg.

Albon® Tablets
(Sulfadimethoxine)

Roche

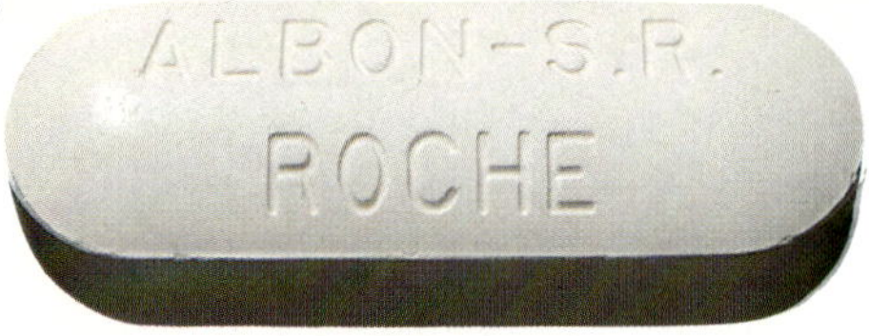

Albon S.R. Bolus (Sulfadimethoxine)

Solvay

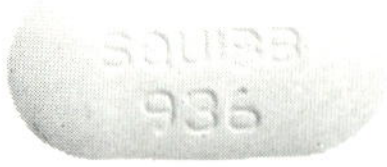

Princillin® Boluses
(Ampicillin trihydrate)

Roche

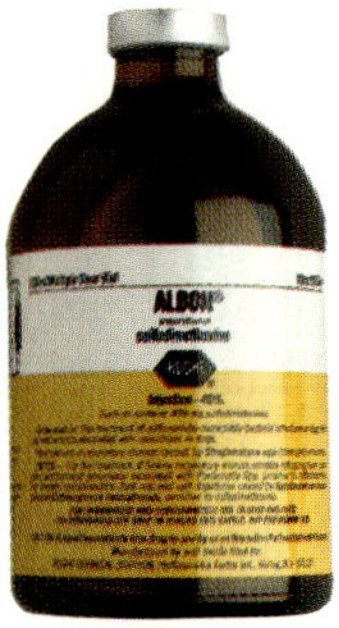

100 ml.
or 250 ml.

Albon® Injection 40%
(Sulfadimethoxine)

Solvay

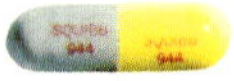

125 mg. 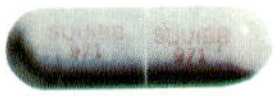 250 mg. 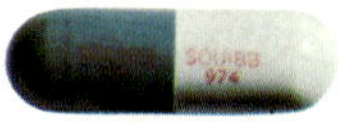 500 mg.

Princillin® Capsules
(Ampicillin trihydrate)

Solvay

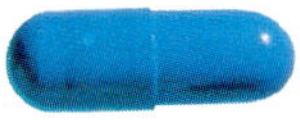

#5
68 mg.

#10
136 mg.

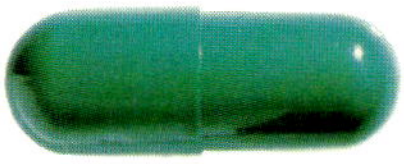

#15
204 mg.

Task®
(Dichlorvos)

Roche

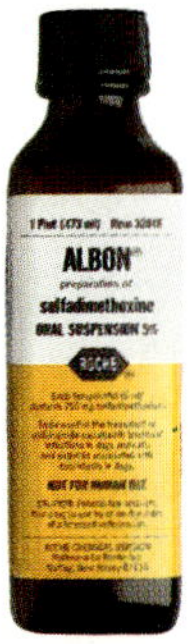

2 oz.
or 16 oz.

Albon® Oral Suspension 5%
(Sulfadimethoxine)

Solvay

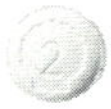

#2
10 mg.

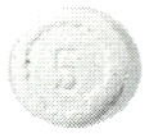

#5
25 mg.

Task® Tabs
(Dichlorvos)

SOLVAY

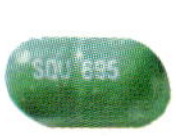

50 mg. 100 mg.

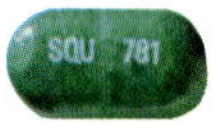

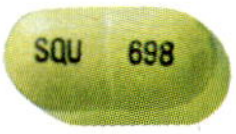

200 mg. 300 mg.

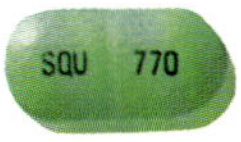

Dirocide® Tablets
(Diethylcarbamazine citrate)

Solvay

0.5 mg. 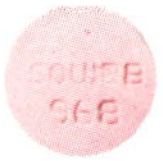 1.5 mg.

Vetalog® Tablets
(Triamcinolone acetonide)

Solvay

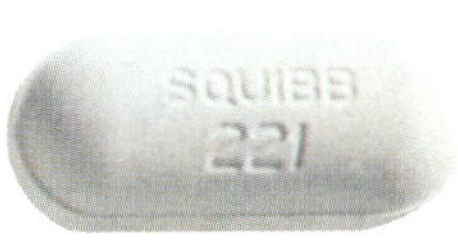

Vetisulid® Boluses
(Sulfachlorpyridazine)

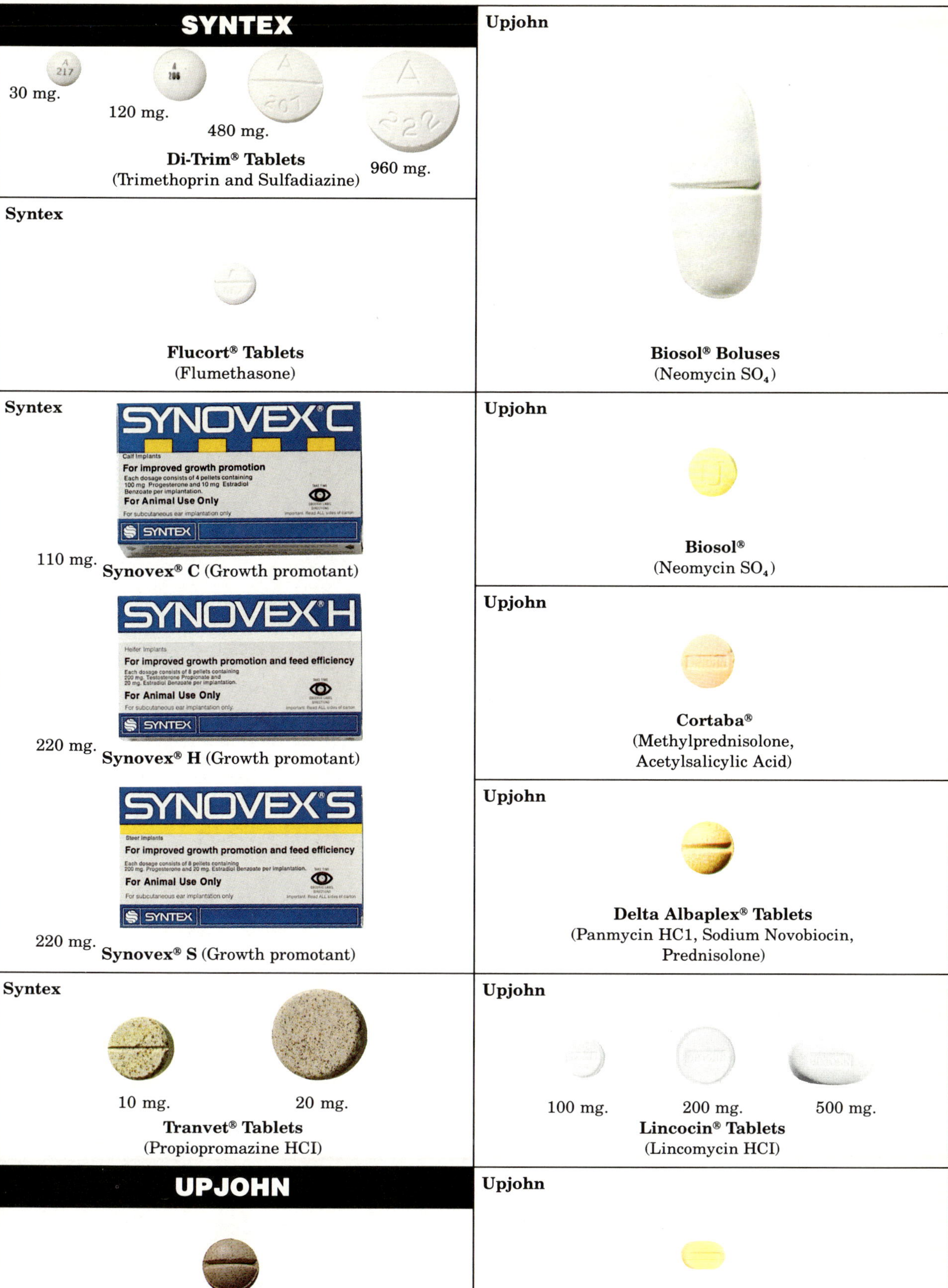

SYNTEX

30 mg. 120 mg. 480 mg. 960 mg.

Di-Trim® Tablets
(Trimethoprin and Sulfadiazine)

Syntex

Flucort® Tablets
(Flumethasone)

Syntex

110 mg. **Synovex® C** (Growth promotant)

220 mg. **Synovex® H** (Growth promotant)

220 mg. **Synovex® S** (Growth promotant)

Syntex

10 mg. 20 mg.

Tranvet® Tablets
(Propiopromazine HCI)

UPJOHN

Albaplex
(Sodium)

Upjohn

Biosol® Boluses
(Neomycin SO_4)

Upjohn

Biosol®
(Neomycin SO_4)

Upjohn

Cortaba®
(Methylprednisolone,
Acetylsalicylic Acid)

Upjohn

Delta Albaplex® Tablets
(Panmycin HC1, Sodium Novobiocin,
Prednisolone)

Upjohn

100 mg. 200 mg. 500 mg.

Lincocin® Tablets
(Lincomycin HCI)

Upjohn

Medrol® Tablets
(Methylprednisolone)

Upjohn

Panmycin® Hydrochloride Boluses
(Tetracycline HCl)

Upjohn

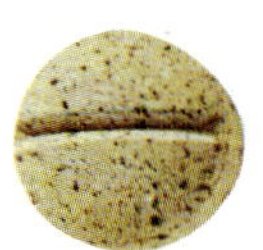

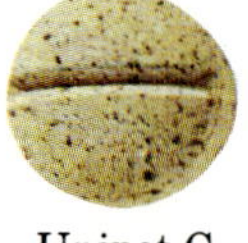

Unipet-C

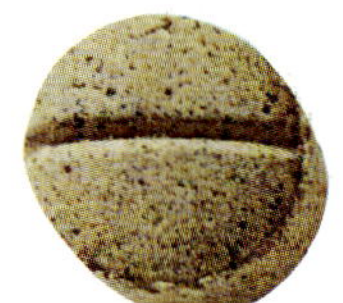

Unipet

Unipet-Senior

Unipet®
(Vitamin, Mineral, Protein Supplement)

No practice is complete without a new edition of VETERINARY PHARMACEUTICALS AND BIOLOGICALS. VPB is the veterinarian's professional reference. It offers quick and easy access to comprehensive information on drugs and dosages.

VET-A-MIX

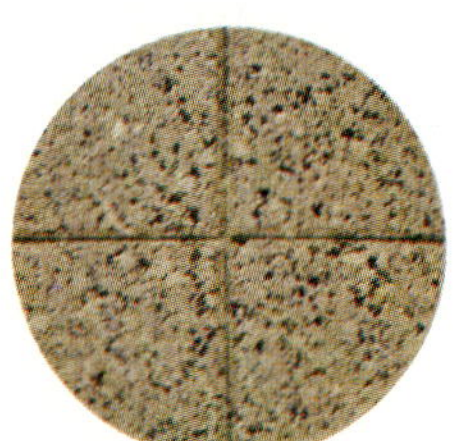

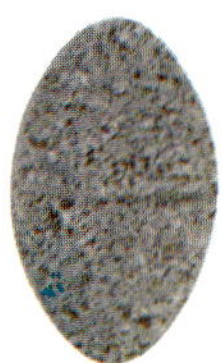

150 mg. 45 mg.

Diro-Form
(Diethylcarbamazine Citrate)

Vet-A-Mix

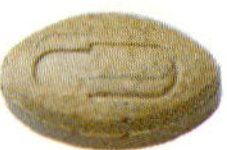

Felo-Form Chewable Tablet
(Feline Vitamin, Mineral Supplement)

Vet-A-Mix

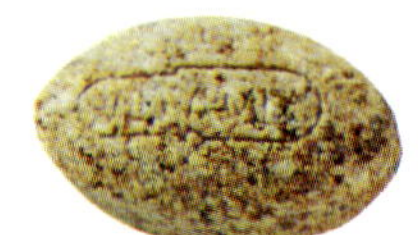

Lipo-Form
(Choline, Multivitamins)

Vet-A-Mix

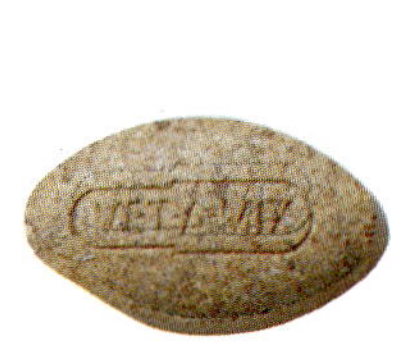

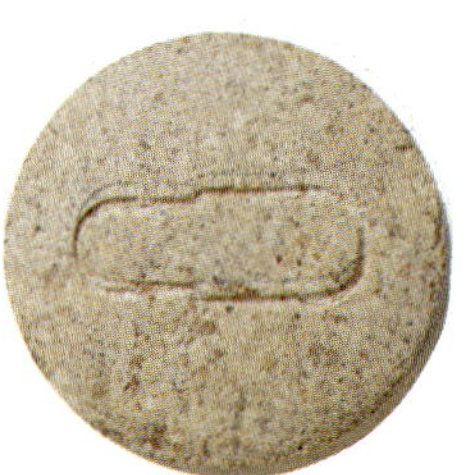

MEq-10 **MEq-30**

Chewable Tablets
(DL-Methionine & Ammonium Chloride)

Vet-A-Mix

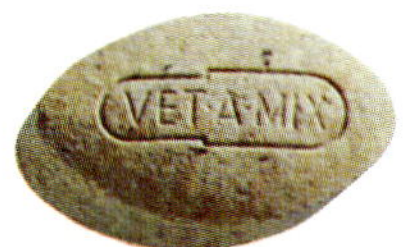

Methio-Form
(D L-Methionine)

Vet-A-Mix

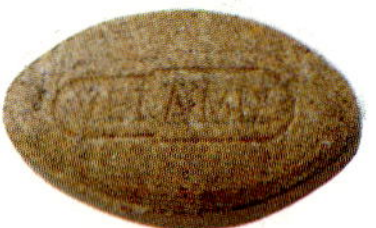

Nutri-Form G Chewable Tablet
(Geriatric Vitamin-Mineral Supplement)

Vet-A-Mix

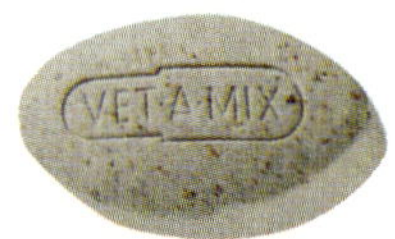

Osteo-Form 181
(Calcium, Phosphorous, Multivitamins)

Vet-A-Mix

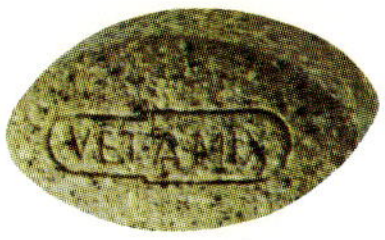

Pet-Form
(Multivitamins, Minerals)

Vet-A-Mix

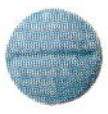

50 mg. 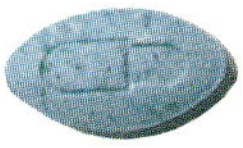 250 mg.

Pipa-Tabs
(Piperazine Dihydrochloride)

Vet-A-Mix

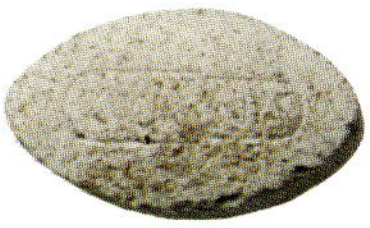

Predni-Form Chewable Tablet
(5 mg. Prednisolone)

Vet-A-Mix

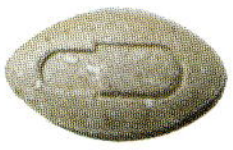

0.2 mg. 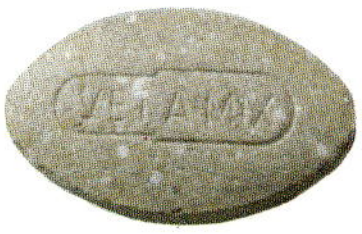 0.8 mg.

Thyro-Form Chewable Tablet
(Levothyroxine Sodium)

Vet-A-Mix

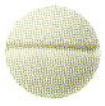

0.1 mg. 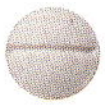 0.2 mg. 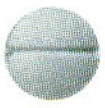 0.3 mg.

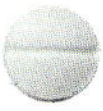

0.5 mg. 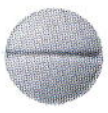 0.8 mg.

Thyro-Tabs
(Levothyroxine Sodium)

Vet-A-Mix

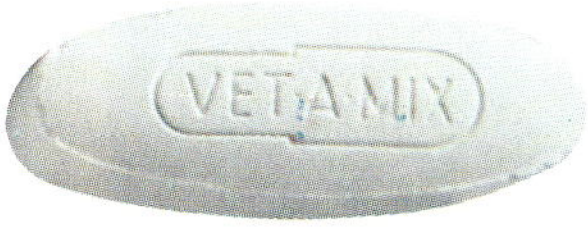

5 gm.

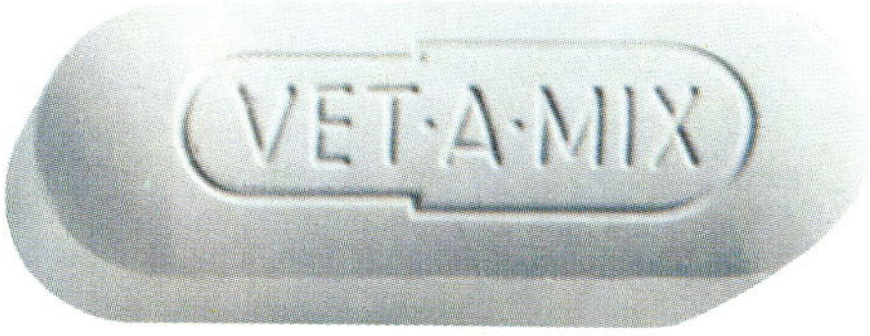

15 gm.

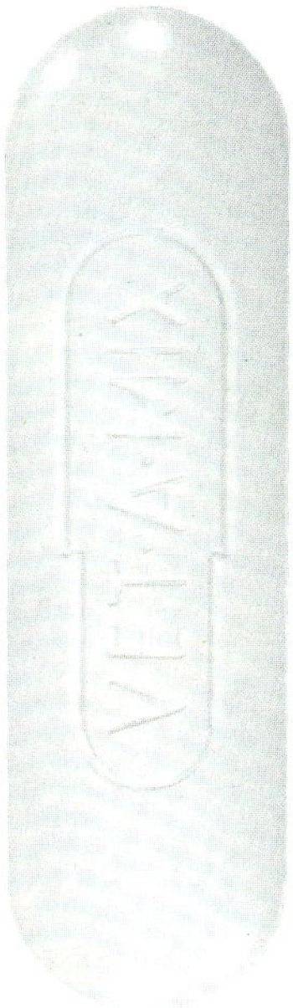

25 gm.

Veta-Meth
(Sulfamethazine)

WINTHROP

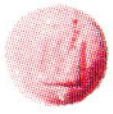

Winstrol®-V Tablet 2 mg.
(Brand of Stanozolol)

Winthrop

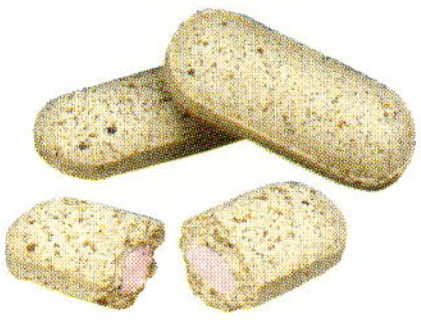

Winstrol®-V Chewable Tablet 2 mg.
(Brand of Stanozolol)

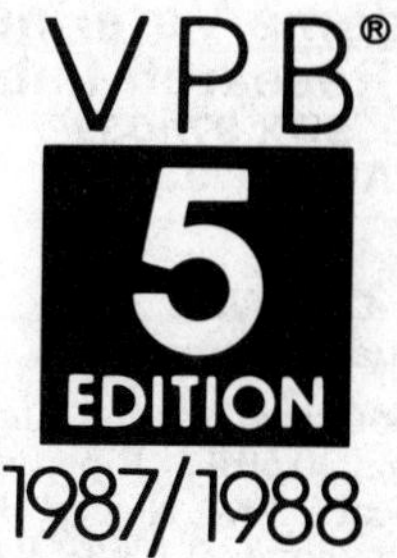

SECTION 6

Product Information

The information in this section was supplied directly by the manufacturer and is designed to provide a convenient reference on pharmaceuticals, biologicals, fluids and electrolytes, parasiticides, and other products employed in the practice of veterinary medicine. Products are arranged alphabetically under the name of the manufacturer.

The Publisher has emphasized to manufacturers the necessity of describing products comprehensively so that veterinarians will have access to all information essential for intelligent and informed prescribing. In organizing and presenting the material in this edition of VETERINARY PHARMACEUTICALS & BIOLOGICALS, the Publisher is providing all the information made available to VPB by manufacturers.

In presenting the following material, the Publisher is not necessarily advocating the use of any product listed.

A

Adams Veterinary Research Labs., Inc.

P.O. BOX 971039
MIAMI, FL 33197

ANTI-CRAWL®
Residual Insecticide

Composition: Active Ingredients, Pyrethrins 0.50%, Piperonyl Butoxide, technical 0.10%, N-octyl Bicycloheptene Dicarboxamide 0.166%, Baygon:2-(1 Methylethoxy) Phenol Methylcarbamate 0.10%, Petroleum Distillate 42.134%, Inert Ingredients 56.55%. (Baygon is Reg. TM of Farbenfabriken Bayer GmbH, Leverkusen, U.S. Pat. No. 3,111,539.)
Indications: Insecticide for surface spray application (not space spray), to kill and control crawling insects including ants, fleas, ticks, roaches, mites, crickets, earwigs, millipedes, scorpions, silver fish, sowbugs, spiders and grain beetles. Has immediate knock-down killing action and leaves a residual spray residue after drying.
Administration: Spray into cracks, crevices, around baseboards, carpets, furniture and other places where these insects hide. Apply behind and beneath cabinets, refrigerators, sinks, stoves and in and around waste containers. Spray animal quarters and areas that pets frequent and their bedding. Spray surfaces of screens, doors, window frames, foundations, patios and other places where insects may enter; spray anthills and runways.
Caution: Keep out of reach of children. Harmful if swallowed or inhaled. Avoid contact with eyes, skin or clothing. If in eyes, wash with large amounts of potable water for 10–15 minutes. If on skin or clothing, wash thoroughly with soap and warm water. Do not allow humans or animals to contact treated surfaces until they are completely dry. Avoid contamination of food, food utensils and food preparation areas. Do not use in area where food is exposed or commercially prepared. Do not spray animals, foodstuffs, house plants or vegetation.
Warning: Flammable, keep away from heat and open flame. Do not spray into or near open flame. Do not apply to painted or finished wood surfaces.
Note to Physician: If symptoms of cholinesterase inhibition appear, atropine is antidotal.
How Supplied: 32 oz. and 1 gallon plastic bottles with trigger sprayers. Sold only through licensed veterinarians.

ANTI-CRAWL® ROOM FOGGER
Residual Insecticide Fogger

Composition: Active Ingredients: 2-(1-Methylethoxy) Phenyl Methylcarbamate* 1.00%, 2,2-Dichlorovinyl Dimethyl Phosphate** 0.47%, Related Compounds 0.03%, Inert Ingredients 98.5%. (*Baygon is the Reg. TM of Farbenfabriken Bayer GmbH, Leverkusen, and ** Vapona is a Reg. TM of the Shell Oil Company.)
Indications: To kill fleas, houseflies, mosquitoes, black carpet beetles, sawtooth grain beetles, rice weevils, small flying moths, brown dog ticks, spiders, crickets, centipedes, sowbugs, and silver fish by fogging of homes, apartments, attics, basements, campers, boats, garages, plants, warehouses, boxcars, trucks, farms, kennels and pet sleeping areas. Aids in control of cockroaches.
Administration: Use one 6 oz. canister for each 5,000 cu.ft. of unobstructed area. Use additional units for remote rooms or where free flow of the mist is not assured. Cover exposed foods, dishes, and food handling equipment. Open cabinets and doors to areas to be treated. Shut off fans and air conditioners. Put out all open flames except pilot light. Remove pets and cover fish tanks or fish bowls with paper, or remove from area. Close exterior doors and windows.
Caution: Keep out of reach of children. Harmful if swallowed. Avoid inhalation of vapors. Avoid contact with skin, eyes or clothing. Wash contaminated skin promptly with soap and warm water. For eyes, flush with plenty of water. Get medical attention if irritation persists. Avoid contamination of food and foodstuffs. Wash hands with soap and water after using and before eating or smoking.
Do not use in commercial food processing, preparation or serving areas or in household storage areas. In home, all food processing surfaces and utensils should be covered during treatment or thoroughly washed before use. Cover or remove exposed food.
Remove pets, birds, and cover fish aquariums before spraying.
For barns-Remove animals before applying. Do not treat animals. Do not contaminate milk or milking utensils. Ventilate before allowing animals to reoccupy buildings.
Warning: Contents under pressure. Do not use near heat or open flame. Do not puncture or incinerate container. Exposure to temperature above 130° may cause bursting.
How Supplied: 6 oz. cans. Sold only through licensed veterinarians.

ANTI-SEPT
Lotion Soap, Skin Cleaner and Shampoo.

Composition: Deionized Water, Sodium Lauryl Sulfate, Tea Lauryl Sulfate, Aloe Vera Gel, Propylene Glycol USP, Ethylene Glycol Monosteareate, Peg 75 Lanolin, Cocamide Dea, Quaternium 19, Coconut Extract, Fragrance, U. S. Certified Colors and Preservatives.
Indications: For external use as a cleansing and deodorizing soap on dogs and cats, as a routine hand soap and cleaner. Contains emolients and conditioners that allow repeated washing without adverse side effects. Lathers quickly and cleans even in hard water.
Caution: Keep out of reach of children. Avoid contact with eyes. In case of contact, flush immediately with water.
How Supplied: 6 and 12 oz. and 1 gallon plastic bottles. Sold only through licensed veterinarians.

CANIDERM MIST®
Insecticide, Repellent, Deodorant With Skin and Coat Conditioners Water-Base Spray for Rapid Kill of Fleas, Ticks and Lice on Dogs.

Composition: Active Ingredients: Pyrethrins 0.2%, Piperonyl Butoxide, technical 0.75%, N-octyl Bicycloheptene Dicarboxamide 2.0%, 2,3,4,5-bis(2 Butylene) Tetrahydro-2-Furaldehyde 0.5%, Inert Ingredients 96.55%.
Indications: Caniderm Mist® provides rapid killing of fleas, ticks and lice on dogs, and temporarily repels fleas, ticks, mites, gnats, biting flies, lice and mosquitoes. It's water-base with aloe vera and lanolin, skin and coat conditioners are designed for dogs with sensitive skin problems that may be irritated by alcohol-base products.
Administration: Cover the dog's eyes with hand and with a firm fast stroke spray the entire body surface, spraying against the natural lay of the hair and ruffling the coat immediately in front of the spray. Make sure the spray thoroughly wets ticks.
Caution: Avoid treatment of nursing puppies. If treatment is necessary, spray on tips of fingers and rub into coat. Keep out of reach of children. Harmful if swallowed or inhaled. Avoid breathing mist. Avoid contamination of foods. Wash hands with soap and water after washing.
How Supplied: 12, 16 and 32 oz. plastic bottles with sprayers. Sold only through licensed veterinarians.

FELIDERM MIST®
Insecticide, Repellent, Deodorant with Skin and Coat Conditioners Water-Base Spray for Rapid Killing of Fleas, Ticks and Lice on Cats.

Composition: Active Ingredients: Pyrethrins 0.2%, Piperonyl Butoxide, technical 0.75%, N-octyl Bicycloheptene Dicarboxamide 2.0%, 2,3,4,5-bis(2-Butylene) Tetrahydro-2-Furaldehyde 0.5%, Inert Ingredients 96.55%.
Indications: Feliderm Mist® provides rapid killing of fleas, ticks, and lice on cats, and temporarily repels fleas, lice, ticks, mites, gnats, biting flies and mosquitoes. It's water-base with aloe vera and lanolin. Skin and coat conditioners are designed for use on cats that may be irritated by alcohol-base products, and especially those with sensitive skin problems.
Administration: Cover the cat's eyes with hand and with a firm fast stroke spray the entire body surface against the natural lay of the hair and ruffling the coat immediately in front of the spray. Make sure the spray thoroughly wets ticks.
Caution: Avoid treatment of nursing kittens. If treatment is necessary, spray on tips of fingers and rub into coat. Keep out of reach of children. Harmful if swallowed or inhaled. Avoid breathing mist. Avoid contamination of foods. Wash hands with soap and water after using.

How Supplied: 12, 16 and 32 oz. plastic bottles with sprayers. Sold only through licensed veterinarians.

FLEA OFF™ DIP
Kills Fleas, Ticks, Lice and Sarcoptic Mange Mites on Dogs and Cats.

Composition: Active Ingredients: Malathion (0,0-Dimethyl Phosphorodithioate of Diethyl Mercaptosuccinate) 53.0%, Xylene 15.0% Inert Ingredients 32.0%.
Indications: To kill and repel fleas ticks and sarcoptic mange mites on dogs and cats.
Administration: Thoroughly mix ½ fl. oz. (1 tablespoon) of Flea Off™ Dip with 1 gallon of warm water. Bathe animal with a good cleaning shampoo. Rinse with warm water and while still wet, sponge or dip the animal with the diluted dip solution, making sure all areas are soaked. Do not rinse off. Let dip dry on animal. For outside dogs or in resistant flea areas, use 1 oz. (2 tablespoons) to 1 gallon of water. Do not use on cats at this concentration. Do not use more than once every 1–3 weeks or as directed by your veterinarian.
Caution: Keep out of reach of children. Harmful if swallowed, inhaled or absorbed through the skin. Avoid contamination of feed or feed products. Wash hands with soap and water after use and before smoking or eating.
Avoid treatment of nursing animals. Do not treat kittens or puppies under three months of age. Do not treat tranquilized or anesthetized animals or animals that are taking any type of medication or using any other type of flea or tick control product without first consulting your veterinarian.
Keep away from heat and open flame. Concentrate is harmful to painted surfaces.
To Physician: Flea Off™ Dip is a cholinesterase inhibitor. Atropine is antidotal.
How Supplied: 4 oz. and half gallon bottles. Sold only through licensed veterinarians.

FLEA OFF™ DUST II
Residual Insecticide Powder for Fleas, Ticks and Lice

Composition: Active Ingredients: Pyrethrins 0.10%, Piperonyl Butoxide, technical 1.0%, Carbaryl: (1-Napthyl N-Methylcarbamate) 12.50%, Silica Gel 10.0%, Petroleum Distillate 1.90%, Inert Ingredients 74.50%.
Indications: Odorless, residual insecticide powder for cats, kittens, dogs and puppies over 4 weeks of age. Kills fleas, ticks and lice on contact and provides residual killing action for 7–10 days.
Administration: Apply powder liberally to body of animal, working in dust by rubbing against the lay of the hair until dust penetrates to the skin. Avoid getting dust in eyes, nose and mouth. Repeat treatment as necessary. For kennels and living quarters dust bedding and floor at the rate of 1 oz. per 50 sq. ft. of surface. Repeat as necessary.
Caution: Harmful if swallowed or inhaled. Avoid breathing dust. Wash thoroughly after handling. Wash hands before eating or smoking. Avoid contamination of food. Keep out of reach of children. Do not use on nursing animals or kittens or puppies under 4 weeks of age.
How Supplied: 3 and 6 oz. plastic bottles. Sold only through licensed veterinarians.

FLEA OFF™ EAR MITE LOTION
Kills and Temporarily Repels Ear Mites, Flies, Mosquitoes, Gnats, Fleas, Ticks, Chiggers and Lice on Dogs and Cats.

Composition: Active Ingredients: Pyrethrins 0.15%, Piperonyl Butoxide, technical 1.50%, N-octyl Bicycloheptene Dicarboxamide 0.50%, 2,3,4,5-bis(2-Butylene) Tetrahydro-2-Furaldehyde 0.50%, Di-n-propyl Isocinchomeronate 0.50%, Petroleum Distillate 0.60%, Inert Ingredients 96.25%.
Administration: Clean ears with Adams Pan-Otic Ear Cleaner to remove dirt and wax. Dry ear and apply a thin film of Flea Off™ Ear Mite Lotion. Make sure lotion covers ticks. To use as a repellent spread lotion lightly on outer and inner surfaces of the ear and between the toes before the animal enters infested areas. May be applied daily or as directed by your veterinarian.
Caution: Keep out of reach of children. Harmful if swallowed. Avoid breathing vapors. Avoid contact with eyes. In case of contact immediately flush eyes with plenty of water. Do not use on meat or milk producing animals. Wash hands with soap and water after using.
How Supplied: 2 oz. plastic bottles. Sold only by licensed veterinarians.

FLEA OFF™ MIST
Insecticide, Repellent and Deodorant Spray For Rapid Kill of Fleas, Ticks and Lice on Dogs and Cats
Repels Flies, Gnats and Mosquitoes.

Composition: Active Ingredients: Pyrethrins 0.15%, Piperonyl Butoxide, technical 1.5%, N-octyl Bicycloheptene Dicarboxamide 0.5%, 2,3,4,5-bis(2-Butylene) Tetrahydro-2-Furaldehyde 0.5%, Petroleum Distillate 0.6%, Inert Ingredients 96.75%.
Indications: Flea Off™ Mist provides rapid flushing and killing of fleas, ticks, lice, gnats, biting flies and mosquitoes.
Administration: Use only in a well ventilated area. Cover animal's eyes with hand and with a firm fast stroke to get a proper mist, spray systematically over the entire surface, except face. For best penetration, direct spray against the natural lay of the hair and ruffle the hair in front of the spray. Make sure spray thoroughly wets ticks. With fingertips rub spray into face around mouth, nose and eyes. Spray pet's bed and bedding. Repeat as often as necessary.
Caution: Avoid treatment of nursing kittens and puppies. If treatment is necessary, spray on tips of fingers and rub into coat. Keep out of reach of children. Harmful if swallowed or inhaled. Avoid breathing mist. Avoid contamination of foods. Wash hands with soap and water after using.
Warning: Flammable, keep away from heat and open flame.
How Supplied: 12, 16 and 32 oz. plastic bottles with sprayers, 16, 32 oz and 1 gallon plastic refill bottles. Sold only through licensed veterinarians.

FLEA OFF™ 14 DAY RESIDUAL MIST
Residual Insecticide and Repellent Spray For Rapid Flushing and Killing of Fleas
Residual Killing and Repelling of Fleas, Ticks, Lice, Mites, Gnats, Biting Flies and Mosquitoes.

Composition: Active Ingredients: Pyrethrins 0.1%, Piperonyl Butoxide, technical 0.37%, N-octyl Bicycloheptene Dicarboxamide 0.61%, 2,3,4,5-bis(2-Butylene) Tetrahydro-2-Furaldehyde 0.2%, Di-n-propyl Isocinchomeronate 0.2%, Inert Ingredients 98.52%.
Indications: Flea Off™ 14 Day Residual Mist provides rapid flushing and killing of fleas on dogs and cats and kills ticks, and lice. The polymer system (U.S. Patent Pending) provides residual killing and repellency of fleas, ticks, lice, mites, gnats, biting flies and mosquitoes for up to 14 days.
Administration: Use only in a well ventilated area. Cover animal's eyes with hand and with a firm fast stroke to get a proper mist, spray systematically over the entire body surface, except face. For best penetration, direct spray against the natural lay of the hair and ruffle the hair in front of the spray. Make sure spray thoroughly wets ticks. With fingertips rub spray into face around mouth, nose and eyes. Spray pet's bed and bedding. Repeat as often as necessary.
Caution: Avoid treatment of nursing kittens and puppies. If treatment is necessary, spray on tips of fingers and rub into coat. Keep out of reach of children. Harmful if swallowed or inhaled. Avoid breathing mist. Avoid contamination of foods. Wash hands with soap and water after using.
Warning: Flammable, keep away from heat and open flame. Do not apply to painted or finished wood surfaces.
How Supplied: 12, 16 and 32 oz. plastic bottles with sprayers, and 1 gallon plastic refill bottle. Sold only through licensed veterinarians.

FLEA OFF™ SHAMPOO
Kills and Repels Fleas, Lice and Ticks on Dogs and Cats
Repels Gnats, Mosquitoes and Biting Flies.

Composition: Active Ingredients: Pyrethrins 0.15%, Piperonyl Butoxide, technical 1.50%, N-octyl Bicycloheptene Dicarboxamide 0.50%, 2,3,4,5-bis(2-Butylene) Tetrahydro-2-Furaldehyde 0.50%, Petroleum Distillate 0.50%, Inert Ingredients 96.75%.

Continued on next page

Adams—Cont.

Indications: A concentrated lathering shampoo enriched with coconut extract and lanolin. Removes loose dandruff, dust and scales, leaves the coat soft and shiny. Kills fleas, lice and ticks and repels gnats, biting flies and mosquitoes.
Administration: Thoroughly soak animal with warm water taking 2–3 minutes to wet hair. Apply Flea Off™ Shampoo systematically and lather over the whole body. Let animal stand 3–5 minutes then rinse thoroughly. Use every 7–10 days or as directed by your veterinarian.
Caution: Do not use on puppies or kittens less than 6 weeks of age. Keep out of reach of children. Harmful if swallowed. Avoid contact with eyes. In case of contact, flush with water. Avoid contact with food and serving areas. Wash thoroughly after using with soap and water.
How Supplied: 6, 12 oz. and 1 gallon plastic bottles. Sold only through licensed veterinarians.

KLEAN SHAMPOO
Enriched Shampoo for Cats and Dogs

Composition: Contains Deionized Water, Sodium Lauryl Ether Sulfate, Triethanolamine Lauryl Sulfate, Coconut Diethanolamide, Propylene Gylcol USP, Peg 75 Lanolin, Quaternium 19, Diazolidinyl Urea, Fragrance, U. S. Certified Colors and Preservatives.
Indications: For external use for normal and dry skin and coats of dogs, cats, horses. Humectifies and removes loose dandruff, dirt and scales. Leaves the skin and coat soft, shining and clean smelling.
Administration: Throughly soak animal with warm water 2–3 minutes to wet hair. Apply systematically, lathering over the entire body. Let stand 3–5 minutes then rinse thoroughly.
Caution: Keep out of reach of children. Avoid contact with eyes. In case of contact, flush immediately with water.
How Supplied: 12 oz, 1 and 5 gallon containers. Sold only through licensed veterinarians.

LIQUID EAR DESSICANT

Composition: Contains Aloe Vera Gel, Propylene Glycol USP, Colloidal Sulfur, Magnesium Aluminum Silicate, Dioctyl Sodium Sulfosuccinate, Xanthan Gum, Diazolidinyl Urea and Preservatives.
Indications: For dogs and cats to create a dry environment conducive to healing in cases of otitis externa and seborrhea oleosa.
Administration: Shake well before using. Clean ear canal and outer ear with Adams Pan Otic Ear Cleaner. Remove excess ear cleaner. Squeeze an adequate amount of Ear Dessicant into ear canal to adequately cover all surfaces. Massage ear canal to spread throughout the affected area. Repeat daily or as recommended by veterinarian. May be used once or twice weekly as preventative measure. If local irritation occurs, discontinue use and consult your veterinarian.
Caution: Keep out of reach of children. For external use only. Avoid contact with eyes. If contact occurs, flush immediately with fresh water.
How Supplied: 2 and 12 oz. plastic bottles. Sold only through licensed veterinarians.

LOTION OF SULFUR

Composition: Contains: Deionized Water, Propylene Glycol USP, Colloidal Sulfur, Magnesium Aluminum Silicate, Dioctyl Sodium Sulfosuccinate, Diazolidinyl Urea and Preservatives.
Indications: For external use as an aid in the treatment of hot spots, bacterial, fungal, parasitic and non-specific dermatoses on dogs and cats.
Administration: Shake well before using. Wash area thoroughly with Sulfur or Sulfur Tar Shampoo and dry, then apply Lotion of Sulfur to affected areas once or twice daily. May be used as a sulfur bath by adding 4 to 8 oz. to 10 gallons of water.
Caution: Keep out of reach of children. For external use only. Avoid contact of the concentrate with eyes. If contact occurs, flush immediately with fresh water. Local irritation from excessive and prolonged topical application of sulfur has been reported. Some patients are intolerant to concentrations of sulfur acceptable to others; in such cases dilute Lotion of Sulfur in half with water. If irritation continues, discontinue use and consult your veterinarian.
How Supplied: 4 oz. and 1 gallon plastic bottles. Sold only through licensed veterinarians.

PAN-OTIC
Aloe Vera Gel Ear Cleaner for Dogs and Cats.

Composition: Contains: Aloe Vera Gel, Glycerine USP, Tea Lauryl Sulfate, Dioctyl Sodium Sulfosuccinate, Preservative and U. S. Certified Colors.
Indications: Ear Cleaner for dogs, cats, puppies and kittens to aid in cleaning ears characterized by pus, seborrhea oleosa and excess wax.
Administration: Apply sufficient amount to fill canal and completely wet the affected area. Grasp base of canal and massage upwards. Remove exudate. Repeat until ear is clean; allowing ear to remain wet with product. Repeat once or twice daily.
Caution: Keep out of reach of children. Avoid contact with eyes. In case of contact, flush immediately with fresh water. In case of irritation or inflammation of ears, discontinue use and consult your veterinarian.
How Supplied: 2 and 12 oz. plastic bottles. Sold only through licensed veterinarians.

PAN-SAN
Disinfectant

Composition: Active Ingredients: Octyl Decyl Dimethyl Ammonium Chloride 3.750%, Dioctyl Dimethyl Ammonium Chloride 1.875%, Didecyl Dimethyl Ammonium Chloride 1.875%, Alkyl (C14, 50%; C_{12}, 40%; C_{16}, 10%) Dimethyl Benzyl Ammonium Chloride 5.000%, Tetrasodium EDTA 3,420%, Inert Ingredients 84.080%.
Indications: A highly concentrated germicide based on a unique blend of quaternaries with organic soil load tolerance. Cleaner, disinfectant, deodorizer, fungicide, virucide, sanitizer for hospital and institutional use. Effective in the presence of blood serum and organic matter on porous and non-porous environmental surfaces.
Use: Dilute ½ ounce per gallon of water. Prepare a fresh solution daily or when solution becomes visibly dirty. Treated surfaces must remain wet for 10 minutes.
Caution: Keep out of reach of children.
Danger: Corrosive. Causes severe eye and skin damage. Do not get in eyes, on skin or on clothing. Wear goggles or face shield and rubber gloves when handling. Harmful or fatal if swallowed. Do not contaminate water, food or feed by storage or disposal.
Statement of Practical Treatment: In case of contact, immediately flush eyes or skin with plenty of water for at least 15 minutes. For eyes, call a physician. Remove and wash contaminated clothing before re-use.
If swallowed, drink promptly a large quantity of milk, egg whites, gelatin solution; or if these are not available, drink large quantities of water. Avoid alcohol. Call a physician immediately.
Note to Physician: Probable mucosal damage may contraindicate the use of gastric lavage. Measures against circulatory shock, as well as oxygen and measures to support breathing manually or mechanically may be needed. If persistent, convulsions may be controlled by the cautious intravenous injection of a short-acting barbiturate drug.
How Supplied: One gallon plastic bottles. Sold only through licensed veterinarians.

SKIN CONDITIONER AND SOFTENER

Composition: Contains: Water, Aloe Vera Gel, Dioctyl Sodium Sulfosuccinate, Peg 75 Lanolin, Propylene Glycol USP, Coconut Extract, Preservatives and U. S. Certified Color.
Indications: To lubricate and soften dry scaly skin in puppies, dogs, cats and kittens. Skin Conditioner and Softener is an aqueous solution of lighty perfumed, highly refined lanolin oil and special hair and skin conditioners to soften and lubricate dry, scaly skin associated with chronic allergic dermatoses, callouses and seborrhea.
Administration: Using a fine mist, wet the affected area thoroughly. Massage until the sudsing effect disappears. Set for 3–5 minutes then towel off excess and air or blow dry. Repeat daily or as needed.
Caution: Keep out of reach of children. Avoid contact with eyes. If contact occurs flush immediately with fresh water.

How Supplied: 16 oz. plastic bottle with trigger sprayer and 1 gallon bottle. Sold only through licensed veterinarians.

SULFUR SHAMPOO
Cleansing Shampoo with Colloidal Sulfur and Aloe Vera Gel for Dogs and Cats.

Composition: Contains: Deionized Water, Sodium Lauryl Ether Sulfate, Aloe Vera Gel, Cocamide Dea, Propylene Glycol USP, Peg 75 Lanolin, Colloidal Sulfur, Magnesium Aluminum Silicate, Fragrance, Preservatives and U.S. Certified Colors.
Indications: For external use as a cleansing shampoo and as an aid in the treatment of bacterial, fungal, parasitic and nonspecific dermatoses of dogs and cats.
Administration: Shake well before using. Thoroughly soak hair with warm water, apply Sulfur Shampoo and work into a lather for several minutes. Avoid getting concentrated shampoo in the eyes. Rinse well with warm water and dry.
Caution: Keep out of reach of children. For external use only. Do not use on animals under 4 weeks of age.
Avoid contact of the concentrate with eyes. If contact occurs flush immediately with fresh water. Rinse hands thoroughly after using. Local irritation from excessive and prolonged topical application of sulfur has been reported. In some cases it may be necessary to dilute sulfur shampoo in half with water. If irritation continues, discontinue use and consult your veterinarian.
How Supplied: 6 and 12 oz. and 1 gallon plastic bottles. Sold only through licensed veterinarians.

SULFUR TAR SHAMPOO
Neutral pH Cleansing Shampoo with Sulfur and Coal Tar for Dogs.

Composition: Contains 3% USP Coal Tar Solution, Deionized Water, Sodium Lauryl Ether Sulfate, Aloe Vera Gel, Cocamide Dea, Propylene Glycol USP, Peg 75 Lanolin, Colloidal Sulfur, Magnesium Aluminum Silicate, Fragrance, Preservatives and U.S. Certified Color.
Administration: Shake well before using. Thoroughly soak hair coat with warm water, apply shampoo, lather and let set for 10 minutes. Rinse well and dry. Repeat as directed by your veterinarian.
Caution: Keep out of reach of children. For external use only. Do not use on cats. Do not use on puppies under 4 weeks of age. Avoid getting concentrated shampoo in eyes. If contact occurs, flush immediately with fresh water.
How Supplied: 6 and 12 oz. and 1 gallon plastic bottles. Sold only through licensed veterinarians.

SURFACE SPRAY
Water-Base Residual Insecticide Spray.

Composition: Active Ingredients: d-trans Allethrin 0.05%, Related Compounds 0.004%, N-octyl Bicycloheptene Dicarboxamide 0.40%, 0,0,-diethyl 0-(3,5,6-trichloro 2-pyridyl phosophorothioate)* 0.50%, Aromatic Petroleum Distillate 0.282%, Petroleum Distillate 0.002%, Inert Ingredients 96.72%, (*Chlorpyrifos U.S. Patent No. 3,244,586, Dow Chemical Co.)
Indications: Residual water-base insecticide spray for application to surfaces to kill fleas, ticks, roaches and ants. For use in homes, kennels, veterinary clinics, commercial buildings, warehouses, theaters, office buildings, schools, motels, restaurants, hotels and food processing facilities. May be used around plants and vegetation.
Administration: Spray surfaces with a coarse spray until wet. Spray into areas where pests are found or may hide, including dark corners of rooms and closets, cracks and crevices, and walls, around baseboards and door and window frames, beneath and behind sinks, stoves, refrigerators and cabinets, around garbage cans, plumbing and other utility installations. Thoroughly apply as a spot treatment to infested areas for control of brown dog ticks and fleas, such as pet beds and resting quarters, nearby cracks and crevices and localized areas of floor and floor coverings where these pests may be present.
Caution: Keep out of reach of children. Harmful if swallowed, inhaled or absorbed through the skin. Avoid breathing spray mist and provide adequate ventilation of areas being treated. Avoid contact with skin, eyes and clothing. Do not allow children to touch treated surfaces until spray has dried. Wash thoroughly with soap and water after handling. Do not use in commercial food processing or preparation areas. In home, all food processing surfaces and utensils should be covered during treatment or thoroughly washed before use. Cover exposed food. Remove pets, birds and cover fish aquaria before spraying. Do not spray pets or allow pets to contact treated surfaces until spray has dried.
Note to Physician: Chlorpyrifos is a cholinesterase inhibitor. Treat symptomatically. Atropine by injection is an antidote of choice.
How Supplied: 32 oz. plastic bottles with trigger sprayers and 1 gallon plastic bottles. Sold only through licensed veterinarians.

IDENTIFICATION PROBLEM?
Consult the
Product Identification Section
where you'll find
products pictured
in full color.

American Hoechst Corporation
See HOECHST-ROUSSEL AGRI-VET COMPANY

Anthony Products Company
5600 PECK ROAD
ARCADIA, CA 91006

DEXAMETH-A-VET INJECTION
(brand of Dexamethasone)

Actions: Dexamethasone is a synthetic corticosteroid and possesses glucocorticoid activity. It is especially designed for intravenous use in situations requiring a rapid and intense glucocorticoid and/or anti-inflammatory effect.
Indications: Dexamethasone is indicated for use in situations in which a rapid adrenal glucocorticoid and/or anti-inflammatory effect is indicated.
Dosage and Administration: For Intravenous Use Only:
Horses—The usual intravenous dosage is 2.5 to 5 mg. as the initial dosage in shock and shock-like states followed by equal maintenance doses at 1, 3, 6 or 10 hour intervals as determined by the condition of the patient.
If permanent corticosteroid effect is required, oral therapy with dexamethason tablets may be substituted. When therapy is to be withdrawn after prolonged corticosteroid administration, the daily dose should be reduced gradually over a number of days, in stepwise fashion.
Contraindications: Do not use in viral infections. Except when used for emergency therapy, dexamethasone is contraindicated in animals with tuberculosis, and chronic nephritis. Existence of congestive heart failure, osteoporosis and diabetes are relative contraindications. In the presence of infection, appropriate anti-bacterial agents should also be administered and should be continued for at least 3 days after discontinuance of the hormone and disappearance of all signs of infection.
Precautions: Because of the anti-inflammatory action of corticosteroids, sign of infection may be hidden and it may be necessary to stop treatment until diagnosis is made. Overdosage of some glucocorticoids may result in sodium retention, potassium loss and weight gains. In infections characterized by overwhelming toxicity, dexamethasone therapy in conjunction with indicated antibacterial therapy is effective in reducing mortality and morbidity. It is essential that the causative organism be known and an effective antibacterial agent be administered concurrently. The injudicious use of adrenal hormones in animals with infections can be hazardous.
Side Effects: The therapeutic use of Dexameth-A-Vet (brand of dexamethasone) is unlikely to cause undesired accentuation of metabolic effects. However, if continued corticosteroid therapy

Continued on next page

Anthony—Cont.

is anticipated, a high protein intake should be provided to keep the animal in positive nitrogen balance. A retardant effect on wound healing has not been encountered, but such a possibility should also be considered when it is used in conjunction with surgery. Euphoria or an improvement of attitude, and increased appetite are usual manifestations. Side reactions such as glycosuria, hyperglycemia, diarrhea, polydipsia and polyuria have been observed in some species.
Warning: Clinical and experimental data have demonstrated that corticosteroids administered orally or parenterally to animals may induce the first stage of parturition when administered during the last trimester of pregnancy and may precipitate premature parturition followed by dystocia, fetal death, retained placenta and metritis.
Not for use in horses intended for food.
Caution: Federal law restricts this drug to sale by or on the order of a licensed veterinarian.
How Supplied: Dexameth-A-Vet is supplied in:
30 ml., 50 ml. and 100 ml. vials, containing 2 mg. of dexamethasone per ml.
Ingredient Statement: Injection 30 ml., 50 ml. and 100 ml. vials, 2 mg of dexamethasone per ml. Each ml. of sterile aqueous solution contains 2 mg. of dexamethasone, polyethylene glycol 400, 500 mg., benzyl alcohol 9 mg., methylparaben 1.8 mg., propylparaben 0.2 mg., alcohol 0.05 ml., Purified Water, USP.

DEX-A-VET INJECTION
(brand of Dexamethasone Sodium Phosphate)

Actions: Dexamethasone is a synthetic corticosteroid and possess glucocorticoid activity. Dexamethasone sodium phosphate is a salt of dexamethasone that is particularly suitable for intravenous administration because it is highly water soluble, permitting administration of relatively large doses in a small volume of diluent. It is especially designed for intravenous use in situations requiring a rapid and intense glucocorticoid and/or anti-inflammatory effect.
Indications: Dexamethasone sodium phosphate is indicated for use in situations in which a rapid adrenal glucocorticoid and/or anti-inflammatory effect is indicated.
Dosage and Administration: For Intravenous Use Only.
Horses—The usual intravenous dosage is 2.5 to 5 mg.
If permanent corticosteroid effect is required, oral therapy with dexamethasone tablets may be substituted. When therapy is to be withdrawn after prolonged corticosteroid administration, the daily dose should be reduced gradually over a number of days, in stepwise fashion.
Contraindications: Do not use in viral infections. Except when used for emergency therapy, dexamethasone sodium phosphate is contraindicated in animals with tuberculosis and chronic nephritis. Existence of congestive heart failure and osteoporosis are relative contraindications.
In the presence of infection, appropriate anti-bacterial agents should also be administered and should not be continued for at least 3 days after discontinuance of the hormone and disappearance of all signs of infection.
Precautions: Because of the anti-inflammatory action of corticosteroids, signs of infection may be hidden and it may be necessary to stop treatment until diagnosis is made. Overdosage of some glucocorticoids may result in sodium retention, fluid retention, potassium loss and weight gains.
In infections characterized by overwhelming toxicity, dexamethasone sodium phosphate therapy in conjunction with indicated antibacterial therapy is effective in reducing mortality and morbidity. It is essential that the causative organism be known and an effective antibacterial agent be administered concurrently. The injudicious use of adrenal hormones in animals with infections can be hazardous.
Side Effects: The therapeutic use of Dex-A-Vet is unlikely to cause undesired accentuation of metabolic effects. However, if continued corticosteroid therapy is anticipated, a high protein intake should be provided to keep the animal in positive nitrogen balance. A retardant effect on wound healing has been encountered, but such a possibility should also be considered when it is used in conjunction with surgery. Euphoria, or an improvement of attitude, and increased appetite are usual manifestations.
Side reactions such as glycosuria, hyperglycemia, diarrhea, polydipsia and polyuria have been observed in some species.
Warning: Clinical and experimental data have demonstrated that corticosteroids administered orally or parenterally to animals may induce the first stage of parturition when administered during the last trimester of pregnancy and may precipitate premature parturition followed by dystocia, fetal death, retained placenta and metritis.
Not for use in horses intended for food.
Caution: Federal law restricts this drug to sale by or on the order of a licensed veterinarian.
How Supplied: Dex-A-Vet is supplied in:
30 ml., 50 ml., and 100 ml. vials, 4 mg. of dexamethasone sodium phosphate per ml. Each ml. of sterile aqueous solution contains 4 mg. of dexamethasone sodium phosphate, 10 mg. sodium citrate, 0.2% sodium bisulfite, 1.5% benzyl alcohol, sodium hydroxide to adjust the pH between 7.5–8.5. Purified Water USP.

DIURIDE
(furosemide)
INJECTION

A diuretic-saluretic for prompt relief of edema.
CAUTION: Federal law restricts this drug to use by or on the order of a licensed veterinarian.
Description: Diuride (furosemide) is a chemically distinct diuretic and saluretic pharmacodynamically characterized by the following:
1) A high degree of efficacy, low-inherent toxicity and a high therapeutic index.
2) A rapid onset of action and of comparatively short duration.[1]
3) A pharmacological action in the functional area of the nephron, i.e., proximal and distal tubules and the ascending limb of the loop of Henle.[3,4]
4) A dose-response relationship and a ratio of minimum to maximum effective dose range greater than tenfold.[1]
5) It is administered parenterally. The intravenous route produces the most rapid diuretic response.

Diuride (furosemide), a diuretic, is an anthranilic acid derivative with the following structural formula:

Generic Name: Furosemide (except in United Kingdom—Frusemide)
Chemical Name: 4-chloro-N-furfuryl-5 sulfamoylanthranilic acid.
Actions: The therapeutic efficacy of Diuride (furosemide) is from the activity of the intact and unaltered molecule throughout the nephron, inhibiting the reabsorption of sodium not only in the proximal and distal tubule but also in the ascending limb of the loop of Henle. The prompt onset of action is a result of the drug's rapid absorption and poor lipid solubility. The low lipid solubility and a rapid renal excretion minimize the possibility of its accumulation in tissues and organs or crystalluria. Diuride (furosemide) has no inhibitory effect on carbonic anhydrase activity in the distal tubule.[2,3,4,5]
Indications: Horses: Diuride (furosemide) is indicated for the treatment of acute non-inflammatory tissue edema.
Precautions: Concurrent therapy for the treatment of the condition causing the edema (pulmonary congestion, ascites, cardiac insufficiency) should be instituted.
The continued use of heart stimulants, such as digitalis or its glycosides is indicated in cases of edema involving cardiac insufficiency.
Diuride (furosemide) is a highly effective diuretic-saluretic which if given in excessive amounts may result in dehydration and electrolyte imbalance. Therefore, the dosage and schedule may have to be adjusted to the patient's needs. The animal should be observed for early signs of electrolyte imbalance, and corrective measures administered. Early signs of electrolyte imbalance are: increased thirst, lethargy, drowsiness or restlessness, fatigue, oliguria, gastrointestinal disturbances and tachycardia. Special attention should be given to potassium levels. Diuride (furosemide) may lower serum calcium levels and cause tetany in

rare cases of animals having an existing hypocalcemic tendency.[6,7,8,9,10]
Electrolyte balance should be monitored prior to surgery in patients receiving Diuride (furosemide). Imbalances must be corrected by administration of suitable fluid therapy.
Contraindications: Diuride (furosemide) is contraindicated in anuria. Therapy should be discontinued in cases of progressive renal disease if increasing azotemia and oliguria occur during the treatment. Sudden alterations of fluid and electrolyte imbalance in an animal with cirrhosis may precipitate hepatic coma, therefore observation during period of therapy is necessary. In hepatic coma and in states of electrolyte depletion, therapy should not be instituted until the basic condition is improved or corrected. Potassium supplementation may be necessary in cases routinely treated with potassium-depleting steroids.
Although diabetes mellitus is a rarely reported disease in animals, active or latent diabetes mellitus may on rare occasions be exacerbated by Diuride (furosemide). While it has not been reported in animals, the use of high doses of salicylates, as in rheumatic diseases, in conjunction with Diuride (furosemide) may result in salicylate toxicity because of competition for renal excretory sites.
Warnings: Do not use in horses intended for food.
Diuride (furosemide) is a highly effective diuretic and if given in excessive amounts, as with any diuretic, may lead to excessive diuresis which could result in electrolyte imbalance, dehydration and reduction of plasma volume enhancing the risk of circulatory collapse, thrombosis and embolism. Therefore, the animal should be observed for early signs of fluid depletion with electrolyte imbalance, and corrective measures administered. Excessive loss of potassium in patients receiving digitalis or its glycosides may precipitate digitalis toxicity. Caution should be exercised in animal administered potassium-depleting steroids. It is important to correct potassium deficiency with dietary supplementation. Caution should be exercised in prescribing enteric-coated potassium tablets.
There have been several reports in human literature, published and unpublished, concerning nonspecific small-bowel lesions consisting of stenosis, with or without ulceration, associated with the administration of enteric-coated thiazides with potassium salts. These lesions may occur with enteric-coated potassium tablets alone or when they are used with nonenteric-coated thiazides, or certain other oral diuretics. These small-bowel lesions may have caused obstruction, hemorrhage and perforation. Surgery was frequently required and deaths have occurred. Available information tends to implicate enteric-coated potassium salts, although lesions of this type also occur spontaneously. Therefore, coated potassium-containing formulations should be administered only when indicated and should be discontinued immediately if abdominal pain, distention, nausea, vomiting or gastrointestinal bleeding occurs.
Human patients with known sulfonamide sensitivity may show allergic reactions to furosemide; however, these reactions have not been reported in animals. Sulfonamide diuretics have been reported to decrease arterial responsiveness to pressor amines and to enhance the effect of tubocurarine. Caution should be exercised in administering curare or its derivatives to patients undergoing therapy with "Diuride" and it is advisable to discontinue "Diuride" for one day prior to any elective surgery.
Dosage and Administration: Administer 0.5 mg. per pound of body weight (approximately 1.0 mg. per kg.) once or twice daily at 6 to 8 hour intervals either intravenously or intramuscularly. A prompt diuresis usually ensues from the initial treatment. Diuresis may be initiated by the parenteral administration of "Diuride" Injection. The dosage should be adjusted to the individual's response. In severe edematous or refractory cases, the dose may be doubled or increased by increments of 1 mg. per pound of body weight. The established effective dose should be administered once or twice daily. The daily schedule of administration can be timed to control the period of micturition for the convenience of the client or veterinarian. Mobilization of the edema may be most efficiently and safely accomplished by utilizing an intermittent daily dosage schedule, i.e. every other day or 2 to 4 consecutive days weekly.
Diuretic therapy should be discontinued after reduction of the edema, or maintained after determining a carefully programmed dosage schedule to prevent recurrence of edema. For long term treatment, the dose can generally be lowered after the edema has once been reduced. Re-examination and consultations with the client will enhance the establishment of a satisfactorily programmed dosage schedule. Clinical examination and serum BUN, CO_2 and electrolyte determination should be performed during the early period of therapy and periodically thereafter, especially in refractory cases. Abnormalities should be corrected or the drug temporarily withdrawn.
How Supplied: Parenteral: Diuride Injection 5% (50 mg. per ml.). Each ml. contains 50 mg. furosemide as a diethanolamine salt, myristyl-gamma-picolinium chloride 0.02%, EDTA sodium 0.1%, sodium sulfite 0.1%, sodium chloride 0.2%, water for injection. pH adjusted with sodium hydroxide.
Available in 30 ml., 50 ml., and 100 ml., multiple dose vials.
TOXICOLOGY *Acute Toxicity:* The following table illustrates low acute toxicity of furosemide in three different species. (Two values indicate two different studies) LD_{50} of furosemide in mg/kg body weight.

SPECIES	INTRAVENOUS
Mouse	308
Rat	680
Dog	>300 and >464

Toxic doses lead to convulsions, ataxia, paralysis and collapse. Animals surviving toxic dosages may become dehydrated and depleted of electrolytes due to the massive diuresis and saluresis.
Chronic Toxicity: Chronic toxicity studies with furosemide were done on a one-year study in rats and dogs. In a one-year study in rats, renal tubular degeneration occurred with all doses higher than 50 mg/kg. A six-month study in dogs revealed calcification and scarring of the renal parenchyma at all doses above 10 mg/kg.
Reproductive Studies:
Reproductive studies were conducted in mice, rats and rabbits. Only in rabbits administered high doses (equivalent to 10 to 25 times the recommended average dose of 2 mg/kg) of furosemide during the second trimester period did unexplained maternal deaths and abortions occur. The safety of Diuride (furosemide) in breeding animals or in pregnant mares has not been investigated. Therefore, do not use in stallions at stud or in pregnant mares.
References:

1. Timmerman, R.J.; Springman, F.R., and Thomas, R.K.; Evaluation of Furosemide, a New Diuretic Agent. Current Therapeutic Research 6 (2): 88–94, February 1964.
2. Muschaweck, R., and Hajdu, P.: Die salidiuretische Wirksamkeit der Chlor-N-(2-furylmethyl)-5-sulfamyl-anthranilsaure. Arzneimittel-Forschung 14:44–47, 1964. (The Saluretic Action of 4-Chloro-N-(2-furylmethyl)-5-sulfamyl-anthranilic acid).
3. Suki, W.; Rector, Jr., F.C., and Seldin, D.W.: The Site of Action of Furosemide and Other Sulfonamide Diuretics in the Dog. Journal of Clinical Investigation 44(9): 1458–1469, 1965.
4. Deetjen, P.: Mikropunktionsuntersuchungen zur Wirkung von Furosemid. Pflugers Archiv fuer die Gesamte Physiologie 284: 184–190, 1965 (Micropuncture Studies of the Action of Furosemide).
5. Berman, L.B., and Ebrahimi, A.:- Experiences with Furosemide in Renal Diease. Proceedings of the Society for Experimental Biology and Medicine 118:333–336, February 1965.
6. Antoniou, L.D.; Eisner, G.M.; Slotkoff, L.M., and Lilienfield, L.S.; Sodium and Calcium Transport in the Kidney. Clinical Research 15(4):476, December 1967.
7. Duarte, C.G.: Effects of Furosemide (F) and Ethacrynic Acid (ETA) on the Renal Clearance of Phosphate (Cp), Ultrafilterable Calcium (CUfCa) and Magnesium (CUfMg). Clinical Research 15(2):357, April 1967.

Continued on next page

Anthony—Cont.

8. Duarte, C.G.: Effects of Ethacrynic Acid and Furosemide on Urinary Calcium, Phosphate and Magnesium. Metabolism 17:867–876, October 1968.
9. Nielsen, S.P.; Andersen, O., and Steven, K.E.: Magnesium and Calcium Metabolism during Prolonged Furosemide Administration to Normal Rats. Acta Pharmacol. et Toxicol. 1969, 27:469–479.
10. Reimold, E.W.: The Effect of Furosemide on Hypercalcemia Due to Dihydrotachysterol. Metabolism 21 (7), July 1972.

FURA-SEPTIN
(Brand of Nitrofurazone Soluble Dressing)
For use only on dogs, cats and horses

Description: An Antibacterial preparation for topical application. Contains: 0.2% Nitrofurazone in a water soluble base of Polyethylene Glycols.
Indications: For the prevention or treatment of surface bacterial infections of wounds, burns, cutaneous ulcers. For use only on dogs, cats and horses.
Administration: Apply directly on the lesion with a spatula or first place on a piece of gauze. Application of a bandage is optional.
This preparation should be in contact with the lesion for at least 24 hours. The dressing may be changed several times daily or left on for a longer period.
Caution: In case of deep or puncture wounds or serious burns consult veterinarian. If redness, irritation or swelling persists or increases, discontinue use and consult veterinarian.
Warning: Do not use on horses intended for food.
Avoid exposure to excessive heat or direct sunlight and strong fluorescent lighting.
How Supplied: Fura-Septin is supplied in 4 oz. and 1 pound jars.

OXYTOCIN INJECTION
20 USP UNITS/ML
For Veterinary Use Only
For Horses and Cows
Sows and Ewes
Dogs and Cats

Description: Oxytocin is a highly purified oxytocic principle prepared by synthesis or obtained from the posterior lobe of the pituitary gland of healthy domestic animals used for food by man. Each ml contains: oxytocic activity equivalent to 20 USP posterior pituitary units, chlorobutanol (chloral derivative) 5 mg., acetic acid 0.25%, water for injection q.s.
Actions: Oxytocin is a hormone of the pituitary with pronounced uterine-contracting and milk-releasing actions.
Oxytocin acts directly on the smooth musculature of the uterus in all species to produce rhythmic contraction. The degree of uterine activity elicited by oxytocin depends to a great extent on the stage of the reproductive cycle. Most authorities agree that the level of estrogen and progesterone in the various phases of pregnancy is the main controlling factor of the activity that oxytocin has on the uterus. During the early phases of normal pregnancy, the uterus is relatively insensitive to oxytocin; in the late phase of pregnancy, the sensitivity is increased.
Oxytocin has an integral relationship with the letdown of milk. The mechanism by which milk is discharged from mammary glands is not definitely known, but oxytocin is presumed to act on certain smooth muscle elements in the gland. It has been clearly demonstrated, however, that oxytocin will promote a prompt milk-ejecting effect.
Indications: Oxytocin may be used as a uterine contractor to precipitate and accelerate normal parturition and postpartum evacuation of uterine debris. In surgery, it may be used postoperatively following Caesarean section to facilitate involution and resistance to the large inflow of blood.
Contraindications: Do not use in dystocia due to abnormal presentation of fetus until correction is accomplished.
Precautions: For prepartum usage, full relaxation of the cervix should be acomplished either naturally or by the administration of estrogen prior to oxytocin therapy.
Dosage and Administration: Oxytocin injection may be injected intravenously, intramuscularly, or subcutaneously under aseptic conditions as indicated. The following dosages are recommended and may be repeated as conditions require:
[See table below].
How Supplied: 10 ml, 30 ml, and 100 ml sterile, multiple dose vials.
Storage: Store in refrigerator at between 2°–8°C (36°–46°F). Do not freeze.
Caution: Federal law restricts this drug to use by or on the order of a licensed veterinarian.
Rev. 11/84

ANTHONY PRODUCTS CO.
ARCADIA, CALIF. 91006 U.S.A.

For Obstetrical Use	USP Units	ml
Horses and Cows	100	(5 ml)
Sows and Ewes	30 to 50	(1.5 to 2.5 ml)
Dogs	5 to 30	(0.25 to 1.5 ml)
Cats	5 to 10	(0.25 to 0.5 ml)
For Milk Letdown		
Cows	10 to 20	(0.5 to 1.0 ml)
Sows	5 to 20	(0.25 to 1.0 ml)

PHEN-BUTA-VET
Tablet or Injection

Description: Phenylbutazone is the accepted generic name for the drug known chemically as 4-Butyl-1,2diphenyl-3-5-pyrazolidinedione.
Phenylbutazone is a white crystalline solid, slightly soluble in water, and soluble in some organic solvents. It has no odor and a slightly bitter taste.
Background Pharmacology: Phenylbutazone is a non-hormonal anti-inflammatory agent. It is unrelated to the corticosteroid anti-inflammatory agents.
The anti-inflammatory activity of phenylbutazone has been shown in lower animals (1) and in man (2). The greatest amount of data of efficacy is in man (3–6). Studies in horses have reported useful anti-inflammatory activity (7–10). Metabolic studies in horses have shown that the drug is well absorbed when administered orally with a balling gun. The apparent half-life is 3.5 hours (11,12).
Indications: Phenylbutazone is used for the relief of inflammatory conditions of horses associated with the musculoskeletal system.
Contraindications: Use with caution in patients who have a history of drug allergy.
Precautions: In the treatment of inflammatory conditions associated with infections specific anti-infective therapy is required.
Warning: Not for use in horses intended for food.
Side Effects: Doses of phenylbutazone higher than those recommended have been shown to produce intestinal ulcerative lesions (12). Necrotizing phlebitis in the portal vein has been observed in horses receiving high doses for extended periods of time (13).
Dosage and Administration—Injection: The intravenous dose for horses is 5 to 10 ml. (1 to 2 grams) per 1000 lbs. per day. The injection should be administered slowly. Intravenous administration should be limited to 5 consecutive days. An initial high dose is recommended to obtain a prompt effect. As the symptom regresses, the dose should be reduced.
Dosage and Administration—Tablets: The oral dose for horses is 2 to 4 tablets (2 to 4 grams) per 1000 lbs. per day. The total daily dose should be limited to 4 tablets per day. Because of the relatively short half-life of the drug, administration every eight hours is the most satisfactory schedule.
Response to phenylbutazone is usually prompt. If there is no significant clinical effect in 5 days, a re-evaluation of the diagnosis and treatment should be made.
Supplied: Phenylbutazone is supplied in:
30 ml. vials, 50 ml. vials and 100 ml. vials containing 200 mg. of phenylbutazone per ml. Bottles of 100 tablets, each tablet containing 1 gram of phenylbutazone.
Caution: Federal (USA) law restricts this drug to use by or on the order of a licensed veterinarian.
Ingredient Statement:—Injection: 30 ml., 50 ml. and 100 ml. vials, 200 mg. of phenylbutazone per ml. Each ml. of sterile aqueous solution contains 200 mg. of phenylbutazone, 1.5% benzyl alcohol as preservative, sodium hydroxide to adjust the pH, purified water, USP.
Store product in a cool place (46° to 59°F) or alternatively store in a refrigerator.

References
1. Lieberman, L. L.: Jour. Amer. Vet. Med. Assoc. 125:128, 1954.
2. Kusell, W.C., Schaffarzick, R.W., Naugler, W.G., and Mankle, E.A.: A.M. Arch. Int. Med. 92:646, 1953.
3. Payne, R.W., Shetlar, M.R., Farr, C. Hellbaum, A.A. and Ishmael W.K.T.: J. Lab. Clin. Med. 45:331, 1955.
4. Fleming, J., and Will. G.: Ann. Rheumat. Dis. 12:95, 1953.
5. Denko, C.W., and Ruml, D.: Amer. Practit. 6:1865, 1955.
6. Yourish, N., Paton, B., Brodie, B.B., and Burns, J.J.: A.M.A. Arch. Ophth. 53:264, 1955.
7. Camberos, H.R.: Rev. Med. Vet (Buenos Aires). 39:9, 1956.
8. Sutter, M.D.: Vet. Med. 53:83 (Feb.), 1958.
9. Oehme, F.W.: Vet. Med. 57:229, 1962.
10. Davidson, A.H., Franks W.C., Mod. Vet. Practice 47:46, 1966.
11. Piperno, E. et al.: Jour. Amer. Vet. Med. Assoc. 153:195, 1968.
12. Finnochio, E.J. et al.: Jour. Amer. Vet. Med. Assoc. 156:454, 1970.
13. Gabriel K. and J.E. Martin: Jour. Amer. Vet. Med. Assoc. 140:337, 1962.

Barry Laboratories, Inc.

Veterinary Division
461 N.E. 27TH ST.
POMPANO BEACH, FL 33064

ALLERGENIC EXTRACT

Description: The vial contains an allergenic extract of individual or mixed allergens from one of the following categories:

1. mixed trees	5. mixed molds
2. mixed grasses	6. mixed inhalants
3. mixed weeds	7. mixed epidermals
4. mixed ragweed	8. house dust

Note: The prefix "mixed" was used for product licensing purposes. Only individual allergens and botanically related mixtures will be produced.
It is a dilution of allergen(s) as labelled in a buffered saline menstruum pH 7.4, containing: 0.5% Sodium Choloride; 0.8% Dibasic Sodium Phosphate; 0.145% Monobasic Potassium Phosphate; 50% Glycerine and 0.4% Phenol as preservative; intended for use in the treatment of canines.
Actions: The mechanism of allergenic extracts is under investigation at this time. However, in sensitive canines, probable actions are as follows:
a. Intradermal injections of antigen causes the release of histamine and other chemical mediators from mast cells as a result of its interaction with lgE skin-sensitizing antibody.
b. Subcutaneous injection of antigen initiates the production of lgG blocking antibody and the reduction of serum lgE concentration.
Indications: Concentrated allergenic extracts, when properly diluted, are indicated for the diagnosis and treatment of canine inhalant dermatitis and contact dermatitis.
How Supplied: They are supplied in 1.0 ml; 10 ml; and 30 ml vials at a dilution of 1:20 05% w/v).

ALLERGENIC EXTRACT, FLEA ANTIGEN

Description: The vial contains an aqueous allergenic extract of fleas commonly found on canines (Ctenocephalides spp.). It is a dilution of allergen as labelled in a buffered saline menstruum ph 7.4, containing: 0.5% Sodium Chloride; 0.8% Dibasic Sodium Phosphate; 0.145% Monobasic Potassium Phosphate; and 0.4% Phenol as preservative.
Actions: The mechanism of allergenic extract (flea antigen) is under investigation at this time.
Indications: The use of allergenic extract (flea antigen) is indicated as an aid in reducing the pruritus and erythema which accompanies fleabite allergic dermatitis. Its use should be in conjunction with a total flea control program.
How Supplied: It is in sterile 10.0 ml vials only at a concentration of 1:60 dilution, unless otherwise specified.

ALLERGENIC EXTRACT
Prescription Product

Description: The treatment set contains a dilution series of an allergenic extract(s) from one or more of the following categories in ready to use form for immunotherapy

1. mixed trees	5. mixed molds
2. mixed grasses	6. mixed inhalants
3. mixed weeds	7. mixed epidermals
4. mixed ragweed	8. house dust

It is a dilution of allergen(s) as labelled in a buffered saline menstruum pH 7.4, containing: 0.5% Sodium Chloride; 0.8% Dibasic Sodium Phosphate; 0.145% Monobasic Potassium Phosphate; 0.4% Phenol as preservative and may contain up to 50% Glycerine; intended for use in the treatment of canines.
Actions: The mechanism of allergenic extracts used for immunotherapy is under investigation at this time. It is probably due to the production of lgG blocking antibody which reduces the effective concentration of antigen that can react with cell bound lgE antibody. There is also a slight reduction in the concentration of serum lgE levels.
Indications: Allergenic Extract, Prescription Product when compounded on the basis of positive skin tests and positive history, is indicated in the treatment of canine inhalant dermatitis.
How Supplied: The Prescription Product is supplied as a sterile 3 Vial dilution series at concentrations of: 1:20, 1:100, 1:1,000 w/v in 5 ml vials. The maintenance dose dilution is supplied in 5 ml and 10 ml vials at a concentration of 1:20 dilution w/v unless otherwise specified.

Products are cross-indexed by generic and chemical names in the **Active Ingredients Section**

Beecham Laboratories

501 FIFTH STREET
BRISTOL, TN 37620

AMOXI-DROP®
(amoxicillin)
Veterinary Oral Suspension
For Use in Dogs and Cats

Composition: Amoxi-Drop® (amoxicillin) is a semi-synthetic antibiotic with a broad spectrum of activity. It provides bactericidal activity against a wide range of common Gram-positive and Gram-negative pathogens. Chemically, it is D-(-)α-amino-p-hydroxy-benzyl penicillin trihydrate.
Indications: *In Dogs*—Amoxi-Drop is indicated in the treatment of susceptible strains of the organisms causing the following infections:
Respiratory Tract Infections (Tonsillitis, Tracheobronchitis) due to *Staphylococcus aureus, Streptococcus spp., E. coli,* and *Proteus mirabilis.*
Genitourinary Tract Infections (Cystitis) due to *Staphylococcus aureus, Streptococcus spp., E. coli,* and *Proteus mirabilis.*
Gastrointestinal Tract Infections (Bacterial gastroenteritis) due to *Staphylococcus aureus, Streptococcus spp., E. coli,* and *Proteus mirabilis.*
Bacterial Dermatitis due to *Staphylococcus aureus, Streptococcus spp.,* and *Proteus mirabilis.*
Soft Tissue Infections (abscesses, lacerations and wounds) due to *Staphylococcus aureus, Streptococcus spp., E. coli,* and *Proteus mirabilis.*
In Cats—Amoxi-Drop is indicated in the treatment of susceptible strains of the organisms causing the following infections:
Upper Respiratory Tract infections due to *Staphylococcus aureus, Staphylococcus spp., Streptococcus spp., Hemophilus spp., E. coli, Pasteurella spp.,* and *Proteus mirabilis.*
Genitourinary Tract Infections (Cystitis) due to *Staphylococcus aureus, Streptococcus spp., E. coli, Proteus mirabilis* and *Corynebacterium spp.*
Gastrointestinal Tract Infections due to *E. coli, Proteus spp., Staphylococcus spp.,* and *Streptococcus spp.*
Skin and Soft Tissue Infections (abscesses, lacerations, and wounds) due to *Staphylococcus spp., E. coli, and Pasteurella multocida.*
Contraindications: The use of this drug is contraindicated in animals with a history of an allergic reaction to penicillin.
Action: Amoxi-Drop is stable in the presence of gastric acid and may be given without regard to meals. It is rapidly absorbed after oral administration. It diffuses readily into most body tissues and fluids with the exception of brain and spinal fluid except when meninges are inflamed. Most of amoxicillin is excreted unchanged in the urine.
Amoxicillin is similar to ampicillin in its bactericidal action against susceptible organisms. It acts through the inhibition

Continued on next page

Beecham—Cont.

of biosynthesis of cell wall mucopeptide. *In vitro* and/or *in vivo* studies have demonstrated the susceptibility of most strains of the following Gram-positive and Gram-negative bacteria: alpha and beta-hemolytic streptococci, non-penicillinase-producing staphylococci, *Streptococcus faecalis, Escherichia coli,* and *proteus mirabilis.* Because it does not resist destruction by penicillinase, it is not effective against penicillinase-producing bacteria, particularly resistant staphylococci. All strains of Pseudomonas and most strains of Klebsiella and Enterobacter are resistant.

Adverse Reactions: Amoxicillin is a semisynthetic penicillin and has the potential for producing allergic reactions. If an allergic reaction occurs, administer epinephrine and/or steroids.

Dosage and Administration:-
Dogs—the usual dosage is 5 mg per pound of body weight. Administer twice daily for 5-7 days. Continue for 48 hours after all symptoms have subsided.
Cats—the usual dosage is 50 mg (5-10 mg/lb).. Administer once daily for 5-7 days. Continue for 48 hours after all symptoms have subsided.

Directions for Mixing Oral Suspension: Add 12 ml or 23 ml of water to the 15 or 30 ml bottle and shake vigorously. Each ml of suspension will contain 50 mg of amoxicillin as the trihydrate.

Note: Any unused portion of the reconstituted suspension must be discarded after 14 days. Refrigeration preferable, but not required.

Caution: Federal law restricts this drug to use by or on the order of a licensed veterinarian.

Warnings: For use in dogs and cats only. Not for use in animals which are raised for food production.

How Supplied: Amoxi-Drop (amoxicillin) is supplied in 15 or 30 ml bottles containing 0.75 gm or 1.5 gm of amoxicillin activity. When reconstituted with 12 or 23 ml ml of water, each ml. contains 50 mg of amoxicillin as the trihydrate.

AMOXI-INJECT®
For Use In Cattle

Description: Amoxi-Inject (amoxicillin) is a semisynthetic antibiotic with a broad spectrum of activity. Amoxicillin provides bactericidal activity against a wide range of common Gram-positive and Gram-negative pathogens. Chemically, it is D-(-)α-amino-p-hydroxybenzyl penicillin trihydrate.

Action: Amoxi-Inject (amoxicillin) is rapidly absorbed following intramuscular or subcutaneous administration. It diffuses readily into most body tissues and fluids with the exception of brain and spinal fluid except when meninges are inflamed. Most of amoxicillin is excreted unchanged in the urine.
Amoxicillin is a bactericidal antibiotic. It acts through the inhibition of biosynthesis of cell wall mucopeptide. *In vitro* and/or *in vivo* studies have demonstrated the susceptibility of most strains of the following Gram-positive and Gram-negative bacteria; alpa- and beta-hemolytic streptococci, non-penicillinase- producing staphylococci, *Streptococcus faecalis, Escherichia coli,* and *Proteus mirabilis.* Because amoxicillin does not resist destruction by penicillinase, it is not effective against penicillinase-producing bacteria, particularly resistant staphylococci. All strains of Pseudomonas and most strains of Klebsiella and Enterobacter are resistant.

Indications: Amoxi-Inject® (amoxicillin) is indicated in the treatment of susceptible strains of the organisms causing the following infections in cattle (non-lactating).

Respiratory Tract Infections: (Shipping fever, pneumonia) due to *Pasteurella multocida, Pasteurella hemolyticus,* Hemophilus spp., Staphylococcus spp., and Streptococcus spp.
As with all antibiotics, appropriate *in vitro* culturing and susceptibility testing of samples taken before treatment should be conducted.

Adverse Reactions: Amoxicillin is a semisynthetic penicillin and has the potential to produce an allergic reaction. If an allergic reaction occurs, administer epinephrine and/or steroids.

Dosage and Administration: The dosage of Amoxi-Inject (amoxicillin)for veterinary aqueous injection will vary according to the animal being treated, the severity of infection, and the animal's response.
The recommended dosage for cattle (non-lactating) is 3–5 mg per pound of body weight once daily by intramuscular or subcutaneous injection. Treatment should be continued 48 to 72 hours after the animal has become afebrile or asymptomatic. Do not continue treatment beyond 5 days. Maximum volume per injection site should not exceed 30 ml.

Directions: Amoxi-Inject (amoxicillin) is packaged as a multi-dose dry filled vial and requires reconstitution prior to use. It should be reconstituted to the desired concentration by adding the recommended amount of Sterile Water for Injection, U.S.P. according to labeled directions.

Warnings: For use in non-lactating cattle only. Treated animals must not be slaughtered for food during treatment and for 25 days after the last treatment. Treatment should not exceed 5 days.

Caution: Federal law restricts this drug to use by or on the order of a licensed veterinarian.

How Supplied: Amoxi-Inject (amoxicillin) is supplied in vials containing 25 grams of amoxicillin activity as the trihydrate.

AMOXI-INJECT®
Sterile Amoxicillin for Suspension For Veterinary Aqueous Injection For Use In Dogs and Cats

Description: Amoxi-Inject (amoxicillin) is a semisynthetic antibiotic with a broad spectrum of activity. It provides bactericidal activity against a wide range of common Gram-positive and Gram-negative pathogens. Chemically it is D-(-)-α-amino-p-hydroxybenzyl penicillin trihydrate.

Actions: Amoxi-Inject is rapidly absorbed following intramuscular or subcutaneous administration. It diffuses readily into most body tissues and fluids with the exception of brain and spinal fluid except when meninges are inflamed. Most of amoxicillin is excreted unchanged in the urine.
Amoxicillin is a bactericidal antibiotic. It acts through the inhibition of biosynthesis of cell wall mucopeptide. *In vivo* and /or *in vitro* studies have demonstrated the susceptibility of most strains of the following Gram-positive and Gram-negative bacteria: alpha- and beta-hemolytic streptococci, non-penicillinase-producing staphylococci, Streptococcus spp., *Escherichia coli,* and *Proteus mirabilis.* Because amoxicillin does not resist destruction by penicillinase, it is not effective against penicillinase-producing bacteria, particularly resistant staphylococci. All strains of Pseudomonas and most strains of Klebsiella and Enterobacter are resistant.

Indications:
In Dogs —Amoxi-Inject is indicated in the treatment of susceptible strains of the organisms causing the following infections: Respiratory Tract Infections (Tonsillitis, Tracheobronchitis) due to *Staphylococcus aureus, Streptococcus* spp., *E. coli,* and *Proteus mirabilis.* Genitourinary Tract Infections (Cystitis) due to *Staphylococcus aureus,*Streptococcus spp., *E. coli,* and *Proteus mirabilis.* Gastrointestinal Tract Infections (Bacterial gastroenteritis) due to *Staphylococcus aureus,* Streptococcus spp., *E. coli,* and *Proteus mirabilis.* Bacterial Dermatitis due to *Staphylococcus aureus,* Streptococcus spp., and *Proteus mirabilis.* Soft Tissue Infections (Abscesses, lacerations and wounds) due to *Staphylococcus aureus,* Streptococcus spp., *E. coli,* and *Proteus mirabilis.*
In Cats —Amoxi-Inject is indicated in the treatment of susceptible strains of the organisms causing the following infections: Upper Respiratory Tract Infections due to *Staphylococcus aureus,* Staphylococcus spp., Streptococcus spp., Hemophilus spp., *E. coli,* Pasteurella spp., and *Proteus mirabilis.* Genitourinary Tract Infections (Cystitis) due to *Staphylococcus aureus,* Streptococcus spp., *E. coli, Proteus mirabilis,* and Corynebacterium spp. Gastrointestinal Tract Infections due to *E. coli,* Proteus spp., Straphylococcus spp., and Streptococcus spp. Skin And Soft Tissue Infections (abscesses, lacerations, and wounds) due to *Staphylococcus aureus,* Staphylococcus spp., Streptococcus spp., *E. coli,* and *Pasteurella multocida.*
As with all antibiotics, appropriate *in vitro* culturing and susceptibility testing of samples taken before treatment should be conducted.

Contraindications: The use of this drug is contraindicated in animals with a history of allergic reaction to penicillin.

Adverse Reactions: Amoxicillin is a semisynthetic penicillin and has the potential to produce an allergic reaction. If

an allergic reaction occurs, administer epinephrine and/or steroids. Possible minor irritation at the injection site may occur.
Dosage: The recommended dosage for dogs and cats is 5 mg per pound of body weight. Administer once daily for up to 5 days by intramuscular or subsutaneous injection. Treatment should be continued for 48 hours after the animal has become afebrile or asymptomatic. If no improvement is seen within 5 days, review the diagnosis and change therapy.
Directions for Use: Amoxi-Inject (amoxicillin) is packaged as a multi-dose dry-filled vial and requires reconstitution prior to use. It should be reconstituted to the desired concentration by adding the recommended amount of Sterile Water for Injection, U.S.P. according to labeled directions.
100 mg/ml Concentration —Add 27 ml of Sterile Water for Injection
250 mg/ml Concentration —Add 9 ml of Sterile Water for Injection
After reconsititution, the product is stable for 12 months under refrigeration or 3 months at room temperature (72°F.). Date and concentration should be noted on the label at the time of reconstitution.
Warning: For use in dogs and cats only.
Caution: Federal law restricts this drug to use by or on the order of a licensed veterinarian.
How Supplied: Amoxi-Inject (amoxicillin) is supplied in vials containing 3 grams of amoxicillin activity as the trihydrate.

AMOXI-SOL® /AMOXI-BOL®

Description: Amoxi-Sol (amoxicillin trihydrate soluble powder) and Amoxi-Bol (amoxicillin) are semisynthetic penicillins with a broad spectrum of activity. Amoxicillin provides bactericidal activity against a wide range of common Gram-positive and Gram-negative pathogens. Chemically, it is D-(-)-α-amino-p-hydroxybenzyl penicillin trihydrate.
Indications: Amoxi-Sol (amoxicillin) and Amoxi-Bol (amoxicillin) are indicated in the treatment of bacterial enteritis when due to susceptible *Escherichia coli* organisms in non-ruminating calves. As with all antibiotics, appropriate *in vitro* culturing and susceptibility testing of samples taken before treatment should be conducted.
Adverse Reactions: Amoxicillin is a semisynthetic penicillin and has the potential for producing allergic reactions. If an allergic reaction occurs, administer epinephrine and/or steroids.
Contraindications: The use of these drugs is contraindicated in animals with a history of an allergic reaction to penicillin.
Action: Amoxicillin is stable in the presence of gastric acid and is not significantly influenced by gastric or intestinal contents. It is rapidly absorbed following oral administration and diffuses readily into most body tissues and fluids with the exception of brain and spinal fluid, except when meninges are inflamed. Most of amoxicillin is excreted unchanged in the urine.
Amoxicillin is bactericidal in action and acts through the inhibition of biosynthesis of cell wall mucopeptide against susceptible organisms. *In vitro* and/or *in vivo* studies have demonstrated the susceptibility of most beta-hemolytic strepto cocci, *Diplococcus pneumoniae,* non-penicillinase-producing staphylococci, *Streptococcus faecalis, Haemophilus influenza, Escherichia coli* and *Proteus mirabilis.* Because it does not resist destruction by penicillinase, it is *not* effective against penicillinase producing bacteria, particularly resistant staphylococci. All strains of Pseudomonas and most strains of Klebsiella and Enterobacter are resistant. Dosage and Aministration: Recommended dose: 400 mg per 100 pounds of body weight twice a day. Treatment should be continued for 48 hours after all symptoms have subsided, but not beyond 5 days. Administer Amoxi-Sol (amoxicillin) by drench or by mixing with water.
Warnings: These products are intended for use in non-ruminating calves only, not for use in other animals which are raised for food production. Treated animals must not be slaughtered for food during treatment or for 20 days after the last treat ment.
Caution: Federal law restricts these drugs to use by or on the order of a licensed veterinarian.
How Supplied: Amoxi-Sol (amoxicillin) is supplied in trays containing 6 individual dose bottles, each dose containing amoxicillin trihydrate equivalent to 400 mg amoxicillin dispersed in an inert carrier. Amoxi-Bol (amoxicillin) is supplied in strip packs of 50 boluses. Each bolus contains amoxicillin trihydrate equivalent to 400 mg of amoxicillin activity.

AMOXI-TABS®
(amoxicillin)

Composition: Amoxi-Tabs (amoxicillin) is a new semisynthetic antibiotic with a broad spectrum of activity. It provides bactericidal activity against a wide range of common Gram-positive and Gram-negative pathogens. Chemically, it is D-(-)-α-amino-p-hydroxybenzyl penicillin trihydrate.
Indications: *In Dogs* —Amoxi-Tabs is indicated in the treatment of susceptible strains of the organisms causing the following infections:
Respiratory Tract Infections (Tonsillitis, Tracheobronchitis) due to *Staphylococcus aureus, Streptococcus spp., E. coli,* and *Proteus mirabilis.*
Genitourinary Tract Infections (Cystitis) due to *Staphylococcus aureus, Streptococcus spp., E. coli,* and *Proteus mirabilis.*
Gastrointestinal Tract Infections (Bacterial Gastroenteritis) due to *Staphylococcus aureus, Streptococcus spp., E. coli,* and *Proteus mirabilis.*
Bacterial Dermatitis due to *Staphylococcus aureus, Streptococcus spp.,* and *Proteus mirabilis.*
Soft Tissue Infections (Abscesses, lacerations and Wounds) due to *Staphylococcus aureus, Streptococcus spp., E. coli,* and *Proteus mirabilis.*
In Cats —Amoxi-Tabs (amoxicillin) is indicated in the treatment of susceptible strains of the organisms causing the following infections:
Upper Respiratory Tract Infections due to *Staphylococcus aureus, Streptococcus spp.,* and *E. coli.*
Genitourinary Tract Infections (cystitis) due to *Staphylococcus aureus, Streptococcus spp., E. coli,* and *Proteus mirabilis.*
Gastrointestinal Tract Infections *due to E. coli.*
Skin and Soft Tissue Infections (abscesses, lacerations and wounds) due to *Staphylococcus aureus, Streptococcus spp., E. coli,* and *Pasteurella multocida.*
As with all antibiotics, appropriate *in vitro* culturing and susceptibility testing of samples taken before treatment should be conducted.
Contraindications: The use of this drug is contraindicated in animals with a history of an allergic reaction to penicillin.
Action: Amoxi-Tabs (amoxicillin) is stable in the presence of gastric acid and may be given without regard to meals. It is rapidly absorbed after oral administration. It diffuses readily into most body tissues and fluids with the exception of brain and spinal fluid except when meninges are inflamed. Most of amoxicillin is excreted unchanged in the urine.
Amoxicillin is similar to ampicillin in its bactericidal action against susceptible organisms. It acts through the inhibition of biosynthesis of cell wall mucopeptide. *In vitro* and/or *in vivo* studies have demonstrated the susceptibility of most strains of the following Gram-positive and Gram-negative bacteria: alpha-and beta-hemolytic streptococci, non-penicillinase-producing staphylococci, *Streptococcus faecalis, Escherichia coli, and Proteus mirabilis.* Because it does not resist destruction by penicillinase, it is *not* effective against penicillinase-producing bacteria, particularly resistant staphylococci. All strains of Pseudomonas and most strains of Klebsiella and Enterobacter are resistant.
Adverse Reactions: Amoxicillin is a semisynthetic penicillin and has the potential for producing allergic reactions. If an allergic reaction occurs, administer epinephrine and/or steroids.
Dosage and Administration: Dogs—The recommended dosage: 5 mg per pound of body weight twice a day.
Cats—The recommended dosage: 50 mg —(5-10 mg/lb) once a day.
Dosage should be continued for 5-7 days or 48 hours after all symptoms have subsided.
If no improvement is seen in 5 days review diagnosis and change therapy.
Warnings: For use in dogs and cats only.
Caution: Federal law restricts this drug to use by or on the order of a licensed veterinarian.

Continued on next page

Beecham—Cont.

How Supplied: Amoxi-Tabs (amoxicillin) tablets are supplied in four concentrations: 50 mg, 100 mg, 200 mg and 400 mg.

AMP-EQUINE®
(sterile ampicillin sodium)
For Use in Horses Only

Description: Amp-Equine (ampicillin sodium) is a semisynthetic penicillin with a broad spectrum of activity. Ampicillin is derived from the penicillin nucleus, 6-aminopenicillanic acid (6 APA) isolated by Beecham. Chemically it is D(-)α-aminobenzyl penicillin sodium salt.
Indications: Amp-Equine (ampicillin sodium) is indicated in the treatment of susceptible strains of the organisms causing the following infections in the horse:
Respiratory tract infections (pneumonia and strangles) due to Staphylococcus spp., *Streptococcus equi,* Streptococcus spp., *E. coli,* and *Proteus mirabilis.*
Skin and soft tissue infections (abscesses and wounds) due to Staphylococcus spp., Streptococcus spp., *E. coli,* and *Proteus mirabilis.*
As with all antibiotics, appropriate in-vitro culturing and susceptibility testing of samples taken before treatment should be conducted.
Contraindications: The use of this drug is contraindicated in animals with a history of an allergic reaction to penicillin.
Action: Amp-Equine (ampicillin sodium) provides bactericidal activity against a wide range of common Gram-positive and Gram-negative pathogens. Ampicillins activity occurs during the stage of active multiplication of the pathogen and acts through inhibition of biosynthesis of cell wall mucopeptide. *In vivo* studies have demonstrated the susceptibility of many strains of the following Gram-positive bacteria: Staphylococcus spp., *Streptococcus equi,* Streptococcus spp. *In vivo* studies have also demonstrated the susceptibility of many strains of the following Gram-negative bacteria: *E. coli* and *Proteus mirabilis.* Because it does not resist destruction by penicillinase, it is not effective against penicillinase-producing bacteria, particularly resistant staphylococci. Most strains of Pseudomonas, Klebsiella and Aerobacter are resistant.
Amp-Equine (ampicillin sodium) diffuses readily into all body tissues and fluids, with the exception of brain and spinal fluid except when the meninges are inflamed. It produces high and persistent blood levels. Most of the ampicillin is excreted unchanged in the urine.
Adverse Reactions: Ampicillin is a semisynthetic penicillin and has the potential for producing allergic reactions. If an allergic reaction occurs, administer epinephrine and/or steroids. Possible minor irritation at the injection site may occur.
Dosage and Administration: Horses—The recommended dose is 3 mg per pound of body weight administered twice a day. Amp-Equine (ampicillin sodium) may be administered by either the intravenous or intramuscular route. Treatment should be continued 48 hours after all symptoms have subsided. If no response is seen in 4–5 days, diagnosis should be re-evaluated.
Directions for Use: The dry filled vials should be reconstituted immediately before use by the addition of 7.6 ml of Sterile Water for Injection, USP which results in a final concentration of 300 mg per ml.
Stability studies with the concentrated product (300 mg/ml) demonstrated that ampicillin is stable for 1 hour at room temperature and 3 hours under refrigeration.
Caution: Federal law restricts this drug to use by or on the order of a licensed veterinarian.
Warnings: Amp-Equine (ampicillin sodium) is for use in horses only. Not for use in horses or other animals raised for food production.
How Supplied: Amp-Equine (ampicillin sodium) is supplied in vials containing 3 grams of ampicillin activity.

ATROBAC-P™
Bordetella Bronchiseptica-Pasteurella Multocida Bacterin

Composition: Atrobac-P consists of standardized cultures of *Bordetella bronchiseptica* and *Pasteurella multocida,* Type A.
The cultures are grown in specially formulated media resulting in high yields of immunizing antigen. *Bordetella bronchiseptica* is inactivated with formaldehyde. A special inactivating process reduces the endotoxin level of the *Pasteurella multocida* fraction and thimerosal is added as a preservative. The cultures are blended with a high quality aluminum hydroxide adjuvant to provide products which possess outstanding potency and safety in each immunizing dose.
Each serial is tested for purity, safety, potency and efficacy. The *Bordetella bronchiseptica* fraction is tested in animals by an approved government potency test. The *Pasteurella multocida,* Type A fraction is tested in accordance with government regulation 9 CFR, 113.106.
Indications: ATROBAC-P. For use in healthy swine to aid in the control or prevention of disease due to *Bordetella bronchiseptica* and *Pasteurella multocida* infections. Colostral antibody protection against *B. bronchiseptica* has been demonstrated in baby pigs.
Use Directions: Shake well. Dosage: Inject 2 ml subcutaneously or intramuscularly. Sows and gilts: Vaccinate approximately 5 and 3 weeks prior to farrowing and 3 weeks prior to subsequent farrowings to stimulate adequate antibodies in colostrum for passive protection of baby pigs during the first weeks of life. Baby pig protection depends upon immediate and frequent nursing of colostrum after birth. Pigs: For active immunity, vaccinate at weaning and 3 weeks later.
Caution: Store at 35°–45°F. (1.5°–7°C.). Do not freeze. Do not vaccinate within 21 days before slaughter. Use entire contents when first opened. Anaphylactoid reactions may occur following use of biological products. Symptomatic therapy should be provided, including epinephrine.
How Supplied: 50 dose plastic vials. Species and color-coded labels for easy product identification.

ATROBAC-R™
Bordetella Bronchiseptica Bacterin

Composition: Atrobac consists of standardized cultures of *Bordetella bronchiseptica.*
The cultures are grown in specially formulated media resulting in high yields of immunizing antigen. *Bordetella bronchiseptica* is inactivated with formaldehyde. The cultures are blended with a high quality aluminum hydroxide adjuvant to provide products which possess outstanding potency and safety in each immunizing dose.
Each serial is tested for purity, safety, potency and efficacy. The *Bordetella bronchiseptica* fraction is tested in animals by an approved government potency test.
Indications: ATROBAC-R: For use in healthy swine to aid in the control or prevention of disease due to *Bordetella bronchiseptica* infection. Colostral antibody protection against *B bronchiseptica* has been demonstrated in baby pigs.
Use Directions: Shake well. Dosage: Inject 2 ml subcutaneously or intramuscularly. Sows and gilts: Vaccinate approximately 5 and 3 weeks prior to farrowing and 3 weeks prior to subsequent farrowings to stimulate adequate antibodies in colostrum for passive protection of baby pigs during the first weeks of life. Baby pig protection depends upon immediate and frequent nursing of colostrum after birth. Pigs: For active immunity, vaccinate at weaning and 3 weeks later.
Caution: Store at 35°–45°F. (1.5°–7°C.). Do not freeze. Do not vaccinate within 21 days before slaughter. Use entire contents when first opened. Anaphylactoid reacitons may occur following use of biological products. Symptomatic therapy should be provided, including epinephrine.
How Supplied: 50 dose plastic vials. Species and color-coded labels for easy product identification.

BENZA-PEN®
(sterile benzathine penicillin G and procaine penicillin G in aqueous suspension)
Veterinary Injection
For Veterinary Use in Beef Cattle, Horses and Dogs

Composition: Each ml. of Benza-Pen contains: Benzathine Penicillin G. 150,000 units; Procaine Penicillin G, 150,000 units, Sodium Formaldehyde Sulfoxylate, 3.0 mg; Lecithin, 14.0 mg; Methylparaben (as preservative), 1.20 mg; Propylparaben (as preservative), 0.14 mg; Tween 40, 7.0 mg; Span 40, 10.0

mg; Sodium Citrate, 10.0 mg; Procaine Hydrochloride, 20.0 mg; Sodium Carboxymethylcellulose, 1.5 mg; Povidone, 3.5 mg; Sorbitol Solution, 0.15 ml; and Water for Injections, q.s.

Indications: Benza-Pen is indicated for treatment of the following bacterial infections in dogs, horses and beef cattle due to penicillin G susceptible microorganisms that are susceptible to the serum levels common to this particular dosage form, such as:

1. Bacterial Pneumonia *(Streptococcus spp., Corynebacterium pyogenes, Staphylococcus aureus)*
2. Upper Respiratory Infections such as Rhinitis or Pharyngitis *(Corynebacterium pyogenes)*
3. Equine Strangles *(Streptococcus equi)*
4. Blackleg *(Clostridium chauvoei)*
5. Anthrax *(Bacillus anthracis)*
6. Prophylaxis of Bovine Shipping Fever in 300–500 pound beef calves.

Contraindications: Benza-Pen is contraindicated in patients which have shown hypersensitivity to penicillin.

Action: Penicillin G is an antibiotic which shows a marked bactericidal effect against certain organisms during their growth phase. It is relatively specific in its action against Gram positive bacteria but is usually ineffective against Gram-negative organisms.

When treating an animal for a bacterial infection, it is advisable to isolate and identify the causative organism and conduct appropriate in vitro susceptibility tests. In cases where organisms other than those susceptible to penicillin are present, reevaluation of treatment should be made. Organisms normally considered susceptible to penicillin include *Clostridium septicum, Corynebacterium pyogenes, Staphylococcus aureus, Streptococcus canis, Streptococcus equi* and *Streptococcus pyogenes.*

It is normally recommended that any bacterial infection be treated as early as possible and with a dosage which will give effective blood levels. Although the recommended dosage of Benza-Pen will give longer detectable penicillin blood levels than procaine penicillin G alone, it is recommended that a second dose be administered at 48 hours when treating a penicillin-susceptible bacterial infection.

Packaging: 100 and 250 ml multi-dose vials.

CLAVAMOX®
amoxicillin trihydrate/ clavulanate potassium
Veterinary, Tablets

Description: CLAVAMOX (amoxicillin trihydrate/clavulanate potassium) is an orally administered formulation comprised of the broad-spectrum antibiotic AMOXI (amoxicillin trihydrate) and the β-lactamase inhibitor, clavulanate potassium (the potassium salt of clavulanic acid).

Amoxicillin trihydrate is a semi-synthetic antibiotic with a broad spectrum of bactericidal activity against many Gram-positive and Gram-negative microorganisms. It does not resist destruction by β-lactamases; therefore, it is not effective against β-lactamase producing bacteria. Chemically, it is D(-)-α-amino-p-hydroxybenzyl-penicillin trihydrate.

Clavulanic acid, an inhibitor of β-lactamase enzymes, is produced by the fermentation of *Streptomyces clavuligerus.* Clavulanic acid by itself has only weak antibacterial activity. Chemically, clavulanate potassium is potassium z-(3R, 5R)-2-β-hydroxyethylidene clavam-3- carboxylate.

Action: CLAVAMOX is stable in the presence of gastric acid and is not significantly influenced by gastric or intestinal contents. The two components are rapidly absorbed resulting in amoxicillin and clavulanic acid concentrations in serum, urine and tissues similar to those produced when each is administered alone.

Amoxicillin and clavulanic acid diffuse readily into most body tissues and fluids, with the exception of brain and spinal fluid, which amoxicillin penetrates adequately when meninges are inflamed. Most of the amoxicillin is excreted unchanged in the urine. Clavulanic acid's penetration into spinal fluid is unknown at this time. Approximately 15% of the administered dose of clavulanic acid is excreted in the urine within the first 6 hours.

CLAVAMOX combines the distinctive properties of a broad spectrum antibiotic and a β-lactamase inhibitor to effectively extend the antibacterial spectrum of amoxicillin to include β-lactamase as well as non-β-lactamase producing organisms.

Microbiology: Amoxicillin is bactericidal in action and acts through the inhibition of biosynthesis of cell wall mucopeptide of susceptible organisms. The action of clavulanic acid extends the antimicrobial spectrum of amoxicillin to include organisms resistant to amoxicillin and other β-lactam antibiotics. Many strains of the following organisms, including β-lactamase producing strains, isolated from veterinary sources, were found to be susceptible to amoxicillin/clavulanate *in vitro* but the clinical significance of this activity has not been demonstrated for some of these organisms in animals:

*Staphylococcus aureus**, β-lactamase producing *Staphylococcus aureus** (penicillin resistant), Staphylococcus species*, *Streptococcus faecalis,* Streptococcus species*, *Bordetella bronchiseptica, Corynebacterium pyogenes, Streptococcus suis, Escherichia coli*,* Proteus species, Enterobacter species, *Klebsiella pneumoniae, Salmonella dublin, Salmonella typhimurium, Pasteurella multocida, Pasteurella hemolytica,* Pasteurella species* and *Erysipelothrix rhusiopathiae.*

*The susceptibility of these organisms has also been demonstrated in *in vivo* studies.

<u>SUSCEPTIBILITY TEST:</u> The recommended quantitative disc susceptibility method (FEDERAL REGISTER 37: 20527–29; Bauer, A. W., Kirby, W. M.M., Sherris, J. C., Turck, M., "Antibiotic Susceptibility Testing by Standardized Single Disc Method." *American Journal of Clinical Pathology* 45: 493, 1966) utilized 30 mcg AUGMENTIN (AMC) discs for estimating the susceptibility of bacteria to CLAVAMOX Tablets.

Indications: CLAVAMOX Tablets are indicated in the treatment of:

CANINE:

<u>Skin and Soft Tissue Infections</u> such as wounds, abscesses, cellulitis, superficial/juvenile and deep pyoderma due to susceptible strains of the following organisms:

β-lactamase producing *Staphylococcus aureus,* non-β-lactamase producing *Staphylococcus aureus,* Staphylococcus spp., Streptococcus spp., and *E. coli.*

FELINE:

<u>Skin and Soft Tissue Infections</u> such as wounds, abscesses and cellulitis/dermatitis due to susceptible strains of the following organisms:

β-lactamase producing *Staphylococcus aureus,* non-β-lactamase producing *Staphylococcus aureus,* Staphylococcus spp., Streptococcus spp., *E. coli* and Pasteurella spp.

<u>Urinary Tract Infections</u> (cystitis) due to susceptible strains of *E. coli.*

Therapy may be initiated with CLAVAMOX prior to obtaining results from bacteriological and susceptibility studies. A culture should be obtained prior to treatment to determine susceptibility of the organisms to CLAVAMOX. Following determination of susceptibility results and clinical response to medication, therapy be reevaluated.

Contraindications: The use of this drug is contraindicated in animals with a history of allergic reaction to any of the penicillins or cephalosporins.

Warnings: Safety of use in pregnant or breeding animals has not been determined.

Store at room temperature 15° to 30°C. (59° to 86°F.) and away from moisture.

Caution: Federal law restricts this drug to use by or on the order of a licensed veterinarian.

Adverse Reactions: CLAVAMOX contains a semi-synthetic penicillin (amoxicillin) and has the potential for producing allergic reactions. If an allergic reaction occurs, administer epinephrine and/or steroids.

Dosage and Administration

Dosage and directons for use:

CANINE:

The recommended dosage is 6.25 mg per pound of body weight twice a day. Skin and soft tissue infections: abscesses, cellulitis, wounds and superficial/juvenile pyoderma should be treated for 5 to 7 days or for 48 hours after all signs have subsided. If no response is seen after 5 days of treatment, therapy should be discontinued and the case re-evaluated. Deep pyoderma may require treatment for 21 days; the maximum duration of treatment should not exceed 30 days.

FELINE:

The recommended dosage is 62.5 mg twice a day. Skin and soft tissue infections: abscesses, cellulitis/dermatitis

Continued on next page

Beecham—Cont.

should be treated for 5 to 7 days or for 48 hours after all signs have subsided. If no response is seen after 3 days of treatment, therapy should be discontinued and the case re-evaluated. Urinary tract infections may require treatment for 10 to 14 days or longer. The maximum duration of treatment should not exceed 30 days.

Dispensing Instructions: Clavulanic acid is sensitive to moisture so CLAVAMOX Tablets must be dispensed in plastic or glass vials. Dispensing containers must be tightly closed at all times. Do not dispense in paper or cardboard containers. Animals should be re-examined and additional medication dispensed if necessary.

How Supplied: CALVAMOX Tablets are supplied in three concentrations:
62.5 mg—50 mg amoxicillin/12.5 mg clavulanic acid
125 mg—100 mg amoxicillin/25 mg clavulanic acid
250 mg—200 mg amoxicillin/50 mg clavulanic acid

CLAVAMOX® DROPS
amoxicillin trihydrate/ clavulanate potassium Veterinary Oral Suspension

Description: CLAVAMOX (amoxicillin trihydrate/clavulante potassium) is an orally administered formulation comprised of the broad-spectrum antibiotic AMOXI (amoxicillin trihydrate) and the β-lactamase inhibitor, clavulanate potassium (the potassium salt of clavulanic acid).
Amoxicillin trihydrate is a semi-synthetic antibiotic with a broad spectrum of bactericidal activity against many Gram-positive and Gram-negative microorganisms. It does not resist destruction by β-lactamases; therefore, it is not effective against β-lactamase producing bacteria. Chemically, it is D-(-)-α-amino-p-hydroxybenzyl-penicillin trihydrate.
Clavulanic acid, an inhibitor of β-lactamase enzymes, is produced by the fermentation of *Streptomyces clavuligerus*. Clavulanic acid by itself has only weak antibacterial activity. Chemically, clavulanate potassium is potassium z-(3R, 5R)-2-β-hydroxyethylidene clavam-3- carboxylate.

Actions: CLAVAMOX is stable in the presence of gastric acid and is not significantly influenced by gastric or intestinal contents. The two components are rapidly absorbed resulting in amoxicillin and clavulanic acid concentrations in serum, urine and tissues similar to those produced when each is administered alone.
Amoxicillin and clavulanic acid diffuse readily into most body tissues and fluids, with the exception of brain and spinal fluid, which amoxicillin penetrates adequately when meninges are inflamed. Most of the amoxicillin is excreted unchanged in the urine. Clavulanic acid's penetration into spinal fluid is unknown at this time. Approximately 15% of the administered dose of clavulanic acid is excreted in the urine within the first 6 hours.
CLAVAMOX combines the distinctive properties of a broad spectrum antibiotic and a β-lactamase inhibitor to effectively extend the antibacterial spectrum of amoxicillin to include β-lactamase as well as non-β-lactamase producing organisms.
MICROBIOLOGY: Amoxicillin is bactericidal in action and acts through the inhibition of biosynthesis of cell wall mucopeptide of susceptible organisms. The action of clavulanic acid extends the antimicrobial spectrum of amoxicillin to include organisms resistant to amoxicillin and other β-lactam antibiotics. Many strains of the following organisms, including β-lactamase producing strains, isolated from veterinary sources, were found to be susceptible to amoxicillin/-clavulanate *in vitro* but the clinical significance of this activity has not been demonstrated for some of these organisms in animals:
*Staphylococcus aureus**, β-lactamase producing *Staphylococcus aureus* (penicillin resistant)*, Staphylococcus species*, *Staphylococcus epidermidis, Staphylococcus intermedius, Streptococcus faecalis,* Streptococcus species*, *Bordetella bronchiseptica, Corynebacterium pyogenes,* Corynebacterium species, *Streptococcus faecalis, Escherichia coli**, *Proteus mirabilis,* Proteus species, Enterobacter species, *Klebsiella pneumoniae, Salmonella dublin, Salmonella typhimurium, Pasteurella multocida**, *Pasteurella hemolytica,* Pasteurella species* and *Erysipelothrix rhusiopathiae.*
*The susceptibility of these organisms has also been demonstrated in *in vivo* studies.
SUSCEPTIBILITY TEST: The recommended quantitative disc susceptibility method (FEDERAL REGISTER 37: 20527–29; Bauer, A. W., Kirby, W. M.M., Sherris, J. C., Turck, M., "Antibiotic Susceptibility Testing by Standardized Single Disc Method." *American Journal of Clinical Pathology* 45: 493, 1966) utilized 30 mcg AUGMENTIN (AMC) discs for estimating the susceptibility of bacteria to CLAVAMOX Tablets and drops.

Indications: Drops are indicated in the treatment of:
CANINE:
Skin and Soft Tissue Infections such as wounds, abscesses, cellulitis, superficial/juvenile and deep pyoderma due to susceptible strains of the following organisms:
β-lactamase producing *Staphylococcus aureus,* non-β-lactamase producing *Staphylococcus aureus,* Staphyloccus spp., Streptococcus spp., and *E. coli.*
FELINE:
Skin and Soft Tissue Infections such as wounds, abscesses and cellulitis/dermatitis due to susceptible strains of the following organisms:
β-lactamase producing *Staphylococcus aureus,* non-β-lactamase producing *Staphylococcus aureus,* Staphylococcus spp., Streptococcus spp., *E. coli, Pasteurella multocida* and Pasteurella spp.
Therapy may be initiated with CLAVAMOX prior to obtaining results from bacteriological and susceptibility studies. A culture should be obtained prior to treatment to determine susceptibility of the organisms to CLAVAMOX. Following determination of susceptibility results, and clinical response to medication, therapy may be reevaluated.

Contraindications: The use of this drug is contraindicated in animals with a history of allergic reaction to any of the penicillins or cephalosporins.

Warnings: Safety of use in pregnant or breeding animals has not been determined. For use in dogs and cats only.

Caution: Federal law restricts this drug to use by or on the order of a licensed veterinarian.

Adverse Reactions: CLAVAMOX contains a semi-synthetic penicillin (amoxicillin) and has the potential for producing allergic reactions. If an allergic reaction occurs, administer epinephrine and /or steroids.

Dosage and Administration
Dosage and directons for use:
CANINE:
The recommended dosage is 6.25 mg per pound of body weight (1 ml/10 pounds) twice a day. Skin and soft tissue infections: abscesses, cellulitis, wounds and superficial/juvenile pyoderma should be treated for 5 to 7 days or for 48 hours after all signs have subsided. Deep pyoderma may require treatment for 21 days, not to exceed 30 days. If no response is seen after 5 days of treatment, therapy should be discontinued and the case re-evaluated.
FELINE:
The recommended dosage is 62.5 mg (1 ml) twice a day. The duration of treatment should be 48 hours after all symptoms have subsided, not to exceed 30 days. If no response is seen after 3 days of treatment, therapy should be discontinued and the case re-evaluated.

Reconstitution Instructions—Oral Suspension: Add 14 ml of water to the 15 ml (0.9375 Gm) bottle and 27 ml to the 30 ml (1.875 Gm) bottle and shake vigorously. Each ml of suspension will contain 50 mg of amoxicillin activity as the trihydrate and 12.5 mg of clavulanic acid activity as the potassium salt.

Note: Any unused portion of the reconstituted suspension must be discarded after 10 days. Refrigeration of the reconstituted suspension is required.

How Supplied: CLAVAMOX Drops are supplied in two sizes:
15 ml bottle (0.9375 Gm)—50 mg amoxicillin/12.5 mg clavulanic acid per ml
30 ml bottle (1.875 Gm)—50 mg amoxicillin/12.5 mg clavulanic acid per ml

COLI-BOVIS™
Escherichia Coli Bacterin

Composition: Coli-Bovis consists of a genetically engineered strain of *E. coli* which produces high yields of the K-99 epilus antigen.
Through the use of Beecham Laboratories' Ultraferm™ process, the temperature and pH are electronically controlled, and the fermentation process is

rigidly monitored. This results in high quality yields.
Inactivation of the cultures is performed in such a manner as to assure antigenicity and immuno genicity. Coli-Bovis is formulated by blending, concentrating and adjuvanting selected *E. coli* cultures to provide a highly efficacious product.
Protection for the newborn calf is provided by maternal antibodies contained in the dam's colostrum. It is therefore important that the newborn calf nurse its vaccinated mother immediately after birth to obtain protection.
Indications: For use in healthy, pregnant cattle as an aid in the prevention of calf scours due to infection with enteropathogenic *E.coli.*
Dosage and Administration: Shake well. For subcutaneous or intramuscular use. To stimulate high levels of antibody in the colostrum, vaccinate pregnant heifers and cows with 2 doses (2 ml) approximately 6 and 3 weeks prior to calving. Administer 1 dose (2 ml) approximately 3 weeks prior to each subsequent calving.
Precautions: Store at 35 to 45 F. (1.5 to 7 C.). Protect from freezing. Use entire contents when container is first opened. Do not vaccinate within 21 days before slaughter. Temporary swelling may occur at the injection site. Anaphylactoid reactions, although rare, may occur. *Antidote: Epinephrine.*
How Supplied: 10 and 50 dose plastic vials. Species coded label for easy product identification.

COLI-SUIS™

Description: Coli-Suis consists of inactivated whole cell cultures. Genetically engineered *E. coli* strains were selected for their ability to produce the K-88 and K-99 antigens and for low levels of capsule production. A 987P clinical isolate was also selected for its ability to produce 987P antigens. Whole cell cultures were used instead of purified pili to prevent cell disruption with resultant release and solubilization of toxic endotoxin. Optimal potency is assured on each serial by laboratory pili titer determination techniques.
Indications: Coli-Suis is indicated for use in healthy, pregnant swine as an aid in the prevention of baby pig scours due to enteropathogenic *E. coli.*
Dosage and Administration: Shake well. Inject 2 ml subcutaneously or intramuscularly. To stimulate high antibody levels in the colostrum, vaccinate pregnant sows and gilts approximately 6 and 3 weeks prior to farrowing and 3 weeks prior to subsequent farrowings.
Precautions: Store at 35–45F. (1.5 to 7C.). Do not freeze. Do not vaccinate within 21 days before slaughter. Use entire contents when container is first opened. Anaphylactoid reactions may occur following the use of products of this nature. Symptomatic treatment should be provided. *Antidote: Epinephrine.*
How Supplied: 20 ml (10 dose) plastic vial. 100 ml (50 dose) plastic vial.

DARICLOX®
(sodium cloxacillin)
Lactating Cow Formula
Intramammary Infusion

Composition: Dariclox® (Sodium cloxacillin) is a stable, non-irritating suspension of sodium cloxacillin containing the equivalent of 200 mg of cloxacillin per disposable syringe.
Sodium cloxacillin is the monohydrate sodium salt of 5-methyl-3-(o-chlorophenyl)-4- isoxazolyl penicillin. Cloxacillin is a semi-synthetic penicillin derived from the penicillin nucleus, 6amino-penicillanic acid discovered by Beecham Research Laboratories.
Indications: Dariclox® (sodium cloxacillin) is indicated in the treatment of bovine mastitis in lactating cows due to *Streptococcus agalactiae* and *Stapyhlococcus aureus,* non-penicillinase producing organisms. Clinical experience indicates that antibiotic efficacy in the treatment of mastitis in lactating cows is directly related to the duration of infection. Therefore treatment should be instituted as early as possible after detection.
Action: Dariclox® (sodium cloxacillin) is bactericidal in action against susceptible organisms during the stage of active multiplication. It acts through the inhibition of biosynthesis of cell wall mucopeptide. Sodium cloxacillin is active against most Gram-positive organisms associated with mastitis. It is effective against *Streptococcus agalactiae* and *Staphylococcus aureus,* nonpenicillinase producing organisms and there is laboratory evidence that indicates cloxacillin is resistant to destruction by penicillinase producing organisms.
Dosage and Administration: Clean and disinfect the teat after milking with alcohol swabs provided in carton. Remove the syringe tip cover and insert the syringe tip into the teat orifice. Express the suspension into the quarter with gentle and continuous pressure. Withdraw the syringe and grasp the end of the teat firmly. Massage the medication up into the milk cistern.
For optimum response the drug should be administered by intramammary infusion in each infected quarter, as described above. Treatment should be repeated at 12-hour intervals for a total of three doses. The treated quarter should be milked out at the next routine milking.
Each carton contains 12 alcohol swabs to facilitate proper cleaning and disinfecting of teat orifice.
Storage: While refrigeration is not required this product should be stored in a cool place (46°-59°F).
Caution: Federal law restricts this drug to use by or on the order of a licensed veterinarian.
Warning: Milk taken from treated animals within 48 hours (4 milkings) after the latest treatment should not be used for food. Animals treated should not be slaughtered for food purposes within 10 days after the latest treatment.
How Supplied: Dariclox® (sodium cloxacillin) is supplied in cartons of 12 syringes with 12 sterile alcohol swabs. Each 10 ml single dose disposable syringe contains sodium cloxacillin equivalent to 200 mg of cloxacillin.

FARROWGEN™

Composition: FARROWGEN consists of inactivated, standardized cultures of *B. bronchiseptica, Cl. perfringens* Type C toxoid and *Escherichia coli* (K-88, K-99, and 987P pilus antigens). Highly antigenic strains were selected for seed cultures. Standardized cultures provide for a consistently safe and highly efficacious antigen dose serial after serial. These cultures are grown in a special media under the rigid electronic control of Beecham Laboratories' ULTRAFERM™ process. This state-of-the-art fermentation process optimizes the production of high quality antigens for best protection. Cultures and toxins are inactivated and blended with a high quality aluminum hydroxide gel. This adjuvant boosts the immune response resulting in higher serum and colostral titers. These high titers are necessary for maximum protection. Each serial is tested for safety, purity, potency and efficacy beyond U.S.D.A. requirements.
Indications: For use in healthy pregnant swine to aid in the control or prevention of disease in baby pigs caused by *B. bronchiseptica, Cl. perfringens* Type C enterotoxemia and scours due to enteropathogenic *E. coli.*
Use Directions: Shake well. Aseptically inject 5 ml intramuscularly. Sows and Gilts: Vaccinate approximately 5 and 3 weeks prior to farrowing and 3 weeks prior to subsequent farrowings to stimulate adequate antibodies in colostrum for passive protection of baby pigs during the first weeks of life. Baby pig protection depends upon immediate and frequent nursing of colostrum after birth. Pigs: For active immunity against *B. bronchiseptica* and *Cl. perfringens* Type C, vaccinate at weaning and approximately 3 weeks later.
Precautions: Store at 35–45°F. (1.5–7°C.) Do not freeze. Do not vaccinate within 21 days before slaughter. Use entire contents when first opened. Anaphylactoid reactions may occur following use of biologicals. Symptomatic therapy should be provided, including epinephrine.
How Supplied: 20-dose plastic vials. Species and color-coded label for easy product identification.

GRANULEX®-V
Aerosol Spray

Composition: Each gram delivered to the wound site contains: Trypsin, crystalline, N.F., 0.12 mg; Balsam Peru, N.F., 87.0 mg; Castor Oil, U.S.P., 788.0 mg. With an emulsifier and propellants (Water Dispersible).
Description: An aerosol or liquid treatment for wounds which assist heal-

Continued on next page

Beecham—Cont.

ing through debridement and stimulation of epithelial tissue.
Indications: For use as an aid in the treatment of external wounds of dogs, cats, horses and cattle.
Directions: For best results, shake well before first and every use. Hold can upright approximately 12 inches from the area to be treated. Press valve and coat rapidly. Wound may be left unbandaged or apply a wet dressing. Apply twice daily or as often as necessary. To remove, wash gently with warm water.
Warnings:
Do not use on fresh arterial clots.
Avoid spraying in eyes and nostrils.
Keep out of reach of children.
Use only as directed.
Intentional misuse by deliberately concentrating and inhaling the contents can be harmful or fatal.
Warning: FLAMMABLE, do not use near fire or open flame.
Contents under pressure, do not puncture or incinerate.
Do not expose to temperature above 120°F.
How Supplied: 1 oz. liquid
4 oz. aerosol
For Veterinary Use Only

IBR/BVD/PI$_3$
Bovine Rhinotracheitis-Virus Diarrhea-Parainfluenza 3 Vaccine

Composition: This vaccine is a combination of antigens for convenient use in healthy beef and dairy cattle for the prevention of bovine rhinotracheitis, bovine virus diarrhea and bovine parainfluenza 3. The NADL strain of bovine virus diarrhea virus is used for vaccine production. This combination product is lyophilized modified by selection and serial passage so it is not virulent for cattle but has retained its capacity for stimulating immunity to the respective disease. The safety and antigenicity of the virus strains have been demonstrated by vaccination and challenge tests in healthy susceptible cattle. It has been shown that vaccinal virus will not transmit to contact controls. Only a 2 ml dose is required to produce specific and durable protection.
Indications: For the immunization of healthy beef and dairy cattle against bovine rhinotracheitis, bovine virus diarrhea and bovine parainfluenza 3 infections.
Dosage and Administration: Aseptically rehydrate the vaccine with accompanying diluent. Using aseptic technique, inject 2 ml intramuscularly.
For calves vaccinated under 6 months of age, revaccinate at 6 months or older when the possible influence of maternal antibody is decreased. Nonpregnant brood cattle should be vaccinated 3 to 4 weeks before breeding. Do not use in pregnant cows or in calves nursing pregnant cows.
How Supplied: 10 and 50 dose vials with sterile diluent. Species coded label for easy product identification.

IBR/PI$_3$/SOMUBAC™
IBR/PI$_3$/SOMUBAC-P™
Bovine Rhinotracheitis—Parainfluenza-3 Vaccine, Haemophilus Somnus Bacterin and Bovine Rhinotracheitis—Parainfluenza-3 Vaccine, Haemophilus Somnus—Pasteurella Haemolytica—Multocida Bacterin

Composition: The bacterin diluents each consist of three chemically inactivated strains of *Haemophilus somnus.* Each strain was specifically selected for its origin in the disease complex. The Somubac-P diluent provides additional respiratory protection against *Pasteurella haemolytica,* Type 1 and *Pasteurella multocida,* Type A. The bacterin cultures are grown utilizing Beecham Laboratories' ULTRAFERM™ process. This state-of-the-art process assures maximum safety and efficacy through the use of modern, electronically monitored and microprocessor controlled production fermenters. The bacterins are produced serum-free to reduce the possibility of anaphylactoid reactions. The final product is formulated by carefully blending and adjuvanting each antigen for maximum protection.
IBR-PI$_3$ consists of attenuated virus strains which are produced under the exacting requirements of Beecham Laboratories' FROZEN STABLE CELL BANK™ system. The use of this special cell system ensures freedom from unwanted and potentially harmful adventitious agents. The vaccine viruses are blended with the Bemapar® stabilizer and presented in lyophilized form. The final product is tested for purity, potency, safety and efficacy in accordance with USDA regulations.
Indications: IBR-PI$_3$/Somubac: For use in healthy cattle for the prevention of infectious bovine rhinotracheitis, parainfluenza-3 and disease caused by *Haemophilus somnus.*
IBR-PI$_3$/Somubac-P: For use in healthy cattle for the prevention of infectious bovine rhinotracheitis, parainfluenza-3, disease called by *Haemophilus somnus* and pasteurellosis.
Dosage and Administration: To rehydrate, aseptically add the contents of the accompanying vial of Somubac (Somubac-P) to the vial of lyophilized IBR-PI$_3$ using a sterile syringe and needle (do not chemically sterilize). This may be accomplished in one step by using a sterile transfer needle. Shake well to rehydrate. After rehydration, the entire contents should be used immediately.
The recommended dose for each animal is 2 ml injected intramuscularly. For animals vaccinated before 6 months of age, revaccinate at 6 months or at weaning. Revaccination with Somubac (Somubac-P) is recommended 2–4 weeks later. Revaccinate annually to maintain a high level of immunity.
Caution: Store at 35–45°F. (1.5–7°C.). Do not freeze. Do not vaccinate pregnant cows or calves nursing pregnant cows. Do not vaccinate within 21 days before slaughter. The product contains permissible levels of Polymyxin B, Neomycin and Amphotericin B as preservatives. Anaphylactoid reactions may occur following the use of biological products. Symptomatic treatment should be provided. Antidote: Epinephrine. Burn all containers and unused contents.
Packaging: 10 dose (20 ml) and 50 dose (100 ml) packages.

IMATHAL® EQUINE
(pyrantel pamoate)
Equine Anthelmintic Suspension

Composition: Imathal Equine is a suspension of pyrantel pamoate in a palatable caramel-flavored vehicle.
Each ml contains 50 mg of pyrantel base as pyrantel pamoate.
Pyrantel pamoate is a compound belonging to a family classified chemically as tetrahydropyrimidines. It is a yellow, water-insoluble crystalline salt of the tetrahydropyrimidine base and pamoic acid containing 34.7% base activity. The chemical name is, (E)-1,4,5,6-Tetrahydro-1-methyl-2[2-(2-thienyl) vinyl]pyrimidine 4,4'methylenebis [3-hydroxy-2-naphthoate](1:1).
Indications: For the removal and control of mature infections of large strongyles (*Strongylus vulgaris, S. edentatus, S. equinus);* small strongyles *(Trichonema,* sp., *Triodontophorus*); pinworms (*Oxyuris*); and large roundworms (*Parascaris*) in horses and ponies.
Dosage: Administer 3 mg pyrantel base per pound of body weight (6 ml Imathal Equine per 100 lbs body weight).
Directions for Use: Imathal Equine may be administered by means of a stomach tube, dose syringe or by mixing into the feed.
Stomach tube —Measure the appropriate dosage of Imathal Equine and mix in the desired quantity of water. Protect drench from direct sunlight and administer to the animal immediately following mixing. Do not attempt to store diluted suspension.
Imathal Equine is inactive against the common horse bot (*Gastrophilus* sp.). However, Imathal Equine may be administered concurrently with carbon disulfide observing the usual precautions with carbon disulfide.
Dose Syringe —Draw the appropriate dosage of Imathal Equine into a dose syringe and administer to the animal. Do not expose Imathal Equine to direct sunlight.
Feed —Mix the appropriate dosage of Imathal Equine in the normal grain ration. Fasting of animals prior to or following treatment is not required.
Caution: THIS PRODUCT IS A SUSPENSION AND AS SUCH WILL SEPARATE. TO INSURE UNIFORM RE-SUSPENSION AND TO ACHIEVE PROPER DOSAGE, IT IS EXTREMELY IMPORTANT THAT PRODUCT BE SHAKEN AND STIRRED THOROUGHLY BEFORE EVERY USE.
Efficacy: Critical (worm count) studies in horses demonstrated that Imathal Equine administered at the recommended dosage was efficacious against mature infections of Strongylus vulgaris (>90%), S. edentatus (69%), S. equinus

(> 90%), Oxyuris equi (81%), Parascaris equorum (> 90%), and small strongyles (> 90%).
Safety: Imathal Equine (pyrantel pamoate) is well tolerated by horses and ponies of all ages. No adverse drug response was observed when dose rates up to 60 mg pyrantel base per pound of body weight were administered by stomach tube nor when 3 mg base per pound was given by intra-tracheal injection. The reproductive performance of pregnant mares and stud horses dosed with Imathal Equine has not been affected.
Warning: NOT FOR HORSES OR PONIES INTENDED FOR FOOD. KEEP OUT OF REACH OF CHILDREN.
Caution: Federal law restricts this drug to use by or on the order of a licensed veterinarian.
It is recommended that severely debilitated animals not be treated with this preparation.
Recommended Storage: Store below 86°F (30°C).
How Supplied: Imathal Equine is available in plastic quart bottles.

LEPTOMUNE-5™
Leptospira Canicola-Grippotyphosa-Hardjo-Icterohaemorrhagiae-Pomona Bacterin

Composition: Leptomune-5 consists of chemically inactivated concentrated cultures of *Leptospira grippotyphosa, hardjo, pomona, icterohaemorrhagiae* and *canicola* grown in a special medium and under conditions to assure optimum antigenicity and potency. The cultures are produced individually to obtain greater antigenicity. This fermentation process provides growth parameters which insure maximum antigen yields. The high antigenic cell mass is assured by the most accurate method available-the direct cell count. These high antigen levels have not caused immune blockage in laboratory or host animals. Leptomune-5 is adjuvanted with aluminum hydroxide to provide greater long-term protection. There is no formaldehyde used in production and each serial is tested to assure it does not contain antiviral properties. The *grippotyphosa, hardjo, pomona, icterohaemorrhagiae* and *canicola* fractions are tested in accordance with U.S. Department of Agriculture regulations wherein 1:800th of a field dose must protect hamsters. The hardjo fraction is being tested in accordance with the outline of production and USDA approved regulations.
Indications: For the prophylactic immunization of healthy cattle against leptospirosis due to *Leptospira grippotyphosa, hardjo, pomona, icterohaemorrhagiae* and *canicola.*
Dosage and Administration: Shake well before using. Animals should be vaccinated intramuscularly or subcutaneously at 4 to 6 months of age.
Dosage: Cattle—one 2 ml dose; **Swine**—two doses (2 ml each) 4 to 6 weeks apart. Revaccinate annually to maintain a high level of immunity. Recent information indicates that in open herds, revaccination every 6 months may be the most effective procedure in preventing disease problems.
Precautions: Store at 35°F to 45°F (1.5°C to 7°C). Use the entire contents when the container is first opened. Do not vaccinate within 21 days before slaughter. This product contains a permissible level of thimerosal as a preservative. Anaphylactoid reactions may occur following the use of products of this nature. Symptomatic treatment should be provided. *Antidote:* Epinephrine.
How Supplied: Available in 10 and 50 dose plastic vials.

LEPTOPAR®
Parvovirus Vaccine, Killed Virus, Porcine Cell Line Origin-Leptospira Canicola-Grippotyphosa-Hardjo-Icterohaemorragiae-Pomona Bacterin

Composition: Leptopar consists of an inactivated porcine parvovirus propagated in a stable cell line of porcine origin. The cell cultures are produced under the rigid requirements of Beecham's Frozen Stable Cell Bank System™. The vaccine virus was subjected to multiple purification procedures to ensure the highest degree of purity. The stocks of purified virus are maintained under ultra-cold condition (—196°C.) and serve as master seed virus (MSV) for PPV. Inactivation of the vaccine is performed in such a manner as to retain the maximum antigenicity of the product. The product is then formulated by carefully blending and adjuvanting each antigen in proper proportions under constant agitation.
All cells and seed virus used for production have been extensively pretested for bacteria, fungi, mycoplasma, and extraneous viruses to ensure the highest degree of purity. All serials of final product are tested in accordance with USDA procedures.
Each serial is tested for safety in cell culture and laboratory animals to ensure the product is completely inactivated and will not cause any untoward reactions.
Each antigen in each serial is tested for potency to ensure that only high quality components are used in the product. Each fraction is tested by an approved USDA test.
Indications: For use in healthy swine for prevention of porcine parvovirus infections and leptospirosis caused by the organisms listed on the label.
Dosage and Administration: Shake well before using. Use sterile syringe and needle. Do not chemically sterilize. Inject intramuscularly. Administer two doses (5 ml each) 7 and 3 weeks prior to first breeding, and one 5 ml dose at each subsequent breeding.
Caution:
Store at 35°–45°F. (1.5°-7°C.) Do not freeze. Use entire contents when container is first opened. Do not vaccinate within 21 days before slaughter. Leptopar contains permissible levels of Penicillin, Streptomycin and Amphotericin B as preservatives. Anaphylactoid reactions may occur following the use of products of this nature. Symptomatic treatment should be provided. Antidote: Epinephrine.
How Supplied: 10 and 50 dose plastic vials. Species and color-coded label for easy product identification.

MYCODEX® AQUA-SPRAY
Water-Based Natural Insecticide

Composition:
Active Ingredients:

Pyrethrin	0.20%
Piperonyl butoxide, tehnical	2.00%
Petroleum distillate	0.96%
2, 3, 4, 5-Bis(2-butylene) Tetrahydro-2-Furaldehyde	0.05%
Inert Ingredients	96.34%
Total	100.00%

Indications: A non-alcohol based, long-acting aqueous spray which kills fleas, ticks, and lice on dogs and cats.
Direction for
Use: It is a violation of Federal law to use this product in a manner inconsistent with its labeling.
Cats and Dogs: Cover animal's eyes with hand and with a firm fast stroke, to get a proper spray mist, spray head, ears and chest until damp. With finger tips rub into face and around mouth, nose, and eyes. Then spray neck, middle and hind quarters, finishing legs last. For best penetration of spray to the skin, direct against the natural lay of the hair. On long-haired dogs, rub your hand against the lay of the hair, spraying the ruffled hair directly behind the hand. Make sure spray throughly wets ticks. Repeat treatment as needed.
Puppies and Kittens: Treat same as cats and dogs except nursing puppies and kittens, spray only along back or on your finger tips and rub in with your finger tips.
Pets Sleeping Quarters: Spray around base boards, windows, door frames, wall cracks and local area of floors. If mosquitoes, gnats, or flies are present, spray into the air. Repeat as needed. The pet's bedding should be sprayed, making sure the area beneath the bedding is sprayed, too. After spray has dried, remove old bedding and replace with fresh bedding. Treat pets with one of our registered Flea and Tick Control products before allowing them to enter treated area. Precautions and
Warnings:
Human: Harmful if swallowed or inhaled. Avoid breathing mist. Avoid contamination of food. Wash hands with soap and water after using.
Animal: Avoid treatment of nursing kittens and puppies. If treatment is necessary spray on tips of fingers and rub into coat.
Environment Hazards: This product is toxic to fish. DO NOT APPLY DIRECTLY TO WATER.
Storage and Disposal:
Storage: Store in a cool, dry area away from heat or open flame.
Disposal: Do not reuse empty container. Wrap container and put in trash collection.

Continued on next page

Beecham—Cont.

Caution: Keep out of reach of children.
How Supplied: 16 oz plastic bottle with trigger sprayer

B

MYCODEX® CREME HC

Composition:

Phenylmercuric Acetate	0.05%
Hydrocortisone Acetate	1.00%
Vanishing Creme Base	98.95%

The antimicrobial activity in combination with hydrocortisone provides effectiveness against fungi and bacteria as well as exerting an anti-inflammatory and antipruritic effect.
Indications: Mycodex Creme HC is particularly useful in the control of both acute and chronic inflammatory processes of the skin of dogs and cats complicated with bacterial or fungal infections. It is of value in treating exudative or dry dermatitis, contact dermatitis, seborrheic dermatitis and otitis externa. Other responsive conditions include interdigital dermatitis, anal gland infections in dogs and as additional therapy for dermatitis associated with external parasitic infections.
Contraindications: Mycodex Creme HC is contraindicated in cases of ruptured tympanic membrane and otitis media as well as deep seated infections or abscesses.
Dosage and Administration: The severity of the condition will dictate the frequency of administration. Mild inflammation frequently responds to daily application. It may be applied three to four times daily if necessary. Infected lesions should be properly cleaned before application. Treatment is facilitated by clipping the hair. Since Mycodex Creme HC has a non-greasy base, it may be massaged into the skin without an oily residue remaining.
Precautions: If improvement is not noted within two or three days after initiation of treatment, or if redness, irritation, or swelling persists or increases, the diagnosis should be redetermined with the administration of appropriate therapy.
Adverse Reactions: Side effects are not ordinarily encountered with topically applied steroids; however, as with all drugs, a few animals may react unfavorably under certain conditions.
If such reactions or idiosyncrasies are encountered, Mycodex Creme HC should be discontinued and appropriate steps taken.
How Supplied: Mycodex Creme HC is supplied in 12.5 Gm tubes.
Caution: Federal law restricts this drug to use by or on the order of a licensed veterinarian.

MYCODEX®
Flea & Tick Spray
An Insecticide Spray
For Rapid Kill of Fleas on Dogs and Cats
and Ticks on Dogs

Composition: Active Ingredients: o-Isopropoxy phenyl Methylcarbamate* 0.25%. Inert Ingredients 99.75%.
Indications: Mycodex Flea & Tick Spray provides rapid kill of fleas on dogs and cats and of ticks on dogs. For more prolonged insect control, the animal's bedding should also be treated to help prevent reinfestation.
Dosage and Administration: Read entire label before using.
Hold container 6 to 10 inches from the animal and spray lightly over the entire body. Do not spray in eyes or on scrotum. For best penetration of spray to the skin, direct spray against the natural lay of the hair to cause fluffing of the coat.
Treat a 5 pound cat for 3–5 seconds or a 10 pound cat for 5–10 seconds. Apply enough to dampen hair and skin. Keep can in motion while spraying. Wet ticks thoroughly. Controls ticks for up to 1 week and fleas for up to 4 weeks. Treat a 15 pound dog for 10–20 seconds or a 24 pound dog for 20–30 seconds.
Repeat as necessary but not more often than once weekly.
Warning: Harmful if swallowed, inhaled, or absorbed through the skin. Avoid breathing of spray mist and provide adequate ventilation of treated area. Contact with skin, eyes, or clothing should also be avoided. Wash thoroughly with soap and warm water after handling. Avoid contamination of food, utensils, and food preparation areas. If poisoning should occur, obtain prompt medical aid.
To Physician: Large doses of active ingredient will result in cholinesterase depression. Atropine is antidotal. Do not give morphine. Watch for delayed pulmonary edema in cases of serious poisoning. In this case, use oxygen therapy and treat symptomatically.
Notice: When used in accordance with these directions Mycodex Flea & Tick Spray is effective. However, because of the wide range of conditions under which the product may be used even though these directions are followed, the user accepts all risks and responsibilities.
Warning: Contents under pressure. Do not puncture. Do not use or store near heat or open flame. Exposure to temperature over 130F may cause bursting. Never throw container into fire or incinerator.
How Supplied: 15 oz aerosol

MYCODEX® MINI-FOG™
Whole House Fogging Kit™
(4× Strength)

Composition:
Active Ingredients:
d-trans Allethrin (allyl homolog Cinerin 1) 1.200%
Related Compounds 0.092%
*3 Phenoxybenzyl d-cis and trans** 2, 2 dimethyl-3-(2 methylpropenyl) cyclopropanecarboxylate 0.746%
*Other isomers 0.036%
Petroleum distillate 28.954%
Inert Ingredients 68.954%
*d(cis,trans) phenothrin
**cis/trans isomer ratio: max. 25% (+ or −) cis; min. 75% (× or −) trans
Indications: A concentrated individual room fogger which kills fleas, ticks, and many other household pests.
Directions for Use: It is a violation of Federal Law to use this product in a manner inconsistent with its labeling.
Product is designed to be used in each room where fleas, ticks, and other pests are found. Read, and follow, all directions contained on and in the Whole House Fogging Kit.™
Used according to directions, and in conjunction with other animal and premise parasiticides, MYCODEX® MINI-FOG™ will control your pest problems.
Warning: This product is hazardous to humans and domestic animals.
Caution: Harmful if swallowed or absorbed through skin. Avoid contact with skin. Avoid breathing vapors. In case of contact, immediately flush skin with plenty of water.
Do not use in commercial food processing or preparation areas. In the home, all food processing surfaces and utensils should be covered during treatment or thoroughly washed before use. Cover exposed food.
Remove pets, birds and cover fish aquariums before spraying.
First Aid: In case of eye contact, flush with plenty of water; get medical attention if irritation persists.
Physical Hazards: Contents under pressure. Do not use or store near heat or open flame. Do not puncture or incinerate container. Exposure to temperature above 130°F. may cause bursting.
Storage and Disposal: Store in a cool, dry area away from heat or open flame. Do not re-use empty container. Wrap container and put in trash collection.
Caution: Keep out of the reach of children. Carefully read DIRECTIONS FOR USE shown on carton.
How Supplied: Handy "Whole House Fogging Kit" containing 4 aerosol containers, each of which contains 1.5 ounces and covers up to 5,000 cubic feet of unobstructed space.

MYCODEX® PEARLESCENT GROOMING SHAMPOO

Composition: A deep-cleansing shampoo formulation incorporating a unique cationic polymer which is substantive to protein substrates, such as hair.
Indications: A routine cleansing and grooming shampoo for dogs and cats, especially those with dry or damaged coats. Mycodex Pearlescent Grooming Shampoo improves the appearance and feel of damaged hair.
Directions for Use: Thoroughly wet the entire hair-coat of the dog or cat with warm water, then apply enough shampoo to make a lather and work well into

the coat. Rinse thoroughly. For damaged or "brittle" hair, leaving the lather on for 5 or 10 minutes before rinsing will enhance the manageability characteristics of the shampoo.
Bathing may be repeated as often as necessary. As a precaution, a bland ophthalmic ointment may be placed in the eyes prior to bathing to prevent irritation.
How Supplied: Clear plastic 8 oz bottles with flip-up spout, and gallon size with pump dispenser on request.

MYCODEX® PET SHAMPOO with PYRETHRINS

Composition:
Active Ingredients:
Pyrethrins 0.05%
Technical Piperonyl Butoxide* 0.5%
Sodium Lauryl Sulfate 12%
Lauramide DEA 5%
Polyethylene Glycol "600" Distearate 1%
Polyoxyethylene Lanolins 2%
Inert Ingredients 79.45%
Total 100%
*Equivalent to 0.4 of (burylcarbityl) (6-propylpiperonyl) ether and to 0.1 of related compounds.
Indications: As a routine cleansing shampoo to restore natural luster to the hair-coat of dogs and cats. Kills fleas and lice. Deodorizes.
As a precaution, a bland ophthalmic ointment may be placed in the eyes prior to bathing to prevent possible irritation.
Dosage and Administration: Thoroughly wet the entire hair-coat with warm water and then apply enough shampoo to make a lather and work thoroughly into the hair-coat. For best effects, allow lather to remain in contact with skin for five minutes or longer before rinsing. Repeat twice weekly or weekly, depending upon severity of affliction and response.
How Supplied: Plastic 6-oz bottle and gallon size with pump dispenser on request.

MYCODEX® PET SHAMPOO with ALLETHRIN

Composition:
Active Ingredients:
d-trans Allethrin (allyl homolog of Cinerin 1) 0.12%
Related Compounds 0.0092%
Piperonyl Butoxide, Technical* 0.50%
Inert Ingredients
Total 100.00%
*Equivalent to 0.4% of (butylcarbityl) (6-propylpiperonyl) ether and to 0.1% of related compounds.
Caution: Keep out of reach of children.
Indications: A routine cleansing shampoo to restore natural luster to the hair-coat of dogs and cats. Kills fleas and lice, deodorizes.
Precautionary Statements
Hazards to Humans and Domestic Animals
Caution: Harmful if swallowed. Avoid contact with eyes. In cases of contact, immediately flush eyes with plenty of water. Obtain medical attention if irritation persists.
Storage and Disposal
Storage: Store at room temperature.
Disposal: Do not reuse empty container. Wrap container and put in trash collection.
Dosage and Administration:
It is a violation of Federal law to use this product in a manner inconsistent with its labeling. As a precaution a bland ophthalmic ointment may be placed in the eyes prior to bathing to prevent possible irritation.
Thoroughly wet the entire hair-coat with warm water and then apply enough shampoo to make a lather and work thoroughly into hair-coat. For best therapeutic effects, allow lather to remain in contact with skin for five minutes before rinsing. Rinse thoroughly.
Repeat semiweekly or weekly, depending on severity of affliction and response.
How Supplied: Plastic 6-oz. and 16 oz. bottles and gallon size with pump dispenser on request.

MYCODEX® Pet Shampoo with Carbaryl

Description: Mycodex Pet Shampoo with Carbaryl is a professional veterinary shampoo which is safe for both cats and dogs, cleans thoroughly, kills fleas, lice and ticks, imparts a pleasing fragrance to the pet, conditions the coat, and adds extra luster to light colored pets.
Composition:

Carbaryl (1-Naphthyl N-Methylcarbamate)	0.50%
Ammonium Lauryl Ether Sulfate	18.75%
Polyoxyethylene Lanolins	2.00%
Disodium Edatate	0.10%
Denatured Ethyl Alcohol	10.00%
Inert Ingredients	68.65%
Total	100.00%

Indications: A routine cleansing shampoo to restore natural luster to the coat of dogs and cats. Kills fleas, lice, and ticks.
Dosage and Administration: Thoroughly wet the entire hair-coat with warm water and apply enough shampoo to make a lather and work thoroughly into the hair-coat. For best effects, allow lather to remain in contact with the skin for five minutes before rinsing. Use no more than once weekly. Do not allow to get into eyes or on scrotum.
Contraindications: Do not treat kittens or puppies under 4 weeks of age.
Precautions: Keep out of the reach of children. Wash thoroughly after handling. For external use only. Harmful if swallowed or inhaled.
Do not reuse empty container. Rinse thoroughly with water and discard.
How Supplied: Plastic 6 oz and quart bottles, and gallon size with pump dispenser on request.

MYCODEX® PET SHAMPOO with 3X PYRETHRINS
For Use On Dogs Only

Active Ingredients: Pyrethrins 0.15%; Piperonyl butoxide, technical* 1.50%; Inert ingredients 98.35%; Total 100.00%.
*Equivalent to 1.2% (butylcarbityl) (6-propyl-piperonyl) ether and to 0.3% of related compounds.
KEEP OUT OF REACH OF CHILDREN.
FOR EXTERNAL USE ONLY
Indications: Kills fleas, ticks and lice on dogs. A shampoo which cleanses, restores and maintains natural luster of the hair-coat.
Cautions: May be harmful if swallowed or absorbed through skin. May cause eye irritation. Avoid contact with skin, eyes or clothing. Wash thoroughly after handling. Obtain medical attention if irritation persists. Do not use for lactating or very young animals.
Directions: It is a violation of Federal law to use this product in a manner inconsistent with its labeling. As a precaution, a bland ophthalmic ointment should be placed in the eyes prior to bathing to prevent possible irritation.
FOR USE ON DOGS ONLY.
Thoroughly wet the entire hair-coat with warm water and then apply enough shampoo to make a lather and work thoroughly into the coat and skin. For best results allow lather to remain in contact with skin for five minutes before rinsing. Rinse thoroughly. Product contains emollient and may be repeated semiweekly or weekly as required.
How Supplied: Plastic 6 oz. bottles and gallon size with pump dispenser on request.

MYCODEX® POWDER PLUS KILLS FLEAS, TICKS & LICE ON DOGS AND CATS

Composition:
Active Ingredients:
Carbaryl (l-naphthyl N-methylcarbamate)......................................5.0%
Pyrethrins 0.1%
Piperonyl Butoxide Technical* 1.0%
INERT INGREDIENTS................93.9%
100.0%
*Equivalent to 0.8% (butylcarbityl) (6-propyl-piperonyl) ether and 0.2% related compounds.
Caution: Keep out or reach of children.
Indications: Designed for the control of Dog Ticks, Fleas and Lice. Pleasantly scented to aid in the elimination of "animal odors."
Precautionary Statements
Hazards to Humans and Domestic Animals
Caution: Avoid breathing of dust when you apply powder. May be harmful if swallowed. Wash hands with soap and water after dusting animals. Do not treat puppies and kittens under 4 weeks of age. Keep out of reach of children.
Notice to Physician: Carbaryl is a moderate reversible cholinesterase inhibitor. Atropine sulfate is antidotal.

Continued on next page

B

Beecham—Cont.

Statement of Practical Treatment: IF IN EYES: Flush with plenty of water. If irritation persists see Physician.
Dosage and Administration: It is a violation of Federal Law to use this product in a manner inconsistent with its labeling.
For control of fleas, ticks and lice, dust pet liberally by rubbing into animals hair. Begin at tail and work toward the head. Take care not to get dust in animals eyes, nose or mouth. Be sure to dust paws and between toes. Dust bedding, kennels and sleeping quarters regularly. Apply at least once weekly for best results.
Disposal: Do not reuse empty container. Wrap in newspaper and put in trash collection.
How Supplied: 6 oz. plastic shaker bottle.

MYCODEX® Room and Carpet Accu–Spray™
KILLS FLEAS, BROWN DOG TICKS, MITES, LICE AND OTHER LISTED INSECTS IN HARD-TO-REACH AREAS.

ACTIVE INGREDIENTS:

Pyrethrins	0.025%
*Piperonyl butoxide, Technical	0.050%
**N-Octyl bicyclohepteene dicarboximide	0.084%
Petroleum distillate	1.017%
Chlorpyrifos [0, 0-diethyl 0-(3,5,6-trichloro-2-pyridyl) Phosphorothioate]	0.500%
INERT INGREDIENTS	98.324%
	100.000%

*Equivalent to 0.04% (butycarbityl) (6-propylpiperonyl) ether and 0.01% related compounds.
**MGK-264 Synergist

Directions for Use:
Shake well before using. Move furniture away from walls. Hold container 18–24 inches from carpeting and, with a sweeping motion, spray at the rate of one foot per second or until surface is wet. Thoroughly spray cracks, crevices, along and behind baseboards and door frames. Allow carpet to dry before replacing furniture or place foil under furniture legs to prevent staining. After replacing furniture, spray balance of carpeting as above. Leave treated areas and do not return for at least one hour. Do not allow children or pets to walk on treated surfaces until they are completely dry. Do not spray pets with this product. Treat pets with a registered flea and tick control product to control the source of infestation.
It is a violation of Federal law to use this product in a manner inconsistent with its labeling.
Important:
This water-based insecticide has no strong kerosene odor; is nonstaining and won't damage carpets, rugs, floors or baseboards.
However, care should be taken not to "soak" fabric-covered furniture or carpeting which has dark colored padding or draperies with dark linings. Discoloration could occur if fabric is too wet.
Caution:
KEEP OUT OF REACH OF CHILDREN. May be harmful if swallowed, inhaled or absorbed through the skin. Avoid breathing spray mist and provide adequate ventilation of area being treated. Avoid contact with skin, eyes and clothing. In case of contact immediately flush skin and eyes with plenty of water. Wash thoroughly with soap and water after handling. If poisoning occurs, get prompt medical aid. Do not allow children to play, lie or sleep in treated areas until at least six hours following treatment. Do not allow children or pets to contact treated surfaces until dry.
Do not use in commercial food processing or preparation areas. In the home, all food processing surfaces and utensils should be covered during treatment or thoroughly washed before use. Cover exposed food. Remove pets, birds and cover fish aquariums before spraying.
Chlorpyrifos is a cholinesterase inhibitor. Treat symptomatically. Atropine, by injection, is antidote of choice.
Warning:
Contents under pressure. Do not use near heat or open flame. Do not puncture or incinerate container. Exposure to temperatures above 130° F. may cause bursting. Replace cap and discard empty container in trash.
Sold exclusively to veterinarians.

MYCODEX® ROOM FOGGER

Indications: Kills exposed fleas, ticks, and other household pests.
FOR USE ONLY WHEN BUILDING IS VACATED BY HUMANS AND PETS.
Directions: Use at least one canister for each 10,000 cubic feet of unobstructed area. Use additional units for remote rooms or where free flow of mist is not assured.
Consult package label for ingredients, complete directions, and precautions for use of products of this nature.

MYCODEX®
Tar & Sulfur Pet Shampoo

Composition: Mycodex Tar & Sulfur Shampoo contains: coal tar, 0.5%; colloidal sulfur, 5%; salicylic acid, 1%; p-chloro-m-xylenol, 1%; combined with the cleansing action of surface active agents.
Directions: Thoroughly wet the entire hair-coat with warm water and apply enough shampoo to make a lather, and work thoroughly into the hair-coat. For best therapeutic response the pet should be bathed a second time and the lather should be left on the animal for 10 to 15 minutes before rinsing, or as directed by your veterinarian. Use Only as Directed.
Warning: FOR EXTERNAL USE ONLY. KEEP OUT OF REACH OF CHILDREN. DO NOT USE ON CATS.
As a precaution, a bland ophthalmic ointment may be placed in the eyes prior to bathing to prevent possible irritation.
Shake Well Before Using.
How Supplied: 6 oz, quart, and gallon plastic containers.

NASAMUNE-IP®
Bovine Rhinotracheitis–Parainfluenza-3 Vaccine

Composition: **NASAMUNE-IP** consists of attenuated strains of infectious bovine rhinotracheitis virus and parainfluenza-3 virus propagated in a cell line, which are produced under the rigid requirements of Beecham's **"FROZEN STABLE CELL BANK™"** system. The use of this special cell system in producing **NASAMUNE-IP** ensures freedom from unwanted and potentially harmful adventitious agents. The vaccine virus is blended with a special stabilizer (Bemapar™) and presented in a lyophilized form. The product is tested for purity, safety, potency, and efficacy in accordance with the regulations of the United States Department of Agriculture and was found to be safe for use in pregnant animals.
Indications: For intranasal use in the immunization of healthy cattle for *Infectious Bovine Rhinotracheitis* (IBR) and *Parainfluenza-3* (PI-3) virus infections.
Dosage and Administration: To rehydrate, add the contents of the accompanying vial of sterile diluent to the vial of lyophilized vaccine using a sterile syringe and needle (do not chemically sterilize). This may be accomplished in one step by using a sterile transfer needle. Shake well before using. Use entire contents when the container is first opened. The recommended dose for each animal is 2 ml. Administer 1 ml in each nostril using the syringe applicator provided with the product. For animals vaccinated before 6 months of age, revaccinate at 6 months or at weaning. Pregnant animals may be vaccinated.
Precautions: Store at 35°F to 45°F (1.5°C to 7°C). FOR INTRANASAL USE ONLY! Do not vaccinate within 21 days before slaughter. The product contains permissible levels of Penicillin, Streptomycin and Amphotericin B as preservatives. Anaphylactoid reactions may occur following the use of products of this nature. Symptomatic treatment should be provided. *Antidote: Epinephrine.* Burn all containers and unused contents.
How Supplied: **NASAMUNE-IP®** is provided in single packages of 10×1, 1×10, 1×25, or 1×50 dose vials of vaccine with accompanying sterile diluent and syringe applicators.

ORBENIN-DC®
(benzathine cloxacillin)

Composition: Orbenin-DC is a stable, nonirritating, suspension of benzathine cloxacillin containing the equivalent of 500 mg of cloxacillin per disposable syringe.
Benzathine cloxacillin is the benzathine salt of 6-[3,2-chlorophenyl)-5-methyl-isoxazolyl-4-carboxamidol] penicillanic acid.
Cloxacillin is a semisynthetic penicillin derived from the penicillin nucleus, 6-amino-penicillanic acid discovered by Beecham Research Laboratories in 1957.

The low solubility of Orbenin-DC (benzathine cloxacillin) results in an extended period of activity. Therefore, directions for use should be followed explicitly.
Actions: Orbenin-DC (benzathine cloxacillin) is bactericidal in action against susceptible organisms during the stage of active multiplication. It acts through the inhibition of biosynthesis of cell wall mucopeptide. Orbenin-DC is active aginst Gram-positive organisms associated with mastitis such as *Streptococcus agalactiae* and *Staphylococcus aureus* and because of its resistance to penicillinase, penicillin G-resistant staphylococci which may be the cause of mastitis.
Indications: Orbenin-DC is indicated in the treatment and prophylaxis of bovine mastitis in nonlactating cows due to *Staphylococcus aureus* and *Streptococcus agalactiae*.
Appropriate laboratory tests should be conducted, including *in vitro* culturing and susceptibility tests on pretreatment milk samples collected aseptically.
Dosage and Administration: At the last milking of lactation, milk the cow out normally. Clean and disinfect the teats, infuse one syringe of Orbenin-DC, which has been warmed to room temperature, into each quarter. Do not milk out. The cow may be milked as usual when she calves.
The extent of subclinical and latent mastitis in a herd is frequently greater than suspected. In untreated herds a significant buildup of subclinical mastitis may occur during the dry period, which results in clinical severity after a few lactations. The adverse influence of subclinical mastitis on milk yield, the risk of crossinfection and the chance of clinical mastitis flare-up make it necessary to treat the matter as a herd problem. Clinical studies have proven the value of treating all the cows in heavily infected herds as they are dried off. When the herd infection has been reduced, it may be desirable to be more selective in treating infected quarters.
Contraindications: Since benzathine cloxacillin is relatively insoluble, Orbenin-DC's activity will be prolonged. Therefore, Orbenin-DC should not be used for the occasional cow which may have a dry period of less than 4 weeks. This precaution will avoid residues in the milk following removal of the colostrum.
Precautions: Because it is a derivative of 6-amino-penicillanic acid, Orbenin-DC (benzathine cloxacillin) has the potential for producing allergic reactions. Such reactions are rare; however, should they occur, the subject should be treated with the usual agents (antihistamines, pressor amines, corticosteroids).
Warning:
1. For use in dry cows only.
2. Not to be used within 4 weeks (28 days) of calving.
3. Treated animals must not be slaughtered for food within 4 weeks (28 days) of treatment.

Caution: Federal law restricts this drug to use by or on the order of a licensed veteriniarian.
Storage: While refrigeration is not required, this product should be stored in a cool place, i.e. 46°-59°F.
How Supplied: Orbenin-DC is supplied in cartons of 12 syringes. Each 10 ml disposable polyethylene syringe contains the equivalent of 500 mg of cloxacillin as the benzathine salt.

OTI-CLENS™
Multicleanse Solution

Composition: A clear, colorless liquid with an approximate pH of 2.3 prepared from the following active ingredients: Propylene glycol; Malic acid; Benzoic acid; Salicylic acid; Alcohol, 0.45%.
Indications: For use in otitis externa, wounds and abrasions, when healing is impaired by the presence of necrotic tissue, debris, or wax.
Directions: Routine ear cleaning: Apply liberally to ear. Massage the base of the ear. Clean accessible portion of the ear with a cotton ball. Repeat if necessary.
Otitis Externa: Follow above directions for routine cleansing; repeating 1–3 times daily over several days according to your veterinarian's specific directions.
Wounds: Apply liberally. Repeat application 2–3 times daily as necessary.
Action: OTI-CLENS Multicleanse Solution performs unique action due to a low pH. At 2.3, the pH is ideal to produce the maximum degree of swelling. Necrotic tissue swells at a faster rate than healthy tissue causing the two to separate. Dead tissue is removed gently and painlessly; underlying tissue remains undamaged providing a healthy environment for healing. Oti-Clens also gently softens ear wax for easier removal.
How Supplied: 4 ounce plastic bottles with otic applicator tip.

PANACINE® RC
Feline Rhinotracheitis-Calici-Panleukopenia Vaccine
Modified Live Virus

Composition: The Feline Rhinotracheitis portion of this combination package consists of a naturally attenuated strain, designated the AL strain, which is propagated in a feline line. The Feline Calicivirus portions consists of an attenuated strain of feline calicivirus propagated in a feline cell line. The vaccines are blended with a special stabilizer and lyophilized. The Feline Panleukopenia portion is a stable liquid vaccine with Bemapar® stabilizer consisting of an attenuated strain of feline panleukopenia (distemper) designated the Alpha-PL strain virus, propagated in a feline cell line and is used to rehydrate the lyophilized Feline Rhinotracheitis-Calici Vaccine. The Feline Rhinotracheitis-Calici and Feline Panleulopenia Vaccine fractions are all produced under the rigid requirements of Beecham's "FROZEN STABLE CELL BANK™" system. The vaccine viruses have undergone extensive purification studies ensuring the highest degree of purity. There is no sting or discomfort on administration. The product meets USDA requirements for purity, safety, potency and efficacy.
Indications: For use in healthy cats for the prevention of feline rhinotracheitis, feline calici and feline panleukopenia infections.
Administration: To rehydrate, aseptically add the contents of an accompanying vial of Feline Panleukopenia Vaccine to a vial of lyophilized Feline Rhinotracheitis-Calici Vaccine. Shake well to rehydrate. After rehydration, the entire contents should be used immediately. PANACINE RC is recommended for vaccination of healthy cats. For intramuscular or subcutaneous use. Administer 2 doses (1 ml each) 3 to 4 weeks apart. For cats vaccinated before 9 weeks of age, revaccinate every 3 to 4 weeks until at least 12 weeks of age. Revaccinate annually with a single dose to maintain a high level of immunity.
Precautions: Store at 35–45°F. (1.5–7°C.). Do not vaccinate pregnant cats. Use sterile syringe and needle (do not chemically sterilize). Use the entire contents when the container is first opened. The vaccine contains permissible levels of Polymyxin B, and Neomycin as preservatives. Anaphylactoid reactions may occur following the use of products of this nature. Provide symptomatic therapy which should include epinephrine. Burn all containers and unused contents.
How Supplied: Packages of 25×1 dose vials. The packages are color-coded for easy identification.

PANAVAC®
Feline Panleukopenia Vaccine
Killed Virus

Composition: Panavac consists of a new strain of feline distemper (panleukopenia) virus propagated in a feline cell line produced under the rigid requirements of our Frozen Stable Cell Bank System and chemically inactivated in such a manner as to retain maximum antigenicity. The use of a feline cell line from our "Frozen Stable Cell Bank System™" in producing the feline distemper vaccine ensures freedom from unwanted and potentially harmful feline disease agents. Chemical inactivation of the vaccine is accomplished rapidly and a soft kill assures the highest degree of antigenicity and a no-sting character for the vaccine. The vaccine is presented in a liquid form as a small 1 ml dose for one dose protection. This killed virus vaccine is tested for purity, safety, potency and efficacy in accordance with the regulations of the United States Department of Agriculture.
Indications: For use in the prevention of feline panleukopenia (distemper) in healthy cats.
Dosage and Administration: Vaccinate healthy cats of any age with one dose (1 ml) except that if the animal is less than 12 weeks of age, a second dose should be given at 12 to 16 weeks of age. Annual revaccination with a single dose

Continued on next page

B

Beecham—Cont.

is recommended. The vaccine may be injected either intramuscularly or subcutaneously. Pregnant cats may be vaccinated.
Precautions: Store at 35°F. to 45°F. (1.5°to 7°C.). Use sterile syringe and needle. Do not chemically sterilize. Use the entire contents when the container is first opened. The vaccine contains permissible levels of Polymyxin B, and Neomycin as preservatives. Anaphylactoid reactions may occur following the use of products of this nature. Provide symptomatic therapy which should include epinephrine.
How Supplied: Package of 25 ×1 dose vials. The package is color coded for easy identification.

PANAVAC®RC
Feline Rhinotracheitis-Calici-Panleukopenia Vaccine Modified Live and Killed Virus Feline Cell Line Origin

Composition: The Feline Rhinotracheitis portion of this combination package consists of a naturally attenuated strain, designated the AL strain, which is propagated in a feline cell line. The Feline Calicivirus portion consists of an attenuated strain of feline calicivirus propagated in a feline cell line. The vaccines are blended with a special stabilizer and lyophilized. The Feline Panleukopenia portion consists of an inactivated strain of feline panleukopenia (distemper) designated the Alpha-PL strain virus propagated in a feline cell line and is used to rehydrate the Feline Rhinotracheitis-Calici Vaccine. The Feline Rhinotracheitis-Calici and Feline Panleukopenia Vaccine fractions are all produced under the rigid requirements of Beecham's "FROZEN STABLE CELL BANK™" system. The vaccine viruses have undergone extensive purification studies ensuring the highest degree of purity.
There is no sting or discomfort on administration. The product meets USDA requirements for purity, safety, potency and efficacy.
Administration: To rehydrate, aseptically add the contents of an accompanying vial of Feline Panleukopenia Vaccine to a vial of lyophilized Feline Rhinotracheitis-Calici Vaccine. Shake well to rehydrate. After rehydration, the entire contents should be used immediately. PANAVAC®RC is recommended for vaccination of healthy cats. For intramuscular or subcutaneous use. Administer 2 doses (1 ml each) 3 to 4 weeks apart. For cats vaccinated before 9 weeks of age, revaccinate every 3 to 4 weeks until at least 12 weeks of age. Revaccinate annually with a single dose to maintain a high level of immunity.
Indications: For use in healthy cats for the prevention of feline rhinotracheitis, feline calici and feline panleukopenia infections.
Precautions: Store at 35–45°F. (1.5–7°C.). Do not vaccinate pregnant cats. Use sterile syringe and needle (do not chemically sterilize). Use the entire contents when the container is first opened. The vaccine contains permissible levels of Polymyxin B and Neomycin as preservatives. Anaphylactoid reactions may occur following the use of products of this nature. Provide symptomatic therapy which should include epinephrine. Burn all containers and unused contents.
How Supplied: Packages of 25×1 dose vials. The packages are color-coded for easy identification.

PENICILLIN G PROCAINE AQUEOUS SUSPENSION

Description: Each ml contains 300,000 units of penicillin G procaine; sodium citrate 10 mg; povidone 5 mg; lecithin 6 mg; sodium carboxymethylcellulose 1 mg; methyl paraben 1.3 mg; propyl paraben 0.2 mg; sodium formaldehyde sulfoxylate 0.2 mg; procaine hydrochloride 20 mg and Water for Injection, q.s.
Indications for Use: For the treatment of cattle and sheep for bacterial pneumonia (shipping fever) caused by *Pasteurella multocida;* swine for erysipelas caused by *Erysipelothrix rhusiopathiae (insidiosa);* AND horses for strangles caused by *Streptococcus equi.*
Warnings: Not for use in horses intended for food.
Milk that has been taken from animals during treatment and for 72 hours (6 milkings) after the last treatment must not be used for food.
Treatment should not exceed 4 consecutive days.
Discontinue use of this drug for the following time periods before treated animals are slaughtered for food: Cattle—10 days, Sheep—9 days, Swine—7 days.
Dosage: The dosage for cattle, sheep, swine and horses is 3000 units per pound of body weight or one ml for each 100 pounds of body weight once daily. Continue treatment at least 1 day after symptoms disappear (usually 2 or 3 days). Treatment should not exceed 4 consecutive days. If improvement is not observed, consult your veterinarian.
How Supplied: Penicillin G Procaine Suspension, 300,000 units per ml is available in 100 ml and 250 ml multiple dose vials.

PET-DEC®
(Diethylcarbamazine Citrate) Chewable Tablets

Composition: Each PET-DEC contains 60 mg, 120 mg or 180 mg of diethylcarbamazine citrate in a chewable tablet base.
Indications: PET-DEC are indicated for use in the prevention of infection of *Dirofilaria immitis* (heartworm disease), and as an aid in the treatment of ascarid (*Toxocara canis* and *Toxascaris leonina*) infections in dogs. PET-DEC may be given to dogs of all ages, including bitches, throughout the reproductive period and following whelping.
Dosage and Administration: PET-DEC are chewable tablets that are palatable to most dogs. Tablets may be fed free choice or crumbled and placed on food. PET-DEC are quarter-scored for convenience in adjusting dosage.
Prevention of Heartworm Disease in Dogs: PET-DEC are given orally once-a-day at a dosage rate to 3 mg diethylcarbamazine citrate per pound of body weight. Young dogs may be started on the preventive program at 2 months of age. Administration of PET-DEC in heartworm endemic areas should start 1 month before the beginning of the mosquito season and be continued daily throughout the mosquito season and for approximately 2 months thereafter. Continuous administration during the mosquito season effectively prevents the maturation of recently inoculated heartworm larvae into adults *(D. immitis).*
Treatment of Ascarid Infection in Dogs: PET-DEC are given as a single, oral dose at the rate of 25–50 mg of diethylcarbamazine citrate per pound of body weight. Fasting or a laxative after treatment is not necessary. To reduce the possibility of vomiting which occasionally occurs, it is preferable to administer PET-DEC with food or directly after feeding. Repeat the dosage in 10–20 days to remove immature ascarids which may enter the intestine from the lungs after the first treatment.
Precautions and Side Effects: The use of diethylcarbamazine citrate is not recommended in dogs with active *D. immitis* infections. Inadvertent administration to heartworm infested dogs may cause adverse reactions due to pulmonary occlusion or shock.
A dog on prophylactic therapy should be examined for the presence of microfilariae every 6 months.
Overdosage may cause emesis. The compound causes no accumulative toxic effects.
Warnings: Dogs with established heartworm infections should not receive PET-DEC until they have been converted to a negative status by use of an adulticidal and microfilaricidal drug.
Caution: Federal law restricts this drug to use by or on the order of a licensed veterinarian.
Do Not Use in Dogs That May Be Harboring Adult Heartworms or Microfilariae.
Keep Out of Reach of Children.
How Supplied: PET-DEC (diethylcarbamazine citrate) are quarter-scored and supplied in three concentrations: 60 mg, 120 mg and 180 mg in 120 count bottles.

PET-DERM,® III
Chewable Tablets (dexamethasone) For Dogs Only

Description: Dexamethasone is an analogue of prednisolone with a more potent (20 times) anti-inflammatory action. Corticosteroids have numerous and diversified effects on hormonal and metabolic actions within the animal. Animals receiving a high dose of dexamethasone and on a limited or low protein diet may exhibit nitrogen loss. Dexamethasone will not cause significant sodium or water retention.
Indications: Pet-Derm, III Chewable Tablets are indicated for supportive therapy in dogs in nonspecific dermatosis

such as summer eczema and atopy. Primary etiology should be determined and therapy instituted to correct it. Pet-Derm, III Chewable Tablets may be used as supportive therapy in inflammatory conditions such as acute arthritic conditions.

Dosage and Administration:

Dogs —0.25 mg to 1.25 mg per day.

Dosage may be administered as a single dose or in two divided doses, until desired therapeutic response is attained or 7 days have elapsed. When desired therapeutic response is attained, dosage should be gradually reduced by 0.125 mg per day until maintenance level is achieved.

Tablets may be administered free choice or crumbled over food.

Diagnosis should be redetermined if no therapeutic response is noted within 7 days.

Therapy should be individualized with PetDerm, III Chewable Tablets, as with any other potent corticosteroid according to the severity of the condition being treated, anticipated duration of steroid therapy and the animals threshold or tolerance for steroids.

Pet-Derm, III Chewable Tablets, may be substituted for treatment with any other corticosteroid with proper adjustment dosage.

Contraindications: Pet-Derm, III Chewable Tablets should not be used in animals with tuberculosis, chronic nephritis, cushingoid syndrome, and peptic ulcers. Existence of congestive heart failure, diabetes and osteoporosis are relative contraindications. Corticosteroids should not be used in animals with an active viremia.

Precautions: Close observation of animals receiving Pet-Derm, III Chewable Tablets is required. Signs of infection may be masked because of the anti-inflammatory action of corticosteroids. Diagnosis should be established prior to use of corticosteroids. Corticosteroids will cause sodium retention, fluid retention, potassium loss and weight gain if overdosed. Providing the infections are controlled with appropriate antibiotic or chemotherapeutic agents, Pet-Derm, III Chewable Tablets may be administered to animals with acute or chronic bacterial infections.

Warning: Clinical and experimental data have demonstrated that corticosteroids administered orally or parenterally to animals may induce the first stage of parturition when administered during the last trimester of pregnancy and may precipitate premature parturition followed by dystocia, fetal death, retained placenta, and metritis. Additionally, corticosteroids administered to dogs, rabbits and rodents during pregnancy have resulted in cleft palate in offspring. Corticosteroids administered to dogs during pregnancy have also resulted in other congenital anomalies, including deformed forelegs, phocomelia and anasarca.

Side Effects: Corticosteroids may cause weight loss, anorexia, polydipsia, and polyuria.

Caution: Federal law restricts this drug to use by or on the order of a licensed veterinarian.

How Supplied: Pet-Derm, III Chewable Tablets, 0.25 mg, scored, in dispensing bottles of 30 tablets.

PNEUMOSUIS® II
Haemophilus Pleuropneumoniae Bacterin

Composition: Pneumosuis II consists of inactivated concentrated cultures of highly antigenic strains of *H. pleuropneumoniae.* These strains are selected to provide protection against serotypes 1, 3, 4, and 5.

The adjuvanted product is a concentrated 2 ml dose for use either subcutaneously or intramuscularly. The strains are grown utilizing the Ultraferm process, in specially formulated media. The Ultraferm process employs the use of modern electrically controlled and rigidly monitored production fermenters resulting in high quality antigen yields.

Inactivation of each strain is performed in such a manner as to retain the maximum antigenicity of the product. The product is formulated by carefully concentrating, blending and adjuvanting each antigen in proper proportions under constant agitation.

Indications: For use in healthy swine for the prevention of pneumonia caused by *Haemophilus pleuropneumoniae.*

Dosage and Administration: The recommended dose is 2 ml injected either subcutaneously or intramuscularly.

For adequate protection, both sows and baby pigs should be vaccinated according to the following directions.

Sows and Gilts: Vaccinate at approximately 4 and 2 weeks prior to first farrowing and at 2 to 4 weeks prior to each subsequent farrowing.

Pigs: Vaccinate at weaning with a revaccination 3 to 4 weeks later.

Caution: Store at 35–45°F. (1.5–7°C.). Do not freeze. Do not vaccinate within 21 days before slaughter. Use entire contents when first opened. Anaphylactoid reactions may occur following the use of biological products. Symptomatic treatment should be provided. Antidote: Epinephrine.

How Supplied: 50 dose plastic vials. Species and color-coded label for easy product identification.

PORCI-RAB®
Porcine Pseudorabies Vaccine, Killed Virus

Composition: Porci-Rab consists of a highly immunogenic field strain of pseudorabies virus. This virus strain has been adapted to and propagated in a porcine cell line, which is produced under the precise conditions of Beecham's FROZEN STABLE CELL BANK™ system.

The most modern and technologically advanced techniques are used in manufacture and testing to ensure the product is pure, safe, potent and efficacious. Careful chemical inactivation of the pseudorabies virus and a unique blend of adjuvants provide maximum antigenic response.

Each serial of Porci-Rab is tested for purity, safety, potency and efficacy beyond USDA requirements.

Indications: For use in healthy swine for the prevention of pseudorabies.

Dosage and Administration: Shake well. DOSAGE: Aseptically inject one dose (2 ml) subcutaneously. If pigs are vaccinated prior to weaning, revaccinate approximately 3 weeks after the initial dose. Semi-annual revaccination is recommended for animals retained for breeding purposes. Safe for use at any stage of pregnancy.

Caution: Pseudorabies vaccination will result in a seropositive response. Consider state and local regulations before use. Store at 35–45°F. (1.5°C.). Do not freeze. Do not vaccinate within 21 days before slaughter. Use entire contents when first opened. Porci-Rab contains permissible levels of Polymyxin B, Neomycin and Amphotericin B as preservatives. Anaphylactoid reactions may occur following the use of biological products. Symptomatic treatment should be provided. Antidote: Epinephrine.

Packaging: 50 ml (25 dose) plastic vial. Coded for easy species identification.

RABCINE®
Rabies Vaccine
Killed virus

Composition: Rabcine® consists of the High Cell Passage Kissling Strain of rabies virus propagated in a hamster stable cell line produced under the rigid requirements of Beecham's "Frozen Stable Cell Bank System™" and chemically inactivated to retain maximum antigenicity. The hamster stable cell line and the High Cell Passage Kissling Strain used in the manufacture of this product have undergone studies ensuring the highest degree of purity. The vaccine is blended with a special adjuvant and presented in a liquid form. There is no sting or discomfort on administration. The product is tested in accordance with the regulations of the U.S. Department of Agriculture.

Indications: For use in the prevention of rabies in healthy dogs and cats.

Dosage and Administration: Recommended for vaccination of dogs and cats. Inject a full 1 ml dose intramuscularly at one site in the thigh at 3 months of age. Revaccinate annually to maintain a high level of immunity.

Precautions: Store at 35°F. to 45°F. (1.5°C. to 7°C.). Do not freeze. Use sterile syringe and needle. Do not chemically sterilize. Use the entire contents when the container is first opened. The product contains permissible levels of antibiotics as preservatives. Anaphylactoid rections may occur following the use of products of this nature. Provide symptomatic therapy which should include epinephrine.

General Information:

Purity of the Vaccine virus—Studies conducted on the Rabies Vaccine Master

Continued on next page

Beecham—Cont.

B

Seed Virus demonstrated no extraneous viruses, Bacteria, Fungi, Mycoplasma, or other adventitious agents.
Purity of the Cell Culture—Master Cell Stocks of the Hamster Stable Cell Line were prepared and pretested prior to use in vaccine production, and demonstrated no Bacteria, Fungi, Mycoplasma, or other adventitious viral agents such as Canine Distemper, Infectious Canine Hepatitis, Bovine Rhinotracheitis, Parainfluenza-3, Bovine Virus Diarrhea, Simian Virus-5, Reovirus 1, Reovirus X, Canine Herpes, and hemadsorbing and hemagglutinating viruses, assuring a vaccine of the highest purity.
Antigenicity (Potency Evaluation in Dogs and Cats) —Serological studies performed in 48 cats, which were initially seronegative, varying in age from 3 months to 21 years of age showed the average serum neutralizing antibody titer elicited to be ≥ 1:207 one month post-vaccination. Serological studies performed in 46 dogs which were initially seronegative, showed the average serum neutralizing antibody titer elicited to be R 1:276 one month post-vaccination. In serological studies on 46 dogs and 48 cats, a positive response was demonstrated in all of the animals vaccinazed.
Safety Studies in Dogs and Cats —The High Cell Passage Kissling Strain of Vaccine Virus was shown to be safe for use in dogs and cats. At exaggerrated dosage levels, the vaccine proved to be safe with no untoward effects. During studies at Beecham Laboratories and in the field, hundreds of dogs and cats of various ages have been vaccinated with no adverse effects.
How Supplied: 10 dose vial.

RABMUNE®-3
Rabies Vaccine, Killed Virus

Indications: For the immunization of healthy dogs and cats against rabies.
Dosage and Administration: Shake well before use. Using aseptic technique, inject 1 ml intramuscularly at one site in the thigh.
Dogs: Administer one dose at 3 months of age or older. Dogs vaccinated under 6 months of age should be revaccinated at 1 year of age. Revaccinate every 3 years.
Cats: Administer one dose at 3 months of age or older. Revaccinate annually.
Precautions: Store at 2° to 7° C (35° to 45°F). Do not freeze. Use entire contents when first opened. Anaphylactoid reactions may occur following use of biologicals. Symptomatic therapy should be provided, including epinephrine. Gentamicin and Amphotericin B added as preservatives.
How Supplied: Package of 10 × 10 dose vials.
Rabmune®-3 is a registered trademark of Schering Corporation.

RE-SORB®
Oral Hydration
Electrolyte Product

The three main causes of calf scours and resulting dehydration are bacteria (*E. coli* and Salmonella, etc.), viruses and nutritional factors. In all cases, there is a loss of water and electrolytes due to the scours, which can lead to severe dehydration and death. Generally, whatever the cause of the scours, dehydration is the main cause of death. When fecal loss of water exceeds the water intake, dehydration occurs. This can be corrected with administration of either oral or intravenous fluids. In the severely dehydrated calf, intravenous administration is the route of choice.
Oral rehydration is of particular value as it permits the livestock owner to start rehydration therapy at the initial signs of scours which, in many cases, will reduce the severity of the condition. **RE-SORB** also provides the owner with a practical method of following up intravenous therapy.
RE-SORB formula contains the following ingredients: sodium chloride 8.82 grams, potassium phosphate 4.20 grams, citric acid, anhydrous 0.5 grams, potassium citrate 0.12 grams, aminoacetic acid (glycine) 6.36 grams and glucose 44.0 grams. Osmolarity of the reconstituted solution is approximately 315 mOsm per kg. The pH of the reconstituted solution is approximately 4.3
Action: Oral glucose/glycine compounds have been used with excellent success to treat dehydration accompanying human cholera for many years (1, 2, 3). The rationale for oral rehydration therapy is based upon the active absorption of glucose and glycine when given orally to scouring animals. Their absorption is linked to the simultaneous absorption of sodium and water. This principle has been verified in scouring animals (4). *E. coli* produces scours by secreting toxins in the small intestine. These toxins, while causing profuse secretion of water and electrolytes, have no effect on glucose/glycine absorption in the calf(5). When **RE-SORB** is administered, the glucose/glycine along with the water and sodium are absorbed resulting in a net gain in water thereby correcting the dehydration.
In diarrhea caused by viruses, the disease process causes a flattening of the intestinal mucosa which reduces digestion and absorption of milk. The undigested milk passes into the colon where bacterial fermentation results in additional diarrhea (6). The replacement of milk with **RE-SORB** for two days followed by a gradual re-introduction of milk mixed with **RE-SORB,** provides an opportunity for the gastrointestinal mucosa to rest.
Since **RE-SORB** is readily absorbed, it provides the livestock owner with an ideal first feed for the stressed or newly purchased calf. It is widely believed that it is often beneficial to starve or only provide half of the initial feeding of milk to newly purchased calves to reduce stress on the gastrointestinal system. **RE-SORB** may be given as the initial feeding following by a 50:50 mixture of **RE-SORB** and milk at the second feeding to reduce stress on the gastrointestinal tract.
Indications: RE-SORB is a readily absorbed source of fluids and electrolytes. It is a convenient and effective means of increasing absorption of water, energy sources and electrolytes. **RE-SORB** is indicated for use in the control of dehydration associated with diarrhea (scours) in calves. **RE-SORB** may be used by the livestock owner as an early treatment at the first signs of scouring. It may also be used as follow-up treatment for the dehydrated calf following intravenous fluid therapy.
RE-SORB, because of its ready source of fluid and electrolytes, makes it an ideal first feed (upon arrival) for newly purchased or severely stressed calves.
Precautions: RE-SORB should not be used in animals with severe dehydration (down, comatose, or in a state of shock). Such animals need intravenous fluids since oral therapy in these cases is too slow. A veterinarian should be consulted in such severely scouring calves or in cases requiring antibacterial therapy.
Antibacterial therapy is often indicated in bacterial scours due to *E. coli* and/or Salmonella, **RE-SORB** does not contain antibacterial agents.
Adequate colostrum intake during the first 12 hours is essential for healthy, vigorous calves.
RE-SORB is not nutritionally complete if administered by itself for long periods of time. It should not be administered beyond the recommended treatment period without the addition of milk or milk replacer.
Warning For use in calves only.
Dosage/Directions Mixing Directions:
Add the contents of one packet (both sides) to two quarts of warm water. Stir until dissolved.
Scouring Calves:
Feed two quarts of **RE-SORB** solution made up as directed, twice daily for two days (four feedings). No milk or milk replacer should be fed during this period. For the next four feedings (days 3 and 4), use one quart of **RE-SORB** solution together with one quart of milk replacer. Thereafter feed as normal.
Newly Purchased Calves:
Feed two quarts of **RE-SORB** solution made up as directed, instead of milk as the first feed upon arrival. For the next scheduled feeding, use one quart of **RE-SORB** solution mixed together with one quart of milk or milk replacer. Thereafter feed as normal.
How Supplied: RE-SORB is supplied in boxes containing 12 packets (double sided).

NDC 0029-3615-39

1. Nalin, D. R. GUT 11: 768–772 (1970)
2. Pierce, N. F. and Hirshhorn, N., WHO CHRONICLE 31: 87–93 (1977)
3. JOHN HOPKINS MEDICAL JOURNAL, 132: 197–205 (1973)

4. Bywater, R., AJVR, 38: 1983 (1977)
5. Bywater, R., J. COMP. PATH., 80: 565 (1970)
6. Halpin, C. S. and Caple, I. W., AUSTRALIAN VET. JOURNAL, 52: 438 (1976)

RIPERCOL® PIPERAZINE
(Levamisole hydrochloride, piperazine dihydrochloride)
Horse Anthelmintic, Ready-to-use Solution

Composition: Each fl oz contains 0.36 g levamisole hydrochloride and piperazine dihydrochloride equivalent to 4.0 g of piperazine base.
The drug contains two safe, well established anthelmintics (levamisole hydrochloride and piperazine dihydrochloride) in a formulation designed to provide a broad spectrum of activity while allowing an adequate margin of safety.
Indication: RIPERCOL®-PIPERAZINE Anthelmintic Ready-To-Use Solution is indicated for the treatment of horses infected with intestinal parasites. Critical test data demonstrate efficacy against the following:

Large Strongyles:	
Strongylus vulgaris	96%
S. edentatus	63%
Small Strongyles:	96%

Including: *Cylicocercus* spp., *Cylicocyclus* spp., *Cylicodontophorus* spp., *Cylicostephanus* spp., *Cylicotetrapedon* spp.

Ascarids:	
Parascaris equorum	100%
Pinworms:	
Oxyuris equi	
Immature	61%
Mature	90%

For most effective results retreat animals in 6–8 weeks. For animals maintained on premises where reinfection is likely to occur, additional retreatment may be necessary.
Dosage and Administration: SHAKE WELL BEFORE USING
Administer one fluid ounce per 100 lb body weight. This dosage supplies 3.6 mg/lb levamisole hydrochloride and 39.8 mg/lb of piperazine dihydrochloride. Levamisole-piperazine liquid is designed to be administered by stomach tube, or as a drench.
At the recommended dose of 1 fl oz per 100 lb, it is highly effective against all of the aforementioned genera. Preconditioning horses by fasting is not necessary or recommended when using the liquid formulation. The formulation is inactive against bots (*Gastrophilus spp.*). However, the preparation is compatible with carbon disulfide and may be given concurrently if desired. Cautions ordinarily observed with carbon disulfide should be observed.
Warning: Do not treat horses intended for food.
It has been reported that horses with onchocerciasis may show transient skin lesions following treatment with this product.
Caution: Federal law restricts this drug to use by or on the order of a licensed veterinarian.
How Supplied: 1 gallon bottles

SALMONELLA BACTERIN
Salmonella Choleraesuis Bacterin

Composition: This product consists of an inactivated culture of *Salmonella choleraesuis.* The strain was selected because of its highly antigenic characteristics. The cultures are grown in a medium under constant agitation utilizing Beecham Laboratories' ULTRAFERM™ process.
The temperature and pH are electronically controlled, and the fermentation process is rigidly monitored. The final bacterin is highly antigenic, pure, safe and uniform from batch to batch. The final bacterin is adjuvanted with aluminum hydroxide to provide greater long-term protection.
Indications: For use in healthy swine for the prevention of disease caused by *Salmonella choleraesuis.*
Dosage and Administration: Shake well. Inject 2 ml subcutaneously or intramuscularly at weaning, with a revaccination approximately 3 weeks later. Annual vaccination is recommended to maintain a high level of immunity. To stimulate high antibody levels in colostrum, administer a booster dose to pregnant sows 4 to 6 weeks prior to farrowing.
Caution: Store at 35–45°F. (1.5–7°C.). Do not freeze. Use entire contents when the container is first opened. Do not vaccinate within 21 days before slaughter. Anaphylactoid reactions may occur following the use of biological products. Sympomatic treatment should be provided. Antidote: Epinephrine.
Packaging: 100 ml (50 dose) plastic vial. Coded for easy species identification.

SENTRYPAR®
Parvovirus Vaccine
Modified Live Virus

Composition: SENTRYPAR consists of a canine parvovirus, isolated from a clinical infection, that has been attenuated and is propagated in a feline cell line, produced under rigidly controlled production requirements. The vaccine is presented in a liquid form. The product has been tested for purity, safety, potency, and efficacy in accordance with regulations of the United States Department of Agriculture.
Indications: For use in healthy dogs for the prevention of canine parvovirus disease.
Dosage and Administration: One dose (1 ml) at 14 weeks of age or older. For dogs vaccinated before 14 weeks of age, revaccinate every 2 weeks until at least 14 weeks of age. Revaccinate annually with a single dose to maintain a high level of immunity.
Shake well before using. Aseptically inject either subcutaneously or intramuscularly. Maternal antibody may interfere with successful vaccination of dogs less than 14 weeks of age.
Precautions: Store at 35–45°F. (1.5–7°C.). Use sterile syringe and needle (do not chemically sterilize). Use the entire contents when the container is first opened. This vaccine contains permissible levels of Polymyxin B and Neomycin as preservatives. Anaphylactoid reactions may occur following the use of products of this nature. Provide symptomatic therapy which should include epinephrine. Burn all containers and unused contents.
How Supplied: Packages of 25×1 Dose Vials. The packages are color-coded for easy identificaton.

SENTRYPAR® DHP
Canine Distemper-Hepatitis-Parainfluenza-Parvovirus Vaccine
Modified Live Virus

Composition: SENTRYPAR DHP consists of lyophilized attenuated strains of canine distemper virus and canine parainfluenza virus propagated in a canine cell line, infectious canine hepatitus virus (CAV-1) propagated in a porcine cell line, and a canine isolate parvovirus propagated in a feline cell line, which are produced under rigidly controlled production requirements. The vaccine viruses are blended with a special stabilizer and presented in a lyophilized form. The product has been tested for purity, safety, potency and efficacy in accordance with regulations of the United States Department of Agriculture.
Indications: For use in healthy dogs of any age for the prevention of canine distemper, hepatitis, parainfluenza and parvovirus.
Dosage and Administration: Administer 2 doses (1 ml each) 2 to 3 weeks apart. For dogs vaccinated before 14 weeks of age, revaccinate every 2 to 3 weeks until at least 14 weeks of age. Revaccinate annually with a single dose to maintain a high level of immunity.
To rehydrate, aseptically add the contents of an accompanying vial of Sterile Diluent to a vial of lyophilized Canine Distemper-Hepatitis-Parainfluenza-Parvovirus Vaccine. Shake well to rehydrate. After rehydration, the entire contents should be used immediately. For intramuscular or subcutaneous use. **SENTRYPAR DHP** is recommended for the immunization of healthy dogs against canine distemper, canine hepatitis, canine parainfluenza and canine parvovirus. Maternal antibodies may interfere with successful immunization with any of the MLV components of the vaccine. It is recommended that a one ml dose be administered at approximately 9 weeks of age with repeat vaccinations at 2 to 3 week intervals until at least 14 weeks of age.
Precautions: Store at 35–40°F. (1.5–7°C.). Use sterile syringe and needle (do not chemically sterilize). **SENTRYPAR DHP** contains permissible levels of Polymyxin B and Neomycin as preservatives. Anaphylactoid reactions may occur following the use of products of this nature. Provide symptomatic therapy which should include epinephrine. Burn all containers and unused contents. Occasionally transient corneal opacity may occur following the administration of

Continued on next page

Beecham—Cont.

this product. This is due to the canine hepatitis fraction, however, the strain used by Beecham Laboratories has been used extensively in the field and appears to involve a very low incidence of corneal opacity.

Supplemental Information: SENTRYPAR DHP has been extensively tested in susceptible puppies at Beecham Laboratories. Studies conducted at Beecham Laboratories have shown that puppies were protected against challenge with virulent canine distemper, canine hepatitis, canine parainfluenza and canine parvo viruses after vaccination with the virus strains used in the **SENTRYPAR DHP** vaccine. Protective antibodies against all four viruses were demonstrated following vaccination. Studies also demonstrated that there was no interference between the canine distemper, hepatitis, parainfluenza, or the parvo virus fractions. The vaccine proved to be safe and efficacious, and did not cause untoward reactions in vaccinated dogs.

How Supplied: Packages of 25×1 Dose Vials. The packages are color-coded for easy identification.

SENTRYPAR®DHP/L
Canine
Distemper-Hepatitis-Parainfluenza-Parvovirus Vaccine
Modified Live Virus
Leptospira Bacterin

Composition: SENTRYPAR DHP/L consists of lyophilized attenuated strains of canine distemper virus and canine parainfluenza virus propagated in a canine cell line, infectious canine hepatitis virus (CAV-1) propagated in a porcine cell line, and a canine isolate parvovirus propagated in a feline cell line; accompanied by liquid inactivated *Leptospira canicola-icterohaemorrhagiae* bacterin as the diluent, which are produced under rigidly controlled production requirements. The vaccine viruses are blended with a special stabilizer and presented in a lyophilized form. The product has been tested for purity, safety, potency, and efficacy in accordance with regulations of the United States Department of Agriculture.

Indications: For use in healthy dogs of any age for the prevention of canine distemper, hepatitis, parainfluenza, parvovirus, and leptospirosis caused by *Leptospira canicola* and *Leptospira icterohaemorrhagiae.*

Dosage and Administration: Administer 2 doses (1 ml each) 2 to 3 weeks apart. For dogs vaccinated before 14 weeks of age, revaccinate every 2 to 3 weeks until at least 14 weeks of age. Revaccinate annually with a single dose to maintain a high level of immunity.

To rehydrate, aseptically add the contents of an accompanying vial of Leptospira Bacterin to a vial of lyophilized Canine Distemper-Hepatitis-Parainfluenza-Parvovirus Vaccine. Shake well to rehydrate. After rehydration, the entire contents should be used immediately. For intramuscular or subcutaneous use. SENTRYPAR DHP/L is recommended for the immunization of healthy dogs against canine distemper, canine hepatitis, canine parainfluenza, canine parvovirus, and leptospirosis caused by *Leptospira canicola* and *Leptospira icterohaemorrhagiae.* Maternal antibodies may intefere with successful immunization with any of the Modified Live Virus components of the vaccine. It is recommended that a one ml dose be administered at approximately 9 weeks of age with repeat vaccinations at 2 to 3 weeks intervals until at least 14 weeks of age.

Precautions: Store at 35–45°F. (1.5–7°C.). Use sterile syringe and needle (do not chemically sterilize). SENTRYPAR DHP/L contains permissible levels of Polymyxin B and Neomycin as preservatives. Anaphylactoid reactions may occur following the use of products of this nature. Provide symptomatic therapy which should include epinephrine. Burn all containers and unused contents. Occasionally transient corneal opacity may occur following the administration of this product. This is due to the canine hepatitis fraction, however the strain used by Beecham Laboratories has been used extensively in the field and appears to involve a very low incidence of corneal opacity.

Supplemental Information: SENTRYPAR DHP/L has been extensively tested in susceptible puppies at Beecham Laboratories. Studies conducted at Beecham Laboratories have shown that puppies were protected against challenge with either virulent canine distemper, canine hepatitis, canine parainfluenza or canine parvo viruses after vaccination with the virus strains used in the SENTRYPAR DHP/L vaccine. Protective antibodies against all four viruses were demonstrated following vaccination. Studies also demonstrated that there was no interference between the canine distemper, hepatitis, parainfluenza, parvo virus or the Leptospira fractions. The vaccine proved to be safe and efficacious, and did not cause untoward reactions in vaccinated dogs. The Leptospira Bacterin diluent contained with the SENTRYPAR DHP/L has been extensively tested in susceptible dogs. Agglutinating antibodies were present in susceptible dogs in 8 days after being vaccinated with a single dose of the Leptospira Canicola-Icterohaemorrhagiae Bacterin. Non-vaccinated dogs showed clinical symptoms such as leptospiremia, leptospiruria, and leptospirae isolation from kidney tissue after challenge with virulent leptospirae. All vaccinated dogs remained healthy and free of clinical symptoms, including renal shedding, after challenge with virulent leptospirae. Studies performed have shown that there is no viricidal activity when the Leptospira Bacterin diluent is used to rehydrate the virus vaccine.

How Supplied: Packages of 25×1 dose vials. Packages are color-coded for easy identification.

SENTRYVAC–DHP™
Canine
Distemper-Hepatitis-Parainfluenza Vaccine
Modified Live Virus

Composition: SENTRYVAC-DHP consists of lyophilized attenuated strains of canine distemper virus and canine parainfluenza virus propagated in a canine cell line, infectious canine hepatitis virus (CAV-1) propagated in a porcine cell line, which are produced under precisely controlled production conditions. The vaccine viruses are blended with a special stabilizer and presented in a lyophilized form. The product is tested for purity, safety, potency, and has been tested for efficacy in accordance with the regulations of the United States Department of Agriculture.

Indications: For use in healthy dogs for the prevention of canine distemper, canine hepatitis and canine parainfluenza.

Dosage and Administration: To rehydrate, aseptically add the contents of an accompanying vial of Sterile Diluent to a vial of lyophilized Canine Distemper-Hepatitis-Parainfluenza Vaccine. Shake well to rehydrate. After rehydration, the entire contents should be used immediately. SENTRYVAC-DHP is recommended for the immunization of healthy dogs against canine distemper, canine hepatitis, and canine parainfluenza. Maternal antibody may interfere with successful vaccination of dogs less than 9 weeks of age. For intramuscular or subcutaneous use.

Administer 2 doses (1 ml each) 3 to 4 weeks apart. For dogs vaccinated before 9 weeks of age, revaccinate every 3 to 4 weeks until at least 12 weeks of age. Revaccinate annually with a single dose to maintain a high level of immunity.

Precautions: Store at 35–45°F. (1.5–7°C.). Use sterile syringe and needle (do not chemically sterilize). The product contains permissible levels of Polymyxin B and Neomycin as preservatives. Anaphylactoid reactions may occur following the use of biological products. Provide symptomatic therapy which should include epinephrine. Burn all containers and unused contents. Occasionally transient corneal opacity may occur following the administration of this product. This is due to the canine hepatitis fraction, however the strain used by Beecham Laboratories has been used extensively in the field and appears to involve a very low incidence of corneal opacity.

How Supplied: Packages of 25×1 dose vials. Packages are color-coded for easy identification.

SENTRYVAC–DHP/L™
Canine
Distemper-Hepatitis-Parainfluenza Vaccine
Modified Live Virus
Leptospira Bacterin

Composition: SENTRYVAC-DHP/L consists of lyophilized attenuated strains of canine distemper virus and canine parainfluenza virus propagated in a canine cell line, infectious canine hepatitis virus (CAV-1) propagated in a porcine cell line, accompanied by liquid inactivated leptospira canicola-icterohaemorrhagiae bacterin as the diluent, which are produced under precisely controlled production conditions. The vaccine viruses are blended with a special stabilizer and presented in a lyophilized form. The combination product is tested for purity, safety, potency, and has been tested for efficacy in accordance with the regulations of the United States Department of Agriculture.

Indications: For use in healthy dogs for the prevention of canine distemper, canine hepatitis, canine parainfluenza and leptospirosis caused by *Leptospira canicola* and *Leptospira icterohaemorrhagiae.*

Dosage and Administration: To rehydrate, aseptically add the contents of an accompanying vial of Leptospira Canicola-Icterohaemorrhagiae Bacterin to a vial of lyophilized Canine Distemper-Hepatitis-Parainfluenza Vaccine. Shake well to rehydrate. After rehydration, the entire contents should be used immediately. SENTRYVAC-DHP/L is recommended for the immunization of healthy dogs against canine distemper, canine hepatitis, canine parainfluenza, and leptospirosis caused by *Leptospira canicola* and *icterohaemorrhagiae.* Maternal antibody may interfere with successful vaccination of dogs less than 9 weeks of age. For intramuscular or subcutaneous use. Administer 2 doses (1 ml each) 3 to 4 weeks apart. For dogs vaccinated before 9 weeks of age, revaccinate every 3 to 4 weeks until at least 12 weeks of age.

Precautions: Store at 35–45°F. (1.5–7°C.). Use sterile syringe and needle (do not chemically sterilize). The product contains permissible levels of Polymyxin B and Neomycin as preservatives. Anaphylactoid reactions may occur following the use of biological products. Provide symptomatic therapy which should include epinephrine. Burn all containers and unused contents. Occasionally transient corneal opacity may occur following the administration of this product. This is due to the canine hepatitis fraction, however the strain used by Beecham Laboratories has been used extensively in the field and appears to involve a very low incidence of corneal opacity.

How Supplied: Packages of 25×1 dose vials. Packages are color-coded for easy identification.

SOMUBAC™
Haemophilus Somnus Bacterin

Composition: Somubac is prepared from three selected strains of *Haemophilus somnus.* The strains are grown *serum-free* in an environmentally controlled fermentation system using a highly nutritious liquid medium and inactivated in such a manner as to maintain the immunogenic integrity. The product is adjuvanted on aluminum hydroxide. Each serial is tested for purity, safety, and potency before release.

Indications: For use in the prevention of disease caused by *Haemophilus somnus* in healthy cattle and calves.

Dosage and Administration: Shake well before using. Animals should be vaccinated at 3 months of age or older. The recommended dose is 2 ml injected either subcutaneously or intramuscularly, with a revaccination 2 to 4 weeks later. Revaccinate annually to maintain a high level of immunity.

Precautions: Store at 35°–45°F(1.5°–7°C). Do not freeze. Use the entire contents when the container is first opened. Do not vaccinate within 21 days before slaughter. Somubac contains permissible levels of Penicillin, Streptomycin and Amphotericin B as preservatives. Anaphylactoid reactions may occur following the use of products of this nature. Symptomatic treatment should be provided. *Antidote: Epinephrine.*

How Supplied: 10 and 50 dose plastic vials species and color-coded for easy identification.

SOMUBAC-P™
Haemophilus Somnus-Pasteurella Haemolytica-Multocida Bacterin

Composition: Somubac-P consists of inactivated cultures of *Haemophilus somnus, Pasteurella haemolytica,* Type 1 and *Pasteurella multocida,* Type A, grown in special medias to assure optimum antigenicity. The cultures are grown *serum-free* in an environmentally controlled process. The bacterin is adjuvanted with aluminum hydroxide. The product is tested for purity, safety and potency before release.

Indications: For use in the prevention of disease caused by *Haemophilus somnus* and pasteurellosis in healthy cattle and calves.

Dosage and Administration: Shake well before using. Animals should be vaccinated at 3 months of age or older. The recommended dose is 2 ml injected either subcutaneously or intramuscularly, with a revaccination 2 to 4 weeks later. Revaccinate annually to maintain a high level of immunity.

Precautions: Store at 35°–45°F (1.5°–7°C). Do not freeze. Use the entire contents when the container is first opened. Do not vaccinate within 21 days before slaughter. Somubac-P contains permissible levels of Penicillin, Streptomycin and Amphotericin B as preservatives. Anaphylactoid reactions may occur following the use or products of this nature, particularly in calves under 3 months of age. Symptomatic treatment should be provided. *Antidote: Epinephrine.*

How Supplied: 10 and 50 dose plastic vials species and color-coded for easy identification.

TICILLIN®
(Sterile ticarcillin disodium)
FOR INTRAUTERINE INFUSION
FOR USE IN HORSES ONLY

Description: TICILLIN (ticarcillin disodium) is a semisynthetic penicillin derived from the penicillin nucleus, 6-amino-penicillanic acid. Chemically, it is α-carboxy-3-thienyl-methylpenicillin disodium salt. It is supplied as a white to pale yellow powder for reconstitution. The reconstituted solution is clear, colorless or pale yellow having a pH of 6.0–8.0. Ticarcillin disodium is very soluble in water. Its solubility is greater than 600 mg/ml.

Action: *MICROBIOLOGY:* Ticarcillin disodium is bactericidal and demonstrates substantial *in vitro* activity against both Gram-positive and Gram-negative organisms. Many strains of the following organisms were found to be susceptible to ticarcillin *in vitro,* but the clinical significance of this action has not been demonstrated in animals: *Pseudomonas aeruginosa* (and other species), *Escherichia coli, Proteus mirabilis, Proteus morganii, Proteus rettgeri, Proteus vulgaris, Enterobacter* spp., *Haemophilus influenzae, Neisseria* spp., *Salmonella* spp., *Staphylococcus aureus* (nonpenicillinase producing), *Staphylococcus albus, beta-hemolytic Streptococci* (Group A), *Streptococcus faecalis* (Enterococcus), and *Streptococcus pneumoniae.* The following anaerobic bacteria have been shown to exhibit *in vitro* susceptibility: *Bacteroides* spp. (including *B. fragilis), Fusobacterium* spp., *Veillonella* spp., *Clostridium* spp., *Eubacterium* spp., *Peptococcus* spp., and *Peptostreptococcus* spp.

Ticarcillin disodium is not stable in the presence of penicillinase.

The 75 mcg ticarcillin antibiotic disc should be used for antibiotic susceptibility testing. If the ticarcillin disc is not available, the 100 mcg carbenicillin disc can be used as a guide for susceptibility to ticarcillin. It should be remembered that these susceptibility methods are based upon expected serum levels in man and do not necessarily reflect susceptibility in certain tissues where the drug is concentrated (urine) or in local infusion where the drug is concentrated.

Safety: Toxicity of TICILLIN (ticarcillin disodium) was evaluated in horses by administering intravenously 100 mg/lb twice a day for 15 days with no significant adverse reactions. Ticarcillin disodium exhibits the same low degree of toxicity as other penicillins.

Histological evaluation of pre- and post-treatment uterine biopsies during the clinical studies revealed no increase in inflammation (irritation) of the endometrium following treatment with TICILLIN.

Adequately controlled studies have not been conducted to support the administration of ticarcillin at the time of breeding.

Indications: TICILLIN (ticarcillin disodium) is indicated for the intrauterine treatment of endometritis in mares caused by *beta-hemolytic streptococci.*

Dosage and Administration: RECOMMENDED DOSAGE AND DIRECTIONS FOR USE: 6 grams intrauterine per day for 3 days during estrus. Reconstitute with 25 ml of Sterile Water for Injection, USP or Sodium Chloride Injection, USP.

Continued on next page

Beecham—Cont.

B

When dissolved, dilute further to desired volume (100 to 500 ml) with Sterile Water for Injection, USP or Sodium Chloride Injection, USP and aseptically infuse into the uterus.
STABILITY: Reconstituted ticarcillin disodium is stable when stored at room temperature for 24 hours. If stored under refrigeration, ticarcillin disodium is stable for 72 hours following reconstitution. If ticarcillin is diluted to a concentration of 100 mg/ml or less with Sterile Water for Injection, USP or Sodium Chloride Injection, USP, these solutions can be frozen (approximately 0°F.) and stored for up to 30 days. The stability of the thawed solutions is similar to the unfrozen solutions (72 hours under refrigeration). Unused solutions should be discarded after time periods mentioned above.
Contraindications: A history of allergic reaction to any of the penicillins is the only known contraindication.
Adverse Reactions: No adverse reactions were reported in the clinical trials conducted with ticarcillin.
Warnings: TICILLIN (ticarcillin disodium) is for use in horses only. Not for use in horses or other animals which are raised for food production.
Ticarcillin is a semisynthetic penicillin and has the potential for producing allergic reactions. If an allergic reaction occurs, administer epinephrine and/or steroids.
Caution: Federal law restricts this drug to use by or on the order of a licensed veterinarian.
How Supplied: TICILLIN (ticarcillin disodium) is supplied in 50 ml vials containing 6 grams of ticarcillin activity.
NDC 0029-6561-26 ....6 gram vial

Beecham laboratories
DIV. OF BEECHAM INC. BRISTOL, TENN. 37620
Rev. Sept., 1984 7517/D

ULTRABAC-CD™
Clostridium Perfringens Types C& D Bacterin —Toxoid

Composition: Ultrabac CD consists of killed and toxoided cultures of *Cl. perfringens* Types C and D grown in special media to assure optimum growth and antigenicity. The cultures are grown in electronically controlled and rigidly monitored fermentation equipment to enhance uniformity of the product from batch to batch. The product is precipitated and adjuvanted. The product is tested in accordance with regulations of the US Department of Agriculture.
Indications: For the prophylactic immunization of healthy cattle and sheep for *Clostridium perfringens* Types C and D bacterial infections (enterotoxemia).
Dosage and Administration: Shake well. For intramuscular or subcutaneous use. The recommended dose is 2 ml for cattle and 1 ml for sheep, and revaccinate 4 to 6 weeks later. Revaccinate pregnant dams 2 weeks prior to parturition. Revaccinate annually to maintain a high level of immunity.
Precautions: Store at 35° to 45°F. Shake well. Use entire contents when container is first opened. Do not vaccinate within 21 days before slaughter. Anaphylactoid may occur following the use of biological products. Symptomatic treatment should be provided including epinephrine.
How Supplied: 10 and 50 dose plastic bottles. Color-coded labels.

ULTRABAC–CS™
Clostridium Chauvoei-Septicum Bacterin

Composition: Ultrabac-CS consists of killed cultures of *Cl. chauvoei* and *Cl. septicum* grown in special media to assure optimum growth and antigenicity. These cultures are grown under constant agitation utilizing the Beecham Ultraferm process. The temperature and pH are electronically controlled and the fermentation process is rigidly monitored. The final bacterin product is highly antigenic, pure, safe and uniform from batch to batch. The bacterin is adjuvanted with aluminum hydroxide.
Indications: For the prophylactic immunization of healthy cattle, calves, sheep and lambs against blackleg (Cl. chauvoei) and malignant edema (Cl. septicum).
Dosage and Administration: To resuspend the bacterin, shake well before use. The recommended dose is 2 ml injected subcutaneously or intramuscularly for cattle and calves and 1 ml for sheep and lambs and revaccinate 4 to 6 weeks later. Revaccinate annually to maintain a high level of immunity.
Precautions: Store at 35°to 45°F (1.5°to 7°C). Protect from freezing. Use entire contents when first opened. Do not vaccinate within 21 days before slaughter. Anaphylactoid reactions may occur following use of biological products: *Antidote: Epinephrine.*
How Supplied: 10 and 50 dose plastic vials. Color-coded labels.

ULTRABAC–CSNS™
Clostridium Chauvoei-Septicum-Novyi-Sordellii Bacterin-Toxoid

Composition: Ultrabac-CSNS consists of killed (formalin), whole cell cultures and toxins of *Clostridium chauvoei, Clostridium septicum, Clostridium novyi* and *Clostridium sordellii* grown in special media to assure optimum growth and antigenicity. These cultures are grown under constant agitation utilizing the Beecham Ultraferm process. The temperature and pH are electronically controlled and the fermentation process is rigidly monitored. The final bacterin product is highly antigenic, pure, safe and uniform from batch to batch. The bacterin is adjuvanted with alum. Ultrabac CSNS is tested in accordance with the regulations of the US Department of Agriculture.
Indications: For use in the prevention of blackleg *(Cl. chauvoei),* malignant edema *(Cl. septicum),* black disease *(Cl. novyi),* and *Clostridium sordellii* infections in healthy cattle, and sheep.
Dosage and Administration: Shake well before using. The recommended dose is 5 ml injected subcutaneously or intramuscularly for cattle and 2½ ml for sheep, and revaccinate 4 to 6 weeks later. Revaccinate annually to maintain a high level of immunity.
Precautions: Store at 35° to 45°F (1.5° to 7°C). Do not vaccinate within 21 days before slaughter. Use the entire contents when the container is first opened. Anaphylactoid reactions may occur following the use of biological products. Symptomatic treatment should be provided. *Antidote: Epinephrine.*
How Supplied: 10 and 50 dose plastic vials. Color-coded labels.

ULTRABAC–CSNS™/SOMUBAC™

Composition: ULTRABAC-CSNS/SOMUBAC consists of 3 killed strains of *Haemophilus somnus,* whole cell cultures and toxoids of highly antigenic strains of *Cl. chauvoei, Cl. septicum, Cl. novyi,* and *Cl. sordellii.*
Cultures are grown in a special media to assure optimum growth and antigenicity. Beecham Laboratories' ULTRAFERM™ process employs rigid electronic control over this culturing process. This state-of-the-art fermentation procedure optimizes the production of cellular and toxoid antigens for best protection. The process also assures antigenicity, purity, safety and uniformity from batch to batch.
Indications: For use in healthy cattle for the prevention of blackleg *(Cl. chauvoei),* malignant edema *(Cl. septicum),* black disease *(Cl. novyi), Clostridium sordellii* infection, and disease caused by *Haemophilus somnus.*
Dosage and Administration: Shake well. Aseptically inject 5 ml subcutaneously or intramuscularly, with a revaccination 4 to 6 weeks later. Revaccinate annually to maintain a high level of immunity.
Precautions: Store at 35–45°F. (1.5–7°C.) Do not freeze. Do not vaccinate within 21 days before slaughter. Use entire contents when first opened. Anaphylactoid reactions may occur following use of biological products. Symptomatic therapy should be provided, including epinephrine.
How Supplied: 10- and 50-dose plastic vials with color-coded labels.

ULTRABAC–CSP™
Clostridium Chauvoei—Septicum—Pasteurella Haemolytica—Multocida Bacterin

Composition: Ultrabac-CSP consists of killed cultures of *Cl. chauvoei, Cl. septicum* and *Pasteurella haemolytica,* Type 1 and *Pasteurella multocida,* Type A grown in a special media to assure optimum growth and antigenicity. These cultures are grown under constant agitation utilizing the Beecham Ultraferm process. The temperature and pH are electronically controlled and the fermenta-

tion process is rigidly monitored. The final bacterin product is highly antigenic, pure, safe and uniform from batch to batch. Ultrabac-CSP is adjuvanted with aluminum hydroxide and is tested for purity, safety, potency, and efficacy in accordance with the regulations of the US Department of Agriculture.
Indications: For use in the prevention of blackleg, malignant edema, and pasteurellosis in healthy cattle, calves, sheep, and lambs.
Dosage and Administration: To resuspend the bacterin, shake well before use. The recommended dose is 5 ml injected subcutaneously or intramuscularly for cattle and calves, and 2½ml for sheep and lambs and revaccination 4 to 6 weeks later. Revaccinate annually to maintain a high level of immunity.
How Supplied: 10 and 50 dose plastic vials. Color-coded labels.

ULTRABAC–7™
Clostridium Chauvoei—Septicum—Novyi—Sordellii—Perfringens Types C & D Bacterin—Toxoid

Composition: Ultrabac–7 consists of killed, whole cell cultures and toxins of *Clostridium chauvoei, Clostridium septicum, Clostridium novyi, Clostridium sordellii* and *Clostridium perfringens* Type C and Type D grown in special media to assure optimum growth and antigenicity. These cultures are anaerobically grown under constant agitation utilizing the Beecham Ultraferm process. The temperature and pH are electronically controlled and the fermentation process is rigidly monitored. The final bacterin product is highly antigenic, pure, safe and uniform from batch to batch. The adjuvanted bacterin is tested in accordance with the regulations of the United States Department of Agriculture.
Indications: For use in the prevention of blackleg *(Cl. chauvoei),* malignant edema *septicum),* black disease *(Cl. novyi), Clostridium sordellii* infections and *Clostridium perfringens* Types C and D enterotoxemia in healthy cattle, calves, sheep and lambs. Although *Cl. perfringens* Type B is not a significant problem in the USA, immunity may be provided against the beta and epsilon toxins elaborated by *Cl. perfringens* Type B. This immunity is derived from the combination of Type C (beta) and Type D (epsilon) fractions.
Dosage and Administration: Shake well before using. For subcutaneous use or intramuscular use. The recommended dose is 5 ml for cattle and calves and 2-½ ml for sheep and lambs with a revaccination 4 to 6 weeks later. Revaccinate annually to maintain a high level of immunity.
Precautions: Store at 35°F to 45°F (1.5°C to 7°C). Do not vaccinate within 21 days before slaughter. Use the entire contents when the container is first opened. Anaphylactoid reactions may occur following the use of products of this nature. Symptomatic treatment should be provided, including epinephrine.
How Supplied: 10, 50 and 200 dose plastic vials.

VIBROMUNE®
Vibrio Fetus Bacterin

Composition: Vibromune consists of chemically killed whole cultures of *Campylobacter fetus (Vibrio fetus).*
Recent research has demonstrated that heat labile surface antigens are the antigens responsible for eliciting a protective immune response in cattle. Vibromune utilizes a unique strain which contains five of the heat labile surface antigens —thus furnishing protection against the strains that have been implicated as causative agents of bovine vibrosis.
Additional studies determined that some of these heat labile surface antigens can be lost from an isolate upon animal passage and also through repetitive media passages. Beecham Laboratories has taken extra precautions to maintain seed stocks and has instituted special procedures to preclude this occurrence. These procedures have been proven effective in retaining the full antigenic spectrum of the strain.
Vibromune contains a high antigenic mass in each dose. Extensive studies suggest the need for high antigen levels to elicit high titer responses and to provide the sustained exposure required for producing the types of antibodies capable of migrating to the areas of infection. Beecham uses a standardized formulation to ensure a more concentrated antigenic mass on a consistent basis.
Campylobacter fetus cultures are grown in a special media under constant agitation utilizing Ultraferm process. The temperature and pH are electronically controlled and the fermentation process is rigidly monitored. Beecham Laboratories Soft-Kill process assures complete sterility without the use of formalin. The final bacterin product is highly antigenic, pure, safe and uniform from batch to batch.
Vibromune is adjuvanted with a highly refined aluminum hydroxide gel. This allows either subcutaneous or intramuscular administration with minimal site reactions and abscesses which may occur with the use of oil or emulsion type bacterins. The product is readily absorbed within a brief period, leaving no permanent nodules or tissue damage.
Indications: For use in the prevention of infertility, delayed conception, or abortion caused by vibriosis in healthy cattle.
Dosage and Administration: Shake well before using. Animals should be vaccinated subcutaneously or intramuscularly with a 2 ml dose 2 to 6 weeks prior to breeding. Revaccinate annually to maintain a high level of immunity.
Precautions: Store at 35°–45°F (1.5°–7°C). Do not freeze. Use the entire contents when the container is first opened. Do not vaccinate within 21 days before slaughter. This product contains a permissible level of thimerosal as a preservative. Anaphylactoid reactions may occur following the use of products of this nature. Symptomatic treatment should be provided. Antidote: Epinephrine.
How Supplied: 25 dose plastic vials. Species coded for easy product identification.

B

VIBROMUNE/5L®
Vibrio Fetus-Leptospira Canicola-Grippotyphosa-Hardjo-Icterohaemorrhagiae-Pomona Bacterin

Composition: Vibromune/5L consists of chemically killed whole cultures of *Campylobacter fetus (Vibrio fetus), Leptospira canicola, Leptospira grippotyphosa, Leptospira hardjo, Leptospira icterohaemorrhagiae,* and *Leptospira pomona.*
Recent research has demonstrated that heat labile surface antigens are the antigens responsible for elicting a protective immune response in cattle. Vibrome/5L utilizes a unique strain which contains five of the heat labile surface antigens, thus furnishing protection against the strains that have been implicated as causative agents of bovine vibrosis.
Additional studies determined that some of these heat labile surface antigens can be lost from an isolate upon animal passage and also through repetitive media passages. Beecham Laboratories has taken extra precautions to maintain seed stocks and has instituted special procedures to preclude this occurrence. These procedures have been proven effective in retaining the full antigenic spectrum of the strain.
Vibromune/5L contains a high antigenic mass in each dose. Extensive studies suggest the need for high antigen levels to elicit high titer responses and to provide the sustained exposure required for producing the types of antibodies capable of migrating to the areas of infection. Beecham uses a standardized formulation to ensure a more concentrated antigenic mass on a consistent basis.
Vibrio cultures are grown in a special media under constant agitation utilizing Beecham Laboratories Ultraferm process. The temperature and pH are electronically controlled and the fermentation process is rigidly monitored. Beecham Laboratories Soft Kill process assures complete sterility without the use of formalin. The final bacterin product is highly antigenic, pure, safe and uniform from batch to batch.
Vibromune/5L is adjuvanted with a highly refined aluminum hydroxide gel. This allows either subcutaneous or intramuscular administration with minimal site reactions and abscesses which may occur with the use of oil or emulsion type bacterins. The product is readily absorbed within a brief period, leaving no permanent nodules or tissue damage.
The leptospira fractions of Vibromune/5L are propagated in a medium which does not contain whole serum but utilizes Bovine Albumin Fraction under strict laboratory methods introduced by Beecham Laboratories to produce high antigenic yields and pure leptospiral cultures.

Continued on next page

Beecham—Cont.

Indications: For use in the prevention of vibriosis caused by *Campylobacter fetus* and leptospirosis caused by *Leptospira canicola, L. grippotyphosa, L. hardjo, L. icterohaemorrhagiae* and *L. pomona* in healthy cattle.
Dosage and Administration: Shake well before using. Animals should be vaccinated subcutaneously or intramuscularly with a 5 ml dose 2 to 6 weeks prior to breeding. Revaccinate annually to maintain a high level of immunity.
Precautions: Store at 35°-45°F (1.5°-7°C). Do not freeze. Use the entire contents when the container is first opened. Do not vaccinate within 21 days before slaughter. This product contains a permissible level of thimerosal as a preservative. Anaphylactoid reactions may occur following the use of products of this nature. Sympotomatic treatment should be provided. *Antidote:* Epinephrine.
How Supplied: 10 and 50 dose plastic vials. Species and color-coded for easy product identification.

Bio-Ceutic
2621 NORTH BELT HIGHWAY
ST. JOSEPH, MO 64502

BAR-1 BVD
Bovine Virus Diarrhea Vaccine
Killed Virus

Indications: Recommended for use in healthy susceptible cattle against disase caused by bovine virus diarrhea.
Administration: Inject 2 ml intramuscularly. Repeat in 21 days and once annually.
Precautions:
- Store out of direct sunlight at a temperature not over 45° F.
- Avoid freezing.
- Shake well.
- Use entire contents when first opened.
- Do not vaccinate within 21 days before slaughter.

Anaphylactoid reactions may occur.
ANTIDOTE: Administer epinephrine.
Packaging: Available in 10 and 50 dose vials.
Product Information: Bar-1 BVD is safe for use in pregnant cows, feeder calves, veal calves and bulls.
Bar-1 BVD, a killed virus vaccine, cannot produce disease and cannot shed BVD-causing organisms to other animals. Studies conducted with Bar-1 BVD show vaccinates experienced no significant reduction in white blood cells. Bar-1 BVD is not immunosuppressive.
Bar-1 BVD elicits an excellent blood antibody titer response with two doses but does not cause an abnormal temperature response. In company tests where calves were directly challenged with BVD virus, the 20 animals vaccinated with a production lot of Bar-1 BVD remained healthy in comparison to the 5 unvaccinated controls. In the study, 20 calves were vaccinated with Bar-1 BVD. Twenty-one days later, they received a second dose. Fourteen days after the booster dose, they were challenged with BVD virus (NY-1 BVD strain).
The average white blood cell level of the vaccinates remained constant while the average white blood cell counts of the unvaccinated controls showed significant decline after challenge. Temperature response monitored in the same study showed that vaccinated animals showed no spike in average body temperature while unvaccinated controls did exhibit fever.

BAR-3
Bovine Rhinotracheitis-Virus Diarrhea-Parainfluenza$_3$ Vaccine
Killed Virus

Indications: Recommended for the immunization of healthy, susceptible, immunocompetent cattle against disease caused by bovine rhinotracheitis, bovine virus diarrhea and parainfluenza$_3$.
Composition: Chemically inactivated bovine rhinotracheitis, virus diarrhea and parainfluenza$_3$ viruses. Contains neomycin and thimerosal as preservatives.
Dosage: 5 ml injected intramuscularly. Repeat in 21 days. Calves vaccinated under six months of age should be revaccinated at six months or weaning. A 5 ml booster dose is recommended annually or prior to time of stress or exposure.
Precautions: It is possible that healthy appearing cattle can be persistently infected or incubating virulent BVD virus at the time of vaccination and may experience disease associated with BVD. Cattle that are immunotolerant and are incapable of an immune response to BVD will not produce antibodies in response to vaccination and will exhibit disease signs of BVD upon exposure to virulent BVD virus.
Store out of direct sunlight at a temperature not over 45° F. Avoid freezing. Shake well. Use entire contents when first opened. Do not vaccinate within 21 days before slaughter. Anaphylactoid reactions may occur.
Antidote: Administer epinephrine.
Packaging: 10 dose and 50 dose vials.

BAR-3/SOMNUS
Bovine Rhinotracheitis-Virus Diarrhea-Parainfluenza$_3$ Vaccine
Killed Virus
Haemophilus somnus Bacterin

Indications: Recommended for the immunization of healthy, susceptible, immuno-competent cattle against disease caused by bovine rhinotracheitis, bovine virus diarrhea, parainfluenza$_3$ and *Haemophilus somnus.*
Composition: Chemically inactivated bovine rhinotracheitis, virus diarrhea and parainfluenza$_3$ viruses and *Haemophilus somnus* bacterin. Contains thimerosal and neomycin as preservatives.
Dosage: 5 ml injected intramuscularly. Repeat in 21 days. Calves vaccinated under six months of age should be revaccinated at six months or weaning. A 5 ml booster dose is recommended annually or prior to time of stress or exposure.
Precautions: It is possible that healthy appearing cattle can be persistently infected or incubating virulent BVD virus at the time of vaccination and may experience disease associated with BVD. Cattle that are immunotolerant and are incapable of an immune response to BVD will not produce antibodies in response to vaccination and will exhibit disease signs of BVD upon exposure to virulent BVD virus.
Store out of direct sunlight at a temperature not over 45° F. Avoid freezing. Shake well. Use entire contents when first opened. Do not vaccinate within 21 days before slaughter. Anaphylactoid reactions may cccur.
Antidote: Administer epinephrine.
Packaging: Available in 10 and 50 dose vials

BIO-MYCIN®
(oxytetracycline HCl injection in povidone)

Composition: Each ml contains 50 mg of oxytetracycline base as oxytetracycline hydrochloride; magnesium chloride hexahydrate 2.5% w/v; sodium formaldehyde sulfoxylate 0.5% w/v; povidone 10% w/v; dimethylpolysiloxane emulsion up to 0.035% w/v; monoethanolamine to adjust pH; water for injection qs. Povidone is used as a carrier for oxytetracycline as it aids in reducing post injection inflammation.
Indications: For the treatment of diseases due to oxytetracycline-susceptible organisms in beef cattle, nonlactating dairy cattle, and swine.
Beef Cattle and Nonlactating Dairy Cattle: For the treatment of pneumonia and shipping fever complex associated with *Pasteurella* sp., *Hemophilus* sp., *Klebsiella* sp., foot rot and diphtheria caused by *Spherophorus necrophorus,* bacterial enteritis (scours) caused by *Escherichia coli,* wooden tongue caused by *Actinobacillus lignieresi,* leptospirosis caused by *Leptospira pomona,* acute metritis, anaplasmosis caused by *Anaplasma marginale,* and wound infections caused by Staphylococcal and Streptococcal organisms. In some forms of foot rot surgical procedures may be indicated when recovery is not satisfactory.
Swine: Indicated in the treatment of bacterial enteritis (scours, colibacillosis) caused by *Escherichia coli,* pneumonia caused by *Pasteurella multocida,* and leptospirosis caused by *Leptospira pomona.*
Sows: For aid in control of infectious enteritis (baby pig scours, colibacillosis) in suckling pigs, caused by *Escherichia coli.*
Dosage and Administration: *Beef Cattle and Nonlactating Dairy Cattle:* The intramuscular or intravenous injection of 3 to 5 mg of oxytetracycline per lb of body weight per day (6 to 10 ml of Bio-Mycin per 100 lb of body weight) is the recommended dosage. In severe forms of foot rot, anaplasmosis, and other severe disease forms 5 mg per lb of body weight is indicated (10 ml of Bio-Mycin per 100 lb of body weight). In disease treatment

the daily dose of Bio-Mycin should be continued 24 to 48 hours following remission of disease symptoms, not to exceed a total of 4 days. When given intramuscularly the volume administered per injection site should be reduced according to age and size so that only 0.5 to 2 ml is injected in the case of smaller animals. No more than 10 ml should be injected intramuscularly per site in adult cattle.
Swine: In swine administer 3 to 5 mg oxytetracycline per lb body weight intramuscularly daily [6 to 10 ml of Bio-Mycin per 100 lb body weight]. No more than 5 ml of Bio-Mycin should be injected intramuscularly per site in swine.
Sows: Administer 3 mg oxytetracycline per lb of body weight (6 ml of Bio-Mycin per 100 lb of body weight) intramuscularly to the sow approximately 8 hours before farrowing or immediately after completion of farrowing. Not more than 5 ml of Bio-Mycin should be injected per site in sows.
Precautions: As with any intramuscular injection, some local tissue irritation may result, manifested by temporary swelling and discoloration at site of injection. Pain can be minimized by injecting the solution at body temperature and by avoiding faulty injection technique.
Administer slowly by intravenous injection.
Reactions of an allergic or anaphylactic nature, sometimes fatal, have been known to occur in hypersensitive animals following the injection of oxytetracycline solution, but such reactions are not common. At the first sign of any adverse reaction or anaphylactic shock the product should be discontinued. Epinephrine Solution, corticosteroids, and antihistimines at the recommended dosage levels should be administered.
Because bacteriostatic drugs interfere with the bactericidal action of penicillin, do not give penicillin in conjunction with oxytetracycline hydrochloride.
As with other antibiotics, use of this drug may result in overgrowth of nonsusceptible organisms. If any unusual symptoms occur, discontinue use immediàtely.
Caution: Do not inject more than 10 ml per site intramuscularly in cattle or 5 ml per site intramuscularly in swine. If no improvement occurs within 48 hours the diagnosis should be redetermined. Do not use for more than 4 days.
When administered intramuscularly to animals within 20 days of slaughter, muscle discoloration may necessitate trimming of the injection site(s) and surrounding tissues during the dressing procedure.
Exceeding the highest recommended dosage level or duration of treatment (not more than 4 days) may result in antibiotic residues beyond the withdrawal time.
Warning: Not for use in lactating dairy cattle. Discontinue use 18 days in cattle and 26 days in swine before slaughter to permit elimination of the drug from edible tissues. Do not use for more than 4 days.
How Supplied: Bio-Mycin is available in 100-ml and 500-ml bottles containing 50 mg oxytetracycline base as oxytetracycline hydrochloride per ml.
Caution: Store product below 86° F (30° C) in a dark place. Keep from freezing.
Caution: Federal law restricts this drug to use by or on the order of a licensed veterinarian.
Keep out of reach of children.
For Veterinary Use Only

BIO–MYCIN® C
(oxytetracycline HCl injection in povidone)

Composition: Each ml contains: 100 mg of oxytetracycline base as oxytetracycline hydrochloride; magnesium chloride hexahydrate 5% w/v; sodium formaldehyde sulfoxylate 0.5% w/v; povidone 18% w/v; monoethanolamine to adjust pH; water for injection qs.
Povidone is used as a carrier for oxytetracycline as it aids in reducing post injection inflammation.
Indications: Bio-Mycin C may be used for the treatment of diseases due to oxytetracycline-susceptible organisms in beef cattle and non-lactating dairy cattle and swine.
Beef cattle and Nonlactating Dairy Cattle: Bio-Mycin C is indicated in the treatment of pneumonia and shipping fever complex associated with *Pasteurella* sp., *Hemophilus* sp., *Klebsiella* sp., footrot and diphtheria caused by *Spherophorus necrophorus,* bacterial enteritis (scours) caused by *Escherichia coli,* wooden tongue caused by *Actinobacillus lignieresi,* acute metritis, anaplasmosis caused by *Anaplasma marginale,* and wound infections caused by Staphylococcal and Streptococcal organisms. In some forms of footrot surgical procedures may be indicated when recovery is not satisfactory.
Swine: Bio-Mycin C is indicated in the treatment of bacterial enteritis (scours, colibacillosis) caused by *Escherichia coli,* pneumonia caused by *Pasteurella multocida,* and leptospirosis caused by *Leptospira pomona.*
In sows Bio-Mycin C is indicated for aid in control of infectious enteritis (baby pig scours, colibacillosis) in suckling pigs caused by *Escherichia coli.*
Dosage and Administration: *Beef Cattle and Nonlactating Dairy Cattle:* The injection of 3 to 5 mg of oxytetracycline intramuscularly per lb of body weight per day (3 to 5 ml of Bio-Mycin C per 100 lb of body weight) is the recommended dosage. In severe forms of footrot, anaplasmosis, and other severe disease forms 5 mg per lb of body weight is indicated (5 ml of Bio-Mycin C per 100 lb of body weight).
In disease treatment the daily dose of Bio-Mycin C should be continued 24 to 48 hours following remission of disease symptoms, not to exceed a total of 4 days.
The volume administered per injection site should be reduced according to age and size so that only 0.5 to 2 ml is injected in the case of smaller animals. No more than 10 ml should be injected per site in adult cattle.
Swine: In swine administer 3 to 5 mg oxytetracycline per lb of body weight intramuscularly daily [3 to 5 ml of Bio-Mycin C per 100 lb body weight]. No more than 5 ml of Bio-Mycin C should be injected intramuscularly per site in swine.
For sows administer 3 mg oxytetracycline per lb of body weight [3 ml of Bio-Mycin C per 100 lb of body weight] intramuscularly to the sow approximately 8 hours before farrowing or immediately after completion of farrowing. No more than 5 ml of Bio-Mycin C should be injected intramuscularly per site in sows.
Warning: Not for use in lactating dairy cattle. Discontinue use 18 days in cattle and 26 days in swine before slaughter to permit elimination of the drug from edible tissues. Do not use for more than 4 days. Do not inject more than 10 ml per site intramuscularly in mature cattle.
Caution: If no improvement occurs within 48 hours the diagnosis should be redetermined.
Do not use for more than 4 days.
When administered to cattle within 20 days of slaughter muscle discoloration may necessitate trimming of the injection site(s) and surrounding tissues during the dressing procedure.
Exceeding the highest recommended dosage level or duration of treatment (not more than 4 days) may result in antibiotic residues beyond the withdrawal time.
For veterinary use only.
Caution: Federal law restricts this drug to use by or on the order of a licensed veterinarian.
Precautions: As with any intramuscularly injection, some local tissue irritation may result, manifested by temporary swelling and discoloration at the site of injection. Pain can be minimized by injecting the solution at body temperature and by avoiding faulty injection technique.
Reactions of an allergic or anaphylactic nature, sometimes fatal, have been known to occur in hypersensitive animals following the injection of oxytetracycline solution, but such reactions are not common. At the first sign of any adverse reaction or anaphylactic shock the product should be discontinued. Epinephrine solution, corticosteroids, and antihistimines at the recommended dosage levels should be administered.
Because bacteriostatic drugs interfere with the bactericidal action of penicillin, do not give penicillin in conjunction with oxytetracycline hydrochloride.
As with other antibiotics, use of this drug may result in overgrowth of nonsusceptible organisms. If any unusual symptoms occur, discontinue use immediately.
How Supplied: 500 ml. bottle.
Caution: Store product below 86° F (30° C) in a dark place. Keep from freezing.
Keep out of the reach of children.

BIO–TAL®
(Thiamylal Sodium for Injection, USP)

Description: Bio-Tal (Thiamylal Sodium for Injection, USP) is the thiobarbiturate analogue of secobarbital [so-

Continued on next page

Bio-Ceutic—Cont.

dium 5-allyl-5-(1-methyl-butyl)-2-thiobarbiturate] mixed with anhydrous Sodium Carbonate. It is a pale yellow, hygroscopic powder, with a disagreeable odor. It is available as the dry powder in air-tight vials containing 1 gram or 5 grams of buffered Thiamylal Sodium for Injection, USP.

Indications: For anesthesia of dogs, cats, swine, horses, and cattle to accomplish interferences and examinations of short duration (10 to 15 minutes), for induction of anesthesia, and for anesthesia in major surgery by administration of additional amounts as necessary.

Contraindications: Any condition interfering with the intake and distribution of oxygen.

Thiamylal sodium should not be used to induce anesthesia in dogs who are also receiving Diathal™. Cardiac arrhythmias, potentially fatal, have been observed in dogs where the products were used concurrently.

CAUTION: Federal (U.S.A.) law restricts this drug to use by or on the order of a licensed veterinarian.

Precautions:

1. Discard solution that is cloudy or precipitated. Solution retained for longer than 48 hours, even if stored at refrigerated temperature, may become cloudy, or precipitate. Discard any solution that exhibits these changes.
2. Do not force air from syringe into the solution.
3. Do not administer to animals with hepatic disease or respiratory disturbances or in traumatic shock.
4. Extravascular injection may cause pain, ulceration, and necrosis.
5. Intra-arterial injection is dangerous and may produce gangrene of an extremity.
6. Do not administer intrapleurally or intraperitoneally.
7. Additional care should be employed when anesthetizing anemic or hypovolemic animals or animals with cardiac or respiratory problems.
8. Liver pathology may delay detoxification.
9. Elevated urea nitrogen or electrolyte imbalances may prolong anesthesia.
10. Prolonged recovery may occur in hypothermia or in malnourished animals and following continuous use for prolonged surgical procedures.
11. The following adverse reactions may occur: Circulatory depression, thrombophlebitis, pain at injection site, respiratory depression including apnea, laryngospasm, bronchospasm, salivation, emergence delirium, injury to nerves adjacent to injection site, skin rashes, urticaria, nausea, and emesis.
12. In case of overdosing, if cyanosis occurs or if respiration becomes excessively depressed, stop injection of Bio-Tal (Thiamylal Sodium for Injection, USP). Institute artificial respiration and give oxygen and analeptics as needed.
13. Maintain free air passageways at all times.

Warning: Emergence excitement in dogs and emergence delirium in horses may occur following barbiturate anesthesia. Intracarotid injections may result in direct cerebrovascular endothelial injury with subsequent edema and ischemic necrosis in the brain, especially in the horse.

Administration and Dosage:

PREPARATION OF SOLUTION

Aseptically add the necessary amount of Sterile Water for Injection USP, or Sodium Chloride Injection USP (DO NOT USE ANY OTHER SOLVENTS) to prepare the solution of desired concentration. (See table.)

There should not be any other substances in the solvent, as they tend to cause precipitation.

QUANTITIES OF SOLVENT REQUIRED TO PREPARE BIO-TAL (THIAMYLAL SODIUM FOR INJECTION, USP) SOLUTIONS OF PERCENTAGE SHOWN.

[See table below].

Use aseptic techniques in handling the solution, as it does not contain preservatives.

Bio-Tal (Thiamylal Sodium for Injection, USP) solution may be retained for up to 48 hours after preparation if stored at refrigerator temperature.

USE ONLY CLEAR SOLUTIONS.

DOSAGE

DOGS AND CATS

The dosage of Bio-Tal (Thiamylal Sodium for Injection, USP) to use is determined by the effect produced and varies with each animal. The average single dose is about 8 mg. of Bio-Tal (Thiamylal Sodium for Injection, USP) per lb. of body weight. **When pre-anesthetic agents such as morphine are used the dose of Bio-Tal (Thiamylal Sodium for Injection, USP) is generally one-half (4 mg. per lb. of body weight).** Dosages tend to be lower for larger and older animals, for those in poor condition, and for brachiocephalic breeds of dogs.

Younger and smaller animals may require more anesthetic.

The animal should be weighed and the approximated dose of 8 mg. per lb. of body weight (1 ml. of a 4% solution per 5 lb. of body weight) plus an excess amount of solution should be drawn into the syringe. For very small animals (under 5 lb.) it is recommended that the more dilute 2% solution be used (approximated dose, 1 ml. per 2½ lb. of body weight). To maintain the stage of surgical anesthesia for longer than 15 to 20 minutes additional amounts of Bio-Tal (Thiamylal Sodium for Injection, USP) may be administered by taping the needle and syringe to the leg and retaining access to the vein. The additional dosage needed is usually about one-fourth the original dose. See ACTION AND USES in package insert for additional details.

SWINE

In swine Bio-Tal (Thiamylal Sodium for Injection, USP) may be injected either into the anterior vena cava (small pigs) or into the external-ear vein (larger hogs). Recommended dosage is 40 mg. per 5 lb. of body weight (1 ml. of a 4% solution per 5 lb. of body weight). This usually provides satisfactory anesthesia for all types of surgery, but dosage should be adjusted to effect.

HORSES

In horses Bio-Tal (Thiamylal Sodium for Injection, USP) injections are usually made into the jugular vein. Recommended dosage for light anesthesia is 1 gram for animals from 500 to 1100 lb. (200 ml. of an 0.5% solution).

Recommended dosage for deeper anesthesia is 40 mg. per 12 lb. of body weight (1 ml. of a 4% solution) or 1 gram per 300 lb. of body weight (25 ml. of a 4% solution). Surgical anesthesia is present for 10 to 25 minutes, with recovery in 30 to 90 minutes. Supplemental volatile liquid or gas may be used to prolong anesthesia, if desired.

CATTLE

In cattle Bio-Tal (Thiamylal Sodium for Injection, USP) injections are usually made into the jugular vein. Recommended dosage for anesthesia of shorter duration is 20 mg. per 5 lb. of body weight (1 ml. of a 2% solution). Recommended dosage for anesthesia of a longer duration is 40 mg. per 7 lb. of body weight (1 ml. of a 4% solution). Surgical anesthesia is present for about 15 minutes, with recovery in 30 to 120 minutes. Longer periods of anesthesia can be maintained by additional doses.

ADMINISTRATION

Administer intravenously. The first one-third to one-half of the calculated dose should be administered rather rapidly to carry the patient through the excitement state. Should apnea or severe respiratory depression occur, suspend injection of Bio-Tal (Thiamylal Sodium for Injection, USP) until rhythmic respiration resumes. Then continue to slowly inject Bio-Tal (Thiamylal Sodium for Injection, USP) until the desired stage of surgical anesthesia is reached, as determined by lack of appropriate reflexes. For best results Bio-Tal (Thiamylal Sodium for Injection, USP) should be administered to fasted animals, since emesis may occasionally occur.

See ACTION AND USES for additional details.

Percent Solution	Calculated mg/cc	BIO-TAL (Thiamylal Sodium for Injection, USP) 1 gram	5 grams
0.5%	5	200 ml.	1000 ml.
2.0%	20	50 ml.	250 ml.
2.5%	25	40 ml.	200 ml.
4.0%	40	25 ml.	125 ml.

Hazardous—Not for human use.
Caution: Keep out of the reach of children.
Supplied: 1-gram and 5-gram vials.
For intravenous injection only.
For veterinary use only.

BREED–BACK–10
**Bovine Rhinotracheitis-
Virus Diarrhea-
Parainfluenza$_3$ Vaccine
Haemophilus somnus-Campylobacter fetus-
Leptospira canicola-
grippotyphosa-hardjo-
icterohaemorrhagiae-pomona
Bacterin**

Indications: Recommended for the immunization of healthy susceptible cattle 4 months of age or older against bovine rhinotracheitis, virus diarrhea, parainfluenza$_3$, *Haemophilus somnus, Campylobacter fetus, Leptospira canicola, L. grippotyphosa, L. hardjo, L. icterohaemorrhagiae,* and *L. pomona.*
Administration: Administer a 5 ml dose intramuscularly. Repeat bacterin dose in 14 to 21 days and once annually. See label for complete directions.
Precautions

- Store out of direct sunlight at a temperature not over 45° F.
- Use entire contents when first opened.
- Burn container and all unused contents.
- Do not use on pregnant cows or calves nursing pregnant cows.
- Do not vaccinate within 21 days before slaughter.
- Avoid freezing.
- Anaphylactoid reactions may occur.

ANTIDOTE: Administer epinephrine.
**Health Programming
Replacement Heifers, Bulls, Beef & Dairy Cows**
Administer a 5 ml dose intramuscularly in healthy cattle 4 months of age or older. Repeat the bacterin dosage in 14 to 21 days. Booster annually with a single dose of Breed-Back-10.
Product Information: BREED-BACK-10 is an exclusive combination product which permits broad protection against many, major bovine respiratory and reproductive disease agents. It is recommended for use in healthy cattle as (1.) an aid in the prevention of IBR, BVD, and PI$_3$ (2.) for the prevention of disease caused by *Haemophilus somnus* (3.) in the prevention of infertility, delayed conception or abortion caused by *Campylobacter fetus* var. *venerealis;* (4.) and for the prevention of leptospirosis due to *Leptospira grippotyphosa, L. hardjo, L. pomona, L. canicola,* and *L. icterohaemorrhagiae.*
Because BREED-BACK-10 combines protection for several disease agents, it also reduces the number of injections and syringes needed thus decreasing the labor and handling required. In addition, it reduces the number of carrier cows within a herd which can transmit the reproductive and respiratory diseases to healthy animals.
Bio-Ceutic's IBR vaccine offers the same rapid protection . . . 48 hours . . . as intranasal vaccines but is more easily and more accurately administered. Bio-Ceutic's IBR is a low passage virus. This means it has high antigenicity for long-term protection.
Bio-Ceutic's BVD is effective, causes no shedding, and provides long-term immunity.
Packaging: Available in 5 and 20 dose vials.

BUZZ OFF
**(pyrethrin, piperonyl butoxide, methoxychlor, butoxypolypropylene glycol)
Equine Spray and Rub-On**

Composition: An insecticide formulation containing two effective insecticides, pyrethrin (0.05%) and methoxychlor (0.5%) plus the insect repellent butoxypolypropylene glycol (10.0%). Also contains piperonyl butoxide (0.5%) as a synergist and Petroleum hydrocarbons 88.95%.
Indications: Use on horse and pony show stock to kill and repel horn flies, stable flies, house flies, face flies, deer flies, horse flies, mosquitoes and gnats. May also be used to spray adjacent stable areas for more effective fly control.
Dosage and Administration: Buzz Off has been specifically formulated for use on horse and pony stock. Do not use on meat animals. The product may be sprayed or wiped onto the animal's coat and will protect the animal from biting insects. The product will also impart a bright sheen to the animal's coat. Apply regularly during fly season.
As a spray: Select a hand sprayer which will apply the product in a fine mist or fog. Use one to two oz per animal per day. Also treat adjacent stable areas for more effective insect control. Do not wet the animal's skin. After application, brush the coat to give overall coverage. Make sure that legs and ankles are treated. For face area. treat as a wipe-on application.
As a wipe-on product: Rub the animal down and remove dirt. Pour a small amount (1 oz) into a soft cloth and wipe on against the hair grain.
Avoid treating animals during cold, stormy weather.
Avoid treating overheated or sick animals.
Caution: Harmful if swallowed. Keep out of the reach of children. Do not contaminate feed or feeding utensils. Cover or remove feed before spraying. Do not use on meat or dairy animals.
This product is toxic to fish. Keep out of lakes, streams, or ponds. Do not apply where runoff is likely to occur. Do not contaminate water by cleaning of equipment, or disposal of wastes. Apply this product only as specified on this label.
DO NOT USE OR STORE NEAR HEAT OR OPEN FLAMES.
See label for additional Cautions.
How Supplied: 1 quart and 1 gallon bottles.

CATRON II
Screwworm and Ear Tick Spray

Description: Gamma Isomer of BHC from Lindane 3.0%.
Product Information: CATRON II contains the gamma isomer of benzene hexachloride (BHC) from lindane which is a white crystalline powder.
CATRON II is essentially a contact poison showing residual activity. It may be used directly on beef cattle, horses, swine, sheep, and goats to kill screwworms and treat ear ticks. Basically, it works by interfering with the metabolism of the insect thereby causing its death.
CATRON II contains a blue color to aid the user by marking treated areas and is easy to use. New superficial wounds should be sprayed promptly to aid in preventing screwworm infestations. For minor wounds such as slight wire cuts, docking shear cuts, tick bites, abrasions, etc., spray thoroughly as directed.
Indications: For the treatment and/or prevention of screwworms and ear ticks.
Administration: For external use only. See label for complete use directions.
General Directions: Remove safety cap. Point nozzle at wound; then, hold can about 4 to 6 inches from area to be treated. Spray the area until it is completely wet (three to ten seconds are usually enough). This product is not recommended for use in deep wounds. Use as directed on superficial (surface) wounds or as an ear tick treatment. Some strains of screwworms may develop resistance to lindane and not respond to treatment.
Cautions:
Avoid inhalation.
May be absorbed through skin. Do not apply to household pets or humans. If sprayed on skin or in eyes, wash thoroughly. Harmful if swallowed.
Do not use on lactating dairy animals or in dairy barns or milk rooms.
Do not use on newborn (very young) animals or calves under 3 months old.
Areas near eyes should be treated with extreme caution.
Avoid contamination of feed or foodstuffs. Use minimum amount of material to treat wounds.
Do not allow children to handle or apply this product.
Flammable. Contents under pressure. Keep away from fire, sparks, or flame. Do not puncture or incinerate container.
REFER TO LABEL FOR COMPLETE USE DIRECTIONS AND CAUTIONS.
Packaging: CATRON II is available in 10 oz aerosol cans.

D–VAC–7
**Canine Distemper-Hepatitis-
Parainfluenza-Parvovirus Vaccine
Modified Live Virus
Leptospira canicola-
icterohaemorrhagiae Bacterin
For Use In Dogs Only**

Description: D-VAC-7 is a combination of highly antigenic, attenuated strains of Canine Distemper, Canine Parainfluenza virus propagated in monkey cell line tissue cultures, Canine Hepatitis virus propagated in porcine cell line tissue culture and Parvovirus propagated

Continued on next page

Bio-Ceutic—Cont.

in feline cell line tissue culture. The accompanying liquid diluent is Parvovirus Vaccine-*Leptospira canicola-icterohaemorrhagiae* Bacterin.
The CD Virus fraction has been manipulated in the laboratory through various tissue culture cell systems which has resulted in a canine-attenuated, but ferret-virulent virus. It has been proven to be avirulent, non-shedding, safe and highly immunogenic when injected into susceptible dogs.
Similarly, the ICH and Parainfluenza fractions have been propagated in several tissue culture cell systems which has resulted in the development of an avirulent, safe and immunogenic vaccine.
The Infectious Canine Hepatitis (CAV-1) fraction stimulates production of antibodies that cross-protect against respiratory disease caused by CAV-2. The three attenuated virus vaccines are blended in proper proportions with a non-protein stabilizer and freeze-dried.
The *Leptospira canicola-icterohaemorrhagiae* fraction contains an inactivated highly antigenic mixture of *Leptospira canicola* and *Leptospira icterohaemorrhagiae* harvested when cellular growth is at a maximum level. The cultures are inactivated in such a manner that the high degree of antigenicity is not impaired.
Directions: The dry Distemper-Hepatitis-Parainfluenza Vaccine is rehydrated with 1 ml of liquid Parvovirus Vaccine-*Leptospira canicola-icterohaemorrhagiae bacterin.* Shake well and use entire contents when first opened.
Dosage: 1 ml injected intramuscularly or subcutaneously. Repeat dosage in 3 to 4 weeks. Annual revaccination with a single dose is recommended. Puppies vaccinated before 9 weeks of age should be revaccinated at 3 to 4 week intervals until 14 to 16 weeks of age. Regardless of age all dogs should receive 2 doses of vaccine in order to insure adequate levels of immunity against canine parainfluenza and parvovirus.
Precautions: Store out of direct sunlight at a temperature not over 45°F. Avoid freezing. Do not vaccinate pregnant animals. Burn containers and all unused contents. Under no circumstances is this product recommended for use in ferrets or mink. An occasional transitory corneal opacity may occur following administration of the vaccine. This will disappear without untoward effect on the animal. Anaphylactoid reactions may occur.
Antidote: Administer epinephrine.
Available in: 10 × 1 dose and 10 × 1 dose vials.

DYBELON
Clostridium perfringens Antitoxin
Types C and D
Equine Origin

Composition: Prepared from the blood of horses hyperimmunized with toxins of *Clostridium perfringens* Types C and D.
Indications: Recommended for the prevention and treatment of enterotoxemia caused by the above named organisms in calves, cattle, lambs, sheep and baby pigs.
Dosage: (Prophylactic) Calves—10 ml; cattle—30; suckling lambs—3 ml; all other sheep—10 ml injected subcutaneously or intravenously. Baby pigs—2 ml administered orally or injected subcutaneously. (Therapeutic) Increase dosage 100%.
Caution:
Store out of direct sunlight at a temperature not over 45° F.
Avoid freezing
Shake well before using
Use entire contents when first opened
Do not administer within 21 days before slaughter
How Supplied: 250 ml vial.

EAR FORCE™ TAGS
For use on dry or lactating dairy and beef cattle and calves to control horn flies, face flies, gulf coast ticks, spinose ear ticks; and as an aid to control lice, stable flies and houseflies.

Active Ingredients:
Permethrin (3-phenoxyphenyl) methyl (±)-cis, trans-3-(2,2-dichloroethenyl)-2, 2-dimethylcyclopropane-carboxylate* 10.00%
Inert Ingredients 90.00%
TOTAL 100.00%
*Cis/trans ratio: Min 35% (±) cis, and max. 65% (±) trans isomers.
Directions For Use
General Use Classification
It is a violation of Federal Law to use this product in a manner inconsistent with its labeling.
CAUTION: KEEP OUT OF REACH OF CHILDREN
See label for additional cautions.
Attach one tag per animal in the spring to control horn flies for a full summer season. Tags are easy to apply or replace, if necessary. Attach two tags per animal to control face flies, gulf coast ticks, spinose ear ticks and as an aid in the control of lice, stable flies, and houseflies.
EAR FORCE TAGS are easy to attach using a variety of methods. They may be punched through an existing ear tag using the ALLFLEX tagging system. However, tags punched through adult sized identification tags on young calves may result in tearing the ear and loss of the tags. Tags may also be positioned across entryways where animals are forced to use them as they gain access to barns, feeders, waterers or milking areas.
Calves and cows may mutilate tags by sucking and chewing. While the active ingredient in EAR FORCE TAGS is relatively non-toxic when ingested, severe mutilation may result in reduced effectiveness or tag loss. The effect of EAR FORCE TAGS in controlling hornflies may be reduced in those areas where resistance to synthetic pyrethroids has developed.

PRECAUTIONARY STATEMENTS HAZARDS TO HUMANS AND DOMESTIC ANIMALS
Caution: Wash thoroughly with soap and water after handling and before eating or smoking.
The effectiveness of Ear Force Tags may be reduced in those areas where resistance to synthetic pyrethroids has developed.
STATEMENT OF PRACTICAL TREATMENT: In case of eye contact, immediately flush eyes with plenty of water. Get medical attention if discomfort persists.
ENVIRONMENTAL HAZARDS: This pesticide is toxic to fish. Do not apply directly to water.
PHYSICAL OR CHEMICAL HAZARDS: Do not use or store near heat or open flame.

Storage and Disposal: Open as needed. Keep container sealed when not in use. Do not contaminate water, food or feed by storage or disposal. Remove tags before slaughter. Wrap used tags and dispose of in trash container. Triple rinse (or equivalent). Then offer for recycling or reconditioning, or puncture and dispose of in a sanitary landfill, or incineration, or, if allowed by state and local authorities, by burning. If burned, stay out of smoke.
Wastes resulting from the use of this product may be disposed of on site or at an approved waste disposal facility.

Available in: packages of 24's and 48's.

FERMICON-4
Clostridium chauvoei-septicum-novyi sordellii Bacterin-Toxoid
Chemically Inactivated

Composition: Prepared from cultures of *Clostridium chauvoei, Clostridium septicum, Clostridium novyi,* and *Clostridium sordellii.*
Indications: This product is recommended for the immunization of healthy susceptible cattle and sheep against disease caused by *Clostridium chauvoei, Clostridium septicum, Clostridium novyi,* and *Clostridium sordellii.*
Dosage and Administration: Inject subcutaneously or intramuscularly cattle 5 ml. sheep 2.5 ml. Repeat in 21 to 28 days and once annually.
Precautions: Store out of direct sunlight at a temperature not over 45° F. Avoid freezing. Shake well before using. Use entire contents when first opened. Do not vaccinate within 21 days before slaughter.
Anaphylactoid reactions may occur.
Antidote: Administer epinephrine.
How Supplied: 50 ml and 250 ml vials.

FERMICON-7
Clostridium
chauvoei-septicum-novyi
sordellii-perfringens
Types C and D
Bacterin-Toxoid
Alum Precipitated

Composition: Prepared from cultures of the above named organisms.
Indications: This product is recommended for the immunization of healthy susceptible cattle and sheep against disease caused by *Clostridium chauvoei, Clostridium septicum, Clostridium novyi, Clostridium sordellii,* and *Clostridium perfringens* Types C and D.
Although *Clostridium perfringens* Type B is not a significant problem in the U.S.A., immunity may be provided against the beta and epsilon toxins elaborated by Clostridium perfringens Type B. This immunity is derived from the combination of Type C (beta) and Type D (epsilon) fractions.
Dosage and Administration: Inject subcutaneously or intramuscularly, cattle 5 ml, sheep 2.5 ml. Repeat in 21 to 28 days and once annually.
Caution: Store out of direct sunlight at a temperature not over 45° F. Avoid freezing. Shake well before using. Use entire contents when first opened. Do not vaccinate within 21 days before slaughter.
Anaphylactoid reactions may occur.
Antidote: Administer epinephrine.
How Supplied: Fermicon-7 (CSNSCD) is available in 50 ml, 250 ml, and 1000 ml vials (5 ml cattle dose, 2.5 ml sheep dose)

FERMICON-7/SOMNUGEN
Clostridium
chauvoei-septicum-novyi-sordellii
perfringens Types C and D
Haemophilus
somnus Bacterin-Toxoid
Alum Precipitated

Composition: Prepared from cultures of the above-named organisms.
Indications: Recommended for the immunization of cattle against disease caused by *Clostridium chauvoei, Cl. septicum, Cl. novyi, Cl. sordellii, Cl. perfringens* Type C and D, and *Haemophilus somnus.*
Dosage and Administration: 5 ml injected intramuscularly. Repeat in 21 to 28 days and once annually.
Precautions:
Store out of direct sunlight at a temperature not over 45° F.
Do not freeze.
Shake well before using.
Use entire contents when first opened.
Do not vaccinate within 21 days before slaughter.
Anaphylactoid reactions may occur.
Antidote: Administer epinephrine.
How Supplied: 10, 50 and 200 dose vials.

HEIFER-oid™
Heifer Implants
Testosterone Propionate USP 200 mg
Estradiol Benzoate USP 20 mg

Description: Each Magnum Multi-Dose Cartridge Belt holds 20 individual dose units of HEIFER-oid implants. Each dose unit (8 implant pellets) contains a total of 200 mg Testosterone Propionate USP plus 20 mg of Estradiol Benzoate USP.
Indications: For use in heifers weighing 400 lbs or more for growth promotion and improved feed efficiency.
Administration: The Magnum Multi-Dose Cartridge Belt is designed so that after each dose is administered, the next dose can be automatically positioned for implant.
Insert plastic cartridge belt as directed into the Magnum Multi-Dose Implanter (either plunger or pistol grip type). Pellets are deposited with the Magnum implanters beneath the skin on the back side of the middle one-third of the ear.
Product Information: HEIFER-oid is a growth-promoting implant for heifers containing a combination of two naturally-occurring hormones: Testosterone Propionate USP (200 mg) and Estradiol Benzoate USP (20 mg). By supplementing the animal's hormonal output, it helps to increase feed conversion efficiency as well as promote increased average daily weight gains. HEIFER-oid does not require withholding before slaughter.
Warning: IMPLANT AND USE ONLY AS DIRECTED
NOT FOR USE IN DAIRY OR BEEF REPLACEMENT HEIFERS. Implant pellets in ear only. Any other site is in violation of Federal Law. Do NOT attempt to salvage implant site for animal feed or human use. KEEP THIS AND ALL OTHER DRUGS OUT OF REACH OF CHILDREN.
Caution: Bulling, vaginal and rectal prolapse, udder development, ventral edema, and elevated tailheads have been reported occasionally in heifers implanted with heifer implants containing Testosterone Propionate USP plus Estradiol Benzoate USP.
Packaging: 100 dose carton (5 × 20-dose cartridge belt)

IBR-PI$_3$/SOMNUGEN-2P
Bovine Rhinotracheitis-
Parainfluenza$_3$ Vaccine
Modified Live Virus
Haemophilus somnus-
Pasteurella haemolytica-
multocida Bacterin
Aluminum Hydroxide Adsorbed

Indications: Recommended for the immunization of healthy susceptible cattle against disease caused by bovine rhinotracheitis and parainfluenza$_3$ viruses and *Haemophilus somnus, Pasteurella haemolytica* and *Pasteurella multocida.*
Directions: Rehydrate the vaccine with the accompanying bottle of bacterin.
Dosage: 2 ml injected intramuscularly. Repeat bacterin dose in 21 days and once annually. Calves vaccinated before 6 months of age should be revaccinated at 6 months of age or at weaning.
Precautions: Store out of direct sunlight at a temperature not over 45° F. Avoid freezing. Shake well. Use entire contents when first opened. Do not use in pregnant cows or in calves nursing pregnant cows. Do not vaccinate within 21 days before slaughter. Burn containers and all unused contents. Anaphylactoid reactions may occur.
Antidote: Administer epinephrine.
Contains neomycin as a preservative.
Available in: 10 dose and 50 dose vials.

LYSIGIN®
Staphylococcus aureus Bacterin

Composition: Lysigin (*Staph. aureus* Bacterin) is a product produced from lysed cells of various phage types of *Staph. aureus* isolated from cases of mastitis in the United States and Canada to be used as a biological aid in the preventive mastitis program against *Staph. aureus* mastitis.
Indications: Lysigin is the product of choice for the prevention and reduction of disease caused by *Staph. aureus* such as mastitis.
Dosage and Administration: Initially administer 5 ml intramuscularly. Repeat the 5 ml dose in 14 days. Follow with a 5 ml booster each five to six months. For best results heifers should be vaccinated at 6 months of age and thereafter.
How Supplied: 50 ml (10 dose), 250 ml (50 dose) vial.

NARAMUNE-2™
Canine Parainfluenza-Bordetella
bronchiseptica Vaccine
Modified Live Virus
Avirulent Live Culture

Description and General Information: Naramune 2, Canine Parainfluenza Vaccine, Modified Live Virus, Bordetella bronchiseptica Vaccine, Avirulent Live Culture is designed to be administered intranasally for convenient, rapid prevention of Canine Upper Respiratory Disease (Kennel Cough). Both of these organisms are widespread, common etiologic agents of this syndrome which appears as a mild, self-limiting disease involving the trachea and bronchi of dogs of any age. It spreads rapidly among dogs that are closely confined as in hospitals, kennels and pet stores. The disease is highly contagious and is transmitted via the airborne route. The incubation period is 5 to 10 days. The outstanding symptom is a harsh dry cough which is aggravated by activity or excitement. The coughing occurs in paroxysms, followed by retching or gagging in attempts to clear small amounts of mucus from the throat. The body temperature is normal in the early stages but may be moderately elevated as secondary bacterial invasion takes place. Both of these

Continued on next page

Bio-Ceutic—Cont.

organisms have been demonstrated to be avirulent so that they can be safely administered intranasally without producing signs of disease. By instilling these organisms into the nasal passages, it becomes possible for these agents to infect target cells of the nasal-pharyngeal region, mimicking the pathogenesis of natural field infection, without producing clinical illness.

Because of this infection, local cellular interference and the production of local secretory antibodies (IgA) occurs to provide resistance to subsequent exposure to virulent organisms. Neomycin is added as a preservative.

Indications: For immunization of healthy susceptible dogs and puppies against Canine Upper Respiratory Disease (Kennel Cough) caused by Canine parainfluenza and *Bordetella bronchiseptica.*

Rehydration: Rehydrate with companion bottle of diluent. Shake well and use immediately.

Dosage and Administration: 1 ml administered intranasally. The vaccine is administered in the anterior nares as the animal inhales. Annual revaccination is recommended.

Caution: Store out of direct sunlight at a temperature not over 45° F. Shake well before using. Use entire contents when first opened. Do not vaccinate pregnant animals. Burn vials and all unused contents.

Anaphylactoid reactions may occur. **Antidote:** Administer Epinephrine.

How Supplied: Available in: 10 × 1 dose and 100 × 1 dose vials.

PERMECTRIN™ Pet, Yard, & Kennel Spray

10% EMULSIFIABLE INSECTICIDE LONG LASTING PET AND PREMISE SPRAY

Active Ingredients

Permethrin (3-phenoxyphenyl) methyl (±)-cis, trans-3-(2,2-dichloroethenyl)-2 2-dimethylcyclopropane-carboxylate* 10.00%

Inert Ingredients 90.00%

TOTAL 100.00%

*Cis/trans ratio: Min. 35% (±) cis, and max. 65% (±) trans isomers.

Contains 0.75 lbs. permethrin per gallon.

Caution: Keep out of the reach of children. See label for additional cautions.

PRECAUTIONARY STATEMENTS

HAZARDS TO HUMANS

Caution: May be harmful if swallowed, inhaled or absorbed through skin. Avoid breathing spray mist. Avoid contact with skin, eyes or clothing. In case of eye contact, immediately flush eyes with plenty of water. In case of skin contact, wash skin with soap and water. Get medical attention if irritation persists. If swallowed call a physician. Vomiting should be supervised by a physician because of possible pulmonary damage due to aspiration of the solvent.

ENVIRONMENTAL HAZARDS

This pesticide is extremely toxic to fish. Use with care when applying to areas adjacent to any body of water. Do not apply directly to water. Do not contaminate water by cleaning of equipment or disposal of wastes. Apply this product only as specified on this label.

PHYSICAL OR CHEMICAL HAZARDS

Do not use or store near heat or open flame.

Directions For Use

GENERAL USE CLASSIFICATION

IT IS A VIOLATION OF FEDERAL LAW TO USE THIS PRODUCT IN A MANNER INCONSISTENT WITH ITS LABELING.

For use on pets and their premises for control of flies, fleas, lice, mites and ticks. Mix PERMECTRIN™ Pet, Yard & Kennel Spray and apply the use-diluted material to animals and pest breeding or resting surfaces at the rates shown below. These dilutions and rates will provide most efficient pest control under conditions of heavy pressure when good contact is achieved. Timing and frequency of application should be based on pest populations reaching nuisance levels, but accompanying manure removal and sanitation practices should precede sprays. Do not spray feed, food, or water. Retreat as needed but not more often than once every two weeks.

[See table below].

Available in: 8 oz plastic containers.

Product Use	Dilution for Use	Application
Fleas, lice, ticks, mange mites. Pests on small animals (dogs and cats).	Mix 8 oz in 25 gal or 1 oz in 3 gal of clean water for area or spot applications.	Spray or dip diluted spray to apply 1 pint per medium-sized dog. For lice or mites repeat treatment 1–2 weeks later.
Spraying kennels, Dog houses, runs and yards.	Mix 8 oz in 6.3 gal or 1⅓ oz in 1 gal of clean water.	Spray all surfaces to run off with diluted spray using 1 gal per 750 sq ft.

PERMECTRIN™ II

(permethrin)

10% Emulsifiable Insecticide LONG LASTING LIVESTOCK and PREMISE SPRAY

Composition:

ACTIVE INGREDIENTS

Permethrin (3-phenoxyphenyl) methyl (±)-cis, trans-3-(2,2-dichloroethenyl)-2, 2-dimethylcyclopropanecarboxylate* 10.00%

INERT INGREDIENTS 90.00%

TOTAL 100.00%

*Cis/trans ratio: Min. 35% (±) cis, and max. 65% (±) trans isomers.

Contains 0.75 lbs. permethrin per gallon.

For use on horses, beef and dairy cattle, swine, poultry and pets and their premises for control of flies, lice, mites and ticks.

Administration: Mix PERMECTRIN™ II and apply the use-diluted material to animals and pest breeding or resting surfaces at the rates shown below. These dilutions and rates will provide most efficient pest control under conditions of heavy pressure when good contact is achieved. Timing and frequency of application should be based on pest populations reaching nuisance levels, but accompanying manure removal and sanitation practices should precede sprays. Do not spray feed, food, or water. Retreat as needed but not more often than once every two weeks. Wash udders thoroughly before milking.

[See table on next page].

Do not ship swine for slaughter within 5 days of last treatment.

Warning:

Keep out of reach of children.

Harmful if swallowed. May be harmful if swallowed, inhaled or absorbed through skin.

Avoid breathing spray mist. Avoid contact with skin, eyes or clothing.

In case of eye contact, immediately flush eyes with plenty of water.

Wash skin with soap and water.

Get medical attention if irritation persists. If swallowed call a physician. Vomiting should be supervised by a physician because of possible pulmonary damage due to aspiration of the solvent.

Do not contaminate water, food or feed by storage or disposal. See label for additional precautions and environmental hazards.

How Supplied: 1 quart and 8 oz plastic containers

IT IS A VIOLATION OF FEDERAL LAW TO USE THIS PRODUCT IN A MANNER INCONSISTENT WITH ITS LABELING.

PSEUDORABIES VACCINE

Pseudorabies vaccine

Modified Live Virus

Description: A pseudorabies vaccine prepared from a modified live PRV strain K-61 that is cytopathic in tissue culture and immunogenic in susceptible swine of all ages.

The K-61 strain of vaccine virus is propagated in a monkey cell line, thus minimizing the potential for contamination with adventitious porcine agents. The virus is stabilized, dispensed into amber, light-restricting bottles and freeze dried to preserve the maximum concentration of viable vaccine virus at the time of use.

Indications: For the immunization of swine of all ages for protection against disease caused by pseudorabies virus.

Dosage: 2 ml of rehydrated vaccine.
Administration: Inject 2 ml injected intramuscularly.
Cautions:
- Store out of direct sunlight at a temperature not over 45° F.
- Use entire contents when first opened.
- The vaccine should be refrigerated at all times.
- Do not vaccinate within 21 days of slaughter.
- Burn this container and all unused contents.
- Anaphylactoid reactions may occur.

ANTIDOTE: Administer epinephrine.
Health Programming*: At time of initial outbreak, it may be desirable to vaccinate all swine on premises.
Boars: Vaccinate initially at any time. Booster annually.
Sows: At initial herd vaccination, vaccinate all sows and gilts. Thereafter, booster three weeks before each farrowing.
Nursing Pigs: Pigs nursing non-immune dams may be vaccinated at 3–5 days. Pigs nursing vaccinated dams should be vaccinated at 3–4 weeks of age and boostered 4–12 weeks after initial dose when maternal antibody levels have declined.
Feeder Pigs: Vaccinate susceptible pigs at any age with a single dose.
Replacement Gilts: Booster at 6 months of age before breeding.
NOTE: Vaccinated animals will be positive to the serum neutralization (SN) test and therefore will create a problem for herds requiring a negative SN test.
*As recommended by the Bio-Ceutic Professional Services Department.
Packaging: Available in 10-dose and 25-dose amber vials.
Product Information: PSEUDORABIES VACCINE is prepared from a modified live PRV Hungarian strain (K-61) that is cytopathic in tissue culture and highly immunogenic in susceptible swine of all ages. This PRV variant strain has been used exensively in Hungary for more than twenty years and was selected from virus isolated from a clinical outbreak of the disease in pigs. The K-61 strain differs from virulent virus because it forms small, uniform plaques in pig kidney cells and has no virulence for domestic animals.[5] It is thus safe to use around all domestic animals.
Safety of the K-61 strain has been demonstrated in limited experimental work using the strain as a live virus vaccine. In these studies, the K-61 strain was passaged in chick embryo or calf testicle culture and given intramuscularly as a vaccine virus to pigs. Results demonstrated that the live virus vaccine was safe for pigs and did not spread to two, susceptible, contact pigs.[5]
PSEUDORABIES VACCINE (Bio-Ceutic) is a modified live vaccine which is propagated in an established monkey cell line in order to produce a final product that is safe and free from adventitious porcine agents. PSEUDORABIES VACCINE is safe to use with all ages of swine including neonates, young pigs, and pregnant sows. The 2-ml dose is administered intramuscularly and does not produce injection site reactions.
Studies with Bio-Ceutic PSEUDORABIES VACCINE have established that it is safe and free of shock reaction. Swine reinoculated with monkey cell antigen were free of shock reaction or interference with vaccinal immune response.
PSEUDORABIES VACCINE is nonshedding and will not revert to virulence in multiple, forced backpassages. Study results show there is no evidence that the vaccine virus spread to non-vaccinated contact pigs.
There are no post-vaccinal reactions with Bio-Ceutic PSEUDORABIES VACCINE. In safety tests using both intramuscular and intranasal administration, there was no evidence of post-vaccinal reaction.
Bio-Ceutic PSEUDORABIES VACCINE is available in 10-dose and 25-dose amber vials. The protective, Sun-Screen packaging is a special feature of Bio-Ceutic Laboratories. The amber bottles filter out harmful light rays to ensure that the potency of the vaccine is maintained.

PESTS	PERMECTRIN II DILUTIONS FOR USE	HOW TO APPLY
PESTS ON FARM PREMISES (Barns, Dairies, Feedlots, Stables, Poultry and Livestock Housing)		
Houseflies, Stableflies, Lesser houseflies and other manure breeding flies. Aids in control of cockroaches, mosquitoes and spiders.	Mix 1 qt in 25 gal of clean water.	Spray all surfaces to runoff with diluted emulsion using 1 gal per 750 sq. ft.
	Use undiluted in mist blower as space spray. Use 1 qt in 25 gal of oil*	Mist or fog 4 oz per 1000 sq. ft.
PESTS ON LARGE ANIMALS (Dairy or Beef Cattle and Horses)		
Faceflies, Hornflies, Horseflies	Mix 1 qt in 20 gal oil* to charge backrubbers	Animals self apply. Recharge backrubber or oiler as needed.
Faceflies, Hornflies, Horseflies, Stableflies, Mosquitoes, Lice, Mites, Ticks	Mix 1 qt in 200 gal clean water for whole body and area spraying.	Spray to thoroughly cover entire animal. For Lice or Mites a second treatment is recommended 14–21 days later.
Ear Ticks, Faceflies, Hornflies	Mix 2 oz in 1 gal oil* or clean water for spot applications	Apply ½ oz per ear or 2–4 oz per face or 12–16 oz along the backline.
PESTS ON SWINE, POULTRY, AND SMALL ANIMALS		
Mange mites	Mix 1 qt in 100 gal water.	Spray or dip animals. Retreat after 14 days spraying walls and floor and replace bedding to kill late hatching, developing stages.
Mosquitoes, Hog lice, Fleas, Ticks	Mix 1 qt in 100 gal clean water for area or spot applications.	Spray, paint, or dip to apply 1 pint per dog or pig, especially around ears.
Poultry mites	Mix 1 qt in 50 gal clean water to spray birds and cages.	Spray 1–2 oz per bird, or 1 gal per 100 birds, directed toward vent area.

*Diesel fuel or other non-irritating organic oil.

QUADRAPLEX/SOMNUGEN
Bovine Rhinotracheitis-Parainfluenza$_3$ killed virus Vaccine and Haemophilus somnus-Pasteurella haemolytica-multocida Bacterin

Composition: Contains chemically inactivated bovine rhinotracheitis and parainfluenza$_3$ viruses grown in bovine tissue culture combined with *Haemophilus somnus* and *Pasteurella haemolytica-multocida* bacterin.
Indications: Recommended for use in healthy susceptible cattle as against disease caused by bovine rhinotracheitis and parainfluenza$_3$ viruses, *Pasteurella*

Continued on next page

Bio-Ceutic—Cont.

haemolytica-multocida and *Haemophilus somnus.*
Administration: Administer 5 ml intramuscularly. Repeat in 14 to 28 days.
Cautions:
- Store out of direct sunlight at a temperature not over 45° F.
- Avoid freezing.
- Shake well before use.
- Use entire contents when first opened.
- Do not vaccinate within 21 days before slaughter.
- Anaphylactoid reactions may occur.
- Antidote: Administer epinephrine.
- Consult label for full directions and cautions.

Packaging: Available in 10 dose and 50 dose vials.
Product Information: Quadraplex/Somnugen is a combination of an inactivated bovine rhinotracheitis and parainfluenza$_3$ vaccine plus a *Haemophilus somnus-Pasteurella haemolytica-multocida bacterin.*
Quadraplex/Somnugen offers an alternative to the modified live virus vaccines. It is formulated for slow absorption which means that the immune stimulation continues after the initial stress of shipping and processing has diminished. In contrast, many of the modified live virus vaccines provide an immune stimulus for a relatively-short time. If calves vaccinated with a MLV vaccine are severely-stressed throughout the entire shipping and processing period, they may not be able to respond adequately. Quadraplex/Somnugen protects the livestock producer's investment when the stale, stressed animals are most susceptible to disease. In addition, Quadraplex/Somnugen does not produce any additional reduction in the white cell count, and thus, it does not create the additional stress produced by some other modified live virus vaccines.
Quadraplex/Somnugen can be used during any stage of pregnancy. Results of studies have shown that neither the IBR nor PI$_3$ virus was isolated from selected fetuses obtained from cows vaccinated in the first three months of pregnancy. Vaccination with Quadraplex/Somnugen during this time produced no adverse effects in the cow or fetus.
Modified live virus vaccines containing IBR virus are contraindicated for use in pregnant cows because the virus has been associated with abortions. However, because Quadraplex/Somnugen contains an inactivated IBR virus, it can be used safely in beef or dairy cattle including pregnant or lactating animals.
The safety of single injections of Quadraplex/Somnugen has been demonstrated in animals of all ages. Because Quadraplex/Somnugen is non-transmissible, it can be given to all unweaned calves running beside their pregnant dams. There is no fear of the pregnant dams aborting because of virus shedding from the vaccinated calves. In addition, newborn calves from cows vaccinated with Quadraplex/Somnugen acquire protective antibodies against *H. somnus* and IBR and PI$_3$ viruses through the first milk.
Quadraplex/Somnugen offers multiple benefits of economy, safety, ease of administration, and broad protection against the common bovine respiratory disease agents. The easy-to-administer injections assure an accurate dose. In addition, no milk withdrawal is needed.

QUATRACON-2X
Corynebacterium pyogenes-Escherichia coli-Pasteurella multocida-Salmonella typhimurium Antiserum Bovine Isolates and Origin Concentrate

Composition: Prepared from the blood of cattle hyperimmunized with *Corynebacterium pyogenes, Pasteurella multocida, Carter's Serotype A, Escherichia Coli Serotype 78:K80:NM, and Salmonella typhimurium.* In addition, the cattle receive repeated injections of viruses of bovine virus diarrhea, bovine rhinotracheitis, bovine parainfluenza, *Haemophilus somnus,* and *Pasteurella multocida.* Contains cresol 0.2% and thimerosal 0.01% as a preservative.
Indications: This product is recommended for the prophylaxis and treatment of disease caused by *Corynebacterium pyogenes, Pasteurella multocida, Escherichia coli,* and *Salmonella typhimurium* in cattle.
Dosage and Administration: Prophylactic: 15 ml per 50 lbs body weight administered subcutaneously as soon as possible after birth; Therapeutic: 30 ml per 50 lbs body weight (depending upon condition of the animal), repeat each 12 to 24 hours until improvement is satisfactory.
Caution: Store out of direct sunlight at a temperature not over 45° F. Avoid freezing. Shake well before using. Use entire contents when first opened. Do not vaccinate within 21 days before slaughter. Do not vaccinate with bovine virus diarrhea vaccine, bovine rhinotracheitis vaccine, or bovine parainfluenza$_3$ vaccine within 21 days after use of this serum.
How Supplied: 250 ml vials.

SECTILIN
with Pyrethrins Insecticidal Shampoo

Composition:
ACTIVE INGREDIENTS:
Pyrethrins 0.06%
Technical piperonyl butoxide (Consists of 0.096% butylcarbityl) (6-propylpiperonyl) ether and 0.024% related compounds 0.12%
N-octyl bicycloheptene dicarboximide 0.20%
INERT INGREDIENTS: 99.62%
Composed of triethanolamine salt of cocoylpolypeptide condensate, triethanolamine alkyl sulfate, lauric diethanolamide, petroleum hydrocarbons, perfume oil, pigment, water.
Indications: A cleansing, soothing shampoo for use on dogs, cats and horses to control fleas, lice* and ticks. Promotes luster and manageability. Contains protein base Surfactant.
*Not approved for sale in California.
Dosage and Administration: Thoroughly wet the entire animal with warm water. Apply just enough shampoo to produce a lather. For best effects on fleas, lice* and ticks, allow lather to remain on animals for approximately five minutes before rinsing.
Rinse thoroughly with warm water. May be repeated once or twice weekly.
How Supplied: 8 oz and gallon.
See label for additional precautions.
It is a violation of Federal Law to use this product in a manner inconsistent with its labeling.

SOW-PLEX-3
Clostridium Perfringens Type C—Erysipelothrix rhusiopathiae—Escherichia coli Bacterin—Toxoid Alum Precipitated

Composition: Prepared from chemically detoxified cultures of *Clostridium perfringens* Type C, *Erysipelothrix rhusiopathiae* and *Escherichia coli.*
Indications: Recommended for the immunization of healthy susceptible swine breeding stock against diseases caused by *Clostridium perfringens* Type C, *Erysipelothrix rhusiopathiae* and enterotoxigenic *Escherichia coli.*
Protection against *Clostridium perfringens* Type C enterotoxemia and *Escherichia coli* scours in the newborn piglet is provided by the maternal antibodies in colostrum. Therefore, piglets should receive colostrum from the vaccinated sow as soon as possible after birth.
Dosage: 5 ml injected intramuscularly into sows and gilts 2 to 3 weeks prior to breeding. Repeat with a second 5 ml dose 2 to 3 weeks prior to farrowing and prior to each subsequent farrowing.
Packaging: Available in 10 and 50 dose vials.
Precautions:
- Store out of direct sunlight at a temperature not over 45° F.
- Avoid freezing.
- Shake well. Use entire contents when first opened.
- Do not vaccinate within 21 days before slaughter.
- Anaphylactoid reactions may occur.

ANTIDOTE: Administer epinephrine.
In just one product, SOW-PLEX-3 provides protection against three major swine diseases. This combination features protection against enterotoxemia, a highly-fatal disease of newborn piglets caused by *Cl. perfringens* Type C bacteria. The *E. coli* fraction in SOW-PLEX-3 is an inactivated, whole-cell culture containing pilus and somatic antigens. It contains the four major *E. coli* pilus antigens which are associated with colibacillosis (K88ab, K88ac, K99 and 987P). These pilus antigens stimulate antibodies to prevent disease-causing *E. coli* from attaching to the gut wall, thereby keeping them from multiplying and releasing toxin.

With SOW-PLEX-3, protection against *Cl. perfringens* Type C enterotoxemia and *E. coli* scours in the newborn piglet are provided by the maternal antibodies in the sow's colostrum. Therefore, piglets should receive colostrum from the vaccinated sow as soon as possible after birth.
SOW-PLEX-3 is recommended for healthy sows and gilts. The first dose (5 ml administered intramuscularly) should be given 2 to 3 weeks prior to breeding with a second 5 ml dose 2 to 3 weeks prior to farrowing and prior to each subsequent farrowing.

STEER-oid™
Steer Implants
Progesterone U.S.P. 200 mg
Estradiol benzoate U.S.P. 20 mg

Description: Each STEER-oid Cartridge Belt holds 20 doses of STEER-oid implants. Each dose of 8 pellets contains a total of 200 mg progesterone USP plus 20 mg estradiol benzoate U.S.P.
Indications: For use in steers weighing 400 lbs or more to improve weight gain and feed efficiency for up to a 150 day feeding or grazing period.
Administration: Insert plastic cartridge belt as directed into the pellet-implanter applicator. Pellets are deposited with the pellet-implanter beneath the skin on the back side of the middle one-third of the ear toward the center.
Product Information: STEER-oid is a growth-promoting implant for steers containing a combination of two naturally-occurring hormones: progesterone U.S.P. (200 mg) and estradiol benzoate U.S.P. (20 mg). By supplementing the animal's hormonal output, it helps to increase feed conversion efficiency as well as promote increased average daily weight gains. STEER-oid does not require withholding before slaughter.
Caution: Bulling, rectal prolapse, ventral edema, and elevated tailheads have been reported occasionally in steers implanted with steer implants containing progesterone U.S.P. plus estradiol benzoate U.S.P.
Warning: IMPLANT AND USE ONLY AS DIRECTED.
Implant pellets in ear only. Any other site is in violation of Federal Law. Do NOT attempt to salvage implant site for animal feed or human use. KEEP THIS AND ALL OTHER DRUGS OUT OF REACH OF CHILDREN.
Packaging: 100 dose carton (5 × 20-dose cartridge belt)

VIBO-5/SOMNUGEN
Campylobacteriosis (Vibriosis) leptospirosis-Haemophilus somnus Bacterin
Haemophilus somnus-Campylobacter fetus-Leptospira canicola-grippotyphosa-hardjo-icterohaemorrhagiae-pomona Bacterin

Description: Inactivated adjuvanted whole cultures of the above named organisms. Contains neomycin as a preservative.
Indications: Recommended for use in healthy susceptible cattle four months of age or older against disease caused by *Haemophilus somnus;* the prevention of infertility, delayed conception or abortion due to *Campylobacter fetus* var. *venerealis;* and against leptospirosis due to *Leptospira canicola, L. grippotyphosa, L. hardjo, L. icterohaemorrhagiae,* and *L. pomona.*
Administration: Administer 5 ml intramuscularly. Repeat in 14 to 21 days and once annually.
Cautions:
- Shake well before using.
- Use entire contents when first opened.
- Store out of direct sunlight at a temperature not over 45° F.
- Avoid freezing.
- Do not vaccinate within 21 days before slaughter.

Anaphylactoid reactions may occur.
ANTIDOTE: Administer epinephrine.
Health Programming:
Replacement Heifers, Bulls, Beef & Dairy Cows: Administer a 5 ml dose intramuscularly in healthy cattle 4 months of age or older. Repeat the dosage in 14 to 21 days. Administer a single 5 ml booster dose annually.
Packaging: Available in 10 dose and 50 dose vials.
Product Information: VIBO-5/SOMNUGEN is an exclusive combination product which permits broad protection against many, major bovine respiratory and reproductive disease agents. It is recommended for use in healthy susceptible cattle as (1.) an aid in the prevention of infertility, delayed conception or abortion due to *Campylobacter fetus* var *venerealis;* (2.) for the prevention of leptospirosis due to *Leptospira grippotyphosa, L. hardjo, L. pomona, L. canicola,* and *L. icterohaemorrhagiae;* (3.) and for the prevention of disease caused by *Haemophilus somnus.*
Because VIBO-5/SOMNUGEN combines protection for several disease agents, it reduces labor and handling. In addition, it also reduces the number of carrier cows within a herd which can transmit the reproductive and respiratory diseases to healthy animals.

VIROSAN CONCENTRATE TEAT DIP
(chlorhexidine with glycerin)

Composition: A concentrated solution containing chlorhexidine digluconate —4% w/w and glycerin 48% w/w.
Indications: For use in preparation of a 0.5% chlorhexidine solution for dipping teats as an aid in the control of mastitis-causing bacteria on teats. Contains a chlorhexidine solution in combination with glycerin whose emollient qualities help soften and soothe tissues.
Dosage and Administration: See label for complete directions for dilution and use.
Cautions:
Dilute with proper amount of water before use as a teat dip.
Do not use the concentrate as a teat dip.
Avoid contamination of feed and foodstuffs.
Do not allow to freeze.
Store at room temperature.
May be harmful if swallowed. Keep out of reach of children.
May be irritating to eyes and mucous membranes. If contact occurs, flush with copious amounts of water.
Call a physician for treatment of eyes.
How Supplied: Available in one pint plastic container; 12 per case.

VIROSAN SOLUTION
(chlorhexidine)

Composition: A concentrated solution containing chlorhexidine digluconate —2.0% w/w and isopropyl alcohol 1%.
Indications: For use in preparation of a 0.5% chlorhexidine solution for dipping teats as an aid in control of mastitis-causing bacteria on teats.
Dosage and Administration: Dip each teat into the 0.5% solution immediately after each milking. Thoroughly wash teats and udder immediately prior to next milking. Teat dipping should start at least one week before the cow freshens and continue until four days or more after drying off.
Directions for Dilution: To prepare 1 gallon of a 0.5% solution for dipping teats as an aid in controlling mastitis-causing bacteria, such as *Streptococcus agalactiae, Streptococcus dysgalactiae, Streptococcus uberis, Staphylococcus aureus, E. coli* and *Pseudomonas aeruginosa* on teats, mix 32 fluid ounces (1 qt) of Virosan Solution with 96 fluid ounces of clean water* or distilled water in a clean 1-gallon container.
Alternately, mix 32 fluid ounces (1 qt) of Virosan Solution with 90 fluid ounces of clean water* or distilled water and 6 fluid ounces of glycerin in a clean 1-gallon container.
*Precipitate may occur with certain types of water used for dilution. It is preferable to use distilled water or deionized water.
Warning: Dilute with the proper amount of water before use as a teat dip. Do not use the concentrate as a teat dip.
Caution: May be irritating to eyes and mucous membranes. If contact occurs, flush with copious amount of water. Call a physician for treatment of eyes. May be harmful if swallowed. Avoid contamination of feed and foodstuffs. Rinse empty container thoroughly with water and properly destroy by crushing or burial.
Store at room temperature.
Do not allow to freeze.
Warning: Keep out of the reach of children.
How Supplied: Available in one gallon plastic containers for ease of diluting to use concentration.

VOREN® Sterile Suspension
(brand of dexamethasone-21-isonicotinate)

Description: Voren is defined chemically as 9-Fluoro-11β,17,21-trihydroxy-16α-methyl-pregna-1,4-diene-3,20 dione 21-(4-pyridinecarboxylate) (dexametha-

Continued on next page

B

Bio-Ceutic—Cont.

sone-21-isonicotinate). It is a white to slightly yellowish, electrostatically charged crystalline powder. It is almost odorless and tasteless.

Voren suspension is an aqueous suspension containing 1.0 mg. of dexamethasone-21-isonicotinate per milliliter with 0.9% sodium chloride, 0.1% polysorbate 80, (methyl paraben 0.18% w/v and propyl paraben 0.02% w/v as preservatives), sodium hydroxide to adjust pH.

Indications: Voren is indicated in the treatment of various inflammatory conditions associated with the musculoskeletal system of the dog, cat and horse.

Pharmacological Activity:
Since Voren is an ester of dexamethasone, some comparative studies were made with the two compounds.

1. Glucocorticoid Effect
   a. Voren (dexamethasone-21-isonicotinate) was compared with dexamethasone in 24-hour fasted rats by measuring the increase in liver glycogen. Measurements were made following a single intramuscular injection of equimolecular amounts of the two substances. Dexamethasone caused a peak of 25 mg/g of liver at 24 hours. The duration of effect was 47–72 hours. Voren caused a peak of 40 mg/g of liver at 48 hours and the duration of effect was 120–144 hours.
   b. The same comparison was made in adrenalectomized rats with similar results, but the glycogen increase obtained from Voren was 3 times that from dexamethasone.
   c. Comparing Voren with dexamethasone orally, the results were almost identical with each other.
2. Anti-inflammatory Effect
   a. Granuloma pouch technique in rats. This is a measurement of anti-exudative action in response to an irritant (croton oil) injected into an artifically created air sac.
   Results:
   (1) Orally: Voren=dexamethasone
   (2) Intramuscularly: Voren=2 times dexamethasone
   (3) Locally: Voren=10 times dexamethasone
   b. Egg-white edema test on rat's paw. This is also a measurement of anti-exudative action as reflected by edema following injection of egg white into a rat's paw.
   Results:
   (1) Orally: Voren=dexamethasone
   (2) Intramuscularly: Voren=6 times dexamethasone
   (3) Locally: Voren=28 times dexamethasone
3. Effect on Lymphatic Tissues—a 14-day test to determine comparative involution rate of thymus. This test showed Voren and dexamethasone to be equivalent in effect.
4. Catabolic Effect—a growth rate study. Both Voren and dexamethasone caused a decreased rate of growth following daily subcutaneous injections, the action being approximately equal.
5. Pituitary Inhibition—a 14-day test to determine any atrophic effect on the hypophyseal gland. The results were very similar with Voren exerting a slightly less inhibiting effect than dexamethasone.
6. Survival Test—a study of dose/effect (D/E) calculated by determining the mean daily subcutaneous dose to cause 50% survival of adrenalectomized mice over a 14-day period. Results: The substitution capacity of Voren (dexamethasone-21-isonicontinate) is 1.7 times that of dexamethasone.
7. Effect on Electrolyte Metabolism—measured by sodium and potassium excretion test on adrenalectomized rats. Voren causes a slight naturesis and kaluresis equal to that of dexamethasone.

Precautions and Side Effects: The usual precautions and contraindications for adrenocorticoid hormones are applicable with this compound. The close observation of animals, under treatment with this drug, is necessary, since the usual signs of adrenocorticoid overdosages which include sodium retention, potassium loss, fluid retention, weight gain, etc., may not be readily observed.
The most commonly observed side effect with corticosteroid therapy in animals is polydipsia, polyuria, and on occasion, a gain in weight. An increased appetite may be evidenced. If this is undesirable, such as in obese animals, dietary management may be necessary. Under clinical and experimental trials with Voren only a few such side effects have been noted. If they occur, the veterinarian should be prepared to take the necessary steps to correct them, which consist of temporarily discontinuing therapy with the drug until the effects disappear, when therapy may be resumed at a lower dose level.
When long-term therapy with corticosteroids is necessary in the dog and cat, the dose should be individually adjusted so that the minimum maintenance dose is used to keep the condition being treated under control. In dogs and cats on long-term therapy with these drugs, a protein-rich diet is useful to counteract nitrogen loss, if it should occur. Similarly, a small amount of potassium chloride, daily on the diet, will counteract excessive potassium loss, if this is present. Experimentally it has been demonstrated that corticosteroids, especially at high dose levels, may result in delayed wound healing. An increase in the incidence of osteoporosis may be noted, mainly in the old animals, with the prolonged use of these compounds. Their use in older dogs, cats and horses during the healing stages of a bone fracture is not indicated for the reason listed above.
In man, corticosteroid therapy, especially of a prolonged nature, has been reported to induce a number of side effects. These include: hypertension or elevation of blood pressure, obesity of the Cushingoid type, plethora, weakness, striae, hirsutism in females, virilism, psychotic states, osteoporosis, ankle edema, purpura, exophthalmos, posterior subcapsular cataracts, peptic ulcers, etc. Side effects of a similar nature during or following corticoid therapy in animals have rarely, if ever, been reported. The veterinarian, however, should be aware of the possible occurrence of such drug induced changes, in animals on long-term corticosteroid therapy.
Continuous therapy with Voren, especially at high dose levels, may result in suppression of adrenal cortical function. In such cases, temporary suspension of therapy and stimulation of the adrenal cortex by the use of ACTH may be advisable. Following prolonged therapy with the drug, it is recommended that the drug be withdrawn gradually. If such animals are later subjected to stressful situations (trauma, surgery, etc.), it is advisable to institute a temporary course of therapy with Voren (dexamethasone-21-isonicotinate).
Voren may be administered to animals with bacterial diseases provided that specific and appropriate antibacterial therapy with antibiotic or chemotherapeutic drugs is administered simultaneously. In the absence of specific concomitant antimicrobial therapy, the prolonged use of corticosteroids is likely to lead to the spread of pathogenic micro-organisms. The use of corticosteroids in such situations is not indicated. It should be borne in mind that Voren, like cortisone, through its anti-inflammatory action, may mask the usual signs of an infection such as pyrexia, inappetence, lassitude, etc. In the course of therapy with Voren, should the question of determining the presence of an infectious disease arise, the drug should be withheld temporarily until a diagnosis or rediagnosis establishes the facts.

WARNING: Not for use in horses intended for food. Voren (dexamethasone-21-isonicotinate) is not to be used in food producing animals since no data are available to indicate the period of time following administration required for edible animal products to be free of residual drug.

WARNING: Clinical and experimental data have demonstrated that corticosteroids administered orally or by injection to animals may induce the first stage of parturition if used during the last trimester of pregnancy and may precipitate premature parturition followed by dystocia, fetal death, retained placenta and metritis. Additionally, corticosteroids administered to dogs, rabbits, and rodents during pregnancy have resulted in cleft palate in offspring. Corticosteroids administered to dogs during pregnancy have also resulted in other congenital anomalies including deformed forelegs, phocomelia, and anasarca.

Dosage and Administration: Administer by the intramuscular route. For use *only* in dogs, cats and horses.

SHAKE WELL BEFORE USING.

Dog—0.25 to 1 mg (0.25 to 1 ml).
Cat—0.125 to 0.5 mg (0.125 to 0.5 ml).
The dose may be repeated in dogs and cats for 3–5 days.

Horse—5 to 20 mg (5 to 20 ml). This dosage may be repeated.
CAUTION: U.S. Federal law restricts this drug to use by or on the order of a licensed veterinarian. Not for human use.
Storage: Store in a tight container. Do not freeze.
Caution: Keep out of reach of children.
How Supplied: 10 ml and 50 ml vials.
Licensed under U.S. Pat. No. 3,314,854
For Veterinary Use Only

Bristol Veterinary Products

Bristol Laboratories
Division of Bristol-Myers Company
P.O. BOX 4755
SYRACUSE, NY 13221-4755

AMFOROL®
Veterinary Oral Suspension and Tablets

Composition:
Each teaspoonful (5 ml) of suspension or each tablet contains:

Kanamycin activity (as the sulfate)	100.0 mg
Aminopentamide hydrogen sulfate	0.033 mg
Pectin	25.0 mg
Bismuth subcarbonate	250.0 mg
Activated attapulgite	500.0 mg

Therapeutic Action of Ingredients:
Kanamycin Sulfate (Kantrim ®): Kanamycin is active against Salmonella, Shigella, *Alcaligenes faecalis, E. coli, Proteus,* and *Staphylococcus aureus,* all species associated with bacterial enteric infections. It is not absorbed from the gastrointestinal tract, providing bactericidal action at the site of infection.
Aminopentamide Hydrogen Sulfate: Aminopentamide is an antispasmodic-anticholinergic agent capable of adequately inhibiting gastrointestinal motility.
Pectin: Pectin is a gastrointestinal detoxifying agent whose detoxifying properties are due to its high content of galacturonic acid, which produces conjugation products with many toxins, thus converting them to non-toxic substances.
Bismuth Subcarbonate: Acts as an adsorbent, protecting the gastrointestinal mucosa, neutralizing gastric acids, and helping to normalize the consistency of stools.
Activated Attapulgite: An activated clay mineral, 5 to 8 times superior to Kaolin as an adsorbent for bacteria, viruses, and toxins.
Indications: Amforol (Veterinary Oral Suspension and Tablets) is indicated for the treatment of bacterial enteritis in dogs (caused by organisms susceptible to kanamycin) and the symptomatic relief of the associated diarrhea.
Dosage: Dogs—The following dosage schedule is recommended, based upon a simple estimation of animal size:
Oral Suspension: Five ml (5 ml) per 20 lbs body weight every 8 hours. Maximum dose, 15 ml every 8 hours. For animals under 10 lbs, 2.5 ml every 8 hours.
Tablets: One tablet per 20 lbs body weight every 8 hours. Maximum dose, three tablets every 8 hours. For animals under 10 lbs, one-half tablet every 8 hours.
It is recommended that an initial loading dose precede the above schedule, consisting of twice the amount of a single dose.
Precautions: Because of the bactericidal activity of kanamycin prolonged treatment may permit overgrowth of nonsusceptible organisms (e.g., fungi). If remission of symptoms is not evident after 3 to 4 days treatment, the diagnosis should be reestablished.
How Supplied: Amforol® Veterinary Oral Tablets and Suspension are supplied as follows:
Tablets: List NDC 0015-2006-60-100 tablet bottle
Suspension: List NDC 0015-2003-60-480 ml (16 oz) List NDC 0015-2003-45-120 ml (4 oz)

AMIGLYDE-V®
(amikacin sulfate)
Veterinary Solution

Description: Amikacin sulfate is a semi-synthetic aminoglycoside antibiotic derived from kanamycin. It is $C_{2}2H_{4}3N_{5}0_{1}32H_{2}SO_{4}$, D-Streptamine, 0-3-amino-3-deoxy—D-Glucopranosyl-(1 6)-0-6-amino-6-deoxy-D-glucopyranosyl-(14)-N^{1}-(4-amino-2-hydroxy-1-oxobutyl)-2-deoxy-, (S)-, sulfate (1:2) (salt).
The dosage form supplied is a sterile, colorless to light straw-colored solution. The solution contains, in addition to amikacin sulfate, 2.5% sodium citrate with pH adjusted to 4.5 with sulfuric acid and 0.66% sodium bisulfite added.
Action: *Antibacterial Activity:* The effectiveness of Amiglyde-V (amikacin sulfate) in infections caused by *Escherichia coli, Pseudomonas* sp, and *Klebsiella* sp has been demonstrated clinically in the horse. In addition, the following microorganisms have been shown to be susceptible to amikacin in vitro[1], although the clinical significance of this action has not been demonstrated in animals:
Enterobacter sp
Proteus mirabilis
Proteus sp (indole positive)
Serratia marcescens
Salmonella sp
Shigella sp
Providencia sp
Citrobacter freundii
Listeria monocytogenes
Staphylococcus aureus (both penicillin resistant and penicillin sensitive)
The aminoglycoside antibiotics in general have limited activity against Gram-positive pathogens, although *Staphylococcus aureus* and *Listeria monocytogenes* are susceptible to amikacin as noted above.
Amikacin has been shown to be effective against many aminoglycoside-resistant strains due to its ability to resist degradation by aminoglycoside inactivating enyzmes known to affect gentamicin, tobramycin and kanamycin[2].
Clinical Pharmacology: *Endometrial Tissue Concentrations:* Comparisons of amikacin activity in endometrial biopsy tissue following intrauterine infusion with that following intramuscular injections of Amiglyde-V (amikacin sulfate) in mares demonstrate superior endometrial tissue concentrations when the drug is administered by the intrauterine route.
Intrauterine infusion of 2 grams Amiglyde-V (amikacin sulfate) daily for three consecutive days in mares results in peak concentrations typically exceeding 40 mcg/g of endometrial biopsy tissue within one hour after infusion. Twenty-four hours after each treatment amikacin activity is still detectable at concentrations averaging 2–4 mcg/g. However, the drug is not appreciably absorbed systemically following intrauterine infusion. Endometrial tissue concentrations following intramuscular injection roughly parallel, but are typically somewhat lower than corresponding serum concentrations of amikacin.
Safety: Amiglyde-V (amikacin sulfate) is nonirritating to equine endometrial tissue when infused into the uterus as directed (see "Dosage and Administration"). In laboratory animals as well as equine studies, the drug was generally found not to be irritating when injected intravenously, subcutaneously or intramuscularly.
Although amikacin, like other aminoglycosides, is potentially nephrotoxic, ototoxic and neurotoxic, parenteral (intravenous) administration of Amiglyde-V (amikacin sulfate) twice daily at dosages of up to 10 mg/lb for 15 consecutive days in horses resulted in no clinical, laboratory or histopathologic evidence of toxicity.
Studies *in vitro* have shown that amikacin is not spermicidal when added to stallion or bull semen extender at concentrations as high as 1,000 mcg/ml. In reproductive studies, all mares artificially inseminated with extended semen containing Amiglyde-V (amikacin sulfate) at a concentration of 100 mcg/ml became pregnant. Intrauterine infusion of 2 grams of Amiglyde-V (amikacin sulfate) 8 hours prior to breeding by natural service did not impair fertility in mares.
Indications: Amiglyde-V (amikacin sulfate) is indicated for the treatment of uterine infections such as endometritis, metritis and pyometra in mares, when caused by susceptible organisms including *Escherichia coli, Pseudomonas* sp, and *Klebsiella* sp. The use of Amiglyde-V (amikacin sulfate) in eliminating infections caused by the above organisms has been shown clinically to improve fertility in infected mares.
While nearly all strains of *Escherichia coli, Pseudomonas* sp and *Klebsiella* sp, including those that are resistant to gentamicin, kanamycin or other aminoglycosides, are susceptible to amikacin at levels achieved following treatment, it is recommended that the invading organ-

Continued on next page

Bristol—Cont.

ism be cultured and its susceptibility demonstrated as a guide to therapy. Amikacin susceptibility discs, 30 mcg, should be used for determining *in vitro* susceptibility.

Contraindications: There are no known contraindications for the use of Amiglyde-V (amikacin sulfate) in horses other than a history of hypersensitivity to amikacin.

Adverse Reactions: No adverse reactions or other side effects have been reported.

Dosage and Administration: For treatment of uterine infections in mares, 2 grams of Amiglyde-V (amikacin sulfate), mixed with 200 ml 0.9% Sodium Chloride Injection USP and aseptically infused into the uterus daily for three consecutive days, has been found to be the most efficacious dosage.

Precautions: Although Amiglyde-V (amikacin sulfate) is not absorbed to an appreciable extent following intrauterine infusion, concurrent use of other aminoglycosides should be avoided because of the potential additive effects.

Warning: Not to be used in horses intended for food.

How Supplied: Amiglyde-V (amikacin sulfate) Veterinary Solution is supplied as a colorless solution which is stable at room temperature. At times the solution may become pale yellow in color. This does not indicate a decrease in potency.

NDC 0015-2330-20 4 ml vial, 250 mg/ml
NDC 0015-2330-95 6 x 4 ml vials, 250 mg/ml
NDC 0015-2332-20 48 ml vial, 250 mg/ml

References:

1. Price, K,E., *et al:* Microbiological Evaluation of BB-K8, a New Semisynthetic Aminoglycoside. *J. Antibiot.* 25: 709–731, 1972.
2. Davies, J., Courvalin, P.: Mechanism of Resistance to Aminoglycosides. *Am J Med* 62: 868–872, 1977.

AMPHODERM®
Kanamycin Sulfate-Calcium Amphomycin-Hydrocortisone Acetate OINTMENT

Description: AMPHODERM (kanamycin sulfate-calcium amphomycin-hydrocortisone acetate) is a dermatological preparation available as a freely flowing ointment. It contains two antibiotics, kanamycin sulfate and calcium amphomycin, plus hydrocortisone acetate in a vanishing base. This combination of two bactericidal antibiotics and hydrocortisone acetate provides a broad antibacterial spectrum as well as anti-inflammatory, anti-allergic, and anti-pruritic activity in a non-irritating, non-staining, water miscible ointment.

Kanamycin sulfate is a bactericidal antibiotic, mainly active against Gram-negative pathogens and most strains of staphylococci, including strains resistant to other antibiotics. Kanamycin sulfate is water soluble, locally nontoxic, and well tolerated by both healthy and damaged tissue.

Calcium amphomycin is a polypeptide antibiotic with bactericidal activity against Gram-positive bacteria; its antibacterial spectrum is similar to that of penicillin. Calcium amphomycin is stable in aqueous solution, locally nontoxic, and not absorbed into the blood stream following topical application.

Hydrocortisone acetate is a well known anti-inflammatory corticosteroid with anti-allergic and antipruritic properties.

Each gram of AMPHODERM (kanamycin sulfate-calcium amphomycin-hydrocortisone acetate) ointment contains 5 mg kanamycin activity as the sulfate, 5 mg amphomycin activity as the calcium salt, and 10 mg hydrocortisone acetate.

Action: The AMPHODERM (kanamycin sulfate-calcium amphomycin-hydrocortisone acetate) combination of antibacterial agents and hydrocortisone exerts an antibacterial, anti-inflammatory, anti-allergic, and antipruritic effect. The stability of the ingredients makes it possible to combine them in an oil-in-water base. This base allows intimate contact of the kanamycin sulfate, calcium amphomycin, and hydrocortisone acetate with the skin, due to their high concentration in the external phase (water phase) of the ointment. The oil-in-water base is miscible with the secretions of the skin thus ensuring intimate contact of the active ingredients with the injured tissue.

Kanamycin is active against many Gram-negative pathogens. These include coliforms, **Aerobacter, Salmonella,** strains of **Proteus, Neisseria,** and **Pasteurella multocida.** Kanamycin's Gram-positive spectrum includes **Bacillus anthracis, Staphylococcus albus,** and **Staphylococcus aureus,** including many strains resistant to other antibiotics. Kanamycin is a bactericidal antibiotic. Bacterial resistance develops very slowly among most sensitive organisms tested, particularly among the staphylococci. Topically applied, it is not absorbed to any appreciable extent into the blood stream, thus precluding any systemic toxicity.

Amphomycin is bactericidal against Gram-positive bacteria. Its bacterial spectrum is very similar to penicillin and bacitracin. It is not absorbed into the blood stream when applied topically. It is non-irritating and has a low sensitizing potential.

AMPHODERM (kanamycin sulfate-calcium amphomycin-hydrocortisone acetate) offers a combination of two antibiotics and a corticosteroid that effectively counteracts inflammatory and infectious changes of the skin.

Indications: Use of AMPHODERM (Kanamycin sulfate-calcium amphomycin-hydrocortisone acetate) OINTMENT is primarily indicated in the treatment of the following conditions when caused by bacteria susceptible to one or both of the antibiotics.

Furunculosis	Acute Otitis Externa
Folliculitis	Erythema
Pruritus	Decubital Ulcer
Anal Gland Infections	Superficial Wounds
	Superficial Abscess

Treatment with AMPHODERM (kanamycin sulfate-calcium amphomycin-hydrocortisone acetate) alone is usually sufficient. However, it may be desirable in some cases to supplement with adjunctive parenteral therapy.

Contraindications: A history of allergic reactions to the active ingredients should be considered a contraindication for use of this agent.

Precautions: AMPHODERM (kanamycin sulfate-calcium amphomycin-hydrocortisone acetate) is well tolerated and does not cause irritation. As with any antibiotic preparation, prolonged use may result in overgrowth of nonsusceptible micro-organisms. If this should occur, appropriate corrective steps should be taken.

Warning: FOR USE IN DOGS ONLY

Adverse Reactions: No adverse reactions have been noted.

Dosage: AMPHODERM (kanamycin sulfate-calcium amphomycin-hydrocortisone acetate) should be applied to the affected areas of the skin at least twice daily. In severe or wide-spread lesions it may be desirable to apply the ointment more than twice a day. After some improvement is observed, treatment can usually be reduced to once a day.

Before application, hair in the affected area should be closely clipped and the area thoroughly cleansed of crusts, scales, dirt, or other detritus prior to treatment.

When treating infections of the anal glands, the drug should be introduced into the orifice of the gland and not through any fistulous tract.

If no response is seen in seven days, diagnosis and therapy should be re-evaluated.

Supply: AMPHODERM (kanamycin sulfate-calcium amphomycin-hydrocortisone acetate) OINTMENT is supplied in plastic tubes containing 7.5 grams (.25 oz) or 15 grams (.50 oz), and plastic squeeze bottles containing 227 grams (8 oz). Each gram of ointment contains 5 mg kanamycin activity as the sulfate, 5 mg amphomycin activity as the calcium salt, and 10 mg hydrocortisone acetate.

Store at controlled room temperature (15°–30°C, 59°–86°F).

Avoid excessive heat.

AMPHODERM OINTMENT
NDC 0015-2304-07— 7.5 g (.25 oz) plastic tube
NDC 0015-2304-15— 15 g (.50 oz) plastic tube
NDC 0015-2304-24— 227 g (8 oz) plastic bottle)

CEFA-DRI®
(cephapirin benzathine)
For Intramammary Infusion into the Dry Cow

Composition: Cefa-Dri® (cephapirin benzathine) for Intramammary Infusion into the Dry Cow is a product which provides a wide range of bactericidal activity against Gram-positive and Gram-negative organisms. It is derived biosynthetically from 7-aminocephalosporanic acid.

Each 10 ml. disposable syringe contains 300 mg. of cephapirin activity in a stable peanut oil gel.
Store at room temperature 59°–86°F; avoid excessive heat.
Action: In the non-lactating mammary gland, Cefa-Dri (cephapirin benzathine) provides bactericidal levels of the active antibiotic, cephapirin, for a prolonged period of time. This prolonged activity is due to the low solubility of the cephapirin benzathine and to the slow release gel base.
Cephapirin is bactericidal to susceptible organisms; it is known to be highly active against *Streptococcus agalactiae* and *Staphylococcus aureus* including strains resistant to penicillin.
To determine the susceptibility of bacteria to cephapirin in the laboratory, the class disc, Cephalothin Susceptibility Test Discs 30 mcg. should be used.
Indications: For the treatment of mastitis in dairy cows during the dry period. Cefa-Dri (cephapirin benzathine) has been shown by extensive clinical studies to be efficacious in the treatment of mastitis in dry cows, when caused by *Streptococcus agalactiae* and *Staphylococcus aureus* including penicillin resistant strains.
Treatment of the dry cow with Cefa-Dri (cephapirin benzathine) is indicated in any cow known to harbor any of these organisms in the udder at drying off.
Dosage and Directions for Use: Cefa-Dri (cephapirin benzathine) is for use in dry cows only.
Infuse each quarter at the time of drying off with a single 10 ml syringe. Use no later than 30 days prior to calving.
Completely milk out all four quarters. The udder and teats should be thoroughly washed with warm water containing a suitable dairy antiseptic and dried, preferably using individual paper towels. Carefully scrub the teat end and orifice with 70% alcohol, using a separate swab for each teat.
Allow to dry.
Remove the protective cap from the syringe, insert the teat tube fully into the orifice and expel the contents into the quarter. Withdraw the syringe and gently massage the quarter to distribute the medication.
Precautions: Cefa-Dri (cephapirin benzathine) should be administered with caution to subjects which have demonstrated some form of allergy, particularly to penicillin. Such reactions are rare; however, should they occur, consult your veterinarian.
Warning:
1. *For use in dry cows only.*
2. Not to be used within 30 days of calving.
3. Milk from treated cows must not be used for food during the first 72 hours after calving.
4. Any animal infused with this product must not be slaughtered for food until 42 days after the latest infusion.

How Supplied: Cefa-Dri (cephapirin benzathine) for Intramammary Infusion into the Dry Cow.
Cephapirin benzathine equivalent to 300 mg. cephapirin activity per syringe.
NDC 0015-2726-10—one 10 ml. syringe.
NDC 0015-2726-13—carton containing 12 x 10 ml. syringes.

CEFA–LAK®
(cephapirin sodium)
For Intramammary Infusion

Composition: Cefa-Lak® (cephapirin sodium) is a cephalosporin which possesses a wide range of antimicrobial activity against Gram-positive and Gram-negative organisms. It is derived biosynthetically from 7-aminocephalosporanic acid.
Each 10 ml. disposable syringe contains 200 mg. of cephapirin activity in a stable peanut-oil gel.
Store at room temperature: 59°–86°F.; avoid excessive heat.
Action: Cephapirin is bactericidal to susceptible organisms; it is known to be highly active against *Streptococcus agalactiae* and *Staphylococcus aureus* including strains resistant to penicillin.
To determine the susceptibility of bacteria to cephapirin in the laboratory, the class disc, Cephalothin Susceptibility Test Discs, 30 mcg., should be used.
Indications: *For Lactating Cows Only.* For the Treatment of Bovine Mastitis.
Cefa-Lak (cephapirin sodium) for Intramammary Infusion should be used at the first signs of inflammation or at the first indication of any alteration in the milk. Treatment is indicated immediately upon determining, by C.M.T. or other tests, that the leucocyte count is elevated, or that a susceptible pathogen has been cultured from the milk.
Cefa-Lak (cephapirin sodium) for Intramammary Infusion has been shown to be efficacious in the treatment of mastitis in lactating cows caused by susceptible strains of *Streptococcus agalactiae* and *Staphylococcus aureus* including strains resistant to penicillin.
Dosage: Infuse the entire contents of one syringe into each infected quarter immediately after the quarter has been completely milked out. Repeat once only in 12 hours. If definite improvement is not noted within 48 hours after treatment, the causal organism should be further investigated. Consult your veterinarian.
Directions for Use: Milk out udder completely, wash udder and teats thoroughly with warm water containing a suitable dairy antiseptic. Dry thoroughly. Saturate a small piece of cotton with 70% alcohol and wipe off end of teat, using a separate piece of cotton for each teat to be treated. Remove cap from tip of syringe and insert tip into teat canal; push plunger to dispense entire contents. Massage the quarter to distribute the suspension up into the milk cistern. Do not milk out for 12 hours.
Reinfection —The use of antibiotics, however effective, for the treatment of mastitis will not significantly reduce the incidence of this disease in the herd unless their use is fortified by good herd management, and sanitary and mechanical safety measures are practiced to prevent reinfection.
Precautions: Cefa-Lak (cephapirin sodium) should be administered with caution to subjects which have demonstrated some form of allergy, particularly to penicillin. Such reactions are rare; however, should they occur, discontinue treatment and consult your veterinarian.
Warning:
1. Milk that has been taken from animals during treatment and for 96 hours (8 milkings) after the last treatment must not be used for food.
2. Treated animals must not be slaughtered for food until 4 days after the last treatment.
3. Administration of more than the prescribed dose may lead to residue of antibiotic in milk longer than 96 hours.

How Supplied: Cefa-Lak (cephapirin sodium) for Intramammary Infusion, Cephapirin sodium equivalent to 200 mg of cephapirin activity per syringe.
NDC 0015-2723-21—one 10 ml syringe.
NDC 0015-2723-13—carton containing 12 x 10 ml. syringes.

CEFA–TABS®
(Cefadroxil)
VETERINARY
FILM-COATED TABLETS

CEFA-TABS (cefadroxil) is a semi-synthetic cephalosporin antibiotic intended for oral administration.
Chemistry: Cefadroxil is a member of a group of semisynthetic derivatives of cephalosporin C, found among the metabolic products of the fungus **Cephalosporium acremonium.** The cephalosporins are structurally related to the penicillins in that both contain a 4-member beta-lactam ring. Cefadroxil is a 7-amino cephalosporanic acid substituted at the 7 position to form a molecule designated chemically as (6R,7R)-7-[(R)-2-Amino-2-(p-hydroxyphenyl)acetamido]-3-methyl-8-oxo-5-thia-1-azabicyclo [4.2.0] oct-2-ene-2-carboxylic acid monohydrate:

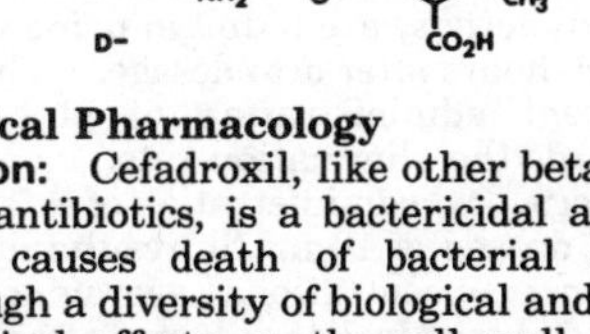

Clinical Pharmacology
Action: Cefadroxil, like other beta-lactam antibiotics, is a bactericidal agent that causes death of bacterial cells through a diversity of biological and biochemical effects on the cell wall. The spectrum of antibacterial activity includes many Gram-negative organisms since cefadroxil, like other cephalosporins, has the ability to penetrate the outer envelope of Gram-negative bacilli, thereby gaining access to cell wall target sites. Cefadroxil is generally not broken down by penicillinases such as those produced by penicillin-resistant staphylococci, although cephalosporinases have been identified that can inactivate the molecule.

Continued on next page

Bristol—Cont.

Microbiology: The effectiveness of CEFA-TABS (cefadroxil) in skin and soft tissue infections caused by **Staphylococcus aureus,** (including penicillin-resistant strains) and in urinary tract infections caused by **Staphylococcus aureus, Escherichia coli,** and **Proteus mirabilis,** has been demonstrated clinically in the dog. In cats the effectiveness of cefadroxil in skin and soft tissue infection caused by susceptible pathogens such as **Pasteurella multocida, Staphylococcus aureus, Staphylococcus epidermidis,** and **Streptococcus** spp. has also been demonstrated. In addition, cefadroxil has a broad spectrum of activity against both Gram-positive and Gram-negative human isolates. Although the clinical significance of **in vitro** data is unknown in the target species, the following human isolates are generally susceptible to cefadroxil at the indicated concentrations[1].

Organism (No. of Isolates)		Minimum Inhibitory Concentration (mcg/ml) Range	MIC_{90}*
Streptococcus pyogenes	(24)	0.063-0.125	0.11
Streptococcus agalactiae	(27)	0.25-1	0.92
Streptococcus pneumoniae	(29)	0.5-2	1.2
Staphylococcus aureus, penicillin sensitive	(16)	2-16	3.2
Staphylococcus aureus, penicillin resistant	(63)	1-32	6.2
Staphylococcus epidermidis	(28)	0.125-4	2.13
Escherichia coli	(59)	4->125	16.0
Proteus mirabilis	(62)	4->125	15.6
Klebsiella pneumoniae	(61)	4-16	7.85
Salmonella spp.	(22)	4-8	7.19
Shigella spp.	(12)	2-8	6.98
Pasteurella multocida	(2)		1.4

*Concentration at which 90% of the isolates are susceptible

The susceptibility of organisms to cefadroxil should be determined using the cephalosporin class disc, 30 mcg. Specimens for susceptibility testing should be collected prior to the initiation of antibiotic therapy.

Pharmacokinetics: Cefadroxil is stable in gastric acid and only moderately bound to serum proteins (approximately 20%). Cefadroxil is well absorbed from the gastrointestinal tract even when administered with food. The drug is excreted largely unchanged by the kidney. In humans, high concentrations of cefadroxil activity are found in urine within three hours after oral dosage.[2] The concurrent administration of probenecid retards the elimination rate.

In dogs, oral administration of cefadroxil at a dosage of 10 mg/lb results in peak serum concentrations averaging 18.6 mcg/ml within 1 to 2 hours after treatment.[3] The serum half life (T½) following oral administration is approximately 2 hours. Over 50% of an orally administered dose is excreted unchanged in the urine of dogs within 24 hours. Serum concentration time profiles in dogs following oral administration are illustrated graphically in Figure 1.

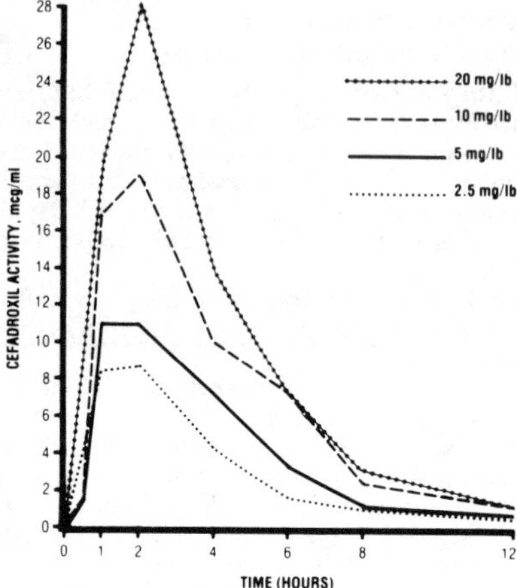

Figure 1: Cefadroxil Serum Concentration Curves in Dogs[3]

In cats, oral administration of cefadroxil at a dosage of 10 mg/lb results in mean peak serum concentrations of 17.4 mcg/ml within 1 to 2 hours after treatment. The serum half-life (T½) following oral administration to cats is 2½ to 3 hours. Serum concentration-time profiles in cats following oral administration are illustrated graphically in Figure 2.

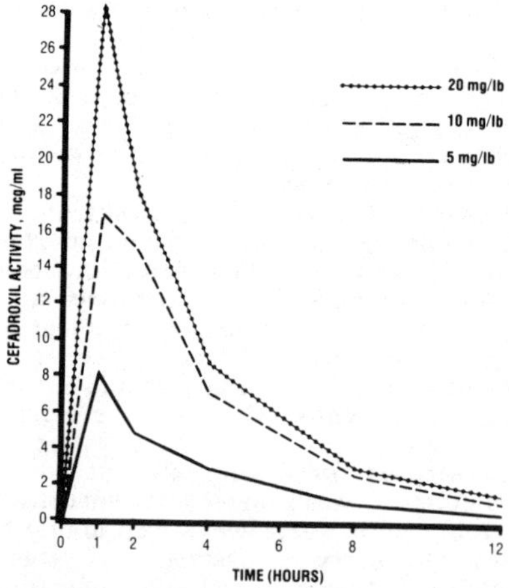

Figure 2: Cefadroxil Serum Concentration Curves in Cats

Indications: CEFA-TABS (cefadroxil) is indicated for the treatment of the following conditions:

Dogs: Genitourinary tract infections (cystitis) caused by susceptible strains of **Escherichia coli, Proteus mirabilis,** and **Staphylococcus aureus.**

Skin and soft tissue infections including cellulitis, pyoderma, dermatitis, wound infections and abscesses caused by susceptible strains of **Staphylococcus aureus.**

Cats: Skin and soft tissue infections including abscesses, wound infections, cellulitis and dermatitis caused by susceptible strains of **Pasteurella multocida, Staphylococcus aureus, Staphylococcus epidermidis,** and **Streptococcus** spp.

Contraindications: CEFA-TABS (cefadroxil) should not be administered to dogs or cats with a known allergy to cephalosporins. In penicillin-allergic animals, CEFA-TABS (cefadroxil) should be used with caution.

Warnings: For use in dogs and cats only. Not to be used in animals which are raised for food production. Safety for use in pregnant female dogs and cats or in breeding males has not been determined (see Animal Toxicology).

Animal Toxicology: The LD_{50} in the dog has been shown to be greater than 500 mg/kg following oral administration. In subacute studies, dogs administered 100, 200 or 400 mg/kg per day for 13 weeks showed no consistent or distinct treatment-related histopathologic changes. In chronic toxicity studies, dogs receiving doses as high as 600 mg/kg/day for six months showed no discernible treatment-related effects, with the exception of emesis in dogs receiving a 400 mg/kg/day dose at one time. No distinct or consistent meaningful drug-related changes in the hematologic, coagulation, or urinalysis test results or in histologic examination of tissues were observed when compared to controls.

In cats oral administration of cefadroxil at a dosage of 240 mg/kg/day divided into two equal doses (ten times the recommended daily dosage) for 21 consecutive days produced no clinical chemistry, pathological or other signs of toxicity other than reduced food consumption, vomiting and diarrhea.

No teratogenic or antifertility effects were seen in reproductive studies done in mice and rats receiving dosages as high as nine times the maximum recommended canine dosage.

Adverse Reactions: Occasional nausea and vomiting have been reported following CEFA-TABS (cefadroxil) therapy. Administration with food appears to decrease nausea. Diarrhea and lethargy have been occasionally reported.

Caution: Federal law restricts this drug to use by or on the order of a licensed veterinarian.

Dosage:

Dogs: CEFA-TABS (cefadroxil) should be administered orally at a dosage of 10 mg per pound of body weight twice daily. Dogs with skin or soft tissue infections

should be treated for a minimum of three days. Genitourinary tract infections should be treated for a minimum of seven days with cefadroxil. Maximum duration of therapy should not exceed 30 days.
Cats: CEFA-TABS (cefadroxil) should be administered orally at a dosage of 10 mg per pound body weight once daily. Maximum duration of therapy should not exceed 21 days.
In both species, drug treatment should continue for at least 48 hours after the animal is afebrile or asymptomatic. If no response is observed after three days of treatment, therapy should be discontinued and the case should be re-evaluated.
Supply: CEFA-TABS (cefadroxil) VETERINARY FILM-COATED TABLETS
NDC 0015-2350-80—50 mg tablets, bottles of 500
NDC 0015-2351-80—100 mg tablets, bottles of 500
NDC 0015-2352-70—200 mg tablets, bottles of 250
References:

1. Leitner, F., et al: Comparative antibacterial spectrum of cefadroxil. *J. Antimicrob. Chemother. 10, Suppl. B,* 1 (1982).
2. Hartstein, A. L., et al: Comparison of pharmacological and antimicrobial properties of cefadroxil and cephalexin. *Antimicrob. Agents Chemother.* 12, 93 (1977).
3. Gingerich, D. A.: Clinical pharmacology of the cephalosporins and their present use in veterinary medicine. *College of Veterinary Medicine Review,* Mississippi State University, 2, 93 (1982).

CENTRINE®
(aminopentamide hydrogen sulfate) Veterinary Injection and Tablets

Composition: Centrine® (aminopentamide hydrogen sulfate) is a potent antispasmodic agent. As a cholinergic blocking agent for smooth muscle, its action is similar to atropine.
Action: Centrine (aminopentamide hydrogen sulfate) effectively reduces the tone and amplitude of colonic contractions to a greater degree and for a more extended period than does atropine.
Centrine (aminopentamide hydrogen sulfate) effects a reduction in gastric secretion, a decrease in gastric acidity, and a marked decrease in gastric motility.
The mydriatic and salivary effects of Centrine (aminopentamide hydrogen sulfate) are less than those produced by atropine at similar dosage, permitting the control of vomiting and diarrhea with less distress to the animal due to dryness of the mouth and blurred vision.
Indications: Centrine (aminopentamide hydrogen sulfate) is indicated in the treatment of acute abdominal visceral spasm, pylorospasm or hypertrophic gastritis and associated nausea, vomiting and/or diarrhea.
Contraindications: Centrine (aminopentamide hydrogen sulfate) should not be used in animals with glaucoma because of the occurence of mydriasis.
Warning: For Use In Dogs and Cats Only.

Centrine Dosage Table Weight of Animal	Amount to be Administered Every 8 to 12 Hours		
	Dosage	Injectable Volume	Oral Tablets
10 lbs. or less	0.1 mg.	0.2 ml.	½ Tab.
11 lbs. to 20 lbs.	0.2 mg.	0.4 ml.	1 Tab.
21 lbs. to 50 lbs.	0.3 mg.	0.6 ml.	1½ Tabs.
51 lbs. to 100 lbs.	0.4 mg.	0.8 ml.	2 Tabs.
Over 100 lbs.	0.5 mg.	1.0 ml.	2½ Tabs.

Precautions: Dryness of the mouth is the most commonly reported side effect. Blurring of vision may occur and dryness of the eyes may occur if larger (greater than therapeutic) doses are used. Centrine (aminopentamide hydrogen sulfate) should be used cautiously, if at all, in pyloric obstruction because of its action in delaying gastric emptying. These effects frequently decrease with continued administration of the drug. Disturbances in urination are relatively infrequent. They vary from slight hesitancy in initiating urination to complete inability to urinate; the latter is an indication for discontinuing the drug. After a day or two, it may be resumed at a lower dosage level.
Dosage and Administration: Centrine (aminopentamide hydrogen sulfate) may be administered by subcutaneous or intramuscular injection or by oral tablets according to the following schedule. If the desired effect is not obtained, the dosage may be gradually increased up to a maximum of 5 times the doses listed. When the condition has been brought under control by parenteral medication, treatment can be continued, if desired, with 0.2-mg. scored tablets according to the dosage schedule. [See table above].
How Supplied: NDC 0015-2401-10—10 ml. vials Centrine (aminopentamide hydrogen sulfate) Veterinary Injection, 0.5 mg./ml.
NDC 0015-2400-60—0.2 mg. Centrine (aminopentamide hydrogen sulfate) Veterinary Tablets, bottles of 100.

DRY-CLOX®
(cloxacillin benzathine) For Intramammary Infusion into the Dry Cow

Composition: Dry-Clox® (cloxacillin benzathine) for Intramammary Infusion into the Dry Cow is a product which provides bactericidal activity against Gram-positive bacteria. The active agent, cloxacillin benzathine, is a sparingly soluble salt of the semisynthetic penicillin, cloxacillin. Cloxacillin is a derivative of 6-aminopenicillanic acid, and, therefore, is chemically related to other penicillins. It has however, the antibacterial properties described below, which distinguish it from certain other penicillins.
Each 10-ml. disposable syringe contains cloxacillin benzathine equivalent to 500 mg. of cloxacillin activity in a stable peanut-oil gel.
Action: In the non-lactating mammary gland Dry-Clox (cloxacillin benzathine) provides bactercidal levels of the active antibiotic, cloxacillin, for a prolonged period of time. This prolonged activity is due to the low solubility of the cloxacillin benzathine and to the slow-release oil-gel base. This prolonged contact between the antibiotic and the pathogenic organism enhances the probability of a bacteriological cure.
Cloxacillin is not destroyed by the enzyme, penicillinase, and therefore, is active against penicillin-resistant strains of *Staphylococcus aureus.* It is also active against non-penicillinase-producing *Staphylococcus aureus* as well as *Streptococcus agalactiae.*
The class disc, Methicillin 5 mcg., should be used to estimate the *in vitro* susceptibility of bacteria to cloxacillin.
Indications: For the treatment of mastitis in dairy cows during the dry period. Dry-Clox (cloxacillin benzathine) has been shown by extensive clinical studies to be efficacious in the treatment of mastitis in dry cows, when caused by *Streptococcus agalactiae,* and *Staphylococcus aureus,* including penicillin-resistant strains.
Treatment of the dry cow with Dry-Clox (cloxacillin benzathine) is indicated in any cow known to harbor any of these organisms in the udder at drying off, or which has had repeated attacks of mastitis during the previous lactation, or is affected with mastitis at drying off, if caused by susceptible organisms.
Dosage For Dry Cows: Infuse the contents of one syringe into each infected quarter following the last milking, or early in the dry period. See 'Directions for Use'.
Directions for Use: Dry-Clox (cloxacillin benzathine) is for use in dry cows only. Administer immediately after the last milking, or early in the dry period. *Use no later than 30 days prior to calving.* Completely milk out all four quarters. The udder and teats should be thoroughly washed with warm water containing a suitable dairy antiseptic and dried, preferably using individual paper towels. Carefully scrub the teat end and orifice with 70% alcohol, using a separate swab for each teat. *Allow to dry.* Remove the protective cap from the syringe, insert the teat tube fully into the orifice and expel the contents into the quarter. Withdraw the syringe and gently massage the quarter to distribute the medication.
Precautions: Because it is a derivative of 6-amino-penicillanic acid, Dry-Clox (cloxacillin benzathine) has the potential for producing allergic reactions. Such

Continued on next page

Bristol—Cont.

reactions are rare; however, should they occur, the subject should be treated with antihistamines or pressor amines, such as epinephrine.

B

Warnings:

1. For use in dry cows only.
2. Not to be used within 30 days of calving.
3. Any animal infused with this product must not be slaughtered for food until 30 days after the latest infusion.

Caution: Federal law restricts this drug to use by or on the order of a licensed veterinarian.

How Supplied: Dry-Clox (cloxacillin benzathine) for Intramammery Infusion into the dry cow. Cloxacillin benzathine equivalent to 500 mg cloxacillin activity per syringe.

NDC 0015-2722-10—one 10 ml syringe.

NDC 0015-2722-13—carton containing 12 × 10 ml syringes.

FLO-CILLIN®

(sterile penicillin G benzathine and penicillin G procaine in aqueous suspension)

Veterinary Injection

For veterinary use in beef cattle, horses and dogs.

Composition: Each milliliter of Flo-Cillin contains:

penicillin G benzathine	150,000 units
penicillin G procaine	150,000 units
sodium formaldehyde sulfoxylate	1.75 mg.
lecithin	11.70 mg.
methylparaben (as preservative)	1.20 mg.
propylparaben (as preservative)	0.14 mg.
Tween 40	8.91 mg.
Span 40	11.30 mg.
sodium citrate	3.49 mg.
procaine hydrochloride	20.00 mg.
sodium carboxymethyl-cellulose	1.04 mg.
povidone	3.12 mg.
water for injection	q.s.

Sodium hydroxide and/or hydrochloric acid may be added to adjust pH.

Action: Penicillin G is an antibiotic which shows a marked bactericidal effect against certain organisms during their growth phase. It is relatively specific in its action against Gram-positive bacteria but is usually ineffective against Gram-negative organisms.

When treating an animal for a bacterial infection, it is advisable to isolate and identify the causative organism and conduct appropriate *in vitro* susceptibility tests. In cases where organisms other than those susceptible to penicillin are present, re-evaluation of treatment should be made. Organisms normally considered susceptible to penicillin include *Clostridium septicum, Corynebacterium pyogenes, Staphylococcus aureus, Streptococcus canis, Streptococcus equi* and *Streptococcus pyogenes.*

It is normally recommended that any bacterial infection be treated as early as possible and with a dosage which will give effective blood levels. Although the recommended dosage of Flo-Cillin will give longer detectable penicillin blood levels than penicillin G procaine alone, it is recommended that a second dose be administered at 48 hours when treating a penicillin- susceptible bacterial infection.

If no definite improvement is noted following the second dose of Flo-Cillin, the diagnosis should be re- evaluated and use of another chemotherapeutic agent considered.

Indications: Flo-Cillin is indicated for treatment of the following bacterial infections in dogs, horses and beef cattle due to penicillin G susceptible micro-organisms that are susceptible to the serum levels common to this particular dosage form such as:

1. Bacterial Pneumonia *(Streptococcus spp., Corynebacterium pyogenes, Staphylococcus aureus)*
2. Upper Respiratory infections such as Rhinitis or Pharyngitis *(Corynebacterium pyogenes)*
3. Equine Strangles *(Streptococcus equi)*
4. Blackleg *(Clostridium chauvoei)*
5. Anthrax *(Bacillus anthracis)*
6. Prophylaxis of Bovine Shipping Fever in 300–500 pound beef cattle.

Contraindications: Flo-Cillin is contraindicated in patients which have shown hypersensitivity to pencillin.

Warning: Beef cattle should be withheld from slaughter for food for 30 days following last treatment. Treatment in beef cattle must be limited to two (2) doses. Not to be used in horses intended for food purposes.

Caution: Federal law restricts this drug to use by or on the order of a licensed veterinarian.

Adverse Reactions: Anaphylactic reactions have been reported in cattle given penicillin. Treated animals should be closely observed and if allergic or anaphylactic reactions occur, administer epinephrine or antihistamines immediately.

Administration: Flo-Cillin should be given by intramuscular injections to horses. In beef cattle the recommended dosage should be administered by *subcutaneous injection only.* Dogs may be injected by either the intramuscular or subcutaneous route.

Dosage: *Horses:* 2 ml per 150 lb body weight given intramuscularly (2,000 units penicillin G procaine and 2,000 units penicillin G benzathine per lb body weight). Treatment should be repeated in 48 hours.

Beef Cattle: 2 ml per 150 lb body weight given *subcutaneously only* (2,000 units procaine penicillin G and 2,000 units benzathine penicillin G per lb body weight). Treatment should be repeated in 48 hours.

IMPORTANT: Treatment in beef cattle should be limited to two (2) doses of Flo-Cillin, given by *subcutaneous injection only.*

Dogs: 1 ml per 10 to 25 lb body weight given intramuscularly or subcutaneously (6,000 to 15,000 units penicillin G procaine and 6,000 to 15,000 units penicillin G benzathine per lb body weight). Treatment should be repeated in 48 hours.

Shake the multiple-dose vial gently to avoid entrapped air bubbles before withdrawing the desired dose. Keep in a cool place—store below 15°C (59°C).

How Supplied: Flo-Cillin Veterinary Injection is supplied in multiple-dose vials of aqueous suspension. Each ml of suspension contains: 150,000 units of penicillin G benzathine and 150,000 units of penicillin G procaine.

NDC 0015-2016-52, 100 ml

NDC 0015-2020-59, 250 ml

HETACIN®–K

(hetacillin potassium)

For Intramammary Infusion

Composition: Hetacin-K (hetacillin potassium) is a broad-spectrum agent which provides bactericidal activity against a wide range of common Gram-positive and Gram-negative bacteria. It is derived from a 6-amino penicillanic acid and is chemically related to ampicillin.

Each 10-ml. disposable syringe contains hetacillin potassium equivalent to 62.5 mg. ampicillin activity in a stable peanut-oil gel.

Action: Hetacillin provides bactericidal levels of the active antibiotic, ampicillin. *In vitro* studies have demonstrated susceptibility of the following organisms to ampicillin: *Streptococcus agalactiae, Streptococcus dysgalactiae, Staphylococcus aureus* and *Escherichia coli.*

Indications: For Lactating Cows Only: For the treatment of acute, chronic or subclinical bovine mastitis. Hetacin-K for Intramammary Infusion should be used at the first signs of inflammation or at the first indication of any alteration in the milk. Subclinical infections should be treated immediately upon determining, by C.M.T. or other tests, that the leucocyte count is elevated, or that a susceptible pathogen has been cultured from the milk.

Hetacin-K for Intramammary Infusion has been shown to be efficacious in the treatment of mastitis in lactating cows caused by susceptible strains of *Streptococcus agalactiae, Streptococcus dysgalactiae, Staphylococcus aureus* and *Escherichia coli.*

Polycillin® (ampicillin) Susceptibility Test Discs, 10 mcg., should be used to estimate the *in vitro* susceptibility of bacteria to hetacillin.

Dosage and Administration: Infuse the entire contents of one syringe into each infected quarter. Repeat at 24-hour intervals until a maximum of three treatments has been given.

If definite improvement is not noted within 48 hours after treatment, the causal organism should be further investigated.

Precautions: Because it is a derivative of 6-aminopenicillanic acid, Hetacin-K (hetacillin potassium) has the potential for producing allergic reactions. Such reactions are rare; however, should they occur, treatment should be discontinued and the subject treated with the usual

agents antihistamines, pressor amines such as Epinephrine, or corticosteroids. The drug does not resist destruction by penicillinase and, hence, is not effective against strains of staphylococcus resistant to penicillin G.
Warning: Milk that has been taken from animals during treatment and for 72 hours (6 milkings) after the latest treatment must not be used for food. Treated animals must not be slaughtered for food until 10 days after the latest treatment.
Caution: Federal law restricts this drug to use by or on the order of a licensed veterinarian.
How Supplied: Hetacin-K (hetacillin potassium) for Intramammary Infusion. Hetacillin potassium equivalent to 62.5 mg. ampicillin activity per syringe.
NDC 0015-2713-10—one 10-ml. syringe.
NDC 0015-2713-13—Carton containing 12 × 10-ml. syringes.

HETACIN®-K
(hetacillin potassium)
Veterinary Film-Coated Tablets/Oral Liquid

Composition: Hetacin-K (hetacillin potassium) is a new broad-spectrum agent which provides bactericidal activity against a wide range of common Gram-positive and Gram-negative bacteria. It is derived from 6- aminopenicillanic acid and is chemically related to ampicillin.
Action: Hetacillin provides bactericidal levels of the active antibiotic, ampicillin. Following administration, hetacillin is found in the blood as hetacillin, as well as in the form of its hydrolysis product, ampicillin. The rate of hydrolysis varies depending upon pH and route of administration. The antibacterial spectrum provided by hetacillin is identical to that of ampicillin. This drug is stable in the presence of gastric acid, and peak serum levels in dogs and cats are reached approximately one hour following the recommended oral dose.
In vitro studies have demonstrated susceptibility of the following organisms to ampicillin: Gram-positive bacteria—alpha-and beta-hemolytic streptococci, staphylococci (non-penicillinase-producing), Bacillus anthracis, and most strains of enterococci and clostridia; Gram-negative bacteria—*Proteus mirabilis, E. coli,* and many strains of Salmonella, and *Pasteurella multocida.*
The drug does not resist destruction by penicillinase and, hence, is not effective against strains of staphylococcus resistant to penicillin G. Polycillin® (ampicillin) Susceptibility Test Disc, 10 mcg., should be used to estimate the *in vitro* susceptibility of bacteria to hetacillin.
Indications: Hetacin-K (hetacillin potassium) has proved effective in the treatment of many infections previously beyond the spectrum of penicillin therapy. This drug is particularly indicated in the treatment of susceptible strains of organisms causing the following infections:
Respiratory-Tract Infections: upper respiratory infections, tonsillitis, and bronchopneumonia due to hemolytic streptococci, *Staphylococcus aureus. Escherichia coli, Proteus mirabilis,* and *Pasteurella* spp.
Urinary-Tract Infections due to *Proteus mirabilis, Escherichia coli, Staphylococcus* spp., hemolytic streptococci and *Enterococcus* spp.
Gastrointestinal Infections due to *Enterococcus* spp., *Staphylococcus* spp., and *Escherichia coli.*
Skin, Soft-Tissue, and Post-Surgical Infections: abscesses, pustular dermatitis, cellulitis, infections of the anal gland, etc., due to *Escherchia coli, Proteus mirabilis,* hemolytic streptococci, *Staphylococcus* spp., and *Pasteurella* spp.
Contraindications: A history of allergic reactions to penicillin, cephalosporins, or their analogues should be considered a contraindication for the use of this agent.
Precautions: Because it is a derivative of 6-amino-penicillanic acid, Hetacin-K (hetacillin potassium) has the potential for producing allergic reactions. Such reactions are rare with oral therapy; however, if they should occur, Hetacin-K (hetacillin poatssium) should be discontinued and the subject treated with the usual agents (antihistamines, pressor amines, corticosteroids).
Intravenous administration of potassium hetacillin in doses in excess of 5 mg./kg. has been noted to enhance the vasopressor effect of epinephrine in dogs.
Oral forms of the drug should be administered in a fasting state to ensure maximum absorption.
Warning: For use in dogs and cats only. Not to be used in animals which are raised for food production.
Caution: Federal law restricts this drug to use by or on the order of a licensed veterinarian.
Adverse Reactions: Slightly softer than normal stools have been noted shortly after dosing dogs with single oral doses of 3000 mg./kg.
Dosage: The dosage of Hetacin-K (hetacillin potassium) will vary according to the animal being treated, the severity of the infection, and the animal's response.
The minimum recommended dose for dogs is 5 mg. per pound of body weight administered twice daily.
In severe infections involving respiratory tract, gastrointestinal tract, skin, soft tissue, or those infections following surgery, the frequency of the dosage may be increased to three times daily or, alternatively, larger doses of up to 10 mg. per pound of body weight may be administered on a twice-daily schedule.
For stubborn urinary-tract infections, the dose may be increased to 20 mg. per pound of body weight twice-daily.
The recommmended dose for cats is 50 mg. twice daily.
Treatment should be continued for 48 to 72 hours after the animal has become afebrile or asymptomatic. The oral drug should be adminstered 1 to 2 hours prior to feeding to ensure maximum absorption. In stubborn infections, therapy may be required for several weeks.
Note: The oral liquid should be shaken well before the desired dose is poured.
How Supplied: Hetacin-K (hetacillin potassium) Veterinary Film-Coated Tablets or Oral Liquid. Hetacillin potassium equivalent to 50 mg., 100 mg., and 200 mg. of ampicillin activity per tablet in bottles of 100 and 500.
Oral Liquid—Hetacillin potassium equivalent to 50 mg., of ampicillin activity per milliliter in 10 ml. dropper bottles and pint bottles.

B

KANTRIM®
(kanamycin sulfate)
Veterinary Injection

Composition: Kanamycin is a water-soluble antibiotic produced through fermentation by *Streptomyces kanamyceticus.* Kantrim (kanamycin sulfate) Veterinary Injection is supplied as an aqueous solution of kanamycin sulfate, buffered with sodium citrate, preserved with methylparaben, propylparaben, sodium bisulfite, and sulfuric acid used to adjust pH. Kanamycin is active against many Gram-negative pathogens. These include coliforms, Aerobacter, Salmonella, strains of Proteus, Neisseria, *Pasteurella multocida,* and Mima. Kanamycins Gram-positive spectrum includes corynebacteria. *Bacillus anthracis, Staphylococcus albus,* and *Staphylococcus aureus* —including many strains resistant to other antibiotics. Bactericidal serum concentrations are obtained by average dosage. Bacterial resistance to kanamycin develops slowly among most susceptible organisms so far tested, particularly among the staphylococci.
Action: The drug is rapidly absorbed after subcutaneous or intramuscular injection. Peak serum levels are obtained approximately one hour after injection. Kanamycin diffuses readily into most body fluids (synovial fluid, bile, pleural and peritoneal fluids, bronchial secretions) but, under normal circumstances, poorly into spinal fluid. Kanamycin is poorly absorbed following oral administration. Systemic infections are preferably treated by subcutaneous injection; the drug may also be administered intramuscularly. Excretion of the drug is almost entirely by glomerular filtration. Virtually no tubular reabsorption of the drug occurs so that high concentrations are reached within the renal tubules. Renal excretion is rapid, approximately one-half of the injected dose clears the kidney within four hours in subjects with normal renal function, and excretion is complete in 24 to 48 hours. Subjects with impaired renal function excrete kanamycin much more slowly—roughly in proportion to the extent of renal damage, and such subjects must be well hydrated. Excessive accumulation of the drug greatly increases the risk of ototoxicity.
Indications: This drug has been used successfully in the treatment of bacterial infections due to kanamycin-susceptible organisms. Among these infections are:

Continued on next page

Bristol—Cont.

B

Urinary—Tract Infections: acute and chronic cystitis, nephritis, pyelonephritis, and prostatitis.
Respiratory—Tract Infections: sinusitis, tracheitis, lobar- and bronchopneumonia, lung abscesses, and tonsillitis.
Bacterial Complications of Canine Distemper, and Feline Pneumonitis.
Skin, Soft-Tissue, and Post-Surgical Infections: abscesses, wound infections, cellulitis, pustular dermatitis.
Osteomyelitis, Septic Arthritis, Periostitis, Septicemia, and Bacteremia.
Gastrointestinal Infections: amebiasis, salmonellosis, gastroenteritis, and staphylococcal enterocolitis.
Endometritis—Mastitis—Otitis Media-Pancreatitis.
While nearly all strains of *Staphylococcus aureus,* and the majority of strains of Proteus, *E. coli,* and *A. aerogenes* are highly suspectible to kanamycin, the invading organisms should be cultured and its susceptibility demonstrated as a guide to therapy.

Warning: In subjects with normal renal function, when recommended precautions and dosage are followed, the incidence of toxic reactions is negligible. However, prolonged use of this antibiotic at doses in excess of those recommended may result in:

a) Ototoxicity from damage to both cochlear and vestibular portions of the auditory nerve. Such damage can be minimized by immediate withdrawal of the drug as soon as any evidence of eighth nerve injury (ataxia, incoordination) is noticed. In cats, weight loss often precedes ototoxicity.
b) Renal injury as evidenced by urinary sediments observed by pyuria, hematuria, proteinuria and cylindruria, which frequently cease shortly after kanamycin therapy is stopped. Older patients and those with renal insufficiency show increased rates of kanamycin-related renal injury as is also the case with ototoxicity. Subjects should be thoroughly hydrated to reduce kanamycin levels in the nephron as much as possible.

When injected intramuscularly, Kanamycin may cause moderately severe but transient pain

For Use in Dogs and Cats Only.

Contraindications: Kanamycin should not be used following high doses or prolonged therapy with other antibiotics that may cause similar toxic reactions, e.g., streptomycin, neomycin. A history of allergic response to this drug is a contraindication. The use of concurrent drugs, other than analgesics, is not recommended. Do not administer to subjects undergoing general anesthesia.

Dosage: The usual dose is 5 mg per lb of body weight per day in equally divided doses at 12-hour intervals (see dosage table below). Kanamycin preferably should be administered by subcutaneous injection, but may be given by the intramuscular route if desired. The remarks regarding excessive dosage under **WARNING** should be noted. If definite clinical response dose not occur within five days, therapy should be stopped and the antibiotic susceptibility pattern of the pathgogenic organism rechecked. Failure of the infection to respond may be due to the presence of a resistant organism or septic foci requiring surgical drainage.

DOG and CAT DOSAGE GUIDE
Amount to be given every 12 hours
VIAL CONCENTRATION 50 mg/ml

Weight in lbs	Dosage every 12 hrs in mg	Dosage every 12 hrs in ml
2	5 mg	0.1 ml
4	10 mg	0.2 ml
6	15 mg	0.3 ml
8	20 mg	0.4 ml
10	25 mg	0.5 ml
15	37.5 mg	0.75 ml
20	50 mg	1.0 ml
25	65.5 mg	1.25 ml
30	75 mg	1.5 ml
35	87.5 mg	1.75 ml
40	100 mg	2.0 ml
45	112.5 mg	2.25 ml
50	125 mg	2.5 ml

How Supplied: Kantrim® (kanamycin sulfate) Veterinary Injection, 50 mg per ml.
NDC 0015-2014-50—2.5 Grams in 50 ml. Vial.

DOG and CAT DOSAGE GUIDE
Amount to be Given every 12 hours
VIAL CONCENTRATION 200 mg/ml

Weight in lbs	Dosage every 12 hrs in mg	Dosage every 12 hrs in ml
20	50 mg	0.25 ml
40	100 mg	0.5 ml
60	150 mg	0.75 ml
80	200 mg	1.0 ml
100	250 mg	1.25 ml
120	300 mg	1.5 ml

How Supplied: Kantrim® (kanamycin sulfate) Veterinary Injection, 200 mg per ml.
NDC 0015-2015-50—10.0 Grams in 50 ml Vial.
Unopened vials may occasionally darken during storage. This change of color does not affect potency.

KETASET®
(ketamine hydrochloride) Veterinary Injection For Intramuscular Use

Composition: Ketaset® (ketamine hydrochloride) is a rapid-acting non-narcotic, nonbarbiturate agent for anesthetic use in cats and for restraint in subhuman primates. It is chemically designated dl (2-o-chlorophenyl)-2-(methylamino) cyclohexanone hydrochloride and is supplied as a slightly acid (pH 3.5 to 5.5) solution for intramuscular injection in a concentration containing the equivalent of 100 mg ketamine base per ml and contains 0.1 mg/ml benzethonium chloride as a preservative.

Action: Ketaset (ketamine hydrochloride) is a rapid-acting agent whose pharmacologic action is characterized by profound analgesia, normal pharyngeal-laryngeal reflexes, mild cardiac stimulation and respiratory depression. Muscle tone is variable in that it may be normal, enhanced or diminished. The anesthetic state produced does not fit into the conventional classification of stages of anesthesia; but instead, Ketaset (ketamine hydrochloride) produces a state of unconsciousness which has been termed "dissociative" anesthesia in that it appears to selectively interrupt association pathways to the brain before producing somesthetic sensory blockade.
In contrast to other anesthetics, protective reflexes, such as coughing and swallowing, are maintained under ketamine anesthesia. The degree of muscle tone is dependent upon level of dose; therefore, variations in body temperature may occur. At low dosage levels there may be an increase in muscle tone and a concomitant slight increase in body temperature. However, at high dosage levels there is some diminution in muscle tone and a resultant decrease in body temperature, to the point where supplemental heat may be advisable.
In cats, there is usually some transient cardiovascular stimulation, increased cardiac output with slight increase in mean systolic pressure, with little or no change in total peripheral resistance. At higher doses respiratory rate is usually decreased.
The assurance of a patent airway is greatly enhanced by virtue of maintained pharyngeal-laryngeal reflexes. Although some salivation is occasionally noted, the persistence of the swallowing reflex aids in minimizing the hazards associated with excessive salivation. Salivation may be effectively controlled with atropine sulfate in dosages of 0.04 mg/kg (0.02 mg/lb) in cats and 0.01 to 0.05 mg/kg (0.005 to 0.025 mg/lb) in subhuman primates.
Other reflexes, e.g., corneal, pedal, etc., are maintained during ketamine anesthesia and should not be used as criteria for judging depth of anesthesia. The eyes normally remain open with the pupil dilated. It is suggested that a bland ophthalmic ointment be applied to the cornea if anesthesia is to be prolonged.
Following administration of recommended doses, cats become ataxic in about 5 minutes, with anesthesia usually lasting from 30 to 45 minutes at higher doses. At the lower doses, complete recovery usually occurs in 4 to 5 hours, but with higher doses recovery time is more prolonged and may be as long as 24 hours.
In studies involving 14 species of subhuman primates, represented by at least ten episodes for each species, the median time to restraint ranged from 1.5 [(*Aotus trivigatus* (night monkey) and *Cebus capunchinus* (white-throated capuchin)] to 5.3 minutes [(*Macaca nemestrina* (pig-tailed macaque)]. The median duration of restraint ranged between 20 and 55 minutes in all but five of the species studied. Total time from injection to end of restraint ranged from 43 [(*Saimiri sciureus* (squirrel monkey) to 183 minutes (*macaca nemestrina* (pig-tailed macaque)] after injection. Recovery is generally smooth and uneventful. The duration is dose related.

By single intramuscular injection, Ketaset (ketamine hydrochloride) usually has a wide margin of safety in cats and subhuman primates. In cats, cases of prolonged recovery and death have been reported.

Indications: Ketaset (ketamine hydrochloride) may be used in cats for restraint or as the sole anesthetic agent for diagnostic or minor, brief surgical procedures that do not require skeletal muscle relaxation. It may be used in subhuman primates for restraint.

Warning: For Use in Cats and Subhuman Primates Only.

Ketaset (ketamine hydrochloride) is detoxified by the liver and excreted by the kidneys; therefore, it is not recommended for use in cats and subhuman primates suffering from renal or hepatic insufficiency.

Precautions: In cats, doses in excess of 23 mg/lb (50 mg/kg) during any single procedure should not be used. The maximum recommended dose in subhuman primates is 40 mg/kg.

To reduce the incidence of emergence reactions, animals should not be stimulated by sound or handling during the recovery period. However, this dose not preclude the monitoring of vital signs.

Adverse Reactions: Respitatory depression may occur following administration of high doses of Ketaset (ketamine hydrochloride). If at any time respiration becomes excessively depressed and the animal becomes cyanotic, resuscitative measures should be instituted promptly. Adeqaute pulmonary ventilation with either oxygen or room air are recommended resuscitative measures.

Adverse reactions reported have included emesis, salivation, vocalization, erratic and prolonged recovery, dyspnea, spastic jerking movements, convulsions, muscular tremors, hypertonicity, opisthotonos and cardiac arrest. In the cat, myoclonic jerking and/or mild tonic convulsions can be controlled by ultrashort-acting barbiturates or acepromazine. *These latter drugs must be given intravenously, cautiously and slowly, to effect (approximately 1/6 to 1/4 the normal dose may be required).*

Dosage and Administration: Ketaset (ketamine hydrochloride) is well tolerated by cats and subhuman primates when administered by intramuscular injection.

Fasting prior to induction of anesthesia or restraint with Ketaset (ketamine hydrochloride) is not essential; however, when preparing for elective surgery, it is advisable to withhold food for at least six hours prior to administration of Ketaset (ketamine hydrochloride).

Anesthesia may be of shorter duration in immature cats. Restraint in subhuman primate neonates (less than 24 hours of age) is difficult to achieve.

As with other anesthetic agents, the individual response to Ketaset (ketamine hydrochloride) is somwehat varied, depending upon the dose, general condition and age of the subject, so that dosage recommendations cannot be absolutely fixed.

Dosage: Cats: A dose of 11 mg/kg (5 mg/lb) is recommended to achieve restraint. Dosages from 22 to 33 mg/kg (10 to 15 mg/lb) produces anesthesia that is suitable for diagnostic or minor surgical procedures that do not require skeletal muscle relaxation.

Subhuman Primates: The recommended restraint dosages of Ketaset (ketamine hydrochloride) for the following species are: *Cercocebus torquatus* (white-collard mangebey), *Papio cynocephalus* (yellow baboon), *Pan troglodytes verus* (chimpanzee), *Papio anubis* (olive baboon), *Pongo pygmaeus* (orangutan), *Macaca nemestrina* (pig-tailed macaque), 5 to 7.5 mg/kg; *Presbytis entellus* (entellus languar), 3 to 5 mg/kg; *Gorill gorilla gorilla* (gorilla), 7 to 10 mg/kg; *Aotus Trivigatus* (night monkey), 10 to 12 mg/kg; *Macaca mulatta* (rhesus monkey), 5 to 10 mg/kg: *Cebus capucinus* (white-throated capuchin), 13 to 15 mg/kg; and *Macaca fascicularis* (crab-eating macaque), *Macaca radiata* (bonnet macaque) and *Saimiri sciureus* (squirrel monkey), 12 to 15 mg/kg.

A single intramuscular injection of the recommended dose of ketase (ketamine hydrochloride) achieves a level of restraint suitable for T.B. testing, radiography, physical examination or blood collection.

Clinical Studies: Ketaset (ketamine hydrochloride) has been clinically studied in subhuman primates in addition to those species listed under "Dosage and Administration". Doses for restraint in these additional species, based on limited clinical data, are: *Cercopithecus aethiops* (grivet), *Papio papio* (guinea baboon), 10 to 12 mg/kg; *Erythrocebus patus patus* (patus monkey), 3 to 5 mg/kg; *Hylobates lar* (white-handed gibbon), 5 to 10 mg/kg; *Lemur catta* (ringtailed lemur), 7.5 to 10 mg/kg; *Macaca fuscata* (Japanese macaque), 5 mg/kg; *Macaca speciosa* (stump-tailed macaque), *Miopithecus talapoin* (Mangrove monkey), 5 to 7.5 mg/kg; and *symphalangus syndactylus* (siamangs), 5 to 7 mg/kg.

How Supplied: Ketaset (ketamine hydrochloride) is supplied as the hydrochloride in multi-dose vials of a solution containing 100 mg/ml ketamine (as base equivalent.)

NDC 0015-2012-10—vial 10 ml.

POLYFLEX®
(sterile ampicillin for suspension, veterinary) for Aqueous Injection

Composition: Polyflex (sterile ampicillin for suspension, veterinary) is a broad-spectrum penicillin which has bactericidal activity against a wide range of common Gram-positive and Gram-negative bacteria.

Action: The antimicrobial action of ampicillin is bactericidal, and only a small percentage of the antibiotic is serum-bound. Peak serum levels in dogs and cats are reached approximately one-half hour following subcutaneous or intramuscular injection, and in cattle 1 hour to 2 hours following intramuscular injection.

In vitro studies have demonstrated sensitivity of the following organisms to ampicillin: Gram-positive bacteria—alpha- and beta-hemolytic streptococci, staphylococci (Non-penicillinase-producing), *Bacillus anthracis,* and most strains of enterococci and clostridia; Gram-negative bacteria—*Proteus mirabilis, E. coli* and many strains of Salmonella, and *Pasteurella multocida.*

The drug does not resist destruction by penicillinase and, hence, is not effective against strains of staphylococcus resistant to penicillin G. Susceptibility tests should be conducted to estimate the in vitro susceptibility of bacterial isolates to ampicillin.

Indications: Polyflex (sterile ampicillin for suspension, veterinary) has proved effective in the treatment of many infections previously beyond the spectrum of penicillin therapy. This drug is particularly indicated in the treatment of the following infections caused by susceptible strains of organisms.

Dogs and cats—Respiratory-Tract infections: Upper respiratory infections, tonsillitis and bronchopneumonia due to hemolytic streptococci, *Staphylococcus aureus, Escherichia coli, Proteus mirabilis,* and *Pasteurella* spp.

Urinary-Tract infections due to *Proteus mirabilis, Escherichia coli, Staphylococcus* spp., hemolytic streptococci, and *Enterococcus* spp.

Gastrointestinal infections due to *Enterococcus* spp., *Staphylococcus* spp., and *Escherichia coli.*

Skin, soft-tissue, and post-surgical infections: Abscesses, pustular dermatitis, cellulitis and infections of the anal gland, due to *Escherichia coli, Proteus mirabilis,* hemolytic streptococci, *Staphylococcus* spp., and *Pasteurella* spp.

Cattle—Respiratory-Tract infections: Bacterial pneumonia (shipping fever, calf pneumonia, and bovine pneumonia) cause by *Aerobacter* spp., *Klebiella* spp., *Staphylococcus* spp., *Streptococcus* spp., *Pasteurella multocida* and *E. coli* susceptible to ampicillin trihydrate.

Containdications: A history of allergic reactions to penicillin, cephalosporins, or their analogues should be considered a contraindication for the use of this agent.

Precautions: Because it is a derivative of 6-amino-penicillanic acid, Polyflex (sterile ampicillin for suispension, veterinary) has the potential for producing allergic reactions. If they should occur, Polyflex (sterile ampicillin for suspension, veterinary) should be discontinued and the subject treated with the usual agents (antihistamines, pressor aminies, corticosteroids.

Warning: Do not treat for more than 7 days.

Milk from treated cows must not be used for food during treatment, or for 48 hours (4 milkings) after last treatment.

Treated animals must not be slaughtered for food during treatment, or for 144 hours (6 days) after the last treatment.

Continued on next page

Bristol—Cont.

Caution: Federal law restricts this drug to use by or on the order of a licensed veterinarian.

Dosage and Administration: The dosage of Polyflex (sterile ampicillin for suspension, veterinary) will vary according to the animal being treated, the severity of the infection, and the animal's response.

Dogs and cats—The recommended dose for dogs or cats is 3 mg per pound of body weight administered twice daily by subcutaneous or intramuscular injection.

Cattle—From 2 mg to 5 mg per pound of body weight once daily by intramuscular injection. Do not treat for more than 7 days.

In all species, three days treatment is usually adequate, but treatment should be continued for 48 to 72 hours after the animal has become afebrile or asymptomatic.

Directions for Use: The multiple-dose dry-filled vials should be reconstituted to the desired concentration by adding the required amount of Sterile Water for Injection, U.S.P., according to label directions.

After reconstitution this product is stable for 12 months under refrigeration or for 3 months at 25°C.

At the time of reconstitution the vial should be dated and the concentration noted on the label.

How Supplied: NDC 0015-2013-52—Polyflex (sterile ampicillin for suspension, veterinary). For Aqueous Injection—vial containing 10.0 grams Ampicillin activity as Ampicillin Trihydrate. NDC 0015-2718-53—Polyflex (sterile ampicillin for suspension, veterinary). For Aqueous Injection—vial containing 25.0 grams Ampicillin activity as Ampicillin Trihydrate.

TORBUGESIC®
butorphanol tartrate
VETERINARY INJECTION

Description: Butorphanol tartrate is a totally synthetic, centrally acting, narcotic agonist-antagonist analgesic with potent antitussive activity. It is a member of the phenanthrene series. The chemical name is Morphinan-3, 14-diol, 17-(cyclobutylmethyl)-, (-)-, (S-(R*, R*))-2, 3-dihydroxybutanedioate (1:1) (salt). It is a white crystalline, water soluble substance having a molecular weight of 477.55; its molecular formula is $C_{21}H_{29}NO_2 \cdot C_4H_6O_6$.

Chemical Structure:

Each ml of TORBUGESIC contains 10 mg butorphanol base (as tartrate), 3.3 mg citric acid, USP, 6.4 mg sodium citrate, USP, 4.7 mg sodium chloride, A.R., 0.1 mg benzethonium chloride, USP, q.s. with water for injection, USP.

Clinical Pharmacology

Comparative Pharmacology

In animals, butorphanol has been demonstrated to be 4 to 30 times more potent than morphine and pentazocine (Talwin) respectively.[1] In humans, butorphanol has been shown to have 5 to 7 times the analgesic activity of morphine and 20 times that of pentazocine.[2,3] Butorphanol has 15 to 20 times the oral antitussive activity of codeine or dextromethorphan in dogs and guinea pigs.[4]

As an antagonist, butorphanol is approximately equivalent to nalorphine and 30 times more potent than pentazocine.[1]

Cardiopulmonary depressant effects are minimal after treatment with butorphanol as demonstrated in dogs[5], humans[6,7] and horses.[8] Unlike classical narcotic agonist analgesics which are associated with decreases in blood pressure, reduction in heart rate, and concomitant release of histamine, butorphanol does not cause histamine release.[1] Furthermore, the cardiopulmonary effects of butorphanol are not distinctly dosage related but rather reach a ceiling effect beyond which further dosage increases result in relatively lesser effects.

Reproduction: Studies performed in mice and rabbits revealed no evidence of impaired fertility or harm to the fetus due to butorphanol tartrate. In the female rate, parenteral administration was associated with increased nervousness and decreased care for the newborn, resulting in a decreased survival rate of the newborn. This nervousness was seen only in the rat species.

Equine Pharmacology

Following intravenous injection in horses, butorphanol is largely eliminated from the blood within 3 to 4 hours. The drug is extensively metabolized in the liver and excreted in the urine.

In ponies, butorphanol given intramuscularly at a dosage of 0.22 mg/kg, was shown to alleviate experimentally induced visceral pain for about 4 hours.[9]

In horses, intravenous dosages of butorphanol ranging from 0.05 to 0.4 mg/kg were shown to be effective in alleviating visceral and superficial pain for at least four hours, as illustrated in the following figure:

Analgesic Effects of Butorphanol Given at Various Dosages in Horses with Abdominal Pain

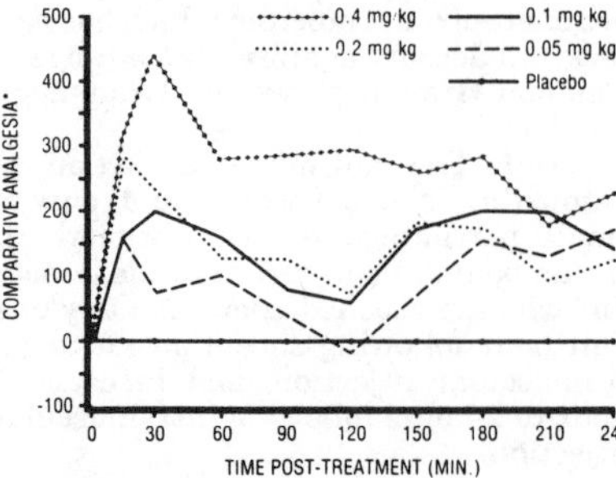

*Pain threshold in butorphanol-treated collicky horses relative to placebo controls.

A definite dosage-response relationship was detected in that butorphanol dosage of 0.1 mg/kg was more effective than 0.05 mg/kg but not different from 0.2 mg/kg in alleviating deep abdominal pain.

Acute Equine Studies

Rapid intravenous, administration of butorphanol at a dosage of 2.0 mg/kg (20 times the recommended dosage) to a previously unmedicated horse resulted in a brief episode of inability to stand, muscle fasciculation, a convulsive seizure of 6 seconds duration, and recovery within three minutes. The same dosage administered after 10 successive daily 1.0 mg/kg dosages of butorphanol resulted only in transient sedative effects. During the 10 day course of administration at 1.0 mg/kg (10 times the recommended use level) in two horses, the only detectable drug effects were transient behavioral changes typical of narcotic agonist activity. These included muscle fasciculation about the head and neck, dysphoria, lateral nystagmus, ataxia, and salivation. Repeated administration of butorphanol at 1.0 mg/kg (10 times the recommended dose) every four hours for 48 hours caused constipation in one of two horses.

Subacute Equine Studies

Horses were found to tolerate butorphanol given intravenously at dosages of 0.1, 0.3, and 0.5 mg/kg every 4 hours for 48 hours followed by once daily injections for a total of 21 days. The only detectable drug effects were slight transient ataxia observed occasionally in the high dosage group. No clinical, laboratory, or gross or histopathologic evidence of any butorphanol-related toxicity was encountered in the horses.

Indications: TORBUGESIC (butorphanol tartrate) is indicated for the relief of pain associated with colic in adult horses and yearlings. Clinical studies in the horse have shown that TORBUGESIC (butorphanol tartrate) alleviates abdominal pain associated with torsion, impaction, intussusception, spasmodic and tympanic colic, and post partum pain.

Warnings: NOT FOR USE IN HORSES INTENDED FOR FOOD. NOT FOR HUMAN USE.

Caution: TORBUGESIC (butorphanol tartrate), a potent analgesic, should be used with caution with other sedative or analgesic drugs as these are likely to produce additive effects.

There are no well controlled studies using butorphanol in breeding horses, weanlings, and foals. Therefore the drug should not be used in these groups.

Adverse Reactions: In clinical trials in horses, the most commonly observed side effect was slight ataxia which lasted 3 to 10 minutes. Marked ataxia was reported in 1.5% of the 327 horses treated. Mild sedation was reported in 9% of the horses.

Dosage: The recommended dosage in the horse in 0.1 mg of butorphanol per kilogram of body weight (0.05 mg/lb) by intravenous injection. This is equivalent to 5 ml of TORBUGESIC (butorphanol tartrate) for each 1000 lbs body weight. The dose may be repeated within 3 to 4 hours but treatment should not exceed 48 hours. Pre-clinical model studies and clinical field trials in horses demonstrate that the analgesic effects of TORBUGESIC (butorphanol tartrate) are seen within 15 minutes following injection and persist for about 4 hours.

Supply: NDC 0015-2033-20—50 ml vials TORBUGESIC (butorphanol tartrate) Veterinary Injection, 10 mg base activity per ml.

CAUTION: Federal law restricts this drug to use by or on the order of a licensed veterinarian.

References

1. Pircio, A. W. *et al:* The Pharmacology of Butorphanol. *Arch Int Pharmacodyn Ther* 220(2): 231–257, 1976.
2. Dobkin, A.B. *et al:* Butorphanol and Pentazocine in Patients with severe Postoperative pain. *Clin Pharmacol Ther* 18: 547–553, 1975.
3. Gilbert, M.S. *et al:* Intramuscular Butorphanol and Meperidine in Postoperative Pain. *Clin Pharmacol Ther* 20: 359–364, 1976.
4. Cavanagh, R.L. *et al:* Antitissue Properties of Butorphanol, *Arch Int Pharmacodyn Ther* 220: 258–268, 1976.
5. Shurig, J.E. *et al:* Effect of Butorphanol and Morphine on Pulmonary Mechanics, Arterial Blood Pressure, and Venous Plasma Histamine in the Anesthesized Dog. *Arch Int Pharmacodyn Ther* 233: 296–304. 1978.
6. Nagashmina, H. *et al:* Respiratory and Circulatory Effects of Intravenous Butorphanol and Morphine. *Clin. Pharm. Ther.* 19: 735–745, 1976.
7. Popio, K.A., *et al:* Hemodynamic and Respiratory Effects of Morphine and Butorphanol. *Clin. Pharm. Ther.* 23:281–287, 1978.
8. Robertson, J.T. and Muir, W.W.: Cardiopulmonary Effects of Butorphanol Tartrate in Horses. *Am J. Vet. Res.* 42: 41–44, 1981.
9. Kalpravidh, M., *et al:* Effects of Butorphanol, Flunixin, Levorphanol, Morphine, Pentazocine and Xylazine in Ponies. *Am J. Vet. Res.* 45: 217–223, 1984.

TORBUTROL®
(butorphanol tartrate)
Veterinary Injection and Tablets

Description: Torbutrol (butorphanol tartrate) is a narcotic antagonist analgesic with potent antitussive activity. It is a member of the phenanthrene series. The chemical name is levo-N-cyclo-butylmethyl-6, 10 α, β-dihydroxy-1,2,3,9,10, 10α-hexahydro-(4H)-10,4a-iminoethanophenanthrene tartrate (1:1). It is a white-crystalline water substance having a molecular weight of 477.56, and its molecular formula is $C_{21}H_{29}NO_2 \cdot C_4H_6O_6$.

Chemical Structure:

[See Formula at top of next column]

HO OH N-CH$_2$ $\cdot C_4H_6O_6$

Clinical Pharmacology: In dogs, the antitussive properties of butorphanol given s.c. were four times more potent than morphine, 10 times more potent than pentazocine, and 100 times more potent than codeine.

Orally butorphanol is approximately 15 to 20 times more active than either codeine or dextromethorphan[1].

Butorphanol given intravenously in large doses (3 mg/kg) to dogs temporarily reduced aortic blood pressure. Aortic pressure returned to baseline control values within 15 to 30 minutes. Changes in cardiac contractile force and cardiac rate were of the same magnitude as the changes in aortic pressure. No appreciable effect on expired carbon dioxide was seen[2]. Studies in anesthetized dogs at equianalgetic doses indicate that butorphanol has less potential than morphine for causing airway constriction, hypotension and histamine release[3]. In conscious dogs butorphanol produced minimal cardiovascular and respiratory effects[4].

The specific site of action of butorphanol is not known. Butorphanol probably exerts analgesic and antitussive effects via the central nervous system (subcortical, possibly the hypothalamus).

Indications: Torbutrol (butorphanol tartrate) is indicated for the relief of chronic non-productive cough associated with tracheobronchitis, tracheitis, tonsillitis, laryngitis and pharyngitis originating from inflammatory conditions of the upper respiratory tract.

Contraindications:

1. The safety of Torbutrol (butorphanol tartrate) has not been determined in dogs afflicted with heartworm disease (Dirofilaria immitus).
2. Torbutrol (butorphanol tartrate) should not be used in dogs with a history of liver disease.
3. Since Torbutrol (butorphanol tartrate) can be effective in totally suppressing cough, it should not be used in conditions of the lower respiratory tract associated with copious mucus production.

Warning: FOR USE IN DOGS ONLY

Precautions:

1. Torbutrol (butorphanol tartrate) has been shown to have potent analgesic activity in rodents; it is undesirable to administer other sedative or analgesic drugs during treatment with Torbutrol (butorphanol tartrate) as these are likely to produce an additive effect.
2. Reproduction studies, performed in mice and rabbits, revealed no evidence of impaired fertility or harm to the fetus due to butorphanol tartrate. In the rat species the female, on parenteral administration, showed increased nervousness and decreased care for the newborn, resulting in a decreased survival rate of the newborn. This nervousness was seen only in the rat species. There are no well-controlled studies in pregnant bitches but, although there is no well-defined risk, the use of Torbutrol (butorphanol tartrate) in pregnant bitches is not recommended.
3. Cough suppression may be accompanied by mild sedation; the degree of sedation is dose related. If sedation is considered undesirable or unneccessary, the dose should be reduced.
4. Toxicity studies indicate that the LD_{50} in dogs by oral administration is greater than 50 mg/kg. In studies of 4.5 and 13 weeks duration, the following effects were noted in some but not all dogs at 4.6 times the recommended therapeutic dose level BID given parenterally: Decreased activity, weight loss, salivation, elevated SGPT and/or SAP and mild proliferative changes of the bile duct epithelium.

Adverse Reactions: The most frequent adverse reaction reported in 264 dogs treated with oral Torbutrol (butorphanol tartrate) was slight sedation in 6 dogs (2.3%). Other less frequent adverse reactions which have been reported include anorexia/nausea and diarrhea (reported incidence less than 1%).

Following the marketing of Torbutrol Veterinary Injection transient sedation and ataxia have been reported rarely as side effects in dogs.

Dosage and Administration: The usual parenteral dose is 0.025 mg of butorphanol base activity per lb of body weight. This is the equivalent of ½ ml (0.5 ml) for each 10 lbs of body weight. It should be administered by subcutaneous injection, and repeated at intervals of 6 to 12 hours as required. If necessary, the dose may be increased to a maximum of 0.05 mg per lb or 1 ml per 10 body weight. Treatment should not normally be required for longer than 7 days.

The usual oral dose of Torbutrol (butorphanol tartrate) is 0.25 mg of butorphanol base activity per pound of body weight. This is the equivalent of one 5 mg tablet per 20 lbs. of body weight. The dose should be repeated at intervals of 6 to 12 hours as required. If necessary, the dose may be increased to a maximum of one 5 mg tablet for each 10 lbs. of body weight. Treatment should not normally be required for longer than seven days.

How Supplied: NDC 0015-2025-60—Bottles of 100 Torbutrol (butorphanol tartrate) Veterinary Tablets—1 mg base activity (per tablet).

NDC 0015-2026-60—Bottles of 100 Torbutrol (butorphanol tartrate) Veterinary Tablets—5 mg base activity (per tablet).

NDC 0015-2027-60—Bottles of 100 Torbutrol (butorphanol tatrate) Veterinary Tablets—10 mg base activity (per tablet).

NDC 0015-2030-19—10 ml vials Torbutrol (butorphanol tartrate) Veterinary Injection, 0.5 mg per ml base activity.

References:

1. Cavanagh, R.L., et al: Antitussive Properities of Butorphanol Archives Internationales de Pharmacodynamie at de Therapie 220 (2): 258–268, 1976.
2. Christie, G.J., et al: Butorphanol Tartrate: A New Antitussive Agent for Use in Dogs. Veterninary Medicine/

Continued on next page

Bristol—Cont.

Small Animal Clinician 75 (10): 1559–1562, 1980.

3. Schurig, J.E. et al: Effects of Butorphanol and Morphine on Pulmonary Mechanics, Arterial Blood Pressure and Venous Plasma Histamine in the Anesthetized Dog. Archives Internationales de Pharmacodynamie et de Therapie 223: 296–304, 1978.
4. Pircio, A.W., et al: The Pharmacology of Butorphanol. Archives Internationales de Pharmacodynamie et de Therapie 220 (2): 231–2576, 1976.

Ceva Laboratories

Professional Veterinary Products
10551 BARKLEY STREET
OVERLAND PARK, KS 66212

14-G ABBOCATH® -T
16-G ABBOCATH® -T
18-G ABBOCATH® -T
20-G ABBOCATH® -T
22-G ABBOCATH® -T

Radiopaque, I.V. Catheter/*Teflon**

Description: 14-G Abbocath-T—Catheter; 14-G, 0.060″ (0.15 cm) I.D., 2″ (6.4 cm) long, also 5½″ long, over 17-G needle.
16-G Abbocath-T—Catheter: 16-G, 0.044″ (0.11 cm) I.D., 2″ (5.1 cm) long, also 5½″ long, over 19-G needle.
18-G Abbocath-T—Catheter: 18-G, 0.034″ (0.09 cm) I.D., 2″ (5.1 cm) long, over 21-G needle.
20-G Abbocath-T—Catheter: 20-G, 0.024″ (0.06 cm) I.D., 1¼″ (3.2 cm) long, over 24-G needle.
22-G Abbocath-T—Catheter: 22-G, 0.022″ I.D., 1¼″ long, over 25-G needle.
Contents sterile and nonpyrogenic in intact unit package.
* Reg. US Pat. Office for DuPont's fluorocarbon resins.

Directions:
1. Prepare site.
2. Remove needle guard.
3. **MAKE VENIPUNCTURE** with needle bevel up. **DO NOT REINSERT NEEDLE IN CATHETER IF VENIPUNCTURE IS UNSUCCESSFUL.**
4. To advance catheter, separate needle from cathether hub and slide catheter forward in vein to desired length. Withdraw needle and connect administration set to catheter hub.
5. **SECURE CATHETER** by taping in place. Discard after use.

Caution: Federal law restricts this device to sale by or on the order of a licensed veterinarian.
Protect from freezing and extreme heat.
Disposable Device—Do not resterilize or reuse.

How Supplied: 20 Units (List Nos. 4535-14/14G; 4535-16/16G; 4535-18/18G; 4535-20/20G; 453522/22G; 4535-84/14G-5½″ long; 4535-76/16G-5½″ long).

A-C-D SOLUTION

Anticoagulant Citrate Dextrose Solution, U.S.P. Formula A
ACD Evacuated Blood Collection Bottle
Sterile, Nonpyrogenic

Composition: Contains 8.4m Eq Sodium
Each 100 ml contains:

Dextrose, hydrous, USP	2.45 g
Sodium citrate, hydrous, USP	2.20 g
Citric acid, hydrous, USP	0.73 g

Indications: For collection of 500 ml blood. Contains 75 ml anticoagulant ACD Solution USP "Formula A"and for collection of 250 ml blood. Contains 37.5 ml anticoagulant ACD Solution USP "Formula A".

Caution:
1. Store blood within a 2° range between 1–6°C.
2. Mix blood thoroughly immediately before use and administer without warming.
3. Infusion set must have fiter.

Caution: Federal (U.S.A.) law restricts this drug to use by or on the order of a licensed veterinarian.

How Supplied: 250 ml bottles containing 37.5 ml anticoagulant (List No. 8683-02), and 500 ml bottles containing 75 ml anticoagulant (List No. 8683-03).

ALCARE™

Foamed Alcohol Skin Sanitizer

Composition: Contains 54% Ethyl alcohol, with emollients.

Indications: For routine hand cleansing and sanitation by operating personnel.

Directions: For general use, apply to hands and massage thoroughly, using sufficient foam to keep hands wet for 30 to 60 seconds. Continue massaging until foam vanishes and hands are dry.

How Supplied: 11-oz.(List No. 6395-36) or 7-oz. (List No. 6395-57) aerosol cans. Packaged 24 cans per shipping case.

AMERSE®

Hospital Instrument Germicide

Composition: Active Ingredients: Vegetable oil soap 11.70%; sodium xylene sulfonate 5.00%; o-benzyl-p-chlorophenol 5.25%; o-phenylphenol 1.00%.
Inert Ingredients: 72.65%

Indications: An instrument disinfectant which is germicidal, fungicidal, pseudomonacidal, staphylocidal, tuberculocidal and virucidal. Will not rust, dull, stain or otherwise attack quality metal instruments. No rust inhibitor required. Recommended for thermometer storage.

Directions: Amerse comes provided with a pump-type dispensing system which accurately delivers ½ oz.per stroke. For instrument disinfection, add ½ fluid oz. (one stroke of pump) to each pint (16 fluid oz.) of water to make 1:32 aqueous use dilution. For cold instrument disinfection, clean instruments, rinse, and immerse articles in a 1:32 aqueous solution for 10 minutes.

Note: A 1:32 solution of Amerse may be used for prolonged storage of all but lensed instruments, woven catheters, plastic or rubber items which may show sensitivity to chemical disinfection or steam or gas sterilization. Exposure time for these items to an Amerse solution should be limited to 10 minutes.

How Supplied: Amerse is a concentrate, packed in unbreakable, ½-gal. plastic containers, six half-gallons per shipping case. Free dispensing pump included with each case. (List No. 6401-16). Also available, 1-oz unit-dose dispenser packs. Pouch makes 1-qt. of solution. 12 pouches per box (List No. 6401-69).

AMINOSYN® 5%

Crystalline Amino Acid Solution

Composition: Each 100 ml contains:
Essential Amino Acids:

Isoleucine	360 mg
Leucine	470 mg
Lysine (acetate)*	360 mg
Methionine	200 mg
Phenylalanine	220 mg
Threonine	260 mg
Tryptophan	80 mg
Valine	400 mg

* Amount cited is for Lysine alone, and does not include acetate salt.
Nonessential Amino Acids:

Alanine	640 mg
Arginine	490 mg
Histidine	150 mg
Proline	430 mg
Serine	210 mg
Tyrosine	44 mg
Glycine (Amino acetic Acid, USP)	640 mg

Indications: Aminosyn is a sterile, non-pyrogenic solution for intravenous infusion. It provides crystalline amine acids to promote protein synthesis and wound healing, and to reduce the rate of endogenous protein catabolism.
Aminosyn given by central venous infusion in combination with concentrated dextrose, electrolytes, vitamins, trace metals, and ancillary fat supplements constitutes total parenteral nutrition (TPN). Aminosyn can also be administered by peripheral vein alone, for 'protein sparing' therapy, or in combination with dextrose and maintenance electrolytes. Intravenous fat emulsion may be substituted for part of the carbohydrate calories during either TPN or peripheral vein administration of Aminosyn.

Warning: Intravenous administration of amino acids may occasionally cause anaphylactoid reactions. Administration of amino acid solutions in the presence of impaired renal function may augment an increasing BUN, as does any protein dietary component.

Cautions: Protect from excessive heat (above 40 degrees C) and freezing. Avoid exposure to light.

How Supplied: 500 ml Abbo-Vac® bottle (List No. 2990-03)

BETA-1200™ ANTITOXIN

Equine Origin

Composition: Contains 1200 I.A.U.s of *Clostridium Perfringens* Type C Antitoxin (equine origin) per each ml of Beta-1200.

Description: An improved product for the management of problem herds of breeding swine where Type C Toxoid immunization programs have not proven effective, and where economic losses from enterotoxemia caused by *Cl. perfringens* Type C infections are running at unacceptably high levels.

The efficacy of Beta-1200 Antitoxin has been extensively tested and demonstrated. Accumulative data from two test sites demonstrated that death rates attributed to clostridial diagnosed infections averaged 3.5 times greater in nontreated controls than in piglets treated with Beta-1200 Antitoxin. Overall survival rates in treated piglets were 1.7 times greater than nontreated, regardless of cause of death or quality of herd management.

The potency of Beta-1200 Antitoxin has been similarly established. In two separate, carefully monitored studies of university-managed closed herds, normal piglets from four sows were treated with the recommended 3 and 5 ml S.C. dosage levels within 20 hours after farrowing. Serum samples were taken from the treated piglets at intervals of 1, 2, 7, 14 and 21 days after treatment and titrated for residual antibody levels.

Results showed that the piglets retained levels greater than 10 I.A.U./ml of serum, a level previously demonstrated to be protective, for a period of at least 14 days post-treatment.

The completed test results show that in those litters treated with Beta-1200 Antitoxin, piglet mortality was held at just 13.2% as opposed to 47.4% among untreated piglets.

Indications: For control of enterotoxemia caused by *Clostridium perfringens* Type C in baby pigs.

Dosage and Administration: Beta-1200 Antitoxin should be administered as a prophylactic treatment to piglets within 20 hours after birth to ensure effective development of passive immunity. Dosage should be 3 to 5 ml subcutaneously.

Precautions:
Store at 35° to 45°F.
Do not freeze.
Use entire contents when first opened.
Do not inject into food-producing animals within 21 days before slaughter.
Allergic reactions may follow use of products of this nature.

How Supplied: 250 ml bottles, shipped 20 per case (List No. 2648-01).

BLOOD ADMINISTRATION SET
With 19 ga. Needle and Nylon Filter

Description: Disposable set for transfusion with any-plug-in type container of blood, plasma or serum.

Fluid path and areas under protective coverings of set are sterile and nonpyrogenic.

Directions: Remove protective coverings as assembly progresses. Close clamp. Swab stopper of blood container with antiseptic solution. Insert piercing cannula through stopper at indentation marked "outlet". Invert and suspend container. Fill drip chamber to level just above filter by compressing chamber. Insert pressure ball valve airintake needle into blood container stopper at indentation marked "air". Attach vein needle to needle adapter. Open clamp to allow blood to expel all air from tubing. Close clamp, make venipuncture. Regulate rate of administration by adjusting clamp. (Approximately 10 drops will deliver 1 ml). Supplemental medication can be injected through gum rubber insert near vein needle.

Caution: Avoid air bubbles in tubing prior to venipuncture. *Discard equipment after use.*

Caution: Federal law restricts this device to use by or on the order of a licensed veterinarian.

Do not store for prolonged periods at extreme temperatures.

Disposable Device—Do not resterilize or reuse.

How Supplied: 1 Unit (List No. 8810-58).

BLOOD COLLECTION SET–36"
With Siliconed Needles

Description: Disposable set for vacuum collection in ACD solution.

Fluid path and areas under protective coverings of set are sterile and nonpyrogenic.

Directions: Remove protective coverings as assembly progresses. Close tubing with hemostat or clamp placed near bottle needle (the shorter needle). Insert bottle needle perpendicularly through swabbed stopper of blood bottle at indenntation marked X. Suspend inverted bottle. Make venipuncture and regulate flow by adjusting hemostat or clamp. For serology, samples can be obtained (1) by transfehng bottle needle into pilot tubes before vein needle has been withdrawn; (2) by draining collection-set tubing into pilot tubes after both needles have been withdrawn. Terminate collection by closing hemostat or clamp, releasing tourniquet and withdrawing needles from vein and bottle. To assure thorough mixing of blood and anticoagulant, replace dust cap and AGITATE bottle for several minutes. Discard equipment after use.

Caution: Federal law restricts this device to use by or on the order of a licensed veterinarian.

Do not store for prolonged periods at extreme temperatures.

Disposable Device—Do not resterilize or reuse.

How Supplied: 1 Unit (List No. 4736-48).

BOVINE RHINOTRACHEITIS VACCINE

Composition: Contains desiccated Bovine Rhinotracheitis Vaccine (modified live virus, bovine tissues culture origin), with sterile diluent.

Contains penicillin, streptomycin and nystatin as preservatives

Indications: For the immunization of healthy cattle against Infectious Bovine Rhinotracheitis.

Dosage and Administration: Rehydrate the vial of desciccated vaccine with the accompanying vial of sterile diluent using aseptic technique, shake well, and administer 2 ml by intramuscular injection.

Precautions: Refrigerate at 35°to 45°F. Use promptly after rehydrating. Do not vaccinate animals under 2 months of age. Revaccinate calves vaccinated before 6 months of age, at 6 months or weaning. Do not use in pregnant cows or in calves nursing pregnant cows. Do not vaccinate within 21 days before slaughter. Use entire contents when first opened. Burn this container and all unused contents. In case of anaphylactoid reaction administer epinephrine or equivalent.

How Supplied: List No.2636-01, one 10-dose vial vaccine (rehydrate to 20 ml) and one 20-ml vial sterile diluent. List No. 2636-02, one 50-dose vial vaccine (rehydrate to 100 ml) and one 100-ml vial sterile diluent.

BOVINE RHINOTRACHEITIS VACCINE WITH LEPTOSPIRA POMONA BACTERIN

Composition: Contains desiccated Bovine Rhinotracheitis Vaccine (modified live virus, bovine tissue culture origin), with Leptospira Pomona Bacterin diluent (aluminum hydroxide adsorbed).

Contains penicillin, streptomycin, nystatin and thimerosal as preservatives.

Indications: For the immunization of healthy cattle against Infectious Bovine Rhinotracheitis and
Leptospira pomona.

Dosage and Administration: Rehydrate the vial of desiccated vaccine with the accompanying vial of *Leptospira pomona* bacterin diluent using aseptic technique, shake well, and administer 2 ml by intramuscular injection.

Precautions: Refrigerate at 35°to 45°F. Use promptly after rehydrating. Do not vaccinate animals under 2 months of age. Revaccinate calves vaccinated before 6 months of age, at 6 months or weaning. Do not use in pregnant cows or in calves nursing pregnant cows. Do not vaccinate within 21 days before slaughter. Use entire contents when first opened. Burn this container and all unused contents. In case of anaphylactoid reaction administer epinephrine or equivalent.

How Supplied: List No. 2643-01, one 10-dose vial vaccine (rehydrate to 20 ml) and one 20-ml vial Leptospira bacterin. List No. 2643-02, one 50-dose vial vaccine (rehydrate to 100 ml) and one 100-ml vial Leptospira Bacterin.

BOVINE RHINOTRACHEITIS–PARAINFLUENZA–3 VACCINE

Composition: Contains desiccated Bovine Rhinotracheitis —Parainfluenza-3 Vaccine (modified live virus, bovine and porcine tissue culture origin). With sterile diluent.

Contains penicillin, streptomycin, nystatin and thimerosal as preservatives.

Continued on next page

C

CEVA—Cont.

Indications: For the immunization of healthy cattle against Infectious Bovine Rhinotracheitis, Parainfluenza-3.
Dosage and Administration: Rehydrate the vial of desiccated vaccine with the accompanying vial of sterile diluent using aseptic technique, shake well, and administer 2 ml by intramuscular injection.
Precautions: Refrigerate at 35°to 45°F. Use promptly after rehydrating. Do not vaccinate animals under 2 months of age. Revaccinate calves vaccinated before 6 months of age, at 6 months or weaning. Do not use in pregnant cows or in calves nursing pregnant cows. Do not vaccinate within 21 days before slaughter. Use entire contents when first opened. Burn this container and all unused contents. In case of anaphylactoid reaction administer epinephrine or equivalent.
How Supplied: List No. 2637-01, one 10-dose vial vaccine (rehydrate to 20 ml) and one 20-ml vial sterile diluent. List No. 2637-02, one 50-dose vial vaccine (rehydrate to 100 ml) and one 100-ml vial sterile diluent.

BOVINE RHINOTRACHEITIS–PARAINFLUENZA–3 VACCINE WITH PASTEURELLA HAEMOLYTICA–MULTOCIDA BACTERIN

Composition: Contains desiccated Bovine Rhinotracheitis —Parinfluenza-3 Vaccine (modified live virus, bovine and porcine tissue culture origin), with Pasteurella Haemolytica-Multocida Bacterin diluent (bovine isolates, aluminum hydroxide adsorbed).
Contains penicillin, streptomycin, nystatin and thimerosal as preservatives.
US Standard of Potency for bovine rhinotracheitis and parainfluenza-3 only.
Indications: For the immunization of healthy cattle against Infectious Bovine Rhinotracheitis, Parainfluenza-3, *Pasteurella haemolytica* and *Pasteurella multocida.*
Dosage and Administration: Rehydrate the vial of desiccated vaccine with the accompanying vial of Pasteurella bacterin diluent using aseptic technique, shake well, and administer 2 ml by intramuscular injection. Repeat Pasteurella vaccination within 14 to 30 days.
Precautions: Refrigerate at 35°to 45°F. Use promptly after rehydrating. Do not vaccinate animals under 2 months of age. Revaccinate calves vaccinated before 6 months of age, at 6 months or weaning. Do not use in pregnant cows or in calves nursing pregnant cows. Do not vaccinate within 21 days before slaughter. Use entire contents when first opened. Burn this container and all unused contents. In case of anaphylactoid reaction administer epinephrine or equivalent.
How Supplied: List No. 2638-01, one 10-dose vial vaccine (rehydrate to 20 ml) and one 20-ml vial Pasteurella Bacterin. List No. 2638-02, one 50-dose vial vaccine (rehydrate to 100 ml) and one 100-ml vial Pasteurella Bacterin.

BOVINE RHINOTRACHEITIS–VIRUS DIARRHEA VACCINE

Composition: Contains desiccated Bovine Rhinotracheitis—Virus Diarrhea Vaccine (modified live virus, bovine and porcine tissue culture origin), with sterile diluent.
Contains penicillin, streptomycin and nystatin as preservatives.
Indications: For the immunization of healthy cattle against Infectious Bovine Rhinotracheitis, Bovine Virus Diarrhea.
Dosage and Administration: Rehydrate the vial of desiccated vaccine with the accompanying vial of diluent aseptic technique, shake well, and administer 2m by intramuscular injection.
Precautions: Refrigerate at 35° to 45°F. Use promptly after rehydrating. Do not vaccinate animals under 2 months of age. Revaccinate calves vaccinated before 6 months of age, at 6 months or weaning. Do not use in pregnant cows or in calves nursing pregnant cows. Do not vaccinate within 21 days before slaughter. Use entire contents when first opened. Burn this container and all unused contents. In case of anaphylactoid reaction administer epinephrine or equivalent.
How Supplied: List No. 2642-01, one 10-dose vial vaccine (rehydrate to 20 ml) and one 20-ml vial sterile diluent. List No. 2642-02, one 50-dose vial vaccine (rehydrate to 100 ml) and one 100-ml vial sterile diluent.

BOVINE RHINOTRACHEITIS–VIRUS DIARRHEA VACCINE WITH LEPTOSPIRA POMONA BACTERIN

Composition: Contains desiccated Bovine Rhinotracheitis-Virus Diarrhea Vaccine (modified live virus, bovine and porcine tissue culture origin), with Leptospira Pomona Bacterin diluent (aluminum hydroxide absorbed).
Contains penicillin, streptomycin, nystatin and thimerosal as preservatives.
Indications: For the immunization of healthy cattle against Infectious Bovine Rhinotracheitis, Bovine Virus Diarrhea and *Leptospira pomona.*
Dosage and Administration: Rehydrate the vial of desiccated vaccine with the accompanying vial of Leptospira pomona bacterin diluent using aseptic technique, shake well, and administer 2ml by intramuscular injection.
Contains penicillin, streptomycin, nystatin and thimerosal as preservatives.
Precautions: Refrigerate at 35° to 45°F. Use promptly after rehydrating. Do not vaccinate under 2 months of age. Revaccinate calves vaccinated before 6 months of age, at 6 months or weaning. Do not use in pregnant cows or in calves nursing pregnant cows. Do not vaccinate within 21 days before slaughter. Use entire contents when first opened. Burn this container and all unused contents. In case of anaphylactoid reaction administer epinephrine or equivalent.
How Supplied: 10-dose Vial Vaccine—rehydrate to 20 ml; 20 ml Vial Bacterin Diluent (List No. 2591-01). 50-dose Vial Vaccine—rehydrate to 100 ml; 100 ml Vial Bacterin Diluent (List No. 2591-02).

BOVINE RHINOTRACHEITIS–VIRUS DIARRHEA–PARAINFUENZA–3 VACCINE

Composition: Contains desiccated Bovine Rhinotracheitis—Virus Diarrhea—Parainfluenza-3 Vaccine (modified live virus, bovine and porcine tissue culture origin), with sterile diluent.
Contains penicillin, streptomycin and nystatin as preservatives.
Indications: For the immunization of healthy cattle against Infectious Bovine Rhinotracheitis, Bovine Virus Diarrhea, and Parainfluenza-3.
Dosage and Administration: Rehydrate the vial of desiccated vaccine with the acompanying vial of sterile diluent using aseptic technique, shake well, and administer 2 ml by intramuscular injection.
Precautions: Refrigerate at 35° to 45°F. Use promptly after rehydrating. Do not vaccinate animals under 2 months of age. Revaccinate calves vaccinated before 6 months of age, at 6 months or weaning. Do not use in pregnant cows or in calves nursing pregnant cows. Do not vaccinate within 21 days before slaughter. Use entire contents when first opened. Burn this container and all unused contents. In case of anaphylactoid reaction administer epinephrine or equivalent.
How Supplied: List No. 2639-04, one 10-dose vial vaccine (rehydrate to 20 ml) and one 20-ml sterile diluent. List No. 2639-03, one 50-dose vial vaccine (rehydrate to 100 ml) and one 100-ml vial sterile diluent.

BOVINE RHINOTRACHEITIS–VIRUS DIARRHEA–PARAINFLUENZA-3 VACCINE WITH PASTEURELLA HAEMOLYTICA–MULTOCIDA BACTERIN

Composition: Contains desiccated Bovine Rhinotracheitis —Virus Diarrhea —Parainfluenza —3 Vaccine (modified live virus, bovine and porcine tissue culture origin), with Pasteurella Haemolytica —Multocida Bacterin diluent (bovine isolates, aluminum hydroxide adsorbed.
Contains penicillin, streptomycin, nystatin and thimerosal as preservatives.
US Standard of Potency for bovine rhinotracheitis, virus diarrhea and parainfluenza-3 only.
Indications: For the immunizaion of healthy cattle against Infectious Bovine Rhinotracheitis, Bovine Virus Diarrhea, and Parainfluenza-3, Pasteurella haemolytica and Pasteurella multocida.
Dosage and Administration: Rehydrate the vial of desiccated vaccine with the accompanying vial of Pasteurella bacterin diluent using aseptic technique, shake well, and administer 2 ml by intra-

muscular injection. Repeat Pasteurella vaccination within 14 to 30 days.
Precautions: Refrigerate at 35° to 45°F. Use promptly after rehydrating. Do not vaccinate animals under 2 months of age. Revaccinate calves vaccinated before 6 months of age, at 6 months or weaning. Do not use in pregnant cows or in calves nursing pregnant cows. Do not vaccinate within 21 days before slaughter. Use entire contents when first opened. Burn this container and all unused contents. In case of anaphylactoid reaction administer epinephrine or equivalent.
How Supplied: List No. 2640-04, one 10-dose vial vaccine (rehydrate to 20 ml) and one 20 ml vial Pasteurella Bacterin. List No. 2640-03, one 50-dose vial vaccine (rehydrate to 100 ml) and one 100-ml vial Pasteurella Bacterin.

BOVINE VIRUS DIARRHEA VACCINE

Composition: Contains Bovine Virus Diarrhea Vaccine (modified live virus, porcine tissue culture origin), with sterile diluent.
Contains penicillin, streptomycin and nyastatin as preservatives.
Indications: For the immunizaion of healthy cattle against Bovine Virus Diarrhea.
Dosage and Administration: Rehydrate by adding the accompanying vial of diluent to the vial of vaccine. Shake thoroughly. Inject 2 ml intramuscularly.
Precautions: Keep refrigerated at 35° to 45°F. Do not vaccinate animals under 2 months of age. Do not vaccinate pregnant animals. Do not vaccinate within 21 days before slaughter. Use entire contents when first opened. Burn this container and all unused contents. In case of anaphylactoid reaction, administer epinephrine or equivalent.
How Supplied: List No. 2632-03, one 10-dose vial vaccine (rehydrate to 20 ml) and one 20-ml vial sterile diluent. List No. 2632-04, one 50-dose vial vaccine (rehydrate to 100 ml) and one 100 ml vial sterile diluent.

BUTTERFLY® 16
BUTTERFLY® 19
BUTTERFLY® 21
BUTTERFLY® 23
BUTTERFLY® 25
INFUSION SETS

Description: Butterfly 16—16-gauge, 1-inch, winged, siliconed thinwall needle (15-gauge bore), with 30-inch tubing.
Butterfly 19—19-gauge, 7/8-inch (2.2 cm), winged, siliconed thinwall needle (18-gauge bore), with 12-inch (30 cm) tubing.
Butterfly 21—21-guage, ¾-inch (1.9 cm) winged, siliconed thinwall needle (20-gauge bore), with 12-inch (30 cm) tubing.
Butterfly 23—23-gauge, ¾-inch (1.9 cm), winged, siliconed thinwall needle (22-gauge bore), with 12-inch (30 cm) tubing.
Butterfly 25—25-gauge, ¾-inch (1.9 cm), winged, siliconed thinwall needle (24-gauge bore), with 12-inch (30 cm) tubing.
Contents sterile and nonpyrogenic in intact unit package.
Directions (Use Aseptic Technique): Attach female adapter to primer I.V. administration set. Open clamp on I.V. set and allow solution to expel air from tubing and needle. Close clamp and proceed with venipuncture.
Caution:
Federal law restricts this device to sale by or on the order of a physician or other licensed practitioner.
Protect from freezing and extreme heat. Disposable Device. Do not resterilize or reuse.
How Supplied: 1 Unit (List Nos. 4716-01/16-G; 4590-01/19-G; 4492-01/21-G; 4565-01/23-G; 4506-01/25-G).

CAPARSOLATE®
(sodium thiacetarsamide)

Composition: Each ml of Caparsolate Sodium 1% solution contains: 10 mg sodium thiacetarsamide with benzyl alcohol 0.9% as a preservative, sodium phosphate as buffer, and sodium chloride sufficient to render solution isotonic. pH adjusted with sodium hydroxide.
Indications: Caparsolate Sodium is an arsenical anthelmintic drug indicated for (intravenous) treatment of canine heartworm disease caused by *Dirofilaria immitis.* When the use of an appropriate larvicidal drug is not practical, Caparsolate Sodium can be used periodically as a preventive measure to kill the young adult heartworms before they have time to cause substantial damage and signs of heartworm disease.
Adverse Reactions: Inflammation and sloughing are common when perivascular leakage occurs.
A cough and temperature elevation are the primary reactions associated with pulmonary emboli formed by dead heartworms.
Commonly occurring reactions associated with liver and/or kidney damage include vomiting, anorexia, lethargy, icterus, bilirubinuria, elevated SGPT, elevated BUN, and other abnormal kidney or liver function test values.
Elevated SGPT values or vomiting have been reported with no other obvious signs of toxicity.
Consult the warnings and precautions sections for additional information.
Dosage and Administration: For the treatment of canine heartworm disease caused by *Dirofilaria immitis,* Caparsolate Sodium is administered intravenously at a rate of 0.1 ml per pound of body weight (1.0 ml for every 10 pounds) twice a day for two days.
Caparsolate Sodium used as a preventive measure is administered intravenously at a rate of 0.1 ml per pound of body weight (1.0 ml for every 10 pounds) twice daily for two days at six-month intervals in areas where mosquitoes exist year round and annually where the mosquito season is limited.
Warnings: The active ingredient in Caparsolate Sodium is a very potent drug. Sodium thiacetarsamide is a potential nephrotoxic and hepatotoxic agent. A thorough pretreatment evaluation, including a detailed physical examination and other tests and procedures as needed, to assess liver, kidney, cardiovascular and pulmonary function is recommended. It is generally advisable to correct reversible pathological conditions before proceeding with Caparsolate Sodium therapy. Any significant impairment of kidney, liver, cardiovascular or pulmonary function not amenable to improvement may justify precluding Caparsolate Sodium therapy.
When the caval syndrome of heartworm disease is diagnosed, Caparsolate Sodium therapy should be delayed until the worms blocking the vena cava are surgically removed (through jugular vein, using local anesthetic). Several weeks following surgery, eliminate the remaining heartworms by administering Caparsolate Sodium, providing the dog can tolerate the therapy.
Close monitoring to detect drug toxicity during and after treatment is recommended. Vomiting sometimes occurs within several hours following drug administration. If no other adverse effects are detected and the appetite remains good, treatment may be continued. Signs suggesting nephrotoxicity, hepatotoxicity or any other significant abnormality are reason to suspend Caparsolate Sodium therapy.
To help avoid the possible serious effects associated with pulmonary emboli formed by dead heartworms, it is imperative that the dog be kept quiet and confined for a period of approximately four to six weeks after Caparsolate Sodium therapy. Following treatment, the adult heartworms gradually die, and are carried into the small pulmonary arteries where they lodge causing obstruction, thrombus formation, inflammation and occasionally death. A temperature elevation and cough are commonly observed signs of pulmonary emboli, and they can be noted starting within the first week after therapy. Temperature should be monitored, and supportive treatment initiated as soon as a reaction is detected. Therapy for a reaction includes corticosteroids to reduce the inflammation and continued restricted activity.
Precautions: Studies have shown considerable variation in effectiveness. The reasons for these variations are presently unknown.
Care must be taken to avoid perivascular leakage because Caparsolate Sodium can cause severe inflammation and sloughing if leakage occurs. Appropriate therapy as soon as perivascular leakage is suspected can minimize the reaction.
Weigh the dog accurately, and measure the amount of drug to be given *precisely,* as overdosage substantially increases the chance of drug toxicity.
When the patient is released to the owner's care, special attention should be given to stress the importance of keeping the dog quiet and confined. Information on how to monitor the dog for signs of pulmonary emboli and signs of drug toxicity is important.

Continued on next page

CEVA—Cont.

Caution: Federal law restricts this drug to use by or on the order of a licensed veterinarian.
Product must be stored in refrigerator at 2° to 8°C (36° to 46°F), and protected from light and freezing. Discard partially-used vials from refrigerator after 3 months.
How Supplied: Caparsolate Sodium is supplied in 50 ml multiple dose, amber containers, 25 per case (List No. 8616-02).

C

CEVAX-8™ BOVINE RHINOTRACHEITIS-VIRUS DIARRHEA-PARAINFLUENZA-3 VACCINE WITH LEPTOSPIRA CANICOLA, GRIPPOTYPHOSA, HARDJO, ICTEROHAEMORRHAGIAE AND POMONA BACTERIN

Composition: Contains desiccated Bovine Rhinotracheitis-Virus Diarrhea-Parainfluenza-3 vaccine (modified live virus, bovine and porcine tissue culture origin), with *Leptospira carnicola, grippotyphosa, hardjo, icterohaemorrhagiae* and *pomona* bacterin diluent (aluminum hydroxide absorbed). Contains penicillin, streptomycin, nystatin and thimerosal as preservatives.
Description: Contains the NADL strain of BVD. Like all CEVA BVD vaccines, the BVD fraction of IRB-BVD-PI_3 is produced from the the NADL virus strain propagated on porcine tissue clutures. The NADL strain (isolated by scientists at the National Animal Disease Laboratory, Ames, Iowa) has been shown not only to provide a high, protective level of immunity against the NADL strain of BVD, but is also effective in stimulating a high level of cross-neutralizing antibodies that will cross-protect against a virulent challenge from field strains and laboratory isolated strains of BVD, including both the Singer and Oregon C24-V strains.
Heterologous Cell
System used in BVD vaccine production: Heterologous Cell Systems (non-bovine systems) have the advantage of being free from potential bovine virus contaminants that are difficult to detect by currently available testing methods. Thus, by utilizing this system, the chances of postvaccinal complications are greatly reduced.
Modified Live Virus utilized: Modified Live Virus vaccines replicate after entering the host animal. This allows a single injection to provide more rapid, longer-lasting protection than is possible with killed virus vaccines. CEVA MLV BVD vaccines have also been shown to be nonshedding and highly antigenic, as demonstrated by serological (antibody measurement) and post-vaccinal challenge studies.
Indications: For the immunization of healthy cattle against Infectious Bovine Rhinotracheitis, Bovine Virus Diarrhea, and Parainfluenza-3, and Leptopsirosis caused by *Leptospira canicola, L. grippotyphosa, L. hardjo, L. icterohaemorrhagiae* and *L. pomona.*
Dosage and Administration: Rehydrate the vial of desiccated vaccine with the accompanying vial of Leptospria Bacterin diluent using aspetic technique, shake well and administer 2 ml by intramuscular injection. In endemic leptospirosis area repeat Leptospira Bacterin vaccination within 3 to 5 weeks.
Precautions: Refrigerate at 2°–7°C (35° to 45°F). Use promptly after rehydrating. Do not vaccinate animals under 2 months of age. Revaccinate calves vaccinated before 6 months of age, at 6 months or weaning. Do not use in pregnant cows or in calves nursing pregnant cows. Do not vaccinate within 21 days before slaughter. Use entire contents when first opened. Burn this container and all unused contents. In case of anaphylactoid reaction administer epinephrine or equivalent.
How Supplied: 10 dose (List No. 2114-01) Rehydrate to 20 ml, 20 ml Vial Bacterin Diluent. 50-Dose (List No. 2114-02) Rehydrate to 100 ml 100 ml Vial Bacterin Diluent.

CLOSTRIDIUM PERFRINGENS ANTITOXIN TYPES C AND D

Composition: Contains Clostridium Perfringens Antitoxin Types C and D (equine origin).
Contains phenol and thymerosal as preservatives.
Indications: For the prevention and treatment of enterotoxemia caused by representative toxins of *Clostridium Perfringens*
Types C and D.
Dosage and Administration:
Prophylactic Treatment:
Calves 10 to 20 ml
Lambs 5 to 10 ml
Administer subcutaneously.
Therapeutic Treatment:
Double serum dosage shown above. For most rapid effect, administer intravenously.
Precautions: Store at 35° to 45°F. Do not freeze. Use entire contents when first opened. Do not inject into food producing animals within 21 days before slaughter. Allergic reactions may follow use of products of this nature. Antidote: Epinephrine or atropine.
How Supplied: List No. 2627-02, one 250-ml vial Clostridium Perfringens Antitoxin Types C and D.

COLIPIG™ *Escherichia coli* Bacterin Porcine Isolates

For the prevention of *E. coli* scours in baby pigs.

Description: Colipig Bacterin contains chemically inactivated cultures of *Escherichia coli,* serotypes K88ab, K88ac, K99 and 987P selected for their ability to produce pilus antigens.
Indications: Colipig is recommended for administration to healthy, pregnant gilts/sows for the prevention of neonatal enteric colibacillosis caused by *E. coli* strains in the antigenic spectrum covered by this bacterin. Protection of the newborn piglet is provided by the maternal antibodies contained in the colostrum of the immune dam's first milk.
Dosage & Administration: Inject 2 ml deep intramuscularly behind ear. A primary vaccination of two 2 ml doses is recommended 5 to 7 weeks and 2 to 3 weeks prior to planned farrowing. Revaccinate with a single 2.0 ml booster 2 to 3 weeks prior to subsequent farrowings provided interval does not exceed 8 months. If farrowing interval exceeds 8 months, repeat 2 dose schedule.
Precautions: Store at 2–7°C (35–45°F). Shake well before using. Do not vaccinate within 21 days before slaughter. Use entire contents when first opened. In case of anaphylactoid reaction, use epinephrine. Thimerosal added as a preservative.
How Supplied: 10 doses/20 ml (List No. 2131-01) and 50 doses/100 ml (List No. 2131-02).

COVERAGE™ 256

Composition: A concentrated germicidal detergent combining three third-generation twin chain quaternary ammonium chloride disinfectants with a synthetic detergent.
Indications: Coverage™ 256 is a broad spectrum disinfectant—fungicidal, virucidal, and germidical in 400 ppm hard water in the presence of 5% organic soil.
Directions: Only ½ ounce per gallon of water delivers a superior detergent-disinfectant cleaner used to simultaneously clean, disinfect, and deodorize animal quarters, runs and cages, and veterinary clinics.
How Supplied: 1 gallon containers, 4 per case (List No. 6360-08). Also available in 55-gallon drums (List No. 6360-01).

CVP MANOMETER

Description: To measure central venous pressure via injection site on any I.V. set connected to properly placed central venous catheter. With 18-G needle. Tubing approximately 51″ length, 0.12″ I.D.
How Supplied: 1 Unit (List No. 4607-01).

CYSTORELIN® (gonadorelin) For Injection

Composition: Cystorelin is a sterile solution containing 50 micrograms of gonadorelin (GnRh) diacetate tetrahydrate per milliliter suitable for intramuscular or intravenous administration. Gonadorelin is a decapeptide composed of the sequence of amino acids –5-oxoPro-His-Trp-Ser-Tyr-Gly-Leu-Arg-Pro-Gly-NH_2—a molecular weight of 1182.32 and empirical formula $C_{55}H_{75}N_{17}O_{13}$. The diacetate tetrahydrate ester has a molecular weight of 1374.48 and empirical formula $C_{59}H_{91}N_{17}O_{21}$.
Gonadorelin is the hypothalamic releasing factor responsible for the release of gonadotropins (e.g., FSH, LH) from the anterior pituitary. Synthetic gonadorelin is physiologically and chemically

identical to the endogenous bovine hypothalamic releasing factor.
Pharmacology and Toxicology: Endogenous gonadorelin is synthesized and /or released from the hypothalamus during various stages of the bovine estrus cycle following appropriate neurogenic stimuli. It passes, via the hypophyseal portal vessels, to the anterior pituitary to effect the release of gonadotropins (e.g., LH, FSH). Synthetic gonadorelin administered intravenously or intramuscularly also causes the release of endogenous LH or FSH from the anterior pituitary.
Gonadorelin diacetate tetrahydrate has been shown to be safe. The LD50 for mouse and rats is greater than 60 mg/kg, and for dogs, greater than 600 mcg/kg, respectively. No untoward effects were noted among rats or dogs administered 120 mcg/kg/day or 72 mcg/kg/day intravenously for 15 days.
It has no adverse effects on heart rate, blood pressure, or ekg to unanesthetized dogs at 60 mcg/kg. In anesthetized dogs it did not produce depression of myocardial or system hemodynamics or adversely affect coronary oxygen supply or myocardial oxygen requirements.
The intramuscular administration of 60 mcg/kg/day of gonadorelin diacetate tetrahydrate to pregnant rats and rabbits during organogenesis did not cause embryotoxic or teratogenic effects.
The intravenous administration of 1000 mcg to normally cycling dairy cattle had no effect on hematology or blood chemistry.
Further, Cystorelin does not cause irritation at the site of intramuscular administration in dogs. The dosage administered was 72 mcg/kg/day for seven (7) days.
Indications: Cystorelin (Gonadorelin) is indicated for the treatment of ovarian folicular cysts in dairy cattle. Ovarian cysts are nonovulated follicles with incomplete luteinization which result in nymphomania or irregular estrus.
Historically, cystic ovaries have responded to an exogenous source of luteinizing hormone (LH) such as human chorionic gonadodotropin. Cystorelin initiates release of endogenous LH to cause ovulation and luteinization.
Dosage and Administration: The recommended intravenous or intramuscular dosage of Cystorelin is 100 mcg/cow.
How Supplied: Cystorelin is available in a concentration of 50 mcg/ml. pH adjusted with potassium phosphate (monobasic and dibasic).
Cystorelin is supplied in single vials containing 2 ml of sterile solution (List No. 8283-02) and multi-dose 10 ml vials of sterile solution (List No. 8283-03).
Write for additional information about Cystorelin.

DEXTRAN 6%
Dextran 75, in Saline

Composition: Dextran 6% (dextran 75)* is a preparation of dextran having an average molecular weight of 75,000, which is offered for intravenous infusion in isotonic saline (sodium chloride injection). Dextran 6% solutions are sterile, non-pyrogenic preparations of partially hydrolyzed dextran which have prolonged stability and do not require refrigeration.
Dextran is prepared by acid hydrolysis of a crude macromolecular polysaccharide produced from the bacterial fermentation of sucrose. The fraction represented by dextran 75 consists of molecules which have a molecular weight ranging from 20,000 to 200,000 (average 75,000) when measured by a light scattering method. The glycosidic linkages in dextran 75 are predominantly those of the 1,6 type, although some are 1,4 and 1,3 linkages.
*This product should not be confused with "low molecular weight" dextrans (eg, dextran 40).
Actions: The colloidal properties of Dextran 6% approximate those of human albumin. Intravenous infusion of dextran results in an expanison of plasma volume slightly in excess of the volume infused and decreases from this maximum over the succeeding 24 hours. This expansion of plasma volume improves the hemodynamic status for 24 hours or longer. Dextran molecules below 50,000 molecular weight are eliminated by renal excretion with approximately 40% appearing in the urine in 24 hours. The remaining dextran is enzymatically degraded to glucose at a rate of about 70 to 90 mg/kg of body weight per day. This is a variable process.
Indications: Dextran 6% (dextran 75) is indicated for use in the treatment of shock or impending shock.
Dextran 6% is intended for emergency treatment only when whole blood or blood products are not available and must not be regarded as a substitute for whole blood or plasma proteins.
Contraindications: Dextran 6% is contraindicated in patients with severe bleeding disorders, with known hypersensitivity to dextran, and with severe congestive cardiac and renal failure.
Warning: Severe and fatal anaphylactoid reactions consisting of marked hypotension have been reported. These reactions occurred in patients not previously exposed to intravenous dextran and early in the infusion period. It is strongly recommended, therefore, that patients not previously exposed to dextran be observed closely during the first minutes of the infusion period.
Because of the seriousness of anaphylactoid reactions, it is recommended that the infusion of intravenous dextran be stopped at the first sign of an allergic reaction provided that other means of sustaining the circulation are available. Resuscitative measures should be readily available for emergency administration in the event such a reaction occurs.
Dextran may interfere to some extent with platelet function, particularly in the dog, and should be used with caution in cases with thrombocytopenia. When large volumes of dextran are administered, plasma protein levels will be decreased.
Precautions: The possibility of circulatory overload should be kept in mind. Special care should be exercised in patients with impaired renal clearance of dextran. When the risk of pulmonary edema and/or congestive heart failure may be increased, dextran should be used with caution.
Because Dextran 6% contains no bacteriostat, partially used bottles of Dextran 6% solution should be discarded.
Adverse Reactions: Allergic reactions include urticaria, nasal congestion, wheezing, tightness of chest, or mild hypotension. Antihistamines may be effective in relieving these symptoms. Other adverse reactions including nausea, vomiting, fever, and joint pains may occur. If a reaction develops, administration of dextran should be discontinued and patient appropriately treated.
Dosage and Administration: Dextran 6% (dextran 75) is administered by intravenous infusion only. Total dosage and rate of infusion depend upon the magnitude of fluid loss and the resultant hemoconcentration.
It is recommended that total dosage not exceed 20 ml/kg of body weight during the first 24 hours.
How Supplied: Abbo-Vac® bottle of 500 ml. (List No. 1505-04). The pH of Dextran 6% (dextran 75) in Saline is adjusted with sodium hydroxide.
Each 500 ml of Dextran 6% (dextran 75) contains 30 g of specially prepared dextran with 0.9% sodium chloride.
Disposable Abbott Equipment of Administering Dextran: Use Venoset to administer Dextran 6% (dextran 75) in Saline, as supplied in the Abbo-Vac® container. To administer solution simultaneously or alternately with another parenteral fluid, use Y-Type Venoset; with blood, use Y-Type Administration Set.

DEXTROSE 2½% IN ½ STRENGTH LACTATED RINGER'S

Composition: Each 100 ml contains:

Dextrose hydrous	2.5 g
Sodium Chloride	300 mg
Sodium Lactate, anhydrous	155 mg
Potassium Chloride	15 mg
Calcium Chloride, USP	10 mg

pH adjusted with hydrochloric acid (approx. 1 mEq/1).
Provides in 1,000 ml (not including ions for pH adjustment):

Dextrose, hydrous	25 g
Sodium	65 mEq
Potassium	2 mEq
Calcium	1 mEq
Total Cations	68 mEq
Chloride	54 mEq
Lactate	14 m Eq
Total Anions	68 m Eq

263 mOsm/l (calc.)
Approx pH 5.0
Indications: Correction of water and electrolyte deficits.
Dosage and Administration: For intravenous use. Contents or such lesser amounts as needed as a single dose.
Caution: Do not administer calcium-containing solutions concurrently with stored blood.

Continued on next page

CEVA—Cont.

Use only if clear and vacuum present.
Warning: Federal law prohibits dispensing without prescription.
How Supplied: Abbo-Vac® bottle of 1000 ml. (List No. 1521-05).

DEXTROSE 2½% IN ½ STRENGTH SALINE
Dextrose and Sodium Chloride Injection, USP
Dextrose 2½% with Sodium Chloride 0.45%

Composition: Each 100 ml. contains:

Dextrose, hydrous	2.5 g
Sodium Chloride	450 mg

Provides in 1000 ml:

Dextrose, hydrous	25.0 g
Sodium	77.0 mEq
Chloride	77.0 mEq

Dosage and Administration: Contents or such lesser amount as determined by the veterinarian as a single dose.
For intravenous or subcutaneous use.
Use only if clear and vacuum present.
Before piercing, cleanse stopper with antiseptic.
Caution: Federal law restricts this drug to use by or on the order of a licensed veterinarian.
How Supplied: Abbo-Vac® bottle of 500 ml. (List No. 1509-03) and 1000 ml. (List No. 1509-05). LifeCare® 1000 ml I.V. bags (List No. 7940-39).

DEXTROSE 5% IN ½ STRENGTH SALINE
Dextrose and Sodium Chloride Injection, USP
Dextrose 5% with Sodium Chloride 0.45%

Composition: Each 100 ml contains: A sterile solution containing 5% Dextrose, hydrous (5g) and Sodium Chloride 450 mg.
Indications: For use as an aid in offsetting tissue dehydration or prevention of postoperative shock. For hydration and re-establishment of renal function. Used also to supplement carbohydrate intake of baby pigs where hypoglycemia is a factor.
Dosage and Administration: Small animals, 10 to 15 ml per pound body weight per day or until adequate renal function is established. Baby pigs, 10 to 15 ml intraperitoneally. Repeat as indicated. This solution contains no preservative.
For intravenous use.
Use only if clear and vacuum present.
Before piercing, cleanse stopper with antiseptic.
Use as a single dose container to avoid contamination.
Caution: Federal law restricts this drug to use by or on the order of a licensed veterinarian.
How Supplied: Abbo-Vac® bottle of 250 ml (List No. 1526-02), 500 ml, (List No. 1526-03) and 1000 ml (List No. 1526-05).

DEXTROSE 5% IN LACTATED RINGER'S

Composition: Each 100 ml contains:

Dextrose, hydrous	5 g
Sodium Chloride	600 mg
Sodium Lactate, anhydrous	310 mg
Potassium Chloride	30 mg
Calcium Chloride, USP	20 mg

pH adjusted with hydrochloric acid (approx 1 mEq/l).
Provides in 1,000 ml (not including ions for pH adjustment):

Dextrose, hydrous	50 g
Sodium	130 mEq
Potassium	4 mEq
Calcium	3 mEq
Total Cations	137 mEq

525 mOsm/l (calc)
Approx pH 5.1
Air in container displaced by inert gas.
Indications: Correction of water and electrolyte deficits.
Dosage and Administration: For intravenous use. Contents or such lesser amounts as determined by the physician as a single dose.
Caution: Do not administer calcium containing solutions concurrently with stored blood.
Caution: Federal law prohibits dispensing without prescription.
How Supplied: Abbo-Vac® bottle of 500 ml. (List No. 1529-03) and 1000 ml (List No. 1529-05). LifeCare® 1000 ml I.V. bags (List No. 7929-39).

DEXTROSE 5% IN SALINE 0.9%
Dextrose and Sodium Chloride Injection, USP

Composition: Each 100 ml contains:

Dextrose, hydrous	5 g
Sodium Chloride	900 mg

Provides in 1,000 ml:

Dextrose, hydrous	50 g
Sodium	154 mEq
Chloride	154 mEq

561 mOsm/l (calc)
Approx pH 4.7
Indications: Correction of water deficits.
Dosage and Administration: For intravenous use. Contents or such lesser amount as determined by the physician as a single dose.
Use only if clear and vacuum present.
Caution: Federal law prohibits dispensing without prescription.
How Supplied: Abbo-Vac® bottle of 500 ml. (List No. 1527-03) and 1000 ml (List No. 1527-05).

DEXTROSE 5% IN WATER
Dextrose Injection, USP

Composition: Each 100 ml contains:
Dextrose, hydrous 5g
253 mOsm/l (calc)
Approx pH 5.0
Indications: Correction of water deficits.
Dosage and Administration: For intravenous use. Contents or such lesser amount as needed as a single dose.
Dextrose solutions without salts should not be used in blood transfusion because of possible rouleau formation.
Use only if clear and vacuum present.
Caution: Federal law prohibits dispensing without prescription.
How Supplied: Abbo-Vac® bottle of 250 ml. (List No. 1522-02), 500 ml (List No. 1522-03) and 1000 ml (List No. 1522-05). LifeCare® 1000 ml I.V. bags (List No. 7922-39).

DEXTROSE INJECTION, USP, 50%

Composition: Dextrose Injection, USP, 50 is a sterile, nonpyrogenic, hypertonic solution of dextrose (D-glucose) in water for injection for intravenous infusion. It provides a maximum number of calories (850) in a minimal amount of solution (500 ml). Dextrose Injection, USP, 50 has the following characteristics:

	Per 500 ml	Per Liter
Dextrose, hydrous USP	250 g	500 g
Caloric value*	850 Cal	1,700 Cal
Tonicity	Hypertonic	
Sp gr	1.171	
pH	4.2 (approx)	

*Caloric value calculated on the basis of 3.4 Cal/g of carbohydrate.
Actions: Dextrose Injection, USP, 50%, acts primarily as a source of carbohydrate calories and restores blood glucose levels in hypoglycemia.
Indications: Dextrose Injection, USP, 50%, is primarily indicated as a parenteral source of carbohydrate calories in patients whose oral intake is restricted or inadequate to maintain nutritional requirements. It may be used alone or in combination with protein hydrolysate solutions for parenteral hyperalimentation, especially in patients suffering from severe malnutrition.
Dextrose Injection, USP, 50%, is also indicated in the treatment of insulin hypoglycemia (hyperinsulinism) to restore blood glucose levels.
Contraindications: A concentrated dextrose solution should not be used when intracranial or intraspinal hemorrhage is present.
Warning: Dextrose Injection, USP, 50%, is extremely hypertonic and may cause phlebitis and thrombosis at the site of influsion. Except in emergencies, it should be given slowly by intravenous catheter into a central vein.
Significant hyperglycemia and possible hyperosmolar syndrome may result from too rapid administration.
Precautions: Prolonged intravenous infusions of sugar solutions may overtax islet production of insulin. To avoid this potential danger and minimize hyperglycemia and consequent glycosuria, it may be necessary to add insulin and make periodic blood determinations. However, when concentrated dextrose infusion is abruptly withdrawn, it is advisable to follow with the administration of Dextrose Injection 5% to avoid hypoglycemic reactions.
Electrolyte deficits, particularly a decrease in serum potassium, may occur during prolonged use of concentrated dextrose solutions. Blood electrolyte monitoring is essential and fluid and electrolyte imbalances should be cor-

rected. Essential vitamins and minerals also should be provided as needed.
If thrombosis should occur during administration, the infusion should be stopped and corrective measures instituted.
Dosage and Administration: Dextrose Injection, USP, 50%, is administered by slow intravenous infusion preferably by intravenous catheter with the tip positioned in a large vein such as the superior vena cava. Dosages should be adjusted to meet the requirements of each individual patient.
For parenteral hyperalimentation, 50% dextrose solution is mixed in varying proportions, according to the needs of the patient, with protein hydrolysate solutions. The amount of dextrose is governed by the ratio of 100 to 200 carbohydrate calories per gram of nitrogen.
Caution: Federal law prohibits dispensing without prescription.
How Supplied: Abbo-Vac® bottle of 500 ml. (List No. 1536-03). Each 100 ml contains dextrose, hydrous, 50 g.

ENVIRON® DISINFECTANT

Composition: A concentrated germicidal detergent combining a proven germicide of the synthetic phenolic class with a compatible synthetic detergent.
Indications: Environ is a concentrated germicidal detergent used for simultaneous cleaning, disinfection and deodorizing of animal quarters, runs and cages, and will destroy a broad range of bacteria, viruses and fungi.
Directions:
1. Preclean and remove all dirt, debris and litter from all surfaces.
2. Scrub down doors, ceilings, rafters, fixtures, ducts, partitions, windows and walls with 1% Environ solution (1 gallon per 100 gallons of water). Inaccessible surfaces should be sprayed throughly with the solution.
3. All stationary equipment such as feeders and water troughs should be cleaned and disinfected with a 1% Environ solution, and rinsed with clean water.
4. After all other surfaces have been cleaned, thoroughly *clean* the floor with a 1% Environ solution. A 2% solution may be used for exceptionally dirty surfaces.
5. Rinse all surfaces after use with clear, fresh water.

Caution: Do not apply to cow's udders or milking utensils.
How Supplied: 1-gallon containers, 4 per case (List No. 9492-08). Also available in 55-gallon drums (List No. 9492-01).

ENVIROQUAT®
Disinfectant Spray and Air Sanitizer

Composition: Active ingredients: n-alkyl dimethyl benzyl ammonium chloride, n-alkyl dimethyl ethybenzyl ammonium chloride, pro pylene glycol, ethanol.
Indications: Spot disinfectant spray wth germicidal, fungicidal, staphylocidal, tuberculocidal, and virucidal properties.
Directions: For general disinfection against bacteria such as mycobacterium tuberculosis, pathogenic fungi, and many viruses, spray surface from a distance of 12 inches for 2 to 3 seconds or until surface is wet.
To deodorize, sanitize and refreshen room air, direct spray upwards toward the center of the room for 3 to 5 seconds. Repeat as necessary.
How Supplied: 20 oz. aerosol can, 24 containers per shipping case. (List No. 6355-72)

ERYSIPELOTHRIX RHUSIOPATHIAE BACTERIN

Composition: Contains chemically inactivated culture of Erysipelothrix Rhusiopathiae (aluminum hydroxide adsorbed).
Indications: For the immunization of healthy swine and turkeys against Erysipelas.
Dosage and Administration: *Swine*—Inject 2 ml subcutaneously at 8 to 12 weeks of age. For breeding animals repeat after 21 days and annually.
Turkeys—For birds under 10 lbs, 0.5 ml, over 10 lbs, 1 ml. Inject subcutaneously in the upper neck region. Repeat dose every three months.
Precautions: Refrigerate at 35°to 45°F. Shake thoroughly before use. Use entire contents when first opened. Do not vaccinate within 21 days before slaughter. In case of anaphylactoid reaction administer epinephrine.
How Supplied: List No. 2628-02, one 50-dose vial Erysipelothrix Rhusiopathiae Bacterin. List No. 5750-04, one 250-dose vial Erysipelothrix Rhusiopathiae Bacterin.

ERYTHRO®-DRY
(erythromycin)
Mastitis Infusion Tube

Composition: Each syringe of Erythro-Dry contains 600 mg of erythromycin.
Description: ERYTHRO-Dry is a clear solution of erythromycin which provides antibacterial activity in the presence of common mastitis-causing microorganisms.
Indications: For the treatment of bovine mastitis in dry cows.
Dosage and Administration: Thoroughly milk out each infected quarter. Clean the udder and teats by washing carefully. Disinfect the teat orifice(s) with cotton soaked in alcohol or other suitable disinfectant (starting with the teats opposite the operator first). Infuse the entire contents of one syringe into each infected quarter starting with the teats nearest the operator if more than one quarter is to be treated. Close the teat orifice with gentle pressure and massage the udder to distribute the medication.
Dosage (One Treatment): Dry Cows Only: Infuse the entire contents of one Erythro-Dry syringe into each infected quarter at the time of drying-off.
Precautions: Milk taken from animals during treatment and for 36 hours (3 milkings) after the latest treatment must not be used for food. Animals treated with this drug must not be slaughtered for food within 14 days from the time of infusion nor within 96 hours after calving. Calves born to treated cows must not be slaughtered for food at less than 10 days of age.
Not for human use. Keep out of the reach of children.
For the treatment of bovine mastitis in DRY COWS only—Restricted drug, use only as directed.
Discard empty container. DO NOT REUSE.
Store at controlled room temperature, 15°-30°C (59°-86°F).
How Supplied: Package Information Erythro-Dry is supplied in 12 ml single dose disposable syringes, twelve syringes per carton. (List No. 8999-01).

ERYTHRO®-36
(erythromycin)
Mastitis Infusion Tube

Composition: Erythro-36 is a clear solution of erythromycin (50 mg/ml), one of the safest and most effective antibiotics for treating gram-positive bacterial infections.
Description: The natural oil vehicle of Erythro-36 rapidly releases erythromycin at high therapeutic levels for highly effective activity against certain *Staphlococcal* and *Streptococcal organisms.*
Erythro-36s natural oil vehicle also prevents separation of the active drug and promotes easy flow even in cold weather. It is a unique product offering effective mastitis control plus the distinct advantages of a short milk-discard time.
Indications: For the treatment of mastitis in lactating cows.
Dosage and Administration: Thoroughly milk out each infected quarter. Clean the udder and teats by washing carefully. Disinfect the teat orifice(s) with cotton soaked in alcohol or other suitable disinfectant (starting with the teats opposite the operator first). Infuse the entire contents of one syringe into each infected quarter starting with the teats nearest the operator if more than one quarter is to be treated. Close the teat orifice with gentle pressure and massage the udder to distribute the medication.
Lactating Cows: Infuse the entire contents of one Erythro-36 syringe into each infected quarter. Repeat after each milking for a total of three consecutive infusions. Discard milk for 36 hours (3 milkings) following the last treatment.
Precautions: Milk taken from animals during treatment and for 36 hours (3 milkings) after the latest treatment must not be used for food. Animals treated with this drug must not be slaughtered for food within 14 days from the time of infusion.
Not for human use. Keep out of reach of children.

Continued on next page

CEVA—Cont.

For the treatment of bovine mastitis in LACTATING COWS only—Restricted drug, use only as directed.
Discard empty container. DO NOT RE-USE.
Store at controlled room temperature, 15°-30°C (59°-86°F).
How Supplied: Eryther-36 is supplied in 6 ml single dose disposal syringes, twelve syringes per carton. List No. (8636-01)

C

ERYTHRO®-100
(erythromycin)
Injectable Antibiotic

Composition: Erythro-100 Injectable—Veterinary is an erythromycin preparation formulated in a sterile solution for intramuscular administration only.
Erythromycin is an antibiotic of low toxicity produced during the growth of the microorganism *Streptomyces erythreus.* The safety of erythromycin and its effectiveness in the treatment of various diseases of both humans and animals are well established. Because of its therapeutic importance, the antibiotic has been marketed for many years in various chemical forms and in numerous dosage forms.
Original studies on erythromycin established the effectiveness of this antibiotic against grampositive organisms. It has a wide range of activity, particularly against staphylococci, streptococci, and pneumococci-including some strains which have become resistant to the aciton of other antibiotics. Scientific studies have established that:

1. Strains naturally resistant to erythromycin are not usually encountered.
2. Cross-resistance and cross-sensitivity do not usually occur between erythromycin and certain broad-spectrum antibiotics.
3. Erythromycin is effective against some organisms that have developed resistance to other antibiotics.

Extensive controlled studies and evaluation under routine conditions by veterinarians have confirmed the value of erythromycin and expanded the indications for its use.
Composition: Erythro-100 (Erythromycin Injectable) is a specially prepared solution in a polyethylene glycol vehicle with 2% butyl aminobenzoate as a local anesthetic. It contains 100 mg. of erythromycin activity per ml.
Indications: Erythro-100 (Erythromycin Injectable) is indicated for prompt and effective treatment of conditions resulting from infections caused by organisms sensitive to erythromycin, as discussed in the following paragraphs.
Cats—Erythro-100 (Erythromycin Injectable) is indicated for treatment of pneumonia, upper respiratory infections (rhinitis, bronchitis), secondary infections associated with panleukopenia ("distemper"), and wound infections.
Dogs—Erythro-100 (Erythromycin Injectable) is indicated for the treatment of pneumonia; upper respiratory infections that may or may not be associated with the "distemper complex"; other respiratory infections, including tonsilitis, bronchitis, tracheitis, pharyngitis, and pleurisy; wound infections and abscesses; metritis and endometritis; and secondary infections associated with virus or virus-like infections.
Sheep—Erythro-100(Erythromycin Injectable) is indicated as an aid in the prevention of "lamb dysentery" and in the treatment of upper respiratory infections.
Swine—Erythro-100 (Erythromycin Injectable) is indicated for treatment of the respiratory syndrome (pneumonia, influenza, "flu", rhinitis, and bronchitis), and as an aid in the management of mastitis, metritis, and leptospirosis in sows at farrowing time and "scours" in young pigs (one week of age or older).
Cattle—Erythro-100 (Erythromycin Injectable) is indicated for the treatment of pneumonia, "shipping fever," intramuscular treatment of mastitis, metritis, infectious pododermatitis ("foot rot"), and as an aid in curtailing weight losses from moving cattle.
Dosage and Administration: *Cats, Dogs, Sheep, Swine and Cattle*—Erythro-100 (Erythromycin Injectable) is designed for intramuscular administration by deep injection into the heavy musculature of the neck or limbs. Where more than one treatment is required, it is advisable to vary the site of the intramuscular injection by alternating legs or alternating leg and neck muscle. It should not be given intravenously or intraperitoneally. Subcutaneous injections should be avoided. For smaller animals (young pigs, cats, and dogs) it is recommended that a 19- or larger 3/4" or 1" needle be used. For larger animals, either a 16- or 18-gauge 2" needle may be used.
Cats—The usual dose is 0.01 to 0.05 ml (1 to 5 mg)/lb of body weight, administered once daily or at two-day intervals as indicated.
Dogs—The usual dose is 0.02 ml (2 mg)/lb of body weight, administered once daily or at two-day intervals as indicated.
Sheep—The usual dose as an aid in the pfrevention of "dysentery"* in newborn lambs is 56 mg/lb of body weight administered once soon after birth as practicable., For the treatment of upper respiratory infections in older animals, the usual dose is 1 mg/lb once daily as indicated. Sheep must not be treated within 48 hours of slaughter for food. (*Where organisms susceptible to erythromycin may be the infective agent.)
Swine—For upper respiratory infections and pneumonia the usual dose is 1 to 3 mg/lb of body weight administered once daily as indicated. Field outbreaks of "scours" in young pigs (one week of age or older) have been reported to respond to a dose of 10 mg/lb of body weight administered in one or more daily doses as indicated by deep intramuscular injection. Swine must not be treated within 48 hours of slaughter for food.
Cattle—The usual dose is 1 to 2 ml/100 lbs of body weight (1 to 2 mg/lb) administered once daily. Milk that has been from animals during treatment and for 72 hours (6 milkings) after the last treatment must not be used for food. Cattle must not be treated within 48 hours of slaughter for food.
Precautions: During extensive clinical investigation of Erythro-100 (Erythromycin Injectable), no significant side effects were reported. Since there may be a transient swelling or soreness at the site of injection, it is advisable, when more than one treatment is required, to vary the site of injection, alternating legs or between the legs and neck muscle. Swelling or soreness encountered at the site of injection is usually mild, transient and disappears in one or two days. Deep intramuscular injections will minimize the incidence of local soreness and swelling.
Special Note:

1. It is imperative that you do not wash syringes with water. We recommened flushing syringes with isopropyl alcohol, rubbing alcohol, or acetone.
2. Erythro-100 (Erythromycin Injectable) is stable at room temperature, prefereably stored at 25°C (70°F to 75°F). Extreme temperatures will vary the viscosity. If very cold weather causes solidification, Erythro-100 (Erythromycin Injectable) can be returned to its normal fluid consistency by placing the bottle in warm water for 15 to 20 minutes bore use. The antibiotic remains fully effective.

Phramacology: Toxicity of Erythro-100 (Erythromycin Injectable) was determined by injection in white rats. Doses of 272 mg/kg, were tolerated without facilities. The LD_{50} for Erythro-100 (Erythromycin Injectable) in rats is 386 mg/kg, with 95% confidence limits of 347 to 429 mg/kg.
Irritation studies were conducted on rabbits. They showed no signs or discomfort during into the gluteal muscles. Areas injected with 1 ml of the solution showed some blanching and some signs of mild irritation. Areas given 0.5 ml did not show any obvious signs of irritation.
Eighty-seven Hereford calves injected in the neck with erythromycin base at 2 mg/lb of body weight showed no sign of irritation, swelling or heat in the area when observed at intervals of 48, 72, and 96 hours.
How Supplied: Erythro-100 (Erythromycin Injectable) is supplied in 100 ml multiple-dose rubber stoppered units. (List No. 8630-03)

ERYTHRO®-200
(erythromycin)
Injectable Antibiotic

Description: Erythromycin Injectable—Veterinary is an erythromycin preparation formulated in a sterile solution for intramuscular administration only.
Erythromycin is an antibiotic of low toxicity produced during the growth of the microorganism, *Streptomyces erythreus.* The safety of erythromycin and its effectiveness in the treatment of various diseases of both humans and animals are

well established. Because of its therapeutic importance, the antibiotic has been marketed for many years in various chemical forms and in numerous dosage forms.
Original studies on erythromycin established the effectiveness of this antibiotic against gram-positive organisms. It has a wide range of activity, particularly against staphylococci, streptococci, and pneumococci—including some strains which have become resistant to the action of other antibiotics. Scientific studies have established that:

1. Strains naturally resistant to erythromycin are not usually encountered.
2. Erythromycin is effective against some organisms that have developed resistance to other antibiotics.

Extensive controlled studies and evaluation under routine conditions by veterinarians have confirmed the value of erythromycin and expanded the indications for its use.
Composition: Erythro-200 Injectable—Veterinary is a specially prepared solution in a polyol diester od short-chain, naturally-derived fatty acids. It contains 200 mg of erythromycin activity per ml.
Indications: Erythro-200 Injectable—Veterinary is indicated for prompt and effective treatment of conditions resulting from infections caused by organisms sensitive to erythromycin, as discussed in the following paragraphs.
Cattle —Erythro-200 Injectable—Veterinary is indicated for the treatment of pneumonia, "shipping fever," intramuscular treatment of mastitis, metritis, infectious pododermatitis ("Foot rot"), and as an aid in curtailing weight losses from moving cattle.
Sheep —Erythro-200 Injectable—Veterinary is indicated as an aid in the prevention of "lamb dysentery" and in the treatment of upper respiratory infections.
Swine —Erythro-200 Injectable—Veterinary is indicated for treatment of the respiratory syndrome (pneumonia, influenza, rhinitis, and bronchitis), and as an aid in the management of mastitis, metritis, and leptospirosis in sows at farrowing time and "scours" in young pigs (one week of age or older).
Dosage and Administration: *Cattle, Sheep, and Swine* —Erythro-200 Injectable—Veterinary is designed for intramuscular administration by deep injection into the heavy musculature of the neck or limbs. Where more than one treatment is required, it is advisable to vary the site of the intramuscular injection by alternating legs or alternating leg and neck muscle. It should not be given intravenously or intraperitoneally. Subcutaneous injections should be avoided. For young pigs, it is recommended that a 19- or 20" gauge 1" needle be used. For larger animals, either a 16- or 18-gauge 2" needle may be used.
Cattle —The usual dose is 0.5 to 1 ml/100 lbs of body weight (1 to 2 mg/lb) administered once daily. Milk that has been from animals during treatment and for 72 hours (6 milkings) after the last treatment must not be used for food. Cattle must not be treated within 14 days of slaughter for food. Temporary tissue irritation follows injection. To avoid excessive trim, do not slaughter beef cattle within 21 days of last injection.
Sheep —The usual dose as an aid in the prevention of "dysentery"* in newborn lambs is 56 mg/lb of body weight administered once soon after birth as practicable. For the treatment of upper respiratory infections in older animals, the usual dose is 0.5 ml(100 mg)/lb once daily as indicated. Sheep must not be treated within 3 days of slaughter for food. Temporary tissue irritation follows injection. To avoid irritation follows injection. To avoid excessive trim, do not slaughter within 10 days of the last injection. (*Where organisms susceptible to erythromycin may be the infective agent.)
Swine —For upper respiratory infections and pneumonia, the usual dose is 1 to 3 mg/lb of body weight administered once daily as indicated. Field outbreaks of "scours" in young pigs (one week of age or older) have been reported to respond to a dose of 10 mg/lb of body weight administered in one or more daily doses as indicated by deep intramuscular injection. Swine must not be treated within 7 days of slaughter for food. Temporary tissue irritation follows injection. To avoid excessive trim, do not slaughter within 10 days of the last injection.
Precautions: During extensive clinical investigation of Erythro-200 Injectable—Veterinary, no significant side effects were reported. Since there may be a transient swelling or soreness at the site of injection, it is advisable, when more than one treatment is required, to vary the site of injection, alternating legs or between the legs and neck muscle. Swelling or soreness encountered at the site of injection is usually mild, transient, and disappears in one or two days. Deep intramuscular injections will minimize the incidence of local soreness and swelling.
Special Note: Thoroughly clean and sterilize syringes and needles before using (needles and syringes may be sterilized by boiling water for 15 minutes).
Use all precautions to prevent contamination of contents of bottle.
Injection site should be disinfected with a suitable disinfectant such as 70% isopropyl alcohol just prior to injecting Erythro-200 Injectable—Veterinary.
How Supplied: Erythro-200 (Erythromycin Injectable) is supplied in 200 ml multiple-dose rubber stoppered vials of 100 ml (List No. 8609-04/12 per case) and 250 ml (List No. 8609-05).

IMMU-COLI-B™
Escherichia coli Bacterin Bovine Isolates
An aid in the prevention of *E. coli* scours

Description: Immu-Coli-B Bacterin contains chemically inactivated cultures of *Escherichia coli* isolates of four serological types formulated for high K99 antigen content, combined with an adjuvant to potentiate the immune response.
Indications: Immu-Coli-B is indicated for use in healthy pregnant cattle as an aid in protecting young calves from severe scours and death caused by the antigenic range of enteropathogenic *E. coli* organisms contained in this bacterin. The protective antibodies for the newborn calf provided by this bacterin are contained in the dam's first milk (colostrum) which must be consumed within 2–4 hours after birth in sufficient quantities by the calf.
Dosage & Administration: Inject two 5 ml doses subcutaneously or intramuscularly 2–4 weeks apart. The first dose should be given about 5–6 weeks before calving and the second dose 2–3 weeks before expected calving date.
Precautions: Store at 2–7°C (35–45°F). Shake well before using. Do not vaccinate within 21 days before slaughter. Use entire contents when first opened. In case of anaphylactoid reaction, use epinephrine. Thimerosal added as a preservative.
How Supplied: Immu-Coli-B is available in 10 dose/50 ml vials (List No. 2500-01).

IONOSOL® T IN D5—W

Composition: Each 100 ml contains:

Dextrose, hydrous	5 g
Sodium Chloride	146 mg
Potassium Lactate, anhydrous	256 mg
Monosodium Phosphate, anhydrous	180.6 mg
Potassium Chloride	111 mg
Sodium Bisulfite added (approx. 2mEq/l)	23 mg
406 mOsm/l (calc.)	Approx. pH 4.7

Provides in 1,000 ml (not including ions in preservative):

Sodium	40 mEq
Potassium	35mEq
Total Cations	75 mEq
Chloride	40 mEq
Lactate	20mEq
Phosphate	15mEq
Total Anions	75mEq

Dosage: For intravenous use. Contents or such lesser amount as determined by the physician as a single dose.
Caution: Federal (U.S.A.) law prohibits dispensing without prescription.
Caution: Rate of administration should not exceed 500 ml per hour.
Air in container displaced by inert gas.
Electrolyte Solution with Dextrose.
How Supplied: IONOSOL T IN D5-W is available in 1000 ml bottles, packages 6 per case (List No. 1552-05).

LACTATED RINGER'S CONCENTRATE

Composition: Each 250 ml of Lactated Ringer's Concentrate contains: Sodium Chloride, 18.0 gm; Sodium lactate, 9.3 gm; Potassium chloride 0.9 gm; Calcium chloride, 0.6 gm.
Description: A sterile solution for replacement of electrolytes, for intravenous or subcutaneous use.
Indications: Solution is a concentrate which must be diluted prior to use. Using

Continued on next page

CEVA—Cont.

2750 ml of sterile water for injection, aseptically dilute contents of each 250 ml vial to 3000 ml. Diluted solution contains the following milliequivalents per 1000 ml (not including ions for adjusting pH):

Sodium	30 mEq
Postasium	4 mEq
Calcium	3 mEg
Total Cations	137 mEq
Chloride	109 mEq
Lactate	28 mEq
Total Cations	137 mEq

Dosage and Administration: 3000 ml of diluted product or such amount as determined by the veterinarian to be needed as a single dose in replacement electrolyte therapy.
Precautions: This product contains no bacteriostat. Solution should be used promptly. Discard unused portion. Protect from freezing.
How Supplied: Lactated Ringer's Concentrate (List No. 1975-02) is supplied in non-breakable, plastic 250 ml containers.

LACTATED RINGER'S SOLUTION
Lactated Ringer's Injection, USP

Composition: Each 100 ml contains:

Sodium Chloride	600 mg
Sodium Lactate, anhydrous	310 mg
Potassium Chloride	30 mg
Calcium Chloride, USP	20 mg
Provides in 1000 ml:	
Sodium	130mEq
Potassium	4 mEq
Calcium	3 mEq
Total Cations	137 mEq
Chloride	109mEq
Lactate	28mEq
Total Anions	137mEq

May contain hydrochloric acid or sodium hydroxide for pH adjustment.
Usual Dose: Contents or such lesser amount as determined by the veterinarian as a single dose.
For intravenous or subcutaneous use.
Use only if clear and vacuum present. Before piercing, cleanse stopper with antiseptic.
For veterinary use only.
Caution: Do not administer calcium-containing solutions concurrently with stored blood.
Federal law restricts this drug to use by or on the order of a licensed veterinarian.
How Supplied: Abbo-Vac® bottle of 250 ml. (List No. 1553-02), 500 ml (List No. 1553-03) and 1000 ml (List No. 1553-05). (LifeCare® 1000 ml I.V. bags (List No. 7953-39) and 3000 ml I.V. bags (List No. 7525-08).

LEPTOSPIRA POMONA BACTERIN

Composition: Contains chemically inactivated cultures of *Leptospira Pomona* (aluminum hydroxide adsorbed).
Indications: For the immunization of healthy swine and cattle against *Leptospira pomona* infection.
Dosage and Administration: Inject 2 ml intramuscularly.
Precautions: Refrigerate at 35° to 45°F. Shake thoroughly before use. Use entire contents when first opened. Do not vaccinate within 21 days before slaughter. In case of anaphylactoid reaction administer epinephrine.
How Supplied: List No. 2630-01, one 10-dose vial Leptospira Pomona Bacterin. List No. 2630-02, one 50-dose vial Leptospira Pomona Bacterin.

5-WAY LEPTOSPIROSIS VACCINE

Composition: Contains chemically inactivated, highly antigenic whole cultures of each of listed serovars.
Description: Effective, long-term protection against all five major lepto strains. Continuously tested to ensure highest standards of antigenicity, uniformity, safety and stability. Each antigenic component has been specially selected for its high antigenic, immunogenic properties in host animals. Highly antigenic whole cultures used in production. Cultures selected to provide optimum potency, while reducing impurities and minimizing potential of anaphylactic shock. Host animal efficacy tests show no renal shedding. May be administered to pregnant animals without fear of abortions.
Indications: For the immunization of healthy cattle against leptospirosos caused by *Leptospira canicola, Leptospira grippotyphosa, Leptospira hardjo, Leptospira icterohaemorrhagiae* and *Leptospira pomona.*
Dosage and Administration: Inject 2 ml intramuscularly. In endemic leptospria areas a second dose is recommnded 3–5 weeks later. Annual revaccination is recommended, or prior to each breeding.
Precautions: Refrigerate at 2–7C (35–45F). Shake thoroughly before use. Use entire contents when first opened.Do not vaccinate animals under 2 months of age. In case of anaphylactic reaction, use epinephrine. Thimerosal added as a preservative.
How Supplied: Packaged in unbreakable plastic bottles capped with specially designed non-leak rubber seals. Size 10-Dose (List No. 2645-01) Size 50-Dose (List No. 2645-02)

3-LITER I.V. SOLUTION BAG

Description: Disposable I.V. solution set for administration of concentrate electrolyte solutions, including Multisol®-R 3X, and Lactated Ringers 3X. 3-liter capacity bag features drip chamber, flow rate regulator, and a triple ziplock seal for easy opening and closing, and leak-tight sealing. Bigbore tubing measures 60″ in length, 0.195″ *i.d.*, 0.275 *o.d.*
How Supplied: 1 Set, 24 sets per case (List No. 1953-01).

LpH® GERMICIDAL DETERGENT

Composition: Active ingredietns: Glycolic acid, 12.6%; o-benzyl-p-chlorophenol, 6.1%; p-tertiary-amylphenol, 3.0%; o-phenylphenol, 0.5%.
Indications: A super concentrated germicidal detergent for manual cleaning and disinfecting of animal and poultry facilties. LpH provides effective control of bacteria, including *Staphylococcus aureus, Streptococcus* spp., *Pseudomonas aeru ginosa, Pseudomonas fragi, Arizona* spp., *Brucella bronchiseptica, Enterobacter* spp., *Escherichia coli, Proteus* spp., *Shigella dysenteriae, Salmonella* spp., *Serratia marcescens,* and *Myco-bacterium tuberculosis.*
LpH quickly destroys *Candila albicans* and *Trichophyton mentagrophytes* fungi, and is effective against the following viruses: Influenza A2, Herpes simplex, Type 2 Adenovirus, Vaccinia, Hog Cholera Virus, and Pseudorabies Virus. It will further destroy the viruses associated with: Marek's Disease, Newcastle Disease, Infectious Bronchitis, Infectious Laryngotracheitis and African Swine Fever.
Directions: Packaged with dispensing pump. Use ½ ounce of LpH (1 stroke of pump) for each gallon of water — 1:256 use solution. Apply with normal techniques, using wiping clothes, sponge or mop. When used as directed, LpH is harmless to fabrics, resilient flooring, tile and varnished surfaces.
Caution: Corrosive to tissues. This concentrate causes eye and skin damage. Harmful or fatal if swallowed.
How Supplied: 1-gallon containers. (List No. 9398-08). Packaged with dispensing pump. Also available in 55-gallon drums (List No. 9398-01).

MALE ADAPTER PLUG

For use in adapting standard venipuncture devices to intermittent administration procedures.
List No. 5878-01.

MEDICATED LOTION SOAP

Composition: Contains: 0.5% p-chloro-m-xylenol in a base containing Sodium Oleate, Potassium Vegetable Oil Soap, Glycerin, Amphoteric-2, TEA-Coco-Hydrolyzed Protein with Sorbitol, DEA Cocamide, Sodium Styrene/PEG-10 Maleate/Nonoxynol-10 Maleate/Acrylate Copolymer with Ammonium Nonoxynol-4 Sulfate, DMDM Hydantoin (presevative) in water with perfume added.
Indications: A medicated lotion soap which is effective against a variety of pathogenic bacteria, fungi and yeast to break the chain of cross infection in critical care areas. Contains 0.5% p-chloro-m-xylenol, a proven antibacterial agent for both Gram positive and Gram negative bacteria. Lathers quickly, even in hard water, and aggressively removes dirt, dead skin and bacteria. Specially blended emollients and skin conditioners help reduce skin trauma, permitting use several times daily.
Directions: Wet hands, dispense a small quantity (1.5 cc) in the palm of one hand, wash thoroughly, rinse completely and dry.
How Supplied: 1-quart containers, 12 per case, including convenient dispenser (List No. 6266-24). 8-oz squeeze bottle, 24 per case (List No. 6266-47).

MULTISOL®-R 3X
Concentrated Replacement Electrolytes

Composition: Each 100 ml contains:

Sodium chloride	15.78 gm
Sodium acetate	6.66 gm
Sodium gluconate	15.06 gm
Potassium chloride	1.11 gm
Magnesium chloride	0.42 gm

Milliequivalents per 100 ml. (not including ions for adjusting pH):

Sodium	140.00 mEq
Potassium	5.00 mEq
Magnesium	3.00 mEq
Total Cations	148.00 mEq
Chloride	98.00 mEq
Acetate	27.00 mEq
Gluconate	23.00 mEq
Total Anions	148.00 mEq

Indications: This isotonic, balanced electrolyte solution is designed for replacement of extracellular fluid losses without disturbing electrolyte balance. It is used as replacement for acute losses which may occur in surgery, trauma, or a variety of clinical disorders. Multisol-R 3X is calcium-free, eliminates the possibility of clotting when administered with citrated blood, and reduces the chance of incompatibilities with certain drugs which may be added to the solution.
Directions: This solution is a concentrate which must be diluted prior to use. Using 2900 ml of sterile water for injection, aseptically dilute contents of this vial (100 ml) to 3000 ml.
Usual Dose: 3000 ml of diluted product or such amount as determined by the veterinarian as a single dose in replacement electrolyte therapy.
Caution:
This product contains no bacteriostat.
Solution should be used promptly.
Discard unused portion.
Protect from freezing.
How Supplied: 100 ml containers, 12 per case (List No. 1923-01). CEVA 3-Liter I.V. Solution Bag for administration also available.

NORMAL SALINE
Sodium Chloride Injection, 0.9%, USP

Composition: Each 100 ml contains:

Sodium Chloride	900 mg

Provides in 100 ml:

Sodium	154 mEq
Chloride	154 mEq

Usual Dose: Contents or such lesser amount as determined by the veterinarian as a single dose.
For intravenous or subcutaneous use.
Use only if clear and vacuum present. Before piercing, cleanse stopper with antiseptic.
For veterinary use only.
Caution: Federal law restricts this drug to use by or on the order of a licensed veterinarian.
How Supplied: Abbo-Vac® bottle of 250 ml (List No. 1583-02), 500 ml (List No. 1583-03) and 1000 ml (List No. 1583-05). LifeCare® I.V. bags (List No. 7983-39) and 3000 ml irrigation bags (List No. 7525-08).

NORMOSOL®-M IN D5-W
Maintenance Electrolytes with Dextrose 5%

Composition: Each 100 ml contains:

Dextrose, hydrous	5 mg
Sodium Chloride	234 mg
Potassium Acetate	128 mg
Magnesium Acetate	21 mg
Sodium Bisulfite added (3 mEq/1)	33 mg

pH adjusted with hydrochloric acid (approx. 1mEq/1).
Milliequivalents per 1000 ml (not including ions for adjusting pH or in preservative):

Sodium	40 mEq
Potassium	13 mEq
Magnesium	3 mEq
Total Cations	56 mEq
Chloride	40 mEq
Acetate	16 mEq
Total Anions	56 mEq

Dosage and Administration: Contents or such lesser amount as determined by the veterinarian as a single dose.
For intravenous use only.
Use only if clear and vacuum present. Before piercing, cleanse stopper with antiseptic.
Air in container displaced by inert gas.
Caution: Federal law restricts this drug to use by or on the order of a licensed veterinarian.
How Supplied: Abbo-Vac® bottle of 500 ml (List No. 1565-03) and 1000 ml (List No. 1565-05). LifeCare® 1000 ml I.V. bags (List No. 7965-39).

NORMOSOL®-R
Replacement Electrolytes in Water

Composition: Each 100 ml contains:

Sodium Chloride	526 mg
Sodium Acetate	222 mg
Sodium Gluconate	502 mg
Potassium Chloride	37 mg
Magnesium Chloride	14 mg

pH adjusted with hydrochloric acid (approx. 1mEq/1).
Milliequivalents per 1000 ml (not including ions for adjusting pH):

Sodium	140 mEq
Potassium	5 mEq
Magnesium	3 mEq
Total Cations	148 mEq
Chloride	98 mEq
Acetate	27 mEq
Gluconate	23 mEq
Total Anions	148 mEq

Dosage and Administration: Contents or such lesser amount as determined by the veterinarian as a single dose.
For intravenous or subcutaneous use.
Use only if clear and vacuum present. Before piercing, cleanse stopper with antiseptic.
Caution: Federal law restricts this drug to use by or on the order of a licensed veterinarian.
How Supplied: Abbo-Vac® bottle of 500 ml (List No. 1567-03) and 1000 ml (List No. 1567-05). LifeCare® 1000 ml I.V. bags (List No. 7967-39) and 3000 ml I.V. bags (List No. 7018-08).

NORMOSOL®-R IN D5-W
Replacement Electrolytes with Dextrose 5%

Composition: Each 100 ml contains:

Dextrose, hydrous	5 g
Sodium Chloride	526 mg
Sodium Acetate, anhydrous	222 mg
Sodium Gluconate	502 mg
Potassium Chloride	37 mg
Magensium Chloride	14 mg
Sodium Bisulfite added (3mEq/1)	33 mg

pH adjusted with hydrochloric acid (approx. 1 mEq/1).
Millieqivalents per 100 ml (not including ions for adjusting pH or in preservative):

Sodium	140 mEq
Potassium	5 mEq
Magnesium	3 mEq
Total Cations	148 mEq
Chloride	98 mEq
Acetate	27 mEq
Gluconate	23 mEq
Total Anions	148 mEq

Dosage and Administration: Contents or such lesser amount as determined by the veterinarian as a single dose.
For intravenous use only.
Use only if clear and vacuum present. Before piercing, cleanse stopper with antiseptic.
Caution: Federal law restricts this drug to use by or on the order of a licensed veterinarian.
How Supplied: Abbo-Vac® bottle of 1000 ml (List No. 1568-05). LifeCare® 1000 ml I.V. bags (List No. 7968-39).

PASTEURELLA HAEMOLYTICA–MULTOCIDA BACTERIN

Composition: Contains chemically inactivated cultures of *Pasteurella multocida* and *Pasteurella haemolytica* (bovine isolates, aluminum hydroxide absorbed).
Contains thimerosal as a preservative.
No US Standard of Potency.
Indications: For the immunization of healthy cattle against *Pasteurella.*
Dosage and Administration: Inject 2 ml intramuscularly. Repeat vaccination within 14 to 30 days.
Precautions: Refrigerate at 35° to 45°F. Shake thoroughly before use. Use entire contents when first opened. Do not vaccinate within 21 days before slaughter. Do not vaccinate animals under 2 months of age. In case of anaphylactoid reaction administer epinephrine.
How Supplied: List No. 2629-01, one 10-dose vial Pasteurella Bacterin. List No. 2629-02, one 50-dose vial Pasteurella Bacterin.

PENTOTHAL® DISPENSING CAP

Screws onto Pentothal® bottles after addition of diluent, to facilitate syringe withdrawal of prepared solution. List No. 6680-03.

Continued on next page

CEVA—Cont.

PENTOTHAL® DISPENSING PIN

Plugs into Pentothal® bottles. Permits addition of diluent from Abbo-Vac bottle via a Secondary Venoset® and syringe withdrawal of prepared solution. List No. 6682-02.

C

POTASSIUM CHLORIDE 20mEq and 40 mEq (2mEq/ml) and 40 mEq (2mEq/ml)

Composition: Potassium Chloride 20 mEq and 40 mEq (2 mEq/ml), is a sterile, nonpyrogenic, *concentrated* solution containing 20 mEq each of K +and Cl—in 10 ml, in water for injection and 40 mEq each of K^+ and Cl^- in 20 ml water for injection. *It should not be administered undiluted.* It is intended only for addition of all or part of the contents of each Abbo-Vial® to other intravenous fluids.
Indications: Potassium Chloride, 20 mEq and 40 mEq (2 mEq/ml), is indicated in the treatment of potassium deficiency states when oral replacement therapy is not feasible.
Contraindications: Potassium chloride, 20 mEq and 40 mEq (2 mEq/ml), is contraindicated in diseases where high potassium levels may be encountered.
Warnings: To avoid potassium intoxication, do not infuse solutions containing potassium chloride rapidly. In patients with severe renal insufficiency or adrenal insufficiency, administration of potassium chloride injection may cause high potassium levels.
Precautions: Potassium should be administered cautiously. Plasma potassium levels are not necessarily indicative of tissue potassium levels.
High plasma concentrations of potassium may cause death through cardiac depression, arrhythmias or arrest.
Potassium Chloride, 20 mEq and 40 mEq (2 mEq/ml), should be used with caution in the presence of cardiac disease, particularly in digitalized patients or in the presence of renal disease.
Adverse Reactions: Vomiting and diarrhea have been reported. The signs and symptoms of potassium intoxication include flaccid paralysis, listlessness, mental confusion, hypotension, cardiac arrhythmias, heart block, electrocardiograph abnormalities such as disappearance of P waves, spreading and slurring of the QRS complex with development of a biphasic curve and cardiac arrest.
Dosage and Administration: Potassium chloride, 20 mEq and 40 mEq (2 mEq/ml), is administered intravenously only after dilution to a larger volume of fluid. (See Directions For Use of Abbo-Vial.®)
The dose and rate of injection are dependent upon the individual needs of each patient. The rate should not exceed 0.5 mEq/kg/hr.
Overdose: In the event of overdose, discontinue the infusion immediately and institute intensive corrective therapy to reduce the serum potassium levels.
How Supplied (For Dilution Only): Potassium Chloride, 20 mEq (2 mEq/ml), is supplied in 10 ml. Abbo-Vial Flip Top container (List No. 6651-71) containing 20 mEq each of K +and Cl—(potassium chloride 1.49 g); pH may be adjusted with hydrochloric acid and 40 mEq (2 mEq/ml) is supplied in 20 ml Abbo-Vial Flip Top container List #6653-06.

RHI-CO-PIG™ Bordetella Bronchiseptica-Escherichia Coli Bacterin

Composition: RHI-CO-PIG contains chemically inactivated cultures of Bordetella bronchiseptica and Escherichia coli serotypes K88ab, K88ac, K99, 987P and F41.
Indications: Recommended for use in healthy pregnant gilts/sows as an aid in control and prevention of disease due to *Bordetella bronchiseptica* infection and neonatal enteric colibacillosis caused by *E. coli* strains in the antigenic spectrum covered by this bacterin. Transfer of passive protection contained in the colostrum of the immune dam's first milk to the newborn piglet has been demonstrated.
Dosage and Administration: Inject 3 ml. deep intramuscularly behind the ear. A primary vaccination of two 3 ml doses is recommended, 5 to 7 weeks and 2 to 3 weeks prior to planned farrowing. Revaccinate with a single 3 ml booster 2 to 3 weeks prior to planned farrowings. For broader protection against atrophic rhinitis, vaccinate all new breeding stock with one dose, 2.0 ml., of Bordetella Bronchiseptica-Pasteurella Multocida Bacterin, RHINIPIG™, at 6 months of age or prior to introduction into vaccinated herds; revaccinate all boars with a single dose annually.
Precautions: Store at 2–7°C (35–45°F). Do Not Freeze. Shake well before using. Transient local reactions may be observed at injection site. Do not vaccinate within 21 days before slaughter. Use entire contents when first opened. In case of anaphylactoid reaction, use epinephrine. Thermerosal added as a preservative.
How Supplied: 10 dose/30 ml (List No. 2713-01) and 25 dose/75 ml (List No. 2713-02).

RHINIPIG™ Bordetella Bronchiseptica-Pasteurella Multocida Bacterin

Composition: Rhinipig™ contains chemically inactivated cultures of Bordetella bronchiseptica and Pasteurella multocida, Type A.
Indications: For use as an aid in the control and prevention of disease due to Bordetella bronchispetica infection and pasteurellosis in healthy swine. Transfer of passive protection to B. bronchiseptica has been demonstrated in piglets.
Dosage and Administration: Inject 2 ml, deep intramuscularly behind ear. *Sows & Gilts:* Two doses (2 ml each) 5 and 3 weeks prior to first farrowing and one dose 3 weeks prior to each subsequent farrowing. Vaccinate all new breeding stock with two doses (2 ml each) at 15 to 21 days intervals, at 6 months of age prior to introduction into vaccinated herds; all boars should be revaccinated with a single dose annually.
Precautions: Store at 2-7°C (35° to 45° F). Do Not Freeze. Shake well before using. Transient local reactions may be observed at the injection site. Do not vaccinate during the last 15 days of gestation. Do not vaccinate within 21 days before slaughter. Use entire contents when first opened. In case of anaphylactoid reaction, use epinephrine. Thimerosal added as a preservative.
How Supplied: 10 doses/20 ml (List No. 2497-01) and 50 Doses/100 ml (List No. 2497-02).

RINGER'S INJECTION, USP

Composition: Each 100 ml contains:

Sodium Chloride	860 mg
Potassium Chloride	30 mg
Calcium Chloride, USP	33 mg

309 mOsm/l (calc)
Approx pH 5.8

Provides in 1,000 ml:

Sodium	147 mEq
Potassium	4 mEq
Calcium	5 mEq
Total Cations	156mEq
Chloride	156mEq
Total Anions	156mEq

Indications: Correction of water and electrolyte deficits.
Dosage and Administration: For intravenous or subcutaneous use. Contents or such lesser amount as needed as a single dose.
Use only if clear and vacuum present.
Caution: Do not administer calcium-containing solutions concurrently with stored blood.
Warning: Federal law prohibits dispensing without presecription.
How Supplied: Abbo-Vac® bottle of 500 ml (List No. 1582-03) and 1000 ml (List No. 1582-05).

SECONDARY VENOSET®

Description: Disposable I.V. set for series hookup.
Fluid path and areas under protective coverings of set are sterile and nonpyrogenic if set covers are in place.
Directions (Use Aseptic Technique): Remove protective coverings as assembly progresses.
Directions for Series Hookup:
1. Prepare Abbo-Vac bottle (or other container).
2. Close slide clamp.
3. With bottle upright, thrust piercing pin straight through stopper center. Do not twist or angle.
4. Immediately invert bottle and check for vacuum by observing rising bubbles.
5. Suspend inverted secondary bottle.
6. Remove fllter from air inlet of primary set and insert adapter of secondary set.
7. Open slide clamp.

Note: Secondary bottle empties first, but some intermixing in primary bottle may occur affecting order in which contents reach patient. Contents must be compatible.

NOT FOR INSERTION INTO BLOOD OR PLASMA CONTAINERS. CHANGE WITHIN 24 HOURS. DISCARD AFTER USE.

Caution: Federal law restricts this device to sale by or on the order of a licensed veterinarian.

Disposable Device. Do not resterilize or reuse.

Do not store at extreme temperatures.

How Supplied: 1 Unit (List No. 1702-48).

SELEEN® SUSPENSION

Composition:

Active ingredient:

Selenium disulfide 0.9 w/w (1 W/V)

Indications: Use on dogs as a cleansing shampoo and for removing skin debris associated with dry eczema, seborrhea and nonspecific dermatoses.

Directions:

1. Instill boric acid ophthalmic ointment into eyes and, in males, cover scrotum well with petrolatum.
2. Wet hair thoroughly with warm water.
3. Shake well before using. Apply 1 to 2 ounces of the suspension and work into the skin of entire body, being careful around the scrotum and eyes. Add sufficient amount of warm water to produce a good lather and continue to wash. Rub especially well into severely affected areas. Three to four ounces may be required in large breeds.
4. Allow suspension to remain in contact with skin for 5 to 15 minutes as indicated.
5. Rinse hair and skin thoroughly using spray type attachment. Treatment should be repeated at 4 to 7 day intervals, as directed.

Protect from freezing.

Caution: Federal law restricts this drug to use by or on the order of a licensed veterinarian.

How Supplied: 5.5 oz container (List No. 8669-01) and 1 gallon container (List No. 8669-02)

SEPTISOL® FOAM
Surgical Hand Scrub

Composition: An emolliented tincture of hexachlorophene dispensed as a foam.

Indications: Bacteriostatic skin cleanser for surgical scrubbing.

Directions: Dispense first foam application and spread over both arms from the wrists to just above the elbow, massaging until the foam is broken. While arms are air drying, dispense second application and rub over hands and wrists. Allow hands to air dry, then don gown and glove. Single application eliminates transient bacteria and reduces resident microflora to levels equal to those normally achieved with conventional scrub procedures.

Caution: Not for use on burned or denuded skin or on mucous membranes. Not for routine prophylactic total body bathing.

How Supplied: 48 6-oz. containers per case (List No. 6288-56). Also available in 20-oz. containers, 24 containers per case (List No. 6288-72). Specially-designed, foot-operated conductive dispenser (List No. 4504-2).

SEPTISOL® SOLUTION
Personnel Handwash

Composition: Contains Irgasan in an aqueous potassium vegetable oil soap, glycerine, propylene glycol, tetraethylene glycol, BHT, EDTA, tertiary butyl hydroperoxide, perfume and certified color added.

Indications: Bacteriostatic skin cleanser for handwashing as part of patient care.

Caution: Not for use on burned or denuded skin or on mucous membranes. Not for routine prophylactic total body bathing. Rinse thoroughly after use.

How Supplied: 1-quart disposible containers, 12 quarts per case, (List No. 6281-24). Also available in 1-gallon containers, four gallons per case (List No. 6281-08). Spring-loaded dispensing pump packaged with each case. Wall-mounted dispenser available.

SODIUM BICARBONATE INJECTION, USP, 5%

Composition: Each 100 ml contains: Sodium Bicarbonate, USP, 5 g (50 mg/ml); Disodium Edetate, anhydrous, added as stabilizer, 90 mg; pH adjusted to approx. 7.6 with CO_2.

1199 mOsm/liter (calc).

Air in container displaced by inert gas. Store at controlled room temperature.

Provides in 500 ml: Sodium 297.5 mEq (approx. 0.6 mEq/ml); Bicarbonate 297.5 mEq (approx 0.6 mEq/ml).

Indications: Correction of metabolic acidosis.

Dosage and Administration: Contents or such lesser amount as needed. Use only if clear and vacuum present.

Caution: Monitor frequently during administration to assure that drip chamber remains at least ⅓ full.

Warning: Federal law prohibits dispensing without prescription.

How Supplied: Abbo-Vac® 500 ml bottle (List No. 1594-03).

SODIUM BICARBONATE INJECTION, USP, 8.4%

Description: Sodium Bicarbonate Injection, USP 8.4% Additive Solution (50 mEq) is a sterile, nonpyrogenic preparation of sodium bicarbonate ($NaHCO_3$), USP, in water for injection. Each 50 ml vial contains 4.2 g of sodium bicarbonate (50 mEq each of sodium and bicarbonate). This concentrated solution has an approximate pH of 7.8.

Actions: Sodium bicarbonate has a valuable role in the treatment of metabolic acidosis due to a wide variety of causes. Sodium bicarbonate therapy increases plasma bicarbonate, buffers excess hydrogen ion concentration, raises blood pH and reverses the clinical manifestations of acidosis.

Indications: Sodium bicarbonate is indicated in the treatment of metabolic acidosis which may occur in severe renal disease, uncontrolled diabetes, circulatory insufficiency due to shock or severe dehydration, cardiac arrest and severe primary lactic acidosis. Sodium bicarbonate also is indicated in severe diarrhea which is often accompanied by a significant loss of bicarbonate.

Contraindications: Sodium bicarbonate is contraindicated in patients who are losing chloride by vomiting or from continuous gastrointestinal suction, and in patients receiving diuretics known to produce a hypochloremic alkalosis.

Precautions: The aim of all bicarbonate therapy is to produce a substantial correction of the low total Co_2 content and blood pH, but the risks of overdosage and alkalosis should be avoided. Hence, repeated fractional doses and periodic monitoring by appropriate laboratory tests are recommended to minimize the possibility of overdosage.

The addition of sodium bicarbonate to parenteral solutions containing calcium should be avoided except where compatibility has been previously established. Precipitation or haze may result from sodium bicarbonate-calcium admixtures, and the resulting solution should not be administered.

Dosage and Administration: Sodium Bicarbonate Injection, USP 8.4% Additive Solution (50 mEq) is administered by the intravenous route.

In general, caution should be observed in emergencies where very rapid infusion of large quantities of bicarbonate is indicated—for example, in cardiac arrest. Sodium bicarbonate solutions are hypertonic and may produce an undesirable rise in plasma sodium concentration in the process of correction of metabolic acidosis. In cardiac arrest, however, the risks from acidosis exceed those of hypernatremia. The contents of four to six 50 ml vials of 8.4% solution may be given undiluted by rapid intravenous infusion, using a needle and syringe.

Sodium Bicarbonate Injection, USP 8.4% Additive Solution (50 mEq in 50 ml) is usually added to other intravenous fluids in the less urgent forms of metabolic acidosis. The amount of bicarbonate to be given over a four-to-eight-hour period is approximately 2 to 5 mEq per kg of body weight—depending upon the severity of the acidosis as judged by the lowering of total CO_2 content, blood pH and clinical condition of the patient. Bicarbonate therapy should always be planned in the stepwise fashion since the degree of response from a given dose is not precisely predictable. Initially an infusion of 2 to 5 mEq per kg of body weight over a period of 4-8 hours will produce a measurable improvement in the abnormal acid-base status of the blood. The next step of therapy is dependent upon the clinical response of the patient. If severe symptoms have abated, then the frequency of administration and the size of the dose may be reduced.

Overdosage: Should alkalosis result, the bicarbonate should be stopped and the patient managed according to the

Continued on next page

CEVA—Cont.

degree of alkalosis present. Sodium chloride injection (0.9%) may be given intravenously; potassium chloride also may be indicated if there is hypokalemia. Severe alkalosis may be accompanied by hyperirritability or tetany, and these symptoms may be controlled by calcium gluconate. An acidifying agent such as ammonium chloride may also be indicated in severe alkalosis.
How Supplied: Sodium Bicarbonate Injection, USP 8.4% Additive Solution (50mEq) is supplied in 50 ml vials, (List No. 6625-03).

SODIUM CHLORIDE INJECTION, BACTERIOSTATIC, U.S.P.

Composition: Each ml contains: Sodium chloride, 9 mg (0.9%), and 9 mg (0.9%) benzyl alcohol added as a preservative, pH adjusted with hydrochloric acid. Sterile, nonpyrogenic.
Indications: For use only as a sterile diluent or solvent for drugs.
Use only if clear. Cleanse stopper with antiseptic.
Caution: Federal (U.S.A.) law prohibits dispensing without prescription.
How Supplied: 30 ml multiple-dose Flip Top Vial (List No. 1966-73).

SODIUM CHLORIDE IRRIGATION, 0.9%
Sodium Chloride Irrigation, USP

Composition: Each 100 ml contains sodium chloride, USP, 0.09 g.
Indications: For irrigation.
Administration: Do not use if not clear or if seal is broken or damaged. Contains no bacteriostat. Discard unused portion. Not for injection.
Warning: Avoid warming to temperatures in excess of 150°F.
Caution: Federal law prohibits dispensing without prescription.
How Supplied: Urogate® semi-rigid containers of 500 ml (List No. 6138-03) and 1000 ml (List No. 6138-09).

SOLUSET® 150 × 60

Description: 150 × 60, 77-inch Microdrip precision volume I.V. set with CAIR Clamp and slide clamps. Includes 150 ml calibrated burette, and Y-injection site 6 inches from the male adapter. (List No. 1882-02)

SPECTAM® INJECTABLE
(spectinomycin)
Injectable Antibiotic

Composition: A clear, sterile solution of spectinomycin (100 mg/ml), from spectinomycin dihydrochloride pentahydrate. Intended for subcutaneous injection of 1- to 3-day-old turkey poults and newly hatched chicks. Stable under normal conditions of storage. Excellent flow characteristics make possible the use of a fine-gauge needle for injection.
Spectinomycin has an extremely low degree of toxicity. Subcutaneous injections of up to 50 mg per poult have caused no detectable ill effects. Doses of 90 mg per poult have produced transient ataxia and coma from which poults recovered in approximately four hours. No local tissue reaction has been observed following the injection of Spectam.
Indications: For use in turkey poults as an aid in the control of airsacculitis associated with *M. meleagridis* sensitive to spectinomycin and as an aid in the control of chronic respiratory disease (CRD) associated with *E. coli.* Also, for newly hatched chicks, as an aid in the control of mortality and to lessen severity of infections caused by *M. synoviae, S. typhimurium, S. infantis* and *E. coli.*
Dosage and Administration: Inject 1- to 3-day-old turkey poults with 0.1 ml (10 mg) subcutaneously in the base of the neck.
Inject newly hatched chicks subcutaneously with Spectam diluted with sterile physiological saline solution to provide 2.5 to 5.0 mg. of spectinomycin in an 0.2 ml. dose.
Thoroughly clean and sterilize syringes and needles before using (needles and syringes may be sterilized by boiling in water for 15 minutes).
Use all precautions to prevent contamination of contents of bottle.
Injection site should be disinfected with a suitable disinfectant such as 70% isopropyl alcohol just prior to injecting Spectam.
Precautions: Produce use data applicable only to 1- to 3-day-old turkey poults and newly hatched chicks. Use only in accordance with directions.
How Supplied: Spectam Injectable, 100 mg/ml, is supplied in 500 cc multiple-dose, rubber-stoppered glass bottles, 12 bottles per case (List No. 5488-01).

SPECTAM® SCOUR-HALT™
(spectinomycin)
Oral Solution Antibiotic

Product Characteristics: Spectam Scour-Halt contains spectinomycin which is a new antibiotic from Abbott research. It is fast-acting and effective against a variety of gram-negative and gram-positive organisms. Spectam Scour-Halt is a convenient dosage form of Spectam for baby pigs.
Indications: Spectam Scour-Halt is indicated for the oral treatment and control of infectious diarrhea (scours) in baby pigs caused by *E. coli,* (Susceptible to spectinomycin.)
Dosage and Administration: The plastic doser supplied in each package with Spectam Scour-Halt makes treatment easy. After inserting the doser in the bottle, screw the top on tightly to avoid spilling. Push the piece of clear plastic tubing over the end of the pump. Then press the plunger a few times to fill the pump and the clear plastic tube with medication. To administer Spectam Scour-Halt, insert the plastic tube in the pigs mouth and press the plunger to obtain the desired dose.
The recommended daily dose is: *Pigs under 10 lbs* —1 pump (1 ml.) twice daily. *Pigs over 10 lbs* —2 pumps (2ml.). twice daily.
Each pump of the plunger delivers 1 ml of solution containing 50 mg of spectinomycin. Treatment may be continued twice daily for 3 to 5 days. If pigs do not improve within 48 hours, rediagnosis is suggested.
Caution: This product is intended for use only on pigs under 4 weeks of age or weighing less than 15 lbs.
Do not administer within 21 days of slaughter.
How Supplied: Spectam Scour-Halt is supplied in 240 ml (List No. 8807-03) multiple-dose plastic bottles. Each bottle is individually packed in a carton with a convenient plastic doser. A 500 ml and 1000 ml refill bottle without the plastic doser is also available (List No. 8807-05 and 8807-06 respectively).

SPECTAM® WATER-SOLUBLE
(spectinomycin)
Water Soluble Antibiotic

Composition: Each gram contains spectinomycin dihydrochloride pentahydrate equivalent to 0.5 gram of spectinomycin activity. Highly water-soluble, it will not clog proportioners. High stability assures effectiveness over extended periods.
Indications: Spectam Water-Soluble Antibiotic is indicated as an aid in the prevention or control of broiler losses due to chronic respiratory disease (CRD) associated with *Mycoplasma gallisepticum* (MG) and infectious synovitis associated with *Mycoplasma synoviae* (MS). It is also indicated as an effective means of increasing rate of weight gain and improving feed efficiency in floor-raised broilers.
Administration: Mix in drinking water according to dosage directions. This mixture should be the only source of water for the first three days of life, and for one (1) day following each vaccination.
Dosage: For CRD associated with MG: add contents of one 200-gram bottle to 50 gallons of water to provide two grams of spectinomycin activity per gallon.
For infectious synovitis associated with MS: add ½ bottle (100 grams) to 50 gallons of water to provide one gram of spectinomycin activity per gallon.
For increased rate of weight gain and improved feed efficiency in floor-raised broiler chickens: dissolve ¼ bottle (50 grams) in 50 gallons of water to provide 0.5 grams of spectinomycin activity per gallon.
Precautions: Warning: *Do not* administer this drug within five (5) days of slaughter.
How Supplied: Spectam Water-Soluble is supplied in:
128-gram screw top, plastic bottles (64 grams, activity per bottle), 12 bottles per case (List No. 5485-03)
1,000-gram screw-top, plastic bottles (500 grams activity per bottle), 6 bottles per case (List No. 5485-02).

STAPHENE®
Disinfectant Spray and Air Sanitizer

Composition: Active ingredients: o-benzyl-p-chlorophenol, p-tertiary amyl-

phenol, o-phenylphenol, n-alkyl dimethyl benzyl ammonium chlorides, n-alkyl dimethyl ethylbenzyl ammonium chlorides, 2,2'-methylenebis (3,4,6-trichlorophenol), propylene glycol, ethanol.
Indications: For general disinfection, including isolation areas and tuberculous disinfection, elimination of fungi and viruses, and air santitization.
Directions: For general disinfection, spray surface from a distance of 12 inches for 2 to 3 seconds, or until surface is wet.
To deodorize, sanitize and refresh the air, direct spray upwards toward the center of room for 3 to 5 seconds.
How Supplied: 20 oz. containers, 24 per case, (List No. 6389-72)

STERILE WATER FOR INJECTION, USP

Use only if clear and vacuum present. Before piercing, cleanse stopper with antiseptic.
For veterinary use only.
Caution: For parenteral use only after addition of suitable solutes to make an approximately isotonic solution.
Caution: This water contains no bacteriostat. Solutions made from this water should be used promptly or sterilized with adequate precautions for maintaining sterility.
Caution: Federal law restricts this drug to use by or on the order of licensed veterinarian.
How Supplied: Abbo-Vac® bottle of 250 ml. (List No. 1590-02) and 1000 ml (List No. 1590-05).

1-STROKE ENVIRON®
Germicidal Detergent

Composition: Super concentrated detergent, free rinsing, biodegradable, hard water-effective. Typical pH (concentrate) 12.3; typical pH (1:256 Dilution) 10.4 Max.
Indications: A broad spectrum, hard-water effective germicidal detergent which quickly destroys many disease-causing germs, fungi and specific viruses. Effective against such organic matter as feces, dried blood and egg albumen, and ideal for disinfecting animal and poultry facilities.
1-Stroke Environ quickly controls both gram positive and gram negative bacteria, including: *Staphylococcus aureus, Streptococcus* spp., *Pseudomonas aeruginosa, Pseudomonas fragi, Arizona* spp. *Brucella bronchiseptica, Entero bacter* spp., *Escherichia coli, Proteus* spp., *Shigella dysenteriae, Salmonella* spp., *Serratia marcescens,* and *Mycobacterium tuberculosis.*
The product provides effective contol of *Candia albicans* and *Trichophyton mentagrophytes* fungi. It also provides activity against a variety of disease-causing viruses, including: Pseudorabies, Influenza A2, Herpes simplex, Type 2 Adenovirus, Vaccinia and Hog Cholera Virus. In addition, it provides activity against the viruses causing or associated with: Marek's Disease, Newcastle Disease, Infectious Bronchitis, Infectious Laryngotracheitis, and African Swine Fever.
Directions: Packaged with dispensing pump. Use ½-ounce of 1-Stroke Environ (1 stroke of pump) for each gallon water—1:256 solution. For heavily soiled areas, use 2 strokes per gallon of water.
Caution: Corrosive to tissues. This concentrate causes eye and skin damage. Harmful or fatal if swallowed.
How Supplied: 1-gallon containers (List No. 9397-08). 1-Stroke Dispensing Pump enclosed with each 4-gallon package. Also available in 55 gallon drums (List No. 9397-01).

SURGEON'S GLOVES
Sterile, Disposable
Sizes: 6, 6½, 7, 7½, 8, 8½, 9

Description: Available in half-sizes; white latex surgeon's gloves assure correct fit with naturally proportioned curved fingers, contoured palm, and snug tapered wrist.
Caution: After donning, remove powder by wiping gloves thoroughly with a sterile wet towel or sponge. Pre-powdered, latex gloves are guaranteed sterile in unopened or undamaged package.
How Supplied: Dispenser boxes of 50 pair each: size 6 (List No. 2556-60); size 6½ (List No. 2556-65); size 7 (List No. 2556-70); size 7½ (List No. 2556-75); size 8 (List No. 2556-80); size 8½ (List No. 2556-85); size 9 (List No. 2556-90).

SYNCRO-MATE B®
Norgestament Implants And Norgestomet/Estradiol Velerate Injection
For Synchronizing Breeding Of Cycling Heifers

Description: SYNCRO-MATE-B is made up of two components: a hydrophilic polymer (Hydron®) ear implant containing norgestomet, a potent progetin; and an injectable solution of norgestomet and estradiol valerate in sesame oil with 10% benzyl alcohol. Each implant contains 6.0 mg of norgestomet and each 2 ml of injectable contains 3.0 mg of norgestomet and 5.0 mg of estradiol valerate.
A treatment is one implant and two ml of injection at the time of implantation.
The implant should be removed from the ear after 9 days.
Indications: SYNCRO-MATE-B is intended to permit synchronized breeding of cycling heifers with or without estrus detection.
Directions for Use:
MANAGEMENT PROCEDURES
Heifers must be of breeding age and weight and showing cycling activity.
They should be on a weight gaining plan of nutrition and free from diseases affecting reproduction.
SYNCRO-MATE-B is not intended to solve infertility, "shy-breeders," and other serious reproductive problems.
Since insemination of treated animals without estrus detection should be conducted 48–54 hours after implant removal, the number treated at one time should be limited to the number that can be inseminated in a 6-hour period without undue stress on cattle or inseminator.
It is essential that insemination be done by skilled, experienced insemination technicians, taking particular care that a technician does not become overtired and therefore less effective.
Where estrus detection is preferred, the animals should be treated in groups of no more than approximately 100 per facility to allow for proper handling during heat detection and insemination.
Only high quality semen that has been properly stored and handled should be used.
Avoid other treatments such as vaccinations, dipping, pour-on grub and louse prevention, spraying, etc., even though it may seem convenient to do so while the animals are restrained.
Be gentle: Do not use electric prods or unduly excite the animals during any of the handling procedures.
Insemination without estrus detection (Timed A.I.)
Synchronized breeding systems allow for maximum possibilities for cattle to become pregnant in a given time period.
Insemination of the entire treated group should be started 48 hours after the last implant has been removed and should be completed within 6 hours.
DO NOT INSEMINATE BEFORE 48 HOURS.
Insemination with estrus detection
Signs of estrus in the herd may begin to appear 24 hours after implant removal. 85% to 100% of treated heifers in good breeding condition and sexually mature may be expected to be in estrus within the next four days with the peak of estrus activity in the herd at 36 hours after implant removal.
Animals should be confined to a relatively small area during this time. Remove individuals to a separate holding pen near the insemination chute as soon as they are detected in estrus. This is necessary to simplify estrus detection in the remainder of the group. It should be done with as little disturbance to the animals as possible.
Insemination should be approximately 12 hours after first detection of estrus. Those detected in the morning should be bred in the evening of the same day. Those detected in the evening should be bred the following morning.
Warning: Do not use in cows producing milk for human consumption.
Keep out of reach of children. For use in animals only—Not for human use.
How Supplied: SYNCRO-MATE B is packed in

25 dose cartons	List #4878-01
10 dose cartons	List #4878-02
Syncromate Implant Gun	List #4877-91

"T" CONNECTOR SET
Tubing Retention: 0.25 ml

For attaching one or more administration sets or syringes at venipuncture site. Short connector with female adapter on

Continued on next page

CEVA—Cont.

one end and T-bar needle adapter/injection site on distal end.

List No.	4612-01
Approx. length	5"
Tubing I.D.	0.54"

TETANUS ANTITOXIN

C

Composition: Contains Tetanus Antitoxin (equine origin) derived from the blood of horses hyperimmunized with the toxin of Clostridium tetani.
Contains phenol and thimerosal as preservatives.
Indications: For use in the prevention and treatment of Tetanus.
Dosage and Administration: The recommended prophylactic dose for horses and other large animals is 1500 units administered intramuscularly or subcutaneously. For therapeutic dose administer 10,000 to 50,000 units intramuscularly or intravenously, and repeat as indicated.
Precautions: Keep refrigerated at 35° to 45°F. Avoid freezing. Entire contents of a vial should be used at time when first opened. Do not inject in food producing animals within 21 days before slaughter. In case of anaphylactoid reactions, administer epinephrine or equivalent.
How Supplied: List No. 2635-01, one 1500-unit vial Tetanus Antitoxin.

THREE-WAY STOPCOCK EXTENSION SET 20-SL

Description: 20-inch three-way stopcock accepts I.V. set and syringe. Optional female adapter under removable rubber reseal. Secure Lock male adapter connects to venipuncture device or other I.V. equipment.
List No. (3230-01)

TRI-KLEAN SOLUTION
Liquid Skin Cleanser

Composition: Active ingredients: 0.25% Triclosan 2,4,4'-trichloro-2'hydroxy diphenyl ether.
Indications: A liquid soap solution with bacteriostatic properties. Frequent and regular use reduces and controls the characteristic microflora of the human skin, including staphylococci, diptheroids, corynebacteria, streptococci and coliform bacteria. Buffered for mildness and wth low potential for irritation, Tri-Klean Solution is ideal for frequent, repeated use.
Directions: Applied to wetted hands and arms, Tri-Klean Solution will lather readily. It may be poured into soap dispensers, or applied directly onto the skin from the shipping container.
How Supplied: 1-gallon containers, 4 per case. (List No. 6299-08).

TrueGrit RAMPAGE®
Rat and Mouse Bait

Composition: A pelleted cereal grain bait containing cholecalciferol (Vitamin D_3) as the rodenticide agent.
Indications: For control of Norway rats, roof rats, and house mice in and around homes, agricultural and poultry buildings.
Directions: Rats—place 2 to 8 RAMPAGE® place packs, usually at intervals of 15 to 30 feet per placement.
Mice—place one RAMPAGE® place pack at intervals of 8 to 12 feet per placement.
Caution: Keep away from humans, domestic animals and pets.
Statement of Practical Treatment: If serum calcium levels are elevated, treatment with calcitonin or cortisone is effective in reducing calcium to normal levels. Continue monitoring serum calcium and treat as necessary for hypercalcemia, with Lasix and fluid therapy.
How Supplied: 30 gram place packs, 50 per pail, 4 pails per case. (List No. 6115-01).

VENOCATH®-14
VENOCATH®-16
VENOCATH®-18
Sterile Peel-Pack

Description: Venocath-14—15 bore 11½" intravenous catheter with 1 ½", 14-G thinwall needle.
Venocath-16—18-G bore 11½" intravenous catheter with 1½" 16-G thinwall needle.
Venocath-18—21-G bore 11½" intravenous catheter with 1½" 18-G thinwall needle.
Contents sterile and nonpyrogenic in unopened, undamaged unit package.
Directions:
1. *Remove From Outer Envelope*—Peel open outer envelope. Do not remove clip on needle hub.
2. *Expose Needle*—While holding blue needle hub and clip with one hand, slide clear plastic ring on needle guard back onto needle hub. Open guard wings, remove and discard protective needle cover.
3. *Enter Vein*—Prepare site and perform venipuncture with needle bevel up. Introduce catheter into the vein to the desired length by "thumbing" through the protective sheath. *Do not exert force if resistance is encountered. Withdraw catheter and needle simultaneously by grasping the needle hub and pulling both out together. Do not attempt to withdraw catheter back through needle with needle still in vein because of danger of severing the catheter.*
4. *Withdraw Needle*—Apply finger pressure over catheter in the vein. Hold it thus while withdrawing the needle.
5. *Close Needle Guard*—Close wings of needle guard over the needle and lock into position by sliding the plastic ring forward to the end of wings. Secure needle hub into white adapter at catheter end.
6. *Attach to I.V. Set*—Remove protective sheath clip and discard sheath. Remove protective cap from white adapter (withdraw stylet) and immediately attach administration set.
7. *Secure Infusion Equipment*—Tape catheter, needle guard and end of administration set for proper immobilization. Do not disconnect without plugging open end of catheter to preclude possible air embolism.

Caution: Federal law restricts this device to sale by or on the order of a licensed veterinarian.
Do not store for prolonged periods at extreme temperatures.
Disposable Device—Do not resterilize or reuse.
How Supplied: 20 Units (List No. 4614-02/14-G. List No. 4816-02/16-G. List No. 4718-02/18-G.

VENOSET® 72

Description: Disposable I.V. set, 72 inch (172 cm) (approx. 15 drops/ml) with latex terminal injection site.
Fluid path and areas beneath undisturbed protective set covers are sterile and nonpyrogenic in unopened, undamaged unit package.
Directions (Use Aseptic Technique): Remove protective coverings as assembly progresses.
1. Prepare Abbo-Vac® bottle (or other I. V. container).
2. Close clamp.
3. With bottle upright, thrust piercing pin straight through stopper center. Do not twist or angle.
4. Immediately invert bottle to automatically establish proper fluid level in drip chamber (half full). Check for vacuum by observing rising bubbles.
5. Attach venipuncture device (not included). Open clamp and allow solution to expel air from tubing and needle. Then close clamp.
6. Make venipuncture adjust flow.

COMPATIBLE MEDICATION may be added by aseptic technique via:
(a) Abbo-Vac stopper before attaching set
(b) air inlet: remove air filter and connect syringe without needle to air vent: after injecting medication, replace filter securely and swirl bottle to mix
(c) latex tubing.

NOT FOR INSERTION INTO BLOOD OR PLASMA CONTAINERS. CHANGE WITHIN 24 HOURS. DISCARD AFTER USE.
Caution: Federal law restricts this device to sale by or on the order of a licensed veterinarian. Disposable Device. Do not resterilize or reuse. Protect from freezing and extreme heat.
How Supplied: 1 Unit, List No. 8962-48.

VENOSET® 78

Description: Disposable I.V. Set. 78 inch (198 cm) with a "Y" injection site 6 inches (15.2 cm) from needle adapter.
Fluid path and areas beneath undisturbed protective set covers are sterile and nonpyrogenic in intact unit package.
Directions (Use Aseptic Technique): Remove protective coverings as assembly progresses.
1. Prepare Abbo-Vac® bottle (or other I.V. container).

2. Close clamp.
3. With bottle upright, thrust piercing pin straight through stopper center. Do not twist or angle.
4. Immediately invert bottle to automatically establish proper-fluid level in drip chamber (half full). Check for vacuum by observing rising bubbles.
5. Attach venipuncture device (not included). Open clamp and allow solution to expel air from tubing and needle. Then close clamp.
6. Make venipuncture and adjust flow.

COMPATIBLE MEDICATION may be added by aseptic technique via:
(a) Abbo-Vac stopper before attaching set
(b) air inlet: remove air filter and connect syringe without needle to air vent: after injecting medication, replace filter securely and swirl bottle to mix
(c) injection site.

NOT FOR INSERTION INTO BLOOD OR PLASMA CONTAINERS CHANGE WITHIN 24 HOURS. DISCARD AFTER USE.

Caution: Federal law restricts this device to sale by or on the order of a licensed veterinarian.
Disposable Device. Do not resterilize or reuse.
Do not store at extreme temperatures.
How Supplied: 1 Unit (List No. 1881-48).

VENOSET® MICRODRIP

Description: Disposable Precision Drop I.V. Set, 70 inch (178 cm). With precision drop orifice, providing approximately 60 drops per ml. "Y" injection site 6 inches (15.2 cm) from needle adapter.
Fluid path and areas under protective coverings of set are sterile and nonpyrogenic if set covers are in place.
Directions (Use Aseptic Technique):- Remove protective coverings as assembly progresses.
1. Prepare Abbo-Vac® bottle (or other I.V. container).
2. Close slide clamp.
3. With bottle upright, thrust piercing pin straight through stopper center. Do not twist or angle.
4. Immediately invert bottle to automatically establish proper fluid level in drip chamber (half full). Check for vacuum by observing rising bubbles.
5. Attach sterile vein needle (not included). Open slide clamp and allow solution to expel air from tubing and needle. Then close screw clamp.
6. Make venipuncture and adjust flow with screw clamp.

COMPATIBLE MEDICATION may be added by aseptic technique via:
(1) Abbo-Vac stopper before attaching set
(b) air inlet: remove air filter and connect syringe without needle to air vent: after injecting medication, replace filter securely and swirl bottle to mix
(c) injection sites.

NOT FOR INSERTION INTO BLOOD OR PLASMA CONTAINERS. CHANGE WITHIN 24 HOURS DISCARD AFTER USE.

Caution: Federal law restricts this device to sale by or on the order of a physician or other licensed practitioner.
Disposable Device—Do not resterilize or reuse.
Do not store at extreme temperatures.
How Supplied: 1 Unit (List No. 1883-48).

VENOSET® Y TYPE
With CAIR® Clamp

Description: Vented Y-Type I.V. set for administration from two I.V. solution containers.
86 inches. 15 drops/ml
Use aseptic technique. Remove protective coverings as assembly progresses.
1. Close all clamps.
2. **For Glass:** Prepare I.V. container. With container upright, thrust one of the piercing pins straight through stopper center or set port. Do not twist or angle. Immediately invert container to check for vacuum by observing rising air bubbles. Repeat with second container. Suspend containers.
For Plastic: Expose outlet of I.V. container. Replace bacterial retentive air filter with piercing pin cover. Insert one piercing pin with twisting motion until shoulder of air filter housing rests against the outlet port flange. Repeat with second container. Suspend containers.
3. Open slide clamp below one of the suspended containers. Open CAIR® clamp and allow fluid to fill tubing leg. Close slide clamp.
4. Repeat procedures with second I.V. container. Close slide clamp and CAIR clamp.
5. Open slide clamp below I.V. container of choice and squeeze drip chamber gently until proper fluid level is established (half full).
6. Open CAIR clamp and allow solution to expel air from tubing. Close CAIR clamp.
7. Attach set to venipuncture device. If device is not indwelling, prime and make venipuncture.
8. Adjust flow with CAIR clamp. 15 drops delivers approximately 1 ml.

To stop flow at CAIR clamp without disturbing setting, lift tubing upward and into shutoff slot.
NOTE: When I.V. tubing is stretched or tugged, all manual flow control clamps may lose flow control effectiveness.
Warning: Never let drip chamber empty, nor operate set unless one slide clamp is tightly closed.
Not for insertion into blood or plasma containers. Change within 24 hours. Discard after use.
US Pat. Nos. 3,893,468; 4,238,108.
Caution: Federal Law restricts this device to sale by or on the order of a physician or licensed practitioner.
How Supplied:
1 unit (List No. 2491-48)

VENOTUBE® 30
Sterile Peel-Pack

Description: Disposable set for syringe attachment or any sterile extension.
Contents sterile and nonpyrogenic in unopened, undamaged unit package.
Note: All I.V. sets shouid be changed within 24 hours. Discard equipment after use.
Caution: Federal law restricts this device to sale by or on the order of a licensed veterinarian.
Do not store at extreme temperatures.
Disposable Device—Do not resterilize or reuse.
How Supplied: 20 Units (List No. 4481-01).

VETERINARY PENTOTHAL® AND VETERINARY PENTOTHAL® KIT
(sodium thiopental for injection)

Composition: Veterinary PENTOTHAL is supplied as 5.0 g of sterile powder in 250 ml size multiple dose containers. Pentothal kit is available with either 1.0 or 5.0 g sodium thiopental with accompanying diluent.
Indications: Pentothal is recommended especially for minor surgery of 10 to 20 minutes duration, reduction of fractures, physical examination, radiography and dentistry. Animals can be completely anesthetized with a single intravenous dose. Since the period of ataxia is short, the patient is able to leave the hospital or office without a prolonged delay.
This type of anesthesia can also be used in prolonged operations, using intermittent or continuous injection appropriate to the species. It is also a valuable induction anesthetic in preparation for a volatile anesthetic which may be required for prolonged operations, particularly in large animals.
Route of Administration: Pentothal is intended for intravenous administration only.
Precautions: Pentothal has little effect upon blood pressure but may depress and slow respiration. In the rare cases of laryngeal spasm, an open air passage must be maintained. Overdosing may cause respiratory failure. In this event artificial respiration and other respiratory stimulants should be used.
In the presence of shock, anemia, liver damage or kidney damage, sodium thiopental must be administered with great care.
Preanesthetic agents, analgesics, some tranquilizers, corticosteroids, and sulfonamides may potentiate the drug and thus reduce the amount necessary to induce a given depth of anesthesia.
Since the placenta is not a protective barrier against sodium thiopental or any other barbiturate, the full anesthetic dose should not be used in pregnant animals. Light doses of this drug may be used as an induction agent in such cases.
To reduce the chance of vomiting and excessive salivation, food should be with-

Continued on next page

CEVA—Cont.

held for 12 hours, when possible, prior to administration.

Multi-Dose Mixing Directions: As with all general anesthetics, occasional hypersensitive animals will respond atypically to this drug.

Weight of Powder	ml. of Solution	Resulting Concentration mg./ml.	%
5 g.	50	100	10
5 g.	77.5	64.8	6.5
5 g.	100	50	5
5 g.	165	30	3
5 g.	250	20	2

Note: This preparation is not indefinitely stable in an aqueous solution. Use within 24 hours after mixing.

Dosage:

Dogs: Range, 6.0 to 12.0 mg (1/10, to ⅕ gr) per pound of body weight. The fatal dose is approximately twice the maximum recommended dose.

For Anesthesia of Short Duration: (8-10 minutes) which may be sufficient for X-ray, physical examination, and minor surgery, 6.0 to 7.5 mg (1/10 to 1/8 gr) lb.

For Anesthesia of Intermediate Duration: (10-15 minutes) such as might be used for dentistry or reduction of fractures, 7.5 to 10 mg (1/8 to 1/6 gr) /lb.

For Major Surgery: requiring anesthesia for long duration (longer than 15 minutes) induce anesthesia with 10 to 12 mg (1/6 to ⅕ gr) per pound of body weight; about half the dose is given rapidly and the balance more slowly, administered over approximately 15 seconds. Depth of anesthesia may be determined by the loss of pedal and eye reflexes. The first stage of anesthesia following the administration of sodium thiopental is commonly evidenced by a deep yawn followed very shortly by loss of reflexes. Although the initial dose may be sufficient for an entire operation, the surgeon should be prepared to administer additional drug as needed. Some clinicians prefer to leave the needle in the vein. Any additional drug should be administered a little more slowly. As much as a third or more of the original dose may be required to produce the depth of anesthesia. Injections should not be at closer than 30 to 60-second intervals.

With Preanesthetic Agents: Preanesthetic agents (such as morphine or a tranquilizer) decrease the dosage requirements of sodium thiopental, provide for smoother induction and recovery, and may prolong the recovery period. Following morphine as a preanesthetic agent, the dose of this drug may be reduced as much as 40 to 50 percent; following a tranquilizer 10 to 25 percent.

The Urinary Bladder: should be emptied immediately after anesthesia is induced, particularly when prolonged anesthesia is anticipated.

Cats: Pentothal use and limitations for cats is similar to that detailed for dogs. The usual dose range is 8 to 12 mg/lb intravenously.

Bovine: Animals 300 Pounds or Over— The recommended dose is 3.7 to 7.0 mg (1/17 to 1/9 gr) per pound of body weight, depending on the depth of anesthesia required, administered rapidly. Rapid administration is defined as injecting the entire specified dose (10 to 30 ml) with a hypodermic syringe in one motion *thrust*. To deliver 5.0 mg/lb of body weight, using a 25% solution would require 2.0 ml. for each 100 pounds of body weight. Should additional drug be required (as in lighter weight animals) it should be injected more slowly, particularly in the obese animal, and the total amount should not exceed 10 mg (1/6 gr) per pound of body weight.

When a phenothiazine tranquilizer is administered intravenously 10 to 15 minutes prior to the injection of sodium thiopental, the lower dose of this drug (3.7 to 4.5 mg (1/17 to 1/15 gr)/lb) should be used. The anesthesia following the tranquilizer is more profound and the righting time is prolonged slightly. *Unweaned Calves* —For unweaned calves, from which food has been withheld 6 to 12 hours prior to anesthesia, no more than 3.0 mg (½2 gr) of Pentothal (sodium thiopental for injection) per pound is required for deep surgical anesthesia.

If a penothiazine tranquilizer is administered to such calves 10 to 20 minutes prior to anesthesia, the dose of sodium thiopental is reduced to 2.0 mg (1/32/gr) per pound of body weight.

Ovine: This preparation has been used successfully for experimental surgery in lambs weighing about 35 lbs. each, at the rate of 4.5 to 6.75 mg/lb, depending on he depth of anesthesia desired.

Increased salivation and ruminal regurgitation in sheep, as in cattle, is a problem with general anesthesia and must be handled as in cattle.

Swine: As in other species, there is an inverse ratio between the dose level and the weight of the animal. The minimum anesthetic dose for healthy animals is shown in the following table:

Dose

Pounds of Body	Weight Mg/lb	ml 5% sol/lb
10-50	5.0	0.1
50-100	4.5	0.09
100-200	4.0	0.08
200-300	3.5	0.07
300-400	3.0	0.06
400-600	2.5	0.05

Slightly over the dose, calculated from the above table, should be drawn into the syringe because an occasional animal may require slightly more. One-half the calculated dose is injected rapidly and the remainder more slowly until the desired anesthesia is obtained; caution should be used with unthrifty animals which may not require, and thus should not receive, the full calculated dose. Only a rare robust animal will require slightly more than the minimum calculated dose. Respiration should be watched, an occasional animal may require artificial respiration.

How Supplied: Veterinary PENTOTHAL® is supplied as sterile powder in 250 ml. size multiple dose containers, 5 g. each in boxes of 12 (List No. 8639-01), without accompanying diluent kits. Sodium carbonate is present as a buffer. Veterinary Pentothal Kits are available in two solution sizes, including a 5-gram, 2.5% solution kit (List No. 8912-01); and 5-gram, 5.0% solution kit (List No. 8913-01). 25 kits each per case.

Each Veterinary Pentothal Kit comes complete with all materials required to prepare a specific Pentothal solution concentration and size, including a squeeze bottle of Pentothal, a partial-fill bottle of sterile water for injection, and pre-gummed transfer label.

WART VACCINE

Composition: Contains a chemically inactivated suspension of Wart Virus Infected Tissue (killed virus, bovine origin).

Contains formaldehyde solution and thimerosal as preservatives.

No US Standard of Potency.

Indications: For use as an aid in the prophylactic treatment of Viral Warts (Papillomas) in cattle only.

Dosage and Administration: Inject 10 ml to 25 ml subcutaneously depending on size of the animal. May be repeated in 10 to 14 days if required. When more than 10 ml is administered, two or more injection sites should be chosen. Disinfect injection site and bottle stopper before puncturing with needle. Use sterile syringes and needles.

Precautions: Refrigerate at 35°to 45°F. Shake well before using, the precipitate is part of the vaccine and must be injected uniformly. Use entire contents when first opened. Do not vaccinate within 21 days before slaughter. In case of anaphylactoid reaction administer epinephrine or equivalent.

How Supplied: List No. 2634-01, one 50-ml vial vaccine.

Colorado Serum Company

4950 YORK STREET
DENVER, CO 80216

ANTHRAX VACCINE

Composition: Colorado Anthrax Spore Vaccine is prepared with a relatively non-pathogenic, uncapsulated variant strain of B. anthracis, originally developed at the Onderstepoort Research Laboratory, Pretoria, South Africa and used with excellent results throughout South Africa, England, India and in many other countries. Extensive use in recent years in the United States has been with most gratifying response. The vaccine consists of viable spores suspended in saponfied diluent. It is fully tested for purity, dissociation, spore count, safety and potency prior to release for sale.

Dosage and Administration: The recommended dose for all domestic farm animals is 1 cc. In heavily contaminated regions a "booster" injection 2 to 3 weeks

after the first dose is administered is recommended.
Anaphylaxis (shock) may sometimes follow the use of products of this nature. Epinephrine, or equivalent, should be available for immediate use in these instances.
Precautions: Do not vaccinate within 60 days before slaughter. If emergency conditions require vaccination of animals reaching market age and condition these should not be offered for slaughter in less than 60 days after administration of the vaccine.
In those areas where anthrax is an annual problem, it is advisable to vaccinate about 4 weeks prior to the time the disease usually appears. If an outbreak occurs, all animals not showing clinical symptoms should be vaccinated. Not all such animals may be fully protected but further spread of the disease may be stopped by promptly following this procedure.
How Supplied: 50 cc, 25 cc, 10 cc; Dosage: 1 cc.

BLUETONGUE
Type 10

Composition: Bluetongue is recommended for the vaccination of healthy sheep and goats against bluetongue infection. This is a tissue culture product.
When to Vaccinate: Incidence of bluetongue is seasonal, with animals contracting the disease mostly in August and September due to the virus being transmitted by biting insects. Treatment is almost totally ineffective and preventive vaccination, late in the spring or in the early summer not only is recommeded but becomes vitally important.
Lambs from immune ewes carry a degree of resistance to bluetongue which may last as long as 3 months. As lambs approach weaning time the "maternal antibody" disappears and the required resistance can break down in the face of field exposure. It is at this time that lambs should be vaccinated. If vaccinated too young the "maternal antibody" may interfere with proper active immune response.
Dosage and Administration: Administer 2 cc of the restored vaccine intramuscular to each animal. The auxillary space (between foreleg and body) is a convenient site. Sterile technique should be used.
Syringes and needles used for administering the vaccine should be sterilized by boiling of water for at least 15 minutes.
Anaphylaxis (shock) may sometimes follow the use of products of this nature. Epinephrine, or equivalent, should be available for immediate use in these instances.
Precautions: Vaccination of pregnant ewes could result in births of abnormal lambs and this practice is definitely not recommended. Instead, all breeding stock should be protected with Bluetongue Vaccine approximately three weeks prior to the breeding season or after lambing.
Do not vaccinate within 21 days before slaughter.
How Supplied: 50 doses; Dosage: 2 cc.

BOVI-SERA
Antiserum

Composition: Prepared from the blood of cattle hyperimmunized with repeated injections of cultures of *Corynebacterium Pyogenes, Escherichia coli, Pasteurella Haemolytica-multocida,* and *Salmonella Typhimurium* of all bovine origin.
Indications: To be used as an aid in the short-term prevention and treatment of enteric and respiratory conditions in calves and cattle when caused by the organisms used to hyperimmunize the cattle in which the antiserum has been produced.
Dosage and Administration: For prevention —*Calves:* 20 cc to 40 cc as soon after birth as possible. *Cattle:* 50 cc to 75 cc.
Dosage and Administration: For treatment —Following dose is to be administered at 12 to 24 hour intervals until improvement is noted: *Calves:* 40 cc to 100 cc. *Cattle:* 75 cc to 150 cc.
All injections should be made either subcutaneously or intramuscularly. Anaphylaxis (shock) may sometimes follow the use of products of this nature. Epinephrine, or equivalent, should be available for immediate use in these instances. Do not vaccinate within 21 days before slaughter.
How Supplied: 250 cc

BRUCELLA ABORTUS VACCINE
Strain 19, Live Culture
Reduced Dose
Restricted to use by or under the direction of a Veternarian

Indications: For use in healthy female cattle only. Age of vaccination and other limitations shall be as directed by proper State authorities.
Dosage and Administration: Rehydrate by adding the accompanying sterile diluent to the dried vaccine. Shake gently to assure proper rehydration and inject subcutaneously 2 ml into each animal. Use immediately after rehydrating.
Precautions: Do not vaccinate within 21 days before slaughter. Anaphylactoid reaction sometimes follows administration of products of this nature. If noted administer adrenalin or equivalent. Use entire contents when bottle is first opened. Burn this container and all unused contents.
Store in dark at 2° to 7°C.
Warning: All distributors are required by the producer and Federal regulations to keep complete records of the disposition on this product.
Accidental Human Exposure: Strain 19, Brucella abortus vaccine can cause brucellosis (undulent fever) in humans. Exposure may occur via injection, ingestion, conjunctiva or broken skin. In the event of accidental exposure, consult a physician.

How Supplied: 5 ds vial
25 ds vial
5 x 1 ds carton
Rehydrate each to 2 ml
For Veterinary Use Only

CAMPYLOBACTER FETUS BACTERIN
Ovine

Composition: Vibrio Fetus Bacterin (Ovine Strains) is an aluminum hydroxide adsorbed culture of killed organisms. Two immunologically different strains of the causative agent, vibrio fetus (intestinalis), have so far been isolated. These have been identified as Type I and Type V. Both of these serotypes are used in the production of the bacterin.
When to Vaccinate: Do not vaccinate within 21 days before slaughter. Two doses of bacterin are recommended. The first should be administered a short time before or shortly after ewes are exposed to rams. The second injection should be made 60 to 90 days later.
Dosage and Administration: Shake the bacterin thoroughly to resuspend the precipitate that may have formed during storage. Aluminum hydroxide added to the bacterin during storage. Aluminum hydroxide added to the bacterin adsorbs the antigenic substances and when injected forms a repository to provide prolonged immunogenic response.
Each of two 5 cc doses should be administered at an interval of 60 to 90 days. Because the adjuvant may cause a slight transitory irritation, it is suggested that the bacterin be injected on the side of the neck or over the rib cage to avoid prime meat areas. All injections should be subcutaneous.
Precautions: Anaphylaxis (shock) may sometimes follow the use of products of this nature. Epinephrine, or equivalent, should be available for immediate use in these instances.
How Supplied: 250 cc, 50 cc,
Dosage: 5 cc.

CAMPYLOBACTER FETUS-LEPTOSPIRA CANICOLA-GRIPPOTYPHOSA-HARDJO-ICTEROHAEMORRHAGIAE-POMONA BACTERIN
Bovib-Lepto 5

General Information: This bacterin is a combination of aluminum hydroxide adsorbed, formalin killed, washed cultures of *Vibrio (Campylobacter) fetus (venerealis)* and whole cultures of five major serotypes of *Leptospira* that are most frequently isolated from cattle. These are *L. canicola, L. grippotyphosa, L. hardjo, L. icterohaemorrhagiae* and *L. pomona.*
Aluminum hydroxide adsorbs and releases the antigens gradually after injection, causing a longer time for complete absorption than would be expected for products that do not contain an adjuvant. This delayed release provides a more significant immune response from a single dose.

Continued on next page

C

Colorado Serum—Cont.

Vibriosis in cattle is an infection of the reproductive organs which can cause infertility, delayed conception, and may sometimes cause abortions. Transmission occurs at breeding time and the disease becomes more virulent as infected females are rebred because of failure to conceive. Many bulls will remain carriers indefinitely unless treatment is successful. Occasionally cows will become chronic carriers and remain infected throughout pregnancy and after calving. Vibriosis can be perpetuated in a herd by just one case that serves to infect clean bulls. Leptospirosis, in breeding cattle, can cause death losses as well as abortions. This combination bacterin can be a valuable aid in eliminating these problems.

When To Vaccinate: Do not vaccinate within 21 days before slaughter. Vaccinate females at least 30 days before being turned in with bulls. Virgin heifers are more susceptible to vibriosis and should be vaccinated 60 days before breeding is started.

Revaccinate on an annual basis using the full recommended dose.

Dosage and Administration: 2.0 ml. administered subcutaneously. A second dose at 3-4 weeks is recommended for exposed animals and in endemic areas.

Precautions: Shake the bacterin well so that the precipitate and micro-organisms are fully resuspended. Use entire contents when the bottle of bacterin is first opened.

Anaphylaxis (shock) may sometimes follow use of products of this nature. Adrenalin or epinephrine should be available for immediate injection in these instances.

How Supplied: 10 ds; 50 ds.

CANINE DISTEMPER-HEPATITIS

This is a combination product that is recommended for the vaccination of healthy dogs against canine distemper and canine hepatitis.

CANINE DISTEMPER-HEPATITIS-LEPTOSPIRA

Composition: This product utilizes multiple antigenic substances and is commonly referred to as a "4 in 1" combination. Canine distemper and hepatitis modified live virus fractions are prepared as a common suspension for filling into a single vial in order that the viruses can be vacuum-dried to insure full retention of the antigenic properties. The bacterin, also in a single vial, likewise contains two antigens. These provide protection against *canicola* and *icterohaemorrhagiae* infections, the serotypes of *Leptospira* most frequently isolated from dogs affected with leptospirosis. When the two vials are combined as directed, a single dose of vaccine results.

When to Vaccinate: For optimum results, vaccinate healthy, unexposed weaned dogs 9-12 weeks of age or older. Puppies vaccinated at an earlier age should be revaccinated within 3 months.

Dosage and Administration: One complete dose of combined vaccine is obtained by restoring the product as directed. Inject this vaccine subcutaneously.

Anaphylaxis (shock) may sometimes follow the use of products of this nature. Epinephrine, or equivalent, should be available for immediate use in these instances.

How Supplied: 1 dose. 5 x 1 dose.

CHLAMYDIA PSITTACI BACTERIN (KILLED CHLAMYDIA)

General Information: This bacterin is produced from cultures of chlamydia psittaci, a filterable bacteria of the psitticosis-lympho-granuloma-trachoma group of micro organisms that cause enzootic abortion of ewes. The cultures are formalin killed.

Enzootic abortion of ewes has been an unidentified problem in a vast area of the western and northwestern United States for many years. Isolation of the causative agent, chlamydia psittaci, is fairly recent, however.

Enzootic abortion of ewes is characterized almost exclusively by loss of lambs late in pregnancy. Weak or dead lambs may be born at full-term. In some instances infected ewes will show no clinical symptoms of any kind and will lamb in a normal manner. Those that do not abort or lamb prematurely are sometimes in poor health showing a rapid deterioration over a short period before lambing. Vaginal discharge is noted after lambing and placenta may be retained for several days. Generally, the ewes will slowly return to normal condition.

The chlamydia is present in fetal membranes and in the uterine discharge. It is at this time that the disease is spread through the flock, being picked up orally by the ewes, to remain inactive until carried to developing placenta during the following pregnancy. In Scotland there is evidence that the chlamydia microorganism can remain in the tissues of a ewe lamb for as long as two years, then cause the animal to abort when she becomes pregnant. It is during the second pregnancy that ewes most often abort or lamb prematurely from the effects of this disease although many are also affected during the first lambing season.

This product is somewhat different than biologics that are familiar to the average user. It is an emulsion and is of heavy consistency because of the oil adjuvant that is used. This adjuvant forms a repository of vaccine to provide prolonged antigenic stimulation. Because of this a granuloma, usually of small to moderate size, may form at the site of injection. This is non-inflammatory and will usually disappear within a reasonable period. Some may become persistent and more permanent in nature but should be no real problem.

This product is sold only on a non-returnable basis and is not eligible for credit at expiration.

When to Vaccinate: Do not vaccinate within 60 days before slaughter. Ewes selected for breeding purposes should be vaccinated 30–60 days prior to exposure to rams. Revaccinate annually.

Dosage and Administration: Shake well. Administer 2 ml subcutaneously on top of the neck about 4 inches from the ear. If small nodules then appear these will be of no consequence in breeding herds and will be less objectionable in the event an occasional animal must be culled from the flock and sold.

Precautions: All biological products should be stored in the refrigerator. Because this is an emulsion, which is very difficult to use when cold, it is suggested that the product be removed from storage a few hours before use so that it will warm slightly. Do not expose to excessive heat or for prolonged periods at room temperature.

Shake the product thoroughly to resuspend any microorganisms that may have precipitated.

Handling of the product, filling of syringes, etc, should be done as aseptically as possible. Great care has been taken to assure the purity of this preparation at the time of release for marketing. Reasonable precaution should be taken in the field to maintain this condition.

Anaphylaxis (shock) may sometimes follow the use of products of this nature. Epinephrine, or equivalent should be available for immediate use in these instances.

CLOSTRIDIUM CHAUVOEI-SEPTICUM BACTERIN
CCS Double Bacterin

Composition: Chemically killed, Aluminum hydroxide, adsorbed, cultures of *Clostridium chauvoei, Clostridium septicum.*

Indications: For vaccinating healthy cattle, sheep, and goats against Blackleg and Malignant Edema.

Dosage and Administration: Inject 2 ml. subcutaneously. Calves vaccinated under 3 months of age should be revaccinated at weaning or 4 to 6 months of age.

How Supplied: 100 cc, 50 cc, 20 cc.

CLOSTRIDIUM CHAUVOEI-SEPTICUM PASTEURELLA BACTERIN
CCSP — Triple Bacterin

Composition: Chemically killed, Aluminum hydroxide adsorbed, cultures of *Clostridium chauvoei, Clostridium septicum,* and *Pasteurella Haemolytica-multocida.*

Indications: For vaccinating healthy cattle, sheep and goats against Blackleg, Malignant Edema and Hemorrhagic Septicum.

Dosage and Administration: *Calves:* Dose is 5 cc.

Calves vaccinated under 3 months of age should be revaccinated at weaning or 4 to 6 months of age.

Sheep & goats: 3 cc injected subcutaneously.

Revaccination with Pasteurella Bacterin is recommended at 2 to 4 weeks.
How Supplied: 250 cc, 50 cc.

CLOSTRIDIUM HAEMOLYTICUM BACTERIN

Description: A formalin inactivated whole culture of *Clostridium haemolyticum.* Aluminum hydroxide adsorbed.
Indications: For vaccination of healthly cattle, sheep and goats to aid in the prevention of Red Water Disease (Bacillary Hemoglobinuria). Dosage & **Administration:** Inject 2 ml subcutaneously or intramuscularly into each animal. In areas where constant exposure is likely animals should be revaccinated each 5 to 6 months. Calves should be vaccinated at 3-4 months of age.
Directions: Shake well to uniformly disperse the adjuvant, which may be slightly precipitated. Store in dark at 2° to 7° C.
Precautions: Do not vaccinate within 21 days before slaughter. Anaphylactoid reaction sometimes follows administration of products of this nature. If noted, administer adrenalin or equivalent. Use entire contents when bottle is first opened.
How Supplied: 10 ds vial
50 ds vial
For Veterinary Use Only

CLOSTRIDIUM PERFRINGENS TYPES C & D ANTITOXIN
Equine Origin

General Information: Antitoxins contain antibodies formed as a result of hyperimmunization with a specific toxin and which are capable of neutralizing that toxin. Almost immediate response is provided at the time of injection. Antitoxins, however, do not actively stimulate the antibody system of the vaccinated animal and the resulting immunity is passive, lasting only until the injected antibodies are eliminated from the system, a period of approximately 14#21 days. This is a potent multivalent antitoxin specific for the temporary prevention of Clostridial entertoxemia in cattle, sheep, and goats caused by Types C & D toxin and in swine when caused by Type C.
Do not vaccinate within 21 days before slaughter. If antitoxin must be used under emergency conditions the animals so treated should be withheld from market for 21 days after injection.
Dosage and Administration: Clostridium Perfringens Types C & D Antitoxin confers a prompt passive immunity lasting about 3 weeks. Administer subcutaneously using aseptic methods. The following doses are recommended:
For prevention:

Suckling Lambs, Goats and Pigs	5 ml.
Suckling Calves	10 ml.
Feeder Lambs and Pigs	10 ml.
Feeder Calves and Cattle	25 ml.

Clostridium Perfringens Type D is not known to cause disease in swine.
Anaphylaxis (shock) may sometimes follow the use of products of this nature. Epinephrine, or equivalent, should be available for immediate use in these instances.
How Supplied: 250 ml

CLOSTRIDIUM PERFRINGENS TYPES C & D—TETANUS TOXOID

Purified formalin detoxified filtrates of highly toxic cultures of *Clostridium perfringens* types C & D micro-organisms and of Tetanus toxin.
For the vaccination of healthy cattle, sheep, goats, and swine as an aid in the prevention of enterotoxemia caused by *Clostridium perfringens* types C & D and for long-term protection against tetanus. Contains thimerosal as a preservative.
Directions: Shake well. Each dose must have proportionate share of precipitate for proper responses. Use entire contents when first opened.
Precautions: Anaphlactoid reaction sometimes follows administration of products of this nature. If noted, administer adrenalin or equivalent. Do not vaccinate within 21 days before slaughter. Store in dark at 2° to 7°C. Do not freeze.
Dosage and Administration: Inject 2 ml subcutaneously or intramuscularly. Repeat full dose in 3 to 4 weeks.
FOR VETERINARY USE ONLY
How Supplied: 100 ml 50 Doses
20 ml 10 Doses

CLOSTRIDIUM PERFRINGENS TYPES C & D TOXOID

Purified formalin detoxified filtrates of highly toxic cultures of Clostridium perfringens types C and D micro-organisms. For the vaccination of cattle, sheep, goats, and swine as an aid in preventing *Clostridial enterotoxemia* cause by *Clostridium perfringens* types C and D. Contains thimerosal as a preservative.
Directions: Shake well. Each dose must have proportionate share of precipitate for proper responses. Use entire contents when first opened.
Precautions: Anaphylactoid reaction sometimes follows administration of products of this nature. If noted, administer adrenalin or equivalent. Do not vaccinate within 21 days before slaughter. Store in dark at 2° to 7° C. Do not freeze.
Dosage and Administration: Inject 2 ml subcutaneously or intramuscularly. Repeat full dose in 3 to 4 weeks.
FOR VETERINARY USE ONLY
How Supplied: 100 ml 50 Doses
20 ml 10 Doses

ENCEPHALOMYELITIS

Composition: Encephalomyelitis Vaccine is prepared from killed cultures of encephalomyelitis viruses propagated in an avian tissue culture system. The vaccine is recommended for the vaccination of horses and mules against encephalomyelitis.
Indications: Antigenically different strains identified as "Eastern" and "Western" types are included in the product.
When to Vaccinate: Because encephalomyelitis virus is spread by mosquitoes, ticks and perhaps other blood sucking insects, to be most effective the vaccine should be administered in the spring or early summer. The incidence of the disease diminishes during cold weather. Annual revaccination of all horses and mules is recommended.
Dosage and Administration: Recommended dose is two intradermal injections of 1 cc each at an interval of 3 weeks. A convenient site of injection is side of the neck.
Precautions: Anaphylaxis (shock) may sometimes follow the use of products of this nature. Epinephrine, or equivalent, should be available for immediate use in these instances.
How Supplied: 10 cc, 10 x 1 cc.

C

ENCEPHALOMYELITIS VACCINE
Eastern and Western, Killed Virus Tetanus Toxoid

General Information: A formalin inactivated and adjuvanted Equine Encephalomyelitis vaccine, Eastern and Western Types, in combination with concentrated Tetanus Toxoid. For the vaccination of healthy equines against Eastern and Western encephalomyelitis and tetanus.
Contains thimerosal, penicillin, and streptomycin as preservatives.
Directions: Store in dark at 2° to 7°C. Shake Well. Each dose must have proportionate share of precipitate for proper response. See Circular for more complete information.
Precautions: Anaphylactoid reaction sometimes follows injection of products of this nature. If noted, administer adrenalin or equivalent. Use entire contents when bottle is first opened. Do not vaccinate within 21 days before slaughter.
Dosage and Administration: Inject 2 ml deep in the muscle. Local reaction may occur if injected subcutaneously. Repeat to 3 to 4 weeks. A booster dose of 2 ml should be administered annually and whenever an epidemic situation develops and exposure is likely.
How Supplied: 10 x 1 ds vials, 10 ds vial
For Veterinary Use Only

ENZABORT EAE-VIBRIO
Ovine Enzootic Abortion Vaccine Killed Chlamydial Chicken Embryo Origin Vibrio Fetus Bacterin Ovine Isolates

General Information: This is a combination vaccine-bacterin prepared for vaccination of ewes to aid in protecting against abortions. The vaccine is produced from cultures of *chlamydia,* a filtrable bacteria of the *psitticosis-lymphogranuloma-trachoma* group of microorganisms that causes an infection generally referred to as *ovine enzootic abortion* or *enzootic abortion in ewes.* The bacterin-fraction consists of cultures of two immunologically different strains of *Campylobacter (Vibrio) fetus intestinalis, serotypes C (I)* and *A-2 (V)* which are known to cause abortion in sheep. Both

Continued on next page

Colorado Serum—Cont.

fractions of the combination vaccine-bacterin are formalin killed.
Enzootic abortion in ewes has been an unidentified problem in a vast area of the western and northwestern sections of the United States for many years. Isolation of the causative agent, a micro-organism of the *psitticosis* group, is fairly recent, however. Occurence of *chlamydial abortion* in association with *vibriosis* has complicated control measures. A combination product providing protection against both diseases, therefore, became highly desirable. Cooperation between research investigators and biological establishments resulted in such a product being offered on an experimental basis.
Enzootic abortion in ewes is characterized almost exclusively by loss of lambs late in pregnancy. Weak or dead lambs may be born at full-term. In some instances infected ewes will show no clinical symptoms of any kind and will lamb in a normal matter. Those that do not abort or lamb prematurely are sometimes in poor health showing a rapid deterioration over a short period before lambing. Vaginal discharge is noted after lambing and placenta may be retained for several days. Generally, the ewes will slowly return to normal condition.
The *chlamydia* is present in fetal membranes and in the uterine discharge. It is at this time that the disease is spread through the flock, being picked up orally by the ewes, to remain inactive until carried to developing placenta during the following pregnancy. In Scotland there is evidence that the *chlamydia* micro-organism can remain in the tissues of a ewe lamb for as long as two years, then cause the animal to abort when she becomes pregnant. It is during the second pregnancy that ewes most often abort or lamb prematurely from the effects of this disease although many are also affected during the first lambing season.
Vibriosis in sheep is sporadic and occurs in many States. Losses from abortion in individual flocks may be substantial. The disease is caused by the micro-organism *Campylobacter (Vibrio) fetus intestinalis.* Two known immunogenically different strains are used in the production of the bacterin fraction of the combination product.
Abortions from *vibriosis* vary from 5% to 75% with a loss of 10% to 20% being common. Occasionally there is a death loss in ewes but this is unusual. As with *ovine enzootic abortion* the principal symptom of vibriosis is abortion usually beginning about 30 to 40 days before lambing is to start. Some infected ewes will carry full term but lambs may be born weak and may not survive. Usually no symptoms are noted before abortion but very close observation may disclose evidence of vaginal discharge several days in advance of abortions and the ewes may not appear to feel well. After aborting the ewe will discharge brownish colored material for several days. *Campylobacter (Vibrio) fetus* can be recovered from the vagina for about a week after abortion. Usually ewes recover rapidly. Source of *Campylobacter (Vibrio) fetus* infection and principal means of transmitting *vibriosis* have not been fully determined. The ram is probably not the chief source. Feed or water carrying the micro-organism could be a factor.
This product is somewhat different than biologics that are familiar to the average user. It is an emulsion and is of heavy consistency because of the oil adjuvant that is used. This adjuvant forms a repository of vaccine to provide prolonged antigenic stimulation. Because of this a granuloma, usually of small to moderate size, may form at the site of injection. This is noninflammatory and will usually disappear within a reasonable period. Some may become persistent and more premanent in nature but should be no real problem.
This product is sold only on a non-returnable basis and it is not eligible for credit at expiration.
When To Vaccinate: Ewes selected for breeding purposes should be vaccinated within 30-60 days of exposure to rams. Revaccinate annually.
Dosage and Administration: Shake well. Administer 2 ml. subcutaneously on top of the neck about 4 inches from the ear. If small nodules then appear these will be of no consequence in breeding herds and will be less objectionable in the event an occasional animal must be culled from the flock and sold.
Precautions: Do not vaccinate within 60 days before slaughter. All biological products should be stored in the refrigerator. Because this is an emulsion, which is very difficult to use when cold, it is suggested that the product be removed from storage a few hours before use so that it will warm slightly. Do not expose to excessive heat or for prolonged periods at room temperature.
Shake the product thoroughly to resuspend any micro-organisms that may have precipitated and inject 2 ml. subcutaneously as recommended above.
Handling of the product, filling of syringes, etc., should be done as aseptically as possible. Great care has been taken to assure the purity of this preparation at the time of release for marketing. Reasonable precaution should be taken in the field to maintain this condition.
Caution:
Store in dark at 2° to 7°C.
Sterilize needles and syringes by boiling in clean water. Do not use chemical disinfectants or detergents for this purpose.
Use entire contents when bottle is first opened.
Anaphylaxis (shock) may sometimes follow the use of products of this nature. Epinephrine, or equivalent, should be available for immediate use in these instances.
Conveniently packaged in 10 dose and 50 dose sizes.
How Supplied: 10 ds 50 ds
For Veterinary Use Only

ERYSIPELAS BACTERIN
Concentrated

Composition: Erysipelas Bacterin is prepared by chemically inactivating whole broth cultures of highly antigenic strains of *E. rhusiopathiae* and adsorbing these cultures with aluminum hydroxide.
Indications: The bacterin, which is supplied in concentrated form, is recommended for the vaccination of healthy swine and turkeys against erysipelas infection.
When to Vaccinate: It is best to vaccinate pigs at 8 to 12 weeks of age. Vaccination of suckling pigs is not recommended. If, under emergency conditions, pigs younger than 8 weeks are vaccinated these animals should be revaccinated at weaning time. Breeding herds should be revaccinated after 21 days and annually.
Turkeys should be vaccinated at 8 to 12 weeks of age. If erysipelas has been a problem on any particular premises, birds should be vaccinated approximately three weeks before infection usually appears and every three months thereafter. If it should be necessary to vaccinate turkeys under 8 weeks, these should be revaccinated within 60 days. In all instances of revaccination the recommended label dose of the bacterin should be administered.
Dosage and Administration: *Swine:* Recommended dose 2 cc. For breeding animals repeat after 21 days and annually.
Turkeys: The dose ½cc for birds weighing less than 10 lbs. and 1 cc for heavier turkeys; Repeat recommended doses every 3 months.
In swine, inject the bacterin in the axillary space. All injections in turkeys should be made beneath the skin in the neck area just behind the head.
Precautions: Anaphylaxis (shock) may sometimes follow the use of products of this nature. Epinephrine, or equivalent, should be available for immediate use in these instances.
Do not vaccinate within 21 days before slaughter. Needle puncture and tissue damage at site of injection could cause condemnation of carcasses.
How Supplied: 100 cc, 50 cc, 20 cc.

LEPTO-5
Leptospira Canicola-Grippotyphosa-Hardjo-Icterohaemorrhagiae-Pomona-Bacterin

Composition: This bacterin is prepared by chemically inactivating whole broth cultures of highly antigenic strains of *Leptospira canicola, Leptospira grippotyphosa, Leptospira hardjo, Leptospira icterohaemorrhagiae,* and *Leptospira pomona.* Aluminum hydroxide is added to the bacterin to enhance its immunizing effect.
Directions —When to Vaccinate: Do not vaccinate within 21 days before slaughter. Vaccination of both cattle and swine at least 3 weeks prior to breeding is recommended (1) on premises having a history of leptospirosis, (2) when the disease exists in the area, and (3) when ani-

mals may have been exposed to carriers of the micro-organisms.
Hogs being raised for market should also be vaccinated if contact with the disease is likely. These animals should not thereafter be offered for slaughter until the full withdrawal time, as shown above, has been observed. Best results are to be expected when the bacterin is administered prior to exposure of the animals. However, if infection has appeared in the herd, isolate the sick animals and vaccinate all those that are apparently unaffected. Some vaccinates may thereafter develop symptoms because immune response from administration of bacterin is not immediate. Vaccination of infected herds is suggested as Leptospira bacterins have been found to be of help in stopping spread of disease and bringing outbreaks under control.
Vaccination is recommended also for healthy herds suspected of having been exposed to leptospirosis and for herds into which replacement stock is periodically introduced. Such replacement stock should be vaccinated as well and held separately until protective immunity is established. Isolation of new stock should be a rigid practice in herd management not only for aid in preventing leptospirosis but other diseases as well.
Revaccinate animals retained for breeding and those held beyond a normal marketing period, on an annual basis. In heavily contaminated areas semi-annually vaccination should be practiced. Occasionally, it may be necessary to vaccinate very young calves. If so, these should be revaccinated at 3-4 months.
Dosage and Administration: Aseptically inject 2 ml intramuscularly or subcutaneously. For swine, a second dose should be administered 2-4 weeks later. Annual revaccination is recommended for both species.
Precautions: Do not vaccinate within 21 days before slaughter. Anaphylactoid reaction sometimes follows administration of products of this nature. If noted, administer adrenalin or equivalent. Use entire contents when bottle is first opened.
How Supplied: 10 ds, 50 ds

NORMAL EQUINE SERUM

Composition: Serum prepared from the blood of healthy animals from the species indicated.
Indications: This serum may be used for nonspecific treatment of horses for anemia, haemorrhage, shock, infections, and any other physically debilitating conditions where blood enrichment is desirable.
Precautions: Anaphylaxis (shock) may sometimes follow the use of products of this nature. Epinephrine, or equivalent, should be available for immediate use in these instances.
Dosage and Administration: 50 cc to 250 cc depending upon age, weight of animal and judgment of administer.
How Supplied: 250 cc, 100 cc.

OVINE ECTHYMA VACCINE

Composition: This package contains one bottle of dried Ovine Ecthyma Vaccine and a bottle of sterile rehydrating fluid labeled as Sterile Diluent. When the vaccine is restored to liquid form by adding the diluent as directed the resulting product is recommended for vaccinating both sheep and goats against "sore mouth" infection.
Directions—When to Vaccinate: Because dried scabs retain the infective virus which is resistant to heat and cold and can be expected to survive from year to year, it is advisable to vaccinate each new lamb and kid crop. Exposure to infection can occur during shipping. Range lambs moving into feed lots should be vaccinated at least 10 days before shipment to prevent possible rapid spread of the disease after arrival.
Normally only healthy animals should be vaccinated but experience has shown that in outbreaks of Sore Mouth vaccination of infected sheep and lambs tends to shorten the course of disease.
This is a live virus vaccine. Do not use within 24 hours of dipping or spraying. Do not vaccinate within 21 days before slaughter.
Dosage and Administration: The bottle of vaccine contains 100 doses. Select a wool free area of skin, such as the inside of the flank or the underside of the tail. Scarify the outer layer of the skin by scratching with the notched handle of the applicator which is furnished as a part of the package, and brush a drop of vaccine well into the scarified area. Do not scratch deep enough to draw blood. Some redness and a slight swelling will be observed on the second or third day after vaccination. This will develop into small raised areas which will rupture and scab over. This reaction indicates a "take".
Precautions: Humans have been accidently infected with Ovine Ecthyma virus. Lesions that have been described in man are most often on the hands and arms. Usually such infections are not serious but all individuals handling the vaccine should take precautions against infecting themselves with the virus.
Brushes and scarifiers should be used only in a single flock of sheep. If there is need to use the instrument a second time it should be sterilized by boiling in water for several minutes.
Caution: Store in dark at a temperature not over 7°C.
Sterilize syringes and needles by boiling clean water.
Use entire contents when bottle is first opened.
Thimerosal has been added to this bacterin as a preservative.
How Supplied: Conveniently packaged in 100 ds size.

PASTEURELLA BACTERIN

Composition: Chemically killed whole cultures of *Pasteurella multocida,* and *Haemolytica,* aluminum hydroxide adsorbed.
Indications: For the vaccination of healthy cattle, sheep, goats against pasteurellosis associated with the organisms contained in the formualtion.
Dosage and Administration: Inject 2 cc subcutaneously into each animal. Vaccination is recommended two weeks before weaning, shipping, or other stress conditions, to allow an increase in resistance against the organisms named in the formulation. A second dose is recommended in 2 to 4 weeks. Do not vaccinate within 21 days before slaughter.
Precautions: Anaphylaxis (shock) may sometimes follow the use of products of this nature. Epinephrine, or equivalent, should be available for immediate use in these instances.
How Supplied: 100 cc, and 20 cc.
Dosage: 2 cc.

RAM EPIDIDYMITIS BACTERIN

Composition: An inactivated aqueous culture of an isolate from the epididymis of an infected ram. Bacterin is adsorbed with aluminum hydroxide.
Indications: For vaccinating rams to stimulate resistance to ram epididymitis. Contains thimersol as a preservative.
Dosage and Administration: Inject 2 ml. subcutaneously. Loose skin behind shoulder or at side of neck are suggested sites. Repeat dose in 30-60 days. Ram lambs at weaning age and mature rams may be vaccinated. Annual revaccination is recommended.
Warning:
Shake well before using.
Store in dark at a temperature not over 7°C.
Do not freeze.
How Supplied: 20 ml 10 doses.
For Veterinary Use Only

RESPIRAGEN
An Antiserum

Composition: Corynebacterium Pyogenes-Pasteurella Haemolytica-Multocida Antiserum, marketed under the trade name or Respiragen, is recommended for use, principally in cattle, but may also be used in sheep and swine for the prevention and as an aid in the treatment of pasteurellosis and diphtheroid infections associated with the isolates contained in the formulation of the hyperimmunizing cultures.
Respiragen is indicated whenever diphtheroid infection is present in combination with pasteurellosis in cattle, sheep and swine. The products can also be used to advantage by administering recommended doses a few days prior to shipping animals as a pre-conditioning procedure. Response is almost immediate, lasting for approximately two to three weeks.
Dosage and Administration:
For Prevention:
Calves: 20 ml to 40 ml as soon after birth as possible.
Cattle: 50 ml to 75 ml.
Sheep and Swine: 10 ml to 15 ml.
For Treatment:
Calves: 40 ml to 100 ml.
Cattle: 75 ml to 150 ml.
Sheep and Swine: 20 ml to 40 ml.

Continued on next page

Colorado Serum—Cont.

Dosage may be repeated according to the judgment of the user.
Injections may be subcutaneous or intramuscular. Multiple sites may be used when injecting large doses.
Precautions: Do not administer antiserum within 21 days before slaughter. Needle punctures and tissue damage may result in condemnation of carcasses.
Because of viral antibodies in Respiragen cattle should not be vaccinated with IBR, BVD, or PI_3 vaccines, or any combination thereof for at least 21 days after injection of the antiserum.
Anaphylaxis may sometimes follow the use of products of this nature. Epinephrine, or equivalent, should be available for immediate use in these instances.
How Supplied: 250 cc, 100 cc

THE RESPIRATORY VACCINES
IBR-Bovine Rhinotracheitis
BVD-Bovine Virus Diarrhea
PI3-Parainfluenza-3
Lepto-Leptospira Pomona
Lepto 5-Canicola, Icterohaemmorghiae, Hardjo, Grippotyphosa, Pomona

Available in the following Combinations:
IBR-BVD-PI_3-Lepto 5
IBR-BVD-PI_3
IBR-BVD
IBR-PI_3
IBR
(Where Lepto is part of the combination it is used in place of the sterile diluent vial.)
General Information: *Bovine rhinotracheitis* is normally sudden and mild in nature. Salivation, congestion of the nasal mucosa, serous nasal discharge, rapid respiration, coughing, and depression, are some of the symptoms frequently observed. Temperature may vary from slightly above normal to as high as 108°F.
Bovine virus diarrhea appears suddenly and most of the animals in herd will become involved. Affected animals develop abnormal temperatures, become depressed, go off feed, and there is a mucous oculonasal discharge with a dry nonproductive cough. Most of the times a diarrhea is noted. Lameness will also develop in a considerable number of the animals.
Parainfluenza$_3$ infection is symptomized by coughing, mucopurulent oculanasal discharge, difficult respiration, and dehydration. Temperatures may range from a little above normal to 104°F. Diarrhea usually is not present. Dry scabs appear on the muzzle.
Leptospirosis symptoms most frequently noted are rapid rise in temperature, depression, and loss of appetite. Urine may become coffee-colored or streaked with blood. Animals become anemic. Milk production drops or ceases. Abortions may occur at any stage of pregnancy but usually in the last one-third. Full-term calves may be dead or weak. Death losses can reach serious proportions in calves a year old or younger.
All three of the above virus infections (IBR, BVD, PI_3) are herd diseases. All produce high morbidity, low mortality. Substantial weight loss is a serious economic factor.
Methods of inactivation and concentration used in the preparation of the Leptospira Bacterin fractions of this combination are improved processes. The method used to inactivate *Leptospira* eliminates any change of killing agent residues that might cause unintentional attenuation of the bovine rhinotracheitis modified live virus when the two products are combined for field use. Inactivation with formalin and associated risks of subsequent possible ineffective neutralization of this agent are avoided. Concentration is by methods other than centrifugation. All of the original antigen is recovered and retained in the concentrate so there is no loss of immunizing effect.
Restoring: One vial contains the modified live virus vaccine(s) in a vacuum-dried state. The other vial contains a sterile diluent or the liquid Leptospira fraction. To mix and rehydrate, withdraw the contents of the liquid vial with a sterile syringe (do not remove stoppers) and transfer it to the vacuum-dried vial. Shake gently.
When to Vaccinate: Cattle should be vaccinated before or at the time of admission to feed lots or dairy areas. Yearly booster injections are recommended for breeding stock. Maternal antibodies in young calves may interfere with development of an active immunity. If emergency conditions require vaccination these calves should be revaccinated one month after weaning.
Precautions: Do not use in pregnant cows or in calves nursing pregnant cows. Be sure that breeding stock is immunized on a regular basis when cows are open. Do not vaccinate within 21 days before slaughter. Needle punctures and tissue damage at the site of injection may cause condemnation of carcasses.
Anaphylaxis (shock) may sometimes follow the use of products of this nature. Epinephrine, or equivalent, should be available for immediate use in these instances.
How Supplied: 50 doses; 10 dose;
Dosage: 2 cc.

SALMONELLA DUBLIN-TYPHIMURIUM BACTERIN
Bovine Isolates

Description: Formalin killed, aluminum hydroxide adsorbed cultures of Salmonella dublin and Salmonella typhimurium, Bovine isolates.
Indications: For vaccination of healthy cattle to induce resistance to Salmonella infections caused by microorganisms named. Contains thimerosal as a preservative.
Directions: Shake well. Each dose must have proportionate share of precipitate for proper response. Store in dark at 2° to 7° C. Do not freeze.
Dosage and Administration: In areas where Salmonella infections have been a problem, adult cattle, pregnant cows and newborn calves should all be given two injections of 2 ml each at an interval of 14-21 days. Boost immunity in pregnant cows with annual 2 ml injection. Vaccinate adult cattle prior to placing on feed and pregnant cows 4 to 6 weeks before calving time. Newborn calves should be left on cows for 7 days at which time bacterin can be administered. All injections should be subcutaneous.
Precautions: Do not vaccinate within 21 days before slaughter. Anaphylactoid reaction sometimes follows administration of products of this nature. If noted, administer adrenalin or equivalent. Use entire contents when bottle is first opened.
How Supplied: 10 ds vial
50 ds vial
For Veterinary Use Only

SWINE ERYSIPELAS ANTISERUM

Composition: Antiserums contain antibodies against specific diseases and are beneficial as a means of providing immediate protection to susceptible animals. Antiserums however, do not actively stimulate the antibody system of the vaccinated animal and the resulting immunity is passive, lasting only until the injected antibodies are eliminated from the system, a period of approximately 14-21 days. This is an anti-serum specific for the treatment and temporary prevention of erysipelas in swine and turkeys. The antibody systems of production animals are stimulated by injections of increasingly large doses of E. rhusiopathiae, which are repeated until a satisfactory titer can be demonstrated in the recovered serum.
Dosage and Administration: *For Prevention:* Pigs weighing less than 50 lbs. — 5 cc. Pigs weighing 50 to 75 lbs. — 10 cc. Pigs weighing 75 to 100 lbs. — 15 cc. Pigs weighing over 100 lbs. — 20 cc.
For Treatment: The dosage shown in the above table should be doubled for treatment of sick animals. Repeat injections may be indicated.
Injections should be made subcutaneously. Avoid fatty tissue and other areas of poor circulation. Small pigs can be vaccinated in the axillary space (armpit.) Larger hogs, sows and boars can be vaccinated in the "pocket" behind the ear. A Colorado Hog Holder can be used to advantage for this purpose.
Precautions: Anaphylaxis (shock) may sometimes follow the use of products of this nature. Epinephrine, or equivalent, should be available for immediate use in these instances.
Do not vaccinate within 21 days before slaughter. Needle puncture and tissue damage may result in condemnation of carcasses.
How Supplied: 250 cc

TETANUS ANTITOXIN AND TETANUS TOXOID

Antitoxin —For quick response of short duration.
Toxoid —Slower acting but long duration.

Composition: *Tetanus Antitoxin* is produced in healthy horses that have been hyperimmunized with repeated large doses of Clostridium tetani toxin. *Tetanus Toxoid* is detoxified toxin precipated with Aluminum potassium sulfate.
Indications: Tetanus is caused by a toxin (poison) produced by growth of *Clostridium tetani,* an anaerobic (lives without air) organism that may be carried into wounds or sites of surgical operations.
When to Use: Meat animals should not be vaccinated within 21 days before slaughter. If *Tetanus Antitoxin* must be used under emergency conditions the animals so treated should be withheld from market for 21 days after injection.
Tetanus Antitoxin is recommended for use whenever an animal suffers a deep penetrating wound that has or may become contaminated with soil. Tetanus Antitoxin should also be administered to livestock following castration and other operations performed on premises where tetanus has been a problem; also to sheep at docking time.
Tetanus Toxoid should be used in non-emergency instances to establish an active immunity against tetanus.
Dosage and Administration: *Tetanus Antitoxin* confers an immediate passive immunity lasting about 7 to 14 days and can be administered in doses of 1500 units for short term prevention.
Tetanus Antitoxin, administered in large doses may provide beneficial response in animals already affected with tetanus. For treatment administer 10,000 to 50,000 units to horses and cattle; 3,000 to 15,000 units to sheep and swine. Animals that suffer slow healing puncture wounds or deep abrasions should be given a second dose of Tetanus Antitoxin in 7 days. Treatment administrations should otherwise be repeated as considered necessary.
Tetanus Toxoid should be administered to cattle and horses in at least 2 doses of 10 cc each at 30 day intervals. For sheep and swine two doses of 1 cc each are recommended with heavier animals being dosed on the basis of 1 cc per hundred pounds bodyweight.
Tetanus Toxoid Concentrated: *Cattle and Horses* 2 doses of 1 ml 30 days apart. *Sheep, goats, and swine* 2 doses of ½ ml 30 days apart. I.M. injection.
Tetanus Toxoid requires 3 to 4 weeks to establish an effective level of protection which will then persist for several months. "Booster" injections should be made on a schedule that provides intervals not longer than one year. In the event of injury to an immunized animal a "booster" dose is advisable regardless of the interval.
Precautions: Anaphylaxis (shock) may sometimes follow the use of products of this nature. Epinephrine, or equivalent, should be available for immediate use in these instances.
How Supplied: *Tetanus Antitoxin:* 10 x 1500 unit; 1500 unit. *Tetanus Toxoid:* 50 cc, 10 cc. (10 cc dose). Concentrated: 10 x 1 ml and 10 ml (1 ml dose).

VESICULAR STOMATITIS VACCINE
Killed Virus

Indications: Formalin killed. For the vaccination of cattle against Vesicular stomatitis.
Dosage and Administration: Shake well to completely resuspend. Aseptically inject 2 ml subcutaneously or intramuscularly. Administer 30 days or more prior to the time the disease usually appears. Repeat the full dose in 21-30 days. Revaccinate annually.
Directions: Store in dark at 2° to 7° C. See circular for more complete directions.
Precautions: Do not vaccinate within 21 days before slaughter. Anaphylactoid reaction may sometimes follow administration of products of this nature. If noted, administer adrenalin or equivalent. Use entire contents when first opened.
Contains thimerosal, penicillin, and streptomycin as preservatives.
How Supplied: 100 ml 50 doses
For Veterinary Use Only

WART VACCINE
Killed Virus
Bovine Origin

Indications: As an aid in the control of warts. Tested for purity and safety in serial lots.
Dosage and Administration: Inject subcutaneously 5 cc to 25 cc depending upon size of animal. May be repeated in 10 to 14 days if necessary.
Precautions: Anaphylaxis (shock) may sometimes follow the use of products of this nature. Epineprine, or equivalent, should be available for immediate use in these instances. Do not vaccinate within 21 days of slaughter.
How Supplied: 50 cc.

Connaught Laboratories, Inc.
ROUTE 611
SWIFTWATER, PA 18370

INFLOGEN®
Equine Influenza Vaccine
Killed Virus

Description: INFLOGEN is a bivalent vaccine derived from the allantoic fluid of embryonated chicken eggs infected with Types A/1 and A/2 equine influenza strains. The vaccine virus strains have been carefully selected and tested for antigenicity. The virus laden fluids are clarified and concentrated by sucrose gradient centrifugation. This process ensures that the final product is virtually free of unwanted protein and ensures the maximum antigenicity of each strain in a 1 ml dose. The virus is then chemically treated and irradiated to ensure complete inactivation. Safety and immunogenicity of this vaccine have been demonstrated by vaccination in susceptible horses. Being an inactivated virus vaccine, it will not cause disease in vaccinated animals.
Indications: For active immunization of healthy horses against equine influenza infection. Influenza is a disease complex caused by two subtypes of related viruses. All equine influenza virus substrains isolated to date have been classified as Type A. Two subtypes of influenza Type A virus have been identified as the cause of equine influenza; these are A/Equi-1 and A/Equi-2. INFLOGEN which contains strains from both subtypes, has undergone extensive field evaluation.
Dosage and Administration: SHAKE WELL before using. Using aseptic technique, vaccinate healthy horses with 1 ml intramuscularly. Administer a second dose 2 to 4 weeks later. Vaccination should be timed to achieve peak antibody response prior to possible exposure. Annual revaccination or revaccination in the event of a threatened epizootic is recommended. To minimize local tissue reaction, ensure that injection is administered in deep muscle tissue.
Precautions: Do Not Freeze. Store at 2-7°C (35-45°F). Use entire contents when first opened. Do not use chemicals to sterilize syringes and needles. In case of anaphylactoid reaction, administer epinephrine. For Veterinary Use Only.
How Supplied: INFLOGEN is supplied in packages containing ten-1 ml doses and one-10 ml (10 dose) vial.
Product information as of October, 1984.
For Veterinary Use Only

INFLOGEN®-T
Equine Influenza
Vaccine–Tetanus Toxoid
Killed Virus

Description: INFLOGEN-T is a bivalent equine influenza vaccine combined with tetanus toxoid. The equine influenza viral antigens are derived from the allantoic fluid of embryonated chicken eggs infected with Types A/1 and A/2 equine influenza strains. The vaccine virus strains have been carefully selected and tested for antigenicity. The virus laden fluids are clarified and concentrated by sucrose gradient centrifugation. This process ensures that the final product is virtually free of unwanted protein and ensures the maximum antigenicity of each strain in a 1 ml dose. The virus is then chemically treated and irradiated to ensure complete inactivation. Safety and immunogenicity of this vaccine have been demonstrated by vaccination in susceptible horses. Being an inactivated virus vaccine, it will not cause disease in vaccinated animals.
The tetanus toxoid component is alum precipitated and highly purified prior to combining with the equine influenza antigens.

Continued on next page

C

Connaught—Cont.

Indications: For active immunization of healthy horses against equine influenza infection and tetanus. Influenza is a disease complex caused by two subtypes of related viruses. All equine influenza virus substrains isolated to date have been classified as Type A. Two subtypes of influenza Type A virus have been identified as the cause of equine influenza; these are A/Equi-1 and A/Equi-2. INFLOGEN-T which contains strains from both subtypes, has undergone extensive field evaluation.
Dosage and Administration: SHAKE WELL before using. Using aseptic technique, vaccinate healthy horses with 1 ml intramuscularly. Administer a second dose 2 to 4 weeks later. Vaccination should be timed to achieve peak antibody response prior to possible exposure. Annual revaccination or revaccination in the event of a threatened epizootic is recommended. To minimize local tissue reaction, ensure that injection is administered in deep muscle tissue.
Precautions: Do Not Freeze. Store at 2-7°C (35-45°F). Use entire contents when first opened. Do not use chemicals to sterilize syringes and needles. In case of anaphylactoid reaction, administer epinephrine.
How Supplied: INFLOGEN-T is supplied in packages containing ten-1 ml doses and one-10 ml (10 dose) vial.
Product information as of October, 1984.
For Veterinary Use Only

TETNOGEN®
Tetanus Toxoid
Alum Precipitated Purified

Description: A sterile suspension of highly purified precipitated tetanus toxoid.
Indications: To confer long-term active immunity against tetanus.
Dosage: Horses, cattle, swine—1 ml; sheep—0.5 ml.
Administration: Inject intramuscularly or subcutaneously using aseptic technique. Repeat in 30 days followed by a single annual dose.
SHAKE WELL before each use.
Caution: Do Not Freeze. Store at 2–7°C (35–45°F). Do not save fractional contents for later use. If used in food animals, do not vaccinate within 21 days before slaughter. Anaphylactoid reactions may occur.
Antidote: Epinephrine.
How Supplied: 1 ml vial (10 per package) and 10 ml vial.
Product information as of March, 1981.
For Veterinary Use Only

TRIPLE-E™
Encephalomyelitis Vaccine
Eastern, Western and Venezuelan, Killed Virus

Description: This is a combination product consisting of Eastern, Western and Venezuelan Equine Encephalomyelitis viruses of cell-line origin. The purified viruses are formalin inactivated and combined with an aluminum hydroxide gel adjuvant.
Indications: For active immunization of healthy horses against Eastern, Western and Venezuelan Encephalomyelitis.
Dosage and Administration: SHAKE WELL before using. Using aseptic technique, vaccinate healthy horses with a 1 ml dose intramuscularly followed by a second 1 ml dose 2 to 4 weeks later. A booster is recommended annually, or in the event of a threatened epizootic.
Precautions: Local reactions following vaccination are rare. To minimize such reactions, ensure that injections are administered in deep muscle tissue. Thimerosal added as a preservative. Contains residual neomycin and streptomycin remaining from cell cultures. Store at 2–7°C (35–45°F). Do Not Freeze. Use entire contents when first opened. Do not use chemicals to sterilize syringes and needles. In case of anaphylactoid reaction, administer epinephrine.
How Supplied: Ten-1 dose (1 ml) prefilled syringes and 10 dose (10 ml) vial.
Product information as of July, 1985.
For Veterinary Use Only.

TRIPLE-E™ FT
Encephalomyelitis-Influenza Vaccine-Tetanus Toxoid
Eastern, Western and Venezuelan, Killed Virus

Description: This is a combination product consisting of Eastern, Western and Venezuelan Equine Encephalomyelitis viruses of cell-line origin, equine influenza viruses types A_1 and A_2 of chicken embryo origin, and tetanus toxoid. The purified viruses are formalin inactivated and combined with Tetanus Toxoid and an aluminum hydroxide gel adjuvant.
Indications: For active immunization of healthy horses against Eastern, Western, and Venezuelan Encephalomyelitis and Tetanus and as an aid in the prevention of equine influenza due to types A_1 and A_2.
Dosage and Administration: SHAKE WELL before using. Using aseptic technique, vaccinate healthy horses with a 1 ml dose intramuscularly followed by a second 1 ml dose 2 to 4 weeks later. A booster is recommended annually, or in the event of a threatened epizootic.
Precautions: Local reactions following vaccination are rare. To minimize such reactions, ensure that injections are administered in deep muscle tissue. Thimerosal added as a preservative. Contains residual neomycin and streptomycin remaining from cell cultures. Store at 2–7°C (35–45°F). Do Not Freeze. Use entire contents when first opened. Do not use chemicals to sterilize syringes and needles. In case of anaphylactoid reaction, administer epinephrine.
How Supplied: Ten-1 dose (1 ml) prefilled syringes and 10 dose (10 ml) vial.
Product information as of July, 1985.
For Veterinary Use Only.

TRIPLE-E™ T
Encephalomyelitis Vaccine-Tetanus Toxoid
Eastern, Western and Venezuelan, Killed Virus

Description: This is a combination product consisting of Eastern, Western and Venezuelan Equine Encephalomyelitis viruses of cell-line origin and tetanus toxoid. The purified viruses are formalin inactivated and combined with Tetanus Toxoid and an aluminum hydroxide gel adjuvant.
Indications: For active immunization of healthy horses against Eastern, Western, and Venezuelan Encephalomyelitis and Tetanus.
Dosage and Administration: SHAKE WELL before using. Using aseptic technique, vaccinate healthy horses with a 1 ml dose intramuscularly followed by a second 1 ml dose 2 to 4 weeks later. A booster is recommended annually, or in the event of a threatened epizootic.
Precautions: Local reactions following vaccination are rare. To minimize such reactions, ensure that injections are administered in deep muscle tissue. Thimerosal added as a preservative. Contains residual neomycin and streptomycin remaining from cell cultures. Store at 2–7°C (35–45°F). Do Not Freeze. Use entire contents when first opened. Do not use chemicals to sterilize syringes and needles. In case of anaphylactoid reaction, administer epinephrine.
How Supplied: Ten-1 dose (1 ml) prefilled syringes and 10 dose (10 ml) vial.
Product information as of July, 1985.
For Veterinary Use Only.

Coopers Animal Health Inc.
520 WEST 21ST ST.
P.O. BOX 419167
KANSAS CITY, MO 64141-0167

A-H™ INJECTION ℞
(doxylamine succinate)
Antihistaminic

Composition: Each ml contains: Doxylamine succinate 11.36 mg; Chlorobutanol (preservative) 5.00 mg; Distilled water q.s.
Action and Uses: Antihistamines can block or replace histamine in its attachment to receptor cells and its effect upon the shock tissues. When administered prophylactically, antihistamines attach to receptor cells before histamines. When administered therapeutically in sufficient concentration, they will replace histamine.
Antihistaminic drugs have been widely used in domestic animals in the management of a variety of conditions in which release of histamine is believed to be a factor, including food allergies, pollinosis, contact allergies, bovine asthma (pulmonary emphysema), simple ulcerative stomatitis, anaphylactoid re-

actions, chronic pulmonary emphysema in horses, laminitis, insect stings, and urticaria.
Indications: For use in conditions in which antihistaminic therapy may be expected to alleviate some signs of disease in horses, dogs, and cats.
Side Effects: Depression of the central nervous system and incoordination may occur at therapeutic dose levels. Disturbances in gastrointestinal function may occur. Overdosage may give rise to excitement, ataxia and convulsions.
Dosage and Administration: Horses: 25 mg (2.2 ml)/100 lb body weight. Dogs and Cats: 0.5 to 1 mg/lb body weight. Doses may be repeated in 8 to 12 hours, if necessary, to produce desired effect. For maintenance therapy, particularly in horses, the oral dosage form is recommended.
Warning: Not for use in horses intended for food.
KEEP OUT OF REACH OF CHILDREN
Caution: Federal (U.S.A.) law restricts this drug to use by or on the order of a licensed veterinarian.
Precautions: Intravenous route is not recommended for dogs and cats and should be injected slowly in horses. Intramuscular and subcutaneous administration should be by divided injection sites.
How Supplied: 250 ml vials.

A-H™ TABLETS ℞
(doxylamine succinate)
Antihistaminic

Composition: Each tablet contains: 100 mg doxylamine succinate.
Actions and Uses: A-H™ Tablets are for more extended antihistamine administration to block the action of, or to replace histamine in its attachment to receptor cells.
It is recommended that treatment be initiated with A-H Injection and that A-H Tablets be used for follow-up therapy.
Indications: For use in conditions in which antihistaminic therapy may be expected to alleviate some signs of disease in horses.
Dosage and Administration: Horses: 1 to 2 mg/lb body weight per day, divided into 3 or 4 equal doses.
Precautions: Depression of the central nervous system and incoordination may occur at therapeutic dose levels. Disturbances in gastrointestinal function may occur. Overdosage may give rise to excitement, ataxia, and convulsions.
Warning: Do not use in horses intended for food.
KEEP OUT OF REACH OF CHILDREN
Caution: Federal (U.S.A.) law restricts this drug to use by or on the order of a licensed veterinarian.
How Supplied: Bottles of 50 (100 mg) tablets.

ANVAX™
Anthrax Spore Vaccine
Nonencapsulated Live Culture

Composition: Anvax™ is a standardized suspension of live spores of nonencapsulated avirulent *Bacillus anthracis* (Sterne's strain). The spores are suspended in a glycerine-saponin diluent. Each serial is tested for purity, potency and safety according to current USDA regulations.
Actions and Uses: Anvax will produce protection against virulent anthrax in ruminants within six to eight days following vaccination. While possessing strong immunogenic qualities, Anvax is safe to use even in highly susceptible animals.
Vaccinate only healthy animals. Previously vaccinated animals should be revaccinated annually in areas where anthrax outbreaks are known to occur.
Indications: For the immunization of healthy cattle, sheep, goats, swine, horses, and mules against anthrax.
Dosage and Administration: Shake well. For aseptic subcutaneous use. Cattle, horses and mules, 1 ml; sheep, swine and goats, 0.5 ml. Vaccinate animals two to four weeks prior to season when anthrax outbreaks may be expected. A second dose administered within three to four weeks enhances the protective titer. Revaccinate annually in areas where anthrax outbreaks are known to occur.
Precautions: Store at not over 45°F or 7°C. Protect from freezing. Use entire contents when first opened. Burn container and all unused contents. Do not vaccinate within 6 weeks of slaughter. Do not vaccinate animals undergoing antibiotic therapy. Contains amphotericin B as preservative. Anaphylactoid reactions may occur following use. **Antidote:** Epinephrine.
For Veterinary Use Only
How Supplied: 10 ml and 50 ml vials.

BRUCELLA ABORTUS VACCINE
Strain 19, Live Culture, Reduced Dose

Description: A desiccated suspension of living *Brucella abortus* Strain 19 with sterile diluent.
Indications: For use in healthy female cattle only. Age of vaccination and other limitations shall be as directed by proper State authorities.
Rehydration: Aseptically add contents of the diluent vial to vaccine. Rotate until completely rehydrated.
Dosage and Administration: Shake well and inject 2 ml of rehydrated vaccine subcutaneously under an area of loose skin. Use sterile syringes and needles.
Accidental Human Exposure: Strain 19 *Brucella abortus* Vaccine can cause Brucellosis (Undulant Fever) in humans. Exposure may occur via injection, ingestion, conjunctiva or broken skin. In the event of accidental exposure, consult a physician.
Warning: All distributors are required by the producer and Federal regulations to keep complete records of the disposition of this vaccine.
Caution: Store at not over 45°F or 7°C. Use entire contents when first opened. Do not use chemical disinfectants to sterilize syringes and needles. Burn container and all unused contents. Do not vaccinate within 21 days of slaughter. Anaphylactoid reactions may occur following use. **Antidote:** Epinephrine. Restricted to use by or under the direction of a veterinarian.
For Veterinary Use Only
How Supplied: 5 dose vial with 10 ml vial sterile diluent, 25 dose vial with 50 ml vial sterile diluent.

BUTAZOLIDIN® ℞
(phenylbutazone)
Veterinary
For horses and dogs only
Anti-inflammatory—Antipyretic compound

Composition: Butazolidin® is a synthetic, non-hormonal anti-inflammatory, antipyretic compound useful in the management of inflammatory conditions. The apparent analgesic effect is probably related mainly to the compound's anti-inflammatory properties.
Chemically, Butazolidin is 4-butyl-1, 2-diphenyl-3,5-pyrazolidinedione. It is a pyrazolon derivative, entirely unrelated to the steroid hormones.
Background Pharmacology: Kuzell, Payne, Fleming, and Denko demonstrated clinical effectiveness of Butazolidin in acute rheumatism, gout, gouty arthritis, and various other rheumatoid disorders in man. Anti-rheumatic and anti-inflammatory activity has been well established by Fabre, Domenjoz, Wilhelmi, and Yourish.
Lieberman reported on the effective use of Butazolidin in the treatment of painful conditions of the musculoskeletal system in dogs, including posterior paralysis associated with intervertebral disc syndrome, painful fractures, arthritis, and painful injuries to the limbs and joints. Joshua observed objective improvement without toxicity following long-term therapy of two aged arthritic dogs. Ogilvie and Sutter reported rapid response to Butazolidin therapy in a review of 19 clinical cases including posterior paralysis, posterior weakness, arthritis, rheumatism, and other conditions associated with lameness and musculoskeletal weakness. Camberos reported favorable results with Butazolidin following intermittent treatment of Thoroughbred horses for arthritis and chronic arthrosis (e.g., osteoarthritis of medial and distal bones of the hock, arthritis of stifle and hip, arthrosis of the spine, chronic hip pains, chronic pain in trapezius muscles, and generalized arthritis). Results were less favorable in cases of traumatism, muscle rupture, strains, and inflammations of the third phalanx. Sutter reported favorable response in chronic equine arthritis, fair results in a severely bruised mare, and poor results in two cases where the condition was limited to the third phalanx.
Indications: For relief of inflammatory conditions associated with the musculoskeletal system in dogs and horses.
Contraindications: Treated animals should not be slaughtered for food purposes.

Continued on next page

Coopers—Cont.

Parenteral injections should be made intravenously only; do not inject subcutaneously or intramuscularly.
Use with caution in patients who have a history of drug allergy.
Dosage and Administration: ***Dogs:*** *Orally*—20 mg per lb of body weight (100 mg/5 lb) in three divided doses daily. Maximum dose is 800 mg per day regardless of weight. Use a relatively high dose for the first 48 hours, then reduce gradually to a maintenance dose. Maintain lowest dose capable of producing desired clinical response.
Intravenously—10 mg per lb of body weight (0.5 ml/10 lb), but not to exceed 800 mg (4 ml) daily regardless of weight. Injection should be given slowly and with care using a 22 or finer gauge needle. Excessive extravascular deposition may result in swelling or necrosis at the injection site. If swelling at the site of injection results, discontinue intravenous administration. Intravenous injections should be limited to two successive days but may be followed by oral Butazolidin dosage forms.
Horses: *Orally*—1 to 2 g per 500 lb of body weight, but not to exceed 4 g daily. Use a relatively high dose for the first 48 hours, then reduce gradually to a maintenance dose. Maintain lowest dose capable of producing desired clinical response.
Intravenously—1 to 2 g per 1,000 lb body weight (5 to 10 ml/1,000 lb) daily. Injection should be made slowly and with care. Limit intravenous administration to a maximum of 5 successive days, but may be followed by oral Butazolidin dosage forms.
Guidelines to Successful Therapy:
1. Use a relatively high dose for the first 48 hours, then reduce gradually to a maintenance dose. Maintain lowest dose capable of producing desired clinical response.
2. Response to Butazolidin therapy is prompt, usually occurring within 24 hours. If no significant clinical response is evident after 5 days, reevaluate diagnosis and therapeutic approach.
3. In animals, Butazolidin is largely metabolized in 8 hours. It is recommended that a third of the daily dose be administered at 8-hour intervals. Reduce dosage as symptoms regress. In some cases, treatment may be given only when symptoms appear with no need for continuous medication. If long-term therapy is planned, oral administration is suggested.
4. In many cases tablets may be crushed and given with feed.
5. Many chronic conditions will respond to Butazolidin therapy, but discontinuance of treatment may result in recurrence of symptoms.

Precautions: Stop medication at first sign of gastrointestinal upset, jaundice, or blood dyscrasia. Authenticated cases of agranulocytosis associated with the drug have occurred in man; fatal reactions, although rare, have been reported in dogs after long-term therapy. To guard against this possibility, conduct routine blood counts at weekly intervals during the early phase of therapy and at intervals of two weeks thereafter. Any significant fall in the total white count, relative decrease in granulocytes, or black or tarry stools, should be regarded as a signal for immediate cessation of therapy and institution of appropriate counter-measures.
In the treatment of inflammatory conditions associated with infections, specific anti-infective therapy is required.
Store injectable in a cool place (46°F to 59°F) or alternatively store in a refrigerator.
Caution: Federal (U.S.A.) law restricts this drug to use by or on the order of a licensed veterinarian.
How Supplied:
Tablets
Bottles of 100—100 mg tablets
Bottles of 500—100 mg tablets
Bottles of 200—400 mg tablets
Bottles of 100—1 g tablets
Bottles of 50—2 g boluses
Boxes of 50—4 g boluses
Injectable
100 ml vials, 200 mg/ml (1 g/5 ml).
Each ml contains 200 mg of phenylbutazone, 10.45 mg of benzyl alcohol as preservative, and sodium hydroxide to adjust pH to 9.5–10.0 and distilled water q.s.
Butazolidin: Registered Trademark, CIBA-GEIGY CORPORATION.

BUTAZOLIDIN® PASTE ℞
(phenylbutazone)
Veterinary—For Horses Only
Anti-inflammatory—Antipyretic compound

Description: Butazolidin® is a synthetic, nonhormonal anti-inflammatory, antipyretic compound useful in the management of inflammatory conditions. The apparent analgesic effect is probably related mainly to the compound's anti-inflammatory properties.
Chemically, Butazolidin is 4-butyl-1, 2-diphenyl-3, 5-pyrazolidinedione. It is a pyrazolone derivative, entirely unrelated to the steriod hormones.
Indications: For relief of inflammatory conditions associated with the musculoskeletal system in horses.
Contraindications: Use with caution in patients who have a history of drug allergy.
Dosage and Administration: Orally—1 to 2 g of phenylbutazone per 500 lb of body weight, but not to exceed 4 g daily. Use a relatively high dose for the first 48 hours, then reduce gradually to a maintenance dose. Maintain lowest dose capable of producing desired clinical response.
Guidelines to Successful Therapy:
1. Use a relatively high dose for the first 48 hours, then reduce gradually to a maintenance dose. Maintain lowest dose capable of producing desired clinical response.
2. Response to Butazolidin therapy is prompt, usually occurring within 24 hours. If no significant clinical response is evident after 5 days, reevaluate diagnosis and therapeutic approach.
3. When administering Butazolidin Paste, the oral cavity should be empty. Deposit paste on back of tongue by depressing plunger that has been previously set to deliver the correct dose.
4. Many chronic conditions will respond to Butazolidin therapy, but discontinuance of treatment may result in recurrence of symptoms.

Warning: Not for use in horses intended for food.
Precautions: Stop medication at first sign of gastrointestinal upset, jaundice, or blood dyscrasia. Authenticated cases of agranulocytosis associated with the drug have occurred in man; fatal reactions, although rare, have been reported in dogs after long-term therapy. To guard against this possibility, conduct routine blood counts at weekly intervals during the early phase of therapy and at intervals of two weeks thereafter. Any significant fall in the total white count, relative decrease in granulocytes, or black or tarry stools, should be regarded as a signal for immediate cessation of therapy and institution of appropriate counter measures.
In the treatment of inflammatory conditions associated with infections, specific anti-infective therapy is required.
Caution: Federal (U.S.A.) law restricts this drug to use by or on the order of a licensed veterinarian.
How Supplied: Syringes containing 6 g and 12 g of phenylbutazone.
Butazolidin: Registered Trademark, CIBA-GEIGY CORPORATION.

CANIHEPTIN™ CAPSULES ℞
Lipotropic Agent

Composition: Each capsule contains: Choline dihydrogen citrate 276 mg; dl-Methionine 110 mg; Inositol 83 mg; In a base of liver concentrate and desiccated liver.
Actions and Uses: Certain poisons, infectious diseases, environmental changes, dietary deficiencies, disturbed fat metabolism and clinical conditions involving one or more of the above factors may result in excessive deposition of fat in the liver. Fibrosis and cirrhosis of the liver and reduced function follow such excessive fat accumulation. Choline and precursors, methionine and betaine, prevent the deposition of or accelerate the removal of fat from the liver.
Indications: A lipotropic agent to aid in the prevention and treatment of liver dysfunctions in dogs due to fatty infiltration or degeneration of the liver such as may occur in infectious hepatitis, cirrhosis, toxemias, obesity, and nutritional deficiencies involving ingredients in this preparation.
Dosage and Administration: One capsule per 20 lb body weight daily. Contents of capsule may be sprinkled on the feed, especially for small dogs requiring less than 1 capsule daily.

KEEP OUT OF REACH OF CHILDREN
Caution: Federal (U.S.A.) law restricts this drug to use by or on the order of a licensed veterinarian.
How Supplied: Bottle of 100 capsules.

CANOPAR® ℞
(thenium closylate)
Anthelmintic

Composition: Canopar® (thenium closylate) has proved to be a safe and effective canine ancylostomicide when given by oral administration to dogs suffering from various degrees of hookworm infestation.
Synthesized by the Wellcome Research Laboratories and reported on by Burrows et al., thenium closylate is a derivative of the bephenium series and is a quaternary ammonium compound chemically described as: N,N-dimethyl-N-(2-phenoxyethyl)-2-thenyl-ammonium p-chlorobenzene sulfonate.
At the recommended dosage levels Canopar has shown excellent efficacy against *Ancylostoma caninum* and *Uncinaria stenocephala.*
One important advantage of Canopar is that it can be administered to severely parasitized dogs without subjecting them to a fasting period. This permits the immediate treatment of the animal, following a positive diagnosis, and eliminates the possibility of creating any additional stress condition in debilitated dogs, by a regimen of starvation.
Some emesis may occur in an occasional animal subsequent to the administration of Canopar. However, it was observed during the clinical development of this product that if vomition was delayed for more than two hours, the effect of the drug was not interfered with and there was no necessity to repeat the dose. In clinical trials, Canopar was administered to over 1,000 infected dogs with consistently effective results.
Of prime concern in assessing the efficacy of Canopar was the measurement of elimination, and percent of clearance of the adult worm from the alimentary canal following treatment. In pursuit of this data, the experimental subjects were sacrificed and a favorable correlation was established between the post-treatment worm elimination count and the number of residual adult hookworms in the intestines.
Indications: A preparation for a single day treatment of canine ancylostomiasis by the removal from the intestines of the adult forms of the species *Ancylostoma caninum* and *Uncinaria stenocephala.*
Dosage and Administration: Since Canopar is insoluble and has a direct action on the adult parasite in situ, a simplified dosage range is based on gut volume rather than the body weight of the animal; consequently, an increase in the amount of drug on a repeated daily dose is unnecessary.
Clinical evidence has indicated that mature dogs respond equally well to a single daily dose as to a divided daily dose. Recently-weaned puppies respond better to Canopar administered twice daily. Canopar should not be given to the unweaned pup or pups weighing less than five pounds.
Regardless of age or weight, it is not necessary to fast the animal or to include a purgative as an aid to Canopar treatment.
The tablets, containing 500 mg of active base, are conveniently scored for administration and dispensing purposes.

Dogs	*Oral Administration*
10 pounds and over	one tablet—single dose
5–10 pounds	one half tablet—twice daily

Give all dosages for one day only. The treatment should be repeated after two or three weeks.
Contraindications: Suckling puppies or recently-weaned puppies weighing less than five pounds should not be treated with Canopar; otherwise, there are no known contraindications for use of this product.
Animals that are severely infected, exhibiting evidence of intestinal hemorrhage, debilitation and anemia; should be given supportive treatment in accordance with recognized forms of therapy.
Precautions
Do not feed milk or other fatty foods during treatment. Canopar must not be administered to unweaned pups because the high fat content of bitch's milk facilitates absorption of thenium with the risk of systemic toxicity. In addition, the vomiting reflex in these pups is poorly developed. Systemic toxicity in unweaned pups is exhibited by depression.
Adverse Reactions: Rare reactions of a toxic or anaphylactic nature, sometimes fatal, have been reported in adult dogs following administration of Canopar. Reports indicate that there is a higher incidence in Airedales than other breeds.
Caution: Federal (U.S.A.) law restricts this drug to use by or on the order of a licensed veterinarian.
Keep out of reach of children.
How Supplied: Each scored tablet contains 500 mg of thenium closylate (in terms of base). Bottles of 100 tablets.

CEPHALOVAC® EWT
Encephalomyelitis Vaccine
Eastern and Western Killed Virus
Tetanus Toxoid

Description: Cephalovac® EWT is a multivalent vaccine comprised of killed eastern (EEE) and western (WEE) equine encephalomyelitis viruses combined with highly purified tetanus toxoid. The EEE and WEE viruses are derived from selected strains propagated in chicken tissue cultures. The virus laden fluids are inactivated to provide maximum safety and are combined in a 2 ml dose for peak antigenicity when administered as directed.
The greater purity inherent in the tissue culture process diminishes the possibility of reaction to the product. This results from virtual elimination of the allergenic egg proteins and particulate material commonly present in products prepared from chicken embryos.
The toxin produced by virulent *Clostridium tetani* has been modified by special treatment so that toxicity is eliminated while the ability to act as an antigen is retained.
Action and Uses: Eastern (EEE) and western (WEE) equine encephalomyelitis are primarily seasonal diseases occurring from June to November and generally reaching epizootic proportions during August and September.
Both viruses, eastern and western, are maintained in nature by arthropod-animal reservoirs from which infections are transmitted to mammalian hosts by biting insects, especially mosquitoes of the species *Aedes, Anopheles, Culex* and *Culiseta,* which serve as the principal biological vectors. Numerous species of domestic and wild birds serve as the major reservoirs for EEE and WEE. However, other mammals, including swine, cattle, dogs, opossums, raccoons and white-tailed deer also develop levels of viremia sufficiently high for mosquito transmission.
The horse may be regarded as a dead-end host for WEE, but with EEE, horses develop viremia sufficient to infect mosquitoes.
Clinical signs of the two viral infections vary in type and severity. Signs include fever, impaired vision, irregular gait, wandering, diarrhea, grinding of teeth, drowsiness, paralysis and death. Mild cases may recover slowly in a few weeks, but severely affected animals die. Case-fatality in horses ranges from 20 to 50% for WEE to 90% and over for EEE.
Indications: For the active immunization of all types and ages of healthy horses against eastern and western equine encephalomyelitis and tetanus.
Dosage and Administration: Shake well before using. Using aseptic technique, inject 2 ml deep intramuscularly. Administer a second 2 ml dose in 4 to 6 weeks, using a different injection site. Only a single annual booster is required. Use a separate, sterile 1½-inch needle for each injection.
Caution: Store at not over 45°F or 7°C. Protect from freezing. Use entire contents when first opened. Contains penicillin and streptomycin as added preservatives. Anaphylactoid reactions may occur following use. **Antidote:** Epinephrine.
How Supplied: 10 one-dose syringes and 10 dose vial.

CEPHALOVAC® V
Encephalomyelitis Vaccine
Venezuelan Modified Live Virus

Composition: Cephalovac® V is a modified live virus vaccine produced in a heterologous cell system. The Trinidad strain of VEE virus has been attenuated by selection and serial passage in fetal guinea pig heart cells. The safety and antigenicity of this virus strain has been demonstrated in susceptible horses.
Indications: For active immunization of equines against Venezuelan equine encephalomyelitis.

Continued on next page

Coopers—Cont.

General Information: Venezuelan equine encephalomyelitis has been demonstrated as the causative agent of intermittent epizootics of fatal encephalitis in the equine populations of Venezuela, Colombia, Ecuador, Central America, Mexico and the United States. The disease is now considered endemic in Mexico. VEE, like eastern and western equine encephalomyelitis is transmitted by mosquitoes, thus the incidence of disease corresponds to the mosquito season. Epidemic VEE strains tend to produce exceptionally high levels of virus in the blood of host animals permitting ready infection of several species of mosquito and maintaining epidemic spread.
The clinical signs of VEE infection in horses vary in type and severity. In experimental infections, the incubation period varies from 24-78 hours. The animal shows a febrile response which may fluctuate between 102° and 106°F, becomes depressed and stops eating. Diarrhea and colic frequently occur, followed by rapid weight loss. In non-fatal cases, the body temperature becomes normal in 2-4 days but convalescence is prolonged. In fatal cases, fever persists. The animal becomes progressively weaker and may die within 2-4 days. The encephalitic form is similar to eastern and western equine encephalomyelitis except that diarrhea more frequently accompanies VEE. Other signs are similar to those seen in the generalized disease—fever, anorexia, colic, depression. The encephalitis is demonstrated in altered personality. Docile animals may become vicious. Other signs include head pressing, grinding teeth, circling, muscle spasms, prostration and convulsions. Convulsions become increasingly frequent terminating in death 2-4 days after initial signs. Mortality approaches 90% in horses that develop encephalitic signs.
Dosage and Administration: Rehydration: Transfer the entire contents of the diluent vial to the vaccine vial using a boiled or autoclaved syringe and needle. Shake gently until the product is in solution. The vaccine is less stable in this form and should be used immediately.
Dosage: Using aseptic technique, inject 1 ml of rehydrated vaccine subcutaneously in the cervical region. Use a separate, sterile needle for each injection.
Precautions: Store at not over 45°F or 7°C. Do not use chemical disinfectants to sterilize syringes and needles. Do not vaccinate pregnant mares or foals under 2 weeks of age. Foals vaccinated at less than 6 months of age should be revaccinated at 6 months of age. Use entire contents when first opened. Burn container and all unused contents. Contains penicillin and streptomycin as added preservatives. Anaphylactoid reactions may occur following use. **Antidote:** Epinephrine
For Veterinary Use Only
How Supplied: 10-1 dose vials with diluent.

CEPHALOVAC® VEW
Encephalomyelitis Vaccine
Eastern, Western and Venezuelan
Killed Virus

Composition: Cephalovac® VEW is a trivalent killed virus vaccine derived from chicken tissue cultures infected with selected strains of eastern and western encephalomyelitis virus, and from porcine cell line cultures infected with an attenuated strain of Venezuelan equine encephalomyelitis virus. The virus laden fluids are inactivated to provide maximum safety and are combined for peak antigenicity in a 2 ml dose when two injections are administered 21 to 28 days apart. The total immunogenicity of Cephalovac VEW is enhanced through a synergistic effect achieved by combining antigens of the three types of encephalomyelitis virus, and from the addition of a specially selected adjuvant. Greater purity, a quality inherent in the tissue culture process, results from virtual elimination of the allergenic egg proteins and particulate material commonly present in products prepared from chicken embryos.
Indications: For active immunization of all types and ages of healthy horses against eastern, western, and Venezuelan equine encephalomyelitis.
Action and Uses: Venezuelan equine encephalomyelitis (VEE) has caused intermittent epizootics of fatal encephalomyelitis in the equine populations of Venezuela, Colombia, Ecuador, Central America, Mexico, and the United States. The disease is considered to be endemic in Mexico.
Eastern (EEE) and western (WEE) equine encephalomyelitis are primarily seasonal diseases occuring from June to November and generally reaching epizootic proportions during August and September.
All three viruses, eastern, western, and Venezuelan, are maintained in nature by an arthropod-animal reservoir from which infections are transmitted to mammalian hosts by biting insects, especially mosquitoes of the species *Aedes, Anopheles, Culex,* and *Culiseta,* which serve as the principal biological vectors. Numerous species of domestic and wild birds serve as the major reservoirs for EEE and WEE and are minor reservoirs for VEE. Small rodents, in particular the cotton rat, are believed to be the most important reservoir for VEE. However, other mammals, including swine, cattle, dogs, opossums, raccoons, and white-tailed deer also develop levels of viremia sufficiently high for mosquito transmission.
The horse may be regarded as a dead-end host for WEE, but with both VEE and EEE, horses develop viremia sufficient to infect mosquitoes. In addition, the horse is recognized as an "amplifying" host for VEE, and, unlike WEE or EEE, under certain conditions VEE can be transmitted between horses by direct contact.
Clinical signs of the three viral infections vary in type and severity. Signs include fever, impaired vision, irregular gait, wandering, diarrhea, grinding of teeth, drowsiness, paralysis, and death. Mild cases may recover slowly in a few weeks, but severely affected animals die. Case-fatality in horses ranges from 20 to 50% for WEE to 90% and over for EEE and VEE.
Dosage and Administration: Using aseptic technique, inject 2 ml deep intramuscularly. Administer a second 2 ml dose in 21 to 28 days, using a different injection site. Only a single annual booster is required. Use a separate, sterile, 1½ inch needle for each injection.
Precautions: Store at not over 45°F or 7°C. Protect from freezing. Use entire contents when first opened. Contains penicillin and streptomycin as added preservatives. Anaphylactoid reactions may occur following use. **Antidote:** Epinephrine.
For Veterinary Use Only.
How Supplied: 10-1 dose syringes and 10 dose vials.

CEPHALOVAC® VEWT
Encephalomyelitis Vaccine —
Eastern, Western and Venezuelan
Killed Virus
Tetanus Toxoid

Composition: Cephalovac® VEWT is a multivalent vaccine comprised of killed eastern (EEE), western (WEE), and Venezuelan (VEE) equine encephalomyelitis viruses combined with highly purified tetanus toxoid. The EEE and WEE viruses are derived from selected strains propagated in chicken tissue cultures, while the VEE virus is derived from an attenuated strain propagated in porcine cell line cultures. The virus laden fluids are inactivated to provide maximum safety and are combined in a 2 ml dose for peak antigenicity when administered as directed. The total immunogenicity of each virus is enhanced through a synergistic effect achieved when the antigens of the three types of encephalomyelitis virus are combined and from the addition of a specially selected adjuvant.
The greater purity inherent in the tissue culture process diminishes the possibility of reaction to the product. This results from virtual elimination of the allergenic egg proteins and particulate material commonly present in products prepared from chicken embryos.
The toxin produced by virulent *Clostridium tetani* has been modified by special treatment so that toxicity is eliminated while the ability to act as an antigen is retained.
Indications: For active immunization of all types and ages of healthy horses against eastern, western and Venezuelan equine encephalomyelitis and tetanus.
Action and Uses: Venezuelan equine encephalomyelitis (VEE) has caused intermittent epizootics of fatal encephalomyelitis in the equine populations of Venezuela, Colombia, Ecuador, Central America, Mexico and the United States. The disease is considered to be endemic in Mexico.
Eastern (EEE) and western (WEE equine encephalomyelitis are primarily seasonal diseases occurring from June to

November and generally reaching epizootic proportions during August and September.

All three viruses, eastern, western and Venezuelan, are maintained in nature by arthropod-animal reservoirs from which infections are transmitted to mammalian hosts by biting insects, especially mosquitoes of the species *Aedes, Anopheles, Culex* and *Culiseta,* which serve as the principal biological vectors. Numerous species of domestic and wild birds serve as the major reservoirs for EEE and WEE and are minor reservoirs for VEE. Small rodents, in particular the cotton rat, are believed to be the most important reservoirs for VEE. However, other mammals, including swine, cattle, dogs, opossums, raccoons and white-tailed deer also develop levels of viremia sufficiently high for mosquito transmission.

The horse may be regarded as a "dead-end" host for WEE, but with both VEE and EEE, horses develop viremia sufficient to infect mosquitoes. In addition, the horse is recognized as an "amplifying" host for VEE, which unlike WEE or EEE, can be transmitted between horses by direct contact under certain conditions.

Clinical signs of the three viral infections vary in type and severity. Signs include fever, impaired vision, irregular gait, wandering, diarrhea, grinding of teeth, drowsiness, paralysis and death. Mild cases may recover slowly in a few weeks, but severely affected animals die. Case-fatality in horses ranges from 20% to 50% for WEE to 90% and over for EEE and VEE.

Dosage and Administration: Shake well. Using aseptic technique, inject 2 ml deep intramuscularly. Administer a second 2 ml dose in 4-6 weeks, using a different injection site. Only a single annual booster is required. Use a separate, sterile 1½ inch needle for each injection.

Precautions: Store at not over 45°F or 7°C. Protect from freezing. Use entire contents when first opened. Contains penicillin and streptomycin as added preservatives. Anaphylactoid reactions may occur following use. **Antidote:** Epinephrine.

For Veterinary Use Only

How Supplied: Ten-1 dose syringes and 10 dose vials.

CO-NAV®

Pesticide For use on Livestock and Dogs

Composition: Co-Nav is an emulsifiable concentrate containing:

Active Ingredient:	
Dioxathion [2,3,p-dioxanedithiol S, S,bis (0,0-diethyl phosphorodithioate)]	20.40%
Inert Ingredients:	79.60%
	100.00%

Indications: Effective as a dip or spray against the following pests.

Dogs —Ticks, fleas, lice; can be used as a premise spray.

Cattle, Sheep, Goats, Swine and Horses —Ticks, horn flies, lice, keds and wool maggots—also helpful in controlling screwworm infestations.

Keep out of reach of children.

Danger Poison

Restricted Use Pesticide: For retail sale to and use only by Certified Applicators or persons under their direct supervision, and only for those uses covered by the Certified Applicator's Certification.

PRECAUTIONARY STATEMENTS

HAZARDS TO HUMANS AND DOMESTIC ANIMALS

DANGER

Poisonous if swallowed. May be fatal if absorbed through skin. Do not get on skin or on clothing. Do not breathe vapors or spray mist. Avoid contact with eyes. Use respirator or goggles if necessary.

Do not contaminate feed or foodstuffs. Food utensils such as teaspoons and tablespoons should not be used for food purposes after use with pesticides.

Do not use concentrations greater than those recommended. Apply this product only as specified on this label.

Do not use on dairy animals or in dairy barns. Do not treat animals under 3 months of age. Do not dip or spray foals. Do not apply to dairy goats. Do not apply to sick, convalescent or stressed animals. Dioxathion is a cholinesterase inhibitor. Do not use this product on animals simultaneously with treatment or exposure to other cholinesterase inhibiting drugs, pesticides or chemicals.

Symptoms of overdosage may include frequent defecation and urination, watering of eyes and muscular twitching followed later by salivation, diarrhea and muscular weakness. At the first sign of adverse reactions consult a veterinarian and thoroughly wash animals to remove excess dip or spray. Brahman/Zebu breeds may be less tolerant than other cattle to organophosphate insecticides such as Co-Nav. Use caution in applying Co-Nav on Brahman/Zebu breeds. Do not use Co-Nav on Brahman/Zebu calves.

Pay strict attention to warning statements on Co-Nav containers.

STATEMENT OF PRACTICAL TREATMENT

If Swallowed: Call a physician/veterinarian or Poison Control Center immediately. DO NOT INDUCE VOMITING, unless under medical supervision. Vomiting may cause aspiration pneumonia.

If Inhaled: Remove victim to fresh air. Apply respiration if indicated.

If On Skin: Wash immediately with plenty of soap and water.

If In Eyes: Immediately flush eyes with plenty of water. Get medical attention if irritation persists.

Note To Physician/Veterinarian: This product contains an organophosphate and petroleum distillates.

ATROPINE IS ANTIDOTAL for the organophosphate ingredient.

ENVIRONMENTAL HAZARDS

This product is toxic to fish, wildlife and birds. Keep out of any body of water. Do not contaminate water by cleaning of equipment or disposal of wastes. Do not apply where runoff is likely to occur.

PHYSICAL OR CHEMICAL HAZARDS

Do not use or store near heat or open flame.

Directions For Use: It is a violation of Federal law to use this product in a manner inconsistent with its labeling.

DOGS

To Kill Ticks, Fleas and Lice: Thoroughly mix at the rate of ½ fl. oz (1 tablespoonful) with 1 gallon of water. Sponge, swab, bathe or dip dog making sure dog is thoroughly wet. Repeat only when necessary but not more frequently than once a week.

Premise Spray for Yards. Kennels: Mix at the rate of 2½ fl. oz (5 tablespoonfuls) with 1 gallon of water. Use 1 gallon of spray per 1,000 sq. ft. of lawn or kennel area. Make sure to spray possible hiding places such as cracks in cement or wood, around dog's bedding and under various pieces of debris.

CATTLE, SHEEP, GOATS, SWINE AND HORSES

To Kill Ticks, Horn Flies, Lice, Keds, Wool Maggots, and Screwworms: Mix at the rate of 1 gallon Co-Nav to 200 gallons of water. Mix thoroughly. Spray or dip as required but not more often than every two weeks. The use of Co-Nav requires no waiting period between last application and slaughter. Co-Nav may be used in quarantine situations for fever tick control.

Long-Lasting Protection: Co-Nav provides long-lasting protection against reinfestation of ticks and 3 weeks protection against horn flies. A single application is usually sufficient for lice and keds. For biting lice on goats, a second application after 21 days may be required for complete clean-up. Co-Nav also aids in controlling screwworm larvae and provides up to 2 months protection against wool maggots.

Spraying: Make sure spray is thoroughly mixed before application. Wet animals thoroughly for best results. Do not allow animals to drink from runoff pools. Prevent oral ingestion. Do not allow young animals to swallow by nursing or licking the insecticide solution on treated animals.

Dipping: Thoroughly mix dip before dipping. Water animals before dipping to prevent drinking of dip wash. Prevent oral ingestion. Do not allow young animals to swallow by nursing or licking the insecticide solution on treated animals.

Replenishment: Add 1 gallon of Co-Nav to each 200 gallons of fresh water added to dipping vat or control replenishment by vatside test.

STORAGE AND DISPOSAL

Do not contaminate water, food or feed by storage or disposal.

Storage: Store in cool, dry place away from heat or open flame.

Pesticide Disposal: Pesticide wastes are acutely hazardous. Improper disposal of excess pesticide spray mixture, or rinsate is a violation of Federal law. If these wastes cannot be disposed of by use according to label instructions, contact

Continued on next page

Coopers—Cont.

your State Pesticide or Environmental Control Agency, or the Hazardous Waste representative at the nearest EPA Regional Office for guidance.
Container Disposal: Triple rinse (or equivalent). Then dispose of in a sanitary landfill or by other approved State and local procedures.
How Supplied: One gallon bottles.

C

CORTISPORIN® OPHTHALMIC OINTMENT—Veterinary
(polymyxin B-bacitracin-neomycin-hydrocortisone)
Antibiotic—Anti-inflammatory ℞

Description: Cortisporin® Ophthalmic Ointment Veterinary is a sterile broad-spectrum antibiotic and anti-inflammatory ointment for ophthalmic use in dogs and cats. Each gram contains: Aerosporin® (Polymyxin B Sulfate) 5000 units, bacitracin zinc 400 units, neomycin sulfate 5 mg (equivalent to 3.5 mg neomycin base), hydrocortisone 10 mg (1%) in a special white petrolatum base, q.s.
Actions: Hydrocortisone, the naturally occuring adrenal corticosteroid affords anti-inflammatory activity. Polymyxin B, neomycin and bacitracin provide anti-bacterial activity against a wide range of bacterial pathogens, both gram-positive and gram-negative.
Indications: For the treatment of acute and chronic conjunctivitis due to organisms susceptible to the antibiotics contained in the ointment. Laboratory tests should be conducted including *in vitro* culturing and susceptibility tests on samples collected prior to treatment.
Contraindications: This product is contraindicated in acute purulent conjunctivitis, fungal or viral lesions, herpes simplex, ulcerative keratitis, deep ulcerative lesions involving the inner layer of the cornea and in those animals showing a sensitivity to any of its components. Corticosteroids may inhibit essential inflammatory responses intrinsic to the fundamental healing mechanism.
Adverse Reactions: Adverse reactions, such as itching, burning or inflammation may occur in animals sensitive to this product.
Dosage and Administration: Properly cleanse area to be treated. Foreign bodies, crusted exudates and debris should be carefully removed. Express a small quantity of ointment into the conjunctival sac beneath the lower eyelid three or four times daily. After application hold the eyelids shut for a short time so that a thin film of ointment covers the cornea.
Precautions: If irritation develops discontinue treatment with this drug. If there is no response to treatment in 2-3 days, discontinue treatment and re-evaluate diagnosis. Prolonged use may result in overgrowth of nonsusceptible organisms, including fungi.
Animals under treatment with this product should be observed for usual signs of corticosteroid overdose which includes polydipsia, polyuria and occasionally an increase in weight.
Care should be taken not to contaminate the applicator tip during administrations of the preparation.
Warning: All topical ophthalmic preparations containing corticosteroids with or without an antimicrobial agent are contraindicated in the initial treatment of corneal ulcers. This should not be used until the infection is under control and corneal regeneration is well under way.
Caution: Federal (U.S.A.) law restricts this drug to use by or on the order of a licensed veterinarian.
How Supplied: 1/8 oz tube with ophthalmic tip.

COVEXIN® 8
Clostridium Chauvoei-Septicum-Haemolyticum-Novyi-Tetani-Perfringens Types C & D Bacterin-Toxoid

Description: A formalin-inactivated, alum-precipitated bacterin-toxoid prepared from highly toxigenic cultures and culture filtrates of *Clostridium chauvoei, Cl. septicum, Cl. haemolyticum* (known elsewhere as *Cl. novyi* Type D), *Cl. novyi, Cl. tetani,* and *Cl. perfringens* Types C and D. Covexin 8 is an Electroferm® product produced by an electronically controlled deep culture process.
The specific toxoids and/or cellular antigens required for optimal disease protection are emphasized in the growth of Electroferm cultures. These cultures are highly concentrated and, when divided for the blending of combination vaccines, make possible the production of the low volume dose. Exacting procedures are employed to help assure that each dose of combination vaccine contains an appropriate amount of each component.
All components of each serial of the final product are tested for potency using USDA-accepted laboratory and/or host animal tests.
The protective value of all components of Covexin 8 has been demonstrated through the most critical test procedures available. Vaccinated sheep withstood the challenge of massive doses of virulent live spores of *Cl. chauvoei, Cl. septicum, Cl. tetani, Cl. novyi* Types B and D. *Cl. perfringens* Types C and D, for which no host-animal direct-challenge test exists, were evaluated by measuring the amount of antitoxin produced by cattle, sheep and laboratory animals.
Indications: For the active immunization of healthy sheep against diseases caused by *Cl. chauvoei, Cl. septicum, Cl. novyi* Type B, *Cl. haemolyticum* (known also as *Cl. novyi* Type D), *Cl. tetani* and *Cl. perfringens* Types C and D.
Although *Cl. perfringens* Type B is not a significant problem in the U.S.A., immunity may be provided against the beta and epsilon toxins elaborated by *Cl. perfringens* Type B. This immunity is derived from the combination of Type C (beta) and Type D (epsilon) fractions.
Caution: Store at not over 45°F or 7°C. Protect from freezing. Use entire contents when first opened. Do not vaccinate within 21 days before slaughter. Anaphylactoid reactions may occur following use. **Antidote:** Epinephrine.
Administration and Dosage: Shake well. Using aseptic technique, inject 5 ml subcutaneously, followed by a 2 ml dose in 6 weeks. Revaccinate annually with 2 ml prior to periods of extreme risk or parturition. For *Cl. novyi* and *Cl. haemolyticum,* revaccinate every 5-6 months. Vaccination should be scheduled so that pregnant ewes receive their second vaccination or annual booster six to two weeks before lambing commences in the flock. Lambs should be given their primary course beginning at 10-12 weeks of age.
How Supplied: 50 ml and 250 ml DuraVial® plastic pouches

CYTORAB®
Rabies Vaccine, Killed Virus,

Description: Cytorab® is an inactivated virus vaccine. The vaccine virus is grown in cultures of a USDA-certified, monkey kidney cell line. Gentamicin has been added. A low level of adjuvant is included to enhance the immune response of vaccinated animals.
The potency of each Cytorab serial is determined by means of the NIH test. Safety tests are conducted in dogs, mice, guinea pigs and rabbits.
The rabies seed virus used for Cytorab is derived from a modified live strain used for many years for the preparation of our ERA Strain® Rabies Vaccine. This virus was chosen because of proven immunogenicity in six animal species, and because it produces high yields of viral antigen in the selected cell line.
Action and Uses: Cytorab is approved for both dogs and cats. One year duration of immunity has been demonstrated through challenge with virulent street virus. The immunogenicity of the vaccine was further seen in the magnitude of initial antibody titers and in the degree of antibody persistence.
The following safety features are inherent in Cytorab; (1) Because vaccine virus is grown in a cell culture system, the potential for myelin reactions associated with nerve-tissue-origin vaccines is eliminated; (2) Use of a continuous cell line provides safeguards against both the propogation and accidental introduction of adventitious pathogens into the vaccine; (3) Humans who are accidentially inoculated are not considered at risk to rabies disease.
Cytorab is a very well tolerated vaccine. Safety studies in over 1,000 dogs and cats showed postvaccinal reactions to be very rare. Its immunogenicity was not affected when used concurrently with other canine and feline vaccines.
Indications: For the active immunization of healthy dogs and cats against rabies.
Dosage and Administration:
Shake well before use. Inject a 1 ml dose intramuscularly at one site in the thigh using aseptic technique. Revaccinate annually. For animals vaccinated under 3 months of age, revaccinate at 3 months of age.

Caution: Store at not over 45°F or 7°C. Do not freeze. Use entire contents when first opened. Contains gentamicin as an added preservative. Anaphylactoid reactions may occur following use. **Antidote:** Epinephrine.
RESTRICTED TO USE BY OR UNDER THE DIRECTION OF A LICENSED VETERINARIAN.
How Supplied: 10 dose vials.

CYTORAB® RCP
Feline Rhinotracheitis-Calici-Panleukopenia-Rabies Vaccine
Modified Live and Killed Virus

Indications: For the active immunization of healthy cats and kittens 12 weeks of age and older against rabies, feline rhinotracheitis, calici and panleukopenia. This vaccine is to be used as an annual booster or as the final dose in a primary immunization series.
Caution: Store at not over 45°F or 7°C. Do not freeze. Do not use chemical disinfectants to sterilize syringes or needles. Burn containers and all unused contents. Do not vaccinate pregnant queens. Contains gentamicin as added preservative. Anaphylactoid reactions may occur following use. **Antidote:** Epinephrine.
Administration and Dosage: Transfer contents of liquid vaccine vial to lyophilized vaccine vial using aseptic technique. Inject 1 ml rehydrated vaccine intramuscularly **at one site in the thigh** using aseptic technique and boiled, autoclaved or sterile disposable syringes and needles.
For primary immunization, two doses of feline rhinotracheitis and calicivirus are required. Revaccinate annually with a single dose of Cytrorab RCP.
Restricted to use by or under the direction of a licensed veterinarian.
How Supplied: 10 (1 dose) vials.

DCM™ SPECIAL WITH PHOSPHORUS ℞
Sterile Solution
Dextrose-Calcium-Magnesium-Phosphorus

Composition:

Contains:	% w/v	mEq/1
Dextrose	15.00%	
Calcium (as calcium borogluconate)	2.15%	1,078
Magnesium (as magnesium hypophosphite)	0.34%	280
Phosphorus (as magnesium hypophosphite)	0.87%	281
Distilled water	q.s.	

Indications: For the treatment of cattle only in deficiencies of:
1. Calcium (milk fever, parturient paresis, hypocalcemia)
2. Magnesium (grass tetany)
3. Magnesium and/or hyperpotassemia (wheat pasture poisoning).

For use in cattle exhibiting the above disease conditions only.
Contraindications: DCM Special with Phosphorus should not be given to animals with elevated blood levels of calcium, magnesium, phosphorus, or glucose.
Do not mix and administer with tetracyclines.
Do not administer to cows showing signs of cardiac distress.
Actions and Uses: Calcium borogluconate is most commonly used in the treatment of parturient paresis (milk fever). Those cases which are accompanied by hypomagnesemia and hypophosphatemia respond better if magnesium and phosphorus are also included. Dextrose is beneficial in those cases complicated by hypoglycemia and hyperketonemia (ketosis).
Adverse Reactions: Cardiac arrest can occur when blood levels of calcium become excessive from improper intravenous administration. Perivascular or subcutaneous deposition of the hypertonic preparation may produce injection site inflammation.
Dosage and Administration: The usual intravenous dose in cattle is 500 ml per 800–1000 lbs (364–455) of body weight. Use a single entry container to avoid contamination.
Precautions: Care must be taken not to overload the circulatory system, especially in cardiac or pulmonary disorders. Strict sterile procedures should be observed.
Intravenous administration of this product must be made slowly to avoid adverse effects, such as heart block or shock. Read insert carefully prior to administration. Keep in cool, dark place. Protect from freezing.
KEEP OUT OF REACH OF CHILDREN.
Caution: Federal (U.S.A.) law restricts this drug to use by or on the order of a licensed veterinarian.
How Supplied: 500 ml bottles.

DERMATHYCIN™ ℞
(thyroid stimulating hormone)

Composition: Dermathycin™ is composed of the highly purified thyrotropic principle of the anterior pituitary gland, significantly free of other active constituents of the hypophysis. Each vial contains 5 International Units (I.U.) of thyrotropic activity, buffered with potassium dihydrogen phosphate, sodium phosphate, dibasic and sodium chloride for isotonicity.
Action and Uses: Dermathycin stimulates all phases of thyroid activity. It possesses marked dermatropic properties.
Indications: For the treatment of acanthosis nigricans and for temporary supportive therapy in hypothyroidism of dogs.
Contraindications: Adrenocortical insufficiency and hyperthyroidism.
Dosage and Administration: Reconstitute with the entire contents of the accompanying vial of Water for Injection. Shake well, and administer 1 to 2 I.U. (1–2 ml) by subcutaneous injection once a day for five days. Refrigerate reconstituted Dermathycin and use within 48 hours.
Caution: Federal (U.S.A.) law restricts this drug to use by or on the order of a licensed veterinarian.
How Supplied: Vials of 5 International Units, with vials of 5 ml of Water for Injection.

DERMATON® DOG COLLAR
Kills Fleas up to 6½ Months and Ticks for up to 4 Months

Composition:
Active Ingredient:

2-chloro-1-(2,4-dichlorophenyl) vinyl diethyl phosphate	15%
Inert Ingredients	85%
	100%

Directions for Use: It is a violation of Federal law to use this product in a manner inconsistent with its labeling.
This product will begin killing fleas in two days and will reach maximum effectiveness in 14 days.
Do not open inner envelope until ready to use. Remove the collar from package and place around dog's neck, adjust for proper fit and buckle in place. Collar must be worn loosely, but securely enough to prevent easy removal and loss. Cut off any excess length, leaving ample length for expansion if the dog grows. Check and adjust collar periodically to assure proper fit.
Results Expected: The flea collar starts killing fleas when it is placed around the dog's neck. The fleas on the dog will be killed and new ones which may temporarily appear on the dog will also be killed during the 6½ months the collar is worn. This product has been shown to provide effective tick control up to 4 months. For continuous protection, replace collar when effectiveness diminishes.
Caution: Keep Out of Reach of Children.
Harmful if ingested. Do not allow children to handle or chew this collar. This collar is intended for use as an insecticide generator and is not to be taken internally by man or animal.
Some animals may be sensitive to this collar. Any collar, when fastened too tightly, may cause skin irritation. If irritation persists after proper adjustment, remove the collar. Consult a veterinarian if irritation persists after collar removal. Do not use on sick or convalescing animals. Do not use on puppies less than three months old. Do not use other cholinestrase inhibiting pesticides on animals wearing this collar.
Do not use on cats.
Statement of Practical Treatment: If ingested: Call a physician immediately. This product contains a cholinesterase inhibitor. **Atropine is antidotal** only if symptoms of cholinesterase inhibition are present.
Storage and Disposal:
Storage: Store in cool, dry place.
Pesticide Disposal: Securely wrap excess or spent collar by wrapping in several layers of newspaper and discard in trash.

Continued on next page

Coopers—Cont.

Container Disposal: Do not reuse empty container. Wrap container and put in trash.
How Supplied: 22-inch collar in individual carton

C

DERMATON® DUST
For dogs
Kills fleas and ticks and protects against reinfestation

Composition:
Active ingredient:
2-chloro-1-(2,4-dichlorophenyl) vinyl diethyl phosphate 0.5%
Inert ingredients 99.5%
100.0%

Keep Out of Reach of Children
PRECAUTIONARY STATEMENTS
HAZARDS TO HUMANS AND DOMESTIC ANIMALS
Warning: Causes eye irritation. Do not get in eyes. May be harmful if swallowed, inhaled, or absorbed through skin. Avoid breathing of dust and contact with skin. DO NOT USE ON CATS. Wash after handling.
Statement Of Practical Treatment:
If Swallowed: Call a physician or Poison Control Center. Drink 1 or 2 glasses of water and induce vomiting by touching back of throat with finger, or, if available, by administering syrup of ipecac. Do not induce vomiting or give anything by mouth to an unconscious person.
If Inhaled: Remove victim to fresh air and apply respiration if needed.
If on Skin: Remove contaminated clothing and immediately wash skin with soap and water.
If in Eyes: Immediately flush eyes thoroughly for at least 5 minutes with plenty of water. Call a physician immediately.
Note to Physician: This product contains an organophosphate. ATROPINE IS ANTIDOTAL.
Directions for Use: It is a violation of Federal law to use this product in a manner inconsistent with its labeling.
To Kill Fleas and Ticks on Dogs: Place the dog on a table or bench, preferably out of doors. Dust entire dog beginning at head, being careful to avoid pet's eyes, and working back, being sure dust penetrates to the skin, especially around feet and legs. Wear gloves or dust mitt when applying on dogs. Each application remains active in coat, killing fleas for up to 21 days and ticks for up to 14 days. Repeat as necessary.
To Control Fleas in Infested Premises: Fleas spend part of their life cycle off the dog, in dust beneath bedding or in cracks or crevices. Dust the dog's living quarters occasionally with Dermaton Dust.
Storage and Disposal:
Storage: Store in cool, dry place.
Pesticide Disposal: Securely wrap original container in several layers of newspaper and discard in trash.
Container Disposal: Do not reuse empty can. Wrap can and put in trash.
How Supplied: 4 oz shaker can.

DERMATON® 3
Kills Ticks and Fleas

Composition:
An emulsifiable concentrate for dogs only
Active Ingredient:
2-chloro-1-(2,4-dichlorophenyl)
vinyl diethyl phosphate 12.25%
Inert Ingredients 87.75%
100.00%

This product contains methylene chloride.
Warning: Keep Out of Reach of Children
Precautionary Statements
Warning:
Hazards To Humans: May be fatal if swallowed, inhaled or absorbed through the skin. Do not breathe spray mist. Causes eye irritation. Do not get in eyes, on skin or on clothing. Children should not be allowed to handle or apply this product. Data indicate this product to be contact allergenic. Hypersensitive individuals should avoid exposure.
Hazards To Domestic Animals: DO NOT USE ON CATS. Do not use at concentrations greater than recommended. Do not allow dogs to drink dip solution.
Statement of Practical Treatment:
If Swallowed: CONSULT A PHYSICIAN OR POISON CONTROL CENTER IMMEDIATELY. NOTE: ATROPINE IS ANTIDOTAL. If swallowed, gastric lavage is indicated. DO NOT INDUCE VOMITING, unless under medical supervision. Vomiting petroleum distillates may produce aspiration pneumonia. If vomiting occurs spontaneously DO NOT let victim lie down. DO NOT allow any material to enter the airway.
If Inhaled: Remove victim to fresh air. Artificial respiration or administration of oxygen may be lifesaving.
If On Skin: Remove contaminated clothing and immediately wash skin thoroughly with soap and water.
If In Eyes: Immediately flush eyes with running water for at least 10 minutes. Get medical attention if irritation persists.
Note to Physician: 2-chloro-1-(2,4-dichlorophenyl) vinyl diethyl phosphate is a cholinesterase inhibitor and treatment of poisoning should include atropine.
Environmental Hazards: This product is toxic to fish, birds and other wildlife. Birds feeding on treated areas may be killed. Do not apply directly to water. Do not apply when weather conditions favor drift from areas treated. Do not contaminate water by cleaning of equipment or disposal of wastes.
Physical or Chemical Hazards: Do not use or store near heat or open flame.
Directions For Use: It is a violation of Federal law to use this product in a manner inconsistent with its labeling.
Ticks and Fleas on Dogs: Thoroughly mix 1 fluid ounce (2 tablespoons) with one gallon of water. Bathe or dip dog, making sure dog is thoroughly wet. Repeat treatment as necessary but not more often than once a week. Use freshly prepared material. Wear rubber gloves while preparing dip and treating dog.
Ticks and Fleas in Yards, Kennels, Etc.: Mix at the rate of 1/2 fluid ounce (1 tablespoon) in one pint of water. Spray or sprinkle solution at the rate of one pint per 100 square feet of yard or kennel area.
Do not treat areas occupied by unprotected humans. Wear rubber gloves while preparing and using spray.
SHAKE OR STIR DIP THOROUGHLY BEFORE USING OR REUSING DILUTED EMULSIONS.
Storage and Disposal Statement: Do not contaminate water, food or feed by storage or disposal.
Storage: Store in cool, dry place away from heat or open flame.
Pesticide Disposal: Pesticide wastes are acutely hazardous. Improper disposal of excess pesticide, spray mixture, or rinsate is a violation of Federal law. If these wastes cannot be disposed of by use according to label instructions, contact your State Pesticide or Environmental Control Agency, or the Hazardous Waste Representative at the nearest EPA Regional Office for guidance.
Container Disposal: 4 oz Bottle - Do not reuse bottle. Rinse thoroughly before discarding in trash. Gallon Drum - Triple rinse (or equivalent). Then offer for recycling or reconditioning, or puncture and dispose of in a sanitary landfill or by other procedures approved by State and local authorities.
How Supplied: 4 oz bottle with child resistant closure. Gallon drum

DEXTROSE SOLUTION, 50% ℞

Composition: Each ml contains: Dextrose 0.5 g; Distilled water q.s.
Indications: As a fluid and nutrient replenisher, Dextrose Solution, 50% is useful for rapid but temporary symptomatic treatment of ketosis and other hypoglycemic conditions.
Dosage and Administration: Cows and horses: 100 to 500 ml. Sheep and swine: 30 to 100 ml. Small animals: 10 to 50 ml.
Administer intravenously. If given intraperitoneally or by split intramuscular or subcutaneous injections, dilute with normal saline solution to a maximum of 5% dextrose content. Repeat as indicated.
Precautions: Contains no preservative. To avoid contamination, use a single-dose container.
KEEP OUT OF REACH OF CHILDREN
Caution: Federal (U.S.A.) law restricts this drug to use by or on the order of a licensed veterinarian.
How Supplied: 500 ml bottles.

DIQUEL®
(ethylisobutrazine hydrochloride)
Tranquilizer ℞

Composition: Diquel® is an amine derivative of phenothiazine with the chemical designation: phenothiazine, 10-[3-(dimethyl-amino)-2- methylpropyl]-3-ethyl-, monohydrochloride.
Each 50 mg tablet contains ethylisobutrazine hydrochloride 50 mg.

Each ml of sterile solution contains ethylisobutrazine hydrochloride 50 mg, in a buffered aqueous vehicle containing sodium chloride 0.6%; with sodium metabisulfite 0.05%, sodium sulfite 0.1% and benzyl alcohol 0.52% as preservatives; distilled water, q.s.

Action: Diquel is one of the amine derivatives of the phenothiazine nucleus, a class of compounds which confer central nervous system depression without marked clinical sedation. The term "tranquilized" describes the condition induced by these compounds, since the effect is more mental than somatic.

Selected solely for its advantages in veterinary medical applications, Diquel possesses central nervous system activity, antiemetic and anesthetic potentiating effects of the same general magnitude as chlorpromazine. It also offers potent antihistaminic and antispasmodic activities, and the convenience of 1 to 3 day activity from a single administration.

In addition to its primary action, Diquel affords marked antihistaminic and antiemetic activity and excellent smooth muscle relaxation to combat many of the physical manifestations (such as pruritus, diarrhea and vomiting) that accompany stress and anxiety states.

Indications: *Dogs:* Diquel can be used as an aid in controlling intractable patients during many common clinical procedures such as examinations, grooming and administration of medications; to control excessive barking in kennels; to control vomiting associated with motion sickness and with administration of anthelmintics; as an aid in the management of pruritus associated with severe dermatoses, especially those with a tendency toward self-mutilation.

Contraindications: Epinephrine is contraindicated for treatment of acute hypotension produced by tranquilizers derived from phenothiazine since further depression of blood pressure can occur. Other pressor amines, such as norepinephrine or phenylephrine, are the drugs of choice.

Tranquilizers are additive in action to the actions of other depressants and will potentiate general anesthesia. They are contraindicated in the presence of preexisting severe central nervous system depression, such as following large doses of barbiturates or opiates.

Do not use this product in conjunction with organophosphates and/or procaine hydrochloride since phenothiazines may potentiate the toxicity of organophosphates and the activity of procaine hydrochloride.

Precautions: Tranquilizers should be administered in smaller doses and with greater care during general anesthesia and also to animals exhibiting symptoms of debilitation, cardiac disease, sympathetic blockage, hypovolemia, or shock.

Tranquilizers are potent central nervous system depressants, and they can cause marked sedation with suppression of the sympathetic nervous system.

Hypotension can occur after rapid intravenous injection, causing cardiovascular collapse.

Tranquilizers can produce prolonged depression or motor restlessness when given in excessive amounts or when given to sensitive animals.

Patients on prolonged therapy should be observed carefully for allergic reactions or blood dyscrasias that have occasionally occurred with other phenothiazine derivatives.

Protect from light and excessive heat. Diquel solution is normally colorless to light yellow or light amber. Discard if any marked deviation from this range is observed.

Dosage and Administration: *Dogs. Orally*—2 to 5 mg per pound body weight, once daily.

Intramuscularly—2 to 5 mg per pound body weight. (0.4 to 1.0 ml/10 lb) for profound tranquilization.

Intravenously—1 to 2 mg per pound body weight (0.2 to 0.4 ml/10 lb) to effect.

Although individual variations will be encountered, the duration and degree of tranquilization may be varied between 6 hours and 72 hours by adjusting dosage. Young animals generally require a lower dosage than adults. When used as a preanesthetic agent, anesthetic dosage should be reduced and administered carefully to effect.

Caution: Federal (U.S.A.) law restricts this drug to use by or on the order of a licensed veterinarian.

How Supplied: Diquel Tablets—Bottles of 50 scored (50 mg) tablets.

Diquel Solution—50 mg/ml in 100 ml vials.

EAS™ ALKALINE PHOSPHATASE TEST KIT

Two-minute test for Alkaline Phosphatase in Heparinized Plasma or Serum.

For use with Coopers EAS (Electronic Animal Sensor)

Product Description: EAS Alkaline Phosphatase Test Kit consists of one pipette, one reagent bottle, disposable vials and enzyme strips for the determination of alkaline phosphatase in heparinized plasma or serum.

EAS Alkaline Phosphatase Test Kit is used with strip carrier that is designated with a yellow arrow.

Test Principle: EAS Alkaline Phosphatase Test Kit is for exclusive use in determination of alkaline phosphatase in heparinized plasma or serum (for concentrations 0–600 IU/l).

Three drops of heparinized plasma or serum are added to an unused vial (provided). Then three drops of alkaline phosphatase reagent are added to the same vial, swirled gently and allowed to react for 1 minute. The test strip is immersed into the solution after 60 seconds countdown on the sensor (buzzer will sound 3 seconds prior to 60-second mark). After an additional 60 seconds, the buzzer sounds and the screen flashes zero, the strip is removed from the vial and excess moisture is removed by *side blotting* as described in WIPE TECHNIQUE. The strip is then inserted into the sensor, the door closed and a value readout appears on the screen. The reflected light intensity is measured as the density of developed color to obtain the alkaline phosphatase concentration in the sample.

REAGENT COMPOSITION FOR EAS ALKALINE PHOSPHATASE

Composition and properties

Phenolphthalein
Monophosphate ....0.09 mg
Buffer 10%
Non-reactive Ingredients..................90%

Warnings and Precautions: EAS Alkaline Phosphatase Kit is for *in-vitro* diagnostic use. The Test Kit should be stored in a secure area away from small children.

Storage and Handling: Kit should be stored under 30°C (86°F) in a dark, dry, cool place. After opening, Test Kit should be kept at 4°C (39°F). Mark the date on the vial when first opened.

Specimen Collection and Preparation: EAS Alkaline Phosphatase Kit is intended for use with heparinized plasma or serum. Citrate and EDTA inhibit alkaline phosphatase and should **NOT** be used. Whole blood should not be used.

Limitations of Procedure: Increases in alkaline phosphatase occur when the specimen is stored at room temperature. Do not use severely hemolyzed specimens.

Performance Characteristics: EAS Alkaline Phosphatase Kit is specific for Serum Alkaline Phosphatase. When used with EAS (Electronic Animal Sensor), readings are comparable to other quantitative methods for Serum Alkaline Phosphatase.

Wipe Technique:

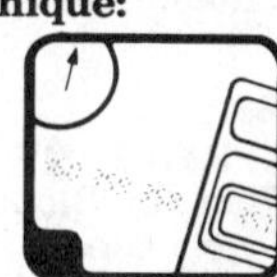

1. Proper timing is critical for this technique. Add strip to reagent and sample mixture at 60 seconds. Begin *side blot* as soon as sensor has completed 120-second count.

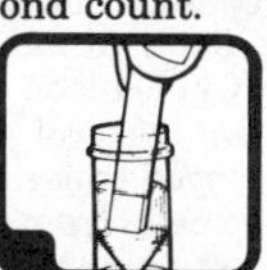

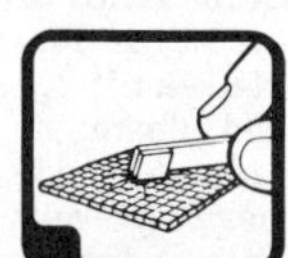

2. Using a piece of cotton gauze as a blotter, remove strip from vial and place side edge of strip gently on gauze. Excess liquid will be removed from pad surface. **DO NOT PLACE PAD FACE DOWN ON GAUZE.**

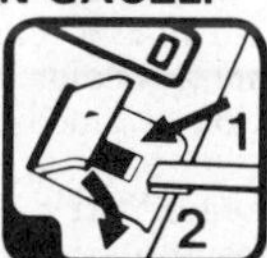

3. Immediately insert the strip into the sensor as directed in the operating manual.

Specifications

1. Range :0–660 IU/l
2. Specimen :Heparinized plasma

Continued on next page

C

Coopers—Cont.

or serum

3. Required Sample Volume :150–200 μl
4. Reaction Time :120 seconds
5. Storage :At room temperatures below 30°C (86°F) in closed container

Caution

1. To prevent the deterioration of sensitivity of EAS Alkaline Phosphatase Test Kit, store in a dark, dry, cool place. Avoid excessive humidity, temperature extremes and direct sunlight.
2. When Test Kit is stored under refrigeration, allow it to return to room temperature before using.
3. Do not touch the test pad area, also avoid contamination with volatile chemicals.
4. Do not remove the desiccant packed in the container.
5. If stored properly, the Test Kit is usable up to the expiration date indicated on the label. Do not use any discolored or mutilated test strips.

Precautions for Specimens

1. Use only heparinized plasma or serum.
2. Use specified amount of sample for testing.
3. The reaction of color development progresses slowly under low temperatures and may result in low measurement values. If frozen serum is used, allow it to return to room temperature before proceeding with the test. It is recommended to conduct measurements at room temperatures between 15°C–30°C (59°F–86°F).

Availability: EAS Alkaline Phosphatase Kit is available in test kits of 25 tests.

EAS™ B.U.N. REAGENT STRIPS

One minute Test for Blood Urea Nitrogen in Whole Blood, Heparinized Plasma or Serum

For use with the COOPERS EAS (Electronic Animal Sensor)

Product Description: EAS B.U.N. Reagent Strips are disposable plastic reagent strips for the determination of blood urea nitrogen in whole blood, heparinized plasma or serum. A semi-permeable membrane is employed to serve as a barrier to prevent blood cells from entering into the reagent test pad area.

EAS B.U.N. Reagent Strips are packaged in a vial with a tight-fitting cap. Each strip is stable and ready for use when removed from the vial. At the beginning of a 60-second time period, one drop of whole blood, heparinized plasma or serum is applied to the reagent test pad area, which changes color in response to the concentration of blood urea nitrogen in the blood.

EAS B.U.N. Reagent Strips are used with strip carrier designated with a green arrow.

Test Principle: EAS B.U.N. Reagent Strip is for exclusive use in determination of blood urea nitrogen (for concentration 5–100 mg/dl).

The reagent pad area of the strip is prepared for optical measuring of the degree of color development which is proportional to the urea nitrogen concentration in the blood sample.

A small amount of whole blood, heparinized plasma or serum is used as the sample, for rapid and accurate measurement of blood urea nitrogen.

The reagent pad area is composed of urease and a pH indicator. It is coated with a substance impermeable to blood cells.

When whole blood, heparinized plasma or serum is applied on the reagent pad area, only low molecule weight components such as urea permeate underneath the surface of the test pad membrane. The area is then enzymatically decomposed by urease to ammonia and carbon dioxide. This ammonia changes to an ammonium hydroxide, and as the pH increases, the color of pH indicator changes. The degree of the color development corresponds to the concentration of urea nitrogen in blood. The blood cell components remaining on the surface of the reagent pad area are removed by wiping with lint-free tissue. A monochromatic light corresponding to the hue of developed color illuminates the reagent area. The reflected light intensity is measured as the density of developed color to obtain the urea nitrogen concentration in blood.

REAGENT COMPOSITION FOR EAS B.U.N. STRIP

Composition and properties

Urease	37.5μg
Bromothymol Blue	22.0μg
Non-Reactive Ingredients	15.0μg

Configuration of EAS B.U.N. Reagent Strip

Reagent Pad

Plastic Strip

Warnings and Precautions: EAS B.U.N. Reagent Strips are for *in vitro* diagnostic use. EAS B.U.N. Reagent Strip should be stored in a secure area away from small children.

Storage and Handling: Store strips at temperatures under 30°C (86°F) in a dark, dry, cool place. Avoid exposing reagent strips to moisture, light and heat to prevent deterioration of reagents. Do not remove the desiccant from the bottle and keep the bottle tightly capped. Do not touch test pad area of the reagent strip. Do not transfer the strips to any other containers. Mark the date the vial was first opened in the space allotted on the label.

Specimen Collection and Preparation: EAS B.U.N. Reagent Strips are intended for use with whole blood, heparinized plasma or serum. If desired, venous whole blood samples with common anticoagulants (citrate, heparin or EDTA) may be used.

Limitation of Procedure: This procedure is free from interference if fresh whole blood, heparinized plasma or serum is used. Whole blood with fluoride as preservative should be avoided. Uric acid and ascorbic acid (when occurring in physiological blood concentrations) do not affect the reaction. Hematocrits greater than 55% can cause lower results.

Performance Characteristics: EAS B.U.N. Reagent Strips are specific for blood urea nitrogen determination. When used with EAS (Electronic Animal Sensor), readings are comparable to other quantitative methods for blood urea nitrogen.

Wipe Technique:

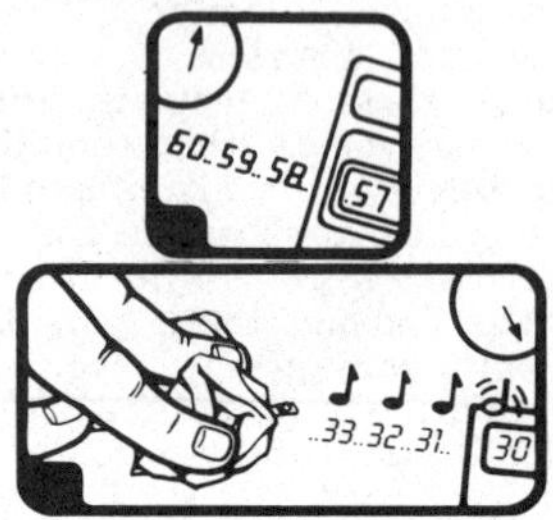

1. Proper timing is critical for this technique. Begin to wipe as soon as the sensor has completed 30 seconds of the 60 second countdown. Improper timing will result in erroneous readings.

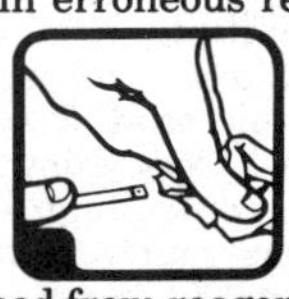

2. Wipe off blood from reagent pad in one forward motion using a lint-free tissue. DO NOT APPLY PRESSURE DIRECTLY ON REAGENT PAD.

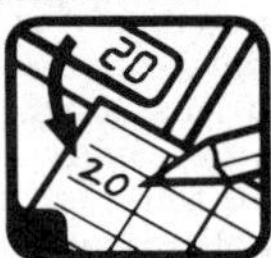

3. When buzzer sounds and zero flashes, immediately insert strip into sensor as directed in the operating manual. B.U.N. Reagent Strip is for exclusive use in determination of blood urea nitrogen (for concentrations 5–100 mg/dl).

The reagent area of the strip is prepared for optical measuring of the degree of color development, which is proportional to the urea nitrogen concentration in the blood sample. A small amount of whole blood, heparinized plasma or serum is used as the sample for rapid, and accurate measurement of blood urea nitrogen.

Specifications

1. Range :5–100 mg/dl
2. Specimen :Whole blood, heparinized plasma or serum
3. Required Sample Volume :about 50μl–100μl
4. Reaction Time :60 seconds
5. Storage :At room temperatures below 30°C (86°F)

Caution

1. To prevent the deterioration of sensitivity of reagent strips, store in a dark, dry, cool place. Avoid excessive humidity, temperature extremes and direct sunlight.
2. If reeagent strips are stored under refrigeration, allow them to return to

room temperature before opening the container and remove only required number of strips and re-cap container immediately.
3. Do not touch the reagent area, also avoid contamination with volatile chemicals.
4. Do not remove the desiccant packed in the container.
5. If stored properly, the reagent strips are usable up to the expiration date indicated on the label. Do not use any discolored or mutilated reagent strips.

Precautions for Specimens
1. Use only whole blood, heparinized plasma or serum.
2. For determination use a sufficient amount of whole blood, heparinized plasma or serum.
3. The reaction of color development progresses slowly under low temperatures and may result in low measurement value. If frozen heparinized plasma or serum is used, allow it to return to room temperature before measurement. It is recommended to conduct measurements at room temperatures between 15°–30°C (59°–86°F).

Availability: EAS B.U.N. Reagent Strips are available in a vial of 25 strips.

EAS™ GLUCOSE REAGENT STRIPS
One minute Test for Glucose in Whole Blood, Heparinized Plasma or Serum For use with the COOPERS EAS (Electronic Animal Sensor)

Product Description: EAS Glucose Reagent Strips are disposable plastic reagent strips for the determination of glucose in whole blood, heparinized plasma or serum. A semi-permeable membrane is employed to serve as a barrier to prevent blood cells from entering into the reagent test pad area.
EAS Glucose Reagent Strips are packaged in a vial with a tight-fitting cap. Each strip is stable and ready for use when removed from the vial. At the beginning of a 60-second time period, one drop of whole blood, heparinized plasma or serum is applied to the reagent test pad area, which changes color in response to the concentration of glucose in the blood.
EAS Glucose Reagent Strips are used with strip carrier designated with a green arrow.

Test Principle: EAS Glucose Reagent Strip chemistry is based on the glucose oxidase/peroxidase reaction. D-glucose is oxidized to gluconic acid and hydrogen peroxide in the presence of atmospheric oxygen and glucose oxidase as a catalyst. In the presence of peroxidase indicators the reagent strip is oxidized to produce various shades of green color.

REAGENT COMPOSITION FOR EAS GLUCOSE STRIP
Composition and properties

ABTS	0.5%
Glucose Oxidase	0.2%
Peroxidase	0.6%
Non-Reactive Ingredients	98.7%

Warnings and Precautions: EAS Glucose Reagent Strips are for *in vitro* diagnostic use. EAS Glucose Reagent Strips should be stored in a secure area away from small children.

Configuration of EAS Glucose Reagent Strip

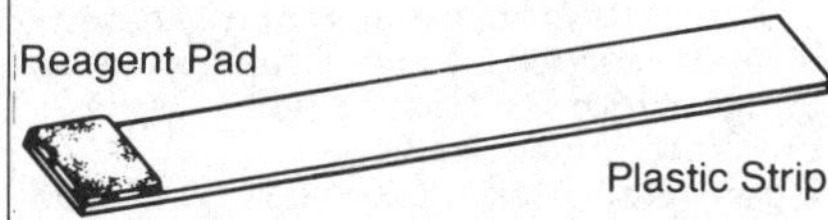

Storage and Handling: Store strips at temperatures under 30°C (86°F) in a dark, dry, cool place. Avoid exposing reagent strips to moisture, light and heat to prevent deterioration of reagents. Do not remove the desiccant from the bottle and keep the bottle tightly capped. Do not touch test pad area of the reagent strip. Do not transfer the strips to any other containers. Mark the date the vial was first opened in the space allotted on the label.

Specimen Collection and Preparation: EAS Glucose Reagent Strips are intended for use with whole blood, heparinized plasma or serum. If desired, venous whole blood samples with common anticoagulants (oxalate, citrate, heparin and EDTA) may be used. Blood glucose undergoes glycolysis rapidly after drawing. To prevent glycolysis, use blood samples immediately.

Limitation of Procedure: This procedure is free from interference if fresh whole blood, heparinized plasma or serum is used. Whole blood with fluoride as preservative should be avoided. Uric acid and ascorbic acid (when occurring in physiological blood concentrations) do not affect the reaction. Hematocrits greater than 55% can cause lower results.

Performance Characteristics: EAS Glucose Reagent Strips are specific for glucose determination. When used with EAS (Electronic Animal Sensor), readings are comparable to other quantitative methods for blood glucose.

Wipe Technique: Please follow exactly:

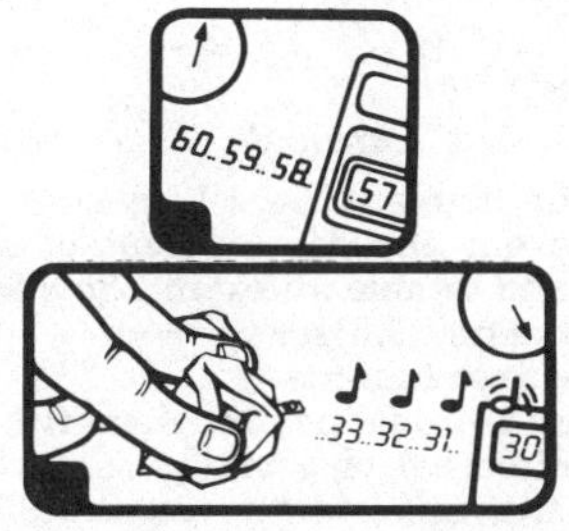

1. Proper timing is critical for this technique. Begin to wipe as soon as the sensor has completed 30 seconds of the 60 second countdown. Improper timing will result in erroneous readings.

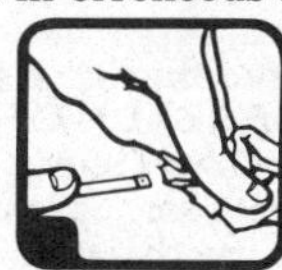

2. Wipe off blood from reagent pad in one forward motion using a lint-free tissue. DO NOT APPLY PRESSURE DIRECTLY ON REAGENT PAD. Countdown continues an additional 30 seconds.

3. When buzzer sounds and zero flashes, immediately insert strip into sensor as directed in the operating manual. Glucose Reagent Strip is for exclusive use in determination of blood glucose (for concentrations 25–250 mg/dl).

The reagent area of the strip is prepared for optical measuring of the degree of color development, which is proportional to the glucose concentration in the blood sample. A small amount of whole blood, heparinized plasma or serum is used as the sample for rapid, and accurate measurement of glucose.

Specifications

1. Range	:25–250 mg/dl
2. Specimen	:Whole blood, heparinized plasma or serum
3. Required Sample Volume	:about 50µl–100µl
4. Reaction Time	:60 seconds
5. Storage	:At room temperature below 30°C (86°F)

Caution
1. To prevent the deterioration of sensitivity of reagent strips, store in a dark, dry, cool place. Avoid excessive humidity, temperature extremes and direct sunlight.
2. If reagent strips are stored under refrigeration, allow them to return to room temperature before opening the container and remove only required number of strips and re-cap container immediately.
3. Do not touch the reagent area, also avoid contamination with volatile chemicals.
4. Do not remove the desiccant packed in the container.
5. If stored properly, the reagent strips are usable up to the expiration date indicated on the label. Do not use any discolored or mutilated reagent strips.

Precautions for Specimens
1. Use only whole blood, heparinized plasma or serum.
2. For determination use a sufficient amount of whole blood, heparinized plasma or serum.
3. The reaction of color development progresses slowly under low temperatures and may result in low measurement value. If frozen heparinized plasma or serum is used, allow it to return to room temperature before measurement. It is recommended that measurements be conducted at room temperatures between 15°–30°C (59°–86°F).

Availability: EAS Glucose Reagent Strips are available in a vial of 25 strips.

ELECTROID® D
Clostridium Perfringens Type D Toxoid

Composition: A "cell-free," formalin-treated toxoid derived from highly toxi-

Continued on next page

Coopers—Cont.

genic (epsilon toxin) culture filtrates of *Clostridium perfringens* Type D.
A product of high antigenicity and small dosage volume is assured through the use of the electronically controlled fermentation process.
The electro-fermentation process employs select strains and optimal culturing conditions to produce high concentrations of specific toxoid-antigen. The toxoid content of the resultant cell-free filtrate is monitored through unique in-process TCP* (total combining power) testing. The final product must meet a standard of not less than 150 TCP units of epsilon toxoid-antigen per sheep dose or 300 TCP units per cattle dose.
Indications: For the active immunization of healthy cattle and sheep against disease caused by *Clostridium perfringens* Type D.
Action and Uses: Enterotoxemia, commonly referred to as "overeating disease" or "pulpy kidney disease" is caused by epsilon toxin of *Clostridium perfringens* Type D. The presence of the organism in the lower bowel of normal animals in conjunction with heavy or rich feeding provides a favorable environment for the rapid microbial growth and toxin formation. The absorption of the lethal toxin causes toxemia and death.
Enterotoxemia caused by Type D epsilon toxin is considered primarily a disease of sheep. Its incidence is widespread throughout the United States, and losses from it have been described as being greater than from all other infectious sheep diseases combined. The role of Type D infection in cattle is not clearly established. Sudden deaths in feedlot cattle have been experienced at several stages of the fattening process. The presence of epsilon toxin in the intestinal contents has been substantiated by laboratory diagnosis in the U.S.A. and Australia. Veterinarians and feedlot operators have reduced these losses through vaccination with Type D toxoids and bacterins and, therefore, believe the organism to be of significance.
The hazards of enterotoxemia can be prevented during periods of heavy feedlot feeding or when animals are moved to fresh, lush pastures by prior immunization. Animals intended for feeding under these conditions should be vaccinated approximately 10 to 14 days before exposure to provide sufficient time for the development of immunity.
Protection for very young suckling animals may be provided by the vaccination of the pregnant females. This has been shown to provide sufficient colostral antitoxin for the protection of suckling lambs for a period of approximately 12 to 16 weeks.
Dosage and Administration: Shake well. Using aseptic technique, inject subcutaneously or intramuscularly. Cattle, 4 ml; sheep, 2 ml, repeated in 3-4 weeks. Revaccinate annually prior to periods of extreme risk or parturition.
Caution: Store at not over 45°F or 7°C. Protect from freezing. Use entire contents when first opened. Do not vaccinate within 21 days before slaughter. Anaphylactoid reactions may occur following use. **Antidote:** Epinephrine.
For Veterinary Use Only
How Supplied: 500 ml vial—125 cattle doses or 250 sheep doses.
*TCP unit represents the amount of toxoid-antigen which will combine with one internationally standardized unit of "epsilon" antitoxin.

ELECTROID® 7
Clostridium Chauvoei - Septicum - Novyi - Sordellii - Perfringens Types C & D Bacterin - Toxoid

Indications: For the active immunization of healthy cattle and sheep against diseases caused by *Cl. chauvoei, Cl. septicum, Cl. sordellii, Cl. novyi* Type B and *Cl. perfringens* Types C and D.
Although *Clostridium perfringens* Type B is not a significant problem in the USA, immunity may be provided against the beta and epsilon toxins elaborated by *Cl. perfringens* Type B. This immunity is derived from the combination of Type C (beta) and Type D (epsilon) fractions.
Administration and Dosage: Shake well. Using aseptic technique, inject subcutaneously or intramuscularly. Dosage: 5 ml, repeated in 3–4 weeks. Revaccinate annually prior to periods of extreme risk, or parturition. For *Cl. novyi*, revaccinate every 5–6 months. Animals vaccinated under 3 months of age should be revaccinated at weaning or 4–6 months of age.
Caution: Store at not over 45°F or 7°C. Protect from freezing. Use entire contents when first opened. Do not vaccinate within 21 days before slaughter. Anaphylactoid reactions may occur following use. **Antidote:** Epinephrine.
For Veterinary Use Only
How Supplied:
50 ml—10 dose
250 ml—50 dose
1000 ml—200 dose

ENDROL™
Equine Oral Larvicide

Contains Rabon® Oral Larvicide
To prevent the development of House Flies and Stable Flies in the Manure from Treated Horses
Active Ingredients
2 chloro-1-(2,4,5-trichlorophenyl) vinyl dimethyl phosphate* 7.76%
Inert Ingredients** 92.24%
100.00%
Rabon® is a registered trademark of Shell Oil Company
*Rabon Insecticide
**Refers only to ingredients which are not larvicidal.
Each pound contains 35 grams Rabon
KEEP OUT OF REACH OF CHILDREN
CAUTION
Directions for Use: It is a violation of Federal law to use this product in a manner inconsistent with its labeling.
Add this product daily to the grain or concentrate portion of the horse's diet to provide 70 mg of Rabon per 100 pounds of body weight. Using the enclosed measuring scoop, this is equivalent to the following: 1 level scoop (2.2g) for a 250 lb. animal; 2 level scoops (4.4g) for a 500 lb. animal; 4 level scoops (8.8g) for a 1000 lb. animal or 8 level scoops (17.6g) for a 2000 lb. animal. Start feeding early in the spring before flies begin to appear and continue feeding throughout the summer and into the fall until cold weather restricts fly activity.
All horses in the stable area should be treated. Endrol Equine Oral Larvicide prevents development of house flies and stable flies in the manure from treated horses but is not effective against existing adult flies.
In some cases, supplemental fly control measures may be needed in and around the stable area to control adult flies which move in from other areas or which breed on decaying vegetable matter elsewhere on the premises.
Do not use on animals intended for slaughter.
In order to achieve optimum fly control Endrol Equine Oral Larvicide should be used in conjunction with other good management and sanitation practices.
PRECAUTIONARY STATEMENTS
HAZARDS TO HUMANS
Caution
Harmful if swallowed. Avoid contact with skin and eyes. Avoid breathing dust. Wash thoroughly with soap and water after handling and before eating or smoking.
If In Eyes: Wash with plenty of water for 15 minutes. If irritation persists, see a physician.
ENVIRONMENTAL HAZARDS
This product is toxic to fish. Keep out of lakes, streams and ponds. Do not contaminate water by cleaning of equipment or disposal of wastes.
STORAGE AND DISPOSAL
Do not contaminate water, food or feed by storage or disposal.
Storage: Store in cool, dry place.
Pesticide Disposal: Wastes resulting from the use of this product may be disposed of on site or at an approved waste disposal facility.
Container Disposal: Triple rinse (or equivalent). Then puncture and dispose of in a sanitary landfill, or incineration, or, if allowed by State and local authorities, by burning. If burned, stay out of smoke.
How Supplied: 4 lb pail

EPIfel® RCP
Feline Rhinotracheitis-Calici-Panleukopenia Vaccine Modified Live and Killed Virus

Indications: For the active immunization of healthy cats and kittens against feline rhinotracheitis, calici and panleukopenia infections.
Caution: Store at not over 45°F or 7°C. Protect from freezing. Do not use chemical disinfectants to sterilize syringes or needles. Burn containers and all unused contents. Do not vaccinate pregnant queens. Contains gentamicin as an added preservative. Anaphylactoid reactions

may occur following use. **Antidote:** Epinephrine.
Administration and Dosage: For use in healthy cats and kittens. Transfer contents of liquid vaccine vial to lyophilized vaccine vial using aseptic technique. Inject 1 ml rehydrated vaccine subcutaneously or intramuscularly using aseptic technique and boiled, autoclaved or sterile disposable syringes and needles.
Kittens should be vaccinated at 9–10 weeks of age with revaccination in 3–4 weeks. Because maternal antibodies may interfere with effective immunization, kittens vaccinated before 9 weeks of age should be revaccinated at 3–4 week intervals with the final dose being given at 12–16 weeks of age. Adult cats should receive a second dose 3–4 weeks after initial vaccination. Annual revaccination with a single dose is recommended.
How Supplied: 10 (1 dose) vials.

EPIVAXINE® DA$_2$P
Canine Distemper-Adenovirus Type 2-Parainfluenza Vaccine Modified Live Virus

Description: EPIvaxine® DA$_2$P is a convenient combination vaccine for the active immunization of healthy puppies and dogs against canine distemper, infectious canine hepatitis (CAV-1), respiratory disease caused by canine adenovirus Type 2 (CAV-2), and canine parainfluenza. EPIvaxine DA$_2$P is a freeze-dried suspension of modified live canine distemper, canine adenovirus Type 2, and canine parainfluenza viruses produced on a USDA-certified canine cell line thus greatly reducing non-protective, potentially allergenic by-products.
Indications: For the active immunization of healthy puppies and dogs against canine distemper, infectious canine hepatitis (CAV-1), respiratory disease caused by canine adenovirus Type 2 (CAV-2), and canine parainfluenza. Data indicate that the development of corneal opacity is not associated with the use of this product.
Dosage and Administration: For use in healthy dogs. Slowly transfer the contents of diluent vial to vaccine vial, using aseptic technique. Inject 1 ml of rehydrated vaccine subcutaneously or intramuscularly immediately after rehydration using aseptic technique and boiled, autoclaved or sterile disposable syringes and needles. Inject entire contents immediately after rehydration.
Dogs 12 weeks of age or older should receive two doses 3–4 weeks apart. If younger dogs are vaccinated, they should be revaccinated at 3–4 week intervals with the final dose being given at 12 weeks or older. Puppies with questionable levels of passive immunity may be vaccinated as early as 2 weeks of age. Annual revaccination is recommended.
Directions For Rehydration: Transfer the entire contents of the diluent vial to the vaccine vial using a sterile syringe and needle. To facilitate rehydration, momentarily disconnect the syringe from the needle while the needle is still penetrating the rubber stopper. This will release the remaining high vacuum and the resulting pressure change will help the diluent penetrate the porous cake. The product then may be shaken as necessary to complete solution.
Use boiled, autoclaved or sterile disposable syringes and needles. The vaccine must contain live virus in order to stimulate effective immunity; therefore, do not use syringes or needles that have been chemically disinfected. The site of injection may be cleaned and disinfected with alcohol and then wiped dry.
Caution: Store at not over 45°F or 7°C. Do not use chemical disinfectants to sterilize syringes and needles. Burn containers and all unused contents. Contains penicillin and streptomycin as added preservatives. Anaphylactoid reactions may occur following use. **Antidote:** Epinephrine.
For Veterinary Use Only
How Supplied: 10 (1 dose) vials vaccine with diluent.

EPIVAXINE® DA$_2$PL
Canine Distemper-Adenovirus Type 2-Parainfluenza Vaccine Modified Live Virus Leptospira Bacterin

Description: EPIvaxine® DA$_2$PL is a convenient combination vaccine for the active immunization of healthy puppies and dogs against canine distemper, infectious canine hepatitis (CAV-1), respiratory disease caused by canine adenovirus Type 2 (CAV-2), canine parainfluenza, and leptospirosis caused by *Leptospira canicola* and *Leptospira icterohaemorrhagiae.* The canine distemper-adenovirus Type 2-parainfluenza component is a freeze-dried suspension of modified live canine distemper, canine adenovirus Type 2, and canine parainfluenza viruses produced on a USDA-certified canine cell line. The leptospira component is prepared from inactivated cultures of *L. canicola* and *L. icterohaemorrhagiae* grown in a low-protein medium. Other non-protective, potentially allergenic by-products of bacterial metabolism are greatly reduced by selective molecular filtration.
Indications: For the active immunization of healthy puppies and dogs against canine distemper, infectious canine hepatitis (CAV-1), respiratory disease caused by canine adenovirus Type 2 (CAV-2), canine parainfluenza, and leptospirosis caused by *L. canicola* and *L. icterohaemorragiae.* Data indicate that the development of corneal opacity is not associated with the use of this product.
Dosage and Administration: For use in healthy dogs. Slowly transfer contents of bacterin vial to vaccine vial, using aseptic technique. Inject 1 ml of rehydrated vaccine subcutaneously or intramuscularly using boiled, autoclaved or sterile disposable syringes and needles. Inject entire contents immediately after rehydration.
Dogs 12 weeks of age or older should receive two doses 3-4 weeks apart. If younger dogs are vaccinated, they should be revaccinated at 3-4 week intervals with the final dose being given at 12 weeks or older. Puppies with questionable levels of passive immunity may be vaccinated as early as 2 weeks of age. Annual revaccination is recommended.
Directions for Rehydration: Transfer the entire contents of the diluent vial to the vaccine vial using a sterile syringe and needle. To facilitate rehydration, momentarily disconnect the syringe from the needle while the needle is still penetrating the rubber stopper. This will release the remaining high vacuum and the resulting pressure change will help the diluent penetrate the porous cake. The product then may be shaken as necessary to complete solution.
Use boiled, autoclaved or sterile disposable syringes and needles. The vaccine must contain live virus in order to stimulate effective immunity; therefore, do not use syringes or needles that have been chemically disinfected. The site of injection may be cleaned and disinfected with alcohol and then wiped dry.
Caution: Store at not over 45°F or 7°C. Do not use chemical disinfectants to sterilize syringes and needles. Burn containers and all unused contents. The viral components of EPIvaxine DA$_2$PL contain penicillin and streptomycin as added preservatives. Anaphylactoid reactions may occur following use. **Antidote:** Epinephrine.
For Veterinary Use Only
How Supplied: 10 (1 dose) vials vaccine with diluent.

EPIVAXINE® DA$_2$PPv
Canine Distemper-Adenovirus Type 2-Parainfluenza-Parvovirus Vaccine Modified Live and Killed Virus

Description: EPIvaxine DA$_2$PPv is a convenient combination vaccine for the active immunization of healthy puppies and dogs against canine distemper, infectious canine hepatitis (CAV-1), respiratory disease caused by canine adenovirus Type 2 (CAV-2), canine parainfluenza, and canine parvovirus. The canine distemper-adenovirus-parainfluenza component is a freeze-dried suspension of modified live canine distemper, canine adenovirus Type 2, and canine parainfluenza viruses produced on a USDA-certified canine cell line. The canine parvovirus component is an inactivated liquid vaccine produced from virus of canine origin grown in a USDA-certified continuous cell line of embryonic feline lung.
Indications: For the active immunization of healthy puppies and dogs against canine distemper, infectious canine hepatitis (CAV-1), respiratory disease caused by canine adenovirus Type 2 (CAV-2), canine parainfluenza, and canine parvovirus. Data indicate that the development of corneal opacity is not associated with the use of this product.
Dosage and Administration: For use in healthy dogs. Invert the liquid vaccine vial several times to resuspend the adjuvant and slowly transfer the contents to

Continued on next page

Coopers—Cont.

the lyophilized vaccine vial using aseptic technique. Inject 1 ml of rehydrated vaccine subcutaneously or intramuscularly immediately after rehydration using aseptic technique and boiled, autoclaved or sterile disposable syringes and needles.

Dogs 12 weeks of age or older should receive two doses 3-4 weeks apart. If younger dogs are vaccinated, they should be revaccinated at 3-4 week intervals with the final dose being given at 12 weeks or older. Puppies with questionable levels of passive immunity may be vaccinated as early as 2 weeks of age. Annual revaccination is recommended.

Directions For Rehydration: Transfer the entire contents of the diluent vial to the vaccine vial using a sterile syringe and needle. To facilitate rehydration, momentarily disconnect the syringe from the needle while the needle is still penetrating the rubber stopper. This will release the remaining high vacuum and the resulting pressure change will help the diluent penetrate the porous cake. The product then may be shaken as necessary to complete solution.

Use boiled, autoclaved or sterile disposable syringes and needles. The vaccine must contain live virus in order to stimulate effective immunity; therefore, do not use syringes or needles that have been chemically disinfected. The site of injection may be cleaned and disinfected with alcohol and then wiped dry.

Caution: Store at not over 45°F or 7°C. Do not use chemical disinfectants to sterilize syringes and needles. Burn containers and all unused contents. The lyophilized component contains penicillin and streptomycin as added preservatives. The liquid component contains gentamicin as a preservative. Anaphylactoid reactions may occur following use. **Antidote:** Epinephrine.

For Veterinary Use Only

How Supplied:
10 (1 does) vials vaccine with diluent.

EPIVAXINE® DA$_2$PPvL
Canine Distemper-Adenovirus Type 2-
Parainfluenza-Parvovirus Vaccine
Modified Live and Killed Virus
Leptospira Bacterin

Description: EPIvaxine® DA$_2$PPvL is a convenient combination vaccine for the active immunization of healthy puppies and dogs against canine distemper, infectious canine hepatitis (CAV-1), respiratory disease caused by canine adenovirus Type 2 (CAV-2), canine parainfluenza, canine parvovirus, and leptospirosis caused by *Leptospira canicola* and *Leptospira icterohaemorrhagiae*. The distemper-adenovirus-parainfluenza component is a freeze-dried suspension of modified live canine distemper, canine adenovirus Type 2, and canine parainfluenza viruses produced on a USDA-certified canine cell line. The canine parvovirus component is an inactivated liquid vaccine produced from virus of canine origin grown in a USDA-certified continuous cell line. The liquid leptospira component is prepared from inactivated cultures of *L. canicola* and *L. icterohaemorrhagiae* grown in a low-protein medium. Other nonprotective, potentially allergic by-products of bacterial metabolism are greatly reduced by selective molecular filtration.

Indications: For the active immunization of healthy puppies and dogs against canine distemper, infectious canine hepatitis (CAV-1), respiratory disease caused by canine adenovirus Type 2 (CAV-2), canine parainfluenza, canine parvovirus and leptospirosis caused by *Leptospira canicola* and *Leptospira icterohaemorrhagiae*. Data indicate that the development of corneal opacity is not associated with the use of this product.

Dosage and Administration: For use in healthy dogs. Invert the liquid vaccine vial several times to resuspend the adjuvant and slowly transfer the contents to the lyophilized vaccine vial using aseptic technique. Inject 1 ml of rehydrated vaccine subcutaneously or intramuscularly immediately after rehydration using aseptic technique and boiled, autoclaved or sterile disposable syringes and needles.

Dogs 12 weeks of age or older should receive two doses 3-4 weeks apart. If younger dogs are vaccinated, they should be revaccinated at 3-4 week intervals with the final dose being given at 12 weeks or older. Puppies with questionable levels of passive immunity may be vaccinated as early as 2 weeks of age. Annual revaccination is recommended.

Directions for Rehydration: Transfer the entire contents of the diluent vial to the vaccine vial using a sterile syringe and needle. To facilitate rehydration, momentarily disconnect the syringe from the needle while the needle is still penetrating the rubber stopper. This will release the remaining high vacuum and the resulting pressure change will help the diluent penetrate the porous cake. The product then may be shaken as necessary to complete solution.

Use boiled, autoclaved, or sterile disposable syringes and needles. The vaccine must contain live virus in order to stimulate effective immunity; therefore, do not use syringes or needles that have been chemically disinfected. The site of injection may be cleaned and disinfected with alcohol and then wiped dry.

Caution: Store at not over 45°F or 7°C. Do not use chemical disinfectants to sterilize syringes and needles. Burn containers and all unused contents. The lyophilized component contains penicillin and streptomycin as added preservatives. The liquid component contains gentamicin as a preservative. Anaphylactoid reactions may occur following use. **Antidote:** Epinephrine.

For Veterinary Use Only

How Supplied: 10 (1 dose) vials vaccine with diluent.

EQUINE INFLUENZA VACCINE
Killed Virus

Description: Equine Influenza Vaccine is a formaldehyde inactivated combination of tissue culture origin Type A_1 and A_2 equine influenza viruses. The virus is blended with the patented adjuvant, to elicit optimum immunization when inoculated into horses.

Indications: For use in healthy equines as an aid in the prevention of equine influenza due to strains A_1 and A_2 virus.

Dosage and Administration: Shake well. Using aseptic technique, inject 1 ml deep intramuscularly. Repeat in 3 to 4 weeks. A single 1 ml booster dose should be given annually or when exposure is anticipated.

Caution: Store the vaccine at 35° to 45°F (2° to 7°C). Protect from freezing. Use entire contents when first opened. Do not vaccinate within 21 days of slaughter. Contains neomycin, polymyxin-B and a fungistat as preservatives. Anaphylactoid reactions may occur following use.

Antidote: Epinephrine.

For Veterinary Use Only.

How Supplied: 10 × 1 ml (1 dose) sterile syringes per box, individually printed plastic bag with 20 ga., 1″ needle.
10 ml (10 doses) vial.

EQUIPAR® EQUINE WORMER PASTE
(oxibendazole)

Description: Equipar Equine Wormer (oxibendizole) Paste is a paste formulation of oxibendazole, a broad spectrum benzimidazole anthelmintic. This formulation has been developed for ease of administration. Each syringe contains 0.85 ounce (24 grams) of paste.

Equipar Equine Wormer contains:
Oxibendazole 22.7%

Indications: Equipar Equine Wormer (oxibendazole) Paste is indicated for removal and control of: large strongylids (*Strongylus edentatus, S. equinus, S. vulgaris*); small strongylids (species of the genera *Cylicostephanus, Cylicocyclus, Cyathostomum, Tridontophorus, Cylicodontophorus,* and *Gyalocephalus*); large roundworms (*Parascaris equorum*); pinworms (*Oxyuris equi*) including various larval stages; and threadworms (*Strongyloides westeri*).

Contraindications: Equipar Equine Wormer is contraindicated in severely debilitated horses or horses suffering from infectious disease, toxemia or colic.

Warning: Not for use in horses intended for food.

Dosage and Administration: The dosage of oxibendizole is 10 mg/kg (2.2 lb) of body weight (15 mg/kg for strongyloides). Each mark on the syringe delivers Equipar Equine Wormer to treat 100 pounds (67 pounds for strongyloides). Horses maintained on premises where reinfection is likely to occur should be retreated in 6 to 8 weeks.

Equipar Equine Wormer is compatible with carbon disulfide, which can be used concurrently for bot control (*Gasterophilus* spp.) when administered by a veteri-

narian. Routine carbon disulfide cautions must be observed.
[See table at right].
Use of Syringe: Determine the weight of the horse and dial the correct setting on the plunger, having the side of the wheel nearest the barrel of the desired mark. Remove the cap from the syringe. Insert the tip of the syringe into the side of the animal's mouth between the incisor and molar teeth, and press the plunger down as far as it will go, depositing the paste on the back of the tongue.
Caution: Consult your veterinarian for assistance in the diagnosis, treatment and control of parasitism.
Keep Out of Reach of Children
How Supplied: Equipar Equine Wormer Paste is supplied in 0.85 ounce (24 gram) syringes.

DOSAGE TABLE

10 mg/kg		15 mg/kg	
Syringe mark	Horse Weight (lb)	Syringe Mark	Horse Weight (lb)
100	100	300	200
200	200	600	400
400	400	900	600
600	600	1200	800
800	800		
1000	1000		
1200	1200		

EQUIPAR® EQUINE WORMER SUSPENSION ℞
(oxibendazole)

Active Ingredient
Oxibendazole 10%
Oxibendazole is a broad spectrum benzimidazole anthelmintic.
Indications: Equipar Equine Wormer (oxibendazole) Suspension is indicated for removal and control of: large strongylids (*Strongylus edentatus, S. equinus, S. vulgaris*); small strongylids (species of the genera *Cylicostephanus, Cylicocyclus, Cyathostomum, Tridontophorus, Cylicodontophorus,* and *Gyalocephalus*); large roundworms (*Parascaris equorum*); pinworms (*Oxyuris equi*) including various larval stages; and threadworms (*Strongyloides westeri*).
Equipar Equine Wormer is compatible with carbon disulfide, which can be used concurrently for bot control (*Gasterophilus* spp.). Routine carbon disulfide cautions must be observed.
Dosage and Administration: The dosage of oxibendazole for the horse is 10 mg/kg body weight (15 mg/kg for strongyloides). Each ml of suspension contains 100 mg of oxibendazole. Administer by stomach tube in 3-4 pints of warm water, or if preferred, by top dressing or mixing into a portion of the normal grain ration. Prepare individual doses to assure that each animal receives the correct amount. Horses maintained on premises where reinfection is likely to occur should be retreated in 6 to 8 weeks.

DOSAGE TABLE

Body Weight (lb)	Dosage of 10% Suspension* 10 mg/kg (ml)	15 mg/kg (ml)
220	10	15
440	20	30
660	30	45
880	40	60
1100	50	75
1320	60	90

*Contains 100 mg oxibendazole per ml of suspension.
Warning: Not for use in horses intended for food.
Keep Out of Reach of Children
Caution: Federal (U.S.A.) law restricts this drug to use by or on the order of a licensed veterinarian.
Protect From Freezing
Shake Well Before Using
How Supplied: 1 gallon and 1 quart

EXPAR® CREAM RINSE FOR DOGS

—Kills fleas, ticks and lice.
—Makes hair coat more manageable.
—Reduces static electricity.
—Helps prevent snarls and tangles.
—Imparts a high sheen to hair coat.

Active Ingredient
Permethrin (3-phenoxyphenyl) methyl (±) cis, trans-3-(2,2-dichloroethenyl)-2, 2-dimethylcyclopropane-carboxylate* 0.5%
Inert Ingredients........................ 99.5%
100.0%
*cis/trans ratio: Max 55% (±) cis and min 45% (±)trans
KEEP OUT OF REACH OF CHILDREN
Caution
PRECAUTIONARY STATEMENTS
HAZARDS TO HUMANS AND DOMESTIC ANIMALS
Caution
For animal use only. Not for use on humans. Harmful if swallowed. Avoid contact with eyes, skin or clothing. Wash thoroughly with soap and water after using.
STATEMENT OF PRACTICAL TREATMENT
If Swallowed: Call a physician immediately. DO NOT INDUCE VOMTING unless under medical attention.
If On Skin: Removed contaminated clothing and wash skin thoroughly with soap and water.
If In Eyes: Immediately flush eyes with water for at least five minutes. Get medical attention if irritation persists.
ENVIRONMENTAL HAZARDS
This product is toxic to fish. Keep out of lakes, ponds or streams. Do not contaminate water by cleaning of equipment or disposal of waste.
Directions for Use
General Classification: It is a violation of Federal law to use this product in a manner inconsistent with its labeling.
Expar Cream Rinse should be used after first bathing the dog. Wet the dog's coat thoroughly. Pour a little Expar Cream Rinse onto dog's coat. Rub all over the dog's wetted coat. Repeat application and massage Expar Cream Rinse thoroughly into the coat. Allow cream rinse to act for five minutes to kill any fleas, ticks or lice that might be present. Lightly rinse with clean water.
Repeat application as required to maintain protection.
STORAGE AND DISPOSAL
Storage: Store in a cool, dry place. **Pesticide Disposal:** Securely wrap original container in several layers of newspaper and discard in trash.
Container Disposal: Do not reuse empty bottle. Wrap bottle and put in trash.
How Supplied: 8 oz. squeeze bottles

EXPAR® EQUINE
Insecticide/Repellent with Silicone
A silicone-based spray or wipe-on for use on horses and ponies.

- Long Lasting
- Fly Insecticide/Repellent
- Kills and repels flies up to 5 days
- Ready-to-use
- Silicone-based formula
- Gives coat gloss and luster
- Non-burning
- Contains 1% permethrin
- No oiliness
- No dust residue

Active Ingredient
Permethrin (3-phenoxyphenyl) methyl (±)-cis, trans-3-(2,2-dichloroethenyl)-2,2-dimethylcyclopropane-carboxylate* 1.0%
Inert Ingredients........................ 99.0%
100.0%
*cis/trans ratio: Max 55% (±) cis and min 45% (±) trans
KEEP OUT OF REACH OF CHILDREN
Caution
Precautionary Statements
Hazards To Humans And Domestic Animals
Caution
For animal use only. Not for use on humans. Harmful if swallowed. Avoid breathing spray mist. Avoid contact with eyes, skin or clothing. Avoid contamination of food. Wash thoroughly with soap and water after handling.
STATEMENT OF PRACTICAL TREATMENT
If Swallowed: Call a physician immediately. DO NOT INDUCE VOMITING unless under medical attention. **If On Skin:** Remove contaminated clothing and wash skin thoroughly with soap and water. **If In Eyes:** Immediately flush eyes with plenty of water. Get medical attention if irritation persists. **Note to Physician:** This product contains petroleum distillates. Vomiting may cause aspiration pneumonia.
ENVIRONMENTAL HAZARDS
This product is toxic to fish. Do not add directly to water. Do not contaminate

Continued on next page

Coopers—Cont.

water by cleaning of equipment or disposal of wastes.
Directions for Use
GENERAL CLASSIFICATION: It is a violation of Federal law to use this product in a manner inconsistent with its labeling.
Not for use on horses intended for human consumption.
Expar Equine Insecticide/Repellent is ready-to-use with no mixing necessary. This non-burning, silicone-based formulation has been developed for use full strength on horses and ponies, and may be applied directly with trigger spray applicator or as a wipe-on.
Expar Equine Insecticide/Repellent will leave your horse's coat lustrously beautiful, shining and soft to the touch—never oily or sticky.
Expar Equine Insecticide/Repellent kills and repels house flies, stable flies, horn flies, face flies, horse flies, deer flies, mosquitoes and gnats. Expar Equine Insecticide/Repellent kills lice and ticks. Kills and repels flies for 3–5 days.
SHAKE WELL BEFORE USING.
DIRECTIONS FOR SPRAY: Apply spray to animal paying special attention to legs, shoulders and neck. For head and eye area, dampen an applicator mitt, cloth or toweling (Turkish) with Expar Equine Insecticide/Repellent and wipe over face. Be especially careful not to get in horse's eyes. Do not soak hair or skin. Repeat as necessary.
DIRECTIONS FOR WIPE-ON: Dampen an applicator mitt, cloth or toweling (Turkish) with Expar Equine Insecticide/Repellent. Rub over hair with special attention to the legs, shoulders, neck and facial areas where flies tend to congregate. Be especially careful not to get in horse's eyes. Repeat as necessary.
STORAGE AND DISPOSAL
Storage: Store in a cool, dry place. **Pesticide Disposal:** Securely wrap original container in several layers of newspaper and discard in trash. **Container Disposal:** Do not reuse empty bottle. Wrap bottle and put in trash.
How Supplied: 28 oz. pump spray.

EXPAR® Home and Carpet Spray

- **Controls cockroaches, fleas, ticks, silverfish and spiders on premises.**
- **Repels* and controls gnats, mosquitoes, biting flies, house flies and ticks on dogs.**
- **Controls fleas, ticks and lice on dogs.**

Active Ingredient
Permethrin (3-phenoxyphenyl) methyl (±)-cis, trans-3-(2,2 dichloroethenyl)-2,2-dimethylcyclopropane-carboxylate** 1.0%
Inert Ingredients 99.0%
100.0%
**cis/trans ratio: Max 55% (±) cis and min 45% (±) trans
KEEP OUT OF REACH OF CHILDREN
CAUTION
Net contents 64 fl. oz (1.893 L)
EPA Est. 6175-LA-1
EPA Reg. No. 59-210
Coopers Animal Health Inc.
Kansas City, MO 64108 U.S.A.
*U.S. Patent No. 4,020,181
56 505280 0
PRECAUTIONARY STATEMENTS
HAZARDS TO HUMANS AND DOMESTIC ANIMALS
CAUTION
Not for use on humans. Harmful if swallowed. Avoid breathing spray mist. Avoid contact with eyes, skin or clothing. Avoid contamination of food. Wash thoroughly with soap and water after handling.
STATEMENT OF PRACTICAL TREATMENT
If Swallowed: Call a physician immediately. DO NOT INDUCE VOMITING unless under medical attention.
If On Skin: Remove contaminated clothing and wash skin with soap and water.
If In Eyes: Immediately flush eyes with plenty of water. Get medical attention if irritation persists.
Note to Physician: This product contains petroleum distillates. Vomiting may cause aspiration pneumonia.
ENVIRONMENTAL HAZARDS
This product is extremely toxic to fish. Do not add directly to water. Do not contaminate water by cleaning of equipment or disposal of wastes.
Directions for Use
GENERAL CLASSIFICATION
It is a violation of Federal law to use this product in a manner inconsistent with its labeling.
Expar Home and Carpet Spray is ready-to-use. No mixing necessary. The non-burning, water-base formulation has been developed to use full strength and may be applied directly with trigger spray applicator.
SHAKE WELL BEFORE USING.
FOR GENERAL SURFACE SPRAY: FOR CONTROL OF FLEAS AND TICKS: Spray infested areas such as pet's beds and resting areas, and areas of floor covering such as carpeting where pests may be present.
FOR GENERAL SURFACE SPRAY: FOR CONTROL OF COCKROACHES*, SILVERFISH*, AND SPIDERS*: Spray baseboards, corners, cracks, crevices and other harborage areas where these pests frequent and hide. Assure that food, feed and food utensils are not contaminated by spray or spray drift.
*Not approved for control in California.
FOR USE ON DOGS: Cover animal's eyes with hand and with a firm fast stroke, to get a proper spray mist, spray head, ears and chest until damp. With fingertips rub into face around mouth, nose and eyes. Then spray neck, middle and hindquarters, finishing legs last. For best penetration of spray to skin, direct spray against the lay of hair. On long haired dogs rub your hand against the lay of hair spraying the ruffled hair directly behind the hand. Make sure spray thoroughly wets ticks.
Old bedding of pets should be removed and replaced with clean fresh bedding after treatment. This product may be used as often as necessary.

Storage and Disposal
Storage: Store in cool, dry place. Protect from freezing.
Pesticide Disposal: Securely wrap original container in several layers of newspaper and discard in trash.
Container Disposal: Do not reuse empty bottle. Wrap container and put in trash.

NOTICE OF WARRANTY
COOPERS ANIMAL HEALTH INC. MAKES NO WARRANTY OF MERCHANTABILITY, FITNESS FOR ANY PARTICULAR PURPOSE, OR OTHERWISE, EXPRESSED OR IMPLIED CONCERNING THIS PRODUCT OR ITS USES WHICH EXTEND BEYOND THE USE OF THE PRODUCT UNDER NORMAL CONDITIONS IN ACCORD WITH THE STATEMENTS MADE ON THIS LABEL.

EXPAR® INSECTICIDE EAR TAG
For Fly and Tick Control on Beef and Dairy Cattle

Compositon:
Active Ingredient:
Permethrin (3-phenoxyphenyl) methyl (±)-cis, trans-3- (2,2-dichloroethenyl)-2,2-dimethyl-cyclopropanecarboxylate* 10%
Inert Ingredients 90%
100%
*cis/trans ratio: Max 55% (±) cis and min 45% (±) trans.
Net wt. 9.5 grams per tag.
Indications: For fly and tick control on cattle. Effective against horn flies and face flies up to 5 months. Provides season-long control of Gulf Coast ticks. Spinose ear ticks also controlled. Aids in control of lice, stable flies and house flies. Permitted for lactating dairy cows. No withdrawal period prior to slaughter.
Action and Uses: Permethrin, the active ingredient in Expar Insecticide Ear Tags, was developed after many years of research by the National Research and Development Corporation of the British government which set out to find a superior synthetic alternative to pyrethrin, a highly effective but short-acting insecticide.
Permethrin is highly active, low in mammalian toxicity and is highly stable in sunlight. Further, it possesses the properties for which natural pyrethrin is well known: a wide spectrum of insecticidal activity and non-persistence in the environment.
The Expar Insecticide Ear Tag is an example of the significance of the permethrin discovery. Permethrin is combined with the compounds making up the tag, establishing a system under which insecticide is available day and night for application by animals themselves. Studies show that tags are highly effective for controlling face flies and horn flies up to five (5) months when used as directed. Gulf Coast ear ticks are controlled season long. Spinose ticks are also controlled.

KEEP OUT OF REACH OF CHILDREN
CAUTION
Precautionary Statement
HAZARDS TO HUMANS AND DOMESTIC ANIMALS
Caution:
Wash thoroughly with soap and water after handling and before eating or smoking. Avoid contamination of feed and foodstuffs.
Environmental Hazards: This pesticide is toxic to fish. Do not add directly to water. Do not contaminate water by disposal of used tags. Use this product only as specified on label.
Directions for Use: It is a violation of Federal law to use this product in a manner inconsistent with its labeling.
For the control of horn flies, attach one tag to one ear of each animal. Tags remain effective up to five months. For season-long control of face flies and Gulf Coast ticks, attach two ear tags per animal (one each ear.) Apply when flies first appear in the spring. Replace as necessary. Apply with the Allflex® Tagging System.
Storage and Disposal:
Do not contaminate water, food or feed by storage or disposal.
Storage: Store in a cool place away from direct sunlight.
Pesticide Disposal: Remove tags before slaughter. Wastes resulting from the use of this product may be disposed of on site or at an approved waste disposal facility.
Container Disposal: Dispose of empty bag in a sanitary landfill or by incineration, or, if allowed by State and local authorties, by burning. If burned, stay out of smoke.
How Supplied: Expar Insecticide Ear Tags are supplied in display cartons of 50 tags (5 packets of 10 tags and buttons). A case contains 4 cartons (200 tags).
Allflex Ear Tag Applicators supplied individually.

EXPAR® INSECTICIDE/REPELLENT FOR DOGS AND HORSES

For control of fleas, ticks and lice on dogs.
Repels* and controls gnats, mosquitoes, biting flies, house flies and ticks on dogs and horses.
Controls cockroaches, fleas, ticks, silverfish and spiders on premises.

Active Ingredient

Permethrin (3-phenoxyphenyl) methyl (±)-cis, trans-3-(2,2 dichloroethenyl)-2,2-dimethylcyclopropane-carboxylate**	1.0%
Inert Ingredients	99.0%
	100.0%

**cis/trans ratio: Max 55% (±) cis and min 45% (±) trans
Keep Out of Reach of Children.
Precautionary Statements
Hazards to Humans and Domestic Animals
Caution: For animal use only. Not for use on humans. Harmful if swallowed. Avoid breathing spray mist. Avoid contact with eyes, skin or clothing. Avoid contamination of food. Wash thoroughly with soap and water after handling.
Statement of Practical Treatment
If Swallowed: Call a physician immediately. DO NOT INDUCE VOMITING unless under medical attention.
If On Skin: Remove contaminated clothing and wash skin thoroughly with soap and water.
If In Eyes: Immediately flush eyes with plenty of water. Get medical attention if irritation persists.
Note To Physician: This product contains petroleum distillates. Vomiting may cause aspiration pneumonia.
Environmental Hazards: This product is extremely toxic to fish. Do not add directly to water. Do not contaminate water by cleaning of equipment or disposal of wastes.
Directions for Use
General Classification: It is a violation of Federal law to use this product in a manner inconsistent with its labeling.
Not for use on horses intended for human consumption.
Expar Insecticide/Repellent For Dogs and Horses is ready-to-use. No mixing necessary. The non-burning, water-base formulation has been developed to use full strength and may be applied directly with trigger spray applicator or as a wipe-on.
Expar Insecticide/Repellent For Dogs and Horses kills fleas, ticks and lice on dogs. Expar also repels and controls house flies, stable flies, horn flies, face flies, horse flies, deer flies, mosquitoes and gnats on dogs and horses; also kills fleas, ticks, cockroaches, silverfish and spiders around premises. Repels flies, mosquitoes and gnats for 3–5 days on horses. **Shake well before using.**
For Use On Dogs: Remove cap and insert sprayer. Cover animal's eyes with hand and with a firm fast stroke, to get a proper spray mist, spray head, ears and chest until damp. With fingertips rub into face around mouth, nose and eyes. Then spray neck, middle and hindquarters finishing legs last. For best penetration of spray to the skin, direct spray against the lay of the hair. On long haired dogs rub your hand against the lay of hair spraying the ruffled hair directly behind the hand. Make sure spray thoroughly wets ticks.
Old bedding of pets should be removed and replaced with clean fresh bedding after treatment. This product may be used as often as necessary.
For Use On Horses
As a Spray: First, remove excess dirt and dust by brushing. Apply spray to animal paying special attention to legs, shoulders, and neck. For head and eye area, dampen an applicator mitt, cloth or toweling (Turkish) with Expar Insecticide/Repellent For Dogs and Horses and wipe over face. Be especially careful not to get in eyes. Do not soak hair or skin. Repeat as necessary.
As a Wipe On: First, remove excess dirt and dust by brushing. Dampen an applicator mitt, cloth or toweling (Turkish) with Expar Insecticide/Repellent For Dogs and Horses. Rub over hair with special attention to the legs, shoulders, neck and facial areas where flies tend to congregate. Be especially careful not to get in eyes. Repeat as necessary.
For General Surface Spray
For Control of Fleas and Ticks: Spray infested areas such as pet's beds and resting areas, and areas of floor covering (such as carpeting) where pests may be present.
For Control of Cockroaches*, Silverfish* and Spiders*: Spray baseboards, corners, cracks, crevices and other harborage areas where these pests frequent and hide. Assure that food, feed and food utensils are not contaminated by spray or spray drift.
Storage and Disposal
Storage: Store in a cool, dry place. Protect from freezing.
Pesticide Disposal: Securely wrap original container in several layers of newspaper and discard in trash.
Container Disposal: Do not reuse empty bottle. Wrap bottle and put in trash.
How Supplied: 16 oz. pump bottle with sprayer and gallon plastic jug refill
*Not approved for control in California.

EXPAR® 3.2% EC

- **Emulsifiable Concentrate**
- **Kills Fleas, Ticks and Lice on dogs**
- **Gives residual protection up to 21 days**

Active Ingredient:

Permethrin (3-phenoxyphenyl) methyl (±) - cis, trans-3-(2,2-dicloroethenyl) -2,2-dimethylcyclopropane-carboxylate*	3.20%
Inert Ingredients	96.80%
	100.00%

*cis/trans ratio: Max 55% (±) cis and min 45% (±) trans
KEEP OUT OF REACH OF CHILDREN
CAUTION
PRECAUTIONARY STATEMENTS
HAZARDS TO HUMANS AND DOMESTIC ANIMALS
CAUTION
Harmful if swallowed or absorbed through skin. Avoid contact with skin, eyes or clothing.
STATEMENT OF PRACTICAL TREATMENT
If Swallowed: Call a physician immediately. DO NOT INDUCE VOMITING unless under medical attention.
If On Skin: Remove contaminated clothing and wash skin thoroughly with soap and water.
If In Eyes: Immediately flush eyes with plenty of water. Get medical attention if irritation persists.
Note to Physician: This product contains petroleum distillates. Vomiting may cause aspiration pneumonia.
Environmental Hazards: This product is toxic to fish. Do not add directly to water. Do not contaminate water by cleaning of equipment or disposal of wastes.
Directions for Use:
General Classification
It is a violation of Federal law to use this product in a manner inconsistent with its labeling.

Continued on next page

C

Coopers—Cont.

This product must be diluted before use. Stir four tablespoonfuls (2 fl. oz) of Expar 3.2% EC into one gallon of water. Dip, sponge or swab dog with this emulsion until thoroughly wet. Allow dog to dry in a warm place without rinsing or toweling.
Expar 3.2% EC gives long-lasting protection against reinfestation, and applications at intervals of two or three weeks will control ticks, fleas and lice on dogs. Repeat application as required.
SHAKE OR STIR PRODUCT THOROUGHLY BEFORE USING OR REUSING DILUTED EMULSION
Storage and Disposal: Do not contaminate water, food, or feed by storage and disposal.
Storage: Store in cool, dry place.
Pesticide Disposal: Wastes resulting from the use of this product may be disposed of on site or at an approved waste disposal facility.
Container Disposal: 8 oz Bottle—Do not reuse empty bottle. Wrap bottle and put in trash. Gallon Drum—Triple rinse (or equivalent). Then offer for recycling or reconditioning, or puncture and dispose of in a sanitary landfill, or by other procedures approved by State and local authorities.
How Supplied: 8 oz bottle with child resistant closure; gallon metal drum

EXPAR® 11% EC
Emulsifiable Concentrate Long-Lasting Insecticidal Spray for Livestock and Their Premises

Composition:
Active Ingredient
Permethrin (3-phenoxyphenyl) methyl (±) cis, trans-3-(2,2-dichloroethenyl)-2, 2-dimethylcyclopropanecarboxylate*..........11.0%
Inert Ingredients.........................89.0%
100.0%
*cis/trans ratio: Max 55% (±) cis and min 45% (±) trans.
This product contains 0.107 lbs. of permethrin per pint.
KEEP OUT OF REACH OF CHILDREN
PRECAUTIONARY STATEMENTS: HAZARDS TO HUMANS & DOMESTIC ANIMALS
CAUTION
Harmful if swallowed or absorbed through the skin. Avoid contact with skin, eyes or clothing.
Statement of Practical Treatment
If Swallowed: Call a physician immediately. DO NOT INDUCE VOMITING unless under medical attention.
If On Skin: Remove contaminated clothing and wash skin thoroughly with soap and water.
If In Eyes: Immediately flush eyes with plenty of water. Get medical attention if irritation persists.
Note to Physician: This product contains petroleum distillates. Vomiting may cause aspiration pneumonia.
Environmental Hazards
This product is extremely toxic to fish. Do not add directly to water. Do not contaminate water by cleaning of equipment or disposal of wastes.
Directions For Use
General Classification
It is a violation of Federal law to use this product in a manner inconsistent with its labeling.
For all sprays intended for direct application to animals and building surfaces, add Expar 11% EC to clean water as directed below, mix thoroughly, and apply as a coarse spray. Spray lactating dairy cows *only* after milking is completed. Repeat applications as needed but not more than once every two weeks.
For Control of Horn Flies on Beef and Dairy Cattle and Horses: Dilute at the rate of one pt. Expar 11% EC to 50 gals of water (3 tbsp/5 gals water) and apply directly to animals at the approximate rate of 1 qt. per animal.
For Control of Face Flies, Stable Flies, House Flies, Horse Flies and Lice on Beef and Dairy Cattle and Horses: Dilute at the rate of 1 pt. Expar 11% EC to 25 gals of water (3 tbsp/2.5 gals water) and apply directly to animals at the approximate rate of two qts per animal, giving particular attention to the face, legs, and underline.
For Control of Ticks and Psoroptic (Scables) Mites on Beef and Dairy Cattle: Dilute at the rate of one pt. Expar 11% EC to 25 gals of water (3 tbsp/2.5 gals water) and apply sufficient spray to thoroughly wet animals and ensure complete coverage. Repeat application in 10 to 14 days for mites.
For Control of Northern Fowl Mites and Lice on Poultry in Cages or Houses: Dilute at the rate of one pt. Expar 11% EC to 25 gals of water (3 tbsp/2.5 gals water) and apply finished spray at the rate of 1 gal. per 100 birds. One application should eliminate an infestation.
For Control of Hog Lice on Swine: Dilute at the rate of one pt. Expar 11% EC to 25 gals of water (3 tbsp/2.5 gals water) and apply spray directly to animals at the approximate rate of 1 pt. per animal. One application should eliminate an infestation.
For Control of Mange Mites on Swine: Dilute at the rate of one pt. Expar 11% EC to 25 gals of water (3 tbsp/2.5 gals water) and apply sufficient spray to thoroughly wet animals and ensure complete coverage. Repeat application in 14 days.
Do not ship swine for slaughter within 5 days of last treatment.
For use in and around Horse, Beef, Dairy, Swine, Sheep and Poultry Premises and ***outside*** *Meat Processing Premises for Control of House Flies, Stable Flies and Little House Flies (Fannia spp.):* Dilute at the rate of one pt. Expar 11% EC to 10 gals of water. For small amounts of finished spray, mix 3 tbsps. in a gal. of water. Apply finished spray to surfaces where flies rest at the rate of 1 gal. per 750–1000 sq. ft., or to the point of runoff.
Timing and frequency of applications should be based upon flies reaching nuisance levels but not more often than once every two weeks. Do not apply dilutions for premise treatment directly on livestock or poultry. Ensure that animals, feed and water are not contaminated by spray drift. Do not use in milk rooms.
Storage and Disposal
Do not contaminate water, food or feed by storage or disposal.
Storage: Store in cool, dry place.
Pesticide Disposal: Wastes resulting from the use of this product may be disposed of on site or at an approved waste disposal facility.
Container Disposal: Triple rinse (or equivalent). Then offer for recycling or reconditioning, or puncture and dispose of in a sanitary landfill, or by other procedures approved by State and local authorities.
How Supplied: Metal cans of 1 pint.

FLAIR™
Insecticide/Repellent For Fleas, ticks, and lice on dogs and cats

Composition:
Active Ingredients:

Pyrethrins	0.06%
Piperonyl butoxide[1], technical	0.48%
Malathion[2]	0.50%
Carbaryl (1-naphthyl N-methylcarbamate)*	0.50%
Butoxypolypropylene glycol**	5.00%
2, 3:4, 5-Bis (2-butylene) tetrahydro-2-furaldehyde***	0.14%
Petroleum distillate	17.85%
Inert Ingredients:	75.47%
	100%

[1] Equivalent to 0.384% (butylcarbityl) (6-propylpiperonyl) ether and 0.096% of related compounds.
[2] 0,0-dimethyl dithiophosphate of diethyl mercaptosuccinate.

Indications: Insecticide and repellent for use against fleas, ticks, lice, flies, mosquitoes and gnats on dogs and cats.
Action and Uses: A pleasantly scented aerosol, Flair™ aids in control of external parasites. The combination of ingredients provides both direct and residual killing action against fleas, ticks and lice; and offers effective repellency against flies, mosquitoes and gnats. Flair is indicated for use on cats as well as dogs.
Pyrethrins potentiated with piperonyl butoxide have rapid "knock-down" action as well as direct killing effect. Malathion and Sevin, insecticides of relatively low toxicity to mammals, provide residual killing action. Two powerful repellents, Stabilene® and MGK® Repellent II, aid in protecting the animal and his bedding between spraying. The inclusion of Sevin in Flair broadens the effectiveness to include insects which have become resistant to other insecticides.
KEEP OUT OF REACH OF CHILDREN
Precautionary Statements
Hazards to Humans and Domestic Animals
Caution: Harmful if swallowed. Avoid inhalation, eye, skin and clothing contact. Wash thoroughly after using. Do not contaminate feed, water or foodstuffs. Avoid spraying in animal's eyes, face, scrotum or open wounds. Do not use near birds or fish. Do not use on pregnant dogs.

Statement of Practical Treatment:
If Swallowed: Call physician immediately. This product contains petroleum distillates. DO NOT INDUCE VOMITING. Vomiting may cause aspiration pneumonia.
If Inhaled: Remove victim to fresh air. Apply respiration if indicated.
If On Skin: Remove contaminated clothing and wash affected areas with soap and water.
If In Eyes: Flush eyes thoroughly with plenty of water. Call a physician immediately.
Chemical or Physical Hazards:
Contents under pressure. Do not use or store near heat or open flame. Do not puncture or incinerate container. Exposure to temperatures above 130°F may cause bursting.
Directions For Use: It is a violation of Federal law to use this product in a manner inconsistent with its labeling.
Hold Flair container about 12 inches from animal and direct spray over entire body until hair is damp. For dogs and cats, apply spray 4 to 6 seconds for each 5 lbs of body weight. Brush back hair while spraying to allow penetration of mist. To kill ticks on long-haired dogs, brush back the hair and spray Flair directly on the ticks.
Repeat treatment not more often than once weekly. To prevent reinfestation, spray sleeping quarters and bedding thoroughly.
Storage and Disposal: *Storage:* Store in cool, dry place away from heat or open flame.
Pesticide Disposal: Securely wrap original container in several layers of newspaper and discard in trash.
Container Disposal: Replace cap and discard container in trash. Do not incinerate or puncture.
How Supplied: 12 oz metal aerosol can.

*Sevin: Registered trademark of Union Carbide Corporation for the active ingredient carbaryl
**Stabilene® Fly Repellent: Registered trademark of Union Carbide Corporation
***MGK® Repellent II

FOGGER 5

Kills exposed fleas and ticks. Also roaches, ants, small flying moths, spiders and scorpions.

Active Ingredients:

2,2-dichlorovinyl dimethyl phosphate	0.47%
Related Compounds	0.03%
Pyrethrins	0.40%
Piperonyl Butoxide* Technical	0.80%
N-octyl bicycloheptene dicarboximide	1.55%
Petroleum Distillate	3.70%
Inert Ingredients	93.05%
	100.0%

*Equivalent to 0.64% (butylcarbityl) (6-propylpiperonyl) ether and 0.16% related compounds.

Keep Out of Reach of Children.
Caution
FOR USE ONLY WHEN BUILDING HAS BEEN VACATED BY HUMAN BEINGS AND PETS.
Precautionary Statements
Hazards to Humans and Domestic Animals
Caution: Harmful if swallowed. Avoid inhalation, eye, skin and clothing contact; wash thoroughly after using. Do not contaminate feed, water or foodstuffs. Food should be removed or covered during treatment. All food processing surfaces should be covered during treatment or thoroughly cleaned before using. When using Fogger 5 in these areas, apply only when the facility is not in operation.
Remove pets and cover fish tanks or fishbowls before using.
Statement of Practical Treatment
If Swallowed: Drink one or two glasses of water and induce vomiting by touching the back of the throat. Repeat until vomit fluid is clear. Call a physician immediately. Do not induce vomiting or give anything by mouth to an unconscious person.
If Inhaled: Remove victim to fresh air. Apply respiration if indicated.
If On Skin: Remove contaminated clothing and wash affected areas with soap and water.
If In Eyes: Flush eyes for at least 15 minutes with water. Call a physician immediately.
Chemical or Physical Hazards: Contents under pressure. Do not puncture. Do not use or store near heat or open flame. Exposure to temperatures above 130°F may cause bursting. Never throw container into fire or incinerator.
Directions For Use: It is a violation of Federal law to use this product in a manner inconsistent with its labeling.
Use one canister for each 5,000 cu. ft. of unobstructed area.
Example: 25′ long × 20′ wide × 10′ high = 5,000 cu. ft. Use additional units for remote rooms or where the free flow of the mist is not assured.
Preparation: Open cabinets and doors to areas to be treated. Shut off fans and air conditioners. Put out all open flames except pilot light. Remove pets and cover fish tanks or fishbowls with paper, or remove from area. Close exterior doors and windows. Solvents may soften some asphalt or synthetic tile floors. If used directly over asphalt or synthetic tile, newspapers should be spread on the floor for several feet around the area of release. Do not use with freshly waxed floors; allow 3 weeks for wax to harden as this product may cause fresh wax to become softened. Some plastics may be affected. Remove or cover plastic items such as eyeglasses, stereo covers, notion boxes.
Cover exposed foods, dishes, and food handling equipment.
To start fogging: Locate Fogger in center of area being treated. Place Fogger on table, chair or stand, at least six feet from pilot light. Place several thicknesses of newspapers under fogger unit for three or four feet around can to prevent staining or marring surfaces. Do not aim directly at furniture. Hold can at arm's length, with top of can pointing away from face and eyes. Push on finger pad until it locks—this will start fogging action. Set canister in upright position on table, etc., and leave building at once.
Do not re-enter building for two hours, then open exterior doors and windows and allow to air for 30 minutes before reoccupying area.
Storage and Disposal
Storage: Store in a cool, dry area away from heat or open flame.
Pesticide Disposal: Securely wrap original container in several layers of newspaper and discard in trash.
Container Disposal: Replace cap and discard container in trash. Do not incinerate or puncture.
How Supplied: 6 oz. metal aerosol can

FOGGER 10

Kills Exposed Fleas and Ticks
Also kills exposed roaches, ants, small flying moths, spiders and scorpions

Composition: Fogger 10 is an aerosol spray containing:
Active Ingredients:

2,2-dichlorovinyl dimethyl phosphate	0.47%
Related Compounds	0.03%
Pyrethrins	0.40%
Technical Piperonyl Butoxide*	0.80%
N-octyl bicycloheptene dicarboximide	1.55%
Petroleum Distillate	3.70%
Inert Ingredients	93.05%
Total	100.00%

*Equivalent to 0.64% (butylcarbityl) (6-propylpiperonyl) ether and 0.16% related compounds.
FOR USE ONLY WHEN BUILDING HAS BEEN VACATED BY HUMAN BEINGS AND PETS.
Precautionary Statements:
Hazards to Humans and Domestic Animals:
Caution: Keep out of the reach of children.
Harmful if swallowed. Avoid inhalation, eye, skin and clothing contact; wash thoroughly after using. Do not contaminate feed, water or foodstuffs. Food should be removed or covered during treatment. All food processing surfaces should be covered during treatment or thoroughly cleaned before using. When using Fogger 10 in these areas, apply only when the facility is not in operation.
Remove pets and cover fish tanks or fishbowls before using.
Statement of Practical Treatment: *If swallowed*—drink one or two glasses of water and induce vomiting by touching the back of the throat. Repeat until vomit fluid is clear. Call a physician immediately. Do not induce vomiting or give anything by mouth to an unconscious person.
If inhaled—remove victim to fresh air. Apply respiration if indicated.

Continued on next page

Coopers—Cont.

If on skin—remove contaminated clothing and wash affected areas with soap and water.
If in eyes—flush eyes for at least 15 minutes with water. Call a physician immediately.
Physical Hazards: Contents under pressure. Do not puncture. Do not use or store near heat or open flame. Exposure to temperatures above 130°F may cause bursting. Never throw container into fire or incinerator.
Directions: It is a violation of Federal law to use this product in a manner inconsistent with its labeling.
Use one canister for each 10,000 cu. ft. of unobstructed area.
Example: 40′ long × 25′ wide × 10′ high = 10,000 cu. ft. Use additional units for remote rooms or where the free flow of the mist is not assured.
Preparation: Open cabinets and doors to areas to be treated. Shut off fans and air conditioners. Put out all open flames except pilot light. Remove pets and cover fish tanks or fishbowls with paper, or remove from area. Close exterior doors and windows. Solvents may soften some asphalt or synthetic tile floors. If used directly over asphalt or synthetic tile, newspapers should be spread on the floor for several feet around the area of release. Do not use with freshly waxed floors; allow 3 weeks for wax to harden as this product may cause fresh wax to become softened. Some plastics may be affected. Remove or cover plastic items such as eyeglasses, stereo covers, notion boxes.
Cover exposed foods, dishes and food-handling equipment.
To start fogging: Locate Fogger 10 in center of room or area being treated. Place Fogger 10 on table, chair, or stand, at least six feet from pilot light. Place several thicknesses of newspapers under fogger unit for three or four feet around can to prevent staining or marring surfaces. Do not aim directly at furniture. Hold can at arm's length, with top of can pointing away from face and eyes. Push on finger pad until it locks—this will start fogging action. Set canister in upright position on table, etc., and leave building at once. *Do not re-enter building for two hours,* then open exterior doors and windows and allow to air for 30 minutes before reoccupying area.
STORAGE AND DISPOSAL:
Storage: Store in cool, dry area away from heat or open flame.
Do not re-use empty container. Wrap container and put in trash collection.
Supply: 12 oz. metal aerosol can

FOOTVAX®
Bacteroides nodosus bacterin

Indications: A multi-strain ovine footrot vaccine for the prevention and treatment of footrot in sheep.
Description: Footvax® contains 10 strains of killed *Bacteroides nodosus* organisms suspended in a water-in-oil emulsion.
Uses: Footvax is designed to stimulate a strong immunological response for the protection from new infection, and treatment of infection already present. It forms an essential part of the recommended footrot control program. Owing to the large differences in flock susceptibility, prevalence of the disease, and seasonal climatic factors in different parts of the United States, a specific control program incorporating Footvax may need to be designed in consultation with your local veterinarian.
The Disease: Footrot in sheep is common in many areas of the United States and is principally caused by the bacterium *Bacteroides nodosus.* The development of footrot is aided by wet conditions when mud and feces may accumulate on the feet, resulting in inflammation between the claws. This inflammatory response facilitates invasion of the hoof by *B. nodosus* organisms. The disease is characterized by a progressive separation of the horny tissues from the soft tissues of the foot due to necrosis of the sensitive laminae. This starts to the rear of the inside of the claw proceeding to the sole and eventually progresses to the outside wall of the claw. In severe cases, there can be almost complete separation of the wall from the underlying structures. Where underrunning is severe the foot may be carried and if both front feet are severely affected the sheep may move about on its knees. There is a characteristic foul odor present.
The Organism: *Bacteroides nodosus,* the organism responsible for footrot in sheep, is separated into groups and strains by the differences in the hairlike structures (or pili) on the surfaces of the bacteria.
The differences between strains can only be identified by laboratory tests. Not all strains are equally pathogenic and the least destructive of them often cause only minor clinical signs. 'Scald' for instance is now thought to be caused by relatively non-proteolytic (non tissue-destructive) and strains of *B. nodosus.* Lameness in a small portion of the flock is usually the first indication of the presence of footrot. The interdigital skin is moist with some erosion and some minor underrunning may occur. Death of the underlying tissues does not occur although the usual footrot odor is present. In most cases of 'scald' there is natural regression and healing. 'Scald' of this nature should be referred to as benign footrot. In fact any infection of the interdigital skin by bacteria such as with *Fusobacterium necrophorum* will present symptoms of 'scald' and it is suggested that this term be used only to describe the early non-specific signs of foot disease of indeterminate origin.
Directions for Use:
Primary Immunization: The primary course of treatment should be initiated prior to the anticipated outbreak period as dictated by local conditions. Following the first (sensitizing) dose, a second inoculation should be administered not sooner than six (6) weeks and not later than six (6) months following the initial dose.
Booster Vaccination: Following the original two dose course of treatment, booster inoculations should be given biannually or just prior to an anticipated outbreak. Protection after vaccination is usually longer than 4 months, but local conditions are known to be very important in affecting this period. Booster inoculations at 4- to 6-month intervals may be beneficial in cases of severe challenge.
Dosage: Aseptically administer 1 ml under the skin in the anterior half of the neck.
Administration: Footvax is very viscous because it contains an oil adjuvant. A considerable excess is included in each vial since some of the product adheres to the sides of the container and cannot be withdrawn. Before use it should be thoroughly shaken. In very cold weather the pack should be immersed in lukewarm water to make the product flow more readily. The use of an 18 gauge × 1 inch needle is recommended, except in cold weather when a 16 gauge × 1 inch needle is recommended. The product can be given through standard automatic syringes that can be set to 1 ml. Sterilize all injection equipment by boiling for at least 10 minutes prior to use. Pre-packed Vaxiguns™ are already sterilized. Maintain maximum cleanliness at all times. Use aseptic technique and change needles frequently (every 20–30 sheep).
Caution: As far as possible, avoid injection of dirty or wet sheep. To reduce injection site contamination use only sharp sterile disposable needles. **INJECT ONLY UNDER THE SKIN, AND NOT INTO THE MUSCLE.** Use entire contents when first opened. Do not vaccinate within 60 days before slaughter.
Footvax contains an oil adjuvant which is likely to cause a localized reaction at the site of injection. This reaction can take the form of either a lump, or a plaque-like swelling or occasionally a sterile abscess may occur. These reactions will normally disappear over a period of 10 weeks. Anaphylactoid reactions may occur following use. **Antidote:** Epinephrine. Store away from light at not over 45° F or 7° C. **Do not freeze.** Use entire contents when first opened.
Accidental Human Exposure: This product does not represent an etiological hazard to humans. Accidental self injection of the vaccine can cause serious local reactions. If accidental injection occurs seek medical attention at once. Inform the doctor that the vaccine contains an oil emulsion.
For Veterinary Use Only.
How Supplied: 50 doses (50 ml), 100 doses (100 ml) and 200 doses (200 ml).

JENCINE® B
Bovine Virus Diarrhea Vaccine
Modified Live Virus

Description: Jencine® B is produced on an established cell line for purity and smoothness. Jencine® B cross-neutralizes five major cytopathic and non-cytopathic BVD strains. The product has remarkable stability for a longer shelf life.

Indications: For the active immunization of healthy cattle against bovine virus diarrhea diseases.
Caution: Store at not over 45°F or 7°C. Use entire contents when first opened. Do not use chemical disinfectants to sterilize syringes or needles. Burn container and all unused contents. Do not vaccinate within 21 days before slaughter. Do not vaccinate pregnant animals. Contains neomycin as an added preservative. Anaphylactoid reactions may occur following use. **Antidote:** Epinephrine.
Administration and Dosage: For use in healthy cattle. Slowly transfer entire contents of diluent vial to vaccine vial, using aseptic technique and sterile syringes and needles. Inject 2 ml intramuscularly into each animal using aseptic technique. Calves vaccinated under 6 months of age should be revaccinated at 6 months or weaning.
For Veterinary Use Only.
How Supplied: 10 and 50 dose vials with diluent.

JENCINE® I
Bovine Rhinotracheitis Vaccine Modified Live Virus

Composition: Bovine Rhinotracheitis Vaccine is a modified live virus vaccine produced by tissue culture methods in cells of bovine origin. Special stabilizing agents are incorporated to assure maximum stability and the vaccine is lyophilized and sealed under vacuum. Attenuation of the virus has been accomplished by serial passage on bovine tissue culture cells. Penicillin and streptomycin are added as preservatives during the manufacturing process.
Indications: For the active immunization of healthy cattle against infectious bovine rhinotracheitis.
Action and Uses: The clinical manifestations of infectious bovine rhinotracheitis (IBR) depend on the tissues affected. The respiratory form is an important part of the Bovine Respiratory Disease Complex. The clinical signs of this form include fever, dyspnea, nasal and ocular discharge, hyperemia of muzzle (red nose), reduced appetite, and weight loss. Morbidity in a herd may range from 25% to 100%, but mortality is low, usually 3% to 5%.
Other disease syndromes associated with the IBR virus are infectious pustular vulvovaginitis (IPV); conjunctivitis and excessive lacrimation; mortality in newborn calves; and abortions.
Maximum protection, as determined by antibody titers, develops 14 to 21 days after vaccination. Field experience indicates, however, that protection against exposure occurs much sooner, probably during the first week following vaccination. Vaccination of healthy cattle is recommended prior to or on arrival at the feedlot or dairy. The vaccine has been shown to be safe, and does not produce the disease in susceptible cattle when used as directed. Maternal antibodies may interfere with the development of protection in calves vaccinated before three to four months of age. Revaccinate such calves at six months of age or weaning.
Dosage and Administration: For use in healthy cattle. Slowly transfer entire contents of diluent vial to vaccine vial, using aseptic technique and boiled or autoclaved syringes and needles. Inject 2 ml intramuscularly into each animal using aseptic technique. Calves vaccinated under six months should be revaccinated at six months or weaning.
Caution: Store at not over 45°F or 7°C. Use entire contents when first opened. Do not use chemical disinfectants to sterilize syringes and needles. Burn container and all unused contents. Do not vaccinate within 21 days before slaughter. Do not vaccinate calves under 2 weeks of age. Do not vaccinate pregnant cows or calves nursing pregnant cows. Contains neomycin as an added preservative. Anaphylactoid reactions may occur following use. **Antidote:** Epinephrine.
For Veterinary Use Only.
How Supplied: 10 dose and 50 dose vials with diluent.

JENCINE® IB
Bovine Rhinotracheitis-Virus Diarrhea Vaccine Modified Live Virus

Description: The components of Jencine® IB are produced on established cell lines for added purity and smoothness. The BVD component cross-neutralizes 5 major cytopathic and non-cytopathic BVD strains. Testing has shown no incompatibility: each fraction works as well or better than when administered alone. The final product has remarkable stability for a longer shelf life.
Indications: For the active immunization of healthy cattle against infectious bovine rhinotracheitis and bovine virus diarrhea diseases.
Caution: Store at not over 45°F or 7°C. Use entire contents when first opened. Do not use chemical disinfectants to sterilize syringes or needles. Burn container and all unused contents. Do not vaccinate within 21 days before slaughter. Do not vaccinate calves under 2 weeks of age. Do not vaccinate pregnant cows or calves nursing pregnant cows. Contains neomycin as an added preservative. Anaphylactoid reactions may occur following use. **Antidote:** Epinephrine.
Administration and Dosage: For use in healthy cattle. Transfer entire contents of diluent vial to vaccine vial, using aseptic technique and sterile syringes and needles. Inject 2 ml intramuscularly into each animal using aseptic technique. Calves vaccinated under 6 months of age should be revaccinated at 6 months or weaning.
For Veterinary Use Only.
How Supplied: 10 and 50 dose vials with diluent.

JENCINE® IBL5
Bovine Rhinotracheitis-Virus Diarrhea Vaccine Modified Live Virus Leptospira Canicola-Grippotyphosa-Hardjo-Icterohaemorrhagiae-Pomona Bacterin

Description: The virus components of Jencine® IBL5 are produced on an established cell line for added purity and smoothness. The leptospirosis fraction (Novalep® 5) is a highly purified, adjuvanted bacterin prepared from inactivated cultures. The BVD component cross-neutralizes 5 major cytopathic and non-cytopathic BVD strains. Testing has shown no incompatibility: each fraction works as well or better than when administered alone. The final product has remarkable stability for a longer shelf life.
Indications: For the active immunization of healthy cattle against infectious bovine rhinotracheitis and bovine virus diarrhea and *Leptospira canicola, L. grippotyphosa, L. hardjo, L. icterohaemorrhagie* and *L. pomona* infections.
Caution: Store at not over 45°F or 7°C. Protect from freezing. Use entire contents when first opened. Do not use chemical disinfectants to sterilize syringes and needles. Do not vaccinate within 21 days before slaughter. Do not vaccinate calves under 2 weeks of age. Do not vaccinate pregnant cows or calves nursing pregnant cows. Combined product contains neomycin as an added preservative. Anaphylactoid reactions may occur following use. **Antidote:** Epinephrine.
Administration and Dosage: For use in healthy cattle. Transfer entire contents of bacterin vial to vaccine vial, using aseptic technique and sterile syringes and needles. Inject 2 ml intramuscularly into each animal using aseptic technique. Calves vaccinated under 6 months of age should be revaccinated at 6 months or weaning.
For Veterinary Use Only.
How Supplied: 10 and 50 dose vials.

JENCINE® IBP
Bovine Rhinotracheitis-Virus Diarrhea-Parainfluenza-3 Vaccine Modified Live Virus

Description: All components of Jencine® IBP are produced on established cell lines for added purity and smoothness. The BVD component cross-neutralizes 5 major cytopathic and non-cytopathic BVD strains. Testing has shown no incompatibility: each fraction works as well or better than when administered alone. The final product has remarkable stability for a longer shelf life.
Indications: For the active immunization of healthy cattle against infectious bovine rhinotracheitis, bovine virus diarrhea and parainfluenza-3 virus.
Caution: Store at not over 45°F or 7°C. Use entire contents when first opened. Do not use chemical disinfectants to ster-

Continued on next page

C

ilize syringes or needles. Burn container and all unused contents. Do not vaccinate within 21 days before slaughter. Do not vaccinate calves under 2 weeks of age. Do not vaccinate pregnant cows or calves nursing pregnant cows. Contains neomycin as an added preservative. Anaphylactoid reactions may occur following use. **Antidote:** Epinephrine.
Administration and Dosage: For use in healthy cattle. Transfer entire contents of diluent vial to vaccine vial, using aseptic technique and sterile syringes and needles. Inject 2 ml intramuscularly into each animal using aseptic technique. Calves vaccinated under 6 months of age should be revaccinated at 6 months or weaning.
For Veterinary Use Only.
How Supplied: 10 and 50 dose vials with diluent.

JENCINE® IBPL5
Bovine Rhinotracheitis-Virus Diarrhea Parainfluenza-3 Vaccine Modified Live Virus Leptospira Canicola-Grippotyphosa-Hardjo-Icterohaemorrhagiae-Pomona Bacterin

Description: All virus components of Jencine® IBPL5 are produced on an established cell line for added purity and smoothness. The leptospirosis fraction (Novalep® 5) is a highly purified, adjuvanted bacterin prepared from inactivated cultures. The BVD component cross-neutralizes 5 major cytopathic and non-cytopathic BVD strains. Testing has shown no incompatibility: each fraction works as well or better than when administered alone. The final product has remarkable stability for a longer shelf life.
Indications: For the active immunization of healthy cattle against infectious bovine rhinotracheitis, bovine virus diarrhea, parainfluenza-3, and *Leptospira canicola, L. grippotyphosa, L. hardjo, L. icterohaemorrhagie* and *L. pomona* infections.
Caution: Store at not over 45°F or 7°C. Protect from freezing. Use entire contents when first opened. Do not use chemical disinfectants to sterilize syringes and needles. Burn container and all unused contents. Do not vaccinate within 21 days before slaughter. Do not vaccinate pregnant cows or calves nursing pregnant cows. Combined product contains neomycin as an added preservative. Anaphylactoid reactions may occur following use. **Antidote:** Epinephrine.
Administration and Dosage: For use in healthy cattle. Transfer entire contents of bacterin vial to vaccine vial, using aseptic technique and sterile syringes and needles. Inject 2 ml intramuscularly into each animal using aseptic technique. Calves vaccinated under 6 months of age should be revaccinated at 6 months or weaning.
For Veterinary Use Only.
How Supplied: 10 and 50 dose vials.

JENCINE® IL
Bovine Rhinotracheitis Vaccine Modified Live Virus Leptospira Pomona Bacterin

Composition: Jencine® IL is a convenient combination of antigens for the active immunization of healthy cattle against infectious bovine rhinotracheitis and leptospirosis.
The bovine rhinotracheitis vaccine is a modified live virus vaccine produced by tissue culture methods in cells of bovine origin. Special stabilizing agents are incorporated to assure maximum stability and the vaccine is lyophilized and sealed under vacuum. The attenuation of the virus has been accomplished by serial passage on bovine tissue culture cells.
The leptospira component of Jencine IL is a highly purified adjuvanted bacterin prepared from inactivated cultures of *Leptospira pomona* grown in a low protein medium. The use of this medium, and the use of selective molecular filtration to further remove many non-protective, potentially allergenic by-products of bacterial metabolism, minimizes the possibility of adverse reactions.
Indications: For the active immunization of healthy cattle against infectious bovine rhinotracheitis and *L. pomona* infections.
Action and Uses: The clinical manifestations of infectious bovine rhinotracteitis (IBR) depend on the tissues affected. The respiratory form is an important part of the Bovine Respiratory Disease Complex. The clinical signs of this form include fever, dyspnea, nasal and ocular discharge, hyperemia of the muzzle (red nose), reduced appetite, and weight loss. Morbidity in a herd may range from 25% to 100%, but mortality is low, usually 3% to 5%.
Other disease syndromes associated with the IBR virus are infectious pustular vulvovaginitis (IPV); conjunctivitis and excessive lacrimation; mortality in newborn calves; and abortions.
Maximum protection against IBR, as determined by antibody titers, develops 14 to 21 days after vaccination. Field experience indicates, however, that protection against IBR exposure occurs much sooner, probably during the first week following vaccination. Vaccination of healthy cattle is recommended prior to or on arrival at the feedlot or dairy. The vaccine has been shown to be safe and does not produce the disease in susceptible cattle when used as directed. Maternal antibodies may interfere with the development of protection in calves vaccinated before three to four months of age. Revaccinate such calves at 6 months of age or weaning.
A single dose of the leptospira component protects cattle against infection and consequent multiplication of the leptospires in both blood and kidney and thus prevents the carrier state and urinary shedding of leptospirosis.
Dosage and Administration: For use in healthy cattle. Transfer entire contents of bacterin vial to vaccine vial, using aseptic technique and boiled or autoclaved syringes and needles. Inject 2 ml intramuscularly into each animal using aseptic technique. Calves vaccinated under six months of age should be revaccinated at six months or weaning.
Caution: Store at not over 45°F or 7°C. Protect from freezing. Use entire contents when first opened. Do not use chemical disinfectants to sterilize syringes or needles. Burn container and all unused contents. Do not vaccinate within 21 days before slaughter. Do not vaccinate calves under 2 weeks of age. Do not vaccinate pregnant cows or calves nursing pregnant cows. Combined product contains neomycin as an added preservative. Anaphylactoid reactions may occur following use. **Antidote:** Epinephrine.
For Veterinary Use Only
How Supplied: 10 and 50 dose vials.

JENOTONE® ℞
(aminopropazine fumarate)
Antispasmodic

Composition: Each ml of sterile aqueous solution contains aminopropazine fumarate, equivalent to 25 mg aminopropazine base; in a vehicle containing citric acid 1.0 mg, sodium citrate 2.0 mg, and sodium chloride 5.0 mg; with potassium metabisulfite 2.0 mg and benzyl alcohol 5.0 mg as preservatives; dissolved in distilled water.
Each tablet contains aminopropazine fumarate, equivalent to 25 mg aminopropazine base.
Background Pharmacology: Jenotone® is a phenothiazine derivative with the chemical designation 10-[2, 3-Bis (dimethylamino) propyl] phenothiazine fumarate. The principal pharmacological action reduces smooth muscle contractions. The spasmolytic activity results from a musculotropic rather than a neurotropic mechanism, permitting control of excessive smooth muscle activity without interruption of glandular secretory activity. Although chemically related to the phenothiazine-derived tranquilizers, Jenotone exhibits only relatively mild sedative action. Clinically, Jenotone acts principally to reduce smooth muscle contractions in the gastrointestinal, respiratory, and genitourinary systems. Jenotone does not exhibit sympatholytic or ganglionic blocking actions. It has only very weak activity on the central nervous system. Although highly active in suppressing uterine motility, Jenotone does not affect the estrous cycle. Biliary secretion is unaffected. Mydriasis and other atropine-like parasympathetic activities are not seen with Jenotone. Unlike other phenothiazine amines, Jenotone demonstrates no antihistaminic activity.
Indications: For reducing excessive smooth muscle contractions, such as occur in urethral spasms associated with urolithiasis in cats and dogs, and colic spasms in horses.
Warning: *Not to be used in animals intended for food purposes.*

Do not inject subcutaneously.
Contraindications: Phenothiazine derivatives may potentiate the action of other central nervous system depressants; do not use with other central nervous system depressants. This drug should not be used in disease conditions where prolonged activity is not desirable, or where it may not be properly metabolized or eliminated.
Do not use this product in conjunction with organophosphates and/or procaine hydrochloride since phenothiazines may potentiate the toxicity of organophosphates and the activity of procaine hydrochloride.
Epinephrine is contraindicated for treatment of acute hypotension produced by phenothiazine derivatives since further depression of blood pressure can occur. Other pressor amines, such as norepinephrine or phenylephrine, are the drugs of choice.
Precautions: Jenotone is a potent drug and must be used with care in patients with history of severe cardiac, renal or hepatic disease or those suffering from any form of shock. The intravenous route is not recommended in such patients.
Jenotone is a phenothiazine derivative and in some cases mild tranquilization or hyperexcitability may occur.
Intramuscular injections should be made deep in a large muscle mass, using alternate sites for subsequent injections.
As with intramuscular injections generally, care must be taken to avoid deposition on or near nerves; deposition on or near major nerves may cause nerve damage.
Intravenous injections should be made slowly, using care to avoid extravascular deposition.
Protect from light and excessive heat. Jenotone solution is normally colorless to light amber. Discard if any marked deviation from this range is observed.
Dosage and Administration: ***Dogs.*** 1 to 2 mg per lb body weight (1 to 2 ml/25 lbs intramuscularly or intravenously; 1 to 2 tablets/25 lbs orally).
Cats. 1 to 2 mg per lb body weight (0.25 to 0.5 ml/6 lbs intramuscularly or intravenously; ¼ to ½ tablet/6 lbs orally).
Horses. 0.25 mg per lb body weight (1 ml/ 100 lbs) intramuscularly or intravenously.
Dosage can be repeated every 12 hours, as indicated.
Caution: Federal (U.S.A.) law restricts this drug to use by or on the order of a licensed veterinarian.
How Supplied: Tablets—25 mg—bottles of 100.
Solution—25 mg/ml—50 ml vials.

KIL-A-MITE™
Controls Sarcoptic Mange

Description:
Active Ingredients

Malathion (0,0-dimethyl dithiophosphate of diethyl mercaptosuccinate)	15.34%
Lindane (gamma isomer of benzene hexachloride)	2.00%
Xylene	12.00%
Mineral Seal Oil	57.46%
Inert Ingredients	13.20%
	100.00%

CAUTION:
KEEP OUT OF REACH OF CHILDREN

PRECAUTIONARY STATEMENTS
Hazards to Humans and Domestic Animals

Caution: Not for human use. Harmful if swallowed or absorbed through skin. Avoid breathing vapors. Avoid contact with skin, eyes or clothing. Use of this product is permitted only for treatment of mites. The use of this product for treatment of other pests is prohibited. Applicators must wear the following protective clothing during the treatment process: elbow-length, waterproof gloves; a waterproof apron; and unlined, waterproof boots. Improper dilution of this product could cause serious injury to your pet. Children should not be allowed to handle or apply this product.
Avoid contamination of food.
Do not use on nursing pups or on bitches nursing pups. DO NOT USE ON CATS.
Never use a solution stronger than recommended. Improper dilution of this pesticide product could cause serious injury to your pet.
Malathion is a cholinesterase inhibitor. Do not use Kil-A-Mite on animals simultaneously or within a few days before or after treatment with or exposure to cholinesterase inhibiting drugs, pesticides or chemicals. Consult a veterinarian at first signs of adverse reaction.
Statement of Practical Treatment:
If Swallowed: Call a physician/ veterinarian immediately. DO NOT INDUCE VOMITING, unless under medical supervision. Vomiting may cause aspiration pneumonia.
If On Skin: Wash immediately with plenty of soap and water.
If In Eyes: Flush eyes for at least 15 minutes with water.
Note to Physician/Veterinarian: This product contains a chlorinated hydrocarbon, an organophosphate and petroleum distillates. ATROPINE IS ANTIDOTAL for the organophosphate ingredient only.
Environmental Hazards: This product is toxic to fish, birds and other wildlife. Do not contaminate water by cleaning of equipment or disposal of wastes. Keep out of any body of water.
Physical or Chemical Hazards: Do not use or store near heat or open flame.
Directions for Use: It is a violation of Federal law to use this product in a manner inconsistent with its labeling.
Sarcoptic Mange: Stir four tablespoonfuls (2 fl. oz) of Kil-A-Mite into one gallon of water. Using a brush, wet dog thoroughly with this emulsion, making sure that mange scabs and lesions are penetrated. Allow dog to dry in a warm place, without rinsing or toweling. Repeat weekly until condition clears up.
SHAKE OR STIR PRODUCT THOROUGHLY BEFORE USING OR REUSING DILUTED EMULSIONS.
Storage and Disposal:
Storage: Store in a cool, dry place away from heat or open flame.
Pesticide Disposal: Securely wrap original container in several layers of newspaper and discard in trash.
Container Disposal: Bottles: Do not reuse empty bottle. Wrap bottle and put in trash. *Drums:* Triple rinse (or equivalent). Then offer for recycling or reconditioning, or puncture and dispose of in a sanitary landfill, or by other procedures approved by State and local authorities.
How Supplied: Bottle of 4 fl oz with child-resistant cap. One gallon drum.

LANOXIN® ELIXIR ℞
—Veterinary (Digoxin)
(A glycoside of *Digitalis lanata*)

Description: Lanoxin (Digoxin) Elixir—Veterinary is a cardiotonic glycoside discovered and developed in 1930 at The Wellcome Research Laboratories. It is derived from the leaves of *Digitalis lanata* Ehrh. (Fam. *Scropuloriacal*). Digoxin contains, on a dry basis, not less than 96 percent of $C_{41}H_{64}O_{14}$.
The physical characteristics of digoxin are clear to white crystals or white crystalline powder. Digoxin is insoluble in water, chloroform and ether, soluble in diluted alcohol.
Pharmacologic Action: As reported by Gold, "Digoxin stands high among digitalis glycosides with respect to the speed and extent of its absorption from the gastrointestinal tract." Doherty utilizing tritium labeled digoxin demonstrated that approximately 90 percent of the drug is uniformly absorbed from the gastrointestinal tract when administered orally. In the failing canine heart, intravenous administration of digoxin has been shown to increase cardiac output, decrease venous pressure, increase the force of the ventricular contractability and, secondarily, to increase the glomerular filtration and renal circulation. Oral preparations of digoxin are more effective than digitoxin or whole-leaf digitalis in controlling heart failure in dogs. Breznock demonstrated that digoxin is absorbed orally within thirty minutes and peak specific activity in the plasma occurs within three hours in the canine.
Advantages: The rapid development of the maximal action of digoxin permits the veterinarian to assess the full effect of the previous dose before administering subsequent doses. The moderately rapid dissipation of the drug permits vigorous therapy without danger of prolonged toxicity. The appearance of early gastrointestinal warning symptoms of toxicity, when overdigitalization with digoxin occurs, lessens the danger of serious arrhythmias and cardiac damage.
Indications: Lanoxin (Digoxin) Elixir—Veterinary is indicated for the treatment of congestive heart failure, atrial fibrillation, atrial flutter, supraventricular tachycardia and premature extrasystoles. Its indications are the same as those for digitalis leaf or other digitalis drugs.
Contraindications: Lanoxin (Digoxin) Elixir—Veterinary is contraindicated in shock, uremia or similar conditions un-

Continued on next page

Coopers—Cont.

less congestive heart failure is present. The use of prophylactic digitalization prior to surgery is contraindicated unless evidence of gross or incipient heart failure is present. In the presence of digoxin or other cardiac glycoside intoxication, Lanoxin (Digoxin) Elixir—Veterinary should not be given. It is usually contraindicated in the presence of ventricular premature contractions and ventricular tachycardia, except when these arrhythmias arise secondarily to decreased cardiac output accompanying congestive heart failure. Heart block is usually a contraindication to the use of digitalis preparations since the glycoside may further increase the degree of heart block and thereby further reduce the ventricular rate. Lanoxin (Digoxin) Elixir—Veterinary may be used in the presence of complete heart block and congestive heart failure; however, extreme caution and electrocardiographic monitoring are recommended.

Dosage and Administration: As with all cardiac glycosides, the dosage of Lanoxin (Digoxin) Elixir—Veterinary must be titrated to the individual patient. Guidelines to dosage are provided by clinical response of the patient.

Digitalization with Lanoxin (Digoxin) Elixir—Veterinary may be accomplished with either a loading-dose schedule or with the daily-maintenance method. When the loading-dose schedule is employed, a total calculated dose of 0.05 mg to 0.10 mg/lb is administered in divided doses over a 48-hour period or *until signs of toxicity appear* (whichever occurs first). After toxic signs appear, additional glycoside therapy is withheld until no toxic signs have been present for 12 to 24 hours. Then maintenance dosage of approximately 0.01 mg/lb/day, divided into two doses every 12 hours, is given. When only the maintenance method for digitalization is used, the patient will be digitalized in 6 to 10 days after therapy is instituted.

The recommended dosages for use of Lanoxin (Digoxin) Elixir—Veterinary are meant as guidelines only and subject to variations to fit individual needs. To achieve the same level of digitalization, proportionately less digitalis per pound is required for large dogs than for smaller dogs. Dogs in atrial fibrillation frequently required higher levels of a cardiac glycoside to slow the ventricular rate.

Lanoxin (Digoxin) Elixir—Veterinary 0.05 mg per ml

Digitalization: Guide* to 48 Hour Loading Dose Method. Digoxin Given Every 12 Hours For 48 Hours.**

[See table below].

Weight in Pounds	Dosage in ml	Dosage in mg
5	1.2 ml–2.4 ml	0.06mg–0.12mg
10	2.4 ml–4.8 ml	0.12mg–0.24mg
15	3.6 ml–7.2 ml	0.18mg–0.36mg
20	4.8 ml–9.6 ml	0.24mg–0.48mg
30	7.8 ml–9.9 ml	0.40mg–0.50mg
40	9.9 ml–15.0 ml	0.50mg–0.75mg
50	15.0 ml	0.75 mg
over 50	19.8 ml	1.0 mg
over 100	30.0 ml	1.5 mg

*Guideline means the approximate amount of the glycoside usually required by dogs in each weight group. Individual variations will occur and must be considered.

**Dosage to be given for four full doses unless intoxication develops first. Signs of digitalis intoxication indicate that full digitalization has been reached, regardless of the dose administered.

Lanoxin (Digoxin) Elixir—Veterinary 0.05 mg per ml

Maintenance: Guide* To Maintenance Dosage. Digoxin Given Every 12 Hours.**

[See table above].

Weight in Pounds	Dosage in ml	Dosage in mg
5	0.45 ml	0.022mg±0.15ml
10	0.90 ml	0.045mg±0.24ml
15	1.50 ml	0.075mg±0.36ml
20	1.80 ml	0.090mg±0.45ml
30	3.00 ml	0.15mg±0.75ml
40	3.60 ml	0.18mg±0.90ml
50	4.50 ml	0.225mg±1.20ml
over 50	6.00 ml	0.30mg±1.50ml
over 100	9.00 ml	0.45mg±3.00ml

*Guideline refers to the approximate amount of the glycoside usually required by dogs in each weight category for daily maintenance therapy. Individual variations require individual titration of the actual dosage.

**Requires twice-daily administration, perferably at 12-hour intervals.

Precautions: If any cardiac glycoside has been used in the previous 10 days, Lanoxin (Digoxin) Elixir—Veterinary dosage must be reduced to avoid digitalis intoxication. Patients with impaired renal and/or hepatic function may require a lower dosage of digoxin due to slower excretion of the glycoside. The margin between the therapeutic and toxic levels of digoxin is often more narrow in dogs with advanced cardiac disease than in healthy dogs.

Serum potassium deficiency increases cardiac irritability and may evoke ventricular arrhythmias. This deficiency also slows impulse conduction and may induce heart block. Serial serum potassium determinations should be made on patients receiving low-potassium diets, corticosteroids, or potassium-depleting diuretic agents. If hypokalemia is present, administration of cardiac glycosides should be stopped temporarily and normal electrolyte levels should be evaluated.

When digitalis glycosides are being given, caution is advised in the use of calcium salts or sympathomimetic amines such as ephedrine or epinephrine. The effectiveness of digoxin is questionable when heart failure occurs secondarily to mechanical causes unrelated to myocardial disease.

Side Effects and Effects of Overdose: The symptoms from overdosage of digoxin are quite similar to those occurring with other digitalis preparations. The most common toxic manifestations are anorexia, nausea, vomiting and various cardiac arrhythmias, including ventricular extrasystoles and paroxysmal supraventricular tachycardia or fibrillation with A-V block. In general, the gastrointestinal manifestations of toxicity with digoxin precede the cardiac arrhythmias occurring from overdose. Furthermore, because of the rapid dissipation of digoxin, manifestations of toxicity are of short duration, usually lasting from a few hours to one to two days.

The most effective method of treating digitalis intoxication is to stop the administration of all cardiac glycosides and maintain fluid electrolyte balance. Potassium-depleting diuretics should also be withheld. Antiemetic agents may be administered parenterally.

In advanced cases of intoxication in which myocardial automatically has developed, potassium chloride may be given orally (up to 1 g daily) or by slow intravenous injection (a maximum of 40 mEq/day) with electrocardiographic monitoring. To avoid accentuation, potassium chloride should be withheld in the presence of heart block.

Caution: Federal (U.S.A.) law restricts this drug to use by or on the order of a licensed veterinarian.

How Supplied: Lanoxin (Digoxin) Elixir—Veterinary, 0.05 mg per ml, bottles of 60 ml, each supplied with a calibrated 1 ml plastic dropper.

LANOXIN® TABLETS-VETERINARY ℞
(Digoxin)
(A glycoside of Digitalis lanata)

Description: Lanoxin® (Digoxin) Tablets-Veterinary is a cardiotonic glycoside discovered and developed in 1930 at The Wellcome Research Laboratories. It is derived from the leaves of *Digitalis lanata* Ehrh. (Fam. *Scropuloriacal).* Digoxin contains, on a dry basis, not less than 96 percent of $C_{41}H_{64}O_{14}$.

The physical characteristics of digoxin are clear to white crystals or white crystalline powder. Digoxin is insoluble in water, chloroform and ether, soluble in diluted alcohol.

Pharmacologic Action: As reported by Gold, "Digoxin stands high among digitalis glycosides with respect to the speed and extent of its absorption from the gastrointestinal tract." Doherty utilizing tritium labeled digoxin demonstrated that approximately 90 percent of the drug is uniformly absorbed from the gastrointestinal tract when administered orally. In the failing canine heart, intravenous administration of digoxin has been shown to increase cardiac output, decrease venous pressure, increase the force of the ventricular contractility and, secondarily, to increase the glomerular filtration and renal circulation. Oral preparations of digoxin are more effective than digitoxin or whole-leaf digitalis in controlling heart failure in dogs. Breznock demonstrated that digoxin is absorbed orally within thirty minutes and peak specific activity in the plasma occurs within three hours in the canine.
Advantages: The rapid development of the maximal action of digoxin permits the veterinarian to assess the full effect of the previous dose before administering subsequent doses. The moderately rapid dissipation of the drug permits vigorous therapy without danger of prolonged toxicity. The appearance of early gastrointestinal warning symptoms of toxicity, when overdigitalization with digoxin occurs, lessens the danger of serious arrhythmias and cardiac damage.
Indications: Lanoxin (Digoxin) Tablets-Veterinary are indicated for the treatment of congestive heart failure, atrial fibrillation, atrial flutter, supraventricular tachycardia and premature extrasystoles. Its indications are the same as those for digitalis leaf or other digitalis drugs.
Contraindications: Lanoxin (Digoxin) Tablets-Veterinary is contraindicated in shock, anemia, uremia or similar conditions unless congestive heart failure is present. The use of prophylactic digitalization prior to surgery is contraindicated unless evidence of gross or incipient heart failure is present. In the presence of digoxin or other cardiac glycoside intoxication, Lanoxin (Digoxin) Tablets-Veterinary should not be given. It is usually contraindicated in the presence of ventricular premature contractions and ventricular tachycardia, except when these arrhythmias arise secondarily to deceased cardiac output accompanying congestive heart failure. Heart block is usually a contraindication to the use of digitalis preparations since the glycoside may further increase the degree of heart block and thereby further reduce the ventricular rate. Lanoxin (Digoxin) Tablets-Veterinary may be used in the presence of complete heart block and congestive heart failure; however, extreme caution and electrocardiographic monitoring are recommended.
Administration and Dosage: As with all cardiac glycosides, the dosage of Lanoxin (Digoxin) Tablets-Veterinary must be titrated to the individual patient. Guidelines to dosage are provided by clinical response of the patient.
Digitalization with Lanoxin (Digoxin) Tablets-Veterinary may be accomplished with either a loading-dose schedule or with the daily maintenance method. When the loading-dose schedule is employed, a total calculated dose of 0.05 mg to 0.10 mg/lb is administered in divided doses over a 48-hour period or *until signs of toxicity appear* (whichever occurs first). After toxic signs appear, additional glycoside therapy is withheld until no toxic signs have been present for 12 to 24 hours. Then maintenance dosage of approximately 0.01 mg/lb/day, divided into two doses every 12 hours is given. When only the maintenance method for digitalization is used, the patient will be digitalized in 6 to 10 days after therapy is instituted.
The recommended dosages for use of Lanoxin (Digoxin) Tablets-Veterinary are meant as guidelines only and subject to variations to fit individual needs. To achieve the same level of digitalization, proportionately less digitalis per pound is required for large dogs than for small dogs. Dogs in atrial fibrillation frequently require higher levels of cardiac glycoside to slow the ventricular rate.
Precautions: If any cardiac glycoside has been used in the previous 10 days, Lanoxin (Digoxin) Tablets-Veterinary dosage must be reduced to avoid digitalis intoxication. Patients with impaired renal and/or hepatic function may require a lower dosage of digoxin due to slower excretion of the glycoside. The margin between the therapeutic and toxic levels of digoxin is often more narrow in dogs with advanced cardiac disease than in healthy dogs.
Serum potassium deficiency increases cardiac irritability and may evoke ventricular arrhythmias. This deficiency also slows impulse conduction and may induce heart block. Serial serum potassium determinations should be made on patients receiving low-potassium diets, corticosteroids, or potassium-depleting diuretic agents. If hypokalemia is present, administration of cardiac glycosides should be stopped temporarily and normal electrolyte levels should be evaluated.
When digitalis glycosides are being given, caution is advised in the use of calcium salts or sympathomimetic amines such as ephedrine or epinephrine. The effectiveness of digoxin is questionable when heart failure occurs secondarily to mechanical causes unrelated to myocardial disease.
Side Effects and Effects of Overdose: The symptoms from overdosage of digoxin are quite similar to those occuring with other digitalis preparations. The most common toxic manifestations are anorexia, nausea, vomiting and various cardiac arrhythmias, including ventricular extrasytoles and paroxysmal supraventricular tachycardia or fibrillation with A-V block. In general, the gastrointestinal manifestations of toxicity with digoxin precede the cardiac arrhythmias occurring from overdose. Furthermore, because of the rapid dissipation of digoxin, manifestations of toxicity are of short duration, usually lasting from a few hours to one to two days.
The most effective method of treating digitalis intoxication is to stop the administration of all cardiac glycosides and maintain fluid electrolyte balance. Potassium-depleting diuretics should also be withheld. Antiemetic agents may be administered parenterally.
In advanced cases of intoxication in which myocardial automaticity has developed, potassium chloride may be given orally (up to 1 g daily) or by slow intravenous injection (a maximum of 40 mEq/day) with electro-cardiographic monitoring. To avoid accentuation, potassium chloride should be withheld in the presence of heart block.
How Supplied: Lanoxin (Digoxin) Tablets-Veterinary, 0.125 mg Scored Tablets (yellow), bottles of 100 and 1000 tablets and Lanoxin (Digoxin) Tablets-Veterinary, 0.25 mg Scored Tablets (white), bottles of 100 and 1000 tablets.
Caution: Federal law restricts this drug to use by or on the order of a licensed veterinarian.

MERC–RED™ BLISTER ℞

Caustic Counterirritant

Composition: Contains: Mercuric iodide 10% in an ointment base.
Action and Uses: Counterirritants enhance healing of some chronic inflammatory processes by conversion into an acute inflammation by an irritation which increases circulation to the affected tissues.
Indications: For use as a blister on horses.
Caution: Do not apply to irritated skin or if excessive irritation develops. Avoid getting into eyes or on mucous membranes. Tie horse securely after treatment to prevent gnawing and irritation of mouth.
Warning: KEEP OUT OF THE REACH OF CHILDREN.
Directions for Use: Clip hair from area to be treated and protect adjacent areas with petrolatum. Apply Merc-Red™ Blister on area to be treated and massage for at least 10 minutes. Do not bandage. Remove remaining blistering agent in 36 to 48 hours by gently bathing treated area with mild, warm soapy water.
Caution: Federal (U.S.A.) law restricts this drug to use by or on the order of a licensed veterinarian.
How Supplied: 397 g (14 oz) jar.

MISTAWAY® EXTRA

For control of fleas, ticks and lice on dogs, cats and horses, and for temporarily repelling gnats, mosquitoes and biting flies.

Active Ingredients

Pyrethrins	0.15%
Piperonyl butoxide, technical*	1.50%
n-Octyl bicycloheptene dicarboximide	0.50%
2,3:4,5-bis (2-butylene) tetrahydro-2-furaldehyde	0.50%

Continued on next page

Coopers—Cont.

Petroleum distillate........................1.35%
Inert Ingredients** 96.00%
100.00%

*Equivalent to 1.2% (butylcarbityl)(6-propyl-piperonyl) ether and 0.3% related compounds.

**Inert ingredients include a grooming agent to ease combing and brushing of coat to remove dead fleas and lice.

C

KEEP OUT OF REACH OF CHILDREN

WARNING

Precautionary Statements

Hazards to Humans and Domestic Animals

Warning

Humans: Harmful if swallowed or inhaled. Avoid breathing spray mist. Avoid contact with skin or eyes. Avoid contamination of feed or foodstuffs.

Animals: Avoid contact with animal's eyes. Do not use on nursing animals.

Statement of Practical Treatment

If Swallowed: Do not induce vomiting. CALL A PHYSICIAN OR POISON CONTROL CENTER IMMEDIATELY.

If In Eyes: Flush with plenty of water. See a physician immediately.

If On Skin: Wash with soap and water. Get medical attention if irritation persists.

Environmental Hazards

This product is toxic to aquatic organisms. Do not apply to water. Do not contaminate water by cleaning of equipment or disposal of wastes.

Physical Or Chemical Hazards

Flammable. Keep away from heat or open flame.

Directions For Use

It is a violation of Federal law to use this product in a manner inconsistent with its labeling.

Cats and Dogs: Remove cap and insert sprayer. Cover animal's eyes with hand and with a firm fast stroke, to get a proper spray mist, spray head, ears and chest until damp. With fingertips rub into face around mouth, nose and eyes. Then spray neck, middle and hindquarters, finishing legs last. For best penetration of spray to the skin, direct spray against the natural layer of the hair. On long-haired dogs rub your hand against the lay of hair, spraying the ruffled hair directly behind the hand. Make sure spray thoroughly wets ticks. Repeat treatment as needed.

Puppies and Kittens: Spray only on back or on your fingertips and rub into coat. Do not use on puppies or kittens under 4 weeks of age.

Pet Sleeping Quarters: Spray around baseboards, windows, door frames, wall cracks and local area of floors. If mosquitoes, gnats or flies are present, spray lightly into the air. Repeat as needed. The bedding should be sprayed and then replaced with fresh bedding for best results.

Horses: To control stable flies, horse flies, deer flies and face flies apply to face, legs, flanks, topline and other body areas commonly attacked by these flies. Repeat as needed.

Storage and Disposal

Storage: Store in cool, dry place away from heat or open flame.

Pesticide Disposal: Securely wrap original container in several layers of newspaper and discard in trash.

Container Disposal: Do not reuse bottle. Rinse thoroughly before discarding in trash.

How Supplied: 16 oz bottles with trigger spray; 1 gallon bottle (refill).

NASALGEN® IP
Bovine Rhinotracheitis-Parainfluenza-3 Vaccine Modified Live Virus, Intranasal

Composition: A modified live virus vaccine produced by tissue culture methods in heterologous cell systems. The bovine rhinotracheitis (IBR) and parainfluenza-3 (PI-3) viruses have been specially attenuated by selection and serial passage. The safety and antigenicity of both virus strains have been demonstrated by vaccination and challenge tests in susceptible cattle.

Indications: For the active immunization of healthy cattle against infectious bovine rhinotracheitis and parainfluenza-3 virus.

General Information: PI-3 and IBR are important causative factors in the Bovine Respiratory Disease Complex (BRD). These viruses, acting alone or in combination with other viruses such as BVD and adenoviruses, may trigger and potentiate secondary bacterial infections. The stress of shipping, handling and climatic changes is also a major factor in the etiology of BRD.

PI-3 infection in cattle is primarily a local infection of the respiratory tract. It has been well demonstrated that such infection stimulates the production of secretory or "local" antibodies in addition to circulating antibodies. In this respect the immune response to infection with PI-3 virus differs from the response to a systemic infection, such as BVD, wherein resistance to infection has been correlated with the development of circulating antibodies. Such correlation has not been consistently demonstrated following intramuscular administration of PI-3 vaccine although levels of circulating antibody are produced.

Neutralizing activity against PI-3 in bovine nasal secretions following intranasal administration of the TELC™ strain (of PI-3) has been reported. Such activity has been shown by Morein to be associated with the IgA class of immunoglobulins. Mach and Pahud had earlier demonstrated the presence of IgA in bovine external secretions, and their work has been confirmed by others. It seems evident, therefore, that the bovine immune response to PI-3 infection is analogous to the response which occurs in humans infected with influenza or parainfluenza viruses, which involves the release of locally produced IgA antibodies in respiratory tract secretions.

Since secretory IgA antibody production appears to be independent of circulating antibody synthesis, these more recent studies provide further evidence of the value of secretory antibody in preventing PI-3 infection in cattle.

Original research conducted at Coopers Animal Health Inc. demonstrated that the TELC strain of PI-3 in Nasalgen® IP, when administered to cattle intranasally, protected them against both laboratory and field challenge. Protection was demonstrated by failure of the challenge virus to establish infection in the respiratory tract. Control animals vaccinated intramuscularly with 10 times the amount of vaccine given intranasally showed no protection. These animals, when exposed to the challenge virus, continued to excrete virus for 10 days after challenge. The postvaccinal, prechallenge circulating antibody levels developed by intranasally vaccinated calves were more than 10 times greater than those developed by the intramuscularly vaccinated calves. Cattle studies conducted by the U.S. Public Health Service Laboratory gave similar results in the comparison of intranasal and intramuscular routes of vaccination.

TELC strain virus has been critically evaluated for safety and potency in colostrum-deprived calves which are generally recognized to be the most sensitive for these tests. In addition, the vaccine has been tested in cattle under a wide range of conditions of husbandry, stress, and climate.

IBR is an acute upper respiratory disease of cattle characterized by sudden onset, high fever, nasal discharge, anorexia, dyspnea, and coughing resulting in severe loss of condition and a marked decrease in production. Morbidity in a herd may range from 25% to 100%, but mortality is low, usually 3% to 5%.

Other disease manifestations which may be associated with the IBR virus are infectious pustular vulvovaginitis (IPV), conjunctivitis, mortality in newborn calves and abortions.

It has been demonstrated that Nasalgen IP protects cattle against challenge with virulent IBR virus as early as 40 to 72 hours following vaccination. This early protection is associated with a high level of vaccine-induced interferon which appears in nasal secretions 40 to 72 hours after vaccination. High levels of interferon are maintained in nasal secretions for 6 to 8 days after which time circulating antibodies first appear. Low levels of circulating interferon also are present in the serum following vaccination.

Interferon present in nasal secretions is apparently produced locally by cells of the respiratory tract in response to vaccine virus replication. In a study designed to evaluate interferon response of calves following administration of intramuscular IBR vaccine, no interferon was detected in nasal secretions or serum during a 14 day postvaccination period. Other investigators detected an extremely low and transitory level of serum interferon after injecting a large dose of IBR virus into a calf by the intramuscular route.

Because the antiviral activity of interferon is not restricted to the virus causing its induction, interferon present in nasal secretions may afford protection against respiratory tract infection by viruses other than IBR. Viruses of virtually every major virus classification have been shown to be sensitive to the inhibitory effect of interferon. The degree of heterologous protection would, nevertheless, be determined by the presence of interferon in the respiratory tract secretions, the sensitivity of different infecting viruses to the inhibitory action of interferon, and by whether or not such viruses replicate initially and/or primarily in the respiratory tract.

In addition to inducing the local production of interferon, Nasalgen IP elicits the production of circulating antibody levels which are equal to or greater than those produced by an effective intramuscular vaccine and also stimulates the elaboration of specific antibodies into respiratory tract secretions. Vaccination of susceptible cattle with Nasalgen IP results, therefore, in early protection mediated by interferon and in long-term protection afforded by specific local and circulating antibodies.

Intramuscular modified live virus IBR and IBR combination vaccines are generally contraindicated for use in IBR-susceptible pregnant cattle because of the potential of inducing abortion. Cattle studies with Nasalgen IP indicate that it will not cause abortion when used in IBR- susceptible cattle at various stages of gestation. In these studies, 306 IBR-susceptible pregnant cows from 15 different herds were vaccinated with either Nasalgen IP or the IBR virus fraction of Nasalgen IP. Certification of pregnancy and stage of gestation was accomplished by rectal palpation at the time of vaccination and again 90 days later.

Dosage and Administration: *For intranasal use only.* For use in healthy cattle. Slowly transfer contents of diluent vial to vaccine vial, using aseptic technique and boiled or autoclaved syringe and needle. Administer 2 ml intranasally—1 ml in each nostril. Use a separate disposable cannula for each animal. Calves vaccinated under 6 months of age should be revaccinated at 6 months or weaning.

Caution: Store at not over 45°F or 7°C. Use entire contents when first opened. Do not use chemical disinfectants to sterilize syringes, needles, or cannulas. Burn container and all unused contents. Do not vaccinate within 21 days before slaughter. Contains polymyxin B and neomycin as added preservatives. Anaphylactoid reactions may occur following use. **Antidote:** Epinephrine.

For Veterinary Use Only

How Supplied: 10-1 dose, 10 dose, 25 dose, and 50 dose vials with diluent.

NEOSPORIN® OPHTHALMIC OINTMENT ℞
Veterinary
(polymyxin B-bacitracin-neomycin)
Sterile
Antibiotic

Composition: Each gram contains: Aerosporin® (polymyxin B sulfate) 5,000 units, bacitracin zinc 400 units, neomycin sulfate 5 mg (equivalent to 3.5 mg neomycin base) in a special white petrolatum base, q.s.

Actions: Polymyxin B is one of a group of closely related substances produced by various strains of *Bacillus polymyxa.* The activity of polymyxin B is sharply restricted to gram-negative bacteria. Neomycin, isolated from *Streptomyces fradiae,* has antibacterial activity *in vitro* against a wide range of gram-negative and gram-postive organisms. Bacitracin, an antibiotic substance derived from cultures of *Bacillus subtilis* (Tracy), exerts antibacterial action *in vitro* against a variety of gram-positive and a few gram-negative organisms.

Indications: This product is indicated for the treatment of superficial bacterial infections of the eyelid and conjunctiva of dogs and cats when due to organisms susceptible to one or more of the antibiotics contained in the ointment.

Laboratory tests should be conducted including *in vitro* culturing and susceptibility tests on samples collected prior to treatment.

Adverse Reactions: Adverse reactions, such as itching, burning or inflammation may occur in animals sensitive to this product.

Dosage and Administration: Properly cleanse area to be treated. Foreign bodies, crusted exudates and debris should be carefully removed. Express a small quantity of ointment into the conjunctival sac beneath the lower eyelid three or four times daily. After application hold the eyelids shut for a short time so that a thin film of ointment covers the cornea.

Precautions: If irritation develops discontinue treatment with this drug. If there is no response to treatment in 2–3 days, discontinue treatment and re-evaluate diagnosis. Prolonged use may result in overgrowth of nonsuspectible organisms, including fungi.

Care should be taken not to contaminate the applicator tip during administrations of the preparation.

Cautions: Federal (U.S.A.) law restricts this drug to use by or on the order of a licensed veterinarian.

How Supplied: ⅛ oz tube with ophthalmic tip.

NOVALEP® 5
Leptospira Canicola-Grippotyphosa-Hardjo-Icterohaemorrhagiae-Pomona Bacterin

Composition: Novalep 5 is a highly purified, adjuvanted bacterin prepared from inactivated cultures of *L. canicola, L. grippotyphosa, L. hardjo, L. icterohaemorrhagiae* and *L. pomona* grown in a low-protein medium. In addition to the use of this medium, other non-protective, potentially allergenic by-products of bacterial metabolism are removed by selective molecular filtration.

Indications: For the active immunization of healthy cattle and swine against *Leptospira canicola, L. grippotyphosa, L. hardjo, L. icterohaemorrhagiae* and *L. pomona* infections.

Dosage and Administration: Shake well. Cattle: 2 ml subcutaneously or intramuscularly. Swine: 2 ml intramuscularly only. Use aseptic technique. Revaccinate annually to maintain a high level of immunity.

Caution: Store at not over 45°F or 7°C. Protect from freezing. Use entire contents when first opened. Do not vaccinate within 21 days before slaughter. Anaphylactoid reactions may occur following use. **Antidote:** Epinephrine.

For Veterinary Use Only

How Supplied: 10 dose (20 ml) vials and 50 dose (100 ml) vials.

PALOSEIN®
brand of orgotein for injection
For intramuscular use in horses and subcutaneous use in dogs.

Description: Palosein, brand of orgotein, is a preparation of superoxide dismutase with anti-inflammatory activity. Palosein is supplied as a lyophilized solid comprising 5 mg orgotein, with 10 mg Sucrose USP per dose. Flame-sealed ampuls of Sodium Chloride Injection USP (pH 6.5–7.0) are provided for dissolving Palosein.

Chemistry: Orgotein, the assigned generic name (USANC) for Palosein, is a naturally occurring copper- and zinc-containing metalloprotein of molecular weight approximately 32,000 purified from bovine liver. Orgotein contains a trace of carbohydrate components. In the Palosein formulation, orgotein displays superoxide dismutase enzymatic activity (>3000 U/mg) and no other significant levels of enzyme activity.

Pharmacology: The toxicity of Palosein, brand of orgotein, is of an extremely low order. Acute, subacute, chronic, and teratologic studies in a number of species have failed to demonstrate any adverse reactions with doses of orgotein varying from 400,000 times the single horse rate (on a mg per kg basis) in acute studies to 200 times the horse dose rate in chronic and reproduction studies. The maximum acute intravenous toxicity dose tested was greater than 10,000 times the recommended intramuscular dose rate in horses. Orgotein showed no demonstrable influence on heart rate or blood pressure. It manifested none of the adverse reactions characteristic of the steroidal or non-steroidal anti-inflammatory agents. Unlike the steroids, it does not interfere with wound healing.

Palosein, brand of orgotein, exhibits anti-inflammatory activity in bioassay models. The efficacy of orgotein as an anti-inflammatory agent in horses and dogs has been demonstrated in controlled clinical trials and in models of induced inflammation. Its mode of action appears to differ from those of synthetic anti-inflammatory agents.

Parenterally administered orgotein is a weak immunogen, however no clinically significant adverse reactions were associated with orgotein treatment in horses or dogs during clinical trials. In subsequent clinical use, sensitization has rarely been

Continued on next page

Coopers—Cont.

reported. A large number of hematological and chemical laboratory tests showed no significant difference in distribution of change from baseline. A slight rise in white cell count, gammaglobulin, and alkaline phosphatase was occasionally seen in horses, with the change, however, always remaining within normal ranges.

Indications: Palosein, brand of orgotein, is indicated for acute and chronic inflammatory conditions.

Equine: Palosein, brand of orgotein, is indicated in the treatment of soft tissue inflammation associated with the musculoskeletal system of horses.

Canine: Palosein is recommended for the relief of inflammation associated with ankylosing spondylitis, spondylosis and disc disease in dogs. When severe nerve damage causes the disability, response to orgotein therapy will occur much more slowly, if at all.

Precautions: Paradoxical transitory exacerbations of symptoms prior to onset of improvement have been reported on occasion in horses.

In the treatment of inflammatory conditions associated with infection, specific anti-infective therapy is additionally required.

Clinical studies with dogs indicate that paraplegia associated with lack of response to painful stimuli exhibits no response to Palosein.

Warning: Not for use in horses intended for food.

Dosage and Administration: Orgotein is supplied as a lyophilized, sterile, nonpyrogenic solid in single-dose vials containing 5 mg of the active medication. The solid should be dissolved immediately prior to administration with the Sodium Chloride Injection provided. No other Sodium Chloride Injection should be used. Since orgotein is freely soluble in Sodium Chloride Injection, as little as 1 ml can be used if desired. Any diluent not used at the time of reconstitution must be discarded, as the special Sodium Chloride Injection pH 6.5–7.0 does not contain a preservative. Palosein dissolves instantly; avoid vigorous shaking of solution.

Equine: Deep intramuscular injection is the only route of administration approved for clinical use.

The dose of orgotein for horses is 5 mg every other day for two weeks and twice weekly for two to three more weeks. For acute conditions, shorter courses of therapy may be worthy of trial. Severe cases, both acute and chronic, may benefit more from daily therapy initially. Dosage may be continued beyond five weeks. If animals relapse or are re-injured, Palosein treatment may be re-instituted. In contrast to orthodox therapy, the animals can be exercised to tolerance during orgotein treatment, except where fractures and/or frank ligamentous tears are present.

Canine: The dose of Palosein for dogs is 5 mg every day for 6 days and thereafter, every other day for 8 days. Administration is by subcutaneous injection. In less severe conditions, shorter courses of therapy may be worthy of trial. If animals relapse or are re-injured, Palosein treatment may be re-instituted.

Adverse Reactions: Rare allergic hypersensitivity reactions associated with the administration of Palosein, including urticaria and pruritus in horses and systemic anaphylaxis in dogs, have been reported.

Contraindications: Use of Palosein is contraindicated in animals that have previously demonstrated hypersensitivity to orgotein or other bovine proteins.

Storage Conditions: Palosein, brand of orgotein, should be stored in a cool, dry place until reconstituted, after which refrigeration at 4°C (40°F) is required. Use only if solution appears clear.

Caution: The unused portion of opened ampuls of Sodium Chloride Injection must be discarded to prevent use at a later time.

How Supplied: Palosein, brand of orgotein, is supplied in single-dose vials. Each contains 5 mg of orgotein and 10 mg of Sucrose USP as lyophilized, sterile, nonpyrogenic solid. Each Palosein vial is provided with an individual 2 ml flame-sealed ampul of Sodium Chloride Injection USP (pH 6.5–7.0, without preservative). Available in package of six each of Palosein with Sodium Chloride Injection.

P.D.C.™
Penicillin G procaine in Dihydrostreptomycin Solution Injectable Antibiotic Preparation

Composition: Each ml of aqueous suspension contains: Penicillin G procaine 200,000 units; Dihydrostreptomycin sulfate, equivalent to dihydrostreptomycin base 0.25 g.

Preservatives: Phenyl 0.25%, Butylparaben 0.015%; Sodium formaldehyde sulfoxylate 0.37%; Procaine hydrochloride 2.0%.

Inert ingredients: Sodium citrate, 1.25%; lecithin, 0.25%; povidone, 0.5%; urea, 0.21%; dibasic sodium phosphite, 2% and sodium hydroxide.

Action and Uses: Penicillin is a potent antibiotic possessing high activity against most gram-positive bacteria. Dihydrostreptomycin sulfate is a highly effective antibiotic possessing activity against most gram-negative bacteria.

P.D.C. represents a combination of penicillin and dihydrostreptomycin antibiotics possessing a high degree of effectiveness against certain bacterial diseases of livestock, pets, and furbearing animals. P.D.C. takes advantage of the synergistic action obtained when dihydrostreptomycin and penicillin are combined, yielding a dosage form with a spectrum of activity including both the gram-negative and gram-positive bacteria.

Indications: P.D.C. is indicated in the following bacterial diseases when caused by organisms that are susceptible to the action of penicillin and dihydrostreptomycin.

Cattle and Calves: Infectious diarrheas, shipping fever, pneumonia, bronchitis, tracheitis, pleurisy, navel infections, footrot, and in bacillary dysentery as supportive treatment.

Swine: Infectious enteritis, pneumonia, bronchitis, pleurisy, tracheitis, erysipelas, mastitis, and bacillary infections associated with pneumonia.

Lambs and Sheep: Scours, shipping fever, pneumonia, navel infections, wound infections, and complications of mastitis.

Horses: Infectious diarrhea, pneumonia, bronchitis, pleurisy, shipping fever, strangles, and bacillary infections associated with pneumonia.

Dogs, Cats, Rabbits, Mink, and Foxes: Otitis externa, infectious diarrhea, pneumonia, bronchitis, tracheitis, pleurisy, and bacillary infections associated with pneumonia.

Turkeys: Erysipelas.

Contraindications:

1. Dihydrostreptomycin is eliminated to a large extent through the kidneys. The use of this product in animals suffering from renal insufficiency or urinary obstruction is therefore contraindicated.
2. Penicillin is a substance of low toxicity. However, allergic or anaphylactoid reactions —sometimes fatal —have been known to occur in animals hypersensitive to penicillin and procaine. The use of this product in such animals is contraindicated. Should anaphylactoid reactions occur, inject epinephrine immediately.

Warning: *Milk that has been taken from animals during treatment and for 48 hours (4 milkings) after the latest treatment must not be used for food. The use of this drug must be discontinued for 30 days before treated animals are slaughtered for food.*

Restricted drug—use only as directed.

Precautions: 1. Store below 15°C (59°F). For ease of administration, warm to room temperature and shake well before using.

2. Do not inject subcutaneously, into blood vessel, or near a major nerve.
3. Most sick animals that have been properly treated with antibiotics show a noticeable improvement within 36 to 48 hours. If improvement is not noted within that period of time, the diagnosis should be reconsidered and proper measures taken.

Dosage and Administration: P.D.C. should be administered by deep intramuscular injection. Shake well. The usual dose is 1 ml for every 100 lb of body weight, except in small animals.

In lactating dairy animals, do not give more than 2,000 units of penicillin or 2.5 mg of dihydrostreptomycin per pound of body weight per day. Injection of more than this dose will cause residue of penicillin and dihydrostreptomycin in milk for longer than 48 hours.

Continue treatment for one or two days after symptoms disappear.

Cattle and Calves: 1 ml for every 100 lb of body wt.

Lambs and Sheep: 8 to 10 lb—0.5 ml; 10 to 20 lb—1 ml; 20 to 50 lb—1 to 2 ml; 50 to 100 lb—2 to 6 ml.

Dogs, Cats, Rabbits, Mink, and Foxes: 2 to 5 lb—0.25 ml; 5 to 10 lb—0.25 to 0.50 ml; 10 to 15 lb—0.50 to 0.75 ml; 15 to 20 lb—0.75 to 1 ml; 20 to 25 lb—1 to 1.5-ml; 25 to 50 lb—2 to 3 ml; 50 to 75 lb—3 to 5 ml.
Swine: 8 to 10 lb—0.5 ml; 10 to 40 lb—1 to 2 ml; 40 to 100 lb—2 to 5 ml; 100 to 200 lb—5 to 8 ml; 200 lb or over—8 to 10 ml.
Horses: Up to 300 lb.—5 to 8 ml; 300 to 600 lb—8 to 10 ml; 600 lb or over—10 to 15 ml.
Turkeys: 5 to 10 lb—0.1 to 0.2 ml; 10 to 20 lb—0.2 to 0.4 ml; 20 to 30 lb—0.4 to 0.6 ml.

For Veterinary Use Only.

How Supplied: P.D.C. is available in 100 ml and 250 ml multiple dose vials.

POLTIS POWDER
Antiphlogistic Agent

Composition: Contains: Colloidal bentonite 99% with aromatics.
Poltis Powder is a finely divided colloidal aluminum silicate, with aromatic oil, possessing the property of absorbing several times its own weight of liquid to form a semi-solid pasty mass.
Action and Uses: The value of Poltis Powder lies in its ability to absorb several times its weight of water forming a gelatinous mass or a firm paste according to the amount of water added. This property is valuable in the reduction of acute inflammatory swellings when applied hot, or as a decongestant when chilled to a low temperature (strains, etc.).
Indications: For external application to help counteract inflammation and reduce swelling. Applied cold, it forms a desirable packing for softening the horny structures of the feet of horses or cattle.
Directions for Use: For use as an antiphlogistic, Poltis Powder is best prepared in a covered earthen vessel. Take any quantity of the product desired, add either hot or cold water and stir thoroughly. Add more water from time to time until the desired consistency is obtained. The prepared poultice mass can be warmed or chilled as indicated. Addition of one ounce of glycerine to each quart of water used will further enhance the antiphlogistic properties. Poltis Powder should be spread thickly and evenly over the affected area with a spatula or fingertips. Heat or cold retention is enhanced by encasement with a wrap of cotton covered by a woolen bandage.
For Veterinary Use Only
How Supplied: 5 lb (454 g) jars.

SCOLABAN® TABLETS ℞
(bunamidine hydrochloride)
Anthelmintic

Composition: Scolaban (bunamidine hydrochloride) a product of The Wellcome Foundation, is one of a series of naphthamidines, selected for its activity as a taeniacide. Bunamidine hydrochloride, N,N-dibutyl-4-(hexyloxy)-1-naphthamidine hydrochloride, is a white, odorless crystalline solid, soluble in methanol and hot water. It has a molecular weight of 419.0 and a melting point of 208–211°C.
Scolaban is an off-white compression-coated tablet with a yellow core. This is a fast disintegrating tablet to allow for maximum efficiency, once administered.
Action: Scolaban is a true taeniacide. It is effective against the tapeworms of dogs: *Dipylidium caninum, Taenia pisiformis,* and *Echinococcus granulosis,* and in cats: *Taenia taeniaeformis* and *Dipylidium caninum.* With Scolaban, the whole tapeworm, including the scolex is quickly destroyed and disintegrates usually before leaving the intestinal tract. Since the worms disintegrate, segments are not usually seen in the feces after treatment.
Advantages: Scolaban in tablet form for oral use provides a simple and effective means of ridding cats and dogs of tapeworms without causing undesirable cathartic effects. Normally, it causes death of the entire parasite and does not, as in the case of some taeniafuges, merely detach the proglottids from scolex and neck thus leaving these portions to restrobilate.
Indications: Scolaban tablets are indicated in common tapeworm infections of dogs and cats. When used as directed, the drug is well tolerated. Some reports indicate that Scolaban may not penetrate thick mucous to exert its effect. A heavy mucous covering (due to enteric pathology) may thus interfere with the efficacy of Scolaban. It is suggested that animals having heavy infections of tapeworms may have catarrhal enteritis and may need retreatment.
Echinococcus granulosus: Scolaban is highly effective for the removal of adult hydatid tapeworms at the recommended dose rate. It is also active against immature stages, the degree depending on the age of the young worms.
For single exposures and infection, the treatment should be repeated in 4–6 weeks.
When treating dogs having continuous access to possibly infected meat or carcasses, repeat treatment at 4–6 week intervals until such exposure is eliminated.
Control of this parasite is of public health importance in areas where it occurs since humans can become infected from dogs.
In control programs the primary focus should be on preventing dogs gaining access to infected carcasses and raw offal.
Dosage and Administration: Scolaban should be given on an empty stomach after a 3 or 4 hour fast. The animal may be fed about 3 hours after treatment. The recommended dosage of 25–50 mg/kg is given as a single dose.
Three tablet sizes are available:
Scolaban 100 contains 100 mg for cats and small dogs.
Cats—½–1 tablet
Dogs—1 tablet per 4½ to 9 lbs bodyweight.
Scolaban 200 contains 200 mg.
Dogs—1 tablet per 9 to 18 lbs bodyweight.
Scolaban 400 contains 400 mg.
Dogs—1 tablet per 18 to 36 lbs bodyweight.
Precautions: The active ingredient of Scolaban, bunamidine hydrochloride, is irritating to the conjunctiva. Where it is necessary to halve a tablet, care should be taken to avoid transferring particles to the eyes. Irritation may also occur to the oral mucous membranes if tablets are crushed in the mouth of the animal. Because of this possibility, the tablets should not be crushed, mixed with food, or dissolved in liquid. Repeat treatments, if necessary, should not be given within 14 days.
Antidote: Wash affected areas with clean water.
Side Effects: Vomiting has been noted occasionally in dogs. In nearly all instances, the animals had food in the stomach. The three hour pretreatment fasting period has reduced the incidence of vomiting almost to nil. Rarely, a mild transient diarrhea has been reported to occur a few hours after treatment.
Toxicology: No significant toxicity was observed in cats given a single dose of 50 mg/kg bunamidine base. Vomiting and diarrhea were observed after single oral doses of 150 or 250 mg/kg bunamidine base.
Idiosyncratic Reactions: There have been reports of rare idiosyncratic reactions characterized by sudden collapse and death following therapeutic doses of Scolaban in dogs. The majority of dogs experiencing these reactions received a dose in excess of 1000 mg of bunamidine hydrochloride. The onset of these reactions is very rapid and not preceded by premonitory symptoms but in some cases has been associated with excitement or exercise. While the exact mechanism of action involved in these rare reactions is not known, it has been postulated that they may result from ventricular fibrillation following sensitization of cardiac muscle to endogenous catecholamines. (Fastier, et al).
Cardiac Effects: Slight, transient changes in the ECG were observed after a single oral dose of 150 mg/kg—3 times the recommended dose. After an oral dose of 250 mg/kg marked changes were observed in the ECG in two of four cats and recovery was incomplete 24 hours after dosing. Slight to severe transient changes in the ECG were observed between the 5th and the 10th dose in cats given daily doses of 50 mg /kg bunamidine base. Recovery was virtually complete by 24 hours after dosing. The ECG changes that were observed after high or prolonged dosing with bunamidine are suggestive of myocardial dysfunction. However, there did not appear to be any permanent damage, nor were there any symptoms associated with cardiac insufficiency.
Spermatogenesis: Snow and Barenfus studied the effect of Scolaban on spermatogenesis in both dogs and cats. At the maximum recommended dose of 50 mg/kg bunamidine, no adverse effect was found in cats. Possible slight interference with spermatogenesis was ob-

Continued on next page

Coopers—Cont.

served in 3 of 8 mongrel dogs after a single oral dose of 50 mg/kg bunamidine. The study was repeated in mature beagles and evidence of reduced spermatogenesis was found in 2 of 3 dogs examined four days after treatment. Groups of three dogs examined at 28 and 50 days after dosing showed no suppression of spermatogenesis.
In a study at the Wellcome Research Laboratories two dogs were given a single oral dose of 100 mg/kg bunamidine hydrochloride. Semen was collected weekly from these dogs and from controls, for several weeks prior to and for 9 weeks after treatment. All samples were normal in volume, color, motility, density and morphology. No evidence of adverse effect on sperm quality or quantity was observed. Three dogs were given 100 mg/kg bunamidine daily for 7 days and semen was collected from these and from 3 controls weekly for 10 weeks. No difference in semen quality or quantity between treated and control animals was detected.
Effects on Pregnancy: Scolaban tablets were given at the dose rate of 100 mg/kg bunamidine base to 10 bitches at varying stages of pregnancy with 10 additional bitches serving as untreated controls. Results showed no differences between the litters.
Hamner concluded that bunamidine hydrochloride has no effect on pregnancy in the cat as measured by the number of cats becoming pregnant, gestation length, weight gain during pregnancy, litter size or survival after birth.
Contraindications: Scolaban should not be given to dogs or cats with a known heart condition.
Male dogs should not be used for breeding purposes within 28 days of treatment.
Do not use butamisole concurrently with Scolaban since an acute toxic reaction, sometimes fatal, may occur.
Avoid use of Scolaban in animals with impaired liver function.
Reports from some countries suggest that Scolaban should not be used in severely debilitated animals.
KEEP OUT OF REACH OF CHILDREN
Caution: Federal (U.S.A.) law restricts this drug to use by or on the order of a licensed veterinarian.
How Supplied: Scolaban 100 Tablets, bottles of 100 tablets; Scolaban 200 Tablets, bottles of 50 tablets; Scolaban 400 Tablets, bottles of 30 tablets.

SITEGUARD® G
Clostridium Perfringens Types C and D Toxoid

Composition: A formalin-inactivated, alum-precipitated toxoid prepared from highly toxigenic culture filtrates of *Clostridium perfringens* Types C and D.
Siteguard G is an Electroferm® product produced by an electronically-controlled deep culture process.
The specific toxoids required for optimal disease protection are emphasized in the growth of Electroferm cultures. These cultures are highly concentrated and when divided for the blending of combination vaccines make possible the production of low volume doses. Exacting procedures are employed in the blending process to assure that each dose of combination vaccine contains an accurate amount of each component.
All components of each serial of the final product are tested for potency using USDA-approved laboratory and/or host animal tests.
Indications: For the active immunization of healthy cattle and sheep against diseases caused by *Cl. perfringens* Types C and D.
Although *Cl. perfringens* Type B is not a significant problem in the USA, immunity may be provided against the beta and epsilon toxins elaborated by *Cl. perfringens* Type B. This immunity is derived from the combination of Type C (beta) and Type D (epsilon) fractions.
Action and Uses: Clostridial organisms fall into groupings based on the primary site at which infection occurs. These sites are muscle, liver and gastrointestinal (GI) tract as shown below.
Primary Infection Sites of Clostridial Organisms of Most Concern in Cattle and Sheep

Organism	Muscle	Liver	GI Tract
Cl. chauvoei	+		
Cl. septicum	+		
Cl. sordellii	+		
Cl. novyi Type B		+	
Cl novyi Type D		+	
Cl. perfringens Type B			+
Cl. perfringens Type C			+
Cl. perfringens Type D			+

Siteguard G contains clostridial organisms that protect against diseases of only the gastrointestinal group. These are listed in the chart above. Information on the action of these organisms is provided below.
Gastrointestinal Group: *Cl. perfringens* Types B, C, and D are normal inhabitants of the intestinal tracts of cattle, sheep and swine. Under anoxic conditions caused by the ingestion of large quantities of concentrated feeds, sudden changes in diet, etc., these organisms multiple rapidly and release destructive toxins. In the very young, this frequently follows the ingestion of large quantities of rich milk. This condition often takes the form of a pure toxemia (enterotoxemia), with toxins being absorbed into the circulation from the intestine and producing destructive effects on vital organs and sudden death. It may in addition cause severe intestinal lesions, particularly in young animals (hemorrhagic enteritis, necrotic enteritis). The management programs of feeding and production operations often predispose animals to this condition.
Protection: Siteguard G contains inactivated toxins (toxoids). Protection results when the immune mechanism responds to toxoids by producing antitoxin. These antitoxins neutralize the toxin produced following the vegetation of inhabitant spores.
The protective value of all components of Siteguard G has been demonstrated through the most critical test procedures available. *Cl. perfringens* Types C and D, for which no host-animal direct-challenge test exists, were evaluated by measuring the amount of antitoxin produced by cattle, sheep and laboratory animals.
Dosage and Administration: Shake well. Using aseptic technique, inject subcutaneously or intramuscularly. Cattle, 4 ml; sheep, 2 ml, repeated in 3–4 weeks. Revaccinate annually prior to periods of extreme risk or parturition.
Caution: Store at not over 45°F or 7°C. Protect from freezing. Use entire contents when first opened. Do not vaccinate within 21 days before slaughter. Anaphlyactoid reactions may occur following use. **Antidote:** Epinephrine.
For Veterinary Use Only
How Supplied: 40 ml—10 cattle doses or 20 sheep doses. 200 ml—50 cattle doses or 100 sheep doses.

SITEGUARD® L
Clostridium Haemolyticum-Novyi Bacterin-Toxoid

Composition: A formalin-inactivated, alum-precipitated bacterin-toxoid prepared from highly toxigenic cultures of *Clostridium novyi* Type B and *Cl. haemolyticum* (known elsewhere as *Cl. novyi* Type D*).
Siteguard L is an Electroferm® product produced by an electronically-controlled deep culture process.
The specific toxoids and/or cellular antigens required for optimal disease protection are emphasized in the growth of Electroferm cultures. These cultures are highly concentrated and when divided for the blending of combination vaccines make possible the production of low volume doses. Exacting procedures are employed in the blending process to assure that each dose of combination vaccine contains an accurate amount of each component.
All components of each serial of the final product are tested for potency using USDA-approved laboratory and/or host animal tests.
Indications: For the active immunization of healthy cattle and sheep against diseases caused by *Cl. novyi* Type B and *Cl. haemolyticum* (known elsewhere as *Cl. novyi* Type D*).
Action and Uses: Clostridial organisms fall into groupings based on the primary site at which infection occurs. These sites are muscle, liver and gastrointestinal (GI) tract as shown below.
Primary Infection Sites of Clostridial Organisms of Most Concern in Cattle and Sheep

Organism	Muscle	Liver	GI Tract
Cl. chauvoei	+		
Cl. septicum	+		
Cl. sordellii	+		
Cl. novyi Type B		+	
Cl. novyi Type D		+	

Cl. perfringens Type B	+
Cl. perfringens Type C	+
Cl. perfringens Type D	+

Siteguard L contains clostridial organisms that protect against diseases of only the liver group. These are listed in the chart above. Information on the action of these organisms is provided below.

Liver Group: Spores of the clostridial organisms whose primary infection site is the liver (*Cl. novyi* Types B and D) are latent residents of such tissue. These spores are acquired from the digestive tract following ingestion of contaminated plants, dust, feed, etc. Some form of liver damage is necessary for their activation and initiation of disease. Precipitating and predisposing factors include abscesses, chemicals, fatty changes, internal parasites, flukes, plant toxins, telangiectasis (sawdust liver) and bacterial hepatitis. The management programs of feedlots and production operations often produce these factors. Powerful toxins produced by the multiplying organisms cause death through destructive effects on vital organs and blood vessels. Fatalities may occur suddenly, as early as 24 hours after onset of infection.

Protection: Siteguard L contains inactivated cellular antigens (bacterins) and inactivated toxins (toxoids). Protection results when the immune mechanism responds to cellular antigens by producing antibodies, and to toxoids by producing antitoxin. These antibodies and antitoxins prevent the bacterial growth and/or neutralize the toxin produced following the vegetation of inhabitant spores. The protective value of all components of Siteguard L has been demonstrated through the most critical test procedures available. Vaccinated cattle withstood challenge with massive doses of virulent live spores of *Cl. novyi* Types B and D.

Dosage and Administration: Shake well. Using aseptic technique, inject subcutaneously or intramuscularly. Dosage: 5 ml, repeated in 3–4 weeks. Revaccinate every 5–6 months and just prior to periods of extreme risk.

Caution: Store at not over 45°F or 7°C. Protect from freezing. Use entire contents when first opened. Do not vaccinate within 21 days before slaughter. Anaphylactoid reactions may occur following use. **Antidote:** Epinephrine.

For Veterinary Use Only

How Supplied: 10 and 50 dose

*Cl. novyi and *Cl. haemolyticum* are generally indistinguishable without extensive biochemical tests. Macheak[1] has stated: *Cl. haemolyticum* and *Cl. novyi* should be regarded in the laboratory as one group since their morphologic and cultural characteristics are closely related . . . All strains of *Cl. novyi* appear to have two somatic antigens in common; one of these is shared with *Cl. haemolyticum*. European scientists have suggested that *Cl. haemolyticum* should be classified as *Cl. novyi* Type D.

1. Macheak, M.E.: Veterinary Medicine/Small Animal Clinician: 73 (2): 197, February 1978.

SITEGUARD® M
Clostridium Chauvoei-Septicum-Sordellii Bacterin-Toxoid

Composition: A formalin-inactivated, alum-precipitated bacterin-toxoid prepared from highly toxigenic cultures and culture filtrates of *Clostridium chauvoei, Cl. septicum* and *Cl. sordellii.*

Siteguard M is an Electroferm® product produced by an electronically-controlled deep culture process.

The specific toxoids and/or cellular antigens required for optimal disease protection are emphasized in the growth of Electroferm cultures. These cultures are highly concentrated and when divided for the blending of combination vaccines make possible the production of low volume doses. Exacting procedures are employed in the blending process to assure that each dose of combination vaccine contains an accurate amount of each component.

All components of each serial of the final product are tested for potency using USDA-approved laboratory and/or host animal tests.

Indications: For the active immunization of healthy cattle and sheep against diseases caused by *Cl. chauvoei, Cl. septicum* and *Cl. sordellii.*

Action and Uses: Clostridial organisms fall into groupings based on the primary site at which infection occurs. These sites are muscle, liver and gastrointestinal (GI) tract as shown below.

Primary Infection Sites of Clostridial Organisms of Most Concern in Cattle and Sheep

Organism	Muscle	Liver	GI Tract
Cl. chauvoei	+		
Cl. septicum	+		
Cl. sordellii	+		
Cl. novyi Type B		+	
Cl novyi Type D		+	
Cl. perfringens Type B			+
Cl. perfringens Type C			+
Cl. perfringens Type D			+

Siteguard M contains clostridial organisms that protect against diseases of only the muscle group. These are listed in the chart above. Information on the action of these organisms is provided below.

Muscle Group: Highly resistant spores of the clostridial organisms whose primary infection site is the muscle (*Cl. chauvoei, Cl. septicum, Cl. sordellii*), are deposited there by the circulation following oral ingestion or contamination of wounds. Under localized anoxic conditions produced by injuries, bruises, etc., these spores vegetate and the resulting organisms multiply. These conditons commonly occur in feedlots and farms during handling, transportation, and animal interaction, i.e., butting and riding. Bacterial growth produces gangrenous myositis. Toxins released by the multiplying organisms and by destroyed cells enter the circulation, producing death through destructive effects on vital organs. Fatalities may occur suddenly, as early as 12 hours from onset of infection.

Protection: Siteguard M contains inactivated cellular antigens (bacterins) and inactivated toxins (toxoids). Protection results when the immune mechanism responds to cellular antigens by producing antibodies, and to toxoids by producing antitoxin. These antibodies and antitoxins prevent the bacterial growth and/or neutralize the toxin produced following the vegetation of inhabitant spores. The protective value of all components of Siteguard M has been demonstrated through the most critical test procedures available. Vaccinated cattle withstood challenge with massive doses of virulent live spores of *Cl. chauvoei* and *Cl. sordellii.* Protection afforded by *Cl. septicum* has been demonstrated by vaccination and challenge studies in sheep, the only host animal species for which a satisfactory experimental challenge method exists.

Dosage and Administration: Shake well. Using aseptic technique, inject subcutaneously or intramuscularly. Dosage: 5 ml, repeated in 3–4 weeks and annually. Animals vaccinated under 3 months of age should be revaccinated at weaning or 4–6 months of age.

Caution: Store at not over 45°F or 7°C. Protect from freezing. Use entire contents when first opened. Do not vaccinate within 21 days before slaughter. Anaphylactoid reactions may occur following use. **Antidote:** Epinephrine.

For Veterinary Use Only

How Supplied: 10 and 50 dose

SITEGUARD® M PLUS PASTEURELLA
Clostridium Chauvoei-Septicum-Sordellii Pasteurella Haemolytica-Multocida Bacterin-Toxoid

Description: A formalin-inactivated, alum-precipitated bacterin-toxoid prepared from highly toxigenic cultures and culture filtrates of *Clostridium chauvoei, Cl. septicum, Cl. sordellii* and *Pasteurella haemolytica* and *P. multocida.*

Cultures produced by improved methods are used for pasteurella components. The *Cl. chauvoei, Cl. septicum,* and *Cl. sordellii* components are produced by an electronically-controlled deep culture process.

The specific toxoids and/or cellular antigens required for optimal disease protection are emphasized in the growth of Electroferm® cultures. These cultures are highly concentrated and when divided for the blending of combination vaccines make possible the production of low volume doses. Exacting procedures are employed in the blending process to assure that each dose of combination vaccine contains an accurate amount of each component.

All components of each serial of the final product are tested for potency using USDA-approved laboratory and/or host animal tests.

Continued on next page

Coopers—Cont.

Indications: For the active immunization of healthy cattle and sheep against diseases caused by *Clostridium chauvoei, Cl. septicum, Cl. sordellii, Pasteurella haemolytica* and *P. multocida.*

Actions and Uses: Clostridial organisms fall into groupings based on the primary site at which infection occurs. These sites are muscle, liver and gastrointestinal (GI) tract as shown below.

Primary Infection Sites of Clostridial Organisms of Most Concern in Cattle and Sheep

Organism	Muscle	Liver	GI Tract
Cl. chauvoei	+		
Cl. septicum	+		
Cl. sordellii	+		
Cl. novyi Type B		+	
Cl. novyi Type D		+	
Cl. perfringens Type B			+
Cl. perfringens Type C			+
Cl. perfringens Type D			+

Siteguard® M *plus* Pasteurella contains clostridial organisms that protect against diseases of only the muscle group. These are listed in the chart above. Information on the action of these organisms is provided below.

Muscle Group: Highly resistant spores of the clostridial organisms whose primary infection site is the muscle (*Cl. chauvoei, Cl. septicum, Cl. sordellii*), are deposited there by the circulation following oral ingestion or contamination of wounds. Under localized anoxic conditions produced by injuries, bruises, etc., these spores vegetate and the resulting organisms multiply. These conditions commonly occur in feedlots and farms during handling, transportation, and animal interaction, i.e., butting and riding. Bacterial growth produces gangrenous myositis. Toxins released by the multiplying organisms and by destroyed cells enter the circulation, producing death through destructive effects on vital organs. Fatalities may occur suddenly, as early as 12 hours from onset of infection.

Protection: Siteguard M *plus* Pasteurella contains inactivated cellular antigens (bacterins) and inactivated toxins (toxoids). Protection results when the immune mechanism responds to cellular antigens by producing antibodies, and to toxoids by producing antitoxin. These antibodies and antitoxins prevent the bacterial growth and/or neutralize the toxin produced following the vegetation of inhabitant spores.

The protective value of all components of Siteguard M *plus* Pasteurella has been demonstrated through the most critical test procedures available. Vaccinated cattle withstood challenge with massive doses of virulent live spores of *Cl. chauvoei* and *Cl. sordellii.* Protection afforded by *Cl. septicum* has been demonstrated by vaccination and challenge studies in sheep, the only host animal species for which a satisfactory experimental challenge method exists.

The use of Siteguard M *plus* Pasteurella should be considered when it is desirable to vaccinate for pasteurellosis at the same time as diseases of the muscle group.

Dosage and Administration: Shake well. Using aseptic technique, inject subcutaneously or intramuscularly. Dosage: 5 ml, repeated in 3–4 weeks and annually. Animals vaccinated under 3 months of age should be revaccinated at weaning or 4–6 months of age.

Caution: Store at not over 45°F or 7°C. Protect from freezing. Use entire contents when first opened. Do not vaccinate within 21 days before slaughter. Anaphylactoid reactions may occur following use. **Antidote:** Epinephrine.

For Veterinary Use Only

How Supplied: 10 and 50 dose

SITEGUARD® MG
Clostridium Chauvoei-Septicum-Sordellii-Perfringens Types C & D Bacterin-Toxoid

Description: A formalin-inactivated, alum-precipitated bacterin-toxoid prepared from highly toxigenic cultures and culture filtrates of *Clostridium chauvoei, Cl. septicum, Cl. sordellii* and*Cl. perfringens* Types C and D.

Siteguard MG is an Electroferm® product produced by an electronically-controlled deep culture process.

The specific toxoids and/or cellular antigens required for optimal disease protection are emphasized in the growth of Electroferm cultures. These cultures are highly concentrated and when divided for the blending of combination vaccines make possible the production of low volume doses. Exacting procedures are employed in the blending process to assure that each dose of combination vaccine contains an accurate amount of each component.

All components of each serial of the final product are tested for potency using USDA-approved laboratory and/or host animal tests.

Indications: For the active immunization of healthy cattle and sheep against diseases caused by *Cl. chauvoei, Cl. septicum, Cl. sordellii* and *Cl. perfringens* Types C and D.

Although *Clostridium perfringens* Type B is not a significant problem in the USA, immunity may be provided against the beta and epsilon toxins elaborated by *Cl. perfringens* Type B. This immunity is derived from the combinations of Type C (beta) and Type D (epsilon) fractions.

Actions and Uses: Clostridial organisms fall into groupings based on the primary site at which infection occurs. These sites are muscle, liver and gastrointestinal (GI) tract as shown below.

Primary Infection Sites of Clostridial Organisms of Most Concern in Cattle and Sheep

Organism	Muscle	Liver	GI Tract
Cl. chauvoei	+		
Cl. septicum	+		
Cl. sordellii	+		
Cl. novyi Type B		+	
Cl. novyi Type D		+	
Cl. perfringens Type B			+
Cl. perfringens Type C			+
Cl. perfringens Type D			+

Siteguard MG contains clostridial organisms that protect against diseases of only the muscle and gastrointestinal groups. These are listed in the chart above. Information on the action of these organisms is provided below.

Muscle Group: Highly resistant spores of the clostridial organisms whose primary infection site is the muscle *(Cl. chauvoei, Cl. septicum, Cl. sordellii),* are deposited there by the circulation following oral ingestion or contamination of wounds. Under localized anoxic conditions produced by injuries, bruises, etc., these spores vegetate and the resulting organisms multiply. These conditions commonly occur in feedlots and farms during handling, transportation, and animal interaction, i.e., butting and riding. Bacterial growth produces gangrenous myositis. Toxins released by the multiplying organisms and by destroyed cells enter the circulation, producing death through destructive effects on vital organs. Fatalities may occur suddenly, as early as 12 hours from onset of infection.

Gastrointestinal Group: *Cl. perfringens* Types B, C, and D are normal inhabitants of the intestinal tract of cattle, sheep and swine. Under anoxic conditions caused by the ingestion of large quantities of concentrated feeds, sudden changes in diet, etc., these organisms multiply rapidly and release destructive toxins. In the very young, this frequently follows the ingestion of large quantities of rich milk. This condition often takes the form of a pure toxemia (enterotoxemia), with toxins being absorbed into the circulation from the intestines and producing destructive effects on vital organs and sudden death. It may in addition cause severe intestinal lesions, particularly in young animals (hemorrhagic enteritis, necrotic enteritis). The management programs of feeding and production operations often predispose animals to this condition.

Protection: Siteguard MG contains inactivated cellular antigens (bacterins) and inactivated toxins (toxoids). Protection results when the immune mechanism responds to cellular antigens by producing antibodies, and to toxoids by producing antitoxin. These antibodies and antitoxins prevent the bacterial growth and/or neutralize the toxin produced following vegetation of inhabitant spores.

The protective value of all components of Siteguard MG has been demonstrated through the most critical test procedures available. Vaccinated cattle withstood challenge with massive doses of virulent live spores of *Cl. chauvoei* and *Cl. sordellii.* Protection afforded by *Cl. septicum* has been demonstrated by vaccination and challange studies in sheep, the only

C

host animal species for which a satisfactory experimental challenge method exists. *Cl. perfringens* Types C and D, for which no host-animal direct-challenge test exists, were evaluated by measuring the amount of antitoxin produced by cattle, sheep and laboratory animals.
Dosage and Administration: Shake well. Using aseptic technique, inject subcutaneously or intramuscularly. Dosage: 5 ml, repeated in 3–4 weeks. Revaccinate annually prior to periods of extreme risk, or parturition. Animals vaccinated under 3 months of age should be revaccinated at weaning or 4–6 months of age.
Caution: Store at not over 45°F ot 7°C. Protect from freezing. Use entire contents when first opened. Do not vaccinate within 21 days before slaughter. Anaphylactoid reactions may occur following use. **Antidote:** Epinephrine.
For Veterinary Use Only
How Supplied: 10 and 50 dose

SITEGUARD® ML
Clostridium Chauvoei-Septicum-Haemolyticum-Novyi-Sordellii Bacterin-Toxoid

Composition: A formalin-inactivated, alum-precipitated bacterin-toxoid prepared from highly toxigenic cultures and culture filtrates of *Clostridium chauvoei, Cl. septicum, Cl. sordellii, Cl. novyi* Type B and *Cl. haemolyticum* (known elsewhere as *Cl. novyi* Type D*).
Siteguard ML is an Electroferm® product produced by an electronically-controlled deep culture process.
The specific toxoids and/or cellular antigens required for optimal disease protection are emphasized in the growth of Electroferm cultures. These cultures are highly concentrated and when divided for the blending of combination vaccines make possible the production of low volume doses. Exacting procedures are employed in the blending process to assure that each dose of combination vaccine contains an accurate amount of each component.
All components of each serial of the final product are tested for potency using USDA-approved laboratory and/or host animal tests.
Indications: For the active immunization of healthy cattle and sheep against diseases caused by *Cl. chauvoei, Cl. septicum, Cl. sordellii, Cl. novyi* Type B and *Cl. haemolyticum* (known elsewhere as *Cl. novyi* Type D*).
Actions and Uses: Clostridial organisms fall into groupings based on the primary site at which infection occurs. These sites are muscle, liver and gastrointestinal (GI) tract as shown below.
Primary Infection Sites of Clostridial Organisms of Most Concern in Cattle and Sheep

Organism	Muscle	Liver	GI Tract
Cl. chauvoei	+		
Cl. septicum	+		
Cl. sordellii	+		
Cl. novyi Type B		+	
Cl. novyi Type D		+	
Cl. perfringens Type B			+
Cl. perfringens Type C			+
Cl. perfringens Type D			+

Siteguard ML contains clostridial organisms that protect against diseases of only the muscle and liver groups. These are listed in the chart above. Information on the action of these organisms is provided below.
Muscle Group: Highly resistant spores of the clostridial organisms whose primary infection site is the muscle (*Cl. chauvoei, Cl. septicum, Cl. sordellii*), are deposited there by the circulation following oral ingestion or contamination of wounds. Under localized anoxic conditions produced by injuries, bruises, etc., these spores vegetate and the resulting organisms multiply. These conditions commonly occur in feedlots and farms during handling, transportation, and animal interaction, i.e., butting and riding. Bacterial growth produces gangrenous myositis. Toxins released by the multiplying organisms and by destroyed cells enter the circulation, producing death through destructive effects on vital organs. Fatalities may occur suddenly, as early as 12 hours from onset of infection.
Liver Group: Spores of the clostridial organisms whose primary infection site is the liver (*Cl. novyi* Types B and D) are latent residents of such tissue. These spores are acquired from the digestive tract following ingestion of contaminated plants, dust, feed, etc. Some form of liver damage is necessary for their activation and initiation of disease. Precipitating and predisposing factors include abscesses, chemicals, fatty changes, internal parasites, flukes, plant toxins, telangiectasis (sawdust liver) and bacterial hepatitis. The management programs of feedlots and production operations often produce these factors. Powerful toxins produced by the multiplying organisms cause death through destructive effects on vital organs and blood vessels. Fatalities may occur suddenly, as early as 24 hours after onset of infection.
Protection: Siteguard ML contains inactivated cellular antigens (bacterins) and inactivated toxins (toxoids). Protection results when the immune mechanism responds to cellular antigens by producing antibodies, and to toxoids by producing antitoxin. These antibodies and antitoxins prevent the bacterial growth and/or neutralize the toxin produced following the vegetation of inhabitant spores.
The protective value of all components of Siteguard ML has been demonstrated through the most critical test procedures available. Vaccinated cattle withstood challenge with massive doses of virulent live spores of *Cl. chauvoei, Cl. sordellii, Cl. novyi* Types B and D. Protection afforded by *Cl. septicum* has been demonstrated by vaccination and challenge studies in sheep, the only host animal species for which a satisfactory experimental challenge method exists.
Dosage and Administration: Shake well. Using aseptic technique, inject subcutaneously or intramuscularly. Dosage: 5 ml, repeated in 3–4 weeks. Revaccinate annually prior to periods of extreme risk. Animals vaccinated under 3 months of age should be revaccinated at weaning or 4–6 months of age. For *Cl. novyi* and *Cl. haemolyticum* revaccinate every 5–6 months.
Caution: Store at not over 45°F or 7°C. Protect from freezing. Use entire contents when first opened. Do not vaccinate within 21 days before slaughter. Anaphylactoid reactions may occur following use. **Antidote:** Epinephrine.
For Veterinary Use Only
How Supplied: 10 and 50 dose
* *Cl. novyi* and *Cl. haemolyticum* are generally indistinguishable without extensive biochemical tests. Macheak[1] has stated: *Cl. haemolyticum* and *Cl. novyi* should be regarded in the laboratory as one group since their morphologic and cultural characteristics are closely related . . . All strains of *Cl. novyi* appear to have two somatic antigens in common; one of these is shared with *Cl. haemolyticum.* European scientists have suggested that *Cl. haemolyticum* should be classified as *Cl. novyi* Type D.

1. Macheak, M.E.: Veterinary Medicine/Small Animal Clinician: 73 (2): 197, February 1978.

SITEGUARD® ML plus NOVALEP® P
Clostridium Chauvoei-Septicum-Haemolyticum-Novyi-Sordellii Leptospira Pomona Bacterin-Toxoid

Composition: A formalin-inactivated, alum-precipitated bacterin-toxoid prepared from highly toxigenic cultures and culture filtrates of *Clostridium chauvoei, Cl. septicum, Cl. sordellii, Cl. novyi* Type B, *Cl. haemolyticum* (known elsewhere as *Cl. novyi* Type D*) and *Leptospira pomona.*
Siteguard ML *plus* Novalep P is an Electroferm® product produced by an electronically-controlled deep culture process.
The specific toxoids and/or cellular antigens required for optimal disease protection are emphasized in the growth of Electroferm cultures. These cultures are highly concentrated and when divided for the blending of combination vaccines make possible the production of low volume doses. Exacting procedures are employed in the blending process to assure that each dose of combination vaccine contains an accurate amount of each component.
Novalep P is a highly purified, adjuvanted bacterin prepared from inactivated cultures of *L. pomona* grown in a low-protein medium. In addition to the use of this medium, the non-protective, potentially allergenic by-products of bacterial metabolism are removed by selective molecular filtration.
All components of each serial of the final product are tested for potency using USDA-approved laboratory and/or host animal tests.

Continued on next page

Coopers—Cont.

Indications: For the active immunization of healthy cattle and sheep against diseases caused by *Clostridium chauvoei, Cl. septicum, Cl. sordellii, Cl. novyi* Type B, *Cl. haemolyticum* (known elsewhere as *Cl. novyi* Type D*), and *Leptospira pomona.*

Actions and Uses: Clostridial organisms fall into groupings based on the primary site at which infection occurs. These sites are muscle, liver and gastrointestinal (GI) tract as shown below.

Primary Infection Sites of Clostridial Organisms of Most Concern in Cattle and Sheep

Organism	Muscle	Liver	GI Tract
Cl. chauvoei	+		
Cl. septicum	+		
Cl. sordellii	+		
Cl. novyi Type B		+	
Cl. novyi Type D		+	
Cl. perfringens Type B			+
Cl. perfringens Type C			+
Cl. perfringens Type D			+

Siteguard ML plus Novalep P contains clostridial organisms that protect against diseases of only the muscle and liver groups. These are listed in the chart above. Information on the action of these organisms is provided below.

Muscle Group: Highly resistant spores of the clostridial organisms whose primary infection site is the muscle *(Cl. chauvoei, Cl. septicum, Cl. sordellii),* are deposited there by the circulation following oral ingestion or contamination of wounds. Under localized anoxic conditions produced by injuries, bruises, etc., these spores vegetate and the resulting organisms multiply. These conditions commonly occur in feedlots and farms during handling, transportation, and animal interaction, i.e., butting and riding. Bacterial growth produces gangrenous myositis. Toxins released by the multiplying organisms and by destroyed cells enter the circulation, producing death through destructive effects on vital organs. Fatalities may occur suddenly, as early as 12 hours from onset of infection.

Liver Group: Spores of the clostridial organisms whose primary infection site is the liver (*Cl. novyi* Types B and D) are latent residents of such tissue. These spores are acquired from the digestive tract following ingestion of contaminated plants, dust, feed, etc. Some form of liver damage is necessary for their activation and initiation of disease. Precipitating and predisposing factors include abscesses, chemicals, fatty changes, internal parasites, flukes, plant toxins, telangiectasis (sawdust liver) and bacterial hepatitis. The management programs of feedlots and production operations often produce these factors. Powerful toxins produced by the multiplying organisms cause death through destructive effects on vital organs and blood vessels. Fatalities may occur suddenly, as early as 24 hours after onset of infection.

Protection: Siteguard ML *plus* Novalep P contains inactivated cellular antigens (bacterins) and inactivated toxins (toxoids). Protection results when the immune mechanism responds to cellular antigens by producing antibodies, and to toxoids by producing antitoxin. These antibodies and antitoxins prevent the bacterial growth and/or neutralize the toxin produced following the vegetation of inhabitant spores.

The protective value of all components of Siteguard ML *plus* Novalep P has been demonstrated through the most critical test procedures available. Vaccinated cattle withstood challenge with massive doses of virulent live spores of *Cl. chauvoei, Cl. sordellii, Cl. novyi* Types B and D. Protection afforded by *Cl. septicum* has been demonstrated by vaccination and challenge studies in sheep, the only host animal species for which a satisfactory experimental challenge method exists.

Dosage and Administration: Shake well. Using aseptic technique, inject subcutaneously or intramuscularly. Dosage: 5 ml, repeated in 3–4 weeks. Revaccinate annually prior to periods of extreme risk. For *Cl. novyi* and *Cl. haemolyticum* revaccinate every 5–6 months. Animals vaccinated under 3 months of age should be revaccinated at weaning or 4–6 months of age.

Caution: Store at not over 45°F or 7°C. Protect from freezing. Use entire contents when first opened. Do not vaccinate within 21 days before slaughter. Anaphylactoid reactions may occur following use. **Antidote:** Epinephrine.

For Veterinary Use Only

How Supplied: 10 and 50 dose

**Cl. novyi* and *Cl. haemolyticum* are generally indistinguishable without extensive biochemical tests. Macheak[1] has stated: *Cl. haemolyticum* and *Cl. novyi* should be regarded in the laboratory as one group since their morphologic and cultural characteristics are closely related ... All strains of *Cl. novyi* appear to have two somatic antigens in common; one of these is shared with *Cl. haemolyticum.* European scientists have suggested that *Cl. haemolyticum* should be classified as *Cl. novyi* Type D.

1. Macheak, M.E.: Veterinary Medicine/Small Animal Clinician: 73 (2): 197, February 1978.

SITEGUARD® MLG
Clostridium Chauvoei-Septicum-Haemolyticum-Novyi-Sordellii-Perfringens Types C and D Bacterin-Toxoid

Composition: A formalin-inactivated, alum-precipitated bacterin-toxoid prepared from highly toxigenic cultures and culture filtrates of *Clostridium chauvoei, Cl. septicum, Cl. sordellii, Cl. novyi* Type B, *Cl. haemolyticum* (known elsewhere as *Cl. novyi* Type D*) and *Cl. perfringens* Types C and D.

Siteguard MLG is an Electroferm® product produced by an electronically-controlled deep culture process. The specific toxoids and/or cellular antigens required for optimal disease protection are emphasized in the growth of Electroferm cultures. These cultures are highly concentrated and when divided for the blending of combination vaccines make possible the production of low volume doses. Exacting procedures are employed in the blending process to assure that each dose of combination vaccine contains an accurate amount of each component.

All components of each serial of the final product are tested for potency using USDA-approved laboratory and/or host animal tests.

Indications: For the active immunization of healthy cattle and sheep against diseases caused by *Cl. chauvoei, Cl. septicum, Cl. sordellii, Cl. novyi* Type B, *Cl. haemolyticum* (known elsewhere as *Cl. novyi* Type D*) and *Cl. perfringens* Types C and D.

Although *Cl. perfringens* Type B is not a significant problem in the USA, immunity may be provided against the beta and epsilon toxins elaborated by *Cl. perfringens* Type B. This immunity is derived from the combination of Type C (beta) and Type D (epsilon) fractions.

Actions and Uses: Clostridial organisms fall into groupings based on the primary site at which infection occurs. These sites are muscle, liver and gastrointestinal (GI) tract as shown below.

Primary Infection Sites of Clostridial Organisms of Most Concern in Cattle and Sheep

Organism	Muscle	Liver	GI Tract
Cl. chauvoei	+		
Cl. septicum	+		
Cl. sordellii	+		
Cl. novyi Type B		+	
Cl. novyi Type D		+	
Cl. perfringens Type B			+
Cl. perfringens Type C			+
Cl. perfringens Type D			+

Muscle Group: Highly resistant spores of the clostridial organisms whose primary infection site is the muscle *(Cl. chauvoei, Cl. septicum, Cl. sordellii),* are deposited there by the circulation following oral ingestion or contamination of wounds. Under localized anoxic conditions produced by injuries, bruises, etc., these spores vegetate and the resulting organisms multiply. These conditions commonly occur in feedlots and farms during handling, transportation, and animal interaction, i.e., butting and riding. Bacterial growth produces gangrenous myositis. Toxins released by the multiplying organisms and by destroyed cells enter the circulation, producing death through destructive effects on vital organs. Fatalities may occur suddenly, as early as 12 hours from onset of infection.

Liver Group: Spores of the clostridial organisms whose primary infection site is the liver (*Cl. novyi* Types B and D) are latent residents of such tissue. These spores are acquired from the digestive tract following ingestion of contaminated plants, dust, feed, etc. Some form of liver damage is necessary for their activation and initiation of disease. Precipitating and predisposing factors include abscesses, chemicals, fatty changes, internal parasites, flukes, plant toxins, telangiectasis (sawdust liver) and bacterial hepatitis. The management programs of feedlots and production operations often produce these factors. Powerful toxins produced by the multiplying organisms cause death through destructive effects on vital organs and blood vessels. Fatalities may occur suddenly, as early as 24 hours after onset of infection.

Gastrointestinal Group: *Cl. perfringens* Types B, C, and D are normal inhabitants of the intestinal tracts of cattle, sheep and swine. Under anoxic conditions caused by the ingestion of large quantities of concentrated feeds, sudden changes in diet, etc., these organisms multiply rapidly and release destructive toxins. In the very young, this frequently follows the ingestion of large quantities of rich milk. This condition often takes the form of a pure toxemia (enterotoxemia), with toxins being absorbed into the circulation from the intestine and producing destructive effects on vital organs and sudden death. It may in addition cause severe intestinal lesions, particularly in young animals (hemorrhagic enteritis, necrotic enteritis). The management programs of feeding and production operations often predispose animals to this condition.

Protection: Siteguard MLG contains inactivated cellular antigens (bacterins) and inactivated toxins (toxoids). Protection results when the immune mechanism responds to cellular antigens by producing antibodies, and to toxoids by producing antitoxin. These antibodies and antitoxins prevent the bacterial growth and/or neutralize the toxin produced following the vegetation of inhabitant spores.

The protective value of all components of Siteguard MLG has been demonstrated through the most critical test procedures available. Vaccinated cattle withstood challenge with massive doses of virulent live spores of *Cl. chauvoei, Cl. sordellii, Cl. novyi* Types B and D. Protection afforded by *Cl. septicum* has been demonstrated by vaccination and challenge studies in sheep, the only host animal species for which a satisfactory experimental challenge method exists. *Cl. perfringens* Types C and D, for which no host-animal direct-challenge test exists, were evaluated by measuring the amount of antitoxin produced by cattle, sheep and laboratory animals.

Dosage and Administration: Shake well. Using aseptic technique, inject subcutaneously or intramuscularly. Dosage: 5 ml, repeated in 3–4 weeks. Revaccinate annually prior to periods of extreme risk, or parturition. For *Cl. novyi* and *Cl. haemolyticum* revaccinate every 5–6 months. Animals vaccinated under 3 months of age should be revaccinated at weaning or 4–6 months of age.

Caution: Store at not over 45°F or 7°C. Protect from freezing. Use entire contents when first opened. Do not vaccinate within 21 days before slaughter. Anaphylactoid reactions may occur following use. **Antidote:** Epinephrine.

For Veterinary Use Only

How Supplied: 10, 50 and 200 dose

**Cl. novyi* and *Cl. haemolyticum* are generally indistinguishable without extensive biochemical tests. Macheak[1] has stated: *Cl. haemolyticum* and *Cl. novyi* should be regarded in the laboratory as one group since their morphologic and cultural characteristics are closely related . . . All strains of *Cl. novyi* appear to have two somatic antigens in common; one of these is shared with *Cl. haemolyticum*. European scientists have suggested that *Cl. haemolyticum* should be classified as *Cl. novyi* Type D.

1. Macheak, M.E.: Veterinary Medicine/Small Animal Clinician: 73 (2): 197, February 1978.

STAPHOID™ A-B
Staphylococcus Aureus Bacterin-Toxoid

Description: This product contains cellular antigens and toxoids derived from quantities of both alpha and beta toxins. Whole cultures of *Staphylococcus aureus* representing bacteriophage typing groups I, III and IV are inactivated with formalin and adsorbed on aluminum hydroxide gel. Each serial is tested in rabbits to assure proper immunologic response.

Indications: For use in healthy cattle as an aid in prevention of infections due to *Staphylococcus aureus*.

Action and Uses: Staphoid A-B stimulates the development of antibodies against somatic antigens, and antitoxins against alpha and beta toxins. Blobel, Derbyshire, Greenberg and other workers have noted that single-strain bacterins will not confer protection against challenge with heterologous strains. In the preparation of Staphoid A-B, over 100 strains of staphylococci were collected from infected udders in dairy herds in the United States and Europe. To assure broad spectrum protection, cultures were selected from the principal phage groups appearing in the collection.

Administration and Dosage: Shake well to produce an even suspension and inject intramuscularly or subcutaneously using aseptic technique.

Staphoid A-B should be given preferably to dry cows and first calf heifers prior to calving. An initial dose of 5 ml is recommended. A second dose of 5 ml is given 2 weeks later. To maintain high antibody levels, additional injections of 5 ml are recommended annually. In heavily infected herds the 5 ml booster dose should be given at intervals of six months. In dairy animals the booster dose should be administered two to four weeks before calving.

Since mature animals appear to respond better, cattle should be at least one year old at the time of initial vaccination. Maximum antibody levels are usually attained approximately two weeks after revaccination.

Contraindications: Staphoid A-B should not be administered to animals with acute mastitis, or animals suffering from acute disease.

Caution:
1. Store at not over 45° For 7°C. Protect from freezing.
2. Use entire contents when first opened.
3. Do not vaccinate within 21 days before slaughter.
4. Anaphylactoid reactions may occur following use. **Antidote:** Epinephrine. Other supportive measures, such as antihistamines and corticosteroids, may be indicated.

Local reactions may occur in some animals. The exact nature of these reactions is not fully understood, but is thought to be a local manifestation of a hypersensitive state. These local reactions most commonly occur after booster vaccinations.

In herds with history of previous hypersensitivity reactions or when the allergic status of the animals is in doubt, a test dose in a few animals several days before complete herd vaccination should be considered.

For Veterinary Use Only

How Supplied: 50 ml—10 dose vials, 250 ml—50 dose vials.

C

STREPVAX® II
Streptococcus Equi Bacterial Extract (Strangles Vaccine)

Description: The active component of Strepvax II is a concentrated, purified M-protein extract of *S. equi*. Extraction of M-protein antigen is accomplished through use of an advanced, patented process developed by Coopers Animal Health Inc., Kansas City (U.S. Patents 3,793,150 and 3,852,420).

The antigenicity is enhanced by adsorption on aluminum hydroxide.

Action and Uses: The serious nature of strangles has motivated scientists around the world to investigate the *S. equi* organism in the search for an efficacious, safe vaccine.

In early research work, the hyaluronic acid capsule was considered the primary virulence factor preventing phagocytosis of the organism. This led to development of whole cell bacterins. These provided some protection, but achieved only limited use because of their unusually high dose volume and the occurrence of frequent, often severe post-vaccination reactions. Subsequent work led to a significant reduction of dose volume.

In the past decade, workers at Coopers Animal Health have concentrated on identifying nonreactive bacterial components capable of producing protection. Their work, and that of others, showed *S. equi* to contain an extractable, antigenic M-protein which fulfilled this objective.

Strepvax II stimulates the production of anti-M-protein antibodies that are believed to promote the phagocytic destruction of virulent *S. equi*. It is well-tolerated by most horses. Horses vaccinated

Continued on next page

Coopers—Cont.

in field trials ranged in age from 3 weeks to 20 years.
Strepvax II is recommended as an *aid* in strangles control because immunity to *S. equi* can be overwhelmed by severe challenge exposure. When used as directed, Strepvax II has been shown to reduce the incidence and/or severity of disease.
The value and limitations of Strepvax II must be well understood by both veterinarians and horse owners if unrealistic expectations and subsequent disappointments are to be avoided. When used in conjuction with good hygiene, appreciable benefits can be obtained.
Horses should be revaccinated at least annually with Strepvax II. Primary and booster immunization may be integrated with other vaccination schedules.
Special emphasis should be placed on horses in herds or stables subject to frequent additions of new animals and/or on animals returning from off-premise use, breeding, etc.
Horses known to have been exposed but not showing signs of disease should be isolated from non-exposed animals. Those showing signs of disease should be further isolated. Surfaces in barns, etc., subject to contamination by exudates from diseased horses should be disinfected.
Indications: For use in healthy horses of all ages as an aid in the prevention of disease (strangles) due to *S. equi* infection.
Dosage and Administration:
Shake well.
Using aseptic technique, inject 1 ml intramuscularly, preferably in the hind quarters. For primary immunization, give 3 doses at intervals of 3 weeks .
Foals vaccinated when less than 3 months of age should receive an additional dose at 6 months or at time of weaning.
Revaccinate annually and prior to anticipated exposure, using a single 1 ml dose.
Use a separate sterile needle for each injection.
Caution: Store at not over 45°F or 7°C.
Protect from freezing.
Use entire contents when first opened.
Field reports suggest certain hypersensitive individuals may demonstrate local or generalized reactions, sometimes severe, following exposure to streptococcal proteins. Field studies indicate that post-vaccinal exercise immediately following each injection will appreciably decrease the incidence and duration of local reactions.
Anaphylactoid reactions may occur following use. **Antidote:** Epinephrine.
For Veterinary Use Only
How Supplied: 10- 1-dose syringes and 10-dose vials.

TETANUS ANTITOXIN
Equine Origin

Composition: Tetanus Antitoxin is prepared from the blood of healthy equines that have been hyperimmunized with repeated doses of *Clostridium tetani* toxin. The product is concentrated and bacteriologically tested for sterility.
Indications: For prophylactic use to confer short-term passive immunity against tetanus and, in larger doses, to aid in early treatment of animals affected with tetanus.
Action and Uses: Horses and sheep are most frequently affected with tetanus, cattle and swine occasionally, carnivorous animals rarely, and birds never. The natural occurrence of tetanus corresponds closely with susceptibility to tetanus toxin.
Tetanus antitoxin is used to confer passive immunity when susceptible animals suffer a wound. An increased prophylactic dose may be indicated in neglected and deep-seated wounds, especially in unvaccinated animals.
Protection gained from antitoxin is limited to approximately two weeks.
When used for treatment in the early stages of the disease, doses much larger than those used prophylactically are employed. However, there can be no assurance that treatment will be successful, since the degree and duration of exposure to the organism are frequently unknown.
Dosage and Administration: Administer subcutaneously or intramuscularly using aseptic technique.
Prophylaxis: 1,500 to 4,500 units for adult cattle and horses. Minimum of 200 units for lambs following surgery. Minimum of 500 units for sheep, calves and pigs.
Treatment: 10,000 units or more. When used for treatment, there can be no assurance of success since the degree and duration of toxemia are frequently unknown.
Caution: Store at not over 45°F or 7°C. Use entire contents when first opened. Do not vaccinate within 21 days before slaughter. Contains cresol as a preservative. This is a heterologous protein for species other than equine. Anaphylactoid reactions may occur following use.
Antidote: Epinephrine.
For Veterinary Use Only
How Supplied: 10-1,500 unit vials. 10,000 unit vials.

THENATOL®
(thenium closylate and piperazine phosphate)
Anthelmintic ℞

Composition: Thenatol 375 tablets contain thenium closylate [N,N-dimethyl-N-(2-phenoxyethyl)-2-thenyl-ammonium-p-chlorobenzenesulfonate] equivalent to 125 mg thenium base and piperazine phosphate equivalent to 250 mg piperazine hexahydrate base.
Thenatol® 750 tablets contain thenium closylate [N,N-dimethyl-N-(2-phenoxyethyl)-2-thenylammonium-p-chlorobenzenesulfonate] equivalent to 250 mg thenium base and piperazine phosphate equivalent to 500 mg piperazine hexahydrate base.
Indications: For removal of immature (4th stage larvae) and adult hookworms (*Ancylostoma caninum, Ancylostoma braziliense* and *Uncinaria stenocephala)* and ascarids (*Toxocara canis*) from weaned pups weighing 2 pounds or more and from adult dogs.
Contraindications: Dogs weighing less than 2 pounds, unweaned pups and pups under 5 weeks of age should not be treated with this product.
Action and Uses: Ascarid infections are common in dogs and, with few exceptions, are universal in pups. The distribution of hookworm infections depends on climatic conditions. In hookworm-enzootic areas dual infections with hookworms and ascarids have been observed in almost three out of every four dogs.
Thenium closylate has been shown to have anthelmintic efficacy in dogs against hookworms (*Ancylostoma caninum, Ancylostoma braziliense* and *Uncinaria stenocephala*), but lower and variable efficacy against ascarids (*Toxocara canis* and *Toxascaris leonina*). Piperazine salts have high anthelmintic efficacy against ascarids (*T. canis* and *T. leonina*) but have negligible activity against two of the canine hookworms (*A. caninum* and *A. braziliense*), and variable or poor activity in normal dosage levels against the third (*U. stenocephala*).
Treatment of dogs with the combination of thenium closylate and piperazine phosphate is efficacious against both hookworms and ascarids. Thenium and piperazine in combination act synergistically since the combination has appreciably increased efficacy over single component values. Thenatol is designed for the treatment of mixed infections of hookworms and ascarids in weaned pups and dogs. In addition to being efficacious against adult hookworms of all three species, the combination has the advantage of being effective against immature (4th stage and immature 5th stage) hookworms of all three species (*A. caninum, A. braziliense* and *U. stenocephala*) on and after the 7th day postinfection, such that the worms may be expelled before they have an opportunity to commence their pathogenic activities.
[See table on next page].
Adverse Reactions: Dogs should not be allowed to chew the tablets because the bitter taste may result in salivation and rejection.
The only side effect observed in dogs treated with the recommended dosage of Thenatol under laboratory and clinical conditions was vomiting. This was observed at the same low rate and intensity in placebo treated controls.
In the event of inadvertent overdosage with Thenatol, vomiting will occur. Dogs that were deliberately overdosed vomited within one hour; some also exhibited diarrhea within five hours. These reactions to overdosage represent a safety feature since signs of systemic toxicity could not be induced.
Thenatol must not be administered to unweaned pups because the high fat content of bitch's milk facilitates absorption of the thenium component with the risk of systemic toxocity. In addition, the vomiting reflex in these pups is poorly developed. Systemic toxicity in unweaned pups is exhibited by depression.

Results of critical controlled tests to measure anthelmintic efficacy of Thenatol tablets against fourth stage, immature and mature hookworms in weaned pups and dogs.

	Study location	Control Values: No. of observations	Control Values: *Worm burdens	Age (days) and stage of worms when treated		No. of dogs treated	Efficacy (% of worms expelled*)
I.	**Ancylostoma caninum**						
	Jensen-Salsbery	17	598±1277	7	4th larvae	13	87±7
	Laboratories	6	112±126	11	Immature adults	6	88±13
	(3 studies)	22	294±1277	13–17	Mature adults	19	97±5
	Cornell University	10	701±236	7	4th larvae	10	85
				11	Immature adults	10	91-98
	Laboratory Research Enterprises, Inc.	12	759±126	7	4th larvae	10	82
				17	Mature adults	8	96
II.	**Ancylostoma brazilinese**						
	Jensen-Salsbery Laboratories	6	686±140	11	Immature adults	5	83
	Laboratory Research Enterprises, Inc.	10	644±79	7	4th larvae	10	82–85
				17	Mature adults	10	91
	University of Georgia	10	568±161	7	4th larvae	10	91
				17	Mature adults	10	97
III.	**Uncinaria stenocephala**						
	Jensen-Salsbery Laboratories	5	40±46	>13	Mature adults	5	86-97
	Cornell University	10	426±55	7	4th larvae	10	85
				11	Immature adults	10	86-97
	Laboratory Research Enterprises, Inc.	12	529±59	7	4th larvae	10	84
				17	Mature adults	8	90

*Values are group mean, range of means or group mean ± standard deviation.

Results of critical controlled tests to measure anthelmintic efficacy of Thenatol tablets against *Toxocara canis* in weaned pups and dogs.

Study location	Worm stage at treatment	No. of worms in dogs	No. of dogs treated	Efficacy (group mean) ±std. deviation: % worms expelled from treated dogs	Corrected for % worms spontेously voided from controls
Jensen-Salsbery Laboratories	Immature	1–9	5	100±0	96
Jensen-Salsbery Laboratories	Mature	1–10	15	80±37	76
University of Missouri	Mature	16–40	5	99±3	90
University of Missouri	Mature	12–49	5	75±26	71

Thenatol is not recommended for use in dogs less than 5 weeks of age or weighing less than 2 pounds because insufficient data have been accumulated to support such use.

For another product containing thenium closylate, rare reactions of a toxic nature, sometimes fatal, have been reported in adult dogs.

Dosage and Administration: Dogs—orally. Maximum anthelmintic efficacy against hookworms necessitates a 2-dose treatment. The interval between the two doses should be at least 4 hours but not more than 24 hours. Administer the first dose in the morning before feeding. Feed the dog between first and second dose. Do not feed milk or other fatty foods during treatment.

Treatment may need to be repeated in 7-28 days as determined by follow-up laboratory fecal examinations or in animals reintroduced to known contaminated quarters.

[See table on next page].

Precautions: Do not feed milk or other fatty foods during treatment.

To reduce the risks of human infection and the potential for visceral larva migrans in children, collect all stools from dogs infected with *T. canis* for the first 48 hours after treatment and destroy by incineration or burying deep in the ground.

Caution: Federal (U.S.A.) law restricts this drug to use by or on the order of a licensed veterinarian.

How Supplied: Thenatol 375—bottles of 100 tablets, Thenatol 750—bottles of 100 tablets.

THIONIUM® SHAMPOO
Cleanser

Composition: A pleasantly scented, biodegradable shampoo for dogs and cats. For routine shampooing of dogs and cats to help maintain healthy skin and a lustrous hair coat. Contains 2% potassium tetrathionate, an active form of sulfur, in a stabilized aqueous detergent solution, with 8% denatured alcohol. Thionum Shampoo is a balanced combination of tetrathionates and detergent.

Continued on next page

Coopers—Cont.

Action and Uses: Thionium Shampoo exerts deep cleansing action. Stable, long-lasting suds which form in either hot or cold water, provide excellent wetting properties. This assures more thorough cleansing with greater penetration and dispersion.
While helping to maintain healthy skin and lustrous hair coat of dogs and cats, Thionium Shampoo leaves no gummy residue and will not stain clothing. Pleasantly scented, Thionium Shampoo is non-irritating, safe and easy to use.
Warning: Keep Out of Reach of Children.
Caution: For external use only. Avoid contact with eyes and metals. Store in a cool place.
Directions for Use: For routine shampooing of dogs and cats.
Wet animal thoroughly with warm water. Apply Thionium Shampoo and massage coat to produce an abundant lather. Rinse with warm water. Repeat as needed.
For Veterinary Use Only
How Supplied: 6 oz. and 1 gallon bottles.

THIONIUM® SHAMPOO WITH EXPAR®

—For dogs.
—Kills fleas and lice.
—Helps maintain healthy skin and lustrous hair coat.
—Exerts deep cleansing action.
—Removes skin debris.

Active Ingredient
Permethrin (3-phenoxyphenyl) methyl (±) cis, trans-3-(2,2-dichloroethenyl)-2,2-dimethylcyclopropane-carboxylate* 0.05%
Inert Ingredients..................... 99.95%**
100.00%
*cis/trans ratio: Max 55% (±) cis and min 45% (±) trans
**Includes 8% denatured alcohol.

A pleasantly scented shampoo containing an active form of sulfur, in a stabilized detergent solution, and Expar brand permethrin.
KEEP OUT OF REACH OF CHILDREN
Caution
PRECAUTIONARY STATEMENTS HAZARDS TO HUMANS AND DOMESTIC ANIMALS
Caution
Avoid contact with eyes. Wash thoroughly with soap and water after using.
Note to Veterinarian: This product has demonstrated dermal sensitization potential. Provide protective equipment such as rubber gloves to applicators. Inform applicators of the sensitization potential of this product and have them discontinue use if symptoms occur. Avoid frequent applications to the same animal. Observe animals closely and discontinue use if symptoms of dermal sensitization occur.
STATEMENT OF PRACTICAL TREATMENT
If In Eyes: Immediately flush eyes with water for at least five minutes. Get medical attention if irritation persists.
ENVIRONMENTAL HAZARDS
This product is toxic to fish. Keep out of lakes, ponds or streams. Do not contaminate water by cleaning of equipment or disposal of wastes.
Directions for Use
General Classification: It is a violation of Federal law to use this product in a manner inconsistent with its labeling.
Wet dog or cat thoroughly. Pour a little Thionium Shampoo with Expar into cup of hand. Rub over animal's wetted coat. Repeat application, adding small amounts of water and rub until coat is covered with lather. Allow lather to act five minutes to kill fleas or lice that might be present. Rinse with clean water.
STORAGE AND DISPOSAL
Storage: Store in cool, dry place.
Pesticide Disposal: Securely wrap original container in several layers of newspaper and discard in trash.
Container Disposal: Do not reuse empty bottle. Wrap bottle and put in trash.
How Supplied: 6 oz. squeeze bottles and 1 gallon jugs.

THIONIUM® SHAMPOO WITH LINDANE
Cleanser-Insecticidal

Composition:
Active Ingredients:
Potassium tetrathionate 2.00%
Lindane (gamma isomer of benzene hexachloride) 0.25%
Inert Ingredients 97.75%*
100%
*Includes 8% denatured ethyl alcohol.

Indications: For routine shampooing of dogs to help maintain natural luster to the hair coat and to aid in control of fleas, ticks, lice and sarcoptic mange mites.
Restricted Use Pesticide: For retail sale to and use only by certified applicators or persons under their direct supervision and only for those uses covered by the certified applicator's certification.
Directions for Use: It is a violation of Federal law to use this product in a manner inconsistent with its labeling.
Wet hair thoroughly with warm water. Apply sufficient Thionium® Shampoo with Lindane to produce an abundant lather. For best results massage thoroughly, and allow lather to remain in contact with the dog's hair and skin for five minutes or longer. Rinse with warm water. Repeat as often as needed, but not more than once weekly.
Keep Out of Reach of Children.
Precautionary Statements
Hazardous to Humans and Domestic Animals.
Harmful if swallowed. May be absorbed through the skin. Avoid contact with the eyes, skin and metals.
Applicators of lindane dog shampoos must wear the following protective clothing during the application process: waterproof, elbow-length gloves; a waterproof apron; unlined, waterproof boots. Wash thoroughly after using. Store in a cool place. Do not use on cats. Do not apply to nursing mothers or to puppies under 3 months of age. Do not use on sick or convalescent animals. Do not use more often than once weekly.
Statement of Practical Treatment
If swallowed: Call a physician or Poison Control Center immediately. Drink one or two glasses of water and induce vomiting by administering syrup of ipecac or by touching back of throat with finger. Repeat until vomit fluid is clear. Do not induce vomiting or give anything by mouth to an unconscious person.
If inhaled: Remove victim to fresh air. Apply artificial respiration if indicated.
If on skin: Remove contaminated clothing and immediately wash skin with soap and water.
If in eyes: Immediately flush eyes with water for at least 15 minutes and get medical attention.
Physician's note: This product contains a chlorinated hydrocarbon.
Environmental Hazards
This product is toxic to fish, birds, and other wildlife. Keep out of lakes, streams or ponds. Do not contaminate water by cleaning of equipment or by disposal of wastes.
Storage and Disposal
Do not contaminate water, food, or feed by storage or disposal.
Pesticide Disposal: Improper disposal of excess pesticide, spray mixture, or rinsate is a violation of Federal law. If these wastes cannot be disposed of by use according to label instructions, contact your State Pesticide or Environmental Control Agency, or the Hazardous Waste representative at the nearest EPA Regional Office for guidance.
Container Disposal: 6 oz Bottle - Do not reuse bottle. Rinse thoroughly before discarding in trash. Gallon Jug - Triple rinse (or equivalent). Then offer for recycling or reconditioning, or puncture and dispose of in a sanitary landfill, or incineration, or, if allowed by State and local authorities, by burning. If burned, stay out of smoke.
For Veterinary Use Only.
How Supplied: 6 oz. bottle and 1 gal. jug

Dosage Schedule

Weight of dog	Number of tablets at each of the two doses	
	Thenatol 375	Thenatol 750
2 lbs but less than 5 lbs	½	—
5 lbs but less than 10 lbs	1	½
10 lbs or heavier	2	1

AVERAGE MINIMUM INHIBITORY CONCENTRATION (MIC-mcg/ml)

Bacteria	TMP Alone	SDZ Alone	TMP/SDZ TMP	TMP/SDZ SDZ
Escherichia coli	0.31	26.5	0.07	1.31
Proteus species	1.3	24.5	0.15	2.85
Staphylococcus aureus	0.6	17.6	0.13	2.47
Pasteurella species	0.06	20.1	0.03	0.56
Salmonella species	0.15	61.0	0.05	0.95
βStreptococcus	0.5	24.5	0.15	2.85

TRIBRISSEN® 60 ORAL SUSPENSION
(trimethoprim and sulfadiazine)
For Use in Dogs ℞

Description: Tribrissen 60 Oral Suspension contains 10 mg trimethoprim* and 50 mg sulfadiazine per ml in a meat-flavored formulation.

Tribrissen is a combination of trimethoprim and sulfadiazine in the ratio of 1 part to 5 parts by weight, which provides effective antibacterial activity against a wide range of bacterial infections in animals.

Trimethoprim is 2,4 diamino-5-(3,4,5-trimethoxybenzyl) pyrimidine.

Actions:

Microbiology: Trimethoprim blocks bacterial production of tetrahydrofolic acid from dihydrofolic acid by binding to and reversibly inhibiting the enzyme dihydrofolate reductase.

Sulfadiazine, in common with other sulfonamides, inhibits bacterial synthesis of dihydrofolic acid by competing with *para*-aminobenzoic acid.

Tribrissen thus imposes a sequential double blockade on bacterial metabolism. This deprives bacteria of nucleic acids and proteins essential for survival and multiplication and produces a high level of antibacterial activity which is usually bactericidal.

Although both sulfadiazine and trimethoprim are antifolate, neither affects the folate metabolism of animals. The reasons are: animals do not synthesize folic acid and cannot, therefore, be directly affected by sulfadiazine; and although animals must reduce their dietary folic acid to tetrahydrofolic acid, trimethoprim does not affect this reduction because its affinity for dihydrofolate reductase of mammals is significantly less than for the corresponding bacterial enzyme.

Tribrissen is active against a wide spectrum of bacterial pathogens, both gram-negative and gram-positive. The following *in vitro* data are available, but their clinical significance is unknown. In general, species of the following genera are sensitive to Tribrissen:

Very Sensitive	**Sensitive**
Escherichia	*Staphylococcus*
Streptococcus	*Neisseria*
Proteus	*Klebsiella*
Salmonella	*Fusiformis*
Pasteurella	*Corynebacterium*
Shigella	*Clostridium*
Haemophilus	*Bordetella*
Moderately Sensitive	**Not Sensitive**
Moraxella	*Mycobacterium*
Nocardia	*Leptospira*
Brucella	*Pseudomonas*
	Erysipelothrix

As a result of the sequential double blockade of the metabolism of susceptible organisms by trimethoprim and sulfadiazine, the minimum inhibitory concentration (MIC) of Tribrissen is markedly less than that of either of the components used separately. Many strains of bacteria that are not susceptible to one or the other components are susceptible to Tribrissen. A synergistic effect between trimethoprim and sulfadiazine in combination has been shown experimentally both *in vitro* and *in vivo* (in dogs).

Tribrissen is bactericidal against susceptible strains and is often effective against sulfonamide-resistant organisms. *In vitro* sulfadiazine is usually only bacteriostatic.

The precise *in vitro* MIC of the combination varies with the ratio of the drugs present, but action of Tribrissen occurs over a wide range of ratios with an increase in the concentration of one of its coomponents compensating for a decrease in the other. It is usual, however, to determine MIC's using a constant ratio of one part trimethoprim in twenty parts of the combination.

The following table shows MIC's, using the above ratio, of bacteria which were susceptible to both trimethoprim (TMP) and sulfadiazine (SDZ). The organisms are those most commonly involved in conditions for which Tribrissen is indicated.

[See table above].

The following table demonstrates the marked effect of the trimethoprim and sulfadiazine combination against sulfadiazine-resistant strains of normally susceptible organisms:

[See table below].

Susceptibility Testing: In testing susceptibility to Tribrissen, it is essential that the medium used does not contain significant amounts of interfering substances which can bypass the metabolic blocking action, e.g., thymidine or thymine.

The standard SxT disc is appropriate for testing by the disc diffusion method.

AVERAGE MINIMUM INHIBITORY CONCENTRATION OF SULFADIAZINE-RESISTANT STRAINS (MIC-mcg/ml)

Bacteria	TMP Alone	SDZ Alone	TMP/SDZ TMP	TMP/SDZ SDZ
Escherichia coli	0.32	>245	0.27	5.0
Proteus species	0.66	>245	0.32	6.2

Pharmacology: Following oral administration, Tribrissen is rapidly absorbed and widely distributed throughout body tissues. Concentrations of trimethoprim are usually higher in tissues than in blood. The levels of trimethoprim are high in lung, kidney and liver, as would be expected from its lipophilic properties.

Studies with labeled trimethoprim in dogs have shown that about two-thirds of the dose is excreted in the urine in 24 hours.

Therapeutic serum levels are detected within one hour after dosing. In dogs, peak blood levels occur one to four hours after oral administration.

Usually, the concentration of an antibacterial in the blood and the *in vitro* MIC of the infecting organism indicate an appropriate period between doses of a drug. This does not hold entirely for Tribrissen because trimethoprim, in contrast to sulfadiazine, localizes in tissues and therefore, its concentration and ratio to sulfadiazine are higher there than in blood. Serum levels following dosing give an indication, however, of the probable duration of effectiveness of a single dose.

The following table shows the average serum concentration of trimethoprim and sulfadiazine in twelve healthy adult beagle dogs following administration of a single oral dose of approximately 30 mg/kg on two separate occasions.

[See table on next page].

Excretion of Tribrissen is chiefly by the kidneys, by both glomerular filtration and tubular secretion. Urine concentrations of Tribrissen are severalfold higher than blood concentrations. Neither trimethoprim nor sulfadiazine interferes with the excretion pattern of the other.

Indications and Usage: Tribrissen 60 Oral Suspension is indicated in dogs where potent systemic antibacterial action against sensitive organisms is required, either alone or as an adjunct to surgery or debridement with associated infection. Tribrissen 60 Oral Suspension is indicated where control of bacterial infections is required during treatment of:

Acute urinary tract infections
Acute bacterial complications of canine distemper
Acute respiratory tract infections
Acute alimentary tract infections
Wound infections and abscesses

Contraindications: Tribrissen 60 Oral Suspension should not be used in dogs showing marked liver parenchymal dam-

Continued on next page

Coopers—Cont.

age, blood dyscrasias or in those with a history of sulfonamide sensitivity.

Adverse Reactions: Conditions reported following use of trimethoprim/sulfadiazine include polyarthritis, urticaria, facial swelling, fever, hemolytic anemia, polydypsia/polyuria, vomiting, anorexia, diarrhea, and seizures. Keratitis sicca possibly due to prolonged use of Tribissen has been reported. This condition has also been associated with the prolonged use of other sulfonamide-containing products.

Hepatitis possibly due to sulfonamide hypersensitivity has been diagnosed following Tribrissen therapy.

Individual animal hypersensitivity may result in local or generalized reactions, sometimes fatal. Anaphylactoid reactions, although rare, may also occur —**Antidote:** Epinephrine.

Precautions: Water should be readily available to dogs receiving sulfonamide therapy.

Toxicity and Side Effects: Toxicity is low. The acute toxicity (LD_{50}) of Tribrissen is more than 5g/kg orally in rats and mice.

No significant changes were recorded in rats given doses of 600 mg/kg per day for 90 days.

Dogs can tolerate up to ten times the recommended therapeutic dose without exhibiting ill effects. Dogs dosed at 300 mg/kg per day for a period of 20 days revealed only slight changes in hematologic values.

Slight to moderate reductions in hematopoietic activity following high, prolonged dosage in several species have been recorded. This is usually reversible by folinic acid (leucovorin) administration or by stopping the drug. During long-term treatment of dogs, periodic platelet counts and white and red blood cell counts are advisable.

Reproduction: Dogs given therapeutic doses (30 mg/kg per day) of Tribrissen continuously and at interrupted intervals throughout pregnancy gave birth to normal progeny. From these studies, it appears that Tribrissen can safely be given to dogs during gestation.

Tribrissen has not been clinically evaluated in stud dogs and therefore cannot be recommended for use.

Dosage and Administration: The recommended dosage for dogs is 1 ml per 5 lb body weight per day. Measure dosage from the pint bottle with a teaspoon (approximately 5 ml), tablespoon (approximately 15 ml) or a measuring spoon. Oral cavity should be empty. Administer proper dose orally in the cheek pouch or mix in food in accordance with the following body weight/dose rate schedule.

Shake well before using.

Weight of Dog	Tribrissen 60 Oral Suspension	Approximate Common Measure
5 lb	1 ml	1/5 teaspoon
10 lb	2 ml	2/5 teaspoon
40 lb	8 ml	1/2 tablespoon
80 lb	16 ml	1 tablespoon

The recommended dose may be given once daily, or one-half the daily dose may be administered every 12 hours.

Continue acute infection therapy for two or three days after clinical signs have subsided.

If no improvement of acute infections is seen in three to five days, re-evaluate diagnosis. Therapy with Tribrissen 60 Oral Suspension is not recommended for more than 14 days. A complete blood count should be done periodically in patients receiving Tribrissen for prolonged periods. If significant reduction in the count of any formed blood element is noted, treatment with Tribrissen should be discontinued.

Tribrissen 60 Oral Suspension may be used alone or in conjunction with Tribrissen 24% Injection.

How Supplied: Tribrissen® 60 Oral Suspension is available in 12-ml syringes, and in pint (473 ml) bottles.

Caution: KEEP OUT OF REACH OF CHILDREN. Federal (U.S.A.) law restricts this drug to use by or on the order of a licensed veterinarian.

*Mfd. under Pat. 3,956,327

Tribrissen 60 Oral Suspension
AVERAGE SERUM CONCENTRATIONS (mcg/ml)

	Trimethoprim (5 mg/kg)				Sulfadiazine (25 mg/kg)			
TMP/SDZ	1 hr	2 hr	4 hr	25 hr	1 hr	2 hr	4 hr	25 hr
(30 mg/kg)	1.83	1.40	.83	<0.04	16.5	19.8	20.3	6.0

TRIBRISSEN®TABLETS ℞
(trimethoprim and sulfadiazine)
Antibacterial

Composition: Tribrissen 30 Tablets
(Each white sugar-coated tablet contains 5 mg trimethoprim* and 25 mg sulfadiazine)
Tribrissen 120 Tablets
(Each white sugar-coated tablet contains 20 mg trimethoprim* and 100 mg sulfadiazine)
Tribrissen 480 Tablets
(Each white scored tablet contains 80 mg trimethoprim* and 400 mg sulfadiazine)
Tribrissen 960 Tablets
(Each white unscored tablet contains 160 mg trimethoprim* and 800 mg sulfadiazine)

Description: Tribrissen is a synthetic antibacterial combination product which provides effective antibacterial activity for a wide range of bacterial infections in animals. The trimethoprim component of Tribrissen was discovered in the Wellcome Research Laboratories.

Tribrissen is a combination of trimethoprim and sulfadiazine in the ratio of 1 part to 5 parts by weight which provides effective antibacterial activity against a wide range of bacterial infections in animals.

Trimethoprim is 2,4 diamino-5-(3,4,5-trimethoxybenzyl)-pyrimidine.

Actions: Microbiology: Trimethoprim blocks bacterial production of tetrahydrofolic acid from dihydrofolic acid by binding to and reversibly inhibiting the enzyme dihydrofolate reductase.

Sulfadiazine, in common with other sulfonamides, inhibits bacterial synthesis of dihydrofolic acid by competing with *para*-aminobenzoic acid.

Tribrissen thus imposes a sequential double blockade on bacterial metabolism. This deprives bacteria of nucleic acids and proteins essential for survival and multiplication and produces a high level of antibacterial activity which is usually bactericidal.

Although both sulfadiazine and trimethoprim are antifolate, neither affects the folate metabolism of animals. The reasons are: animals do not synthesize folic acid and cannot, therefore, be directly affected by sulfadiazine; and although animals must reduce their dietary folic acid to tetrahydrofolic acid, trimethoprim does not affect this reduction because its affinity for dihydrofolate reductase of mammals is significantly less than for the corresponding bacterial enzyme.

Tribrissen is active against a wide spectrum of bacterial pathogens, both gram-positive and gram-negative. In general, species of the following genera are sensitive to Tribrissen:

Very Sensitive	Sensitive
Escherichia	*Staphylococcus*
Streptococcus	*Neisseria*
Proteus	*Klebsiella*
Salmonella	*Fusiformis*
Pasteurella	*Corynebacterium*
Shigella	*Clostridium*
Haemophilus	*Bordetella*
Moderately Sensitive	**Not Sensitive**
Moraxella	*Mycobacterium*
Nocardia	*Leptospira*
Brucella	*Pseudomonas*
	Erysipelothrix

As a result of the sequential double blockade of the metabolism of susceptible organisms by trimethoprim and sulfadiazine, the minimum inhibitory concentration (MIC) of Tribrissen is markedly less than that of either of the components used separately. Many strains of bacteria that are not susceptible to one of the components are susceptible to Tribrissen. A synergistic effect between trimethoprim and sulfadiazine in combination has been shown experimentally both *in vitro* and *in vivo* (in dogs).

Tribrissen is bactericidal against susceptible strains and is often effective against sulfonamide-resistant organisms. *In vitro* sulfadiazine is usually only bacteriostatic.

The precise *in vitro* MIC of the combination varies with the ratio of the drugs present, but action of Tribrissen occurs over a wide range of ratios with an increase in the concentration of one of its components compensating for a decrease in the other. It is usual, however, to determine MICs using a constant ratio of one part trimethoprim in twenty parts of the combination.

The following table shows MICs, using the above ratio of bacteria which were susceptible to both trimethoprim (TMP) and sulfadiazine (SDZ). The organisms are those most commonly involved in conditions for which Tribrissen is indicated.
[See table at right]

Average Minimum Inhibitory Concentration
(MIC-mcg/ml)

Bacteria	TMP Alone	SDZ Alone	TMP/SDZ TMP	TMP/SDZ SDZ
Escherichia coli	0.31	26.5	0.07	1.31
Proteus species	1.3	24.5	0.15	2.85
Staphylococcus aureus	0.6	17.6	0.13	2.47
Pasteurella species	0.06	20.1	0.03	0.56
Salmonella species	0.15	61.0	0.05	0.95
βStreptococcus	0.5	24.5	0.15	2.85

The following table demonstrates the marked effect of the trimethoprim and sulfadiazine combination against sulfadiazine-resistant strains of normally susceptible organisms.
[See table below]

Average Minimum Inhibitory Concentration of Sulfadiazine-Resistant Strains
(MIC-mcg/ml)

Bacteria	TMP Alone	SDZ Alone	TMP/SDZ TMP	TMP/SDZ SDZ
Escherichia coli	0.32	>245	0.27	5.0
Proteus species	0.66	>245	0.32	6.2

Pharmacology: Following oral administration, Tribrissen is rapidly absorbed and widely distributed throughout body tissues. Concentrations of trimethoprim are usually higher in tissues than in blood. The levels of trimethoprim are high in lung, kidney and liver, as would be expected from its physical properties. Studies with labeled trimethoprim in dogs have shown that about two-thirds of the dose is excreted mainly in the urine, as unchanged drug, in 24 hours.
Therapeutic serum levels are detected one to three hours after dosing. In dogs, peak blood levels occur three to four hours after oral administration.
Usually, the concentration of an antibacterial in the blood and the *in vitro* MIC of the infecting organism indicate an appropriate period between doses of a drug. This does not hold entirely for Tribrissen because trimethoprim, in contrast to sulfadiazine, localizes in tissues and, therefore, its concentration and ratio to sulfadiazine are higher there than in blood. Serum levels following dosing give an indication, however, of the probable duration of effectiveness of a single dose.
The following table shows the average serum concentrations of trimethoprim and sulfadiazine in six adult dogs following administration of a single oral dose of 30 mg/kg on two separate occasions.
[See table at bottom of next page]
Excretion of Tribrissen is chiefly by the kidneys, by both glomerular filtration, and tubular secretion. Urine concentrations of Tribrissen are severalfold higher than blood concentrations. Neither trimethoprim or sulfadiazine interferes with the excretion pattern of the other.
Susceptibility Testing: In testing susceptibility to Tribrissen, it is essential that the medium used does not contain significant amounts of interfering substances which can bypass the metabolic blocking action, e.g., thymidine or thymine.
The standard SXT disc is appropriate for testing by the disc diffusion method.
Indications: Tribrissen therapy is indicated in dogs where potent systemic antibacterial action against sensitive organisms is required, either alone or as an adjunct to surgery or debridement with associated infection.
Tribrissen tablets are indicated where control of bacterial infections is required during treatment of:
Acute urinary tract infections
Acute bacterial complications of canine distemper
Acute respiratory tract infections
Acute alimentary tract infections
Wound infections and abscesses
Contraindications: Tribrissen should not be used in dogs showing marked liver parenchymal damage, blood dyscrasias, or in those with a history of sulfonamide sensitivity.
Precautions: Water should be readily available to dogs receiving sulfonamide therapy.
Adverse Reactions: Conditions reported following use of trimethoprim/sulfadiazine include polyarthritis, urticaria, facial swelling, fever, hemolytic anemia, polydypsia, polyuria, vomiting, anorexia, diarrhea and seizures.
Keratitis sicca possibly due to prolonged use of trimethoprim/sulfadiazine has been reported. This condition has also been associated with the prolonged use of other sulfonamide-containing products.
Hepatitis possibly due to sulfonamide hypersensitivity has been diagnosed following trimethoprim/sulfadiazine therapy. Individual animal hypersensitivity may result in local or generalized reactions, sometimes fatal. Anaphylactoid reactions, although rare, may also occur —**Antidote:** Epinephrine.
Toxicity and Side Effects: Toxicity is low. The acute toxicity (LD_{50}) of Tribrissen is more than 5g/kg orally in rats and mice.
No significant changes were recorded in rats given doses of 600 mg/kg per day for 90 days.
Dogs can tolerate up to ten times the recommended therapeutic dose without exhibiting ill effects. Dogs dosed at 300 mg/kg per day for a period of 20 days revealed only slight changes in hematologic values.
Slight to moderate reductions in hematopoietic activity following high, prolonged dosage in several species have been recorded. This is usually reversible by folinic acid (leucovorin) administration or by stopping the drug. During long-term treatment of dogs, periodic platelet counts and white and red blood cell counts are advisable.
Teratology: Dogs given therapeutic doses (30 mg/kg per day) of Tribrissen continuously and at interrupted intervals throughout pregnancy gave birth to normal progeny. From these studies, it appears that Tribrissen can safely be given to gestating dogs.
Dosage and Administration: The schedule below provides for a dose of 30 mg/2.5 lb per day (approximately 30 mg/kg per day).

WEIGHT OF DOG	TRIBRISSEN TABLET
2.5 lb	1 × 30 mg Tablet
10.0 lb	1 × 120 mg Tablet
40.0 lb	1 × 480 mg Tablet
80.0 lb	1 × 960 mg Tablet

The recommended dose may be given once daily, or one-half the daily dose may be administered every 12 hours.
Administer for two to three days after symptoms have subsided.
If no improvement is seen in three to five days, re-evaluate diagnosis.
Tribrissen Tablets may be used alone or in conjunction with Tribrissen 24% Injection.
Therapy with Tribrissen Tablets is not recommended for more than 14 days. A complete blood count should be done periodically in patients receiving Tribrissen for prolonged periods. If significant reduction in the count of any formed blood element is noted, treatment with Tribrissen should be discontinued.
KEEP OUT OF REACH OF CHILDREN
Caution: Federal (U.S.A.) law restricts this drug to use by or on the order of a licensed veterinarian.
How Supplied: Tribrissen 30 Tablets in bottles of 100, Tribrissen 120 Tabrissen 120 Tablets in bottles of 100 and 500, Tribrissen 480 Tablets in bottles of 100 and 250, and Tribrissen 960 Tablets in bottles of 50.
*Manufactured under Pat. 3,956,327.

Continued on next page

Coopers—Cont.

TRIBRISSEN® 24% INJECTION ℞

Sterile
(trimethoprim 40 mg and sulfadiazine 200 mg per ml)
For Use in Dogs

Composition: Tribrissen 24% Injection is a sterile aqueous suspension of trimethoprim* in a solution of the sodium salt of sulfadiazine for subcutaneous administration. Each ml contains: trimethoprim 40 mg and sulfadiazine 200 mg. Vehicle contains the inactive ingredients diethanolamine 6 mg, polyvinylpyrrolidone 25 mg, sodium hydroxide 32.8 mg (additional may be added to adjust pH), polysorbate 80 0.1 mg, sodium metabisulfite 1 mg (at time of manufacture) and water for injection, q.s.

Tribrissen is a combination of trimethoprim and sulfadiazine in the ratio of 1 part to 5 parts by weight, which provides effective antibacterial activity against a wide range of bacterial infections in animals.

Trimethoprim is 2,4 diamino-5-(3,4,5-trimethoxybenzyl) pyrimidine.

Actions: *Microbiology:* Trimethoprim blocks bacterial production of tetrahydrofolic acid from dihydrofolic acid by binding to and reversibly inhibiting the enzyme dihydrofolate reductase.

Sulfadiazine, in common with other sulfonamides, inhibits bacterial synthesis of dihydrofolic acid by competing with *para*-aminobenzoic acid.

Tribrissen thus imposes a sequential double blockade on bacterial metabolism. This deprives bacteria of nucleic acids and proteins essential for survival and multiplication and produces a high level of antibacterial activity which is usually bactericidal.

Although both sulfadiazine and trimethoprim are antifolate, neither affects the folate metabolism of animals. The reasons are: animals do not synthesize folic acid and cannot, therefore, be directly affected by sulfadiazine; and although animals must reduce their dietary folic acid to tetrahydrofolic acid, trimethoprim does not affect this reduction because its affinity for dihydrofolate reductase of mammals is significantly less than for the corresponding bacterial enzyme.

Tribrissen is active against a wide spectrum of bacterial pathogens, both gram-negative and gram-positive. The following *in vitro* data are available, but their clinical significance is unknown. In general, species of the following genera are sensitive to Tribrissen:

Very Sensitive	Sensitive
Escherichia	*Staphylococcus*
Streptococcus	*Neisseria*
Proteus	*Klebsiella*
Salmonella	*Fusiformis*
Pasteurella	*Corynebacterium*
Shigella	*Clostridium*
Haemophilus	*Bordetella*

Moderately Sensitive	Not Sensitive
Moraxella	*Mycobacterium*
Nocardia	*Leptospira*
Brucella	*Pseudomonas*
	Erysipelothrix

As a result of the sequential double blockade of the metabolism of susceptible organisms by trimethoprim and sulfadiazine, the minimum inhibitory concentration (MIC) of Tribrissen is markedly less than that of either of the components used separately. Many strains of bacteria that are not susceptible to one of the components are susceptible to Tribrissen. A synergistic effect between trimethoprim and sulfadiazine in combination has been shown experimentally both *in vitro* and *in vivo* (in dogs).

Tribrissen is bactericidal against susceptible strains and is often effective against sulfonamide-resistant organisms. *In vitro* sulfadiazine is usually only bacteriostatic.

The precise *in vitro* MIC of the combination varies with the ratio of the drugs present, but action of Tribrissen occurs over a wide range of ratios with an increase in the concentration of one of its components compensating for a decrease in the other. It is usual, however, to determine MICs using a constant ratio of one part trimethoprim in twenty parts of the combination.

The following table shows MIC's, using the above ratio, of bacteria which were susceptible to both trimethoprim (TMP) and sulfadiazine (SDZ). The organisms are those most commonly involved in conditions for which Tribrissen is indicated.

[See table above].

Average Minimum Inhibitory Concentration (MIC—mcg/ml)

Bacteria	TMP Alone	SDZ Alone	TMP/SDZ	
			TMP	SDZ
Escherichia coli	0.31	26.5	0.07	1.31
Proteus species	1.3	24.5	0.15	2.85
Staphyloccus aureus	0.6	17.6	0.13	2.47
Pasteurella species	0.06	20.1	0.03	0.56
Salmonella species	0.15	61.0	0.05	0.95
β Streptococcus	0.5	24.5	0.15	2.85

The following table demonstrates the marked effect of the trimethoprim and sulfadiazine combination against sulfadiazine-resistant strains of normally susceptible organisms:

[See table at bottom of next page]

Susceptability Testing: In testing susceptibility to Tribrissen, it is essential that the medium used does not contain significant amounts of interfering substances which can bypass the metabolic blocking action, e.g., thymidine or thymine.

The standard S × T disc is appropriate for testing by the disc diffusion method.

Pharmacology: Following parenteral administration, Tribrissen is rapidly absorbed and widely distributed throughout body tissues. Concentrations of trimethoprim are usually higher in tissues than in blood. The levels of trimethoprim are high in lung, kidney and liver, as would be expected from its physical properties.

Studies with labeled trimethoprim in dogs have shown that about two-thirds of the dose is excreted in the urine in 24 hours.

In dogs, therapeutic levels in serum are detected 30 to 60 minutes after dosing with peak levels occuring two to four hours after parenteral administration.

Usually, the concentration of an antibacterial in the blood and the *in vitro* MIC of the infecting organism indicate an appropriate period between doses of a drug. This does not hold entirely for Tribrissen because trimethoprim, in contrast to sulfadiazine, localizes in tissues and therefore, its concentration and ratio to sulfadiazine are higher there than in blood. Serum levels following dosing give an indication, however, of the probable duration of effectiveness of a single dose.

The following table shows the average serum concentration of trimethoprim and sulfadiazine in five adult dogs following a once daily 30 mg/kg subcutaneous injection of Tribrissen for three consecutive days.

[See table at bottom of next page].

Average Serum Concentration (mcg/ml)

Trimethoprim (5 mg/kg)				Sulfadiazine (25 mg/kg)			
1 hr	3 hr	6 hr	24 hr	1 hr	3 hr	6 hr	24 hr
1.36	1.52	0.51	<0.047	21.6	30.1	27.3	9.8

Excretion of Tribrissen is chiefly by the kidneys, by both glomerular filtration, and tubular secretion. Urine concentrations of Tribrissen are severalfold higher than blood concentrations. Neither trimethoprim nor sulfadiazine interferes with the excretion pattern of the other.

Indications: Tribrissen therapy is indicated in dogs where potent systemic antibacterial action against sensitive organisms is required.

Tribrissen 24% Injection is indicated where control of bacterial infections is required during treatment of:

Acute Urinary Tract Infections
Acute Bacterial Complications of Canine Distemper
Acute Respiratory Tract Infections
Acute Alimentary Tract Infections
Wound Infections and Abcesses
Acute Septicemia due to *Streptococcus zooepidemicus*

Contraindications: Tribrissen should not be used in dogs showing marked liver parenchymal damage, blood dyscrasias, or in those with a history of sulfonamide sensitivity.

Adverse Reactions: An occasional dog may exhibit minor transient pain or discomfort following an injection.

Conditions reported following use of trimethoprim/sulfadiazine include polyarthritis, urticaria, facial swelling, fever, hemolytic anemia, polydypsia/polyuria, vomiting, anorexia, diarrhea and seizures.

Keratitis sicca, possibly due to prolonged use of trimethoprim/sulfadiazine, has been reported. This condition has also been associated with the prolonged use of sulfonamide-containing products.

Hepatitis, possibly due to sulfonamide hypersensitivity, has been diagnosed following Tribrissen therapy.

Individual animal hypersensitivity may result in local or generalized reactions, sometimes fatal. Anaphylactoid reactions, although rare, may also occur - **Antidote:** Epinephrine.

Precaution: Water should be readily available to dogs receiving sulfonamide therapy.

Toxicity and Side Effects: Toxicity is low. The acute toxicity (LD_{50}) of Tribrissen is more than 5g/kg orally in rats and mice.

No significant changes were recorded in rats given doses of 600 mg/kg per day for 90 days.

Dogs can tolerate up to ten times the recommended therapeutic dose without exhibiting ill effect. Dogs dosed at 300 mg/kg per day for a period of 20 days revealed only slight changes in hematologic values.

Slight to moderate reductions in hematopoietic activity following high, prolonged dosage in several species have been recorded. This is usually reversible by folinic acid (leucovorin) administration or by stopping the drug. During long-term treatment of dogs, periodic platelet counts and white and red blood cell counts are advisable.

Teratology: Dogs given therapeutic doses (30 mg/kg per day) of Tribrissen continuously and at interrupted intervals throughout pregnancy gave birth to normal progeny. From these studies, it appears that Tribrissen can safely be given to dogs during gestation.

Dosage and Administration: The recommended dose is 1 ml Tribrissen 24% Injection per 20 lb (9 kg) body weight per day.

Shake well before using.

Administer by subcutaneous injection.

The dose should be given once every 24 hours. Alternatively, for severe infections, the initial dose may be followed by one-half the normal daily dose every 12 hours.

Average Serum Concentration (mcg/ml)

TMP/SDZ (30 mg/kg)	Trimethoprim (5 mg/kg)			Sulfadiazine (25 mg/kg)		
	3 h	6 h	24 h	3 h	6 h	24 h
	0.28	0.24	0.18	38.7	23.7	4.3

Average Minimum Inhibitory Concentration of Sulfadiazine-Resistant Strains (MIC—mcg/ml)

Bacteria	TMP Alone	SDZ Alone	TMP/SDZ TMP	TMP/SDZ SDZ
Escherichia coli	0.32	>245	0.27	5.0
Proteus species	0.66	>245	0.32	6.2

Continue acute infection therapy for two or three days after clinical signs have subsided.

If no improvement of acute infections is seen in three to five days, re-evaluate diagnosis.

Tribrissen 24% Injection may be used alone or in conjunction with oral dosing. Following an initial injection, therapy can be maintained using Tribrissen Tablets.

Therapy with Tribrissen Injection is not recommended for more than 14 days. A complete blood count should be done periodically in patients receiving Tribrissen for prolonged periods. If significant reduction in the count of any formed blood element is noted, treatment with Tribrissen should be discontinued.

KEEP OUT OF REACH OF CHILDREN

Caution: Federal (U.S.A.) law restricts this drug to use by or on the order of a licensed veterinarian.

How Supplied: 30 ml multiple dose vials

*Mfg. Under Pat. 3,956,327

TRIBRISSEN® 48% INJECTION STERILE ℞
(trimethoprim 80 mg and sulfadiazine 400 mg per ml)
For Use in Horses

Description: Tribrissen 48% Injection is a sterile aqueous suspension of trimethoprim* in a solution of the sodium salt of sulfadiazine for intravenous administration. Each ml contains trimethoprim 80 mg and sulfadiazine 400 mg. Vehicle contains the inactive ingredients diethanolamine 6 mg, sodium hydroxide 55 mg (additional may be added to adjust pH), polysorbate 80 0.2 mg, sodium metabisulfite 1 mg (at time of manufacture) and water for injection, q.s.

Tribrissen is a combination of trimethoprim and sulfadiazine in the ratio of 1 part to 5 parts by weight, which provides effective antibacterial activity against a wide range of bacterial infections in animals.

Trimethoprim is 2,4 diamino-5-(3,4,5-trimethoxybenzyl) pyrimidine.

Actions: *Microbiology:* Trimethoprim blocks bacterial production of tetrahydrofolic acid from dihydrofolic acid by binding to and reversibly inhibiting the enzyme dihydrofolate reductase.

Sulfadiazine, in common with other sulfonamides, inhibits bacterial synthesis of dihydrofolic acid by competing with *para*-aminobenzoic acid.

Tribrissen thus imposes a sequential double blockade on bacterial metabolism. This deprives bacteria of nucleic acids and proteins essential for survival and multiplication and produces a high level of antibacterial activity which is usually bactercidal.

Although both sulfadiazine and trimethoprim are antifolate, neither affects the folate metabolism of animals. The reasons are: animals do not synthesize folic acid and cannot, therefore, be directly affected by sulfadiazine; and although animals must reduce their dietary folic acid to tetrahydrofolic acid, trimethroprim does not affect this reduction because its affinity for dihydrofolate reductase of mammals is significantly less than for the corresponding bacterial enzyme.

Tribrissen is active against a wide spectrum of bacterial pathogens, both gram-negative and gram-positive. The following *in vitro* data are available, but their clinical significance is unknown. In general, the species of the genera listed in Table 1 are sensitive to Tribrissen.

[See table on next page].

As a result of the sequential double blockade of the metabolism of susceptible organisms by trimethoprim and sulfadiazine, the minimum inhibitory concentration (MIC) of Tribrissen is markedly less than that of either of the components used separately. Many strains of bacteria that are not susceptible to one of the components are susceptible to Tribrissen. A synergistic effect between trimethoprim and sulfadiazine in combination has been shown experimentally both *in vitro* and *in vivo* (in dogs).

Tribrissen is bactericidal against susceptible strains and is often effective against sulfonamide-resistant organisms. *In vitro* sulfadiazine is usually only bacteriostatic.

The precise *in vitro* MIC of the combination varies with the ratio of drugs present, but action of Tribrissen occurs over a wide range of ratios with an increase in concentration of one of its components compensating for a decrease in the other. It is usual, however, to determine MIC's using a constant ratio of one part trimethoprim in twenty parts of the combination.

Table 2 shows MIC's using the above ratio, of bacteria which were susceptible to both trimethoprim (TMP) and sulfadiazine (SDZ). The organisms are those most

Continued on next page

Coopers—Cont.

commonly involved in conditions for which Tribrissen is indicated.
[See table below]
Table 3 demonstrates the marked effect of the trimethoprim and sulfadiazine combination against sulfadiazine-resistant strains of normally susceptible organisms. [See table at right]

Susceptibility Testing: In testing susceptibility to Tribrissen, it is essential that the medium used does not contain significant amounts of interfering substances which can bypass the metabolic blocking action, e.g., thymidine or thymine.

The standard SxT disc is appropriate for testing by the disc diffusion method.

Pharmacology: Following parenteral administration, Tribrissen is rapidly absorbed and widely distributed throughout body tissues. Concentrations of trimethoprim are usually higher in tissues than in blood. The levels of trimethoprim are high in lung, kidney and liver, as would be expected from its physical properties.

Serum concentrations in horses following intravenous administration indicate rapid dissolution of trimethoprim particles and a steady rate of elimination of both components, with half lives of about three hours and clearance within 24 hours.

Usually, the concentration of an antibacterial in the blood and the *in vitro* MIC of the infecting organism indicate an appropriate period between doses of a drug. This does not hold entirely for Tribrissen because trimethoprim, in contrast to sulfadiazine, localizes in tissues and therefore, its concentration and ratio to sulfadiazine are higher there than in the blood. Serum levels following dosing give an indication, however, of the probable duration of effectiveness of a single dose. Table 4 shows the average serum concentration of trimethoprim and sulfadiazine in eleven adult horses following administration of a single IV dose of 22 mg/kg. [See table on next page].

Excretion of Tribrissen is chiefly by the kidneys, by both glomerular filtration and tubular secretion. Urine concentrations of both trimethroprim and sulfadiazine are severalfold higher than blood concentrations. Neither trimethoprim nor sulfadiazine interferes with the excretion pattern of the other.

Indications and Usage: Tribrissen therapy is indicated in horses where potent systemic antibacterial action against sensitive organisms is required. Tribrissen 48% Injection is indicated where control of bacterial infections is required during treatment of:
Acute Strangles
Respiratory Tract Infections
Acute Urogenital Infections
Wound Infections and Abcesses
Tribrissen is well tolerated by foals.

Contraindications: Tribrissen should not be used in horses showing marked liver parenchymal damage, blood dyscrasias or in those with a history of sulfonamide sensitivity.

Warning: Not for use in horses intended for food.

Adverse Reactions: Transient pruritus has been reported following the first dose in a small number of horses. This resolved spontaneously within 24 hours and did not recur after subsequent doses. Following administration intramuscularly, subcutaneously or by accidental perivascular infiltration, swelling, pain and minor tissue damage have occasionally been observed.

Serious, sometimes fatal, shock-like reactions accompanied by convulsions and collapse occurring within seconds to minutes following injection have been reported.

Individual animal hypersensitivity may result in local or generalized reactions, sometimes fatal. Anaphylactoid reactions, although rare, may also occur —**Antidote:** Epinephrine.

Precaution: Water should be readily available to horses receiving sulfonamide therapy.

Toxicity and Side Effects: Toxicity is low. The acute toxicity (LD_{50}) of Tribrissen is more than 5 g/kg orally in rats and mice. No significant changes were recorded in rats given doses of 600 mg/kg per day for 90 days.

Horses have tolerated up to five times the recommended daily dose for seven days or the recommended daily dose for 21 consecutive days without clinical effects or histopathological changes.

Lengthening of clotting time was seen in some of the horses on high or prolonged dosing in one of two trials. The effect, which may have been related to a resolving infection was not seen in a second similar trial.

Slight to moderate reductions in hematopoietic activity following high, prolonged dosage in several species have been recorded. This is usually reversible by folinic acid (leucovorin) administration or by stopping the drug. During long-term treatment of horses, periodic platelet counts and white and red blood cell counts are advisable.

Teratology: The effect of Tribrissen 48% Injection on pregancy has not been determined. Studies to date show there is no detrimental effect on stallion spermatogenesis with or following the recommended dose of Tribrissen 48% Injection.

Dosage and Administration: The recommended dose is 2 ml Tribrissen 48% Injection per 100 lb (45 kg) body weight per day.
Shake well before using.
Administer by intravenous injection.
The usual course of treamtent is a single, daily dose for 5 to 7 days. The daily dose may be halved and given morning and evening.
Continue acute infection therapy for two to three days after clinical signs have subsided.
A convenient dosage guide is:
250 lb. body weight—5 ml daily
500 lb. body weight—10 ml daily
750 lb. body weight—15 ml daily
1000 lb. body weight—20 ml daily
1250 lb. body weight—25 ml daily
If no improvement of acute infections is seen in three to five days reevaluate diagnosis.
Tribrissen 48% Injection may be used alone or in conjunction with oral dosing. Following an initial injection, therapy

Table 1. Species of Genera Sensitive to Tribrissen

Very Sensitive	Sensitive	Moderately Sensitive	Not Sensitive
Escherichia	*Staphylococcus*	*Moraxella*	*Mycobacterium*
Streptococcus	*Neisseria*	*Norcardia*	*Leptospira*
Proteus	*Klebsiella*	*Brucella*	*Pseudomonas*
Salmonella	*Fusiformis*		*Erysipelothrix*
Pasteurella	*Corynebacterium*		
Shigella	*Clostridium*		
Haemophilus	*Bordetella*		

Table 2. Average Minimum Inhibitory Concentration (MIC—mcg/ml)

Bacteria	TMP Alone	SDZ Alone	TMP/SDZ TMP	TMP/SDZ SDZ
Escherichia coli	0.31	26.5	0.07	1.31
Proteus species	1.3	24.5	0.15	2.85
Staphylococcus aureus	0.6	17.6	0.13	2.47
Pasterurella species	0.06	20.1	0.03	0.56
Salmonella species	0.15	61.0	0.05	0.95
βStreptococcus	0.5	24.5	0.15	2.85

Table 3. Average Minimim Inhibitory Concentration of Sulfadiazine-Resistant Strains (MIC—mcg/ml)

Bacteria	TMP Alone	SDZ Alone	TMP/SDZ TMP	TMP/SDZ SDZ
Escherichia coli	0.32	>245	0.27	5.0
Proteus species	0.66	>245	0.32	6.2

can be maintained using Tribrissen 400 Oral Paste.
A complete blood count should be done periodically in patients receiving Tribrissen for prolonged periods. If significant reduction in the count of any formed blood element should be noted, treatment with Tribrissen should be discontinued.
Caution: Federal (U.S.A.) law restricts this drug to use by or on the order of a licensed veterinarian.
KEEP OUT OF REACH OF CHILDREN
How Supplied: Tribrissen 48% Injection is available in 100 ml multiple dose vials.
*Manufactured under Pat. 3,956,327

TRIBRISSEN® 400 ORAL PASTE
(trimethoprim 67 mg and sulfadiazine 333 mg per gm)
For Use in Horses ℞

Description: Tribrissen® 400 Oral Paste contains 67 mg trimethoprim* and 333 mg sulfadiazine per gram.
Tribrissen is a combination of trimethoprim and sulfadiazine in the ratio of 1 part to 5 parts by weight, which provides effective antibacterial activity against a wide range of bacterial infections in animals.
Trimethoprim is 2,4 diamino-5-(3,4,5-trimethoxybenzyl) pyrimidine.
Actions:
Microbiology: Trimethoprim blocks bacterial production of tetrahydrofolic acid from dihydrofolic acid by binding to and reversibly inhibiting the enzyme dihydrofolate reductase.
Sulfadiazine, in common with other sulfonamides, inhibits bacterial synthesis of dihydrofolic acid by competing with *para-* aminobenzoic acid.
Tribrissen thus imposes a sequential double blockade on bacterial metabolism. This deprives bacteria of nucleic acids and proteins essential for survival and multiplication and produces a high level of antibacterial activity which is usually bactericidal.
Although both sulfadiazine and trimethoprim are antifolate, neither affects the folate metabolism of animals. The reasons are: animals do not synthesize folic acid and cannot, therefore, be directly affected by sulfadiazine; and although animals must reduce their dietary folic acid to tetrahydrofolic acid, trimethoprim does not affect this reduction because its affinity for dihydrofolate reductase of mammals is significantly less than for the corresponding bacterial enzyme. Tribrissen is active against a wide spectrum of bacterial pathogens, both gram-negative and gram-positive. The following *in vitro* data are available, but their clini al significance is unknown. In general, species of the genera sensitive to Tribrissen are listed in Table 1. [See next page]
As a result of the sequential double blockade of the metabolism of susceptible organisms by trimethoprim and sulfadiazine, the minimum inhibitory concentration (MIC) of Tribrissen is markedly less than that of either of the components used separately. Many strains of bacteria that are not susceptible to one of the components are susceptible to Tribrissen. A synergistic effect between trimethoprim and sulfadiazine in combination has been shown experimentally both *in vitro* and *in vivo* (in dogs).
Tribrissen is bactericidal against susceptible strains and is often effective against sulfonamide resistant organisms. *In vitro* sulfadiazine is usually only bacteriostatic.
The precise *in vitro* MIC of the combination varies with the ratio of the drugs present, but action of Tribrissen occurs over a wide range of ratios with an increase in the concentration of one of its components compensating for a decrease in the other. It is usual, however, to determine MIC's using a constant ratio of one part trimethoprim in twenty parts of the combination.
Table 2 shows MIC's, using the above ratio of bacteria which were susceptible to both trimethoprim (TMP) and sulfadiazine (SDZ). The organisms are those most commonly involved in conditions for which Tribrissen is indicated.
Table 3 demonstrates the marked effect of the trimethoprim and sulfadiazine combination against sulfadiazine-resistant strains of normally susceptible organisms: [See next page]
Susceptibility Testing: In testing susceptibility to Tribrissen, it is essential that the medium used does not contain significant amounts of interfering substances which can bypass the metabolic blocking action, e.g., thymidine or thymine.
The standard SxT disc is appropriate for testing by the disc diffusion method.
Pharmacology: Following oral administration, Tribrissen is rapidly absorbed and widely distributed throughout the body tissues. Concentrations of trimethoprim are usually higher in tissues than in blood. The levels of trimethoprim are high in lung, kidney and liver, as would be expected from its physical properties.
Serum trimethoprim concentrations in horses following oral administration indicate rapid absorption of the drug; peak concentrations occur in 2 to 3 hours. The mean serum elimination half-life is 2 to 3 hours. Sulfadiazine absorption is slower, requiring 3 to 6 hours to reach peak concentration. The mean serum elimination half-life for sulfadiazine is about 7 hours.
Usually, the concentration of an antibacterial in the blood and the *in vitro* MIC of the infecting organism indicate an appropriate period between doses of a drug. This does not hold entirely for Tribrissen because trimethoprim, in contrast to sulfadiazine, localizes in tissues and therefore its concentration and ratio to sulfadiazine are higher there than in blood.

Table 4. Average Serum Concentration (mcg/ml)

Trimethoprim (3.6 mg/kg)					*Sulfadiazine (18 mg/kg)*				
1h	3h	6h	8h	24h	1h	3h	6h	8h	24h
1.15	0.64	0.17	0.07	<0.02	27.2	16.4	7.5	4.5	0.09

Table 4 shows the average serum concentration of trimethoprim and sulfadiazine in eleven adult horses observed on Day Three of three consecutive daily doses of Tribrissen 400 Oral Paste.
[See table on next page].
Excretion of Tribrissen is chiefly by the kidneys, by both glomerular filtration and tubular secretion. Urine concentrations of both trimethoprim and sulfadiazine are severalfold higher than blood concentrations. Neither trimethoprim nor sulfadiazine interferes with the excretion pattern of the other.
Indications and Usage: Tribrissen 400 Oral Paste is indicated in horses where potent systemic antibacterial action against sensitive organisms is required. Tribrissen 400 Oral Paste is indicated where control of bacterial infections is required during treatment of:
- Acute Strangles
- Respiratory Tract Infections
- Acute Urogenital Infections
- Wound Infections and Abscesses

Tribrissen is well tolerated by foals.
Contraindications: Tribrissen should not be used in horses showing marked liver parenchymal damage, blood dyscrasias or in those with a history of sulfonamide sensitivity.
Warning: Not for use in horses intended for food.
Adverse Reactions: No adverse reactions of consequence have been noted following administration of Tribrissen 400 Oral Paste. During clinical trials, one case of anorexia and one case of loose feces following treatment with the drug were reported.
Individual animal hypersensitivity may result in local or generalized reactions, sometimes fatal. Analphylactoid reactions, although rare, may also occur. **Antidote:** Epinephrine.
Precaution: Water should be readily available to horses receiving sulfonamide therapy.
Toxicity and Side Effects: Toxicity is low. The acute toxicity (LD_{50}) of Tribrissen is more than 5 g/kg orally in rats and mice. No significant changes were recorded in rats given doses of 600 mg/kg per day for 90 days.
Horses treated intravenously with Tribrissen 48% Injection have tolerated up to five times the recommended daily dose for seven days or the recommended daily dose for 21 consecutive days without clinical effects or histopathological changes.
Lengthening of clotting time was seen in some of the horses on high or prolonged dosing in one of two trials. The effect which may have been related to a resolving infection, was not seen in a second similar trial.
Slight to moderate reductions in hematopoietic activity following high, prolonged

Continued on next page

Coopers—Cont.

dosage in several species have been recorded. This is usually reversible by folinic acid (leucovorin) administration or by stopping the drug. During long-term treatment of horses, periodic platelet counts and white and red blood cell counts are advisable.

Teratology: The effect of Tribrissen 400 Oral Paste on pregnancy has not been determined. Studies to date show there is no detrimental effect on stallion spermatogenesis with or following the recommended dose of Tribrissen 400 Oral Paste.

Dosage and Administration: The recommended dose is 5 g Tribrissen 400 Oral Paste per 150 lb (68 kg) body weight per day. Administer orally once a day by means of the Dial-A-Dose® ** syringe. Each marking on the syringe doses 150 lbs body weight. When administering Tribrissen 400 Oral Paste, the oral cavity should be empty. Deposit paste on back of tongue by depressing plunger that has been previously set to deliver the correct dose.

The usual course of treatment is a single daily dose for five to seven days.

Continue acute infection therapy for two to three days after clinical signs have subsided.

If no improvement of acute infections is seen in three to five days, reevaluate diagnosis.

Tribrissen 400 Oral Paste may be used alone or in conjunction with intravenous dosing. Following treatment with Tribrissen 48% Injection, therapy can be maintained using the oral paste.

A complete blood count should be done periodically in patients receiving Tribrissen for prolonged periods. If significant reduction in the count of any formed blood element is noted, treatment with Tribrissen should be discontinued.

KEEP OUT OF REACH OF CHILDREN

Caution: Federal law (U.S.A.) restricts this drug to use by or on the order of a licensed veterinarian.

How Supplied: 30g Dial-A-Dose®** syringes.

*Mfd. under Pat. 3,956,327

**Trademark—Silver Industries, Inc.

Table 1. Species of the Genera Sensitive to Tribrissen

Very Sensitive	*Sensitive*	*Moderately Sensitive*	*Not Sensitive*
Escherichia	*Staphylococcus*	*Morexella*	*Mycobacterium*
Streptococcus	*Neisseria*	*Nocardia*	*Leptospria*
Proteus	*Klebsiella*	*Brucella*	*Pseudomonas*
Salmonella	*Fusiformis*		*Erysipelothrix*
Pasteurella	*Corynebacterium*		
Shigella	*Clostridium*		
Haemophilus	*Bordetella*		

Table 2. Average Minimum Inhibitory Concentration (MIC—mcg/ml)

Bacteria	*TMP Alone*	*SDZ Alone*	*TMP/SDZ*	
			TMP	*SDZ*
Escherichia coli	0.31	26.5	0.07	1.31
Proteus species	1.3	24.5	0.15	2.85
Staphylococcus aureus	0.6	17.6	0.13	2.47
Pasteurella species	0.06	20.1	0.03	0.56
Salmonella species	0.15	61.0	0.05	0.95
βStreptococcus	0.5	24.5	0.15	2.85

Table 3. Average Minumum Inhibitory Concentration of Sulfadiazine-Resistant Strains (MIC—mcg/ml)

Bacteria	*TMP/SDZ Alone*	*SDZ Alone*	*TMP/SDZ*	
			TMP	*SDZ*
Escherichia coli	0.32	>245	0.27	5.0
Proteus species	0.66	>245	0.32	6.2

Table 4. Average Serum Concentration (mcg/ml)

Trimethoprim (5 mg/kg)					*Sulfadiazine (25 mg/kg)*				
1h	*3h*	*6h*	*10h*	*24h*	*1h*	*3h*	*6h*	*10h*	*24h*
0.71	0.95	0.37	0.04	<0.04	8.0	15.8	9.9	5.6	0.6

TRIRAB®
Rabies Vaccine
Killed Virus

Description: TriRab® is an inactivated virus vaccine. The vaccine virus is grown in cultures of a USDA-certified monkey cell line. Gentamicin has been added. A low level of adjuvant is included to enhance the immune response of vaccinated animals.

The potency of each TriRab serial is determined by means of the NIH test. Safety tests are conducted in dogs, mice, guinea pigs and rabbits.

The seed virus used for TriRab is derived from a modified live strain used for many years for the preparation of ERA Strain® Rabies Vaccine. This virus was chosen because of its accepted immunogenicity in six animal species, and its production of high yields of viral antigen in the selected cell line.

Indications: For the active immunization of healthy dogs and cats against rabies.

Action and Uses: TriRab is approved for use in both dogs and cats. Three years duration of immunity in dogs has been demonstrated through challenge with virulent street virus. TriRab is licensed for one year duration of immunity in cats.

The following safety features are inherent in TriRab: (1) Because vaccine virus is grown in a cell culture system the potential for myelin reactions, associated with nerve tissue origin vaccines, is eliminated; (2) Use of a continuous cell line provides safeguards against both the propagation and accidental introduction of adventitious pathogens into the vaccine; (3) Humans who are accidentally inoculated with an inactivated vaccine are not considered at risk to rabies disease.

Administration and Dosage: Shake vial well before use. Inject 1 ml intramuscularly at one site in the thigh using aseptic technique.

Vaccinate dogs and cats at three months of age or older with a repeat dose one year later. Revaccination is recommended every three years thereafter for dogs and annually for cats.

Caution:

Store at not over 45°F or 7°C. Do not freeze. Use entire contents when first opened. Contains gentamicin as an added preservative. Anaphylactoid reactions may occur following use. **Antidote:** Epinephrine.

Restricted to Use By or Under the Direction of a Licensed Veterinarian.

How Supplied: 10 dose vials.

UNITOX®
Tetanus Toxoid

Composition: A sterile suspension of highly purified precipitated tetanus toxoid. The toxin produced by virulent tetanus bacilli has been modified by special treatment to eliminate its toxicity while still retaining its antigenicity. Thimerosal is added as a preservative.
Indications: To confer long-term active immunity against tetanus.
Action and Uses: Primary immunization consists of 2 injections spaced 30 days apart. To maintain a high degree of immunity, a single booster injection may be given annually. A single booster dose should also be given to previously immunized animals that have been exposed to tetanus from injuries, particularly puncture wounds. Tetanus toxoid is not recommended for use at the time of exposure in animals not previously immunized.

Dosage and Administration: Shake well before use. Administer subcutaneously or intramuscularly, using aseptic technique. **Dosage:** Horses, cattle, swine: 1 ml; Sheep: 0.5 ml. Repeat in 30 days followed by a single annual dose.
Caution: Store at not over 45°F or 7°C. Protect from freezing. Use entire contents when first opened. Do not vaccinate within 21 days before slaughter. Anaphylactoid reactions may occur following use. **Antidote:** Epinephrine.
For Veterinary Use Only
How Supplied: 10 ml vials and ten 1 ml syringes.

VETPRO™-G
Penicillin G Procaine

Description: Each ml of aqueous suspension contains 300,000 units of penicillin G procaine; sodium citrate 10 mg; povidone 5 mg; lecithin 6 mg; sodium carboxymethylcellulose 1 mg; methylparaben 1.3 mg; propylparaben 0.2 mg; sodium formaldehyde sulfoxylate 0.2 mg; procaine hydrochloride 20 mg and water for injection, q.s.
Indications For Use: For the treatment of cattle and sheep for bacteria pneumonia (shipping fever) caused by *Pasteurella multocida;* swine for erysipelas caused by *Erysipelothrix rhusiopathiae* (insidiosa); and horses for strangles caused by *Streptococcus equi.*
Warnings: Not for use in horses intended for food.
Milk that has been taken from animals during treatment and for 72 hours (6 milkings) after the last treatment must not be used for food.
Treatments should not exceed 4 consecutive days.
Discontinue use of this drug for the following time periods before treated animals are slaughtered for food: Cattle—10 days; Sheep—9 days; Swine—7 days.
Precautions: Sensitivity reactions to penicillin or procaine such as hives or respiratory distress, sometimes fatal, have been known to occur in some animals. If signs of sensitivity do occur, stop medication and call your veterinarian. If respiratory distress is severe, the immediate injection of epinephrine may be helpful.
As with any antibiotic preparation, prolonged use may result in the overgrowth of non-susceptible organisms, including fungi. If this condition is suspected, stop medication and consult your veterinarian.
Dosage: The dosage for cattle, sheep, swine and horses is 3000 units per pound of body weight or 1 ml for each 100 pounds of body weight once daily. Continue treatment at least 1 day after symptoms disappear (usually 2 or 3 days). Treatment should not exceed 4 consecutive days. If improvement is not observed, consult your veterinarian.
Directions For Use: VETPRO-G should be injected deep within the fleshy muscles of the hip, rump, round or thigh. Do not inject subcutaneously, into a blood vessel or near a major nerve. The site of each injection should be changed.
Use a 16 or 18 gauge needle, 1½ inches long. The needle and syringe should be washed thoroughly before use and sterilized in boiling water for 15 to 20 minutes before use. The injection site should be washed with soap and water and painted with a disinfectant such as 70% alcohol. Warm the product to room temperature and shake well. Wipe the stopper in the vial with 70% alcohol. Withdraw the suspension from the vial and inject deep into the muscle. Do not inject more than 10 ml into one site.
Storage: VETPRO-G should be stored in a refrigerator (2°–8°C, 36°–46°F).
For Veterinary Use Only
How Supplied: VETPRO-G is available in 100 ml and 250 ml vials.

Products are cross-indexed

by product classifications

in the

Product Category Section

VETSPAN™
(Sterile Penicillin G Benzathine and Penicillin G Procaine)
Antibiotic in Aqueous Suspension ℞

Description: Each ml of aqueous suspension contains 150,000 units penicillin G benzathine, 150,000 units penicillin G procaine; 11.7 mg lecithin; 1.75 mg sodium formaldehyde sulfoxylate; 1.20 mg methylparaben (as preservative); 0.14 mg propylparaben (as preservative); 8.19 mg Tween 40; 11.3 mg Span 40; 3.98 mg sodium citrate anhydrous; 20.0 mg procaine hydrochloride; 1.04 mg sodium carboxymethylcellulose; and water for injection USP q.s.
Action: Penicillin G in VETSPAN is an antibiotic which shows a marked bactericidal effect against certain organisms during their growth phase. It is relatively specific in its action against Gram-positive bacteria but is usually ineffective against Gram-negative organisms.
When treating an animal for a bacterial infection, it is advisable to isolate and identify the causative organisms and conduct appropriate *in-vitro* susceptibility tests. In cases where organisms other than those susceptible to penicillin are present, re-evaluation of treatment should be made. Organisms normally considered susceptible to penicillin include *Clostridium septicum, Corynebacterium pyogenes, Staphylococcus aureus, Streptococcus canis, Streptococcus equi* and *Streptococcus pyogenes.*
It is normally recommended that any bacterial infection be treated as early as possible and with a dosage that will give effective blood levels. Although the recommended dosage will give longer detectable penicillin blood levels than penicillin G procaine alone, it is recommended that a second dose be administered at 48 hours when treating a penicillin-susceptible bacterial infection.
If no definite improvement is noted following the second dose, the diagnosis should be re-evaluated and use of another chemotherapeutic agent considered.
Indications: VETSPAN is indicated for treatment of the following bacterial infections in dogs, horses, and beef cattle due to penicillin susceptible microorganisms that are susceptible to the serum levels common to this particular dosage form, such as:

1. Bacterial Pneumonia *(Streptococcus spp., Corynebacterium pyogenes, Staphylococcus aureus).*
2. Upper Respiratory Infections as rhinitis or pharyngitis *(Corynebacterium pyogenes).*
3. Equine strangles *(Streptococcus equi).*
4. Blackleg *(Clostridium chauvoei).*

Contraindications: VETSPAN is contraindicated in patients which have shown hypersensitivity to penicillin.
Warnings: Beef cattle should be withheld from slaughter for food use for 30 days following last treatment. Treatment in beef cattle must be limited to two (2) doses. Not to be used for horses intended for slaughter for food purposes.
Adverse Reactions: Anaphylactic reactions have been reported in cattle given penicillin. Treated animals should be closely observed and if allergic or anaphylactic reactions occur, administer epinephrine or antihistamines immediately.
Administration: VETSPAN should be given by intramuscular injection to horses. In beef cattle the recommended dosage should be administered by subcutaneous injection only. Dogs may be injected by either the intramuscular or subcutaneous route.

Continued on next page

C

Coopers—Cont.

Dosage
Horses: 2 ml per 150 lbs of body weight given intramuscularly (2,000 units penicillin G procaine and 2,000 units penicillin G benzathine per lb body weight). Treatment should be repeated in 48 hours.
Beef Cattle: 2 ml per 150 lbs body weight given subcutaneously only (2,000 units penicillin G procaine and 2,000 units penicillin G benzathine per lb body weight). Treatment should be repeated in 48 hours. IMPORTANT: Treatment in beef cattle should be limited to two (2) doses given subcutaneous injection only.
Dogs: 1 ml per 10 to 25 lbs body weight given intramuscularly or subcutaneously (6,000 to 15,000 units penicillin G procaine and 6,000 to 15,000 units penicillin G benzathine per lb body weight). Treatment should be repeated in 48 hours.
SHAKE WELL BEFORE EACH USE
STORE UNDER REFRIGERATION BELOW 59°F (15°C)
Caution: Federal law restricts this drug to use by or on the order of a licensed veterinarian.
How Supplied: VETSPAN is available in 100 ml vials (dogs, horses and beef cattle) and 250 ml vials (horses and beef cows only).

VOVAX®
Parvovirus Vaccine
Killed Virus
For Use in Dogs

Description: Vovax® is an inactivated virus vaccine prepared from a canine origin parvovirus. It is grown in a USDA-certified continuous cell line of embryonic feline lung. A low level of adjuvant is included to enhance immunogenicity.
A canine rather than feline virus isolate was selected for Vovax to, as studies show, take advantage of its direct antigenic relationship to the canine disease agent and to provide a more complete and more durable disease protection.
The seed virus used was derived from a dog experiencing acute parvovirus disease. A cell line is also employed. These separately developed components combine ideally to produce the virus yield required for a highly immunogenic inactivated virus vaccine.
Action and Uses: Susceptible puppies vaccinated with Vovax developed exceptionally high initial antibody (SN) titers. These titers ranged up to 1:10,000 and higher, at least 20 times higher than is considered protective. Duration of immunity studies showed the antibody levels at one year after vaccination to be 4 to 5 times higher than that considered protective.
Eight-week-old puppies with maternal antibody titers (SM) of up to 1:100 were protected by vaccination with Vovax. All vaccinates had protective levels of active antibody 7 days after the second dose which had been administered at 11 weeks. They remained free of disease when challenged with virulent CPV three weeks later.
Dogs inoculated with Vovax experienced no change in normal white cell profiles and showed no signs of disease. These findings confirm the efficient method of inactivating vaccine virus. They also indicate that changes characteristic of live virus replication did not occur.
When administered in combination with Coopers live modified vaccines for canine distemper, canine adenovirus, canine parainfluenza and leptospira bacterins (C& I), Vovax did not interfere with the immune responses to these antigens.
The safety features of Vovax include: (1) No post-vaccination shedding of CPV as may occur following use of modified live virus vaccines; (2) well-tolerated upon inoculation—no local or systemic reactions occurred during field studies involving the vaccination of over 1600 dogs; (3) may be administered to pregnant bitches without fear of abortions or fetal anomalies resulting from virus replication; (4) the vaccine virus is grown on a heterotypic cell line which provides high assurance that adventitious, pathogenic agents are not propagated.
Indications: For the active immunization of healthy puppies and dogs against disease caused by canine parvovirus (CPV).
Dosage and Administration: Shake well. For use in healthy puppies and dogs. Inject 1 ml subcutaneously or intramuscularly using aseptic technique and boiled, autoclaved or sterile disposable syringes and needles.
Dogs 12 weeks of age or older should receive 2 doses 3-4 weeks apart. If younger dogs are vaccinated, they should be revaccinated at 3-4 week intervals with the final dose being given at 12 weeks or older. Annual revaccination is recommended.
Caution: Store at not over 45°F or 7°C. Protect from freezing. Use entire contents when first opened.
Contains gentamicin as an added preservative. Anaphylactoid reactions may occur following use. **Antidote:** Epinephrine.
How Supplied: 10 dose vials.
For Veterinary Use Only

Daniels Pharmaceuticals, Inc.
2527 25TH AVENUE NORTH
ST. PETERSBURG, FL 33713

AMMONIL®

Composition: DL-Methionine in 200 mg and 500 mg tablets.
Indications: For use as a urinary acidifier in cats and dogs.
Dosage: The suggested dose of Ammonil 200 mg tablet for adult cats is one (1) tablet per 10 lbs (4.5 kg) body weight 3 or 4 times daily with food. For dogs one tablet per 10 lbs (4.5 kg) body weight once or twice daily with food. Dosage may then be adjusted to attain desired urine pH (approximately 6). Not intended for use in kittens.
The suggested dose of Ammonil 500 mg tablet for adult cats is one (1) tablet per 10 lbs (4.5 kg) body weight once or twice daily with food. For dogs one-half (½) tablet per 10 lbs (4.5 kg) body weight once or twice daily with food. Dosage may then be adjusted to attain desired urine pH (approximately 6). Not intended for use in kittens.
Caution: Federal law restricts this drug to use by or on the order of a licensed veterinarian.
Warning: Do not administer to animals with severe liver or kidney damage or to animals exhibiting acidosis. KEEP THIS AND ALL MEDICATIONS OUT OF THE REACH OF CHILDREN. STORE AT CONTROLLED ROOM TEMPERATURE 15°–30°C (59°–86°F)
How Supplied: Tablets, 200 mg and 500 mg in bottles of 1,000.

BENOXYDERM™ SHAMPOO

Composition: 2.5% Benzoyl Peroxide
Action: Cleansing, antiseptic, removes excess oils.
Indications: Where antiseptic, cleansing or debriding action is desired.
Directions: Lather well into wet coat. Allow to stand 10 minutes. Rinse thoroughly and completely. Use as often as needed contingent upon severity of condition.
Warnings: If irritation occurs, decrease frequency of use or discontinue entirely. In severe conditions or where there is poor therapeutic response, use of systemic antibiotic treatment should be considered.
AVOID CONTACT WITH EYES.
KEEP THIS AND ALL MEDICATIONS OUT OF THE REACH OF CHILDREN.
Store in a Cool Dry Place (Below 80°F).
Caution: Federal law restricts this drug to use by or on the order of a licensed veterinarian.
How Supplied: 6 oz. (180 ml.), 1 Gallon (3.785 Liters)

METHIO PWD™
DL-Methionine Powder

Indication: For use as a urinary acidifier in cats and dogs.
NET WEIGHT
One Pound
(454 grams)
Dosage: The suggested dose of Methio PWD for adult cats is one (1) gram per 10 lbs (4.5 kg) body weight daily in divided doses with food. For dogs one-half (½) gram per 10 lbs (4.5 kg) body weight daily in divided doses with food. Dosage may then be adjusted to attain desired urine pH (approximately 6). Not intended for use in kittens.

Caution: Federal law restricts this drug to use by or on the order of a licensed veterinarian.
Warning:
Do not administer to animals with severe liver or kidney damage or to animals exhibiting acidosis. KEEP OUT OF THE REACH OF CHILDREN. STORE AT CONTROLLED ROOM TEMPERATURE 15°-30°C (59°-86°F)
How Supplied: 1-lb and 5-lb containers.

OXYDENT™

Composition: Sodium Carbonate Peroxyhydrate, Sodium Bicarbonate, Sodium Chloride, Silica, Meat Flavor
Action: An effervescent, non-detergent, antimicrobial dentifrice that helps remove food particles and plaque. Also helps prevent plaque formation by controlling the spread of susceptible organisms by the liberation of oxygen in a pleasant bubbling and foaming action.
Directions: Pour powder on dry surface. Moisten tooth brush and pick up powder on bristle tips. Brush at least every other day according to your veterinarian's directions.
For Veterinary Use Only.
Store in a cool, dry place. (Below 80° F)
How Supplied: 3 oz. puffer.

PANCREZYME™
Tablets 425 mg
Powder

Each 425 mg tablet contains:

Lipase	8,500 USP Units
Protease	52,000 USP Units
Amylase	62,000 USP Units

Each teaspoonful (2.8g) contains:

Lipase	61,000 USP Units
Protease	330,000 USP Units
Amylase	440,000 USP Units

Description: PANCREZYME is an enzymatic concentrate derived from porcine pancreas containing standardized lipase, protease and amylase plus esterases, peptidases, nucleases and elastase.
Indications: For use in animals with exocrine pancreatic insufficiency. As a digestive aid in enzyme replacement therapy where digestion of carbohydrate, protein and fat is inadequate.
Caution: Federal law restricts this drug to use by or on the order of a licensed veterinarian.
Precautions: Discontinue use in animals with symptoms of sensitivity. KEEP THIS AND ALL MEDICATIONS OUT OF THE REACH OF CHILDREN.
Suggested Dosage: Dose should be adjusted according to the severity of the condition and the weight of the animal. Tablets—average dose for adult dogs 3 tablets with each meal. Adult cats 1 tablet with each meal. Powder—Adult dogs 1-1½ teaspoonfuls with each meal. Adult cats ½-¾ teaspoonful with each meal. Mix well with moistened food (canned or dry) and let stand at room temperature for 15–20 minutes before feeding. Frequent feeding, at least 3 times daily is important.
How Supplied: Pancrezyme tablets 425 mg Bottles of 100 and 500.
Pancrezyme Powder Bottles of 4 oz., 8 oz. and 12 oz.

SOLOXINE® (LEVOTHYROXINE SODIUM TABLETS, USP)

Description: Each **SOLOXINE®** (Levothyroxine Sodium, USP) Tablet provides synthetic crystalline levothyroxine sodium (L-thyroxine).
The structural formula for levothyroxine sodium is:

HO–(3,5-diiodophenyl)–O–(3,5-diiodophenyl)–$CH_2CHCOONa$ (NH_2)

Levothyroxine Sodium

Action: Levothyroxine sodium acts, as does endogenous thyroxine, to stimulate metabolism, growth, development and differentiation of tissues. It increases the rate of energy exchange and increases the maturation rate of the epiphyses. Levothyroxine sodium is absorbed rapidly from the gastrointestinal tract after oral administration. Following absorption, the compound becomes bound to the serum alpha globulin fraction. For purposes of comparison. 0.1 mg of levothyroxine sodium elicits a clinical response approximately equal to that produced by one grain (65 mg) of desiccated thyroid.
Indications: Provides thyroid replacement therapy in all conditions of inadequate production of thyroid hormones. Hypothyroidism is the generalized metabolic disease resulting from deficiency of the thyroid hormones levothyroxine (T_4) and liothyronine (T_3). Soloxine (levothyroxine sodium) will provide levothyroxine (T_4) as a substrate for the physiologic deiodination to liothyronine (T_3). Administration of levothyroxine sodium alone will result in complete physiologic thyroid replacement.
Canine hypothyroidism is usually primary, i.e., due to atrophy of the thyroid gland. In the majority of cases the atrophy is associated with lymphocytic thyroiditis and in the remainder it is non-inflammatory and as of yet unknown etiology. Less than 10 percent of cases of hypothyroidism are secondary, i.e., due to deficiency of thyroid stimulating hormone (TSH). TSH deficiency may occur as a component of congenital hypopituitarism or as an acquired disorder in adults dogs, in which case it is invariably due to the growth of a pituitary tumor.
Hypothyroidism in the Dog: Hypothyroidism usually occurs in middle-aged and older dogs although the condition will sometimes be seen in younger dogs of the larger breeds. Neutered animals of either sex are also frequently affected, regardless of age. The following are clinical signs of hypothyroidism in dogs.

Lethargy, lack of endurance, increased sleeping
Reduced interest, alertness and excitability
Slow heart rate, weak apex beat and pulse, low voltage on ECG
Preference for warmth, low body temperature, cool skin
Increased body weight
Stiff and slow movements, dragging of front feet
Head tilt, disturbed balance, unilateral facial paralysis
Atrophy of epidemis, thickening of dermis
Surface and follicular hyperkeratosis, pigmentation
Puffy face, blepharoptosis, tragic expression
Dry, coarse, sparse coat, slow regrowth after clipping
Retarded turnover of hair (carpet coat of boxers)
Shortening or absence of estrus, lack of libido
Dry feces, occasional diarrhea
Hypercholesterolemia
Normochromic, normocytic anemia
Elevated serum creatinine phosphokinase

Contraindications: Levothyroxine sodium therapy is contraindicated in thyrotoxicosis, acute myocardial infarction and incorrected adrenal insufficiency. Use in pregnant bitches has not been evaluated.
Precautions: The effects of levothyroxine sodium therapy are slow in being manifested. Overdosage of any thyroid drug may produce the signs and symptoms of thyrotoxicosis including but not limited to polydipsia, polyuria, polyphagia, reduced heat tolerance and hyperactivity or personality change. Administer with caution to animals with clinically significant heart disease, hypertension or other complications for which a sharply increased metabolic rate might prove hazardous.
Adverse Reactions: There are no particular adverse reactions connected with L-thyroxine therapy at the recommended dosage levels. Overdosage will result in the signs of thyrotoxicosis listed above under precautions.
Dosage: The initial recommended daily dose is 0.1 mg/10 lb body weight. Dosage is then adjusted according to patient's response by monitoring T_4 blood levels at time intervals of four weeks.
Administration: Soloxine tablets may be administered orally or placed in the food.
Dosage forms available: 0.1 mg, 0.2 mg, 0.3 mg, 0.4 mg, 0.5 mg, 0.6 mg, 0.7 mg, 0.8 mg tablets in bottles of 1,000.
Storage: Store at controlled room temperature 15°C to 30°C (59°F to 86°F).

UROEZE® CHEWABLE TABLETS

Composition: Each scored tablet contains: ammonium chloride 400 mg in a palatable amino acid protein base.
Indication: For use as a urinary acidifier in cats and dogs.
Dosage: The suggested dose of Uroeze Chewable Tablets for adult cats and dogs is one (1) tablet per 10 lbs (4.5 kg) body weight twice daily with food. Dosage may then be adjusted to accomplish the desired urine pH (approximately 6). Not intended for use in kittens.

Continued on next page

D

Daniels—Cont.

Caution: Federal law restricts this drug to use by or on the order of a licensed veterinarian.
Administration: Uroeze Chewable Tablets may be fed free choice, from the hand or may be crumbled and mixed into the food.
Warning: Do not administer to animals with severe liver or kidney damage or to animals exhibiting acidosis.
Caution: May cause gastric mucosa irritation. KEEP THIS AND ALL MEDICATIONS OUT OF THE REACH OF CHILDREN. STORE AT CONTROLLED ROOM TEMPERATURE 15°–30°C (59°–86°F).
How Supplied: Bottles of 60 and 200 tablets.

D

UROEZE® POWDER

Composition: Each ¼ level teaspoon (650 mg) contains: ammonium chloride 400 mg in a palatable amino acid protein base.
Indications: For use as a urinary acidifier in cats and dogs.
Dosage: The suggested dose of Uroeze for adult cats and dogs is one-quarter (¼) level teaspoonful per 10 lbs (4.5 kg) body weight twice daily with food. Dosage may then be adjusted to accomplish the desired urine pH (approximately 6). Not intended for use in kittens.
Caution: Federal law restricts this drug to use by or on the order of a licensed veterinarian.
Warning: Do not administer to animals with severe liver or kidney damage or to animals exhibiting acidosis.
Caution: May cause gastric mucosa irritation. KEEP THIS AND ALL MEDICATIONS OUT OF THE REACH OF CHILDREN. STORE AT CONTROLLED ROOM TEMPERATURE 15°–30°C (59°–86°F).
How Supplied: 4 oz and 16 oz powder.

UROEZE® TABLETS

Composition: Each scored tablet contains: Ammonium chloride 400 mg in an amino acid protein base.
Indications: For use as a urinary acidifier in cats and dogs.
Dosage: The suggested dose of Uroeze Tablets for adult cats and dogs is one (1) tablet per 10 lbs (4.5 kg) body weight twice daily with food. Dosage may then be adjusted to accomplish the desired urine pH (approximately 6). Not intended for use in kittens.
Caution: Federal law restricts this drug to use by or on the order of a licensed veterinarian.
Warning: Do not administer to animals with severe liver or kidney damage or to animals exhibiting acidosis.
Caution: May cause gastric mucosa irritation. KEEP THIS AND ALL MEDICATIONS OUT OF THE REACH OF CHILDREN. STORE AT ROOM TEMPERATURE 15°–30°C (50°–86°F).
How Supplied: Bottles of 100 and 500 tablets.

Elanco Products Company

Lilly Corporate Center
INDIANAPOLIS, IN 46285

COBAN® 45
Monensin Sodium
Premix/Medicated

Composition: Active Drug Ingredients: Monensin (as monensin sodium) 45 g per pound.
Ingredients: Light Mineral Oil may be added to Control Dusting.
Indications: For use in Broiler and Replacement Chicken Feeds Only.
As an aid in the prevention of coccidiosis caused by *Eimeira necatrix, E. tenella, E. acervulina, E. brunetti, E. mivati, and E. maxima.*
Important: Must be Thoroughly Mixed in Feeds Before Use.
Mixing Directions: Thoroughly mix the following amounts of Coban® 45 Premix in one ton of feed to provide 90 through 110 grams monensin per ton of feed.

Monensin (grams per ton)	Coban® 45 Premix (lbs. per ton of feed)
90	2.00
95	2.11
100	2.22
105	2.33
110	2.44

Feeding Directions: Feed continuously as the only ration.
Caution: For replacement chickens intended for use as cage layers only.
Warning: Do not feed to laying chickens. Do not feed to chickens over 16 weeks of age. When mixing and handling monensin, use protective clothing and impervious gloves.
Caution: Do not allow horses or other equines access to formulations containing Coban®. Ingestion of Coban® by equines has been fatal.
How Supplied: 50 lb bag.

RUMENSIN® 60
monensin sodium
Premix/Medicated
Do Not Feed Undiluted
For Use in Beef Cattle Feeds Only

Important: Must be thoroughly mixed in feeds before use. This product should be further diluted before mixing in the final feed.
Active Drug Ingredient: Monensin (as monensin sodium) 60 g. per pound.

A. **Feedlot Cattle: Fed in confinement for slaughter**—For improved feed efficiency.

1. *Complete Feeds for Feedlot Cattle*

a. Intermediate Blending: Mix 1 pound of **Rumensin 60 Premix** with 11 pounds of finely ground nonmedicated feedstuff to provide an **Intermediate Premix** containing 5 grams of monensin per pound.
b. Final Blending in Complete Feeds: [See table at top of next page]
c. Feed complete feed (5–30 g/ton) continuously to growing finishing beef cattle to provide not less than 50 nor more than 360 mg monensin per head per day.
d. Rations containing silages or other wet feeds should be corrected to a 90 percent dry matter basis.
e. Labeling for complete feeds must carry the above feeding directions.

2. *Supplements for Feedlot Cattle (Dry and Liquid)*

a. Dry Supplements:
 (1) Intermediate Blending: Mix 1 pound of **Rumensin 60 Premix** with 2 pounds of finely ground nonmedicated feedstuff to provide an **Intermediate Premix** containing 20 grams of Rumensin per pound.
 (2) Final Blending in Supplements for Feedlot Cattle:
 [See table at top of next page]
b. Liquid Supplements:
 (1) Add appropriate amount of **Rumensin 60 Premix** to liquid supplement: [See next page]
 (2) The pH of the supplement must be between 4.3–7.1
 (3) Stored Rumensin Liquid Supplements should be recirculated or agitated for 10 minutes daily.

Caution: Inadequate mixing, (recirculation or agitation), of Rumensin Liquid Supplements has resulted in increased Rumensin concentration which has been fatal to cattle.

c. Thoroughly mix dry or liquid supplement with grain and roughage to provide 5 to 30 g/ton Rumensin in the complete feed.
d. Feed complete feed (5 to 30 g/ton) continuously to growing-finishing beef cattle to provide not less than 50 nor more than 360 mg Rumensin/hd/day.

B. **Pasture Cattle (Slaughter, stocker and feeder Cattle weighing more than 400 pounds)**—For increased rate of weight gain. *Feeding Directions:* Feed at the rate of not less than 50 nor more than 200 mg per head per day in not less than one pound of medicated feed. The concentration of Rumensin in the pasture supplement must be between 25 and 400 grams per ton.

Caution: During the first 5 days, cattle should receive no more than 100 mg per day contained in not less than 1 lb. of feed.
Do not self feed.
Do not exceed the levels of Rumensin recommended in the feeding directions as reduced average daily gains may result.

1. *Feeds and Supplements Requiring No Further Dilution Before Use*

a. Intermediate Blending: Mix 1 pound of **Rumensin 60 Premix** with 2 pounds of finely ground nonmedicated feedstuff to provide an **Intermediate Premix** containing 20 grams of monensin per pound.

b. Final Blending:
[See table below]

2. *Dry Supplements Requiring Further Dilution Before Use. Important:* Rumensin supplements must carry label directions for mixing into feeds in accord with B.1.b., above.

a. Intermediate Blending: Mix 1 pound of **Rumensin 60 Premix** with 2 pounds of finely ground non-medicated feedstuff to provide an **Intermediate Premix** containing 20 grams of Rumensin per pound.

b. Final Blending into Dry Supplements:
[See next page]

c. Dry supplements must be further diluted in feed to produce Rumensin concentrations between 25 and 400 grams per ton.

Warning: Do Not Feed Undiluted. When Mixing and handling Rumensin 60 Premix, use protective clothing, impervious gloves, and a dust mask. Operators should wash thoroughly with soap and water after handling.

Complete Feeds

Pounds of 5 Grams Per Pound **Intermediate Premix** Per Ton of Air-dry Feed	To Achieve a Rumensin Concentration of
1	5 grams/ton
2	10
3	15
4	20
5	25
6	30*

* Maximum approved concentration in complete feeds.

Dry Supplements

Add the following Amounts of 20 Gram Per Pound **Intermediate Premix** Per Ton of Supplement Mixed	Rumensin will be Present in the Supplement at the Following Concentrations
2.5 lbs.	50 g/ton
10	200
18	360
30	600
60	1200*

* Maximum approved supplement concentration

Liquid Supplements

Add the following Amounts of **Rumensin 60 Premix** Per Ton of Supplement Mixed	Rumensin will be Present in the Supplement at the Following Concentrations
3.3 lbs.	200 g/ton
6	360
10	600
20	1200*

* Maximum approved supplement concentration

TYLAN® 10 PLUS SULFA
Tylosin Phosphate and Sulfamethazine Premix/Medicated
For Use in Swine Feeds Only

Composition: Active Drug Ingredients: Tylosin (as tylosin phosphate) (10 g per lb) Sulfamethazine 2.2% (10 g per lb).
Important: Must be Thoroughly Mixed in Feeds Before Use.
Mixing and Feeding Directions: Thoroughly mix 10 pounds Tylan® 10 Plus Sulfa Premix in one ton of complete feed to provide 100 grams of tylosin and 100 grams of sulfamethazine per ton.
For maintaining weight gains and feed efficiency in the presence of atrophic rhinitis—feed 100 grams of tylosin and 100 grams of sulfamethazine per ton of complete feed.
For lowering the incidence and severity of *Bordetella bronchiseptica* rhinitis—feed 100 grams of tylosin and 100 grams of sulfamethazine per ton of complete feed.
For prevention of swine dysentery (vibrionic)—feed 100 grams of tylosin and 100 grams of sulfamethazine per ton of complete feed.
For control of swine pneumonias caused by bacterial pathogens *(Pasteurella multocida and/or Corynebacterium pyogenes)*—feed 100 grams of tylosin and 100 grams of sulfamethazine per ton of complete feed.
Warning: Feeds containing Tylan® 10 Plus Sulfa Premix must be withdrawn 15 days before swine are slaughtered.
How Supplied: 50 lb bag.

Continued on next page

In Feeds Fed at the Rate of	To Achieve a Rumensin Intake of	Add the Following Amonts of 20 Gram Per Pound **Intermediate Premix** Per Ton of Supplement Mixed	Rumensin Will Be Present in the Supplement at the Following Concentrations
1 lb./hd./day	50 mg./hd./day	5 lbs.	100 grams/ton
	100	10	200
	200*	20	400*
2	50	2.5	50
	100	5	100
	200*		200
3	50	1.67	33
	100	3.33	67
	200*	6.67	133
4	50	1.25	25
	100	2.50	50
	200*	5.00	100

* Maximum approved level

Elanco—Cont.

TYLAN® 40
tylosin phosphate
PREMIX/Medicated
For Use in Swine, Beef Cattle, and Chicken Feeds Only

Important: Must be thoroughly mixed in feeds before use. To insure adequate mixing, an intermediate blending step should be used prior to manufacturing a complete feed.
Do not use in any finished feed (supplement, concentrate or complete feed) containing in excess of 2% bentonite.
Active Drug Ingredient:
Tylosin....................................40 g per lb.
(as tylosin phosphate)
Mixing and Feeding Directions for Swine Feeds:
For increased rate of weight gain and improved feed efficiency.
[See table above].
For prevention of swine dysentery (vibrionic), Feed 100 g. of tylosin per ton (2.5 pounds Tylan 40 Premix per ton) of complete feed for at least three weeks. Follow with 40 g. tylosin per ton (1 pound Tylan Premix per ton) of complete feed until pigs reach market weight.
For maintaining weight gains and feed efficiency in the presence of atrophic rhinitis—Feed 100 g. of tylosin per ton (2.5 pounds Tylan 40 Premix per ton) of complete feed. Feed continuously as the only ration.
For the treatment and control of swine dysentery (vibrionic). Treat with Tylan Plus Vitamins (250 mg. tylosin per gallon) in drinking water for 3 to 10 days and follow with 40 to 100 g. tylosin per ton (1 to 2.5 pounds Tylan 40 Premix) of complete feed for two to six weeks.
Mixing and Feeding Directions for Beef Cattle Feeds:
For reduction of incidence of liver abscesses in beef cattle caused by *Sphaerophorus necrophorus* and *Corynebacterium pyogenes.*

Tylan 40 Premix per Ton of Feed	Tylosin per Ton of Feed
0.2 to 0.25 lbs.	8 to 10 g.

To be fed so that each animal receives not more than 90 mg. per head per day and not less than 60 mg. per head per day.
Feed continuously as the only ration.

Feed	Tylan 40 Premix per Ton of Feed	Tylosin per Ton of Feed
Pre-Starter or Starter	0.5 to 2.5 lbs.	20 to 100 g.
Grower	0.5 to 1 lb.	20 to 40 g.
Finisher	0.25 to 0.5 lbs.	10 to 20 g.

Feed continuously as the only ration.

TYLAN® 50 INJECTION
(tylosin)
For Use in Swine, Beef Cattle and Nonlactating Dairy Cattle Only

Description: Tylan 50 Injection is a sterile solution of tylosin base in 50% propylene glycol with 4% benzyl alcohol and purified water. Each ml. contains 50 mg. of tylosin activity (as tylosin base).
Actions: Tylan has an antibacterial spectrum that is essentially gram-positive, but it is also active against certain spirochetes, large viruses, and certain gram-negative organisms (not including coliforms). It has also been found to be active against certain Mycoplasma species.
Indications: In beef cattle and nonlactating dairy cattle, Tylan 50 Injection is indicated for use in the treatment of bovine respiratory complex (shipping fever, pneumonia) usually associated with *Pasteurella multocida* and *Corynebacterium pyogenes;* foot rot (necrotic pododermatitis) and diphteria caused by *Fusobacterium necrophorum* and metritis caused by *Corynebacterium pyogenes.*
In swine, Tylan 50 Injection is indicated for use in the treatment of swine arthritis caused by *Mycoplasma hyosynoviae;* swine pneumonia caused by *Pasteurella spp;* swine erysipelas caused by *Erysipelothrix rhusiopathiae;* acute swine dysentery associated with *Treponema hyodysenteriae* when followed by appropriate medication in the drinking water and/or feed.
Dosage and Administration: Tylan 50 Injection is administered intramuscularly.
Beef Cattle and Nonlactating Dairy Cattle: Inject intramuscularly 8 mg. per pound of body weight one time daily (1 ml. per 6.25 pounds). Treatment should be continued 24 hours following remission of disease signs, not to exceed 5 days. Do not inject more than 10 ml. per site.
Swine: Inject intramuscularly 4 mg. per pound of body weight (1 ml. per 12.5 pounds) twice daily. Treatment should be continued 24 hours following remission of disease signs, not to exceed 3 days. Do not inject more than 5 ml. per site.
Side Effects: Side effects consisting of an edema of the rectal mucosa, anal protrusion, diarrhea, erythema, and pruritus have been observed in some hogs following the use of tylosin. Discontinuation of treatment effected an uneventful recovery from the reaction.
Caution: Do not mix Tylan 50 Injection with other injectable solutions as this may cause a precipitation of the active ingredients.
Precaution: Adverse reactions, including shock and death may result from overdosage in baby pigs.
Do not attempt injection into pigs weighing less than 6.25 pounds (0.5 ml.), nless the syringe is capable of accurately delivering 0.1 ml.
If tylosin medicated drinking water is used as a followup treatment for swine dysentery the animal should thereafter receive feed containing 40 to 100 grams of tylosin per ton for 2 weeks to assure depletion of tissue residues.
Warning:
Discontinue use in cattle 21 days before slaughter.
Discontinue use in swine 14 days before slaughter.
Do not use in lactating dairy cattle.
Store at 72°F (22°C.) or below.
How Supplied: Tylan 50 Injection is supplied in 100 ml. vials with aluminum sealed rubbed stoppers.

TYLAN® 200 INJECTION
(tylosin)
For Use in Swine, Beef Cattle and Nonlactating Dairy Cattle

Descriptions: Tylan 200 Injection is a sterile solution of tylosin base in 50% propylene glycol with 4% benzyl alcohol and purified water. Each ml. contains 200 mg. of tylosin activity (as tylosin base).
Actions: Tylan has an antibacterial spectrum that is essentially gram-positive, but it is also active against certain spirochete, large viruses, and certain gram-negative organisms (not including coliforms). It has also been found to be active against certain Mycoplasma species.
Indications: In beef cattle and nonlactating dairy cattle, Tylan 200 Injection is indicated for use in the treatment of bovine respiratory complex (shipping fever, pneumonia) usually associated with *Pasteurella multocida* and *Corynebacterium pyogenes;* foot rot (necrotic pododermatitis) and diphteria caused by *Fusobacterium necrophorum* and metritis caused by *Corynebacterium pyogenes.*
In swine, Tylan 200 Injection is indicated for use in the treatment of swine arthritis caused by *Mycoplasma hyosynoviae;*

Desired Rumensin Concentration in Supplement to Be Manufactured	Pounds of 27 Gram Per Pound **Intermediate Premix** Per Ton of Supplement Manufactued
600 grams/ton	30
800	40
1000	50
1200*	80

* Maximum approved level

swine pneumonia caused by *Pasteurella spp.*, swine erysipelas caused by *Erysipelothix rhusiopathiae;* acute swine dysentery associated with *Treponema hyodysenteriae* when followed by appropriate medication in the drinking water and/or feed.
Dosage and Administration: Tylan 200 Injection is administered intramuscularly.
Beef Cattle and Nonlactating Dairy Cattle: Inject intramuscularly 8 mg. per pound of body weight one time daily (1 ml. per 25 pounds). Treatment should be continued 24 hours following remission of disease signs, not to exceed 5 days. Do not inject more than 10 ml. per site.
Swine: Inject intramuscularly 4 mg. per pound of body weight (1 ml. per 50 pounds) twice daily. Treatment should be continued 24 hours following remission of disease signs, not to exceed 3 days. Do not inject more than 5 ml. per site.
Side Effects: Side effects consisting of an edema of the rectal muscoa, anal protrusion, diarrhea, erythema, and pruritus have been observed in some hogs following the use of tylosin. Discontinuation of treatment effected an uneventful recovery from the reaction.
Caution: Do not mix Tylan 200 Injection with other injectable solutions as this may cause a precipitation of the active ingredients.
Precaution: Adverse reactions, including shock and death may result from overdosage in baby pigs.
Do not attempt injection into pigs weighing less than 25 pounds (0.5 ml.), with the common syringe. It is recommended that Tylan 500 Injection be used in pigs weighing less than 25 pounds.
If tylosin medicated drinking water is used as followup treatment for swine dysentery the animal should thereafter receive feed containing 40 to 100 grams of tylosin per ton for 2 weeks to assure depletion of tissue residues.
Warning:
Discontinue use in cattle 21 days before slaughter.
Discontinue use in swine 14 days before slaughter.
Do not use in lactating dairy cattle.
Store at 72°F. (22°C.) or below.
How Supplied: Tylan 20 Injection is supplied in 100 ml., and 250 ml. vials with aluminum sealed rubber stoppers.

TYLAN® PLUS NEOMYCIN EYE POWDER
(tylosin)
For treatment of pinkeye (infectious keratoconjunctivitis) in cattle.

Composition: tylosin activity (as the base), 2%; neomycin sulfate (equivalent to 0.25% neomycin base); Metycaine, piperocaine hydrochloride, Lilly, 1%, acriflavine neutral (coloring agent), 0.5%; boric acid, q.s.
Directions: Confine animals. Hold eyelids open. Invert and squeeze container to dust powder into eye. Treat both eyes. Repeat daily up to 7 days depending on severity of infection. Protect infected animals from direct sunlight, dust and flies. In an infected herd, all animals with or without signs of disease should receive at least one treatment.
Warning: In case of severe eye damage, or if condition persists or increases, discontinue drug and consult a veterinarian. Keep out of reach of children.

Essar
See OSBORN

Evsco Pharmaceuticals
Affiliate of Immunogenetics, Inc.
P.O. BOX 209, HARDING HIGHWAY
BUENA, NJ 08310

CARDOXIN®
(digoxin veterinary elixir) 0.15 mg per ml

Composition: Cardoxin® (Digoxin Veterinary Elixir) a glycoside derived from *Digitalis lanata* is a stable solution specially formulated for small animals. Each ml contains 0.15 mg of Digoxin in a flavored base containing 30% alcohol. The custom designed dropper made of plastic prevents accidental glass breakage and provides accurate dosing. The 1.0 ml custom designed dropper is clearly and accurately calibrated in 0.1 ml divisions, each 0.2 ml delivering 0.03 mg of the cardiac glycoside in elixir form.
The effects of Cardoxin are comparable to those of Digoxin in tablet and parenteral form. However, due to the narrow range between the therapeutic and toxic levels of Digoxin, accurate administration is essential. Cardoxin assures accurate oral administration because the Digoxin is evenly dissolved in an alcohol base rather than mixed unevenly in a filler tablet base. The use of oral liquid therapy assures accurate and simple dosing each time whereas with tablet preparations there is a risk of inadequate dosing or overdosing.
Pharmacologic Action: Cardoxin is rapidly absorbed from the gastrointestinal tract. Its pharmacologic effects are the same as those produced by Digoxin in tablet form.
Cardoxin promotes increased inotropic action and thus increases the force of myocardial contraction. In the failing canine heart the intravenous administration of Digoxin has been shown to increase cardiac output, decrease venous pressure, increase the force of ventricular contractability and secondarily to increase the glomerular filtration and renal circulation. (1,2 3) Oral Digoxin preparations in the canine have been demonstrated to be more effective in controlling heart failure than digitoxin or whole leaf digitalis (4,5,6). Cardoxin induces both vagal and extravagal effects thereby slowing the cardiac rate, via increased S-A and A-V nodal refractoriness, and slowing impulse conduction. These effects occur at varying levels of clinical digitalization. It should be emphasized that these effects (decreased heart rate or increased P-R interval) may or may not be present when clinical digitalization has occurred. Increased myocardial automaticity, a toxic response, may result in the development of ventricular premature contractions. (See Digitalis Intoxication).
Indications: Cardoxin is indicated for the treatment of congestive heart failure, regardless of its etiology. In addition, it is indicated for the treatment of atrial and junctional premature beats, supraventricular tachycardias, atrial fibrillation, and atrial flutter. It may be indicated for the treatment of ventricular premature beats or ventricular tachycardia if these result from decreased cardiac output secondary to congestive heart failure (see Contraindications).
Contraindications: Cardoxin is contraindicated in the presence of digoxin (or any other cardiac glycoside) intoxication. It is usually contraindicated in the presence of ventricular premature contractions and ventricular tachycardia, except when these arrhythmias arise secondarily to decreased cardiac output which accompanies congestive heart failure. Heart block is usually a contraindication to the use of digitalis preparations since the glycoside may further increase the degree of heart block thereby further reducing the ventricular rate. Cardoxin may be used in the presence of complete heart block and congestive heart failure; however, extreme caution and electrocardiographic monitoring is recommended.
Dosage and Administration: Cardoxin (Digoxin Veterinary Elixir) is pleasantly flavored and may be administered by inserting the plastic dropper directly into animal's mouth. The dosage of Cardoxin, like all cardiac glycosides, must be individually titrated for each patient. Electrocardiographic, radiographic, and blood chemical analyses provide only guidelines for the clinical use of Digoxin. The dosage of Cardoxin administered to the patient will depend upon the clinical response and requirements of each patient. Clinical response provides some but not all of the information regarding digitalization; thus the patient should be monitored periodically with electrocardiographic and other laboratory tests.
Digitalization with Cardoxin may be accomplished using either the loading dose schedule (see Table I) or the daily maintenance method (see Table II) (1). Using the loading dose method a total calculated dose of 0.05-0.10 mg/lb is administered in divided doses over 48 hours or until toxicity occurs, whichever occurs first. After toxic signs appear, additional glycoside therapy is withheld until the toxic signs have been absent for 12 to 24 hours. Then a maintenance dosage of approximately 0.01 mg/lb/day is administered, divided into two doses given every 12 hours (Table II). Using the maintenance method only for digitalization, the patient will be digitalized in 6–10 days after therapy is instituted. The dosages recommended are meant to be guidelines for the use of Cardoxin. Individual varia-

Continued on next page

Evsco—Cont.

tions necessitate the individual titration of the correct amount for each patient. Larger dogs require proportionately less digitalis per pound body weight than do smaller dogs to effect the same level of digitalization. Dogs in atrial fibrillation frequently require higher levels of cardiac glycoside to slow the ventricular rate.

TABLE I
GUIDELINE* TO DIGITALIZATION—48 HOUR LOADING DOSE

Weight (lbs)	ml of Cardixon (mg) every 12 hours for 48 hrs.**
5	0.4 (0.06mg) to 0.8 (0.12 mg)
10	0.08 (0.12mg) to 1.6 (0.24mg)
15	1.2 (0.18mg) to 2.4 (0.36mg)
20	1.6 (0.24 mg) to 3.2 (0.48 mg)
30	2.6 (0.40 mg) to 3.3. (0.50 mg)
40	3.3. (0.50 mg) to 5.0 (0.75 mg)
50	5.0(0.75 mg)
Over 50	6.6(1.0 mg)
Over 100	10.0 (1.5 mg)

*Guideline means the approximate amount of the glycoside usually required by a dog for each weight group. Individual variations will occur and must be considered.

**Dosage to be given for 4 full doses unless intoxication develops first. The presence of digitalis intoxication indicates the full digitalization has been reached, regardless of the dose administered.

TABLE II
GUIDELINE* TO MAINTENANCE DOSAGE

Weight (lbs)	ml of Cardoxin (mg) every 12 hours**
5	0.5(.022 mg) ± 0.05 ml
10	0.3(.045 mg) ± 0.08 ml
15	0.5(.075 mg) ± 0.12 ml
20	0.6(.090 mg) ± 0.15 ml
30	1.0(0.15 mg) ± 0.25 ml
40	1.2(0.18 mg) ± 0.30 ml
50	1.5(0.225 mg)± 0.40 ml
Over 50	2.0 (0.30 mg) ± 0.50 ml
Over 100	3.0 (0.45 mg) ± 1.00 ml

*Guideline refers to the approximate amount of the glycoside usually required by a dog in each weight category for daily maintenance therapy. Individual variations require individual titration of the actual dosage.

**Requires twice daily administration preferably at 12 hour intervals.

Precautions: Frequent electrocardiographic monitoring is recommended when digitalis clycosides are administered.

Previous use of any cardiac glycoside in the past 10 days requires that the dosage of Cardoxin (Digoxin Veterinary Elixir) be reduced to avoid digitalis intoxication. Patients with impaired renal and/or hepatic function may require a lower dosage of Digoxin due to slower excretion of the glycoside. Dogs with more advanced cardiac disease often have a narrower margin between the therapeutic and toxic levels of Digoxin, than do healthy dogs.

Serum potassium deficiency increases cardiac irritability and may evoke ventricular arrhythmias. Serum potassium deficiency also slows impulse conduction and may induce heart block. Patients on cardiac glycosides, low potassium diets, corticosteroids, or potassium deleting diuretic agents should have serial serum potassium determinations made. Hypokalemia requires that the administration of cardiac glycosides be temporarily stopped and normal electrolyte levels be restored. Patients on any digitalis product demonstrating persistent intoxication should have potassium and other electrolyte levels evaluated.

Cardoxin is not indicated for shock, anemia, uremia, or other conditions unless congestive heart failure is present. When digitalis glycosides are being administered caution is advised in the use of calcium salts or sympathomimetic amines such as ephedrine or epinephrine. Cardoxin is unlikely to be effective when heart failure occurs secondarily to mechanical causes unrelated to myocardial disease. The use of prophylactic digitalization prior to surgery is not indicated unless evidence of gross or incipient heart failure is present.

Side Effects: (Digitalis Intoxication): Digitalis intoxication is an accentuation of the effects of clinical digitalization. The signs of Digoxin intoxication are the same as those of all other glycosides when administered at toxic levels. The clinical signs are depression, anorexia, vomition, diarrhea, severe weakness, dehydration, and cardiac rhythm irregularities. The cardiac arrhythmias most often recognized in the dog include heart block (first and second degrees), ventricular premature contractions, supraventricular tachycardia, ventricular tachycardia, and ventricular fibrillation. It should be emphasized that any abnormal arrhythmia which develops during digitalization should be suspect as a sign of intoxication. In most instances the cardiac arrhythmias induced by digitalis administration are preceded by gastrointestinal signs of Digoxin intoxication.

Because Cardoxin is rapidly broken down in the body, signs of intoxication are usually of short duration. The signs may last from several hours to one or two days, unless the case is complicated by other disease or electrolyte inbalances. The most effective method of treating digitalis intoxication is to cease all cardiac glycoside administration and maintain fluid and electrolyte balance. Potassium depleting diuretics should also be withheld. Antiemtic agents may be administered parenterally.

For more advanced cases of intoxication in which increased myocardial automaticity has developed, potassium chloride may be given orally (up to 1 gram daily) or intravenously (a maximum of 40 mEq per day administered slowly and with electrocardiographic monitoring). Antiarrhytmic agents such as lidocaine hydrochloride or propranolol hydrochloride (Inderal™—Ayerst Labs) may be necessary to treat more advanced conduction abnormalities.

Caution: Federal law restricts this drug to use by or on the order of a licensed veterinarian.

How Supplied: Cardoxin (Digoxin Veterinary Elixir) is supplied in 2 fluid ounce (59.1 ml) bottles, each supplied with a calibrated 1 ml plastic dropper. Cardoxin contains 0.15 mg of Digoxin per ml or 0.03 mg per 0.2 ml calibration.

CARDOXIN® LS
(digoxin veterinary elixir)
0.05 mg per ml

Composition: Cardoxin® LS (Digoxin Veterinary Elixir), a glycoside derived from *Digitalis lanata*, is a stable solution specially formulated for small animals. Each ml contains 0.05 mg of Digoxin in a flavored base containing 15% alcohol. The custom designed dropper made of plastic, prevents accidental glass breakage and provides accurate dosing. The 1.0 ml custom designed dropper is clearly and accurately calibrated in 0.1 ml divisions, each 0.1 ml delivering 0.0005 mg of the cardiac glycoside in elixir form.

The effects of Cardoxin LS are comparable to those of Digoxin in tablet and parenteral form. However, due to the narrow range between the therapeutic and toxic levels of Digoxin, accurate administration is essential. Cardoxin LS assures accurate oral administration because the Digoxin is evenly dissolved in an alcohol base rather than mixed unevenly in a filler tablet base. The use of oral liquid therapy assures accurate and simple dosing each time whereas with table preparations there is a risk of inadequate dosing or overdosing.

Pharmacologic Action: Cardoxin LS is rapidly absorbed from the gastrointestinal tract. Its pharmacologic effects are the same as those produced by Digoxin in tablet form.

Cardoxin LS promotes increased inotropic action and thus increases the force of myocardial contraction. In the failing canine heart the intravenous administration of Digoxin has been shown to increase cardiac output, decrease venous pressure, increase the force of ventricular contractability and secondarily to increase the glomerular filtration and renal circulation. (1, 2,3) Oral Digoxin preparations in the canine have been demonstrated to be more effective in controlling heart failure than Digitoxin or whole leaf digitalis (4, 5, 6).

Cardoxin LS induces both vagal and extravagal effects thereby slowing the cardiac rate, via increased S-A and A-V nodal refractoriness, and slowing impulse conduction. These effects occur at varying levels of clinical digitalization. It should be emphasized that these effects (decreased heart rate or increased P-R interval) may or may not be present when clinical digitalization has occured. Increased myocardial automaticity, a toxic response, may result in the development of ventricular premature contractions. (See Digitalis Intoxication).

Indications: Cardoxin LS is indicated for the treatment of congestive heart failure, regardless of its etiology. In addition it is indicated for the treatment of atrial and junctional premature beats, supraventricular tachycardias, atrail fibrillation, and atrial flutter. It may be indicated for the treatment of ventricular premature beats of ventricular tachycardia if these result from decreased cardiac output secondary to congestive heart failure (See Contraindications).

Contraindications: Cardoxin LS is contraindicated in the presence of Digoxin (or any other cardiac glycoside) intoxification. It is usually contraindicated in the presence of ventricular premature contractions and ventricular tachycardia, except when these arrhythmias arise secondarily to decreased cardiac output which accompanies congestive heart failure. Heart block is usually a contraindication to the use of digitalis preparations since the glycoside may further increase the degree of heart block thereby further reducing the ventricular rate. Cardoxin LS may be used in the presence of complete heat block and congestive heart failure; however, extreme caution and electrocardiographic monitoring is recommended.

Dosage and Administration: Cardoxin LS (Digoxin Veterinary Elixir) is pleasantly flavored and may be administered by inserting the plastic dropper directly into the animal's mouth. The dosage of Cardoxin LS like all cardiac glycosides must be individually titrated for each patient. Electrocardiographic, radiographic, and blood chemical analyses provide only guidelines for the clinical use of Digoxin. The dosage of Cardoxin LS administered to the patient will depend upon the clinical response and requirements of each patient. Clinical response provides some but not all of the information regarding digitalization; thus the patient should be monitored perodically with electrocardiographic and other laboratory tests.

Digitalization with Cardoxin LS may be accomplished using either the loading dose schedule (See Table 1) or the daily maintenance method (See Table 2) (1). Using the loading dose method a total calculated dose of 0.005-0.10 mg/lb is administered in divided doses over 48 hours or until toxicity occurs, whichever occurs first. After toxic signs appear, additional glycoside therapy is withheld until the toxic signs have been absent for 12 to 24 hours. Then a maintenance dosage of approximately 0.01 mg/lb/day is administered, divided into two doses given every 12 hours (Table 2). Using the maintenance method only for digitalization, the patient will be digitalized in 6–10 days after therapy is instituted.

The dosages recommended are meant to be guidelines for the use of Cardoxin LS. Individual variations necessitate the individual titration of the correct amount for each patient. Larger dogs require proportionately less digitalis per pound body weight than do smaller dogs to effect the same level of digitalization. Dogs in atrial fibrillation frequently require higher levels of cardiac glycoside to slow the ventricular rate.

TABLE I
GUIDELINE* TO DIGITALIZATION—48 HOUR LOADING DOSE

Weight (lbs)	ml of Cardoxin LS (mg) every 12 hours for 48 hours**
1	0.25 (0.12 mg) to 0.5 (0.025 mg)
2	0.50 (0.025 mg) to 1.0 (0.50 mg)
3	0.75 (0.037 mg) to 1.5 (0.075 mg)
4	1.00 (0.50 mg) to 2.0 (0.100 mg)
5	1.25 (0.062 mg) to 2.5 (0.125 mg)
6	1.50 (0.75 mg) to 3.0 (0.150 mg)
7	1.75 (0.087 mg) to 3.5 (0.175 mg)
8	2.00 (0.100 mg) to 4.0 (0.200 mg)
9	2.25 (0.112 mg) to 4.5 (0.225 mg)
10	2.5 (0.125 mg) to 5.0 (0.250 mg)

*Guideline means the approximate amount of the glycoside usually required by a dog for each weight group. Individual variations will occur and must be considered.

**Dosage to be given for 4 full doses unless intoxication develops first. The presence of digitalis intoxication indicates that full digitalization has been reached, regardless of the dose administered.

TABLE 2
GUIDELINE* TO MAINTENANCE DOSAGE

Weight (lbs)	ml of Cardoxin LS (mg) every 12 hours
1	0.1(0.0005 mg)
2	0.2(0.10 mg)
3	0.3(0.015 mg)
4	0.4(0.020 mg)
5	0.5(0.025 mg)
6	0.6(0.030 mg)
7	0.7(0.035 mg)
8	0.8(0.040 mg)
9	0.9(0.045 mg)
10	1.0(0.050mg)

*Guideline refers to the approximate amount of the glycoside usually required by a dog in each weight category for daily maintenance therapy. Individual variations require individual titration of the actual dosage.

**Requires twice daily administration preferably at 12 hour intervals.

Precautions: Frequent electrocardiographic monitoring is recommended when digitalis glycosides are administered.

Previous use of any cardiac glycoside in the past 10 days requires that the dosage of Cardoxin LS (Digoxin Veterinary Elixir) be reduced to avoid digitalis intoxication. Patients with impaired renal and/or hepatic function may require a lower dosage of Digoxin due to slower excretion of, the glycoside. Dogs with more advanced cardiac disease often have a narrower margin between the therapeutic and toxic levels of Digoxin than do healthy dogs.

Serum potassium deficiency increases cardiac irritability and may evoke ventricular arrhythmias. Serum potassium deficiency also slows impulse conduction and may induce heart block. Patients on cardiac glycosides low potassium diets, corticosteroids, or potassium depleting, diuretic agents should have serial serum potassium determinations made. Hypokalemia requires that the administration of cardiac glycosides be temporarily stopped and normal electrolyte levels be restored. Patients on any digitalis product demonstrating persistent intoxication should have potassium and other electrolyte levels evaluated.

Cardoxin LS is not indicated for shock, anemia, uremia, or other conditions unless congestive heart failure is present. When digitalis glycosides are being administered caution is advised in the use of calcium salts or sympathomimetic amines such as ephedrine or epinephrine. Cardoxin LS is unlikely to be effective when heart failure occurs secondarily to mechanical causes unrelated to myocardial disease. The use of prophylactic digitalization prior to surgery is not indicated unless evidence of gross or incipient heart failure is present.

Side Effects (Digitalis Intoxication): Digitalis Intoxication is an accentuation of the effects of clinical digitalization. The signs of Digoxin intoxication are the same as those of all other glycosides when administered at toxic levels. The clinical signs are depression, anorexia, vomition, diarrhea, severe weakness, dehydration, and cardiac rhythm irregularities. The cardiac arrhythmias most often recognized in the dog include heart block (first and second degrees), ventricular premature contractions, supraventricular trachycardia, ventricular tachycardia, and ventricular fibrillation. It should be emphasized that any abnormal arrhythmia which develops during digitalization should be suspect as a sign of intoxication. In most instances the cardiac arrhythmias induced by digitalis administration are preceded by gastrointestinal signs of Digoxin intoxication.

Because Cardoxin LS is rapidly broken down in the body, signs of intoxication are usually of short duration. The signs may last from several hours to one or two days, unless the case is complicated by other disease or electrolyte imbalances. The most effective method of treating digitalis intoxication is to cease all cardiac glycoside administration and maintain fluid and electrolyte balance. Potassium depleting diuretics should also be withheld. Antiemetic agents may be administered parenterally.

For more advanced cases of intoxication in which increased myocardial automaticity has developed, potassium chloride may be given orally (up to 1 gram daily) or intravenously (a maximum of 40 mEq per day administered slowly and with electrocardiographic monitoring). Antiarrhythmic agents such as lidocaine hydrochloride or propranolol hydrochloride (Inderal™ —Ayerst Labs) may be necessary to treat more advanced conduction abnormalities.

Caution: Federal law restricts this drug to use by or on the order of a licensed veterinarian.

How Supplied: Cardoxin LS is supplied in 2 fluid ounce (59.1 ml) bottles, each supplied with a calibrated 1 ml plastic dropper, Cardoxin LS contains 0.05

Continued on next page

E

Evsco—Cont.

mg of digoxin per ml or 0.005 mg per 0.1 ml calibration.

CERUMITE®

Composition: Cerumene (Squalane) 25.00%, Pyrethrins 0.05%, Technical Piperonyl Butoxide* 0.50%, inert ingredients 74.45%.

*Equivalent to 0.4% butylcarbityl (6-propyl piperonyl) ether and 0.1% other related com pounds.

Indications: Cerumite provides the penetrating action of Cerumene along with the miticidal action of pyrethrins. It quickly penetrates the wax barrier in the ear and effectively treats the mite infestation.

Dosage and Administration: Clean the ear canal thoroughly. Depending on size of animal, place 5-15 drops in ear daily. Recommended treatment—7 to 10 days, repeat treatment in two weeks if necessary.

How Supplied: ½ fl oz (15 ml) applicator bottles.

E

CHLORASOL®
(Chloramphenicol) 0.5%
Sterile Ophthalmic Solution

Composition: Chloramphenicol 0.5% (5 mg/ml) Chlorobutanol (chloral deriv.) as preservative 0.5% with polyethylene glycol 300, polyoxyl 40 stearate, sodium hydroxide and/or hydrochloric acid if needed to adjust pH and purified water.

Description: Chlorasol is the first commercially available chloramphenicol solution for veterinary use which does not require reconstitution prior to dispensing; possibilities of contamination or compounding errors are thereby reduced. Chlorasol (chloramphenicol) has a wide spectrum of antimicrobial activity and is effective against many Gram-negative and Gram-positive organisms such as *Escherichia coli, Staphylococcus aureus* and *Streptococcus hemolyticus*.

Indications: As an aid in the treatment of bacterial conjunctivitis in dogs and cats caused by organisms susceptible to chloramphenicol.

Contraindications: This chloramphenicol product must not be used in meat, egg, or milk producing animals. The length of time that residues persist in milk or tissues has not been determined.

Warnings: Not for use in animals which are raised for food production. Prolonged use in cats may produce blood dyscrasias. As with other antibiotics, prolonged use may result in overgrowth of nonsusceptible organisms. If superinfection occurs, or if clinical improvement is not noted within a reasonable period, discontinue use and institute appropriate therapy.

Dosage: One or two drops 4 to 6 times a day for the first 72 hours, depending upon the severity of the condition. Intervals between applications may be increased after the first two days. Since the action of the drug is primarily bacteriostatic, therapy should be continued for 48 hours after an apparent cure has been attained. Therapy for cats should not exceed 7 days.

Caution: Federal (U.S.A.) law restricts this drug to use by or on the order of a licensed veterinarian.

How Supplied: Chlorasol (chloramphenicol) is available in 7.5 ml plastic dropper bottles. Refrigerate until dispensed.

CHLORASONE®
(chloramphenicol—prednisolone acetate)
Sterile Ophthalmic Ointment

Composition: Each gram contains Chloramphenicol U.S.P. 10 mg, Prednisolone Acetate U.S.P. 2.5 mg in a light Mineral Oil, White Petrolatum, Polyoxyethylene Sorbitan Monostearate base.

Indications: For use in dogs and cats for the treatment of bacterial conjunctivitis and ocular inflammation caused by organisms susceptible to Chloramphenicol.

Description: Chloramphenicol has a wide spectrum of anti-microbial activity and is effective against many Gram negative and Gram positive organisms such as *Excherichia coli, Staphylococcus aureus* and *Streptococcus hemolyticus*. Prednisolone Acetate exerts a marked anti-inflammatory effect when used topically in the eye.

Dosage and Administration: Apply to affected eye 4-6 times daily for first 72 hours, depending upon the severity of the condition. Continue treatment for 48 hours after eye appears normal. Therapy for cats should not exceed 7 days.

Warning: Not for use in animals which are raised for food production. Prolonged use in cats may produce blood dyscrasias. As with other antibiotics, prolonged use may result in overgrowth of non-susceptible organisms. If superinfection occurs, or if clinical improvement is not noted within a reasonable period, discontinue use and institute appropriate therapy. All topical opthalmic preparations containing corticosteroids with or without an anti-microbial agent. are contraindicated in the initial treatment of corneal ulcers. They should not be used until the infection is under control and corneal regeneration is well under way.

Precautions: When infection is suspected as being the cause of the disease process, particularly in purulent or catarrhal conjunctivitis, attempts should be made to determine what effective antibiotics should be used by sensitivity tests prior to applying opthalmic preparations containing a corticosteroid.

Contraindications: This Chloramphenicol product must not be used in meat, egg, or milk producing animals. The length of time that residues persist in milk or tissues has not be determined.

Caution: Federal Law (U.S.A.) restricts this drug to use by or on the order of a licensed veterinarian.

How Supplied: Available in 1/8 ounce (3.5 gram) ophthalmic tip tubes.

CHLORICOL™
Chloramphenicol 1%
Sterile Veterinary Ophthalmic Ointment

Composition: Each gram contains: Chloramphenicol U.S.P. 10 mg, in a Light Mineral Oil, White Petrolatum, Polyoxyethylene Sorbitan Monostearate base.

Action: Chloramphenicol is a broad-spectrum antibiotic providing rapid clinical response and having therapeutic activity against susceptible strains of a number of gram-positive and gram-negative organisms including *Escherichia coli, Staphylococcus Aureus* and *Streptococcus hemolyticus*.

Indications: Chloricol (Chloramphenicol) Veterinary Ophthalmic, Ointment, 1% is appropriate for use in dogs and cats for the topical treatment of bacterial conjunctivitis caused by pathogens susceptible to chloramphenicol.

Contraindications: Chloramphenicol products must not be used in meat, egg, or milk-producing animals. The length of time that residues persist in milk or tissues has not been determined.

Warning: Not for use in animals which are raised for food production.

Prolonged use in cats may produce blood dyscrasias.

Precautions: Most susceptible bacteria will respond to chloramphenicol therapy in a few days. If improvement is not noted in this period of time, a change of therapy should be considered.

When infection is suspected as the cause of a disease process, especially in purulent or catarrhal conjunctivitis, attempts should be made to determine through susceptibility testing, which antibiotics will be effective prior to applying ophthalmic preparations.

Dosage and Administration: Application of the ointment should be preceded by cleansing to remove discharge and crusts. The ointment is applied every three hours around the clock from 48 hours, after which night instillations may be omitted. A small amount of ointment should be placed in the conjunctival sac. Treatment should be continued for two days after the eye appears normal. Therapy for cats should not exceed 7 days. For Veterinary Use Only.

Caution: Federal law restricts this drug to use on or by the order of a licensed veterinarian.

How Supplied: ⅛ (3.5 g) Sterile Tamper Proof Tubes.

DIFIL® SYRUP
(diethylcarbamazine citrate syrup)

Description: Difil syrup is a taste-acceptable flavored base containing 60 mg diethylcarbamazine citrate U S P per 1 ml.

Actions: Diethylcarbamazine citrate, a relatively non-toxic piperazine derivative, is reported to have no cumulative toxic effect when given at recommended levels. When administered orally to dogs at dosages of 25 to 50 mg/lb, diethylcarbamazine citrate has been found to be highly effective against *Toxocara canis*.

In cats, an oral dosage of 25 to 50 mg/lb has been found effective against *Toxocara canis* and *Toxascaris leonina.* Diethylcarbamazine citrate prevents the development of the infective stage of *Dirofilaria immitis* when given daily at the rate of 3 mg per pound of body weight.
Indications: For the prevention of heartworm disease (*Dirofiaria immitis*) in dogs and as an aid in the treatment of ascarid infection in dogs (*Toxocara canis*) and cats (*Toxocara canis* and *Toxascaris leonina*).
Contraindications: Dogs older than 8 months of age may also be infected with heartworm (*Dirofilaria immitis*), and the use of Difil syrup is CONTRAINDICATED IN DOGS WITH ACTIVE *DIROFILARIA IMMITIS* INFECTION. Ascarid infections are usually limited to immature animals, those exceeding 4-6 months of age are generally not considered candidates for such treatment.
Dogs with established heartworm infections should not receive Difil syrup until they have been converted to a negative status by the use of adulticidal and microfilaricidal drugs.
Dosage and Administration: It is not necessary to fast the animal before treatment.
Difil syrup, diethylcarbamazine citrate, is preferably given with (on) feed or immediately after feeding. This reduces the possibility of vomiting which may occasionally occur if the stomach is empty.
For Prevention of Heartworm: For accurate dosage, use the calibrated dropper. The dosage of 3 mg diethylcarbamazine citrate per pound of body weight may be directly administered orally or placed on the animal's food. Care should be taken to see that all food containing the medication is consumed.
Daily dosage (Based on 3 mg/lb body weight).

60 mg/ml	Body Weight
½ ml	10 lbs
1 ml	20 lbs
1½ ml	30 lbs
2 ml	40 lbs

Administration of Difil syrup should start one month before the mosquito season and continue daily throughout the mosquito season and for two months thereafter.
Dogs on prophylactic therapy should be examined for the presence of microfilariae every six months.
For Ascariasis: Dosage for roundworm treatment based on 25 to 50 mg per pound of body weight:

60 mg/ml	Body Weight
2 to 4 ml	5 lbs
4 to 8 ml	10 lbs
6 to 12 ml	15 lbs
8 to 16 ml	20 lbs

A repeat dose should be given in 10 to 20 days to remove immature worms which may enter the intestine from the lungs after the first dose. Roundworms may be expelled dead or living. They should be promptly removed to prevent reinfestation.
Caution: Federal law (U.S.A.) restricts this drug to use by or on the order of a licensed veterinarian.
Warning: Do not use in dogs that may be harboring adult heartworms. Inadvertent administration to dogs infected with heartworm may cause adverse reactions due to pulmonary occlusion or shock.
How Supplied: Difil syrup is supplied in 8 oz bottles with measuring dropper, and in gallon containers. Bottles of 8 fl oz (236.6 ml) and 1 gallon (3.785 liters).
KEEP OUT OF REACH OF CHILDREN

DIFIL® TABS
(diethylcarbamazine citrate tablets)

Description: Difil tabs are available in 5 tablet sizes as scored tablets containing 50 and 100 mg and as quartered tablets containing 200, 300 and 400 mg diethylcarbamazine citrate.
Actions: Diethylcarbamazine citrate, a relatively non-toxic piperazine derivative, is reported to have no cumulative toxic effect when given at recommended levels. When administered orally to dogs at dosages of 25 to 50 mg/lb, diethylcarbamazine citrate has been found to be highly effective against *Toxocara canis.* In cats, an oral dosage of 25 to 50 mg/lb has been found effective against *Toxocara canis* and *Toxascaris leonina.* Diethylcarbamazine citrate prevents the development of the infective stage of *Dirofilaria immitis* when given daily at the rate of 3 mg per pound of body weight.
Indications: For prevention of heartworm disease *(Dirofilaria immitis)* in dogs and as an aid in the treatment of ascarid infection in dogs *(Toxocara canis)* and cats *(Toxocara canis* and *Toxascaris leonina).*
Contraindications: Dogs older than 8 months of age may also be infected with heartworm disease *(Dirofilaria immitis)* and the use of Difil tabs is CONTRAINDICATED IN DOGS WITH ACTIVE *DIROFILARIA IMMITIS* INFECTION. Ascarid infections are usually limited to immature animals, those exceeding 4–6 months of age are generally not considered candidates for such treatment.
Dogs with established heartworm infections should not receive Difil tabs until they have been converted to a negative status by the use of adulticidal and microfilaricidal drugs.
Dosage and Administration: It is not necessary to fast the animal before treatment. Difil tabs, diethylcarbamazine citrate, is preferably given with (on) feed or immediately after feeding. This reduces the possibility of vomiting which may occasionally occur if the stomach is empty.
Dosage for Prevention of Heartworm Disease: The optimum dosage is 3 mg per pound of body weight, diethylcarbamazine citrate, administered daily.
Administration of Difil tabs should start one month after the mosquito season and continue daily throughout the mosquito season and for two months thereafter.
Dogs on prophylactic therapy should be examined for the presence of microfilariae every six months.
Dosage for Ascariasis: The dosage is 25 to 50 mg/lb body weight in dogs and cats in a single dose.
A repeat dose should be given in 10–20 days to remove worms which may have entered the intestines from the lungs after the first dose. Roundworms may be expelled dead or living. They should be promptly removed to prevent reinfection.
Caution: Federal law (U.S.A.) restricts this drug to use by or on order of a licensed veterinarian.
Warning: Do not use in dogs that may be harboring adult heartworms.
Inadvertent administration to dogs infected with heartworm may cause adverse reactions due to pulmonary occlusion or shock.
KEEP OUT OF REACH OF CHILDREN
How Supplied: Available in bottles of: 500—50 mg tablets, 300—100 mg tablets, 200—200 mg tablets, 100—300 mg tablets and 100—400 mg tablets.

E

GROOM AID® SPRAY
Hair Coat Dressing and Deodorant Cologne Spray

Composition: A coat dressing spray containing lanolin.
Indications: Canine coat dressing and deodorant. Groom Aid contains absorbable lanolin which brings out natural highlights. When used after bathing, makes coat easy to comb, brush and groom. Groom Aid is excellent for use during the winter confinement of animals.
Directions: To operate, remove protective cap from top of can. Hold can upright, about 8 to 12 inches from pet's hair. Point opening on side of valve in desired direction for spray. To release spray, place finger on top of valve and press down. Move the bomb over the entire animal, using a "Zig-Zag" motion, until the coat is slightly damp. It may be advantageous especially on long haired animals to rub the hand against the lay of hair, spraying into the ruffled hair directly behind the hand.
Warning: Contents under pressure. Do not puncture or incinerate container. Do not expose to heat or store at temperature above 130°F. Keep out of reach of children.
Caution: Avoid spraying into animals eyes.
How Supplied: 9 oz (255 grams) spray cans

K-P-SOL™
(kaolin-pectin suspension)
Diarrhea Medicine

Composition: Each fluid ounce contains:

Kaolin	(7g)	108 grs
Pectin	(259 mg)	4 grs

Indications: An aid in the treatment of diarrhea in dogs and cats.
Dosage: One to two teaspoonsful per ten pounds of body weight every six hours or as needed after each loose stool.

Continued on next page

Evsco—Cont.

Treatment may be continued for three to five days.
Warning: If clinical signs persist after two to three days, diagnosis should be redetermined.
Shake Well Before Using
How Supplied: Available in Gallons.

LAXATONE®
Laxative and Lubricant

Composition: Liquid petrolatum, white petrolatum, linoleic acid, linolenic acid, and iron peptonized in a special palatable base.
Indications: A laxative and lubricant for hairball removal with supplemental iron.
Dosage and Administration: *Cats*—for hairballs: ½-1 teaspoonful for two-three days then ¼-½ teaspoonful two-three times a week.
Laxative: ¼-½ teaspoonful two-three times a week. *Dogs*—½ to 1 teaspoonful two-three times a week.
How Supplied: 2½ ounce tubes.

E

LIQUI-BAN™
Brand of Flea Spray for Dogs

Composition: Contains Dursban*
Active Ingredients:
Chlorpyrifos [0,0 -Diethyl 0- (3,5,6- trichloro- 2 pyridyl) phosphorothioate] 0.22%
Xylene Range Aromatic Solvent 0.15%
Inert Ingredients 99.63%
*Trademark of The Dow Chemical Co. U.S. Pat. 3,244,586
Indications: Kills fleas for up to one month:
Directions for Use: It is a violation of Federal Law to use this product in a manner inconsistent with its labeling.
To operate, remove regular cap. Replace with pump. Remove cap from nozzle.
Place dog on a table or bench, preferably out of doors. Hold bottle in an upright position about 3-6 inches from the dog and continue to pump until animal's coat gets an even covering of Liqui-Ban. Spray all over the body against the lay of the coat. Avoid spraying in eyes. Spray to leave coat slightly damp down to the skin level. One treatment will kill fleas and protect against reinfestation for up to one month. Repeat treatment as necessary.
Precautionary Statements: Hazards to Humans and Domestic Animals: May cause eye irritation. Avoid contact with eyes, skin or clothing. May be harmful if swallowed. Avoid inhalation of vapors.
Note to Physician: Chlorpyrifos is a cholinesterase inhibitor. Treat symptomatically. Atropine is an antidote, by injection only.
Statement of Practical Treatment:
If Swallowed: Drink 1 or 2 glasses of water and induce vomiting by touching back of throat with finger.
If On Skin: Wash thoroughly with soap and warm water.
If In Eyes: Flush with plenty of water. Get medical attention if irritation persists.
If Inhaled: Remove from exposure, establish adequate airway, give oxygen or artificial respiration as indicated.
Do not use on cats.
Free bitches from fleas before they bear pups. Do not use on dogs nursing puppies or on pups under 10 weeks old.
Warning: Keep Out of Reach of Children.
Storage and Disposal: Do not store near heat. Store in original container in a safe place. Do not reuse container. Rinse thoroughly and wrap in several layers of newspaper before discarding in trash.
How Supplied: 16 ounces (473 ml) EPA Reg. No. 3134-40 EPA Est. No. 3134-NJ-1

LIQUICHLOR® With Cerumene™ (chloramphenicol—prednisolone—tetracaine—squalane)

Composition: Each ml contains Chloramphenicol 4.2 mg, Prednisolone 1.7 mg, Tetracaine 4.2 mg, cerumene (Squalane) 0.21 ml, in a petrolatum-mineral oil base. Pat. No. 3,821, 375.
Indications: For use in the treatment of acute otitis externa and pyodermas (acute moist dermatitis, vulvar fold dermatitis, lip fold dermatitis, inter-digital dermatitis and juvenile dermatitis) in dogs and cats. Laboratory tests should be conducted, including *in vitro* culturing and susceptibility tests on samples collected prior to treatment.
Actions: Antibacterial. Anti-inflammatory-Anesthetic. The organisms involved in otitis externa which are sensiive to Chloramphenicol are *Staphylococcus aureus, Streptococcus hemolyticum, Pseudomonas aeruginosa, Escherichia coli* and *Proteus vulgaris,* Cerumene (Squalane) speeds up percutaneous penetration, both transfollicular as well as transepidermal, allowing for accelerated penetration of the active ingredients through the horny layer. It is miscible with sebum and epidermal lipids facilitating removal of accumulated ear wax and dirt and permits direct contact between the active ingredients in Liquichlor and the affected area.
Dosage and Administration: 2-3 applications daily or as needed. Severe infections should be supplemented by systemic therapy. Therapy should not exceed 7 days.
Contraindications: Chloramphenicol products must not be used in meat, egg or milk producing animals. The length of time residues persist in milk or tissues has not been determined.
Precaution: Animals under treatment with this product should be observed for the usual signs of corticosteroid overdosage which include polydipsia, polyuria and occasionally an increase in weight.
Side Effects: If signs of irritation or sensitivity develop, discontinue use. Prolonged use of this product may result in overgrowth of nonsusceptible organisms. Constant observation of the patient is essential. If new infections due to bacteria or fungi appear during therapy, appropriate measures should be taken.
Warning: This drug must not be used in the eyes. Not for use in animals which are raised for food production. Prolonged use in cats may produce blood dyscrasias.
Caution: US Federal law restricts this drug to use by or on the order of a licensed veterinarian.
How Supplied: 10 ml Tubes, 12 ounce (355 ml) Bottles.
Shake well before each use.

MEDICOLLAR®

Description: Medicollar is a disposable, protective collar designed to prevent an animal from imposing self-inflicted trauma. Medicollar is lightweight, constructed of heavy coated fiberboard laminated with polyurethane foam.
Product Uses and Indications: Medicollar keeps an animal from reaching his body, and thereby prevents:
1. Licking sores or surgical wounds
2. Removing topical medications
3. Chewing, biting or destroying dressing, splints, casts and bandages
4. Chewing or biting at itching skin conditions
5. Pawing at eye or ear infections or irritation
6. Disturbing cropped ears or docked tails

How Supplied:
Small (dogs & cats 10-30 pounds)
Large (dogs 30-50 pounds)
X-Large (dogs 50 pounds & over).

METHIGEL®
A palatable urinary acidifier for use in cats and dogs

Composition: Each teaspoonful (5 grams) contains Methionine, 400 mg.
Indications: To maintain an acid urine in cats when urethral obstruction is a recurrent problem and for use following the removal of phosphate calculi in dogs. Also aids in the control of urine odors.
Dosage and Administration: Methigel is extremely palatable. To stimulate taste interest, place a small amount of Methigel on animal's nose or directly into mouth. Cats ½- 1 teaspoonful twice daily. Dogs 1 teaspoonful twice daily.
Warning: Methigel should not be administered to animals with severe liver or kidney disease. Methigel should not be administered to animals on an empty stomach. Large doses may cause gastrointestinal upset.
How Supplied: 4½ ounce tubes (120.5 grams).

OPTISONE®
(Neomycin Sulfate with Prednisolone) Sterile Veterinary Ophthalmic Ointment

Composition: Each gram contains: Neomycin Sulfate U.S.P. 5 mg (0.5%) (Equivalent to 3.5 mg of Neomycin base), Prednisolone 2 mg (0.2%), in a Cod Liver Oil-Mineral Oil-Petrolatum Base.
Indications: For use in superficial ocular inflammation or infections limited to the conjunctiva or the anterior segment

of the eye of dogs and cats, such as those associated with allergic reactions or gross irritants. The organisms involved in eye infections which are sensitive to Neomycin are *Escherichia coli, Staphylococcus aureus* and *Streptococcus hemolyticus.*

Contraindications:

a) Viral disease of the cornea and conjunctiva;
b) Fungal disease of the eye;
c) Acute purulent untreated infections of the eye which like other disease caused by microorganisms may be masked or enhanced by the presence of the steroid;
d) Purulent conjunctivitis; and purulent blepharitis;
e) Glaucoma

Dosage and Administration: The recommended dose is one application four times a day for seven days. Insert tip of the tube beneath the lower lid and express a small quantity of Optisone into the conjunctival sac. If clinical improvement is not noted after seven days of treatment, re-evaluation of the diagnosis should be considered.

Precautions: When infection is suspected as being the cause of the disease process particularly in purulent or catarrhal conjunctivitis attempts should be made to determine what effective antibiotics should be used by sensitivity tests prior to applying ophthalmic preparations containing a corticosteroid.

Warning: All topical ophthalmic preparations containing corticosteroids with or without an antimicrobial agent, are contraindicated in the initial treatment of corneal ulcers. They should not be used until the infection is under control and corneal regeneration is well under way. Patient should be observed for signs of adrenocorticoid systemic side reactions due to absorption of Prednisolone. The administration of systemic corticosteroids while patient is under treatment with this product represents a potential hazard.

a) Extended use may cause increased intraocular pressure and it is therefore advisable to check pressure frequently.
b) In those diseases causing thinning of the cornea, perforation has been known to occur with the use of topical steroids.
c) If signs of irritation or sensitivity develop discontinue use.
d) Tip of tube should not come in contact with eye surface.

Caution: Federal law (U.S.A.) restricts this drug to use by or on the order of a licensed veterinarian.

How Supplied: ⅛ ounce (3.5 g.) tube.

SECT-A-CHLOR™

Composition:

Active Ingredient:

Chlorpyrifos (0,0-Diethyl 0-(3,5,6-trichloro-2-pyridyl) Phosphorothioate	0.22%
Inert Ingredients:	99.78%

E.P.A. Registration No. 3134-38AA
E.P.A. Establishment No. 7056-TX-1

Indications: Flea spray for dogs. Kills fleas for up to one month.

Directions: Place dog on a table or bench, preferably out of doors. Hold can in upright position 3-6"from the dog and thoroughly spray all over the body against the lay of the coat. Avoid spraying in eyes. Spray to leave the coat slightly damp down to skin level. Spraying time should be between 30 and 60 seconds on a medium sized dog. This can should provide 8-12 complete treatments.

One treatment will kill fleas and protect against reinfestation for up to one month. Repeat treatment as necessary. Spray bedding and sleeping area.

Free bitches from fleas before they bear pups. Do not use on dogs nursing puppies or on pups under 10 weeks old.

Warning: May cause eye irritation. Avoid contact with eyes, skin or clothing. May be harmful if swallowed. Avoid inhalation of vapors.

Note to Physician: Chlorpyrifos is a cholinesterase inhibitor. Treat symptomatically. Atropine is an antidote, by injection only.

Statement of Practical treatment: If Swallowed: Drink 1 or 2 glasses of water and induce vomiting by touching back of throat with finger.

If On Skin: Wash thoroughly with soap and warm water.

If In Eyes: Flush with plenty of water. Get medical attention if irritation persists.

If Inhaled: Remove from exposure, establish adequate airway, give oxygen or artificial respiration as indicated.

Do not use on cats.

FLAMMABLE.

CONTENTS UNDER PRESSURE. DO NOT USE NEAR FIRE, SPARKS OR FLAME. DO NOT PUNCTURE OR INCINERATE CONTAINER. EXPOSURE TO TEMPERATURE ABOVE 130°F. MAY CAUSE BURSTING.

Caution: Keep Out of Reach of Children

How Supplied: Net Weight: 340 g/12 oz. Aerosol spray cans.

SECT-A-FOG™
Pressurized Fogger

Composition:

Active Ingredients:

O-Isopropoxyphenyl methylcarbamate	1.00%
2,2-Dichlorovinyl dimethyl phosphate	0.47%
Related compounds	0.03%
Inert Ingredients	98.50%
	100.00%

Indications: Sect-a-Fog kills exposed ticks, fleas, roaches, ants, flying moths, spiders and scorpions. The entire contents are released from one spot and fog penetrates throughout area.

Directions for Use: It is a violation of Federal Law to use this product in a manner inconsistent with its labeling. Use at least one canister for each 10,000 cubic feet of unobstructed area. Use additional units for remote rooms or where free flow of mist is not assured.

Important: Locate fogger in center of room or area being treated. Place newspapers under fogger unit and for three or four feet around the can to prevent staining or marring surfaces. Close doors and windows. Remove pets and cover or remove fish bowls. Cover or remove exposed foods and dishes. Open cabinets and doors to areas to be treated. Shut off fans and air conditioners. Put out all open flames except pilot light. Place at least 5 feet away from pilot light. Keep at arms length when releasing. Point top of can away from face and eyes. To start fogging action, press plastic tab on valve down until it clicks. Set in upright position and leave building at once. Leave undisturbed for at least 2 hours. Open doors and windows and thoroughly ventilate for at least 30 minutes longer. Solvents may soften some asphalt or synthetic tile floors. If used directly over asphalt or synthetic tile, newspaper should be spread on floor for several feet around the area of release. Do not use with freshly waxed floors; allow wax to become hardened. Some plastics may be affected. Remove or cover plastic items such as eyeglasses, stereo covers, notion boxes. NOTE: This product may not control hidden crawling insects. It will kill only those insects that come in contact with the mist. Therefore, complete control of an infestation of crawling insects may not be achieved.

Disposal: Do not reuse empty container. Wrap container and put in trash collection.

Precautionary Statements:

Hazards to Humans & Domestic Animals-Caution: Harmful if swallowed. Avoid breathing of mist. Avoid contact with eyes. Avoid contact with skin. Wash hands after handling. Do not contaminate food, water or foodstuffs. Food should be removed or covered during treatment. Do not use in edible product areas of food processing plants, restaurants or other areas where food is commerically processed. Do not use in serving areas while food is exposed.

Physical or Chemical Hazards: Contents under pressure. Do not puncture or incinerate container or throw into fire. Exposure to temperatures above 130°F may cause bursting.

For Use Only When Building Is Vacated By Humans & Pets.

Statement of Practical Treatment: If in *Eyes:* Flush eyes with plenty of water. Get medical attention if irritation persists.

Caution: Keep out of reach of children.

How Supplied: 12 ounce (340 grams)

EPA Est. No. 7056-TX-1
EPA Reg. No. 43288- 12-AA-3134

SECT-A-SPRAY®

Composition: Contains pyrethrins 0.05%, Piperonyl Butoxide, Technical*0.50% Carbaryl (1-naphthyl N-methylcarbamate)** 0.50%, MGK Repellent No. 11.20%, Petroleum distillate 0.20%, inert ingredients 98.55%.

*Equivalent to 0.4% (butylcarbityl) (6-propyl piperonyl) ether and 0.1% related compounds.

Continued on next page

Evsco—Cont.

Indications: Kills fleas, lice and ticks. Excellent residual action. Helps check doggie odor. For use on dogs and cats.
Dosage and Administration: To operate, remove protective cap from top of can. Hold can upright, about 2 to 4 inches from animal's hair. Point opening on side of valve in desired direction for spray. To release spray, place finger on top of valve and *press-down.* Move the bomb over the entire animal, using a "zig-zag" motion, until the coat is slightly damp. It may be advantageous, especially on long-haired animals, to rub the hand against the lay of hair, spraying into the ruffled hair directly behind the hand. 45 seconds is sufficient to treat a 30 lb animal. Repeat treatment as necessary, making sure spray wets ticks. Do not use more often than once every 7 days. Thoroughly spray interior of kennel or other animal sleeping quarters. Also spray bedding or replace with fresh bedding if necessary. Where animal odor is present, spray lightly into the air. This bomb makes a slight hissing sound and causes a temporary cool sensation. Nervous animals may become frightened the first time this bomb is used but soon become accustomed to the treatment.
Warning: May be harmful if swallowed, inhaled or absorbed through the skin. Causes temporary eye injury. *In case of contact,* immediately flush eyes or skin with plenty of water. Get medical attention if irritation persists. *If inhaled* remove from exposure, establish adequate airway, give oxygen or artificial respiration as indicated. *If Swallowed* give 1 tablespoon syrup of ipecac followed by ½ glass of water to induce vomiting or induce vomiting by touching back of throat with finger. Avoid treatment of puppies under four weeks of age and kittens under eight weeks of age.
Extremely Flammable. Contents under pressure. Do not use near fire, sparks or flame. Do not puncture or incinerate container. Exposure to temperature above 130°F may cause bursting.
How Supplied: 13 ounce (384.4 ml) spray cans.
EPA Reg. No. 3134-35AA
EPA Est. No. 10806NJ01

07056TX-01

THERADEX™

Composition:
Active Ingredients:

Sodium Lauryl Sulfate	13.00%
Lauric Diethanolamide	8.00%
Polyoxyethylene Lanolins	5.00%
Propylene Glycol	5.00%
*Technical Piperonyl Butoxide	0.60%
Pyrethrins	0.06%
Total	31.66%
Inert Ingredients	68.34%
Total	100.00%

*Equivalent to 0.48% (butylcarbityl) (6-propylpiperonyl) ether and 0.12% related compounds.
Indications: A cleansing shampoo which aids in restoring the natural lustre of the hair coat of dogs and cats. Kills fleas and ticks.
Dosage and Administration: Apply only as specified on this label. Wet animal completely with warm water. Apply enough Theradex to obtain a good lathering of the entire body. Allow lather to remain in contact with skin for five minutes or longer before rinsing thoroughly with warm water. Use once or twice a week depending on the severity of condition.
Warning: Keep out of reach of children.
Causes eye injury. If in eyes: Flush with plenty of water. Get medical attention. Harmful if swallowed. If swallowed: Drink large quantities of milk, egg whites, gelatin solution, of if these are not available, large quantities of water. Avoid alcohol. Wash hands thoroughly with soap and water after using. Avoid contact with animal's eyes, mouth or other mucous membranes. For external use only.
Do not contaminate water, food or feed by storage or disposal. Rinse thoroughly, wrap empty container in several layers of newspaper and put in trash.
How Supplied: Gallon Bottle (3.785 liters) 6 ounce (177 ml) Bottles.
EPA Reg. No. 3134-28
EPA Est. No. 3134-NJ 1

THIOMAR™

Composition: Pleasantly scented coal tar shampoo for dogs containing 4-Choro-3, 5-Xylenol 0.5%; Salicylic Acid 2.0%; Evtar (Special Form of Coal Tar) 0.5%; in a shampoo base.
Indications: Pleasantly scented coal tar shampoo when excellent cleansing and deodorizing qualities are required. Aids in maintaining and natural lustre and sheen of the animal's hair coat, too.
Directions for Use: Thoroughly wet the animal with warm water. Apply enough shampoo to obtain a good, rich lather. Massage well into the animal's coat. Allow to remain in contact with the skin for 10 minutes before rinsing. Use 2 to 3 times a week or as a weekly shampoo.
Warning:
Not for use on cats.
Avoid contact with eyes.
How Supplied:
Gallon bottles (3.785 liters)
6 oz bottles (177 ml).

IDENTIFICATION PROBLEM?
Consult the
Product Identification Section
where you'll find
products pictured
in full color.

Fort Dodge Laboratories, Inc.
800 FIFTH STREET
FORT DODGE, IA 50501

ANAPLAZ® ℞
Anaplasmosis Vaccine
Killed-Bovine Origin
Bio. 161

Indications: For use in healthy cattle as an aid in prevention of clinical symptoms and economic loss due to bovine anaplasmosis caused by *Anaplasma marginale.*
This product has been potency tested as specified in Fort Dodge Laboratories production manual.
Composition: Anaplaz is composed of *A. marginale* organisms which have been inactivated, concentrated, and lyophilized. A specially prepared adjuvant is used for rehydration to facilitate absorption of the vaccine at a proper rate so as to elicit the maximum antigenic response.
Dosage and Administration: Sterile adjuvant diluent is supplied with each vial of Anaplaz. To rehydrate to a liquid state, aseptically withdraw the entire diluent contents into a clean, sterile syringe and inject directly into the vial of vaccine. Shake vigorously until thoroughly dissolved. Inject 2 ml. of the rehydrated vaccine subcutaneously in the neck or behind the shoulder, using a separate sterile needle for each individual animal.
Do not slaughter vaccinates for food within 60 days after vaccination, to avoid injection site trim-out or possible unwholesomeness of meat.
For primary immunization, it is important to vaccinate cattle twice at not less than four week intervals. Bulls may be vaccinated at anytime. Breeding females should be vaccinated while open. A 2 ml. booster dose should be given the following year. If epidemic conditions exist or the animal has been exposed to anaplasmosis, the veterinarian may, in his judgment, administer an additional booster dose. (Based upon experimental evidence, animals should receive subsequent single booster injections every two years to restore herd protection. (See General Information and Warning.) When vaccinating during an outbreak, simultaneous injection of an appropriate antibiotic may be given with the vaccine.
General Information: Anaplasma complement fixation (CF) antibodies may be expected to persist in vaccinated cattle for up to four months after the second injection. Recent information suggests these CF antibodies may persist in some animals for a considerably longer period of time after a booster dose. This should be considered when scheduling vaccination of cattle which may subsequently be required to pass a CF test.
Laboratory and field studies indicate that two doses at not less than four weeks apart prevent clinical illness and death from anaplasmosis during the subsequent vector season. Vaccination will not alter the existing carrier state in previ-

ously infected and recovered animals, nor will the vaccine produce the carrier state in susceptible animals. The carrier state may occur in vaccinated cattle subsequently exposed to infection; however, clinical symptoms of anaplasmosis, erythrocyte infection, and anemia of such cattle are absent or minimal.

Warning: *Anaplaz* is restricted to use by or under the direction of a veterinarian. *Anaplaz* contains antigens which can stimulate red cell antibody production in cows negative for the respective antigen. Thus Anaplaz can cause the development of Neonatal Isoerythrolysis (N.I.). *Field evidence indicates the vaccination of brood cows with Anaplaz can be a calculated risk and the protective benefits of vaccination should be weighed against the possible risks of N.I.* Decisions should be made by the veterinarian based upon all available information. N.I. is an anemic syndrome of newborn calves caused by antibodies in the colostrum which, when absorbed, destroy the red blood cells of the calf. The onset of the disease is sudden after the intake of the colostrum, with death in acute cases usually occurring by the fourth day. Immunization of the sire is not a factor in the development of N.I. Cows known to produce N.I. calves should not receive *Anaplaz.* Such cows may subsequently produce healthy calves or N.I. calves, since red cell antibody production may be stimulated by sources other than *Anaplaz* vaccine. Based on general immunological knowledge, the risk of N.I. may be reduced by vaccinating cows while open, and by giving only one 2 ml. booster dose following primary immunization. Resistance provided by vaccination will decline and 24 and 30 months after the initial booster dose a significant number of animals will be susceptible. Although the occurrence of N.I. following the administration of *Anaplaz* is infrequent, it may affect a significant number of calves in a herd.

As an aid in prevention of N.I., colostrum could be withheld from newborns for the first 36 hours. The calves may safely nurse their dams after the 36 hour withholding period, provided the dams have been milked out during this time. This colostrum withholding procedure creates substantial risks since the calf is thus deprived of the disease protective benefits of colostrum. Precautions, such as the use of antibiotics, should be taken.

If N.I. is observed, affected calves should be given blood transfusions and corticosteroid therapy. Since in N.I. there is no immediate loss in blood volume, large or rapid transfusions may lead to shock, pulmonary edema, and death. Additional supportive treatment should be used as indicated and undue stresses, such as excitement and handling avoided.

Scientific and field usage data show N.I. to be absent or rare when breeding females receive only the primary series and a single booster dose. Subsequent booster doses increase the N.I. risks and most N.I. occurs in offspring of vaccinates having received multiple booster doses. Although increased resistance to infection remains, protection gradually declines, and a significant number of animals may be susceptible 12 months after primary vaccination or 24 months after a booster dose, if they have not been exposed. When exposed to infection, those animals previously vaccinated will more rapidly respond with increased resistance to challenge than non-vaccinated susceptible animals. Limiting the number and frequency of booster doses further minimizes the risks of N.I. therefore the veterinarian may not wish to administer a booster dose until exposure is imminent or herd symptoms of disease appear.

Recovered animals have immunity or increased resistance to anaplasmosis. Herds in endemic areas ordinarily have a high percentage of older animals which are immune carriers. Animals under 2 years of age rarely suffer fatal anaplasmosis infection. By considering the above together with protection afforded by vaccination the veterinarian can devise an immunization program so as to take advantage of protection afforded by vaccination and herd immune status. Such programs provide protection during periods of greatest disease risks while decreasing the number of vaccine injections and minimizing the risks of N.I.

Caution:

Store in dark at 2° to 7° C. (35° to 45° F.).

Use entire contents without delay after rehydration.

In case of anaphylactoid reaction administer epinephrine.

Neomycin, polymyxin B and a fungistat B added as preservatives.

How Supplied: 10 ml— 5 doses
40 ml—20 doses

ANNUMUNE®
Rabies Vaccine
Killed Virus
Bio. 150

Indications: For the annual immunization of healthy dogs and cats against rabies.

Dosage and Administration: Inject 1 ml. intramuscularly at one site in the thigh, using aseptic technique. Give one dose at 3 months of age or older. Repeat dosage annually.

Caution: Store in the dark at 2° to 7° C. (35° to 45° F.). Do not freeze. Shake well. Use entire contents when first opened. In case of anaplylactoid reaction administer epinephrine.

BPL inactivated, thimerosal, neomycin, polymyxin B and a fungistat added as preservatives.

How Supplied:
10 ml—10 doses

ANTIVENIN ℞
(Crotalidae) Polyvalent
Equine Origin
Bio. 210

Indications: For use in dogs which have received bites from viperene snakes, such as rattlesnakes, copperheads, and cottonmouth water moccasins.

Composition: *Antivenin* is a refined and concentrated preparation of equine serum globulins obtained by fractionating blood from healthy horses that have been immunized with the following venoms: Eastern diamond-back (C. adamanteus), Western diamond-back (C. atrox), Central and South American rattlesnake (C. Terrificus), and fer-de-lance (B. atrox). 0.25% phenol and 0.005% thimerosal (mercury derivative) are added as preservatives.

Antivenin neutralizes the venom of the viperene snakes, including all North American species of rattlesnakes, copperheads, and cottonmouth moccasins. It contains a protective substance against the venoms of the related species in Central and South America, including the bushmaster and the fer-de-lance, and the habu and Mamushi of the Pacific Islands and Asiatic mainland.

Antivenin is standardized by its ability to neutralize in mice the toxic action of a standard venom injected intravenously.

General Information: Antivenin is specific against the viperene class of snakes, whose venom is hemotoxic. The elapine are the second class of poisonous snakes, and include the coral snake, the cobra, and the mamba. Their venom is mainly neurotoxic. Both classes of poisonous snakes contain some neurotoxic and hemotoxic factors. However, horses from which Antivenin is derived have not been immunized against elapine venom.

The death incidence, worldwide, from snakebite is greater in dogs than in any other domestic animal. They most frequently are bitten in the head region; occasionally on the shoulders, thighs, or legs. Fatalities in horses and cattle are less common. However, they do occur, particularly when bitten about the head or neck.

Symptoms from viperene envenomation are swelling, pain, muscular weakness, impaired vision, cyanosis, hemolytic anemia, bleeding tendencies, dyspnea, shock, and subsequently tissue necrosis. Some clinical evaluators of *Antivenin* reported the diamond-back as the most lethal snake to dogs, and the ground or pygmy rattler the least dangerous. Sloughing or tissue necrosis was most frequently associated with, but not limited to, the water moccasin.

Sixteen practicing veterinarians had uniformly successful results with *Antivenin* in patients having mild symptoms at time of treatment. Of 103 dogs treated with acute symptoms, 72% survived following a single 10 ml. dose; there was a higher percentage (83%) of recovery when 20 to 70 ml. was given. Overall, 82% of *Antivenin*-treated animals survived; the majority not receiving *Antivenin* succumbed. The success of *Antivenin* appears to be directly related to the time interval before treatment. Only 45% of dogs survived if there was at least a four-hour lag period between time of bite and Antivenin treatment. The survival rate doubled if less than four hours

Continued on next page

F

elapsed before antivenin was administered.

Dosage and Administration: The dose varies from 10 to 50 ml. (1 to 5 vials), intravenously, of rehydrated antivenin, depending on the severity of symptoms, lapse of time after the bite, size of snake, and size of patient (the smaller the body of the victim, the larger the dose required). Additional doses should be given every 2 hours as required, if symptoms such as swelling and pain persist or recur.

In emergency, when exposure is such that intravenous administration of *Antivenin* is not practical, the product may be administered intramuscularly as close to the site of exposure as practical.

General supportive therapy should be instituted whenever required. Corticosteroids should be given to suppress systemic reactions or delayed serum sickness. They also exert a beneficial effect on shock that invariably accompanies a snake bite. There is no evidence to indicate that corticosteroids will neutralize venom or inhibit the accompanying necrosis. However, they may minimize tissue destruction. Antibiotics, fluid therapy, blood transfusions, and tetanus prophylaxis may be indicated.

Precautions: Attempts should be made to immobilize the patient until treatment is initiated. The use of excessive heat or cold is contraindicated. Antihistamines and tranquilizers are also contraindicated, and may potentiate the effect of snake venom. Sedatives and analgesics should also be employed with discretion, because large doses may mask important clinical signs.

Caution:

Storage temperature not to exceed 98° F. (37° C.).

Use immediately after rehydration.

In case of anaphylactoid reaction, administer epinephrine.

Restricted to use by or under the direction of a veterinarian.

How Supplied: 10 ml—1 dose

This product is not returnable for credit or exchange.

F

ARVAC™
EQUINE ARTERITIS VACCINE
Modified Live Virus
Bio. 170

Composition: **Arvac™**, is a desiccated preparation containing viable modified Equine Arteritis virus propagated on an equine cell line culture system.

This vaccine has been tested and shown to be satisfactory for marketing in accordance with procedures required by the U.S. Department of Agriculture.

Disease Information: Equine Arteritis Virus (EAV) is known to infect only equines. The severity of the disease is variable ranging from highly acute to subclinical in nature. The acute disease is characterized clinically by fever, leukopenia, depression, nasal discharge, lacrimation, conjunctivitis, photophobia, edema of the face, limbs, transient maculopapular skin rash and produces abortion in pregnant mares. The most consistent clinical signs have been hyperthermia, leukopenia and edema of the eye. There may be colic, diarrhea and severe loss of weight with dehydration.

Indications and Dosage: For the vaccination of healthy non-stressed horses to stimulate the development of protection against viral abortion and respiratory infection due to equine arteritis virus. Aseptically rehydrate to liquid form using the diluent supplied. Administer a 1 ml. dose intramuscularly. Vaccinate males and young animals at any time, but stallions should be vaccinated at least 3 weeks prior to breeding. Vaccinate mares preferably as maidens or when open. Mares in foal should not be vaccinated until after foaling and then at least 3 weeks prior to breeding. Maiden and barren mares may be vaccinated anytime but should be vaccinated at least 3 weeks prior to breeding. See section on Cautions. Repeat with annual booster dose.

Cautions: Store in dark at 2° to 7° C. (35° to 45° F.). Use entire contents within 60 minutes after rehydration. Burn container and unused contents. In case of anaphylactoid reaction administer epinephrine.

The vaccinal virus has been modified to the extent that it may be irregularly infective when given by natural portals of entry. A high degree of safety has been demonstrated for horses of any age and pregnant mares.* However, the vaccination of foals under six weeks of age is not recommended except in emergency situations when threatened by natural exposure.

Pregnant mares SHOULD NOT be vaccinated during the last two months of gestation since a few instances of fetal invasion by vaccinal virus have been demonstrated during this period. It is preferable to immunize mares during the maiden or open periods; however, when pregnant mares are threatened by known natural exposure, vaccination may be undertaken with considerably less risk than is inherent in natural infection. Owners are to be advised of the possibility of fetal infection before vaccinating pregnant mares.

Mild post-vaccinal febrile reactions and normal total white counts with mild transient lymphopenia have occurred in some vaccinates. Vaccinated horses will serologically convert, a condition that should be kept in mind in the case of animals intended for export to countries with regulations regarding EAV.

Distribution shall be limited to those States where authorized by proper State officials and under such additional conditions as these authorities may require.

Neomycin, Polymyxin B and a fungistat added as preservatives.

How Supplied: Pkg 10—1 ml—10 doses

*Reference

Development of a Modified Virus Strain and Vaccine for Equine Viral Arteritis. William H. McCollum PhD., JAVMA, Vol. 155 #2, July 15, 1969.

ATROPINE INJECTABLE, L.A. ℞

Dosage and Administration:

Cattle, Horses, Sheep and Swine Only: As a preanesthetic adjuvant or to reduce salivation, bronchial secretions, peristalsis or hypermotility associated with colic, 1 ml/100 lb. bodyweight intravenously, intramuscularly or subcutaneously.

To reverse toxicity from organophosphate insecticides or other cholinergic drugs, 5 ml/100 lb. bodyweight (for ruminants 10 to 15 ml/100 lb. bodyweight) administered to effect and repeated as necessary. Administer 1/4 of dosage intravenously and remainder intramuscularly or subcutaneously.

Composition: Each ml contains 2.0 mg. (1/30 gr. approx.) atropine sulfate, U.S.P. in distilled water with 0.5% chlorbutanol (preservative).

Side Effects: Blurred vision, drowsiness and tachycardia. Toxic dosage may cause ataxia, excitation or confusion.

Contraindications: Glaucoma and tachycardia.

Warning: Keep out of reach of children.

Caution: Federal law restricts this drug to use by or on the order of a licensed veterinarian.

How Supplied: 100 ml.

ATROPINE INJECTABLE, S.A. ℞

Dosage and Administration:

Dogs and Cats Only: As a preanesthetic adjuvant or to reduce salivation, bronchial secretion or peristalsis 1 ml/15 lb. bodyweight, intravenously, intramuscularly or subcutaneously.

To reverse toxicity from organophosphate insecticides or other cholinergic drugs, 1 ml/5 lb. bodyweight, administered to effect and repeated as necessary. Administer 1/4 of dosage intravenously and remainder intramuscularly or subcutaneously.

Composition: Each ml contains 0.5 mg. (1/120 gr. approx.) atropine sulfate, U.S.P. in distilled water with chlorbutanol (0.5%) as a preservative.

Side Effects: Blurred vision, drowsiness, tachycardia. Toxic dosage may cause ataxia, excitation or confusion.

Contraindictations: Glaucoma and tachycardia.

Warning: Keep out of reach of children.

Caution:

Federal law restricts this drug to use by or on the order of a licensed veterinarian.

How Supplied: 50 ml.

CLOSTROID® C-D
Clostridium Perfringens
Types C and D Toxoid
Bio. 280

Indications: For vaccination of healthy cattle and sheep against enterotoxemias due to the toxins of *Cl. perfringens* types C and D. Clostroid C-D stimulates antitoxins that are common to *Cl. perfringens type B*.

Composition: A formalin toxoid prepared from *Cl. perfringens* types C and D cultures.

Dosage:
2 ml. Inject subcutaneously or intramuscularly. Repeat in 10 to 21 days.
Caution:
Store in dark at 2° to 7° C. (35° to 45°F.). Avoid freezing. Shake well.
Use all of this product at time container is first opened.
Do not vaccinate within 21 days before slaughter.
In case of anaphylactoid reaction administer epinephrine.
How Supplied: 20 ml—10 doses
100 ml—50 doses

CLOSTROID® CS
Clostridium Chauvoei-Septicum Bacterin
Bio. 139

Indications: Use in healthy cattle, sheep and goats as an aid in prevention of blackleg and malignant edema.
Composition: Chemically killed clostridium chauvoei and clostridium septicum organisms.
Dosage and Administration:
Cattle: 2 ml. Inject subcutaneously or intramuscularly. Calves vaccinated under three months of age should be revaccinated at weaning or four to six months of age.
Sheep and Goats: 1 ml. Inject subcutaneously or intramuscularly.
Caution:
Store in dark at 2° to 7° C. (35° to 45°F.). Shake well.
Use entire contents when first opened.
Do not vaccinate within 21 days before slaughter.
In case of anaphylactoid reaction administer epinephrine.
How Supplied: 20 ml—10 doses
100 ml—50 doses

Products are cross-indexed

by product classifications

in the

Product Category Section

CLOSTROID® CSNS
Clostridium Chauvoei-Septicum, Novyi-Sordellii Bacterin-Toxoid
Bio. 133

Indications: Use in healthy cattle as an aid in prevention of blackleg, malignant edema, black disease and *Clostridium sordellii* infections.
Composition: Chemically killed *Clostridium chauvoei, Clostridium septicum, Clostridium novyi* and *Clostridium sordellii* organisms.
Dosage and Administration:
Cattle: 5 ml. Inject subcutaneously or intramuscularly. Calves vaccinated under three months of age should be revaccinated at weaning or four to six months of age. Revaccination with Clostridium sordellii bacterin is recommended at two to four weeks. For cattle subject to re-exposure to *Cl. novyi,* repeat the dose every 5–6 months.
Caution:
Store in dark at 2° to 7° C. (35° to 45°F.). Shake well.
Use entire contents when first opened.
Do not vaccinate within 21 days before slaughter.
In case of anaphylactoid reaction administer epinephrine.
How Supplied: 50 ml—10 doses
250 ml—50 doses

CLOSTROID® D
Clostridium Perfringens Type D Toxoid
Bio. 281

Indications: For vaccination of healthy sheep as an aid in prevention of enterotoxemia (pulpy kidney disease).
Composition: A formalin toxoid prepared from Clostridium perfringens type D cultures.
Dosage and Administration: 2 ml. Inject subcutaneously or intramuscularly. Repeat in 14 to 21 days.
Caution:
Store in dark at 2° to 7°C (35° to 45°F).
Avoid freezing.
Shake well.
Use entire contents when first opened.
Do not vaccinate within 21 days before slaughter.
In case of anaphylactoid reaction administer epinephrine.
How Supplied: 20 ml— 10 doses
100 ml—50 doses
250 ml—125 doses

CLOSTROID® D–T
Clostridium Perfringens Type D-Tetanus Toxid
Aluminum Phosphate Adsorbed Refined and Concentrated
Bio. 279

Indications: For vaccination of healthy sheep to protect against enterotoxemia (due to *Cl. perfringens* Type D toxin) and tetanus.
Composition: The tetanus and the *Cl. perfringens* Type D toxoids have been refined and concentrated by a patented process which essentially eliminates the non-specific nitrogen but leaves the antigenic fraction unchanged. Highly purified toxoids are desirable since components responsible for producing allergic or side reactions are practically eliminated.
This product has been tested and shown to be satisfactory for marketing in accordance with existing Standard Requirements set forth by the U.S. Department of Agriculture.
Dosage and Administration: Inject one 2 ml. dose subcutaneously or intramuscularly using aseptic technique. Administer a second 2 ml. dose 2 to 4 weeks after the first dose. Revaccinate annually using one 2 ml. booster dose. Administer in a wool-free area, but do not inject in the axillary space.
The two doses of the initial series or the annual booster dose should be administered to ewes during the last two months of pregnancy. The second dose of the initial series, or the annual booster dose, when administered not later than two weeks before lambing, is recommended to aid in conferring protection to the lamb during the nursing period.
Protective tetanus antibody titers usually occur two weeks after the second injection of the initial series. In the event of injury during the course of the initial vaccination program, or if annual boosters have not been given, a prophylactic dose of at least 1,500 units of tetanus antitoxin should be given.
Caution:
Store in dark at 2° to 7° C. (35° to 45°F.).
Shake vigorously to assure uniform suspension of the precipitate.
Use entire contents when container is first opened.
Do not vaccinate within 30 days of slaughter.
In case of anaphylactoid reaction administer epinephrine.
Transitory local reactions at the injection site may occur.
How Supplied: 20 ml—10 doses
100 ml—50 doses

F

CLOSTROID® 7
Clostridium Chauvoei-Septicum-Novyi-Sordellii-Perfringens Types C and D Bacterin-Toxoid
Bio. 134

Indications: For vaccination of healthy cattle to protect against blackleg, malignant edema, black disease, *sordellii* infections, and *Cl. perfringens* Types C & D related enterotoxemias. Immunity is also provided against beta and epsilon toxins elaborated by *Cl. perfringens* Type B. This immunity is derived from the combination of Type C (beta) and Type D (epsilon) fraction.
Dosage and Administration:
Cattle: 5 ml. Inject subcutaneously or intramuscularly. Repeat in 2 to 4 weeks. Calves vaccinated under 3 months of age should be revaccinated at weaning or 4 to 6 months of age. For animals subject to re-exposure to *Cl. novyi,* repeat the dose every 5 to 6 months. Post-vaccinal tissue reactions occasionally occur at site of injection.
Caution:
Store in dark at 2° to 7°C (35° to 45°F).
Use entire contents when first opened.
Shake well.
Do not vaccinate within 21 days before slaughter.
In case of anaphylactoid reaction administer epinephrine.
How Supplied: 50 ml—10 doses
250 ml—50 doses

Continued on next page

Fort Dodge—Cont.

COLIGEN®
Escherichia Coli
Bacterin
Bovine Isolates Bio. 103

Indications: For vaccination of healthy pregnant cattle to protect calves from severe scours and death caused by the antigenic spectrum of *E. coli* enteropathogenic organisms contained in the bacterin.
The protective response afforded by this bacterin results from colostral antibodies supplied by the dam which must be consumed within 2 to 4 hours after birth and in sufficient amounts by the calf.
Composition: A formalin killed suspension of *Escherichia coli* isolates of four serological types combined with an adjuvant to facilitate absorption of the bacterin at a proper rate to elicit a protective antigenic response.
Dosage and Administration: Administer to healthy pregnant cows using aseptic technique. Inject two 5 ml. doses subcutaneously or intramuscularly 2 to 4 weeks apart. The first dose should be administered about 5 to 6 weeks before calving and the second dose 2 to 3 weeks before the expected calving date. A single annual booster dose is recommended 2 to 6 weeks prior to calving.
Caution:
Store in dark at 2° to 7° C. (35° to 45°F.).
Shake well.
Use entire contents when first opened.
Do not vaccinate within 21 days before slaughter.
In case of anaphylactoid reaction administer epinephrine.
How Supplied: 50 ml—10 doses. 250 ml—50 doses

Products are
indexed alphabetically
in the
Product Name Section

DURAMUNE® Cv-K
Canine Coronavirus Vaccine
Killed Virus
Bio. 147
Canine Coronavirus Vaccine
(MLV and inactivated)
Pat. No. 4,567,043
Inactivated Canine Coronavirus Vaccine
Pat. No. 4,567,042

Product Indication: This product is for the vaccination of healthy dogs against the disease of canine coronavirus infections.
Composition: The canine coronavirus vaccine is composed of a killed virus which has been purified, grown to a high antigen level in a cell line and specially adjuvanted.
The manufacture of an efficacious and safe inactivated antigen is made possible by special production techniques and the use of a unique adjuvant system.
Discussion: Canine coronavirus gastroenteritis—canine coronavirus enteritis (CCv) is a highly contagious disease with world wide distribution. The incidence of CCv disease in family owned dogs has been reported to range from 14.8% to 26%. The incidence in kennel raised dogs ranged upward to 30%. The incidence of gastroenteritis where both canine coronavirus and canine parvovirus were isolated is even higher.[10]
The disease can occur in dogs of any age. CCv gastroenteritis was first observed in 1971 with similar outbreaks of disease having been reported in 1972,[6] in 1976 and 1978.[5] The importance of CCv gastroenteritis has seemingly increased with the outbreak of CPv gastroenteritis.
CCv gastroenteritis is characterized by a number of disease symptoms which have been compiled from the literature as follows: The first signs of disease are lethargy, anorexia and depression. The sudden onset of vomition occurs in which blood can sometimes be found. Diarrhea can range from moderate to severe and projectile in nature. Diarrhea may persist up to 10 days. The fecal material has a yellow-orange color with blood and mucus occasionally found. The fecal material has a marked foul odor. Dehydration, weight loss and death have been reported.[2,4,5,8,9,10,11,12] Protracted or recurring diarrhea may occur 2–3 weeks later.[12]
The severity of the CCv disease syndrome is thought to vary according to age, stress, environmental conditions, breed and concurrent infections.[9,10]
Canine coronavirus has also been associated with respiratory disease symptoms of ocular and nasal discharge.[3,11,12]
Experimentally both respiratory and enteric symptoms of disease have been seen by this laboratory. The symptoms observed include slight ocular discharge, a light nasal discharge, diarrhea, weight losses, anorexia, dehydration, elevated temperatures and slight drops in both white blood cell levels and lymphocyte levels. Intestinal samples of infected dogs demonstrated a significant degree of virus infection occurs following challenge.
Safety: Laboratory test and field studies have shown vaccination with Duramune Cv-K simultaneously or in close time proximity to other vaccine antigens to be safe.
Efficacy: Vaccination-challenge studies demonstrated Duramune Cv-K to provide 99.3% reduction in intestinal infection with Canine coronavirus. Challenge results also indicated that no CCv was found in the meninges of vaccinates whereas controls showed 30% to have CCv present.
Directions for Use:
- **General Directions:** Aseptically remove vaccine and inject 1 ml. subcutaneously or intramuscularly.
- **Primary Vaccination:** All dogs over 12 weeks of age should initially receive one dose of Duramune Cv-K and a second dose 2 to 3 weeks later. Annual revaccination with one dose is recommended.
Puppies of any age can be safely vaccinated. A recommended vaccination should start at or about 6 weeks of age. The presence of maternal antibody is known to interfere with the development of active immunity. Puppies should be revaccinated every 2 to 4 weeks until they are at least 12 weeks of age.
- **Annual Vaccination:** Annual revaccination with one dose is recommended.

Caution: Store in dark at 2° to 7° C. (35° to 45° F.). In case of anaphylactoid reaction administer epinephrine.
Gentamicin, thimerosal, and a fungistat added as preservatives.
How Supplied: 10 ml—10 doses
References:
1. Appel, M., Cooper, B., Greisen, H., Scott, R., Carmichael, L., "Canine Viral Enteritis 1. Status Report on Corona and Parvovirus-like Viral Enteritis." *Cornell Veterinarian,* 1979, Vol. 69, No. 3, pp. 123–133.
2. Appel, M., Meunier, P., Pollock, R., Greisen, H., and Carmichael, L., "Canine Viral Enteritis." *Canine Practice,* 1980, Vol. 7, No. 4, pp. 22–36.
3. Binn, L.N., Alford, J.P., Marchwicki, R.H., Keefe, T.J., Beattie, R.T., and Wall, H.G., "Studies of Respiratory Disease in Random Source Laboratory Dogs: Viral Infections in Unconditioned Dogs." *Laboratory Animal Science,* Feb. 1979, Vol. 29, No. 1, pp. 48–52.
4. Binn, L.N., Lazar, E.C., Keenan, K.P., Huxsoll, D.L., Marchwicki, R.H., and Strano, A.J., "Recovery and Characterization of a Coronavirus from Military Dogs with Diarrhea." Proc. 78th Meeting, U.S. Animal Health Assoc. (Oct. 1974), pp. 359–366.
5. Carmichael, L.E., "Infectious Canine Enteritis Caused by a Corona-like Virus." *Canine Practice,* Vol. 5, No. 4, pp. 25–27, August, 1978.
6. Cartwright, S.F. and Lucas, M., "Vomiting and Diarrhea in Dogs." *Veterinary Record.* 91:571, pp. 571–572, 1972.
7. Helfer-Baker, C., Evermann, J., McKeuman, A., Morrison, W., "Serological Studies on the Incidence of Canine Enteritis Viruses." *Canine Practice,* Vol. 7, No. 3, pp. 37–42, 1980.
8. Keenan, K.P., Binn, L.N., Takeuchi, A., "Animal Model of Human Disease, Acute Non-bacterial Gastroenteritis, Animal Model: Acute Enteritis in dogs infected with Coronavirus." 1-71, *American Journal Pathologists* 94(2) 439–442, 1979.
9. Keenan, K.P., Jervis, H.R., March-

wicki, R.H., Binn, L.N., "Intestinal Infection of Neonatal Dogs with Canine Coronavirus 1-71: Studies by Virologic, Histolgic, Histochemical and Immunofluorescent Techniques." *American Journal Veterinary Resources,* Vol. 37, No. 3, pp. 247–256, March 1976.

10. Miller, J., Evermann, J., Ott, R., "Immunofluorescence Test for Canine Coronavirus and Parvovirus." *Western Veterinarian,* 1980, Vol. 19, No. 1, pp. 14–19.
11. Pollock, R.V.H. and Carmichael, L.E., "Canine Viral Enteritis—Recent Developments." *Modern Veterinary Practice,* Vol. 50, pp. 375–380, May 1979.
12. Vanderghe, J.M., Ducatelle, R., Debock, P. and Hoorens, J., "Coronavirus infection in a Litter of Pups." *The Veterinary Quarterly,* Vol. 2, No. 3, pp. 136–141, 1980.

IDENTIFICATION PROBLEM?

Consult the

Product Identification Section

Where you'll find

products pictured

in full color.

DURAMUNE® DA$_2$P + Pv
CANINE DISTEMPER
ADENOVIRUS TYPE 2
PARAINFLUENZA—PARVOVIRUS
VACCINE
MODIFIED LIVE VIRUS
Bio.149

Product Indication: Duramune®-DA$_2$P + Pv is for the vaccination of healthy dogs against canine distemper, infectious canine hepatitis, respiratory disease caused by canine adenovirus type 2, canine parainfluenza and canine parvovirus infections.

Composition: The canine parvovirus (CPv) fraction of the combination vaccine was the first licensed canine virus isolate which has been modified and attenuated for use in prevention of parvovirus induced enteritis. The virus was extensively purified and modified for safety, yet remains very antigenic and efficacious. A study conducted with Hazelton Research at Vienna, Virginia, demonstrated seroconversion in 95% of the 6 week old vaccinates having SN maternal antibody as high as 1:100. Additional studies were conducted and sample testing by 3 different laboratories confirm the efficacy of this parvovirus vaccine in face of maternal antibody levels.

The canine adenovirus type 2 (CAv-2) fraction is a modified live virus which has been purified and attenuated in a cell line. The adenovirus type 2 fraction provides protection against respiratory disease caused by canine adenovirus type 2 and cross protects against the fatal disease caused by the infectious canine hepatitis virus (CAv-1). The CAv-2 vaccine virus also provides significant safety advantages as specified in the safety and efficacy portion.

The canine distemper (CDv) fraction and the canine parainfluenza (CPI) fraction of the vaccine are modified live viruses which have been purified and attenuated in a cell line.

Safety and Efficacy: Controlled studies demonstrated that **Duramune®-DA$_2$P + Pv** immunized dogs against CD (canine distemper). CAv-2 (canine adenovirus type 2), ICH (infectious canine hepatitis [CAv-1]), CPI (canine parainfluenza), and CPv (canine parvovirus) infections.

Laboratory studies demonstrated that as little as 603 TCID$_{50}$s of the CAv-2 virus fraction provided protection against challenge with CAv-2 and a highly virulent ICH challenge virus. Vaccination challenge studies showed 25 out of 25 vaccinates to be protected against ICH challenge; whereas, 6 out of 6 challenge controls died due to the severity of the challenge. Ninety-five per cent protection against symptoms was afforded vaccinates in the face of a virulent CAv-2 challenge.

The safety advantages of the canine adenovirus type 2 vaccine have been studied and are listed below:

- 5 backpassages in susceptible dogs with no reversion to virulence. An equivalent to 12,000 field doses were administered to each puppy in the initial backpassage.
- The CAv-2 fraction was administered intravenously to 38 susceptible dogs with no adverse effects. Four dogs received 5,000; 15 dogs received 3,000; and 19 dogs received 200 field dose equivalents by the intravenous route of inoculation. Data generated from this study indicate that corneal opacity is not associated with the use of Duramune® DA$_2$P + Pv.
- Field trial studies in over one thousand dogs consisting of 32 breeds and ranging in ages from 5 weeks to 13 years further substantiate the safety of Duramune® DA$_2$P + Pv.
- Tests also have shown that no immunologic interference exists among the fractions of Duramune® DA$_2$P + Pv.

Discussion:

- Canine Parvovirus—causes an enteritis in dogs of all ages with most acute infections occurring in dogs under 6 months of age. Two forms, enteric and myocardial are presented. The enteric form is indicated by signs of depression, inappetence, vomiting, diarrhea, bloody stools, leukopenia and lymphopenia. The less common form, myocardial, is only reported in pups less than 12 weeks of age. Infected pups often cry and vomit, with as high as 50% mortality rate.
- Canine distemper virus—causes a contagious disease in dogs typified by diphasic temperature rise, leukopenia, gastrointestinal and respiratory catarrh with neurological and pneumonic complications. Mortality rates are extremely high.
- Infectious canine hepatitis—causes a disease characterized by signs of temperature rise, congestion, depression, leukopenia and prolonged bleeding time. Simultaneous infection along with distemper sometimes occurs.
- Canine adenovirus type 2—primarily causes respiratory infections indicated by pharyngitis, bronchitis, tonsillitis, and pneumonia.
- Canine parainfluenza has been implicated as a causative agent in the kennel cough complex.

Directions For Use:

- **General Directions:** Aseptically rehydrate vaccine with sterile dilute supplied. Administer 1 ml. subcutaneously or intramuscularly.
- **Primary Vaccination:** All dogs over 12 weeks of age should initially receive one dose of Duramune DA$_2$P + Pv and a second dose 2 to 3 weeks later. Annual revaccination with one dose is recommended.

  Puppies of any age can be safely vaccinated. A recommended vaccination should start at or about 6 weeks of age. The presence of maternal antibody is known to interfere with the development of active immunity. Puppies should be revaccinated every 2 to 4 weeks until they are at least 12 weeks of age.
- **Annual Vaccination:** Annual revaccination with one dose is recommended.

Caution: Store at 2° to 7° C. (35°–45° F.). In case of anaphylactoid reaction, administer epinephrine. Burn this container and all unused contents.

Gentamicin, thimerosal and a fungistat added as preservatives.

How Supplied: 25 × 1 ml—25 doses.

DURAMUNE® DA$_2$LP + Pv
CANINE DISTEMPER
ADENOVIRUS TYPE 2
PARAINFLUENZA—PARVOVIRUS
VACCINE
MODIFIED LIVE VIRUS
LEPTOSPIRA BACTERIN
BIO. 157

Product Indication: Duramune®-DA$_2$LP + Pv is for the vaccination of healthy dogs against canine distemper, infectious canine hepatitis, respiratory disease caused by canine adenovirus type 2, canine parainfluenza, canine parvovirus and leptospira canicola and leptospira icterohaemorrhagiae infections.

Composition: The canine parvovirus (CPv) fraction of the combination vaccine was the first licensed canine virus isolate which has been modified and attenuated for use in prevention of parvovirus in-

Continued on next page

F

Fort Dodge—Cont.

duced enteritis. The virus was extensively purified and modified for safety, yet remains very antigenic and efficacious. A study conducted at the Hazelton Research at Vienna, Virginia, demonstrated seroconversion in 95% of the 6 week old vaccinates having SN maternal antibody as high as 1:100. Additional studies were conducted and sample testing by 3 different laboratories confirm the efficacy of this parvovirus vaccine in face of maternal antibody levels.

The canine adenovirus type 2 (CAv-2) fraction is a modified live virus which has been purified and attenuated in a cell line. The adenovirus type 2 fraction provides protection against respiratory disease caused by canine adenovirus type 2 and cross protects against the fatal disease caused by the infectious canine hepatitis virus (CAv-1). The CAv-2 vaccine virus also provides significant safety advantages as specified in the safety and efficacy portion.

The canine distemper (CDv) fraction and the canine parainfluenza (CPI) fraction of the vaccine are modified live viruses which have been purified and attenuated in a cell line.

The leptospira (L) fractions of this combination vaccine are inactivated cultures of leptospira canicola and icterohaemorrhagiae which have been used extensively and proven effective.

Safety and Efficacy: Controlled studies demonstrated that **Duramune®-DA$_2$LP + Pv** immunized dogs against CD (canine distemper), CAv-2 (canine adenovirus type 2), ICH (infectious canine hepatitis [CAv-1]), CPI (canine parainfluenza), CPv (canine parvovirus) infections and leptospirosis caused by L. canicola and L. icterohaemorrhagiae.

Laboratory studies demonstrated that as little as 603 TCID$_{50}$s of the CAv-2 virus fraction provided protection against challenge with CAv-2 and highly virulent ICH challenge virus. Vaccination challenge studies showed 25 out of 25 vaccinates to be protected against ICH challenge; whereas, 6 out of 6 challenge controls died due to the severity of the challenge. Ninety-five per cent protection against symptoms was afforded vaccinates in the face of a virulent CAv-2 challenge.

The safety advantages of the canine adenovirus type 2 vaccine have been studied and are listed below:

- 5 back passages in susceptible dogs with no reversion to virulence. An equivalent to 12,000 field doses were administered to each puppy in the initial backpassage.
- The CAv-2 fraction was administered intravenously to 38 susceptible dogs with no adverse effects. Four dogs received 5,000; 15 dogs received 3,000; and 19 dogs received 200 field dose equivalents by the intravenous route of inoculation. Data generated from this study indicate that corneal opacity is not associated with the use of Duramune DA$_2$LP + Pv.
- Field trial studies in over one thousand dogs consisting of 32 breeds and ranging in ages from 5 weeks to 13 years further substantiate the safety of Duramune DA$_2$LP + Pv.
- Tests also have shown that no immunologic interference exists among the fractions of Duramune DA$_2$LP + Pv.

Discussion:

- Canine parvovirus—causes an enteritis in dogs of all ages with most acute infections occurring in dogs under 6 months of age. Two forms, enteric and myocardial, are presented. The enteric form is indicated by signs of depression, inappetence, vomiting, diarrhea, bloody stools, leukopenia and lymphopenia. The less common form, myocardial, is only reported in pups less than 12 weeks of age. Infected pups often cry and vomit, with as high as 50% mortality rate.
- Canine distemper virus—causes a contagious disease in dogs typified by diphasic temperature rise, leukopenia, gastrointestinal and respiratory catarrh with neurological and pneumonic complications. Mortality rates are extremely high.
- Infectious canine hepatitis—causes a disease characterized by signs of temperature rise, congestion, depression, leukopenia and prolonged bleeding time. Simultaneous infection along with distemper sometimes occurs.
- Canine adenovirus type 2—primarily causes respiratory infections indicated by pharyngitis, bronchitis, tonsillitis, and pneumonia.
- Canine parainfluenza has been implicated as a causative agent in the kennel cough complex.
- Leptospirosis is an infectious disease characterized by nephritis, hemorrhagic gastroenteritis and icterus. Mortality seldom exceeds 10%.

Directions for Use:

- **General Directions:** Aseptically rehydrate vaccine with leptospira bacterin supplied. Administer 1 ml subcutaneously or intramuscularly.
- **Primary Vaccination:** All dogs over 12 weeks of age should initially receive one dose of Duramune DA$_2$LP + Pv and a second dose 2 to 3 weeks later. Annual revaccination with one dose is recommended.

  Puppies of any age can be safely vaccinated. A recommended vaccination should start at or about 6 weeks of age. The presence of maternal antibody is known to interfere with the development of active immunity. Puppies should be revaccinated every 2 to 4 weeks until they are at least 12 weeks of age.
- **Annual Vaccination:** Annual revaccination with one dose is recommended.

Caution:

Store at 2° to 7° C. (35°–45°F.). In case of anaphylactoid reaction, administer epinephrine. Burn this container and all unused contents.

Gentamicin, thimerosal and a fungistat added as preservatives.

How Supplied: 25 ×1 ml—25 doses

DURAMUNE® PV
Parvovirus Vaccine
Modified Live Virus
For Use in Dogs Only
Bio. 151

Composition: Duramune PV is prepared from a *Canine Virus Isolate* which is the first licensed Canine Virus Isolate which has been modified and attenuated for use in prevention of parvovirus induced enteritis. The virus was extensively purified and modified for safety; yet remains very antigenic and efficacious. Studies conducted at Hazelton Research, Vienna, Virginia, demonstrated seroconversion in 95% of the 6 week old vaccinates having SN maternal antibody as high as 1:100. Testing demonstrated that this CPv vaccine strain does not revert to virulence following six consecutive back passages in susceptible dogs. Also tests have revealed no evidence of immunosuppression.

This product has been tested and shown to be satisfactory by the U.S. Department of Agriculture.

Product Indication: Duramune Pv is for the vaccination of healthy unexposed dogs and puppies as a prophylaxis against the disease symptoms for canine parvovirus induced enteritis.

Discussion: Canine Parvovirus causes an enteritis in dogs of all ages with most acute infections occurring in dogs under 6 months of age. Two forms, enteric and myocardial, are presented. The enteric form is indicated by signs of depression, inappetence, diarrhea, bloody stools, leukopenia and lymphopenia. The less common form, myocardial, is only reported in pups less than 12 weeks of age. Infected pups often cry and vomit, with as high as a 50% mortality rate.

Directions For Use:

- **General Directions:** Administer 1 ml subcutaneously or intramuscularly.
- **Primary Vaccination:** One dose (1 ml) is recommended for dogs 12 weeks of age or older.

  Puppies of any age can be safely vaccinated. A recommended vaccination should start at or about 6 weeks of age. The presence of maternal antibody is known to interfere with the development of active immunity. Puppies should be revaccinated every 2 to 4 weeks until they are at least 12 weeks of age.
- **Annual Vaccination:** Annual revaccination with one dose is recommended.

Caution:

Store at 2° to 7° C. (35°–45°F.).
Shake well.
Use entire contents when first opened.
In case of anaphylactoid reaction administer epinephrine.

Gentamicin, thimerosol and a fungistat added as preservatives.

How Supplied: 10 ml—10 doses

DURSBAN* 44 INSECTICIDE (CPF 44)

Indications: For control of lice and horn flies on beef breed cattle only.
Composition:
Active Ingredients:
Chlorpyrifos [0,0 Diethyl 0-(3,5,6-trichloro-2-pyridyl) phosphorothioate]..........42.2%
Inert Ingredients: 57.8%
Contains 3.8 pounds of chlorpyrifos per gallon.
Contains petroleum distillates. E.P.A. Reg. No. 410-82-1117
KEEP OUT OF REACH OF CHILDREN

WARNING: PRECAUTIONARY STATEMENTS: Hazards to Humans
MAY BE FATAL IF SWALLOWED • MAY BE ABSORBED THROUGH SKIN • MAY BE INJURIOUS TO EYES AND SKIN
Do Not Take Internally • Do Not Get in Eyes or on Skin • Wear Rubber Gloves When Handling • Wash Thoroughly After Handling • Wash Contaminated Clothing Before Reuse • Avoid Breathing Vapors.
Statement of Practical Treatment: *If Swallowed:* Do not induce vomiting • Call a physician immediately. *If On Skin* • In case of contact, remove contaminated clothing and immediately wash skin with soap and water. *If in Eyes* • Flush eyes with plenty of water and get prompt medical attention.
Note to Physician and Veterinarian • Chlorpyrifos is a cholinesterase inhibitor.
Treat symptomatically. Atropine only by injection is an antidote.
Environmental Hazards: This product is toxic to fish, birds and other wildlife. Keep out of any body of water. Do not apply where runoff is likely to occur. Do not contaminate water by cleaning of equipment or disposal of wastes.
Physical or Chemical Hazards: **COMBUSTIBLE** • Do not use, pour, spill or store near heat or open flame.

Agricultural Chemical: Do Not Ship or Store with Food, Feeds, Drugs or Clothing.
Directions For Use: It is a violation of Federal law to use this product in a manner inconsistent with its labeling. FOR COMPLETE USE PRECAUTIONS AND NOTICE OF WARRANTY, READ ENTIRE LABEL.
FORT DODGE DURSBAN 44 Insecticide is a convenient "one-shot" treatment to provide season-long control of biting and sucking lice. *FORT DODGE* DURSBAN 44 is not effective against cattle grubs. Cattle may be treated during any season of the year for lice and horn fly control. *FORT DODGE* DURSBAN 44 provides for control of horn flies up to 6 weeks.
HOW TO APPLY: Wearing rubber gloves, and in a well ventilated area, pour the required dose of *FORT DODGE* DURSBAN 44 in one spot to the top midline area of the animal, just behind the shoulder blades and neck junction.
AMOUNT TO USE: Use *FORT DODGE* DURSBAN 44 for lice and horn fly control at the rate of **2 ml. per 100 lb.** of animal bodyweight up to 800 lb. For animals weighing more than 800 lbs., **use no more than 16 ml.** Due to the small amount of material required, care must be taken to apply the proper dose.
Storage and Disposal:
PROHIBITIONS: Do not contaminate water, food or feed by storage or disposal. Open dumping is prohibited. Do not reuse empty container.
PESTICIDE DISPOSAL: Waste resulting from use of this product may be disposed of on site or at an approved waste disposal facility.
CONTAINER DISPOSAL: Triple rinse (or equivalent). Then offer for recycling or reconditioning, or dispose of in a sanitary landfill, or by incineration if allowed by state and local authorities. If burned, stay out of smoke.
GENERAL: Consult federal, state or local disposal authorities for approved alternative procedures such as limited open burning.
Use Precautions:
DO NOT TREAT • Beef breed animals under 200 lbs. or 12 weeks of age • Bulls over 8 months of age of any breed • Purebred continental or exotic breed cattle such as Simmental, Chianina, Charolais or Gelbvieh, etc. • Dairy-breed cattle of any age • Cows 30 days before or after calving • Veal calves • Sick, convalescent or severely stressed animals • Cattle 10 days before or after shipping, dehorning, castration, vaccination, etc.
Do not slaughter animals within 14 days of treatment. If reinfestation does occur animals may be re-treated but not within 45 days of initial treatment.
FORT DODGE DURSBAN 44 contains a cholinesterase inhibitor. Do not use any drug or other pesticidal chemical having cholinesterase inhibiting activity, either simultaneously or within 45 days before or after treatment with it.
Do not brand animal with a hot iron while treating with *FORT DODGE* DURSBAN 44. The solvent system is combustible and could cause a serious burn to the animal.
Dairy, Brahma, continental or exotic breed cattle crossed with beef breeds (British) may be treated.
Notice: Seller warrants that the product conforms to its chemical description and is reasonably fit for the purposes stated on the label when used in accordance with directions under normal conditions of use, but neither this warranty nor any other warranty of MERCHANTABILITY or FITNESS FOR A PARTICULAR PURPOSE, express or implied, extends to the use of this product contrary to label instructions, or under abnormal conditions, or under conditions not reasonably foreseeable to seller, and buyer assumes the risk of any such use.
How Supplied: Pkg. 12—1 pint

U.S. Patent No. 3,244,586

*Trademark of THE DOW CHEMICAL COMPANY

DYREX® T.F. ℞
(trichlorfon + phenothiazine + piperazine)
Anthelmintic for Horses

Indications: *Dyrex T.F.* (trichlorfon + phenothiazine + piperazine) is indicated for removal of the following equine parasites: bots *(Gastrophilus nasalis, Gastrophilus intestinalis),* ascarids *(Parascaris equorum),* large strongyles *(Strongylus vulgaris),* pinworms *(Oxyuris equi)* and small strongyle species.
Description: This product has been specifically formulated as an equine anthelmintic for administration by stomach tube.
Dosage and Administration: Preferably, all horses should be treated 1 month after the first killing frost and 1 month after being on pasture. The weight of each animal should be estimated carefully and the correct dosage prepared individually. The contents of both of the outer bottle and the inner vial should be mixed together in warm water. Administration is by stomach tube. To minimize the possibility of spillage, it is recommended that a funnel be used in pouring the suspension into the tube. After administration, the suspension remaining in the tube should be rinsed away with fresh water. Do not blow through the tube to empty. Flush unused suspension or powder down the drain or bury.
For removal of bots *(Gastrophilus nasalis, Gastrophilus intestinalis),* ascarids *(Parascaris equorum),* large strongyle *(Strongylus vulgaris),* pinworms *(Oxyuris equi)* and small strongyle species: Contents of one #500 bottle for each 500 lb. bodyweight; contents of one #1000 bottle for each 1000 lb. bodyweight. It is important that precautions be read before administration.
Side Effects: A loosening of the stool may occasionally be seen several hours after treatment. Symptoms of overdosage are colic, diarrhea and ataxia, and appear within 1 to 3 hours after treatment. Such symptoms are usually transient and persist only briefly. Atropine (5 to 10 mg/100 lb. bodyweight), administered to effect and repeated as necessary, is the antidote to aid in the control of these symptoms. Administer ¼ of dosage intravenously and remainder intramuscularly or subcutaneously.
Occasionally a horse will show a reaction within 72 hours in which reduction of packed cell volume and hemoglobin is observed, sometimes accompanied with hemoglobinuria and hematuria. Treatment consists of symptomatic supportive treatment, rest, and avoidance of stress or training until animal has recovered.
Precautions: Field experience with *Dyrex T.F.* (trichlorfon + phenothiazine + piperazine) in pregnant animals

Continued on next page

F

Fort Dodge—Cont.

would indicate no adverse affects. However, such treatment has historically been considered risky with any anthelmintic and, accordingly, treatment of mares in late pregnancy is not recommended.
Surgery or any severe stress should be avoided for at least 2 weeks before or after treatment. Do not administer to sick, toxic or debilitated horses.
Warning: *Dyrex T.F.* (trichlorfon + phenothiazine + piperazine) is a cholinesterase inhibitor. Do not use this product in horses simultaneously or within 2 weeks before or after treatment with, or exposure to, cholinesterase inhibiting drugs, pesticides, or chemicals. Examples of these are succinylcholine, organophosphorus and carbamate insecticides, eserine and prostigmine.
If swallowed by a human, IMMEDIATELY call a physician, poison control center or hospital emergency room. Upon medical advice induce vomiting with ipecac syrup. If ipecac is not available, have person drink a glass of water or milk, then gently try to induce vomiting by tickling back of throat with finger or blunt object—be extremely careful not to damage the throat. Avoid prolonged or repeated contact with skin. Wash hands after use.
NOTE TO PHYSICIAN: Trichlorfon is a cholinesterase inhibitor. Atropine is an antidote; give after cyanosis is overcome. 2-PAM is a supplemental treatment.
Caution: Federal law restricts this drug to use by or on the order of a licensed veterinarian.
Warning: Not to be used in horses intended for use as food. Store at room temperature, avoid storage at temperatures above 30° C. (86° F.).
How Supplied:
Pkg. 12 #500 bottle (one for each 500 lb. bodywt.)
Pkg. 12 #1000 bottle (one for each 1,000 lb. bodywt.)

ENCEPHALOID® I.M.
Encephalomyelitis Vaccine Eastern and Western-Killed Virus Aluminum Phosphate Adsorbed Bio. 169

Indications: For vaccination of healthy equines against equine encephalomyelitis caused by Eastern and Western strains. Inject deep into heavy muscles of the hindquarter.
This product has been tested and shown to be satisfactory for marketing in accordance with existing Standard Requirements set forth by the U.S. Department of Agriculture.
Composition: This vaccine is prepared from virus-bearing chicken tissue culture fluids infected with Eastern and Western types encephalomyelitis virus. The viruses are formalin inactivated and combined with an aluminum phosphate adjuvant so as to provide optimum immunizing efficacy against both types.
Dosage and Administration: Inject one ml. dose intramuscularly using aseptic technique. Administer a second 1 ml. dose 21 days after the first dose. Revaccinate annually using one 1 ml. dose. To insure proper placement and retention of the vaccine, inject deep into the heavy muscles of the hindquarter. Mild exercise to promote absorption is recommended for one week after injection.
Caution:
Store in dark 2° to 7° C. (35° to 45°F).
Shake well.
Use entire contents when first opened.
Transitory local reactions at the injection site may occur if the vaccine leaks back to subcutaneous tissues or is deposited in intramuscular septas.
In case of anaphylactoid reaction administer epinephrine.
Thimerosal, neomycin, polymyxin B and a fungistat added as preservatives.
How Supplied: Pkg. 25, 1 ml. loaded disposable plastic syringes with needles, 25 doses.
10 ml.—10 doses.

EQUIBAC® II ℞
Streptococcus Equi Bacterin (Strangles Bacterin) Bio. 137

Indications: *Streptococcus Equi* Bacterin is indicated for use in healthy equine species, three months of age and older, to protect against infection due to *Streptococcus equi* (Strangles).
Composition: A beta-propiolactone killed suspension of *Streptococcus equi* in Gel 21 (aluminum hydroxide gel), which is added to absorb and concentrate the killed organisms to enhance the immunizing ability of the bacterin. Thimerosal added as a preservative.
Dosage and Administration: Administer three 2 ml. doses at 2 to 4 week intervals. Inject deep into the heavy muscle of the hindquarter, using strict aseptic technique. A single 2 ml. dose should be administered to previously vaccinated animals at yearly intervals.
Caution:
Store in dark at 2° to 7° C. (35° to 45°F.).
Shake well.
Use entire contents when first opened.
In case of anaphylactoid reaction administer epinephrine.
Adjuvants in equine biologicals increase the potential for muscle irritation, resulting in local reactions, such as muscle soreness, local edema, cellulitis, and abscess formation. Systemic symptoms, such as lethargy, depression, and elevated temperatures, may occur in animals sensitized to streptococci antigens or sensitive to adjuvants. These reactions may be minimized by mild exercise after injection.
The simultaneous use of antibiotics has been reported to be of value in reducing abscesses in those animals having a nondetectable or low-grade bacteremia.
Vaccination of animals infected with strangles, or in the incubative stages of the disease is contraindicated.
The administration of more than a single 2 ml. booster dose annually following strangles infection or following an initial vaccination series may result in increased anaphylactoid or local reactions.
Restricted to use by or under the direction of a veterinarian.
How Supplied: 20 ml—10 doses

EQUILOID®
Encephalomyelitis Vaccine-Eastern and Western Killed Virus Tetanus Toxoid Refined and Concentrated Aluminum Phosphate Adsorbed Bio. 276

Indications: For vaccination of healthy equines against Eastern and Western equine encephalomyelitis and tetanus. Inject deep into heavy muscles of hindquarters.
This product has been tested and shown to be satisfactory for marketing in accordance with procedures acceptable to the U.S. Department of Agriculture.
Composition: The encephalomyelitis fraction is prepared from virus-bearing chicken tissue culture fluids infected with Eastern and Western types encephalomyelitis virus. The viruses have been formalin inactivated and combined so as to provide optimum immunizing efficacy against both types.
The tetanus toxoid fraction is refined and concentrated by a patented process which eliminates at least 97% of the nonspecific nitrogen but leaves the antigenic fraction unchanged. Highly purified toxoids are desirable since components responsible for producing allergic or side reactions are practically eliminated.
The two fractions have been combined with an aluminum phosphate adjuvant which provides increased antigenic stimulation.
Dosage and Administration: Inject one 1 ml. dose intramuscularly using aseptic technique. Administer a second 1 ml. dose 4 to 8 weeks after the first dose. Revaccinate annually using one 1 ml dose.
To insure proper placement and retention of the vaccine, inject deep into the heavy muscles of the hindquarter. Mild exercise to promote absorption is recommended for one week after injection.
Protective tetanus antibody titers usually occur two weeks after the second injection of the initial series. In the event of injury during the course of the initial vaccination program, or if annual boosters have not been given, a prophylactic dose of at least 1,500 units of tetanus antitoxin should be given.
Caution:
Store in dark at 2° to 7° C. (35° to 45°F.).
Shake well. Use entire contents when first opened.
Transitory local reactions at the injection site may occur.
In case of anaphylactoid reaction administer epinephrine.
Thimerosal, neomycin, polymyxin B and a fungistat added as preservatives.
How Supplied: 25—1 ml. prefilled disposable plastic syringes with needles—25 doses, 10 ml.—10 doses.

ERSIPELIN®
Erysipelothrix Rhusiopathiae Bacterin
Bio. 117

Indications: Use in healthy swine as an aid in prevention of erysipelas.
Composition: A formalin killed suspension of Erysipelothrix rhusiopathiae, adsorbed with aluminum hydroxide gel.
Dosage and Administration:
Swine: 2 ml. Inject subcutaneously or intramuscularly.
For breeding animals repeat after 21 days and annually.
Caution:
Store in dark at 2° to 7°C (35° to 45°F).
Shake well. Use entire contents when first opened.
Do not vaccinate within 21 days before slaughter. In case of anaphylactoid reaction, administer epinephrine.
How Supplied: 100 ml— 50 doses
250 ml—125 doses

FEL–O–VAX® PCT
Feline Rhinotracheitis-Calici-Panleukopenia Vaccine
Killed Virus
Bio. 162

Indications: For vaccination of healthy cats and kittens to protect against diseases caused by feline rhinotracheitis, calici, and feline panleukopenia viruses.
Composition: Fel-O-Vax® PCT is prepared from viruses of feline rhinotracheitis, calici, and feline panleukopenia which have been grown on feline kidney tissue cell line and inactivated with formaldehyde. The antigens have been combined and an adjuvant added for convenient administration to cats of all ages. Prior to inactivation of the viruses, the tissue culture fluids are filtered to remove cellular debris, often responsible for tissue reactions, and to assist in complete inactivation of the viruses.
This product has been tested and shown to be satisfactory for marketing in accordance with procedures required by the U.S. Department of Agriculture.
Discussion: Feline rhinotracheitis and calici viruses both cause an upper respiratory tract infection in susceptible cats of all ages. The rhinotracheitis virus affects the epithelial surface of the upper respiratory passages and conjunctiva, which frequently causes hypersalivation, coughing and sneezing. Ocular discharge is a common symptom associated with the infection.
Calici virus infections are recognized by ulcerative lesions in the oral cavity, tongue epithelium and the nose. Both rhinotracheitis and calici viruses cause serious, and occasionally fatal, disease in susceptible cats, but are most pronounced in young kittens.
Feline panleukopenia infection usually results in an acute fulminating disease with high mortality, especially in kittens; however, subclinical or mild cases can be common under certain conditions. Symptoms include depression, anorexia, vomiting, weight loss and diarrhea which is frequently accompanied by blood-tinged feces. In young kittens the virus causes cerebellar hypoplasia characterized by incoordination, staggering, and rolling. Such kittens have been exposed in utero or shortly after birth.
Dosage and Administration: Vaccinate healthy cats of any age with one 1 ml dose of Fel-O-Vax PCT, followed by a second 1 ml dose three to four weeks later. Inject intramuscularly or subcutaneously. Cats vaccinated at less than 12 weeks of age should be given an additional 1 ml dose of vaccine at 12 to 16 weeks of age. Annual revaccination with a single dose of vaccine is recommended. Vaccination of pregnant queens has shown no deleterious effect.
Caution: Store in dark at 2° to 7°C (35° to 45°F.) Shake well. In case of anaphylactoid reaction administer epinephrine.
Thimerosal, neomycin, polymyxin B and a fungistat added as preservatives.
How Supplied: 25—1 ml prefilled disposable plastic syringes with needles—25 doses.
10 ml—10 doses

FEL-O-VAX® PCT-R
Feline Rhinotracheitis-Calici Panleukopenia-Rabies Vaccine Killed Virus
Bio. 163

Indications: For vaccination of healthy cats 12 weeks of age or older to protect against feline rhinotracheitis, calici, panleukopenia and rabies.
Dose: 1 ml. intramuscularly using aseptic technique. For rabies, give one dose at 3 months of age or older. Give a second dose one year later. Repeat subsequent doses every 3 years.
For feline rhinotracheitis-calici-panleukopenia vaccinate with Fort Dodge's Fel-O-Vax PCT vaccine 3 to 4 weeks before or after vaccination with Fort Dodge's Fel-O-Vax PCT-R and revaccinate annually.
Caution: Store in dark at 2° to 7° C. (35° to 45°F.)
Do not freeze.
Shake well. Use entire contents when first opened.
In case of anaphylactoid reaction administer epinephrine.
BPL inactivated. Thimerosal, neomycin, polymyxin B and a fungistat added as preservatives.
How Supplied:
25 - 1 ml. prefilled disposable syringes with needles—25 doses.
10 ml — 10 doses.

FLUOTHANE® ℞
(brand of halothane, U.S.P.)
Nonflammable
Nonexplosive
Inhalation Anesthetic

Indications: Fluothane (halothane, U.S.P.) is indicated for the induction and maintenance of general anesthesia for dogs, cats, and other non-food animals.
Composition: Contains 0.01% Thymol (w/w) and up to 0.00025% Ammonia (w/w).
Description: Fluothane, brand of halothane, U.S.P. (2-bromo-2-chloro-1,1,1-trifluoroethane). The specific gravity is 1.872-1.877 at 20° C. and the boiling point (range) is 49° C.–51° C. at 760 mm Hg. The vapor pressure is 243 mm Hg at 20° C. The blood/gas coefficient is 2.5 at 37° C., and the olive oil/water coefficient is 220 at 37° C. Vapor concentrations within the anesthetic range have a pleasant and nonirritating odor. Fluothane is nonflammable and its vapors mixed with oxygen in proportions from 0.5 percent to 50 percent (v/v) are not explosive. Fluothane (halothane, U.S.P.) is twice as potent as chloroform, and four times as potent as ether.
Fluothane does not decompose in contact with warm soda lime.When moisture is present, the vapor attacks aluminum, brass, and lead, but not copper. Rubber, some plastics, and similar materials are soluble in Fluothane; such materials will deteriorate rapidly in contact with Fluothane vapor or liquid. Stability of Fluothane is maintained by the addition of 0.01 percent thymol (w/w), up to 0.00025% ammonia (w/w), and storage is in amber colored bottles. Fluothane should not be kept indefinitely in vaporized bottles not specifically designed for its use. Thymol does not volatilize along with Fluothane and therefore accumulates in the vaporizer, and may, in time, impart a yellow color to the remaining liquid or to wicks in vaporizers. The development of such discoloration may be used as an indicator that the vaporizer should be drained and cleaned, and the discolored Fluothane (halothane, U.S.P.) discarded. Accumulation of thymol may be removed by washing with diethyl ether. After cleaning a wick or vaporizer, make certain all the diethyl ether has been removed before reusing the equipment to avoid introducing ether into the system.
Actions: Fluothane is an inhalation anesthetic. Induction and recovery are rapid, and depth of anesthesia can be rapidly altered.
Fluothane acts first by depressing the higher centers of the brain, then the motor and sensory nerves, and finally, in high concentrations, the vital medullary centers. It is an exceptionally potent anesthetic with rapid, easily reversible action.[1,2,3,4,5,8,11,12]
Fluothane (halothane, U.S.P.) progressively depresses respiration.[1,5,6,7] There may be tachypnea with reduced tidal volume and alveolar ventilation. Fluothane is not an irritant to the respiratory tract, and minimal increase in salivary or bronchial secretions ordinarily occurs.[1,6] Pharyngeal and laryngeal reflexes are rapidly diminished. It causes bronchodilation. Hypoxia, acidosis, or apnea may develop during deep anesthesia.
Fluothane reduces the blood pressure, and frequently results in bradycardia (decreased pulse rate).[1,5,8,9] The greater the concentration of the drug, the more evident these changes become. In those instances where bradycardia is not

Continued on next page

F

Fort Dodge—Cont.

caused by Fluothane administration, but is the result of vagal stimulation, it can be effectively reversed by the use of atropine. Fluothane also causes dilation of the vessels of the skin and skeletal muscles.
Cardiac arrhythmias may occur during Fluothane anesthesia.[7] Fluothane sensitizes the myocardial conduction system to the action of epinephrine and norepinephrine. Fluothane ordinarily produces a satisfactory degree of muscular relaxation for most surgical procedures, including abdominal surgery and bone-pinning operations.[3,4,10,11] Fluothane is a potent uterine relaxant.[10]
Contraindications: Fluothane is not recommended for obstetrical anesthesia except when uterine relaxation is required.
Adverse Reactions: The following adverse reactions have been reported: mild hepatic dysfunction, cardiac arrest, hypotension, hypothermia, respiratory arrest, cardiac arrhythmias, hyperpyrexia, and shivering.[5,8] Nausea and vomiting are relatively uncommon complications observed with Fluothane anesthesia.[1,3,9]
Dosage and Administration:
Caution: Operating rooms should be provided with adequate ventilation to prevent the accumulation of anesthetic gases and vapors.
Fluothane (halothane, U.S.P.) may be administered by the non-rebreathing technique, partial rebreathing, or closed technique. Because of the high potency and other physical and pharmacological properties, these methods all have their advantages and disadvantages. Use of an open or semi-open method using non-rebreathing technique is possible, but is wasteful, costly and permits anesthetic gas to be discharged into the atmosphere. Because of these disadvantages the closed and semi-closed rebreathing methods employing a carbon dioxide absorber have been developed which preferable to the non-rebreathing technique. Fluothane should be used in vaporizers that provide accurate concentrations which can be adjusted in percentage fractions over the entire clinical range of 0.5 to 5.0 percent (v/v). It is important that the anesthetic equipment be in good condition, and that the operator be familiar with inhalation anesthesiology techniques.
The concentration of Fluothane required to induce anesthesia will vary from patient to patient, but will often be between 2.0 to 5.0 percent. Maintenance dose of Fluothane usually will vary between 0.5 and 2.0 percent in the inhaled atmosphere. Fluothane (halothane, U.S.P.) may be administered with either oxygen or a mixture of oxygen and nitrous oxide.
It is absolutely necessary that the vaporizer be placed between the gas supply and breathing bag. If between the bag and the patient over-dosage may result.
Induction should not be hurried, and the concentration of vapor should not be suddenly increased.
When endotracheal intubation is desired, the intubation may be accomplished by using an anesthetic dose of one of the short-acting barbituates.
Maintenance anesthesia using Fluothane should be administered as soon as the intravenous administration is completed.
Precautions: Fluothane increases cerebrospinal fluid pressure. Therefore, in patients with markedly increased intracranial pressure, Fluothane administration should be preceded by measures ordinarily used to reduce cerebrospinal fluid pressure.
Ganglionic blocking agents (muscle relaxants) should be administered cautiously, since their hypotensive effect may be augmented by Fluothane. Epinephrine or norepinephrine should be employed cautiously, if at all, during Fluothane anesthesia, since their simultaneous use may induce cardiac arrhythmias.
Fluothane (halothane, U.S.P.) should be administered cautiously to patients in shock, in those with minimal cardiac reserve, and in those with grossly distributed cardiac rhythm.
Aminoglycoside antibiotics should be employed cautiously, if at all, in patients who are in shock and receiving Fluothane since there is moderate circulatory depression that is attributed to these antibiotics.
After cessation of the Fluothane anesthesia, reflexes are evident within one to two minutes, and sometimes slight muscular tremors occur. Horses, when recovering and semiconscious, do attempt to rise to their feet prematurely. If they are quietly restrained for about one hour, it will help prevent self-injury to the patient.[2,11] Cattle often voluntarily assume breast recumbancy within 15 minutes and rise to their feet unaided in approximately one hour. They show no excitement during recovery and no inhibition of salivation.
The uterine relaxation caused by Fluothane anesthesia may fail to respond to oxytocin. Fluothane produces marked relaxation of the anus during anesthesia, which may result in voiding of feces.[4]
Warning: Fluothane should not be used in pregnant animals, since the safe use of Fluothane has not been established with respect to possible adverse effects upon fetal development.
A condition known as malignant hyperthermia has on rare occasion been reported with the use of Fluothane in dogs, cats, pigs and horses.
Fluothane should be used only in vaporizers that permit a reasonable approximation of output, and preferably of the calibrated type.
It is absolutely necessary that the vaporizer be placed between the gas supply and breathing bag. If between the bag and the patient, overdosage may result.
The patient should be closely observed for signs of overdosage, i.e., depression of blood pressure, pulse rate, and ventilation, particularly during assisted or controlled ventilation. Fluothane should not be used in animals intended for use as food.
Caution: Federal law restricts this drug to use by or on the order of a licensed veterinarian.
How Supplied: Unit packages of Fluothane (halothane, U.S.P.) stabilized with 0.01 percent thymol (w/w), and up to 0.00025% ammonia (w/w). In bottles of 250 ml.
References:

1. Reventos, J.: *Brit. J. Pharmacol.*, 11:394 (Dec.) 1956.
2. Fisher, E.W. and Jennings, S.: *Vet. Rec.*, 70:567 (July) 1958.
3. Lumb, W.V.: *J.A.V.M.A.*, 134:218 (Mar.) 1959.
4. Sims, F.W.: *Vet. Rec.*, 72:617 (July) 1960.
5. Hall, L.W.: *Vet. Rec.*, 69:615 (June) 1957.
6. Kinard, R. and McPherson, C.W.: *Am. J. Vet. Res.* 21:385 (May) 1960.
7. Jones, E.W., Vasko, K.A., Hamm, D. and Griffith, R.W.: *J.A.V.M.A.*, 140:148 (Jan.) 1962.
8. Short, C.E., Keats, A.S., Liotta, D. and Hall, C.W.A.: *Am. J. Vet. Res.* 29:2287 (Dec.) 1968.
9. Luschei, E.S. and Mehaffey, J.J.: *J. Applied Physiol* 22:595 1967.
10. Dhindsa, D.S., Hoverland, A.S. and Kluemple, R.: *Am. J. Vet. Res.*, 31:1897 (Oct.) 1970.
11. Jennings, S.: *Can. Vet. Journal*, 4:86 (April) 1963.
12. Carter, H.E.: *Vet. Rec.*, 76:147 (Feb.) 1964.

FLUVAC®
Equine Influenza Vaccine
Killed Virus
Aluminum Phosphate Adsorbed
Refined and Concentrated
Bio. 156

Indications: For vaccination of healthy equines to protect against equine influenza due to A_1 and A_2 viruses.
Composition: This vaccine is prepared from the virus-bearing allantoic fluid of embryonated chicken eggs infected with types A_1 and A_2 equine influenza virus. The virus is formalin inactivated, concentrated and purified by differential centrifugation, and standardized to provide a chicken blood cell agglutination titer for optimum immunizing efficiency. An adjuvant is added to facilitate the proper rate of vaccine absorption following inoculation.
Dosage and Administration: Inject 1 ml. intramuscularly using aspectic technique. Administer a second dose 2 to 4 weeks after the first dose. A 1 ml. booster dose should be given annually or at any time epidemic conditions exist or when exposure is likely. Mild exercise to promote absorption is recommended.
Caution:
Store in dark at 2° to 7° C. (35° to 45° F.).
Shake well.
Use entire contents when first opened.
Transitory local reactions at the injection site may occur.

In case of anaphylactoid reaction administer epinephrine.
Thimerosal, neomycin, polymyxin B and a fungistat added as preservatives.
How Supplied: Pkg 25—1 ml. prefilled disposable plastic syringes with needles—25 doses. 10 ml—10 doses.

FLUVAC® EHV–1
Equine Rhinopneumonitis
Influenza Vaccine-Killed Virus
Aluminum Phosphate Adsorbed
Bio. 159

Indications: For vaccination of healthy equines against equine rhinopneumonitis caused by EHV-1 and influenza caused by types A Equi-1 and A Equi-2. This product has been tested and shown to be satisfactory for marketing in accordance with procedures required by the U.S. Department of Agriculture.
Composition: Fluvac EHV-1 is a killed virus vaccine of Equine Herpesvirus 1 (equine rhinopneumonitis virus) produced on a cell line and virus bearing allantoic fluid of embryonated chicken eggs infected with types A Equi-1 and A Equi-2 equine influenza virus which has been chemically inactivated with formaldehyde and combined with an aluminum phosphate adjuvant.
Dosage and Administration: Inject one 1 ml intramuscularly using aseptic technique. Administer a second 1 ml dose 4 to 6 weeks after the first dose. For young horses a third 1 ml dose should be administered 4 to 6 weeks after the second dose. A 1 ml booster dose should be given annually or at any time epidemic conditions exist or when exposure is likely. Mild exercise to promote absorption is recommended.
Caution: Store in dark at 2° to 7° C. (35° to 45° F.). Avoid freezing. Shake vigorously to assure uniform suspension of the adjuvant. When used according to instructions, it is unusual for reactions to appear, other than those expected with any vaccination of horses; for example, occasional temporary local swelling. Use entire contents when first opened. In case of anaphylactoid reaction administer epinephrine.
Thimerosal, neomycin, polymyxin B and a fungistat added as preservatives.
How Supplied: Pkg. 25—1 ml prefilled disposable plastic syringes with needles—25 doses.
10 ml—10 doses

FLUVAC® EWT
Encephalomyelitis– Influenza Vaccine
Eastern and Western
Killed Virus
Tetanus Toxoid
Refined and Concentrated
Aluminum Phosphate Adsorbed
Bio. 158

Indications: The antigens in Fluvac EWT are recommended for vaccination of healthy equines to protect against encephalomyelitis due to Eastern and Western viruses, equine influenza due to types A_1 and A_2 viruses, and tetanus. This product has been tested and shown to be satisfactory for marketing in accordance with procedures required by the U.S. Department of Agriculture.
Composition: This vaccine is a combination product consisting of equine encephalomyelitis virus, Eastern and Western strains, chicken tissue culture origin (CTCO), equine influenza virus, types A_1 and A_2, chicken embryo origin (CEO), and Tetanus Toxoid.
Fluvac® EWT is a combination of Fort Dodge Encephalomyelitis Vaccine IM (Encephaloid® IM) and Equine Influenza Vaccine-Tetanus Toxoid (Fluvac® T) produced in a single 2 ml. dose vaccine containing aluminum phosphate adjuvant. The viruses are formalin inactivated and combined with Tetanus Toxoid, which has been refined and concentrated by a patented process which eliminates at least 97 percent of the non-specific nitrogen but leaves the antigenic fraction unchanged.
Dosage and Administration: Inject one 2 ml. dose intramuscularly using aseptic technique. Administer a second 2 ml. dose 4 to 8 weeks after the first dose. A 2 ml. booster dose should be given annually. A booster dose of influenza vaccine, Fort Dodge Fluvac®, should be given any time epidemic conditions exist or when exposure is likely. Mild exercise to promote absorption is recommended for one week after injection.
Protective tetanus antibody titers usually occur two weeks after the second injection of the initial series. In the event of injury during the course of the initial vaccination program, or if annual boosters have not been given, a prophylactic dose of at least 1,500 units of tetanus antitoxin should be given.
Caution:
Store in dark at 2° to 7° C. (35° to 45° F.). Shake well.
Use entire contents when first opened. Transitory local reactions at the injection site may occur. In case of anaphylactoid reaction administer epinephrine.
Thimerosal, neomycin, polymyxin B and a fungistat added as preservatives.
How Supplied: 25—2 ml. prefilled disposable plastic syringes with needles—25 doses
20 ml—10 doses

FLUVAC® T
EQUINE INFLUENZA VACCINE
Killed Virus
TETANUS TOXOID
Aluminum Phosphate Adsorbed
Refined and Concentrated
Bio. 155

Indications: The antigens in Fluvac® T are highly antigenic and recommended for vaccination of healthy equines to protect against equine influenza due to types A_1 and A_2 viruses and tetanus.
This product has been tested and shown to be satisfactory for marketing in accordance with procedures acceptable to the U.S. Department of Agriculture. The influenza fraction is potency tested as specified in Fort Dodge Laboratories production manual. The Tetanus Toxoid fraction has been tested and shown to be satisfactory for marketing in accordance with existing Standard Requirements set forth by the U.S. Department of Agriculture.
Composition: Fluvac T is a combination vaccine containing Equine Influenza types A_1 and A_2 virus with the refined and concentrated Tetanus Toxoid for primary or booster vaccination programs in all equines.
The vaccine fraction is prepared from the virus-bearing allantoic fluid of embryonated chicken eggs infected with types A_1 and A_2 equine influenza virus. The virus is formalin inactivated, concentrated and purified by differential centrifugation, and standardized to provide a chicken blood cell agglutination titer of optimum immunizing efficiency. The inactivated virus is combined with Tetanus Toxoid, Fort Dodge, which has been refined and concentrated by a patented process which eliminates at least 97% of the non-specific nitrogen but leaves the antigenic fraction unchanged.
Dosage and Administration: Inject one 1 ml. dose intramuscularly using aseptic technique. Administer a second 1 ml. dose 4 to 8 weeks after the first dose. A 1 ml. booster dose should be given annually or at any time epidemic conditions exist or when exposure is likely.
Protective tetanus antibody titers usually occur two weeks after the second injection of the initial series. In the event of injury during the course of the initial vaccination program or if annual boosters have not been given, a prophylactic dose of at least 1,500 units of tetanus antitoxin should be given.
Caution:
Store in dark at 2° to 7° C. (35° to 45°F.). Shake well.
Use entire contents when first opened.
Transitory local reactions at the injection site may occur.
In case of anaphylactoid reaction, administer epinephrine.
Thimerosal, neomycin, polymyxin B and a fungistat added as preservatives.
How Supplied: Pkg. 25 - 1 ml. prefilled disposable plastic syringe with needles—25 doses. 10 ml—10 doses

GLUCOSE SOLUTION 50%
Sterile

Indications: Glucose (dextrose) solution for veterinary use in cattle for treatment of Acetonemia (ketosis).
Composition: Each ml. contains: Dextrose U.S.P. 500 mg; Sodium biphosphate with distilled water q.s.
Dosage and Administration: *Cattle:* 25 to 50 ml. per 100 lb. bodyweight. May be repeated after 3 to 5 hours if necessary. Administer intravenously, intraperitoneally or subcutaneously.
To Open Container: Wipe cap, top and neck of bottle with 70% alcohol. Screw down cap until a snap is heard indicating bottle top seal is broken. Carefully unscrew cap removing top of bottle. Attach sterile IV administration unit.
Caution: Unused portion remaining in bottle should be discarded.

Continued on next page

Fort Dodge—Cont.

Warning: Keep out of reach of children.
How Supplied: Pkg. 12—500 ml.

GLYCERIN

Composition: Contains Not Less Than 95% $C_3H_8O_3$
Notice: Glycerin is incompatible with and may result in explosion if mixed with strong oxidizing agents such as chromium trioxide, potassium chlorate and postassium permanganate.
How Supplied: 1 gallon.

KOPERTOX™
Water-Resistant Protection Without Bandaging

Indications: Recommended for use in the treatment of thrush in horses and ponies.
Not for use on horses intended for food.
Composition: Active Ingredient

Copper Naphthenate	37.5%
Inert Ingredients	62.5%
Total	100.0%

F

General Directions: Clean the hoof thoroughly removing debris and necrotic material prior to application of Kopertox. Apply daily to affected hoofs with a narrow paint brush (about 1″) until fully healed. Caution: Do not allow runoff of excess Kopertox onto hair since contact with Kopertox may cause some hair loss. Do not contaminate feed.
Caution:
Combustible Mixture.
Use in a well-ventilated place.
Avoid fire, flame, sparks or heaters.
If swallowed, do not induce vomiting; call physician immediately.
Avoid breathing vapor.
Avoid contact with skin and eyes.
Keep out of reach of children and pets.
Do not use on animals which are raised for food production.
Note: Kopertox is easily removed from hands, clothing, and surfaces with light grade fuel oil or any type of lighter fluid.
How Supplied: 16 oz. (473 ml.), 8 oz. (236 ml.) squeeze bottles.

LONGICIL® FORTIFIED ℞
(sterile benzathine penicillin G and procaine penicillin G suspension)

Indications: Longicil Fortified is indicated for treatment of the following bacterial infections in dogs, horses and beef cattle due to penicillin G susceptible microorganisms that are susceptible to the serum levels common to this particular dosage form, such as:
1. Bacterial Pneumonia (Shipping fever complex) (*Streptococcus spp., Corynebacterium pyogenes, Staphylococcus aureus*)
2. Upper Respiratory Infections such as Rhinitis or Pharyngitis (*Corynebacterium pyogenes*)
3. Equine Strangles (*Streptococcus equi*)
4. Blackleg (*Clostridium chauvoei*)
5. Anthrax (*Bacillus anthracis*)

Composition: Each ml. of suspension contains: 150,000 units penicillin G benzathine; 150,000 units penicillin G procaine; 3.0 mg sodium formaldehyde sulfoxylate; 14.0 mg lecithin; 1.20 mg methylparaben (as preservative); 0.14 mg propylparaben (as preservative); 0.25% Phenol (as preservative); 7.0 mg tween 40; 10.0 mg span 40; 10.0 mg sodium citrate; 20.0 mg procaine hydrochloride; 1.5 mg sodium carboxymethylcellulose; 3.5 mg povidone; 0.15 ml. sorbitol solution; and water for injection q.s.
Action: Penicillin is an antibiotic which shows a marked bactericidal effect against certain organisms during their growth phase. It is relatively specific in its action against gram-positive bacteria but is usually ineffective against gram-negative organisms.
When treating an animal for a bacterial infection, it is advisable to isolate and identify the causative organism and conduct appropriate in vitro susceptibility tests. In cases where organisms other than those susceptible to penicillin are present, re-evaluation of treatment should be made. Organisms normally considered susceptible to penicillin include *Clostridium septicum, Corynebacterium pyogenes, Staphyloccus aureus, Streptococcus canis, Streptococcus equi and Streptococcus pyogenes.*
It is normally recommended that any bacterial infection be treated as early as possible and with a dosage which will give effective blood levels. Although the recommended dosage of Longicil Fortified will give longer detectable penicillin blood levels than procaine penicillin G alone, it is recommended that a second dose be administered at 48 hours when treating a penicillin-susceptible bacterial infection.
If no definite improvement is noted following the second dose of Longicil Fortified, the diagnosis should be re-evaluated and use of another chemotherapeutic agent considered.
Contraindications: Longicil Fortified is contraindicated in patients which have shown hypersensitivity to penicillin.
Adverse Reactions: Anaphylactic reactions have been reported in cattle given penicillin. Treated animals should be closely observed and if allergic or anaphylactic reactions occur, administer epinephrine or antihistamines immediately.
Dosage and Administration:
Horses: 2 ml. per 150 lb. bodyweight given intramuscularly (2,000 units procaine penicillin G and 2,000 units benzathine penicillin G per lb. bodyweight). Treatment should be repeated in 48 hours.
Beef Cattle: 2 ml. per 150 lb. bodyweight given *subcutaneously* only (2,000 units procaine penicillin G and 2,000 units benzathine penicillin G per lb. bodyweight). Treatment should be repeated in 48 hours.
Important: Treatment in beef cattle should be limited to 2 (two) doses of Longicil Fortified, given by *subcutaneous injection only.*
Dogs: 1 ml. per 10 to 25 lb. bodyweight given intramuscularly or subcutaneously (6,000 to 15,000 units procaine penicillin G and 6,000 to 15,000 units benzathine penicillin G per lb. bodyweight). Treatment should be repeated in 48 hours.
Store below 15° C. (59° F.).
Shake Well before using.
Administration: Longicil Fortified should be given by intramuscular injection to horses. In beef cattle the recommended dosage should be administered by *subcutaneous injection only.* Dogs may be injected by either the intramuscular or subcutaneous route.
Warning:
Beef cattle should be withheld from slaughter for food use for 30 days following last treatment.
Treatment in beef cattle must be limited to 2 (two) doses.
Not to be used in horses intended for food purposes.
Caution: Federal law restricts this drug to use by or on the order of a licensed veterinarian.
How Supplied: 100 ml.

MYLEPSIN® ℞
(primidone)

Indications: Use only in dogs to treat:
Idiopathic Epilepsy: Archibald has reported on the use of primidone in the treatment of idiopathic epilepsy in dogs previously treated with other anticonvulsants without success. In his experience, primidone was found to be an effective agent, completely controlling the convulsions in most of the cases studied and reducing the number and severity of seizures in the remaining small percentage.
According to Chappel, effective control of convulsions has been achieved on daily dosages ranging from 30 to 40 mg per kg of bodyweight (or approximately 0.15 grams to 0.2 grams of primidone per 10 lb.). As optimum therapeutic effect was obtained, dosage was gradually reduced to maintenance level, and in some cases, therapy was eventually discontinued.
Epileptiform Convulsions: Clincially, these convulsions are similar to those of true epilepsy. Mylepsin may be useful as a symptomatic treatment of these convulsions of unknown etiology.
Mylepsin provides an effective means of controlling convulsions associated with infectious neuropathies such as virus encephalitis, distemper, and hard pad disease which occurs as a clinically recognizable lesion in certain entities in dogs. Supplementation of therapy with primidone is recommended as soon as diagnosis is made.
This is particularly important in distemper, since early protection against convulsions may help to promote recovery. However, it must be borne in mind that Mylepsin does not correct the primary cause of these disorders, but is a valuable adjunct to therapy, making possible control of seizures without hypnosis or interference with proper nutrition.

The initial dose of Mylepsin is gradually increased until optimum control of convulsions is achieved, and the dosage level necessary to establish this effect is usually maintained. In severe cases, certain workers have found it necessary to utilize higher dosages than those recommended for idiopathic epilepsy and epileptiform convulsions.

Mylepsin has not proved useful in the treatment of chorea.

Description: Primidone [5-ethyldihydro-5-phenyl-4,6 (*1H, 5H*)-pyrimidinedione] is a white crystalline substance. This pyrimidine derivative was discovered in 1949 by Bogue and Carrington, in their search for an anticonvulsant less toxic than those available at that time. These investigators demonstrated the protective action of primidone against both electrically and chemically induced convulsions in laboratory animals, a property also confirmed by Goodman, Swinyard, Brown, Schiffman, *et al.*

Subsequent trials have further substantiated the effectiveness of primidone and its high margin of safety in both dogs and man. No apparent gastrointestinal irritation has been noted. Abortion did not occur in pregnant bitches receiving high therapeutic doses of primidone.

In some cases, improvement in behavior pattern has been observed during primidone therapy, the animals being more alert and easier to manage. Weight gains have been reported.

Actions: Mylepsin acts upon the central nervous system to raise the seizure threshold, hence its value as an anticonvulsant, whether the seizure is induced electrically or is a symptom of a primary disease process.

Warning: For use only in dogs.

Precautions: Do Not Use In Feline Species.

Mylepsin is not recommended for use in the cat, because it appears to have, as do may other compounds, a specific neurotoxicity for this species.

Adverse Reactions: Mylepsin is well tolerated at effective therapeutic levels. Side reactions such as staggering and drowsiness occur infrequently and usually disappear with adjustment in dosage.

One reported case of laboratory-confirmed megaloblastic anemia was successfully treated with folic acid, vitamin B_{12}, and iron.

Dosage and Administration: Usual Daily Dosage—55 mg/kg (25 mg/lb) of bodyweight.

Tablets may be administered whole, or crushed and mixed with food.

When convulsions are frequent, the daily dosage should be divided and administered at intervals. When convulsions occur only every few days, or less often, daily dosage should be given at one time.

Reduction in dosage should always be made gradually, and treatment should never be discontinued abruptly.

Toxicity: In dogs receiving dosages well above effective therapeutic levels, for instance, in excess of 200 mg per kg of bodyweight, postmortem examinations showed no untoward pathologic effects on the alimentary canal, liver, kidneys, spleen, brain, or endocrine glands.

Caution: Federal law restricts this drug to use by or on the order of a licensed veterinarian.

How Supplied: Each tablet contains 250 mg of primidone (scored) in bottles of 100 and 1,000.

NOLVACIDE® INSECTICIDE SHAMPOO
with Conditioner and Nolvasan® (as preservative)

Indications: Use as a shampoo to kill fleas, lice and ticks. Cleans and restores luster to the hair coat of dogs and cats.

Composition:

Active Ingredients:	
Pyrethrin	0.045%
Piperonyl Butoxides Technical [equivalent to 0.072(butylcarbityl) (6-propylpiperonyl) ether and 0.018% related compounds.]	0.090%
N.-octyl bicycloheptane dicarboximide	0.150%
Petroleum Distillate	0.215%
Inert Ingredients:	99.500%
Total	100.000%

Directions for Use: It is a violation of federal law to use this product in a manner inconsistent with its labeling.

Wet dog or cat thoroughly with warm water. Apply enough *Nolvacide Insecticide Shampoo* to make a lather, and starting at the head, massage the wet hair coat and rub over the entire body of the animal. Add additional shampoo and water as necessary to make sufficient lather to cover the animal's body. Allow lather to stand on pet's body for about 5 minutes and then rinse hair coat and skin thoroughly with clean warm water. Dry hair of pet thoroughly.

Storage: Store at room temperature.

Pesticide Disposal: Securely wrap original container in several layers of newspapers and discard in trash.

Container Disposal: Do not reuse container bottles. Rinse thoroughly before discarding in trash.

Caution:

Harmful if swallowed. Avoid contact with eyes.

In case of contact immediately flush eyes with plenty of water.

Get medical attention if irritation persists.

Keep out of reach of children.

How Supplied: 12—8 oz., 1 gallon

NOLVACIDE® MIST
Insecticide Spray with Nolvasan® (as preservative) For Listed Insects on Dogs and Cats Pump Spray

Indications: *On Dogs:* Kills fleas and brown dog ticks.

On Cats: Kills fleas.

Composition:

Active Ingredients:	
Tetramethrin [(1-Cyclohexene-1,2-dicarboximido) methyl 2,2-dimethyl -3-(2-methylpropenyl) cyclopropanecarboxylate]	0.050%
*3-Phenoxybenzyl d-cis and trans** 2,2-dimethyl-3-(2-methylpropenyl) cyclopropanecarboxylate	0.096%
*Other isomers	0.004%
Inert Ingredients:	99.850%
Total	100.000%

*d-(cis, trans) phenothrin

**cis/trans isomer ratio: Max. 25% (+ or −) cis;
Min. 75% (+ or −) trans.

Directions for Use: It is a violation of federal law to use this product in a manner inconsistent with its labeling.

Shake before use. This product will kill fleas on cats and brown dog ticks and fleas on dogs. Spray the animal from a distance of 8–12 inches. Start spraying at the tail, moving the dispenser rapidly and making sure that the animal's entire body is covered, including the legs and under the body. As you spray, fluff the hair so the spray will penetrate to the skin. Make sure spray wets ticks thoroughly. Do not spray into the eyes, face or on genitals. Repeat as needed.

For cats, apply at the rate of one second per pound of body weight. For dogs, apply at the rate of two seconds per pound of body weight for thin or short haired dogs and up to eight seconds per pound of body weight for heavy or long haired dogs.

Storage: Store in a cool area away from heat or open flame.

Pesticide Disposal: Do not re-use empty container. Wrap container and put in trash collection.

Caution:

Hazards to Humans and Domestic Animals: Harmful if swallowed. Avoid breathing vapors. Wash hands with soap and water after use.

In the home, all food processing surfaces, exposed food, and utensils should be covered during treatment, or thoroughly washed before use.

Cover fish aquariums before spraying.

Physical Hazards: Do not use or store near heat or open flame.

How Supplied: 16 oz. spray bottles

NOLVALUBE®

Indications: A ready to use, antiseptic lubricant for topical or intrauterine application. Nongreasy; free from irritating effects; will not injure rubber appliances or surgical instruments.

Composition: A lubricant containing Nolvasan (0.1% chlorhexidine acetate).

Dosage and Administration:

Topical: Remove sufficient amount to cover hand and arm or instruments as required. If desired, a small amount of water can be used.

Intrauterine: Add approximately four ounces of Nolvalube per gallon of warm water and mix well.

Caution:

Keep container tightly closed.

Keep out of reach of children.

How Supplied: 12—8 oz., 8 pound

NOLVASAN® Solution
(chlorhexidine diacetate) Disinfectant

Composition: Active ingredients: 1,1′-Hexamethylenebis [5-(p-chlorophenyl)

Continued on next page

F

Fort Dodge—Cont.

biguanide] diacetate 2%. Inert Ingredients 98%. Total 100%. It is a violation of federal law to use this product in a manner inconsistent with its labeling.
Veterinary or Farm Premises.

Directions:

1. Remove all animals and feed from premises, vehicles, and other equipment.
2. Remove all litter and manure from floors, walls and surfaces of barns, pens, stalls, chutes, and other facilities and fixtures occupied or traversed by animals.
3. Empty all troughs, racks, and other feeding and watering appliances.
4. Thoroughly clean all surfaces with soap or detergent and rinse with water.
5. Saturate all surfaces with the recommended disinfecting solution for a period of 10 minutes.
6. Immerse all halters, ropes, and other types of equipment used in handling and restraining animals, as well as forks, shovels, and scrapers used for removing litter and manure.
7. Ventilate buildings, vehicles, and other closed spaces. Do not house livestock or employ equipment until treatment has been absorbed, set, or dried.
8. Thoroughly scrub all treated feed racks, mangers, troughs, automatic feeders, fountains, and waterers with soap or detergent, and rinse with potable water before reuse.

Indications: For disinfection of official meat, poultry, rabbit and egg establishments.

Directions:

1. All food products and packaging material must be removed from the room or carefully covered and protected.
2. Remove any loose dirt, litter, etc., that might be lying on floor or attached to the equipment.
3. Thoroughly clean all surfaces with soap or detergent and rinse with water.
4. Saturate all surfaces with the recommended disinfecting solution for a period of 10 minutes.
5. Expose or soak all equipment and/or utensils with the recommended disinfecting solution for a period of 10 minutes.
6. After disinfection, all equipments and/ or utensils must be thoroughly rinsed with potable water before operations are resumed.

Indications: For dipping teats as an aid in controlling bacteria that causes mastitis.

Directions: Immediately after the cow is milked dip each teat into the dipping solution. Teat dipping should start one week before the cow freshens. When drying off a cow the teats should continue to be dipped once a day for 3 to 4 days. Udder and teats of the cow must be thoroughly washed before milking.

Recommended Concentration For Use:

1.* For disinfection of inanimate objects to aid in control of canine distemper virus, equine influenza virus, transmissible gastroenteritis virus, hog cholera virus, parainfluenza-3 virus, bovine rhinotracheitis virus, bovine virus diarrhea virus, infectious bronchitis, Newcastle virus, Venezuelan equine encephalitis virus, equine rhinopneumonitis virus, feline rhinotracheitis virus and pseudorabies virus, equine arteritis virus and canine coronavirus —3 ounces (6 tablespoonfuls) per gallon of clean water. Nolvasan Solution has been shown to be virucidal in vitro against rabies virus (CVS strain) in laboratory tests when used as directed above.
2. For disinfection of veterinary or farm premises —1 ounce (2 tablespoonfuls) per gallon of clean water.
3. For disinfection of official meat, poultry, rabbit and egg establishments —1 ounce (2 tablespoonfuls) of Nolvasan Solution to each gallon of clean water.
4. For dipping teats as an aid in controlling bacteria that causes mastitis. Make up a final dipping solution by putting 32 ounces (one quart) of Nolvasan Solution in a clean gallon container, adding 6 ounces of glycerin and then adding clean potable water until you have a total volume of one gallon.

Not effective against Pseudomonas aeruginosa or gram-positive cocci on inanimate surface.*

*According to A.O.A.C. Use Dilution Test Method.

Caution:

Precautionary Statements Hazards To Humans (And Domestic Animals):
May be harmful if swallowed.
May be irritating to eyes or mucous membranes.
In case of contact, immediately flush eyes with plenty of water.
Get medical attention if irritation persists.
Keep out of reach of children.
Environmental Hazards: Keep out of lakes, ponds, or streams. Do not contaminate water by cleaning of equipment or disposal of wastes.

Storage and Disposal: Prohibition: Do not contaminate water, food, or feed by storage or disposal. Open dumping is prohibited. Do not reuse empty container.
Pesticide Disposal: Wastes resulting from use of this product may be disposed of on site or at an approved waste disposal facility.
Container Disposal: Do not reuse containers. Rinse thoroughly with water and discard in trash.
General: Consult federal, state or local disposal authorities for approved alternative procedures such as limited open burning.

How Supplied: 1 gallon, 50 gallon drum—non-returnable in this size.

NOLVASAN® CAP-TABS®
(Chlorhexidine)
Antibacterial Uterine Cap-Tabs

Indications: For prevention or treatment of metritis and vaginitis in cows and mares when caused by pathogens sensitive to chlorhexidine hydrochloride.

Composition: Each cap-tab contains 1 gm. chlorhexidine hydrochloride incorporated in an effervescent base.

Administration: Unattached placental membranes and any excess uterine fluid or debris should be removed from the uterus. The external genitalia should be carefully cleaned and 1 or 2 cap-tabs placed deep into each uterine horn. The operator should wear a clean obstetrical sleeve while inserting the cap-tabs into the uterus so that no contamination is introduced.
In a uterus which contains little or no uterine fluid, the effervescent cap-tab may cause some localized irritation. For treatment of such a uterus, or where the cervix is tightly constricted, the cap-tab should be dissolved in an appropriate amount of clean, boiling water and the solution infused into the uterus using a clean, sterile catheter. Treatment may be repeated in 48 to 72 hours.

Warning: *Keep out of reach of children.*

Caution: Keep bottle tightly closed to avoid deterioration by moisture or heat.

How Supplied: 50 cap-tabs

NOLVASAN® OINTMENT
Antiseptic

Composition: 1.0% Chlorhexidine acetate in a Hydrophilic Ointment base which contains 10% stearyl alcohol.

Suggested Usage:
Dogs, Cats, and Horses: For use as a topical antiseptic ointment for surface wounds. Carefully cleanse the wound area and apply daily.

Caution:
Not to be used in horses intended for use as food.
In case of deep or puncture wounds or serious burns consult veterinarian.
If redness, irritation or swelling persists or increases, discontinue use and consult veterinarian.
Store at room temperature (approximately 25° C. or 77° F.).
Keep out of reach of children.

How Supplied: Pkg 12-1 oz. tubes
Pkg 12-7 oz. jars
16 oz.

NOLVASAN® S
(chlorhexidine diacetate)
Scented
Disinfectant

Composition: Active Ingredient: 1,1'-Hexamethylenebis [5-(p-chlorophenyl) biguanide] diacetate 2%. Inert Ingredients 98%.

Recommended Concentration For Use: For disinfection of inanimate objects to aid in control of canine distemper virus, equine influenza virus, transmissible gastroenteritis virus, hog cholera virus, parainfluenza-3 virus, bovine rhinotracheitis virus, bovine virus diarrhea virus, infectious bronchitis, Newcastle virus, Venezuelan equine encephalitis virus, equine rhinopneumonitis virus, feline rhinotracheitis virus and pseudorabies virus, equine arteritis virus and canine coronavirus—3 ounces (6 tablespoonfuls) per gallon of clean water. Nolvasan has been shown to be virucidal in vitro against rabies virus (CVS strain) in laboratory tests when used as directed above.

For disinfection of veterinary or farm premises—1 ounce (2 tablespoonfuls) per gallon of clean water.

Not effective against *Pseudomonas aeruginosa* or gram-positive cocci on inanimate surface.*

*According to A.O.A.C. Use Dilution Test Method.

Directions for Use: It is a violation of federal law to use this product in a manner inconsistent with its labeling.

Veterinary or Farm Premises:

1. Remove all animals and feed from premises, vehicles, and other equipment.
2. Remove all litter and manure from floors, walls and surfaces of barns, pens, stalls, chutes, and other facilities and fixtures occupied or traversed by animals.
3. Empty all troughs, racks, and other feeding and watering appliances.
4. Thoroughly clean all surfaces with soap or detergent and rinse with water.
5. Saturate all surfaces with the recommended disinfecting solution for a period of 10 minutes.
6. Immerse all halters, ropes, and other types of equipment used in handling and restraining animals, as well as forks, shovels, and scrapers used for removing litter and manure.
7. Ventilate buildings, vehicles, and other closed spaces. Do not house livestock or employ equipment until treatment has been absorbed, set, or dried.
8. Thoroughly scrub all treated feed racks, mangers, troughs, automatic feeders, fountains, and waterers with soap or detergent, and rinse with potable water before reuse.

Precautionary Statements:

Hazards to Humans (And Domestic Animals)

Caution:

May be harmful if swallowed.

May be irritating to eyes or mucous membranes.

In case of contact, immediately flush eyes with plenty of water.

Get medical attention if irritation persists.

Keep out of reach of children.

Environmental Hazards: Keep out of lakes, ponds or streams. Do not contaminate water by cleaning of equipment or disposal of wastes.

Storage and Disposal:

Prohibition: Do not contaminate water, food or feed by storage or disposal. Open dumping is prohibited. Do not reuse empty container.

Pesticide Disposal: Wastes resulting from use of this product may be disposed of on site or at an approved waste disposal facility.

Container Disposal: Do not reuse containers. Rinse thoroughly with water and discard in trash.

General: Consult federal, state or local disposal authorities for approved alternative procedures such as limited open burning.

How Supplied: 1 pint
1 gallon

NOLVASAN® SHAMPOO
With Conditioner

Indications: Nolvasan Shampoo cleans and restores luster to the hair coat of dogs, cats and horses. Nolvasan Shampoo has excellent cleansing and deodorizing properties.

Composition: Contains Chlorhexidine acetate, 0.5%

Directions: Wet animal thoroughly with warm water. Apply enough shampoo to make a lather, adding more water if necessary. Massage into the hair coat for 2-5 minutes. Rinse hair and skin thoroughly with clean water. A second application of shampoo may be applied if necessary. Dry thoroughly.

Caution:

Keep out of reach of children.

Avoid contact with eyes.

Not to be used in horses intended for food.

How Supplied: Pkg. 12—8 oz. bottles, 1 gallon

NOLVASAN®
Skin and Wound Cleanser

Indications: Nolvasan® Skin and Wound Cleanser possesses a wide range of antimicrobial activity and provides a rapid and residual antimicrobial effect.

Composition: Contains 2% (w/v) chlorhexidine acetate in a stable detergent base.

Directions for Use:

General Skin Cleansing: Thoroughly rinse area to be cleansed with water. Apply sufficient Nolvasan Skin and Wound Cleanser and wash gently. Rinse again thoroughly.

Wound Cleansing: Rinse the area to be cleansed with clean water. A moistened gauze pad may be used to apply a small amount of Nolvasan Skin and Wound Cleanser to the affected area. Gently cleanse for 2–4 minutes. Additional water may be needed to obtain adequate sudsing. Repeat cleaning if necessary. Wipe away excess foam with a clean gauze pad. After cleansing, an antiseptic ointment or suitable dressing may be applied.

Caution: In case of deep or puncture wounds or serious burns, contact a veterinarian. If redness, irritation, or swelling persists or increases, consult a veterinarian.

Avoid contact with the eyes and mucous membranes. If contact is made, flush promptly and thoroughly with clean water. Hypersensitivity to Nolvasan is rare; however, if reactions should occur, discontinue use.

For veterinary use only.

Keep out of reach of children. For external use only.

How Supplied: 12—8 oz.
12—4 oz.

NOLVASAN®
SURGICAL SCRUB
(chlorhexidine)

Indications: An antimicrobial skin and wound cleanser. Nolvasan® Surgical Scrub possesses a wide range of antimicrobial activity and provides a rapid and residual antimicrobial effect.

Composition: Contains 2% (w/v) chlorhexidine diacetate in a stable detergent base.

Directions for use: Rinse the area to be cleansed with clean water. Apply 1 to 5 ml of Nolvasan Surgical Scrub to the area and wash with a sponge or brush for 2 to 4 minutes. It may be necessary to apply additional water to obtain adequate sudsing. Wipe away excess foam with sterile sponge.

Caution:

Avoid contact with the eyes and mucous membranes.

If contact is made, flush promptly and thoroughly with clean water.

Hypersensitivity to Nolvasan is rare; however, if reactions should occur discontinue use.

Keep out of reach of children.

For external use only.

How Supplied: 1 pint, 1 gallon

NOLVASAN® SUSPENSION
(chlorhexidine)
Antibacterial

Indications: For prevention and treatment of metritis and vaginitis in cows and mares caused by pathogens sensitive to chlorhexidine hydrochloride.

Composition: Each 28 ml syringe contains 1 Gm chlorhexidine hydrochloride in a special base.

Administration: Unattached placental membranes and any excess uterine fluid or debris should be removed from the uterus. The external genitalia should be carefully cleaned and a clean, sterile inseminating pipette should be passed through the cervix and the Nolvasan® Suspension infused into the uterus. Treatment may be repeated in 48 to 72 hours.

Warning: Keep out of reach of children.

How Supplied: Pkg. 12-28 ml syringe. Plastic pipettes for each order, gratis on request. 1-1610 pipette.

NOLVASAN® TEAT DIP
Concentrate
(chlorhexidine acetate)

Indications: For use as an aid in controlling bacteria that cause bovine mastitis.

Composition: Each pint contains: Active ingredient: Chlorhexidine acetate 4% (18.9 Gm.) Inert Ingredients: q.s. (including 39% glycerin)

Directions: To Prepare 0.5% Teat Dip Solution. One pint of Nolvasan® Teat Dip Concentrate should be reconstituted to 1 gallon of 0.5% teat dip solution.

Continued on next page

Fort Dodge—Cont.

Place entire contents in a clean 1 gallon container and add clean, potable water to give one gallon of teat dip solution. (Use of "hard water" may result in some precipitation. If the 0.5% solution is to be held longer than 1 week, it is advisable to use distilled or deionized water).
Use of 0.5% Teat Dip Solution. Teat dipping should start one week before the cow freshens. During lactation, dip each teat into the 0.5% solution immediately after the cow is milked. When the cow is dried off, the teats should continue to be dipped in the solution once a day for 3 to 4 days. Dip each teat so that the lower one inch of the teat has been covered with the solution.
Udder and teats of the cow should be thoroughly washed before milking.
If minor irritation or chapping of the teats should occur during lactation, it is often helpful to dilute the 0.5% solution half and half with clean water for a couple of days and then gradually return to use of the 0.5% solution.
Caution:
Keep out of reach of children. May be irritating to eyes or mucous membranes. May be harmful if swallowed. Avoid contamination of feed or feedstuffs. If in contact, flush thoroughly with water. Rinse empty container with water and discard.
Warning:
Do not use this solution undiluted. Dip teats only in a properly prepared 0.5% solution as directed. Do not use this solution for cleaning milking equipment. Store at room temperature. Avoid freezing or exposure to excessive heat. *Keep out of reach of children.*
How Supplied: 1 pint.

F

NOLVASAN® 5% TEAT DIP
Concentrate
(chlorhexidine acetate)

Indications: For use as an aid in controlling bacteria that cause bovine mastitis. Refer to directions for preparation of the 0.5% solution and proper use as a teat dip.
Composition: Contains:
Active ingredient:
Chlorhexidine acetate 5% (94.6 Gm.)
Inert Ingredients: q.s.
(including 48.7% glycerin)
Directions: To Prepare 0.5% Teat Dip Solution: This ½ gallon of Nolvasan® (chlorhexidine acetate) 5% Teat Dip Concentrate should be reconstituted to 5 gallons of 0.5% teat dip solution. Place entire contents in a clean 5 gallon container and add clean, potable water to give 5 gallons of teat dip solution. (Use of "hard water" may result in some precipitation. If the 0.5% solution is to be held longer than 1 week, it is advisable to use distilled or deionized water.)
To prepare small quantity of final 0.5% solution, this Nolvasan 5% Teat Dip Concentrate should be used at a dilution of 1 pint per 1¼ gallon clean, potable water.
Use of 0.5% Teat Dip Solution: Teat dipping should start one week before the cow freshens. During lactation, dip each teat into the 0.5% solution immediately after the cow is milked. When the cow is dried off, the teats should continue to be dipped in the solution once a day for 3 to 4 days. Dip each teat so that the lower one inch of the teat has been covered with the solution.
Udder and teats of the cow should be thoroughly washed before milking.
If minor irritation or chapping of the teats should occur during lactation, it is often helpful to dilute the 0.5% solution half and half with clean water for a couple of days and then gradually return to use of the 0.5% solution.
Caution: Keep out of reach of children. May be irritating to eyes or mucous membranes. May be harmful if swallowed. Avoid contamination of feed or feedstuffs. If in contact, flush thoroughly with water. Rinse empty container with water and discard.
Warning: Do not use this solution undiluted. Dip teats only in a properly prepared 0.5% solution as directed. Do not use this solution for cleaning milking equipment. Store at room temperature. Avoid freezing or exposure to excessive heat.
How Supplied: ½ gallon

NOLVASAN® UDDER WASH CONCENTRATE
(chlorhexidine acetate)

Indications: A special formula of surfactant and the antimicrobial agent, chlorhexidine acetate, to be used in washing the udder and teats prior to milking. As an aid in sanitizing; and reducing bacteria from the surface of the udder and teats.
Composition: Contains:
Active ingredient:
Chlorhexidine acetate 4.0%
Inert Ingredients: q.s
Directions: To prepare the final udder wash product add 1 fluid ounce (2 tablespoonfuls) of Nolvasan® Udder Wash Concentrate to two (2) gallons of clean, potable water. Prepare fresh wash for each milking.
To wash the udder and teats use a separate clean paper towel for each cow; soak the paper towel in the prepared udder wash; and thoroughly wash the entire udder and teats of the cow within 2 minutes of applying the milk machine. Discard the paper towel after use. When washing be careful to remove all dirt and debris from the surface of the udder. (If udder or teats are excessively dirty, a second paper towel should be soaked and the udder/teats washed the second time.)
After the udder/teats are washed with the udder wash another paper towel should be used to thoroughly wipe dry the surface of the udder and teats before the milk machine cups are placed on the cow.
Washing of udder/teats should be conducted before each milking. It is also advised to use the Nolvasan Teat Dip to dip all teats after milking. This will aid in control of bacteria that cause bovine mastitis.
Caution: Keep out of reach of children. Concentrate may be irritating to eyes or mucous membranes. May be harmful if swallowed. Avoid contamination of feed or feedstuffs. If in contact, flush thoroughly with water. Rinse empty container with water and discard.
Warning: Do not use this solution undiluted. Wash udder and teats only with properly diluted udder wash and then wipe off udder and teats with clean towel as directed. Do not use this solution for washing of milking equipment.
Store at room temperature. Avoid freezing or exposure to excessive heat.
How Supplied: 12—1 pint

NOMAGEN™
Mycobacterial Cell Wall Fraction Immunostimulant
Bio. 295

Indications: *For the treatment of equine sarcoids and treatment of bovine ocular squamous cell carcinoma.*
Equine. Results of the equine sarcoid field trial are as follows:

Tumor Size	Tumor Diameter	# of Animals Treated	% Regression
Small	2.5 cm	4	100
Medium	2.5–7.0 cm	11	91
Large	7.0 cm	5	80

The average period until complete regression of the tumor was 5.24 months.
Bovine. Results of the bovine ocular carcinoma field trials are as follows: From the table below, correlation of tumor size and prognosis of treatment is evident.

Tumor Size	Tumor Diameter	# of Animals Treated	% Regression
Small	2.5 cm	8	88
Medium	2.5–7.0 cm	23	70
Large	7.0 cm	4	0

The average period until complete regression of the tumor was 2.72 months.
Contraindications: There are no known contraindications to this preparation when used as directed.
Dosage: Dependent on size of tumor. Inject 5 ml for each inch of tumor diameter.
Treatment Schedule: It is strongly recommended that the tumor site be injected twice, two-three weeks apart. Further treatment may be called for, depending on tumor response.
Method of Reconstitution: Using a 20 gauge sterile needle and 10 ml syringe, sterile diluent is injected into vial containing lyophilized preparation. The material is emulsified by repeated injections into the vial and aspirations into the syringe. The procedure should be continued for at least 2 minutes. Syringe and needle remain in the serum vial during this procedure. It may be necessary to warm the vial or the diluent vial in warm water (37° C) prior to emulsification procedure to facilitate emulsification. Emulsion should have cloudy or milky appearance after reconstitution. Failure to reconstitute in the method prescribed may adversely affect efficacy of product.
Method of Injection: The syringe should be fitted with a 25 gauge needle to

prevent loss of material through the site of injection. The emulsion should be injected directly into the tumor, obliquely towards the base of the tumor. The tumor should be completely infiltrated with the emulsion. Often, several injections from different angles are necessary to completely infuse the tumor.
Side Effects: During field trials, local reactions reported were transient erythema, edema and granulomatous reactions. The tumor site may dry up or weep, ulcerate or slough-off tissue. Localized transient edema is the most prevalent reaction noted.
Occasional cases of infection of the tumor site have been observed. Therefore, it is recommended that sterile techniques should be used. If infection develops, treatment with antibiotics is indicated.
Caution: Use of this preparation may affect TB reactivity in **cattle.** Because of the possibility of non-specific reaction resulting from the injection, the supplemental comparative cervical test may not serve to establish the tuberculosis status of a treated animal. It is therefore suggested that a certificate be provided to the animal owner stating that the animal has been injected with the product and the date of injection.
The certificate should establish the identity of the recipient by an alpha numeric ear tag such as a pass tag utilized in routine brucellosis and tuberculosis tests by an accredited veterinarian.
A certificate from the practicing veterinarian, with the unique identification and retained by the owner, would help to clarify the animal status should the animal respond to a tuberculosis test subsequent to treatment. In case of anaphylactoid reaction, administer epinephrine.
How Supplied: 5 ml—1 dose

Produced for:
Fort Dodge Laboratories, Inc.
Fort Dodge, Iowa 50501
Produced by:
Ribi Immunochem Research, Inc.
Hamilton, MT 59840

PENTOBARBITAL SODIUM Ⓒ ℞
Solution (Sterile)
Alcohol 10% by Volume

Composition: Each ml. contains: Pentobarbital sodium 64.8 mg (1 gr.); Distilled water q.s.
Directions: The average dose of 1 ml. (1 gr. or 64.8 mg. pentobarbital sodium) per 5 lb. bodywt. for dogs and cats will vary according to the size, age and health of the animal. In dogs and cats the proper use of a preanesthetic will allow a smoother induction and also reduce the dosage of pentobarbital by 20% to 33%. Always inject sodium pentobarbital intravenously. This must be done SLOWLY. Pause a minute after half the average dose has been injected to avoid overdosing an animal which may be susceptible to the drug. If one-half the average dose does not produce abnormal depression, the balance may be injected or that portion which produces anesthesia. An animal should be anesthetized just to the point where sharply pinching the skin or foot does not cause reflex. Do not go beyond this point. At least two minutes should be taken for intravenous injection, with frequent pauses while the drug is being taken up by the central nervous system.
Precautions: Use additional care when anesthetizing anemic or hypovolemic animals and animals with cardiac or respiratory problems. The following conditions may cause prolonged recovery: (1) liver pathology, (2) elevated urea nitrogen or electrolyte imbalance, (3) hypothermic or malnourished animals, (4) following a prolonged surgical procedure. In general, barbiturates should not be employed for cesarean section because of respiratory depression to the fetus.
Store at room temperature (approx. 25° C.). Do not use if material has precipitated.
Warning: Do not inject perivascularly, because soft tissue irritation will result. Avoid intra-arterial injection. Emergence excitement may occur in dogs following barbiturate anesthesia.
Caution:
Federal law restricts this drug to use by or on the order of a licensed veterinarian.
Keep out of reach of children.
How Supplied: 100 ml. Requires use of DEA order form (DEA-222 C).
This product is not returnable for credit or exchange.

pHos-pHaid
Urinary Acidifier for Dogs and Cats

Composition:

Active ingredients:	.5 Gm	.25 Gm
Ammonium biphosphate	190 mg.	95 mg.
Sodium biphosphate	200 mg.	100mg.
Sodium acid pyrophosphate	110 mg.	55 mg.
Sodium per tablet, less than	1 gr.	½ gr.

Dosage: For .5 gm. tablet: 1 tablet twice daily for each 15-30 lb. bodyweight. For .25 gm. tablet: 2 tablets twice daily for each 15-30 lb. bodyweight.
Caution: *Keep out of reach children.*
How Supplied: Pkg. 12—90 .5 Gm.
Pkg. 12—150 .25 Gm.

PNEUMABORT® K
Equine Rhinopneumonitis Vaccine
Killed Virus
Bio. 287
U.S. Patent No. 4,083,958

Indications: For vaccination of healthy equines to contribute to the maturation of immunity against respiratory disease caused by the EHI Virus and for use in pregnant mares as an aid in the prevention of abortion due to EHI Virus infection. Horses incubating other infections or suffering from malnutrition, parasitism, or other diseases and conditions subjecting them to stress are poor subjects for immunization and may not develop or maintain a serviceable immune response.
Composition: Pneumabort K is a killed virus vaccine of Equine Herpesvirus I (equine rhinopneumonitis virus) which has been chemically inactivated with formaldehyde and combined with a specially prepared oil adjuvant.
This product has been tested and shown to be satisfactory for marketing in accordance with procedures required by the U.S. Department of Agriculture.
General Information: A short duration of serviceable immunity occurs after herpesvirus I infection or vaccination. It is necessary to maintain as high a level of immunity as possible to aid in protection against upper respiratory tract infection and spread of field strains of virus to pregnant mares. Pregnant mares require the highest possible level of protection against infection after the fifth month of pregnancy; this should be maintained throughout pregnancy.
The vaccine is a killed virus preparation and may be administered at any time to horses or mares that may be moved from the premises, or that may be exposed to infection.
Dosage and Administration: For pregnant mares, administer a 2 ml. dose intramuscularly during the 5th, 7th, and 9th months of pregnancy. Revaccinate annually at the 5th, 7th, and 9th months of pregnancy.
For young horses, administer a 2 ml. dose intramuscularly followed by a second 2 ml. dose 3 to 4 weeks later. Revaccinate with a single 2 ml. dose 6 months after the second primary dose and annually thereafter. To insure proper placement and retention of the vaccine, inject deep into the heavy muscles of the hindquarter. Mild exercise to promote absorption is recommended for one week after injection.
Maiden and barren mares kept in barn- or pasture-contact with vaccinated pregnant mares should be vaccinated on the same schedule as the pregnant mares with which they are in contact. Mares more than five months pregnant at the time of arrival on a farm should be vaccinated upon arrival and at two-month intervals until foaling.
Pregnant mares that are in contact with mares that have aborted equine herpesvirus I infected fetuses should be vaccinated. Such vaccination may provide immunity for those mares in the group which are not incubating an abortigenic infection at the time of vaccination.
Caution:
Store in dark at 2° to 7° C. (35° to 45° F.).
Shake well.
Use entire contents when first opened.
Transitory local reactions at the injection site may occur. In case of anaphylactoid reaction administer epinephrine.
Thimerosal, neomycin, polymixin B and a fungistat added as preservatives.
How Supplied: 25—2 ml. prefilled syringes—25 doses. 20 ml—10 doses.

Continued on next page

Fort Dodge—Cont.

PORSIBAC® 2
Escherichia Coli,
Pasteurella Multocida,
Salmonella Choleraesuis Bacterin,
Porcine Isolates
Bio. 102

Indications: For vaccination of healthy swine to protect against conditions attributed to organisms listed in the formula.
Composition: A killed suspension of *Salmonella choleraesuis, Pasteurella multocida* and *Escherichia coli.* Gel 21 (aluminum hydroxide gel) added as an adjuvant.
Each ml. contains at least 7.5 billion killed organisms.
Dosage and Administration:
Mature Swine: 2 ml.
Small Pigs: 1 ml.
Inject subcutaneously or intramuscularly. Repeat in 14 to 21 days.
Caution:
Store in dark at 2° to 7° C. (35° to 45° F).
Shake well.
Use all of this product at time container is first opened.
Do not vaccinate within 21 days of slaughter.
In case of anaphylactoid reaction, administer epinephrine.
How Supplied: 100 ml 50 doses.

PORSIVAC™ Pv 5L
Parvovirus Vaccine
Killed Virus
Leptospira
Canicola-Grippotyphosa-Hardjo-Icterohaemorrhagiae-Pomona Bacterin
Bio. 168

Indications: For vaccination of healthy swine to protect against reproductive failure due to *porcine parvovirus* infection and *leptospira canicola, grippotyphosa, hardjo, icterohaemorrhagiae* and *pomona* infections.
Dose: Gilts and sows, inject one 4 ml. dose intramuscularly or subcutaneously 2–8 weeks before breeding or after 6½ months of age. Boars may be vaccinated to control virus spread in a herd. An annual booster dose is recommended to maintain a high level of immunity.
Caution: Store in dark at 2° to 7° C. (35° to 45° F.). Avoid freezing. Shake well. Use entire contents when first opened. Do not vaccinate within 21 days before slaughter. In case of anaphylactoid reaction administer epinephrine.
Thimerosal, neomycin, polymyxin B and a fungistat added as preservatives.
How Supplied: 40 ml—10 doses
200 ml—50 doses

PORSIVAC T.G.E.®
Transmissible Gastroenteritis Vaccine
Modified Live Virus
Bio. 188

Indications: For vaccination of healthy pregnant sows and gilts to protect against infection and death of baby pigs due to transmissible gastroenteritis. In pregnant sows and gilts it is important to vaccinate well in advance of farrowing to allow adequate time for development of antibodies in the milk, which pass to the suckling pigs and confer a temporary passive immunity. The immunity conferred to the pigs is effective only as long as the pigs continue to nurse and are protected by good management against excessive exposure which may overcome the limited passive protection from the antibodies in the colostrum and milk.
Composition: Porsivac T.G.E.® is a desiccated preparation containing viable modified transmissible gastroenteritis virus propagated on a porcine cell line culture system.
This vaccine has been tested and shown to be satisfactory for marketing in accordance with procedures required by the U.S. Department of Agriculture.
General Information: Transmissible gastroenteritis (TGE) is an infectious and contagious disease of swine. Although the disease affects swine of all ages, it causes most severe losses in baby pigs under ten days of age. The onset of disease in very young pigs is rapid, within 24 to 48 hours, characterized by inappetence, vomiting, profuse watery diarrhea, and dehydration.
Sows, gilts, and feeder pigs may exhibit any of the symptoms which affect baby pigs, but usually to a milder degree. In addition they may show weight loss, and in farrowed sows and gilts, a reduction or cessation of milk flow.
Dosage and Administration: Rehydrate to liquid form using the sterile diluent supplied in the package. Inject 2 ml six (6) to eight (8) weeks prior to farrowing either intramuscularly or intramammarily. Repeat 2 ml dosage one (1) to two (2) weeks prior to farrowing.
Intramuscular: Inject 2 ml into the ham.
Intramammary: Inject 2 ml dose by injecting 1 ml into the base, not the cistern, of each of two hind mammary glands.
Caution:
Store in dark at 2° to 7° C. (35° to 45° F.)
Use entire contents within 30 minutes after rehydration.
Burn container and unused contents.
Do not vaccinate within 21 days before slaughter.
In case of anaphylactoid reaction, administer epinephrine.
Neomycin, polymyxin B and a fungistat added as preservatives.
For Veterinary Use Only
How Supplied: Pkg. 10/2 ml—10 doses
20 ml—10 doses

PORSIVAC T.G.E.®-C
Transmissible Gastroenteritis Vaccine
Modified Live Virus
Clostridium Perfringens Type C Toxoid
Bio. 189

Composition: Porsivac T.G.E.® is a desiccated preparation containing viable modified transmissible gastroenteritis virus propagated on a porcine cell line culture system and clostridium perfringens type C toxoid.
Indications: Porsivac T.G.E.-C combines Porsivac T.G.E. with Clostroid® C in a 2 ml. dose for vaccination of healthy pregnant sows and gilts to protect against infection and death of baby pigs due to transmissible gastroenteritis virus (TGE) and Clostridium perfringens Type C.
General Information: Transmissible gastroenteritis (TGE) is an infectious and contagious disease of swine. Although the disease affects swine of all ages, it causes most severe losses in baby pigs under ten days of age. The onset of disease in very young pigs is rapid, within 24 to 48 hours, characterized by inappetence, vomiting, profuse watery diarrhea and dehydration.
Sows, gilts and feeder pigs may exhibit any of the symptoms which affect baby pigs, but usually to a milder degree. In addition they may show weight loss, and in farrowed sows and gilts, a reduction or cessation of milk flow.
Necrotic Enteritis in Young Pigs Due to Clostridium Perfringens Type C: The newborn pig ingests Clostridium perfringens Type C organisms within minutes to a few hours after birth.[1] These organisms usually cause a highly fatal necrotic enteritis in pigs less than 1 week old, characterized by diarrhea, which is hemorrhagic in acute cases.[2] In a chronic form, pigs to 4 weeks of age may be affected, including weaned pigs. The incidence of affected litters in a herd may vary from less than 10% to 100%.
Clinically, the disease may occur in several forms. In the peracute form, pigs sicken and die by the end of the first or second day of life. They nearly always have a bloody diarrhea. In acute, less severe cases, pigs usually die after 2 days and have a diarrhea with reddish brown liquid feces. They become progressively gaunt and weak.
In milder subacute cases, the pigs have a persistent diarrhea and usually become emaciated and die when 5–7 days old. The feces are soft at first, then change to liquid, containing flecks of gray necrotic debris or "rice water stools". Pigs with the chronic form have a diarrhea with yellow-gray mucoid feces for about a week. Although they remain alert, some may die later and survivors fail to gain weight.
Efficacy Evaluation of Clostroid C Component: Investigators have found that a concentration of antitoxin of 5 IU/ml. or greater, in the colostrum of a sow,[3] protected her pigs from natural infection. Potency tests on the Clostroid C component with vaccinated gilts demonstrated colostrum antitoxin levels above the 5 IU/ml. some more than 10X higher.
Piglets from these vaccinated gilts and from nonvaccinated control gilts were challenged with Clostridium perfringens Type C toxin cultures. The piglets from control gilts had no immunity and were killed by a small amount of toxin given intravenously. On the other hand, the piglets from the vaccinated gilts withstood intravenous challenge with high

levels of toxin, more than 20X that required to kill controls, without showing any signs of illness.

Administration and Dosage: Rehydrate to liquid form using the Clostroid C diluent supplied in the package. Inject 2 ml. intramuscularly deep into the ham six (6) to eight (8) weeks prior to farrowing. Repeat 2 ml. dosage one (1) to two (2) weeks prior to farrowing.

Caution: Store in dark at 2° to 7° C. (35° to 45° F.). Use entire contents within 30 minutes after rehydration. Burn container and unused contents. Do not vaccinate within 21 days before slaughter. In case of anaphylactoid reaction administer epinephrine.

Neomycin, polymyxin B and a fungistat added as preservatives.

How Supplied: 10-2 ml—10 doses
20 ml—10 doses

References:

1 Bergeland, M.E., Clostridial Infections in Disease of Swine, 5th ed., p. 419, edited by A.D. Lemon, et al (1981), Iowa State Univ. Press.
2 Bergeland, M.E., Necrotic Enteritis in Nursing Piglets, Proc. Am. Assoc. Vet. Lab. Diag. (1977), 20, p. 151.
3 Hogh, P., Clostridial Products in Veterinary Medicine. Devel. Biol. Standards (1976), 32, 69 Karger, Basel, Swit.

PROMACE® ℞
(acepromazine maleate) Injectable and Tablets

Indications:

Dogs and Cats: PromAce Injectable and Tablets can be used as an aid in controlling intractable animals during examination, treatment, grooming, x-ray, and minor surgical procedures; to alleviate itching as a result of skin irritation; as an antiemetic to control vomiting associated with motion sickness.

PromAce Injectable is particularly useful as a preanesthetic agent (1) to enhance and prolong the effects of barbiturates, thus reducing the requirements of general anesthesia; (2) as an adjunct to surgery under local anesthesia.

Horses—PromAce Injectable can be used as an aid in controlling fractious animals during examination, treatment, loading and transportation. Particularly useful when used in conjunction with local anesthesia for firing, castration, neurectomy, removal of skin tumors, ocular surgery and applying casts.

Description: Acepromazine maleate, a potent neuroleptic agent with a low order of toxicity, is of particular value in the tranquilization of dogs, cats, and horses. Its rapid action and lack of hypnotic effect are added advantages. According to Baker[1], the scope of possible applications for this compound in veterinary practice is only limited by the imagination of the practitioner.

Actions: PromAce (acepromazine maleate) has a depressant effect on the central nervous system and therefore causes sedation, muscular relaxation, and a reduction in spontaneous activity. It acts rapidly, exerting a prompt and pronounced calming effect.

Contraindications: Phenothiazines may potentiate the toxicity of organophosphates and the activity of procaine hydrochloride. Therefore, do not use PromAce to control tremors associated with organic phosphate poisoning. Do not use in conjunction with organophosphorus vermifuges or ectoparasiticides, including flea collars. Do not use with procaine hydrochloride.

Dosage and Administration: The dosage should be individualized, depending upon the degree of tranquilization required. As a general rule, the dosage requirement in mg/lb. of bodyweight decreases as the weight of the animal increases.

PromAce Injectable: May be given intravenously, intramuscularly, or subcutaneously. The following schedule may be used as a guide to I.V., I.M., or S.C. injections: ***Dogs:*** 0.25–0.5 mg per lb. of bodyweight ***Cats:*** 0.5–1.0 mg per lb. of bodyweight ***Horses:*** 2.0–4.0 mg per 100 lb. of bodyweight.

I.V. doses should be administered slowly, and a period of at least 15 minutes should be allowed for the drug to take full effect.

PromAce Tablets: ***Dogs:*** 0.25–1.0 mg/lb. of bodyweight. Dosage may be repeated as required.

Cats: 0.5–1.0 mg/lb. of bodyweight. Dosage may be repeated as required.

Toxicology: Acute and chronic toxicity studies have shown a very low order of toxicity.

Acute toxicity: The LD_{50} dose of acepromazine maleate in mice was determined by means of a probit transformation with the following results.[2]

Intravenous route	61.37 mg/kg
Subcutaneous route	130.5 mg/kg
Oral route	256.8 mg/kg

Chronic toxicity tests[3] in rats revealed no deleterious effects on renal or hepatic function, or on hemopoietic activity. In several groups of two male and two female beagle hounds treated for six months with daily oral doses of 20 to 40 mg/kg. no untoward effects were encountered. Hematologic studies and urinalysis gave values within normal limits. Another group of four dogs, given gradually increasing oral doses up to a level of 220 mg/kg daily and reaching a total daily dose of 2.2 Gm per dog, showed some signs of pulmonary edema and hyperemia of the internal organs, but no animals died.

When administered intramuscularly, acepromazine maleate causes a brief sensation of stinging comparable with that observed with other phenothiazine tranquilizers.

Clinical Data: Controlled clinical studies in the United States and Canada have demonstrated the effectiveness and safety of acepromazine maleate as a tranquilizer.

Good to excellent results were reported[1,4,5] in dogs, cats, and horses given acepromazine maleate injectable for restraint during examination, treatment and minor surgery, and for preanesthetic sedation. In dogs, the drug reportedly[4] helps control convulsions associated with distemper.

In both dogs and cats, good to excellent results were obtained[4] when acepromazine maleate tablets were used to control nervousness and excessive vocalization, neurotic and excitable behavior, vomiting associated with motion sickness, coughing, and itching caused by dermatitis.

In horses, Bauman[6] had good results using the drug as an aid in the control of painful spasms due to colic.

Other practitioners[7,8] found the drug useful as a preanesthetic sedative for nervous or aggressive horses, but it had to be administered while the animals were quiet and not in an excited state. In a trial[9] on more than 200 horses with a wide variety of disorders, acepromazine maleate injectable proved to be both effective and safe.

Precautions: Tranquilizers are potent central nervous system depressants, and they can cause marked sedation with suppression of the sympathetic nervous system.

Tranquilizers can produce prolonged depression or motor restlessness when given in excessive amounts or when given to sensitive animals.

Tranquilizers are additive in action to the actions of other depressants and will potentiate general anesthesia. Tranquilizers should be administered in smaller doses and with greater care during general anesthesia and also to animals exhibiting symptoms of stress, debilitation, cardiac disease, sympathetic blockage, hypovolemia, or shock. PromAce, like other phenothiazine derivatives, is detoxified in the liver; therefore, it should be used with caution on animals with a previous history of liver dysfunction or leukopenia.

Hypotension can occur after rapid intravenous injection causing cardiovascular collapse.

Epinephrine is contraindicated for treatment of acute hypotension produced by phenothiazine-derivative tranquilizers since further depression of blood pressure can occur. Other pressor amines, such as norepinephrine or phenylephrine, are the drugs of choice.

In horses, paralysis of the retractor penis muscle has been associated with the use of phenothiazine-derivative tranquilizers. Such cases have occurred following the use of PromAce. This risk should be duly considered prior to the administration of PromAce to male horses (castrated and uncastrated). When given, the dosage should be carefully limited to the minimum necessary for the desired effect. At the time of tranquilization, it is not possible to differentiate between reversible protrusion of the penis (a normal clinical sign of narcosis) and irreversible paralysis of the retractor muscle. The cause of this side reaction has not been determined. It has been postulated that such paralysis may occur when a tranquilizer is used in conjunction with testosterone (or in stallions).

Accidental intracarotid injection in horses can produce clinical signs ranging

Continued on next page

Fort Dodge—Cont.

from disorientation to convulsive seizures and death.
Warning: Federal law prohibits the use of this product in animals intended for human consumption.
Caution: Federal law restricts this drug to use by or on the order of a licensed veterinarian.
U.S. Patent No. 3,330,826
How Supplied: 50 ml. vials. Each ml. contains 10 mg acepromazine maleate. (Also contains sodium citrate 0.36%, citric acid 0.075%, benzyl alcohol 1%, and water for injection, U.S.P.)
Each *light orange* tablet contains 5 mg of acepromazine maleate and is available in bottles of 100.
Each *orange* tablet contains 10 mg of acepromazine maleate, and is available in bottles of 100 and 500.
Each *yellow* tablet contains 25 mg of acepromazine maleate, and is available in bottles of 100 and 500.
References:
1. Baker, J.M., Paper presented at the Ontario Veterinary Association meeting, held in Toronto, Canada, 1958.
2. Pharmacology Reports. ClinByla Laboratories, Paris, France.
3. Stegen, M.G.: Pharmacology Report, Ayerst Laboratories, 1958.
4. Veterinary Medical Records, Ayerst Laboratories.
5. Foley, J.T.: Clinical Reports to Ayerst Laboratories, 1963.
6. Bauman, W.G.: Clinical Reports to Ayerst Laboratories, 1963.
7. Ford, R.W., in Equine Panel Report, Mod. Vet Pract. 40:45 (Nov. 1) 1959.
8. Baldwin, R., in Equine Panel Report, Mod. Vet. Pract. 40:46 (Nov. 1) 1959.
9. Dunkin, T.E.: Clinical Reports to Ayerst Laboratories, 1963.

F

PROMAZINE GRANULES ℞
(promazine hydrochloride)
Tranquilizer for Horses

Indications: Promazine Granules (promazine hydrochloride) are indicated in unruly, nervous or intractable horses.
Examples of its uses:
An aid in training horses.
In minor surgical procedures in which anesthesia is not required.
As a preanesthetic to augment action and permit smoother induction and recovery, thus preventing injury.
In non-surgical procedures, such as shoeing and floating teeth.
An aid in handling mares during breeding.
In animals that have wounds which cannot heal due to constant irritation (biting, licking, etc.) by the individual.
Composition: Promazine is a phenothiazine derivative 10-[3- (dimethylamino) propyl] phenothiazine monohydrochloride.
It has established itself as an effective and safe tranquilizer in both men and animals. As an injectable it has been widely acclaimed as being the ataraxic of choice for horses.[1,2,3,4] The oral administration of Promazine Granules now provides an easy and effective method of tranquilizing horses without the excitement and stress often associated with parenteral injection.[5,6]
Each 10.25 oz. of Promazine Granules contains 8 Gm. of promazine hydrochloride in a palatable inert base. Promazine is a potent tranquilizing drug to be used with discretion, but has a relatively wide margin of safety. In animal toxicity studies it compares favorably with other phenothiazine ataraxics, which, as a class of drugs, are quite safe.
Action: *Promazine* exerts its actions on the central nervous system. Clinically animals respond by showing relaxation and less anxiety, while retaining coordination and awareness of environment.
Dosage and Administration: The required dosage of Promazine Granules (promazine hydrochloride) varies somewhat depending upon the individual temperament of the animal, with the effective oral dosage slightly greater than the injectable. The suggested dosage for horses is 1.63 to 3.26 grams Promazine Granules per 100 lb. bodyweight (.45 to .9 mg. promazine hydrochloride per lb. bodyweight).
To facilitate administration in the field use the cap from the Promazine Granules container and carefully measure *1 level capful* per 300 lb. bodyweight. (To assure accurate dosing use knife blade or other straight-edged object to level off the contents in the cap.) This level capful will provide an average of 7.2 g. Promazine Granules (or 0.66 mg. promazine hydrochloride per lb. bodyweight).
Exceeding the recommended dosage will not necessarily intensify the effect. Promazine Granules should be given with an amount of grain or feed that will be readily consumed. The drug's effect will usually begin in 45 minutes, producing maximum effect in 1 to 2 hours. Duration of action varies with the dosage, but usually continues for 4 to 6 hours.
Precautions: Tranquilizers should be administered in lower doses and with greater care to animals exhibiting symptoms of debilitation, cardiac disease, sympathetic blockage, hypovolemia and shock.
Tranquilizers are potent central nervous system depressants and can produce marked sedation with suppression of the sympathetic nervous system. Epinephrine is contraindicated for the treatment of acute hypotension produced by phenothiazine-derivative tranquilizers since further depression of the blood pressure can occur. Other pressor-amines, such as norepinephrine or neosynephrine, are the drugs of choice.
Do not use this product in conjunction with organophosphates and/or procaine hydrochloride since phenothiazine may potentiate the toxicity of organophosphates and the activity of procaine hydrochloride.
Tranquilizers may produce prolonged depression or motor restlessness when given in excessive amounts or to sensitive animals. Tranquilizers are additive to the actions of other depressants and will potentiate general anesthesia.
Warning:
Do not use in horses intended for food use.
Keep out of reach of children.
Caution:
Federal law restricts this drug to use by or on the order of a licensed veterinarian.
How Supplied: Pkg. 12—10.25 oz.
References:
1. Baker, C.W., and English, B., J.A.V.M.A., 134:23, 1959.
2. Stucki, B., Western Vet., 5:15, 1958.
3. Skewes, A.R., Mod. Vet. Prac., 40, 21:45, 1959.
4. Brown, C.W., ibid, 40, 21:47, 1959.
5. Cresswell, M., ibid, 40, 21:45, 1959.
6. Cunningham, J.A., Vet. Rec., 71:395, 1959.

SLEEPAWAY®
Euthanasia Ⓒ ℞ Solution
Sodium Pentobarbital
10% Isopropyl Alcohol
Poison

Composition: Sodium Pentobarbital 26%; Isopropyl Alcohol 10%; Propylene Glycol 20%; Distilled Water, q.s.
Dosage and Administration:
Dogs and Cats: 2 ml intravenously for first 10 lb. bodyweight, 1 ml for each additional 10 lb.
Warning: *Keep out of reach of children.*
Store at room temperature (approx. 25° C.). Do not use if material has precipitated.
Caution: Federal law restricts this drug to use by or on the order of a licensed veterinarian.
How Supplied: 100 ml.
Requires use of DEA order form (DEA-222C)
This product is not returnable for credit or exchange.

SULFASOL®
12.5%
Antibacterial

Indications: Use in beef cattle for the treatment of bovine respiratory disease complex (shipping fever complex) and bacterial pneumonia (associated with *Pasteurella spp.*) and necrotic pododermatitis (foot rot) (associated with *Fusobacterium necrophorum*) where organisms are sensitive to sulfamethazine, sulfathiazole and sulfamerazine.
Composition:

Sulfamethazine*	5.63% w/v
Sulfathiazole*	5.75% w/v
Sulfamerazine*	1.12% w/v

*Equivalent to Sodium salt.
Dosage and Administration: Administer orally 75 ml. of each 100 lb. bodyweight (approximately 1.5 grain/lb.). Repeat at 24 hour intervals using 50 ml./100 lb. (approximately 1 grain/lb.). Treat for 4 days. Oral administration can be made by use of a suitable dose syringe.
Warning: Use of this product must be withdrawn 10 days before treated animals are slaughtered for food.
Caution:
Provide adequate supply of drinking water.

If symptoms persist after using this preparation for 2 or 3 days consult veterinarian.
Keep out of reach of children.
How Supplied: 1 Gallon

TETANUS ANTITOXIN
(Equine Origin)
Bio. 278

Indications: Tetanus Antitoxin is recommended for use in domestic animals for prevention and treatment of tetanus.
This product has been tested and shown to be satisfactory for marketing in accordance with existing Standard Requirements set forth by the U.S. Department of Agriculture.
Composition: This product is prepared from the blood of horses repeatedly injected with large doses of the toxin of *Clostridium tetani.*
Dosage and Administration: 1,500 units, minimum, if injected within 24 hours of exposure. Administer subcutaneously, intravenously or intraperitoneally. Increase dose relative to lapse of time following exposure to as much as 30,000 to 100,000 units in animals which are showing symptoms. Massive initial doses may succeed in effecting a cure where repeated smaller doses of the same aggregate volume may have no value.
It should always be remembered that good nursing and proper supportive treatment, in addition to administration of antitoxin, will improve the patient's chances for recovery.
Caution:
Store in dark at 2° to 7° C. (35° to 45°F.)
Use entire contents when first opened.
Do not administer to food-producing animals within 21 days of slaughter.
In case of anaphylactoid reaction administer epinephrine.
It has been reported that biologicals of equine origin may in some manner be associated with the development of hepatitis (Theiler's Disease)[1,2] when injected into the equine species. The incidence of Theiler's Disease is rare and in affected animals may be manifested as hepatitis, icterus, anorexia, emaciation and death. Consult your veterinarian for additional details and recommendations.
How Supplied: Pkg. 10 × 1,500 units.
10,000 units.
References:

1. Serum Hepatitis in the Horse, Roger J. Panciera, D.V.M., Ph.D., J.A.V.M.A., 155 (July 15, 1969) 408-410.
2. Serum Hepatitis in the Horse, J.A. Rose, R.D. Immenschuh, and Ethel M. Rose, Proc. 20th Ann. Conv. Am. Assoc. Equine Practice, December, 1974.

TETANUS TOXOID
Aluminum Phosphate Adsorbed
Refined and Concentrated
Bio. 277

Indications: For vaccination of healthy horses, sheep and swine against tetanus.
Composition: Tetanus Toxoid, Fort Dodge, is refined and concentrated by a patented process which eliminates at least 97 percent of the non-specific nitrogen but leaves the antigenic fraction unchanged. Highly purified toxoids are desirable since components responsible for producing allergic or side reactions are practically eliminated.
This product has been tested and shown to be satisfactory for marketing in accordance with existing Standard Requirements set forth by the U.S. Department of Agriculture.
Dosage and Administration: Horses, 1 ml. Inject intramuscularly using aseptic technique. Administer a second 1 ml. dose 4 to 8 weeks after the first dose. Revaccinate annually using one 1 ml. dose. For smaller equines, sheep and swine, administer a 0.5 ml. dose according to the above schedule for horses.
Protective tetanus antibody titers usually occur two weeks after the second injection of the initial series. In the event of injury during the course of the initial vaccination program, or if annual boosters have not been given, a prophylactic dose of at least 1,500 units of tetanus antitoxin should be given.
Caution:
Store in dark at 2° to 7° C. (35° to 45°F.).
Shake well.
Use entire contents when first opened.
Transitory local reactions at the injection site may occur.
In case of anaphylactoid reaction administer epinephrine.
Do not vaccinate within 21 days of slaughter.
Formaldehyde solution is used as an inactivating agent.
Formaldehyde solution and thimerosal added as preservatives.
Transistory local reactions at the injection site may occur.
How Supplied: 25-1 ml. prefilled syringes with needles—25 doses. 10 ml-10 doses.

TRIANGLE®-1
Bovine Virus
Diarrhea Vaccine
Killed Virus
Bio. 187

Indications: For vaccination of healthy cattle to protect against bovine virus diarrhea (BVD).
Administration and Dosage:
Cattle: Inject 2 ml. intramuscularly using aseptic technique. May be administered to pregnant animals at any stage of gestation. Repeat in 14 to 28 days. A 2 ml. booster dose is recommended annually or prior to time of stress or exposure. Calves vaccinated under six months of age should be revaccinated at six months or weaning. Protect animals from exposure for at least 14 days after the last dose of vaccine.
Caution:
Store in dark at 2° to 7° C. (35° to 45°F.).
Shake well.
Use entire contents when first opened.
Do not vaccinate within 21 days before slaughter.
In case of anaphylactoid reaction administer epinephrine.
Neomycin, polymyxin B and a fungistat added as preservatives.
How Supplied: 20 ml—10 doses
100 ml—50 doses

TRIANGLE®-1+IBR
Bovine Rhinotracheitis-
Virus Diarrhea Vaccine
Killed Virus
Bio. 181

Indications: For vaccination of healthy cattle to protect against infectious bovine rhinotracheitis (IBR) and bovine virus diarrhea (BVD).
Administration and Dosage: *Cattle.* Inject 2 ml. intramuscularly using aseptic technique. May be administered to pregnant animals at any stage of gestation. Repeat in 14 to 28 days. A 2 ml. booster dose is recommended annually or prior to time of stress or exposure. Calves vaccinated under six months of age should be revaccinated at six months or weaning. Protect animals from exposure for at least 14 days after the last dose of vaccine.
Caution: Store in dark at 2° to 7° C. (35° to 45° F.). Shake well. Use entire contents when first opened. Do not vaccinate within 21 days before slaughter. In case of anaphylactoid reaction administer epinephrine.
Neomycin, polymyxin B and a fungistat added as preservatives.
How Supplied: 20 ml—10 doses
100 ml—50 doses

TRIANGLE®-2
Bovine Rhinotracheitis-
Parainfluenza-3 Vaccine
Killed Virus
Bio. 182

Indications: For vaccination of healthy cattle to protect against infectious bovine rhinotracheitis (IBR) and parainfluenza-3 (Pl-3).
Administration and Dosage:
Cattle: Inject 2 ml. intramuscularly using aseptic technique. May be administered to pregnant animals at any stage of gestation. Repeat in 14 to 28 days. A 2 ml. booster dose is recommended annually or prior to time of stress or exposure. Calves vaccinated under six months of age should be revaccinated at six months or weaning. Protect animals from exposure for at least 14 days after the last dose of vaccine.
Caution:
Store in dark at 2° to 7° C. (35° to 45°F.).
Shake well.
Use entire contents when first opened.
Do not vaccinate within 21 days before slaughter.
In case of anaphylactoid reaction administer epinephrine.
Neomycin, polymyxin B and a fungistat added as preservatives.
How Supplied: 20 ml—10 doses
100 ml—50 doses

Continued on next page

F

Fort Dodge—Cont.

TRIANGLE®-3
Bovine Rhinotracheitis-
Virus Diarrhea-
Parainfluenza-3 Vaccine
Killed Virus
Bio. 190

Indications: For vaccination of healthy cattle to protect against infectious bovine rhinotracheitis (IBR), bovine virus diarrhea (BVD) and parainfluenza-3 (PI-3).
Administration and Dosage: *Cattle.* Inject 5 ml. intramuscularly using aseptic technique. May be administered to pregnant animals at any stage of gestation. Repeat in 14 to 28 days. A 5 ml. booster dose is recommended annually or prior to time of stress or exposure. Calves vaccinated under six months of age should be revaccinated at six months or weaning. Protect animals from exposure for at least 14 days after the last dose of vaccine.
Caution:
Store in dark at 2° to 7° C. (35° to 45° F.).
Shake well.
Use entire contents when first opened.
Do not vaccinate within 21 days before slaughter.
In case of anaphylactoid reaction administer epinephrine.
Neomycin, polymyxin B and a fungistat added as preservatives.
How Supplied: 50 ml—10 doses
250 ml—50 doses

TRIMUNE®
Rabies Vaccine
Killed Virus Murine Origin
Bio. 199

Indications: For vaccination of healthy dogs and cats against rabies.
Dose: Inject 1 ml. intramuscularly using aseptic technique. Give one dose at 3 months of age or older. Give a second dose one year later. Repeat subsequent doses every 3 years.
Caution:
Store in dark 2° to 7°C (35° to 45°F)
Do not freeze.
Shake well.
BPL inactivated.
Anaphylactoid reactions may occur.
Antidote: Epinephrine.
Gentomicin and amphotericin-B added as preservatives.
How Supplied: Pkg. 25 × 1 ml. prefilled disposable plastic syringes with needles—25 doses.
10 ml—10 doses.

TRIVIB®
Campylobacter Fetus
Bovine Isolates Bio. 138

Indications: For vaccination of healthy heifers or cows to protect against *Campylobacter fetus* infections.
Composition: TriVib is prepared from three specially selected antigenic strains of *campylobacter fetus* var. venerealis. These strains are inactivated, concentrated and suspended in a special oil adjuvant which enhances the antigenic response.
Dosage and Administration: ***Heifers and cows.*** Inject 2 ml. subcutaneously under aseptic conditions in the neck or behind the shoulder. In non-infected herds and susceptible animals a second dose should be administered 2 to 4 weeks later. The last injection should precede the breeding season by 4 to 8 weeks. Revaccinate annually.
Caution:
Store in dark at 2° to 7° C. (35° to 45°F.).
Shake well.
Avoid freezing. Use entire contents when first opened.
Do not vaccinate within 60 days before slaughter.
In case of anaphylactoid reaction, administer epinephrine.
How Supplied: 20 ml—10 doses
100 ml—50 doses

TRIVIB 5L®
Campylobacter Fetus
Canicola-Grippotyphosa-Hardjo-Icterohaemorrhagiae-Pomona
Bacterin
Bio. 106

Indications: For vaccination of healthy cattle to protect against *campylobacter fetus, leptospira pomona, hardjo, grippotyphosa, canicola,* and *icterohaemorrhagiae* infections.
Composition: Killed, concentrated cultures of *campylobacter fetus, var. venerealis leptospira pomona, hardjo, grippotyphosa, canicola,* and *icterohaemorrhagiae* organisms suspended in a special adjuvant.
Dosage and Administration: ***Cattle,*** Inject 5 ml subcutaneously under aseptic conditions in the neck or behind the shoulder. In non-infected herds and susceptible animals, a second dose should be administered 2 to 4 weeks later. The last injection should precede the breeding season by 4 to 8 weeks. Revaccinate annually.
Caution:
Store in dark at 2° to 7° C (35° to 45°F). Avoid freezing. Shake well. Use entire contents when first opened. Do not vaccinate within 60 days before slaughter. In case of anaphylactoid reaction, administer epinephrine.
How Supplied: 50 ml—10 doses
250 ml—50 doses

ULTILEP® 5
Leptospira Canicola-Grippotyphosa-Hardjo-Icterohaemorrhagiae-Pomona Bacterin
Bio. 105

Indications: For vaccination of healthy cattle and swine against *L. pomona, hardjo, grippotyphosa, canicola* and *icterohaemorrhagiae* infections.
Composition: Killed, concentrated cultures of *L. pomona, hardjo, grippotyphosa, canicola* and *icterohaemorrhagiae,* adsorbed and aluminum hydroxide Gel 21.
Dosage and Administration:
Cattle: Inject 2 ml subcutaneously or intramuscularly. Booster doses should be given annually and for animals vaccinated as suckling calves, a 6 months' booster is desirable.
Swine: 8 weeks of age or older, inject 2 ml intramuscularly. Booster doses should be given annually.
Caution:
Store in dark at 2° to 7°C. (35° to 45°F).
Avoid freezing.
Shake well.
Use entire contents when first opened.
Do not vaccinate within 21 days before slaughter.
In case of anaphylactoid reaction, administer epinephrine.
How Supplied: 20 ml 10 doses
100 ml 50 doses

WART VACCINE
Killed Virus Bovine Origin
Bio. 160

Indications: For vaccination of cattle as an aid in the prophylactic treatment of viral warts (papillomas).
This product consists of chemically killed bovine wart tissue from otherwise healthy cattle.
Dosage and Administration: Mature cattle 10–20 ml per dose. Calves 10–15 ml per dose. Using aseptic precautions inject subcutaneously (under the skin) preferably on the side of the neck. Do not inject more than 10 ml in any one location. Repeat the dose in 3 to 5 weeks.
Warning: The use of this product will cause indurations (swellings) in some animals at the site of vaccination. These usually disappear in time and will not impair the immune response.
In case of anaphylactoid reaction (shock) administer epinephrine or equivalent.
Shake well before using.
For veterinary use only.
Caution:
Do not vaccinate within 21 days before slaughter.
Store in dark at 2° to 7°C (35° to 45°F).
Use all of this product at time container is first opened.
How Supplied: 50 ml
This product is not returnable for credit or exchange.

Fromm Laboratories
See SOLVAY VETERINARY, INC.

F

Haver
Mobay Corporation
Animal Health Division
SHAWNEE, KS 66201

ALOBAC™-2 WITH HAVLOGEN®
Erysipelothrix Rhusiopathiae Bacterin

Composition: A formaldehyde inactivated and adjuvanted whole culture of *Erysipelothrix rhusiopathiae. Erysipelothrix rhusiopathiae* culture, aluminum hydroxide adsorbed and concentrated.
Indications: For the vaccination of swine against erysipelas.
Dosage and Administration: All weights and ages, 2 ml. Inject subcutaneously or intramuscularly. Pigs vaccinated under six weeks of age should be revaccinated at 8 to 12 weeks of age. For breeding animals, repeat after 21 days and annually.
How Supplied:
Code: 4431 (20 ml) (10 doses)
4433 (100 ml) (50 doses)
4407 (500 ml) (250 doses)

BAYMIX® CRUMBLES (Cutter label)

Composition: Coumaphos (0.32%).
Indications: A feed supplement designed for use as a top-dress to control 5 economically important types of stomach (*Haemonchus contortus, Ostertagia* spp., *Trichostrongylus* spp.) and intestinal worms (*Cooperia* spp., *Nematodirus* spp.) infecting beef and dairy cattle. Milk from treated lactating dairy cows does not have to be withdrawn during or following treatment.
Dosage and Administration: Give 1 oz for each 100 lbs of body weight per day for six consecutive days. Should conditions warrant, treatment should be repeated at 30-day intervals.
Warning: Do not use in conjunction with or within a few days before or after treatment with cholinesterase-inhibiting drugs, pesticides or chemicals.
How Supplied:
Code: 332-31 (50 lbs bag)

CARICIDE®
Oral Liquid - Tablets

Composition: Caricide® Oral Liquid contains 60 mg diethylcarbamazine citrate per ml.
Caricide® Tablets each contain 3 mg of diethylcarbamazine (as citrate) per pound of body weight when administered at the recommended dose.
Indications: Caricide® Oral Liquid and Tablets are recommended as an aid in the control of large roundworms *(Toxocara canis)* in dogs, and for the prevention of heartworm disease *(Dirofilaria immitis)* in dogs.
Dosage and Administration: Caricide® Oral Liquid does not require special preparation prior to or during administration. It is added to daily food ration (once a day) at a dosage rate of 3.0 mg/lb body weight. It may be mixed with either dry or wet foods as follows:

Body Weight	*Caricide® Oral Liquid*
10 lbs	0.5 ml
20 lbs	1.0 ml
30 lbs	1.5 ml
40 lbs	2.0 ml
50 lbs	2.5 ml
60 lbs	3.0 ml
70 lbs	3.5 ml
80 lbs	4.0 ml

Caricide® Tablets - For Heartworm Prevention
Administration of Caricide® in heartworm endemic areas should start one month before the beginning of the mosquito season, continue daily throughout the mosquiito season and for two months thereafter. This regimen prevents heartworm disease by arresting the development of the infective larvae of *Dirofilaria immitis.*
The optimum dosage is 3 mg of diethlycarbamazine citrate per pound of body weight administered daily as follows:

Number of Tablets Daily

Lbs body weight	*50 mg*	*200 mg*	*400 mg*
4	¼		
8	½	½	
16	1		
32	2	½	¼
66		1	½
133		2	1

Dosage for Ascariasis:
The basic dosage is 25–50 mg/lb (55–100 mg/kg). Three tablets sizes are available and directions for use are listed below:
50 mg tablets - ½ to 1 tablet per lb of body weight
200 mg tablets - ½ to 1 tablet for each 4 lb of body weight
400 mg tablets - ½ to 1 tablet for each 8 lbs of body weight
A repeat dosage should be given in 10 to 20 days to remove immature worms which may enter the intestines from the lungs after the first dose.
Caricide® is active against the adult stage of *Toxocara canis.* The majority of mature worms will be passed within the first week of treatment with additional worms passed for several weeks thereafter.
Puppies can be placed on medication as soon as they start to eat solid food; older dogs can be placed on medication at any time and continued throughout life if they are free of adult heartworms.
Contraindications: Do not use in dogs that may be harboring adult heartworms. Dogs with established heartworm infections should not receive Caricide® until they have been converted to a negative status. Inadvertant administration to heartworm infected dogs may cause adverse reactions due to shock or pulmonary occlusion.
Overdose: Caricide® has a high margin of safety. Emesis is rare following administration, but may occur with extreme overdosage.
Precautions: Caricide® will not affect roundworm larvae encysted in tissues. Pups of treated bitches may require individual worming in the first four weeks of life.
Dogs on prophylactic therapy should be examined for the presence of microfilaria every six months. Dogs with established heartworm infections should not receive Caricide® until they have been converted to a negative status by the use of adulticidal and microfilaricidal drugs. Inadvertant administration to heartworm infected dogs may cause adverse reactions due to shock or pulmonary occlusion.
Warnings: Federal law restricts this drug to use by or on the order of a licensed veterinarian.
Caution: Keep out of reach of children.
How Supplied: Caricide® Oral Liquid
Code:
2258 - 8 oz
2260 - 1 gal
Caricide® Tablets
Code:
2250 - (500's) - 50 mg
2252 - (200's) - 200 mg
2254 - (100's) - 400 mg

CLOSTRI-BAC™ 4 with Havlogen®
Clostridium Chauvoei-Septicum-Novyi-Sordellii Bacterin — Toxoid

Composition: A chemically inactivated, detoxified and Havlogen adjuvanted suspension of organisms to immunize healthy cattle and sheep against diseases caused by *Clostridium chauvoei* (Blackleg), *Clostridium septicum* (Malignant edema), *Clostridium novyi* (Black disease) and *Clostridium sordellii.*
Dosage and Administration: Cattle —5 ml., Sheep —3 ml. Inject intramuscularly. Revaccination with a bacterin-toxoid containing Cl. sordellii is recommended at 2 to 4 weeks. Calves vaccinated under 3 months of age should be revaccinated at weaning or 4 to 6 months of age. Repeat the dose every 5 to 6 months in animals subject to re-exposure to *Cl. novyi.* Anaphylactoid reactions may occur. *Antidote:* Epinephrine.
How Supplied:
Code: 50 ml—4577 (10 doses)
250 ml—4579 (50 doses)

CLOSTRI-BAC™ 7 with HAVLOGEN®
Clostridium Chauvoei-Septicum-Novyi-Sordellii-Perfringens Types C and D Bacterin-Toxoid

Composition: A formaldehyde inactivated, detoxified and adjuvanted suspension of organisms listed above.
Indications: For use in healthy cattle and sheep as an aid in preventing diseases caused by *Clostridium chauvoei* (Blackleg), *septicum* (Malignant edema), *novyi* (Black disease), *sordelli* and *perfringens* Types C and D (Enterotoxemia).

Continued on next page

H

Haver—Cont.

Dosage and Administration:
Cattle: 5 ml.,
Sheep: 3 ml. Inject intramuscularly. Revaccinate with *Cl. perfringens* Types C and D at 3 to 5 weeks. Revaccination with a bacterin containing *Cl. sordellii* is recommended at 2 to 4 weeks. Calves vaccinated under 3 months of age should be revaccinated at weaning or 4 or 6 months of age. Repeat the dose every 5 to 6 months in animals subject to reexposure to *C. novyi.*
Caution:
Shake well before using.
Store at 35° to 45°F. (2° to 7°C.)
Use entire contents when first opened.
Do not vaccinate within 21 days of slaughter.
Anaphylactoid reactions may occur.
Antidote: Epinephrine.
Contains formaldehyde as preservative.
How Supplied:
Code: 4592—(50 ml)—10 doses
4593—(250 ml)—50 doses

CLOSTRI-BAC™ 8 w/HAVLOGEN®
Clostridium Chauvoei-Septicum-Haemolyticum-Novyi-Sordellii-Perfringens Types C & D Bacterin Toxoid

Description: A formaldehyde inactivated, detoxified and adjuvanted suspension of organisms listed above.
Indications: For use in healthy cattle and sheep as an aid in preventing diseases caused by *Clostridium chauvoei* (Blackleg), *septicum* (Malignant edema), *haemolyticum* (Bacillary Hemoglobinuria/Red Water), *novyi* (Black disease), *sordellii* and *perfringens* Types C & D (Enterotoxemia).
Administration And Dosage: Cattle 5 ml., Sheep - 3 ml. Inject intramuscularly. Revaccinate with *Cl. perfringens* Types C & D at 3 to 5 weeks. Revaccination with a bacterin containing *Cl. sordellii* is recommended at two to four weeks. Calves vaccinated under three months of age should be revaccinated at weaning or four to six months of age. Repeat the dose every five to six months in animals subject to re-exposure to *Cl. novyi* and *Cl. haemolyticum.*
Caution: Shake well before using. Store at 35° to 40° F (2° to 7° C). Use entire contents when first opened. Do not vaccinate within 21 days before slaughter. Anaphylactoid reactions may occur. Antidote: Epinephrine. Contains formaldehyde as preservative.
Packaging:
Code: 4600 - 250 ml. (50 doses)
4598 - 50 ml. (10 doses)

CLOSTRI-BAC™ C&D WITH HAVLOGEN®
Clostridium Perfringens Types C & D Bacterin-Toxoid

Composition: A formalin detoxified and adjuvanted culture of Clostridium perfringens Types C and D.
Indications: For use in healthy cattle and sheep as an aid in the prevention of enterotoxemia caused by Clostridium perfringens Types C and D.
Dosage and Administration: Dose: Cattle 2 ml, Sheep 1 ml—Inject intramuscularly and repeat in 21 days.
Caution: Store at 35° to 45°F. (2° to 7°C.) Shake well before using. Use entire contents when first opened. Do not vaccinate within 21 days of slaughter. Anaphylactoid reactions may occur.
Antidote: Epinephrine.
How Supplied:
Code: 4542—20 ml—10 doses
4544—100 ml—50 doses

CLOSTRI-BAC™ CS with Havlogen®
Clostridium Chauvoei-Septicum Bacterin with Havlogen® Adjuvant

Composition: A formalin-inactivated and adjuvanted suspension of Clostridium chauvoei and Clostridium septicum organisms for use in healthy cattle and sheep as an aid in the prevention of blackleg and malignant edema.
Dosage and Administration: 2 ml. Inject imtramuscularly. Calves vaccinated under 3 months of age should be revaccinated at weaning or 4 to 6 months of age. Anaphylactoid reactions may occur. *Antidote:* Epinephrine.
How Supplied:
Code: 4572—20 ml—10 doses
4573—100 ml—50 doses

CLOSTRI-BAC™ CSN WITH HAVLOGEN®
Clostridium Chauvoei-Septicum Novyi Bacterin-Toxoid

Composition: Formalin —inactivated and adjuvanted suspension of oraganisms listed above.
Indications: For use in healthy cattle and sheep as an aid in the prevention of blackleg, malignant edema and black disease.
Dosage and Administration: Cattle 5 ml, sheep 3 ml. Inject intramuscularly. Calves vaccinated under three months of age should be revaccinated at weaning or 4 to 6 months of age. Repeat the dose every 5 to 6 months in animals subject to reexposure to *Clostridium novyi* infection.
Caution: Store at 35° to 45°F. (2° to 7°C.). Shake well before using. Use entire contents when first opened. Do not vaccinate within 21 days before slaughter. Anaphylactoid reactions may occur. *Antidote:* Epinephrine.
How Supplied:
Code: 4601—50 ml—10 doses
4603—250 ml—50 doses

CLOSTRI-BAC™ CSP WITH HAVLOGEN®
Clostridium Chauvoei-Septicum Pasteurella Haemolytica-Multocida bacterin

Composition: Chemically-inactivated and adjuvanted suspension of organisms listed above.
Indications: For use in healthy cattle and sheep as an aid in the prevention of blackleg, malignant edema and the diseases caused by the Pasteurella organisms used in this product.
Dosage and Administration: 5 ml. Inject intramuscularly. Calves vaccinated under three months of age should be revaccinated at weaning or 4 to 6 months of age. Revaccination with Pasteurella Bacterin is recommended at 2 to 4 weeks.
Caution: Store at 35° to 45° F. (2° to 7°C.) Shake well before using. Use entire contents when first opened. Do not vaccinate within 21 days before slaughter. Anaphylactoid reactions may occur. Preservative: Formaldehyde. *Antidote:* Epinephrine.
How Supplied:
Code: 4586—50 ml—10 doses
4594—250 ml—50 doses

COMBOT® LIQUID
(trichlorfon)
Equine Anthelmintic and Boticide

Composition: Active Ingredient: Trichlorfon 12.3% w/v, Inert Ingredients: 87.7% w/v.
Indications: For removal and control of Bots (*Gastrophilus* spp.), Ascarids (*Parascaris equorum*), and Pinworms (*Oxyuris equi*) in horses and ponies.
Combot® Equine Anthelmintic is a ready-to-use preparation that requires no further dilution before use in horses and ponies.
Contraindications: Use only as directed and do not exceed recommended dose. Do not treat colts under 4 months of age, mares in the last month of pregnancy, or animals other than horses or ponies. Horses severely debilitated, suffering from diarrhea or severe constipation, infectious disease, toxemia or colic should not be treated until such conditions are corrected with proper therapy.
Combot® is a cholinesterase inhibitor. Do not use this product in horses simultaneously or within 10 days before or after treatment with or exposure to cholinesterase inhibiting drugs, pesticides or chemicals.
Side Effects: Occasional slight transient diarrhea and/or colic may occur soon after administering Combot®. Fasting prior to the administration of Combot® or treatment on an empty stomach will increase the incidence of these side effects.
Note to Veterinarian: Symptoms of overdose in horses are profuse diarrhea, severe colic, muscle tremors and ataxia. Atropine is antidotal.

Dosage and Administration: Administer by stomach tube following consumption of at least a portion of the daily grain ration. Dose at the rate of one-half ounce Combot® per 100 pounds of body weight. This will provide a dosage of 18.2 mg active ingredient per pound of body weight which will effectively control the parasites indicated. Do not administer on an empty stomach. Do not fast animals prior to treatment (see Side Effects).
Use in Conjunction with Other Anthelmintics—In clinical trials, Combot® at the recommended dosage has been used successfully with the recommended rates of mebendazole, thiabendazole, phenothiazine and piperazine. If Combot® is used with these compounds to increase the spectrum of anthelmintic activity, administer simultaneously but do not mix Combot® with any of these products and do not store for future use.
Warning: Not for use in horses intended for food. Not for human use. Keep out of reach of children. Avoid contact with skin. Wash hands with soap and water after use. If swallowed by a human, immediately call a physician, poison control center or hospital emergency room. Upon medical advice induce vomiting with ipecac syrup. If ipecac is not available, have person drink a glass of water or milk, then gently try to induce vomiting by tickling back of throat with finger or blunt object—be extremely careful not to damage the throat.
To Physician: This material is a cholinesterase inhibitor. Atropine is antidotal; give after cyanosis is overcome. 2-PAM is also antidotal but must be administered in conjunction with atropine. Give supportive treatment.
Warning: Not for use in horses intended for food.
Keep out of reach of children.
Do not store product above 77°F. (25°C) for a period exceeding 10 days. Protect from sunlight.
Caution: Federal (U.S.A.) law restricts this drug to use by or on the order of a licensed veterinarian.
How Supplied:
Code: 0157—1 gal

COMBOT® PASTE
(Trichlorfon)
Equine Anthelmintic and Boticide

Description: ComBot Paste Specific Spectrum Equine Anthelmintic and Boticide is designed for easy administration directly into the horse's mouth from the prefilled syringe. The paste has a pleasant brown sugar taste and a consistency that causes it to stick in the horse's mouth. A horse cannot refuse the paste as can occur with a product given in the feed. This provides every animal with the exact amount of medication required.
Indications: ComBot Paste is indicated for the specific control and/or treatment of mouth and stomach stages of bots (*Gasterophilus intestinalis* and *G. nasalis*) mature large roundworms or ascarids (*Parascaris equorum*) and adult pinworms (*Oxyuris equi*) in horses and foals.
Actions: Trichlorfon, the active ingredient in ComBot Paste, is well known as an equine anthelmintic especially for the control of bots, ascarids and pinworms. Until recently, the effect of trichlorfon on the tissue stages of bots (*Gasterophilus sp.*) was unknown. Trichlorfon has been demonstrated to be 100% active against 1st instar bot larvae in the tissues of the mouth, gums and tongue when administered as a liquid formulation via stomach tube or as a paste formulation directly into the mouth. The activity against 1st instars in the mouth when the drug was administered via stomach tube proved conclusively trichlorfon's systemic action against bots.
Precaution: For horses maintained on the premises where reinfections are likely to occur, retreatment may be necessary. For most effective results, retreat horses in 4 to 8 weeks or as recommended by your veterinarian.
Contraindications: Use only as directed. Do not treat horses suffering from colic, diarrhea, constipation or infectious disease until such conditions have been corrected. Do not administer ComBot Paste to stallions standing at stud as fertility studies in stallions have not been completed with this formulation of trichlorfon.
Dosage and Administration: DO NOT ADMINISTER ON AN EMPTY STOMACH. Administer directly from the syringe onto the back of the horses's tongue.
For removal of bots, ascarids and pinworms. Administer 16 mg. trichlorfon/lb. body weight (1 division on plunger/100 lb. body weight).
Partial contents: A partially used syringe, if recapped, may be stored up to four (4) months at temperatures below 86°F provided the expiration date of the product is not exceeded.
Method of Administration:
1. Remove cap from end of syringe.
2. Place dial on zero mark, advance plunger.
3. Determine weight of horse and dial proper dose. Use edge of dial closest to barrel to mark dose (consult use directions for dosage).
4. Check that the horse's mouth is free of any food. Hay or grain in the mouth will allow horse to reject the paste.
5. To administer paste products to horses, it is best to open the mouth of the horse with the syringe. Hold the horse's head either by the halter or the lead rope and insert the barrel of the syringe in the horse's mouth at the space where the bit rides, then direct the syringe tip on top of the tongue and quickly deposit the dose as far back toward the throat as you can reach with the syringe. DO NOT ADMINISTER THE PASTE BETWEEN THE CHEEK AND THE TEETH OR UNDER THE TONGUE.
6. Immediately following administration of the paste on the very back of the tongue, raise the horse's head for a few seconds after dosing by pushing the head upward with one hand on the horse's lower jaw.

Oral Discomfort: Placement of the paste dose under the tongue or in the cheek pouch (rather than far back on the tongue) may result in irritation to the mouth and subsequent salivation. Less frequently, chewing of the tongue and swelling of the lips may be observed. However, this reaction usually subsides within hours, even without treatment. If discomfort is observed, remove the remaining paste from the mouth by flushing with water.
Side Effects: ComBot Paste Specific Spectrum Equine Anthelmintic and Boticide will occasionally cause loose stools. The feces usually will become firm in 1 to 3 days without treatment. If signs persist, consult your veterinarian. On rare occasions, especially in horses with heavy roundworm (ascarid) infections, a horse may develop colic. Should this occur, walk the horse until signs disappear. If signs persist, consult your veterinarian.
Withholding feed prior to dosing increases side effects. DO NOT WITHHOLD FEED PRIOR TO DOSING.
Notice to Veterinarians—Overdosage
Symptoms of overdosage are colic, diarrhea and ataxia, and appear within 1 to 3 hours after treatment. Such symptoms are usually transient and persist only briefly. Surgery or other severe stress should be avoided for at least one week after treatment. Atropine is antidotal.
Pregnancy: ComBot Paste Specific Spectrum Equine Anthelmintic and Boticide may be given to pregnant mares at any time. However, it is unwise to administer any medication to a mare during the last month of pregnancy unless absolutely necessary. Prior to dosing a mare in the last month of pregnancy, consult your veterinarian.
Warning: NOT FOR USE IN HORSES INTENDED FOR FOOD. Trichlorfon is a cholinesterase inhibitor. Do not use this product simultaneously or within a few days before or after treatment with or exposure to cholinesterase inhibiting drugs, pesticides or chemicals. Do not administer in conjunction with or within one week of administration of succinylcholine chloride, phenothiazine-derived tranquilizers, or anesthetics.
Warning: *Keep out of reach of children.* Not for human use. *If swallowed by human,* IMMEDIATELY *call physician, poison control center or hospital emergency room.*
Upon medical advice, induce vomiting with ipecac syrup. If ipecac is not available, have person drink milk or water and gently induce vomiting by tickling back of throat with finger or blunt object. Be careful not to damage throat. Avoid prolonged or repeated contact with skin. Wash hands after use.
Notice to Physician Trichlorfon is a cholinesterase inhibitor. Atropine is an antidote, give after cyanosis is overcome and to effect. 2-PAM is a supplemental treatment.

Continued on next page

Haver—Cont.

Storage: Store below 86°F.
How Supplied:
Code: 0153-40 gm syringe
COMBOTEL (Trichlorfon and Febautel) is also available from HAVER.
See the product insert for detailed information.

COMBOTEL® PASTE (FEBANTEL AND TRICHLORFON)
Broad Spectrum Equine Anthelmintic and Boticide

Description: COMBOTEL®Paste is a Broad Spectrum Equine Anthelmintic and Boticide that provides control of both gastrointestinal nematodes and bots. The dose is administered directly onto the back of the horse's tongue from the prefilled syringe. The paste has a consistency that causes it to remain in the horse's mouth until swallowing takes place, thus providing more accurate dosing.
Active Ingredients:
Each syringe contains: 2.7 g febantel and 16 g trichlorfon in an inert base.
Indications: COMBOTEL® Paste is indicated for the removal of the following parasites in horses, stallions, breeding mares, pregnant mares, foals and ponies: Large Strongyles (*Strongylus vulgaris, Strongylus edentatus, Strongylus equinus);* Ascarids (*Parascaris equorum* — adult and sexually immature forms); Pinworms (*Oxyuris equi* adult and 4th stage larva); Small Strongyles (various); Mouth and stomach stages of bots (*Gasterophilus intestinalis* and *G. nasalis*).
Actions: Febantel is a highly active compound against strongyles, ascarids and pinworms.
Trichlorfon is well known for the control of equine bots as well as removal of ascarids and pinworms. Trichlorfon has been demonstrated to be 100% effective against 1st instar bot larvae in the tissues of the mouth, gums and tongue. The activity against 1st instars in the mouth when the drug was administered via stomach tube proved conclusively trichlorfon's systemic action against bots.
Precaution: For horses maintained on the premises where reinfections are likely to occur, retreatment may be necessary. For most effective results, retreat horses in four to eight weeks or as recommended by your veterinarian.
Contraindications: Use only as directed. Do not treat horses suffering from colic, diarrhea, constipation or infectious disease until such conditions have been corrected.
Use Directions And Dosage: DO NOT ADMINISTER ON AN EMPTY STOMACH. Horses should be fed concentrates one-half to one hour prior to dosing with COMBOTEL®Paste.
Administer directly from the syringe onto the back of the horse's tongue.
For removal of large and small strongyles, ascarids, pinworms and bots administer one division on plunger per 100 lbs. body weight (one syringe for a 1000 lb. horse).
Partial Contents: A partially used syringe, if recapped immediately after use, may be stored up to three (3) months at temperature below 77°F provided the expiration date of the product is not exceeded.
Method Of Administration:
1. Remove cap from end of syringe.
2. Place dial on zero mark, advance plunger.
3. Determine weight of horse and dial proper dose. Use edge of dial closest to barrel to mark dose (one division on plunger per 100 lbs. body weight).
4. Check that the horse's mouth is free of any food. Hay or grain in the mouth will allow horse to reject the paste.
5. To administer paste products to horses, it's best to open the mouth of the horse with the syringe. Hold the horse's head either by the halter or the lead rope and insert the barrel of the syringe in the horse's mouth at the space where the bit rides, then direct the syringe tip on top of the tongue and quickly deposit the dose as far back toward the throat as you can reach with the syringe. DO NOT ADMINISTER THE PASTE BETWEEN THE CHEEK AND THE TEETH OR UNDER THE TONGUE.
6. Immediately following the administration of the paste on the very back of the tongue, raise the horse's head for a few seconds by pushing the head upward with one hand on the horses lower jaw.

Oral Discomfort: Placement of the paste dose under the tongue or in the cheek pouch (rather than far back on the tongue) may result in irritation to the mouth and subsequent salivation. Less frequently, swelling of the tongue and lips may be observed. However, this reaction usually subsides within hours, even without treatment. If discomfort is observed, remove the remaining paste from the mouth by flushing with water.
Side Effects: COMBOTEL® Paste will occasionally cause diarrhea and/or mild colic within one to three hours after treatment. These signs are usually transient, but if they intensify or persist, consult your veterinarian. Atropine as an antidote is not usually indicated if the proper dose was administered. On rare occasions, colic may also develop in horses with heavy roundworm (ascarid) infections. Should this occur, walk the horse until signs disappear. Withholding feed prior to dosing or treatment on an empty stomach increases the incidence of side effects. DO NOT WITHHOLD FEED PRIOR TO DOSING.
NOTICE TO VETERINARIANS-OVERDOSAGE: Cautious clinical judgment is sometimes required to distinguish certain signs of side effects (see above) from symptoms of overdosage. Symptoms of overdosage are profuse diarrhea, severe colic, muscle tremors and ataxia. Atropine is antidotal. Repeated dosing with atropine should be used with extreme caution to prevent unintentional antidote overdosage as bowel stasis, hyperexcitability and caecal bloat can occur. Surgery or other severe stress should be avoided for at least one week after treatment.
PREGNANCY: COMBOTEL® Paste may be given to pregnant mares at any time. However, it is unwise to administer any medication to a mare within the last month of pregnancy unless absolutely necessary. Prior to dosing a mare in the last month of pregnancy, consult your veterinarian.
Warning: NOT FOR USE IN HORSES INTENDED FOR FOOD. DO NOT REUSE CONTAINER. Render syringe inoperable prior to discarding.
Trichlorfon is a cholinesterase inhibitor. Do not use this product simultaneously or within a few days before or after treatment with or exposure to other cholinesterase inhibiting drugs, pesticides or chemicals. Do not administer in conjunction with or within one week of administration of succinylcholine chloride, phenothiazine-derived tranquilizers, or anesthetics.
Warning: Keep out of reach of children. Not for human use. *If swallowed by a human, IMMEDIATELY call physician, poison control center or hospital emergency room.* Upon medical advice, induce vomiting with ipecac syrup. If ipecac is not available, have person drink milk or water and *gently* induce vomiting by tickling back of throat with finger or blunt object. Be careful not to damage throat. Avoid prolonged or repeated contact with skin. Wash hands after use.
Notice to Physician: Trichlorfon is a cholinesterase inhibitor. Atropine is an antidote; give only after cyanosis is overcome. 2-PAM is a supplemental treatment.
Packaging:
Code: 0145—40 gm syringes (12 per box)

CO-RAL® EMULSIFIABLE LIVESTOCK INSECTICIDE (Cutter label)

Composition: Coumaphos: 11.6% Aromatic Petroleum Distillate, 83.4%; Inert ingredients, 5.0%.
Indications: Coumaphos for effective control of cattle grubs, external parasites of cattle and horses, and lice on swine.
Dosage and Administration: Adaptable for spray treatment on beef cattle or horses or backrubber application on beef and dairy cattle. For backrubber application, mix 4 quarts with 13 gallons #2 fuel oil or #2 diesel oil. See label for specific spray treatment recommendations.
Warning: Do not use in conjunction with oral drenches or other internal medications such as phenothiazine, natural or synthetic pyrethyroids or synergists, or other organic phosphates.
How Supplied:
Code: 132-85—1 qt.
132-91—1 gal

CO-RAL® POUR-ON (Cutter label)

Composition: Coumaphos, 4%; Inert ingredients, 96%.
Indications: Insecticide that provides highly effective control of cattle grubs with a single application by killing the grubs inside the cattle before any dam-

age to meat occurs. Reduction of lice may also be obtained.
Dosage and Administration: For most effective control treat cattle early in the grub cycle as soon as possible after heel fly activity has ceased. Apply at the rate of ½fluid ounce per 100 lbs body weight by pouring uniformly along the back line of the animal.
Warning: Do not apply in conjunction with oral drenches or other internal medications such as phenothiazine, natural or synthetic pyrethroids, synegists, or other organic phosphates. Milk not to be used for human consumption for 14 days after treatment. Do not treat animals for 10 days before or after shipping or weaning or exposure to contagious or infectious diseases.
Dippers—Supplied with Pour-Ons
How Supplied:
Code: 132-56—1 gal

CO-RAL® Animal Insecticide (Shaker Can) (Cutter label)

Composition:
Coumaphos phosphorothioate, 1%; Inert ingredients, 99%.
Indications: Coumaphos for control of horn flies and lice on beef and dairy cattle, lice on swine, and horn flies on horses. No milk or meat withdrawal required after use.
Dosage and Administration:
Cattle—apply not more than 2 oz per animal by dusting evenly into the hair over the head, neck, shoulders, back, and tailhead. Repeat as necessary.
Swine—apply not more than 1 oz per animal evenly to the shoulders and back. Repeat as necessary but not more often than every 10 days. Can be combined with bedding treatment in severe infestations.
Bedding treatment—apply 2 oz, uniformly for each 30 sq. ft. of fresh, dry bedding. Repeat as necessary but not more often than every 10 days.
How Supplied:
Code: 132-45—2-lbs can

CO-RAL® LIVESTOCK DUSTER (Cutter label)

Composition: Coumaphos phosphorothioate, 5%; Inert ingredients, 95%.
Indications: Coumaphos recommended as a spot treatment for control of ear ticks and screwworms infesting cattle, horses, swine, sheep and goats. Routine treatment of wounds resulting from injury, dehorning, docking, castration, shearing, etc. is recommended to help prevent screw-worm infestation. No withdrawal required for animals producing meat or milk for food.
Dosage and Administration: For screw-worms treat infested wounds with light but thorough coverage. Dust new wound at once with a light, uniform coat to avoid infestation. Repeat as necessary. For ear ticks dust into the ear and around the adjacent head area. Repeat as necessary.
How Supplied:
Code: 132-35—5 oz plastic bottle

CO-RAL® 25% WETTABLE POWDER (Cutter label)

Composition: Coumaphos phosphorothioate, 25.0%; related organic phosphates, 1.3%; Inert ingredients, 73.7%.
Indications: APHIS approved coumaphos for scabies, screw-worms, and tick control and Federal eradication programs. Also for control of cattle grubs and external parasites of cattle, sheep, goats, swine, horses and poultry.
Dosage and Administration: For use as spray mix not more than 16 pounds per 100 gallons of water. For use as a spray to lactating dairy cattle mix not more than 1 pound per 100 gallons of water. For use in dip vats mix not more than 8 pounds per 100 gallons of water. See label for more complete information.
Warning: Do not use milk for human consumption for 14 days after treatment. Do not apply in conjunction with oral drenches or other internal medication such as phenothiazine. For further contraindications, see label.
How Supplied:
Code: 132-14—4 lb bag (4 per case)
132-17—48 lb drum

DEXABIOTIC™ AQUEOUS SUSPENSION

Composition: Each cc contains: Procaine penicillin G. 200,000 units; Dihydrostreptomycin sulfate, equivalent to 250 mg dihydrostreptomycin base; Dexamethasone, 0.5 mg; Chlorpheniramine maleate, 10 mg; Procaine hydrochloride, 20 mg; Sodium citrate, 10 mg; Lecithin (2% Tricalcium phosphate), 1 mg; Propylparaben sodium 1 mg (as preservative); Water for injection, q.s.
Indications: For use in treating infections in horses, dogs and cats in which the invading organisms are known to be sensitive to penicillin or dihydrostreptomycin and when stress due to infection necessitates the administration of corticosteroid as adjuvant therapy.
Dosage and Administration: Administer by intramuscular injection only:
Horses—1 to 1.5 cc per 100 lbs body weight;
Dogs and cats—under 10 lbs body weight, 0.5 cc; 10 to 20 lbs body weight, 1 cc; 20 to 30 lbs body weight, 1.5 cc; over 30 lbs body weight, 2 cc's.
Warning: Do not use intravenously or subcutaneously. Not for use in horses to be slaughtered for human consumption.
How Supplied:
Code: 3148—100 ml vial

D.N.P.® Anthelmintic for dogs and cats

Composition: 4.5% sodium disophenol in a water-polyethylene glycol vehicle.
Indications: D.N.P. is indicated for the treatment of dogs and cats infected with major hookworms, including *A. caninum, A. braziliense, U. stenocephala,* and *A. tubaeforme.*
Dosage and Administration: Recommended dosage is 0.1 ml per lb body weight (1 ml per 10 lb) injected subcutaneously.
Special pretreatment preparation not required. Intramuscular use is not recommended because pain may be produced at injection site.
Do not repeat treatment within 21 days. Treatment at short intervals will not improve efficacy. Because D.N.P is primarily effective against adult hookworms more than 12 days old, and since animals may harbor worms of all ages, a fecal examination should be conducted 3 days after the injection to determine the effect of the treatment.
It is imperative that each animal be weighed to determine accurate dosage. A tuberculin syringe should be used to administer the drug to animals weighing less than 5 lb body weight.
Precautions: Severe hook worm infection, particularly in puppies and kittens, can result in marked anemia. Supportive therapy in the nature of blood transfusions or injection of iron compounds should accompany treatment with D.N.P. in such cases.
Do not use in conjunction with other anthelmintics.
How Supplied:
Code: 2292—50 ml vial

DRONCIT® INJECTABLE (praziquantel) Injectable Cestocide for Dogs and Cats

Composition: Droncit® Injectable Cestocide is a clear solution containing 56.8 milligrams of praziquantel per ml which has been formulated for subcanteous, or intramuscular use in dogs and cats for removal of cestodes (tapeworms).
Indications: Droncit® (praziquantel) Injectable Cestocide is indicated for the removal of *Dipylidium caninum, Taenia pisiformis,* and *Echinococcus granulosus* from dogs and *Dipylidium caninum* and *Taenia taenaeformis* in cats.
Dosage and Administration: Droncit® (praziquantel) Injectable Cestocide may be administered by either the subcutaneous or intramuscular route to dogs and cats. The recommended dosage of praziquantel varies according to body weight. Smaller animals require a relatively larger dosage. The optimum dosage for each individual animal wil be achieved by utilizing the following dosage schedule.

*Dogs and Puppies***	
Dogs:	
5 lbs and under	0.3 ml
6-10 lbs	0.5 ml
11-25 lbs	1.0 ml
over 25 lbs	0.2 ml/5 lbs body weight to a maximum at 3 ml

Cats and Kittens**	
Cats:	
under 5 lbs	0.2 ml
5-10 lbs	0.4 ml

Continued on next page

H

Haver—Cont.

11 lbs and under	0.6 ml (max dose)

**Not intended for use in puppies less than four (4) weeks of age or kittens less than six (6) weeks of age.

Fasting - The recommended dosage of praziquantel is not affected by the presence or absence of food in the gastrointestinal tract, therefore, FASTING IS NEITHER NECESSARY NOR RECOMMENDED.

Droncit® (praziquantel) Injectable Cestocide may be administered by either the subcutaneous or intramuscular route. The intramuscular route may be preferred due to a brief period of pain that occasionally follows subcutaneous administration.

Anaphylactoid reactions were not observed in clinical trials. However, as with any drug an anaphylactoid reaction can occur with this product and should be treated symptomatically it if occurs.

Retreatment - For those animals maintained on premises where reinfections are likely to occur, clients should be instructed in the steps necessary to prevent reinfection; otherwise, retreatment may be necessary. This is especially true in cases of *Dipylidium caninum* infections where reinfection is almost certain to occur if fleas are not removed from the animal and its environment.

Action: Droncit® (praziquantel) is absorbed, metabolized in the liver and excreted via the bile into the digestive tract. Following exposure to praziquantel, the tapeworm loses its ability to resist digestion by the mammalian host. Because of this, whole tapeworms, including the scolex, are very rarely passed after administration of praziquantel. It is common to see only disintegrated and partially digested pieces of tapeworms in the stool. The majority of tapeworms killed are digested and not found in the feces.

Overdosage: The safety index has been derived from controlled saftey evaluation, clinical trials and prior approved use in foreign countries. Dosages of five times the labeled rate at 14 day intervals to dogs as young as four weeks did not produce signs of clinical toxicity following either intramuscular or subcutaneous injections. No significant clinical chemistry, hematological, cholinesterase or histopathological changes occurred. Symptoms of overdosage (33.8 to 40 times the labeled dosage rate) included vomition, excessive salivation and depression, but no deaths in adult dogs. Symptoms of overdosage (10 to 20 times the labeled dosage rate) in adult cats included vomition, depression, muscle tremors and incoordination. Deaths occurred in five of eight cats treated subcutaneously and in all eight injected intramuscularly at doses greater than 20 times the label rate.

Contraindications: There are no known contraindications to use of praziquantel.

Pregnancy: Droncit® (praziquantel) has been tested in breeding and pregnant dogs and cats. No adverse effects were noted.

Adverse Reaction: Mild side effects were observed in 18 of 189 dogs (9.5%) and 8 of 85 cats (9.4%) administered Droncit® Injectable in field trials. The majority of these were described as brief pain responses following injections to larger dogs (weighing over 50 lbs.) Two dogs exhibited a brief period of mild vomiting and/or drowsy or staggering gait. The eight cats exhibited either diarrhea, weakness, vomition, salivation, sleepiness, burning on injection and/or a temporary lack of appetite. The investigators considered these effects slight or not significant.

Warning: Keep out of reach of children. Not for human use.

How Supplied: Code: 1831 - 10 ml vial

DRONCIT® TABLETS
(praziquantel)
Oral Cestocide for Dogs and Cats

Description: Droncit® (praziquantel) canine and feline cestocide tablets are sized for easy oral administration to either adults dogs or puppies and adult cats or kittens. The tablets may be crumbled and mixed with the feed. The canine tablets contain 34 mg praziquantel and the feline tablets contain 23 mg praziquantel.

Indication: Droncit® (praziquantel) oral cestocide is indicated for the removal of *Dipylidium caninum, Taenia pisiformis,* and *Echinococcus granulosus* from dogs and *Dipylidium caninum* and *Taenia taeniaeformis* in cats.

Dosage and Administration: Droncit® Canine and Feline Tablets may be administered directly per os or crumbled and mixed with the feed. The recommended dosage of praziquantel varies according to body weight. Smaller animals require a relatively large dosage because of their higher metabolic rate. The optimum dose for each individual animal will be acheived by utilizing the following dosage schedule.

*Dogs and Puppies** *(34 mg tablet)*	
5 lbs and under	½ tablet
6-10 lbs	1 tablet
11-15 lbs	1½ tablet
16-30 lbs	2 tablets
31-45 lbs	3 tablets
46-60 lbs	4 tablets
over 60 lbs	5 tablets max.

*Cats and Kittens** *(23 mg tablet)*	
4 lbs and under	½ tablet
5-11 lbs	1 tablet
over 11 lbs	1½ tablet

*Not intended for use in puppies less than four (4) weeks of age or kittens less than six (6) weeks of age.

Fasting - The recommended dosage of praziquantel is not affected by the presence or absence of food in the gastrointestinal tract, therefore, FASTING IS NEITHER NECESSARY NOR RECOMMENDED.

Retreatment - For those animals maintained on premises where reinfections are likely to occur, clients should be instructed in the steps necessary to prevent reinfection; otherwise, retreatment may be necessary. This is especially true in cases of *Dipylidium caninum* infections where reinfection is almost certain to occur if fleas are not removed from the animal and its environment.

Action: Droncit® (praziquantel) is absorbed, metabolized in the liver and excreted in the bile. Upon entering the digestive tract from the bile, cestocidal activity is exhibited.- Following exposure to praziquantel, the tapeworm losses its ability to resist digestion by the mammalian host. Because of this, whole tapeworms, including the scolex, are very rarely passed after administration of praziquantel. In many instances only disintergrated and partially digested pieces of tapeworms will be seen in the stool. The majority of tapeworms killed are digested and are not found in the feces.

Overdosage: The safety index has been derived from controlled safety evaluations, clinical trials and prior approved use in foreign countries. Dosages of five times the labeled rate at 14 day intervals to dogs as young as four weeks and cats as young as 5½weeks did not produce clinical signs of toxicity. No significant clinical chemistry, hematological, or histopathological changes occurred. Symptoms of gross overdosage include vomition, salvation, diarrhea and depression.

Contraindications: There are no known contraindications to the use of prazinquantel in dogs.

Pregnancy: Droncit® (praziquantel) has been tested in breeding and pregnant dogs and cats. No adverse effects were noted.

Adverse Reaction: *Canine Tablets* Seven instances (3.2%) of either vomiting, anorexia, lethargy or diarrhea were reported during the field trials in which 218 dogs were administered Droncit® Canine Cestocide Tablets. The investigators rated these as non-significant.

Feline Tablets - One instance of diarrhea and one of salivation (1.5%) were reported during the field trials in which 135 cats were administered Droncit® Feline Cestocide Tablets.

Warning: Keep out of reach of children. Not for human use.

How Supplied: Code: 1828-(50's)-Canine Tablets
Code: 1829-(50's)-Feline Tablets

ELECTROFIN® POWDER
Balanced electrolyte-trace mineral powder

Composition: The electrolyte ions Sodium Potassium Calcium, Magnesium, Chloride and Bicarbonate (after metabolic conversion) obtained from Sodium chloride (food grade), 50.0%; Potassium chloride (chemical grade), 20.4%; Clacium lactate (food processing grade),

8.7%; Magnesium carbonate, 1.61%; and the trace elements Cobalt, Zinc, Manganese, Copper, and Iron; with certified Color added, in a palatable base.
Indications: For use before stress periods to reduce shipping and dressing losses and to improve meat quality.
Dosage and Administration: Administer over a period of 3 to 7 days. In drinking water—1 ounce per 10 gallons; in feed—1% in place of each 1% salt. ***Individually to cattle, horses, sheep or swine***—½ to 1 ounce per 800 to 1,000 lbs. Provide plenty of drinking water.
How Supplied:
Code: 1885—50 lb pail

ELECTROFIN® TABSULES

Composition: Each tablet contains: The electrolyte ions Sodium Potassium, Calcium, Magnesium, Chloride, and Bicarbonate (after metabolic conversion) obtained from Magnesium citrate soluble, 91.14 mg.; Sodium Chloride (food grade), 2.55 gm.; Potassium Chloride (chemical grade), 1.04 gm.; and Calcium lactate (food processing grade), 462.5 mg.
Indications: For use in the prevention and treatment of electrolyte depletion and dehydration in horses, cattle, sheep and swine.
Dosage and Administration: Dissolve 1 tabsule per 2½ gal. drinking water. Individual treatment: 1 or more tabsules given with balling gun. Dosage may be administered continuously.
US Patent No. 3,241,974.
How Supplied:
Code: 1440—100's bottles

ELTRADD™-4000
Electrolyte Powder

Composition: Sodium chloride 9.68%, Sodium citrate 7.36%, Potassium chloride 1.27%, Calcium lactate (from monohydrate) 1.28%, Magnesium citrate 0.8% and Dextrose 79.8%.
Indications: For making an electrolyte solution of Na,+K,+Mg++, Ca++Cl- and HCO-3 ions with dextrose for oral use in cattle, horses, sheep and swine.
Directions: For oral use dissolve in drinking water at the rate of one package (8 oz) in approximately 20 gallons of drinking water.
Warning: This product contains citrate salts which may in some cases be incompatible with tetracycline antibiotics; therefore, it should not be mixed with or used in close sequence with such antibiotics.
How Supplied:
Code: 1890—8 oz container

ENCEVAC® WITH HAVLOGEN®
Encephalomyelitis Vaccine

Composition: Encevac® is a formalin-inactivated, bivalent vaccine derived from chicken tissue cultures infected with known eastern and western strains of encephalomyelitis virus. This vaccine contains a patented adjuvant, Havlogen®, to provide maximum antigenicity of each strain in a 1 ml. dose. Contains penicillin, streptomycin, and amphotericin-B as preservatives.
Indications: For immunization of healthy equines against encephalomyelitis caused by either the eastern or western strain of the virus.
Dosage and Administration: For primary immunization, aseptically inject 1 ml. intramuscularly and repeat in 3 weeks. A 1 ml. booster should be administered annually.
Caution: Store at 35° to 45°F. (2° to 7°C.) Shake well before using. Local reactions may occur if this product is given subcutaneously. Inject deep into the muscle only. Do not vaccinate within 21 days of slaughter. Use entire contents when first opened. Anaphylactoid reactions may occur.
Antidote: Epinephrine.
How Supplied:
Code: 4652—1 ml syringe
4653—10 ml vial

ENCEVAC®-T WITH HAVLOGEN®
Encephalomyelitis Vaccine
Tetanus Toxoid

Composition: The Eastern and Western Encephalomyelitis viruses are prepared from infected chicken tissue culture fluids. Each virus is formalin inactivated and combined with a purified and concentrated tetanus toxoid. This product contains a patented adjuvant, Havlogen®, which results in an increased response to the vaccine antigens after injection into horses. Penicillin, streptomycin and amphotericin B added as preservatives.
Indications: Encevac®-T is recommended for the immunization of healthy equines against Tetanus and Eastern and Western Encephalomyelitis.
Dosage and Administration: For primary immunization, aseptically inject 2 ml. intramuscularly and repeat in 3 to 4 weeks. A 2 ml. booster dose should be administered annually.
Caution: Store at 35° to 45°F. (2° to 7°C.) Do not freeze. Shake well before using. Do not vaccinate within 21 days of slaughter. Local reactions may occur if this product is given subcutaneously. Inject deep into the muscle only. Injury to the horse should be followed by a 2 ml. booster dose of Encevac®-T or Super-Tet. If the injury occurs during the first two months of primary vaccination or after 12 months without a booster dose, administer at least 1500 tetanus antitoxin units as a prophylactic measure. Anaphylactoid reactions may occur. *Antidote:* Epinephrine.
How Supplied:
Code: 4671—2 ml syringe (1 dose)
4672—20 ml syringe (10 doses)

ENCEVAC® TC-4 WITH HAVLOGEN®
Encephalomyelitis-Influenza Vaccine-Tetanus Toxoid

Composition: Encevac®-4 is a formaldehyde inactivated and adjuvanted polyvalent equine vaccine-toxoid consisting of Eastern and Western Encephalomyelitis virus with concentrated and purified A_1 and A_2 Influenza virus of Canine Cell Line Origin and Tetanus Toxoid. These fractions are blended with a patented adjuvant, Havlogen®, to elicit an increased antigenic response. Neomycin, polymycin B, and a fungistat added as preservatives.
Indications: For immunization of healthy equines against Eastern and Western Encephalomyelitis and Tetanus and as an aid in the prevention of equine influenza due to strains A_1 and A_2 virus.
Dosage and Administration: For primary immunization, aseptically inject 2 ml intramuscularly and repeat in 3 to 4 weeks. A 2 ml booster dose should be administered annually and at any time epidemic conditions exist or are reported and exposure is imminent.
Caution: Store at 35° to 45°F (2° to 7°C). Shake well before using. Do not vaccinate within 21 days of slaughter. Local reactions may occur if this product is given subcutaneously. Inject deep into the muscle only. Injury to the horse should be followed by a 2 ml booster dose of Encevac®-4, Encevac®-T or Super-Tet®. If the injury occurs during the first two months of primary vaccination or after 12 months without a booster dose, administer at least 1500 tetanus antitoxin units as a prophylactic measure. Anaphylactoid reactions may occur. *Antidote:* Epinephrine.
How Supplied:
Code: 4658—2 ml syringe
4659—20 ml syringe

ENE-PET™ SOLUTION

Composition: Each syringe contains 250 mg. Dioctyl Sodium Sulfosuccinate in 5 ml. Glycerine, with Sorbic Acid (as a preservative).
Indications: As an aid in the softening of hardened fecal matter and lubricating the rectal wall.
Administration: Remove cap and gently insert nozzle into rectum. If desired, nozzle can be lubricated prior to insertion. Depress plunger to express contents. Withdraw nozzle and discard syringe. Treatment may be repeated in one hour if indicated.
Dosage Schedule:
Cats—One-half of syringe.
Small Dogs (under 15 pounds)—One-half of syringe
Dogs (15 pounds and over)—one full syringe. May be repeated in one hour to extra large dogs or in severe cases. Do not exceed 3 syringes.
Warning: Do not administer this product if the animal is presently receiving a prescription drug or mineral oil.
Caution: This product should be used only occasionally, but in any event, no longer than daily for one week.
For rectal use only in dogs and cats.
Caution: Keep out of reach of children.
How Supplied: 0883—5 ml syringe (25 per box)

Continued on next page

Haver—Cont.

EQUICINE™ II with HAVLOGEN®
Equine Influenza Vaccine

Indications: For use in healthy equines as an aid in the prevention of equine influenza due to strain A_1 and A_A viruses.
Dosage and Administration: *Horses and foals*— 1 ml injected intramuscularly. A single 1 ml. booster dose should be administered annually and at any time epidemic conditions exist or are repored and exposure is imminent. Repeat in 3 to 4 weeks. Use entire contents when first opened. Store at 35° to 45°F. (2° to 7°C.)
Caution: Do not vaccinate within 21 days of slaughter. See carton for more complete directions.
How Supplied:
Code: 4702—1 ml syringe
4703—10 ml syringe

EQUICINE™-T WITH HAVLOGEN®
Equine Influenza Vaccine Tetanus Toxoid

Indications: For use in healthy equines as an aid in the prevention of equine influenza due to A_1 and $_2$ viruses and Tetanus.
Dosage and Administration: For primary immunization, aseptically inject 2 ml intramuscularly. Repeat in 3 - 4 weeks. A single 2 ml booster dose should be administered annually and at any time epidemic conditions exist or are reported and exposure is imminent.
Caution: Store at 35° to 45°F. (2° to 7°C.). Shake well before using. Do not vaccinate within 21 days of slaughter. Local reactions may occur if this product is given subcutaneously. Inject deep into the muscle only. Anaphylactoid reactions may occur. Antidote: Epinephrine.
How Supplied:
Code: 4695—2 ml syringe
4696—20 ml vial

H

EQUIMATE®
(fluprostenol)
Injectable Prostalgandin Analogue for Mares

Composition: Equimate® is a synthetic staglandin analogue structually related to prostaglandin $F_{2\alpha}$ ($PGF_{2\alpha}$). Each ml of the colorless aqueous solution contains 52.4 mcg of fluprostenol sodium, equivalent to 50 mcg of fluprostenol in a sodium citrate, anhydrous citric acid and sodium chloride buffer.
Action: Equimate® causes regression of the corpus luteum in Mares. This luteolysis usually results in estrus and ovulation with normal fertility. Most mares exhibit behavorial estrus within six days of the injection. As with the natural estrous cycle, ovulation occurs approximately 24 hours prior to the end of estrus. Mares which do not exhibit behavorial extrus ("silent heat") may be bred successfully if follicular development and ovulation are determined by examination of the reproductive tract.
Note: It is advisable to conduct a thorough examination for breeding soundness including rectal palpatation of the reproductive tract before administering this drug. There is a refractory period of 4 to 5 days after ovulation when mare are not responsive to the luteolytic action of prostaglandins.
Indications: Controlling the life span of the corpus luteum makes Equimate® a valuable management aid in:
a) *Successful mare and stallion management.*
Mares may be brought into estrus on a planned timing schedule (singly or in groups) to facilitate a more efficient breeding season. The time at which a mare or a group of mares are bred can be manipulated so that precious time is not lost or so that stallions are not overworked by large numbers of mares being presented for service at an unpredictable time.
b) *Postpartum breeding*
To avoid the reduced fertility associated with breeding at "foal heat", mares may be treated 7 to 9 days after the ovulation at the foal heat to induce an early return to estrus and to offset the risk of lactational anestrus.
Therapeutic aid for
a) *Induction of luteolysis* following early fetal death and resorption
About 8 to 10 percent of all mares which conceive lost the conceptus during the first 100 days of pregnancy. Persistence of luteal function in the ovary precludes an early return to estrus.
b) *Termination of persistent diestrus*
Non-pregnant mares frequently and spontaneously go into and out of periods of prolonged diestrus. A very high proportion of mares in this category i.e., not cycling, are in prolonged diestrus rather than anestrus, particularly in the latter part of the breeding season.
c) *Termination of pseudopregnancy*
Some mares which are bred at normal estrus and subsequently found to be non-pregnant (but not having lost or resorbed a conceptus) display clinical signs of pregnancy. These animals are said to be "Pseudopregnant."
d) *Treatment of lactational anestrus*
Some lactating mares fail to cycle again for several months after exhibiting an early "foal heal."
e) *Estabishing estrous cycles* in barren/ maiden mares
Some mares have a functional corpus luteum and are either suffering from abnormal presistence of luteal function or are simply failing to exhibit normal estrous behavior ("silent heat") while ovarian cyclicity continues.
f) *Determining if a mare is cycling*
Equimate® may be used as a diagnostic aid to determine if a non-pregnant mare is cycling by confirming the presence or absence of a functional corpus luteum. Lack of a cyclic ovarian function (true anestrus) is indicated if a mare does not exhibit behavioral estrus or does not have follicular development after either of two Equimate® injections 10 to 15 days apart.
Contraindications: Adverse reactions have not been seen after the recommended effective dose of Equimate®, and even after dose levels in excess of that which is recommended these are mild and transient—in the form of mild sweating and diarrhea. However, Equimate® should not be administered to:
a) Pregnant mares—since luteolysis at some stages in gestation will result in loss of the fetus.
b) Mares receiving non-steroidal anti-inflammatory drugs since these drugs inhibit the synthesis and release of prostaglandins.
c) Mares suffering from acute or sub-acute disorders of the gastro-intestinal tract.
d) Mares suffering from acute or sub-acute respiratory disease.
Dosage and Administration: Equimate® fluprostenol should be given by intramuscular injection. The dosage of Equimate of 0.55 mcg fluprostenol/kg. Thus, for the average mature mare the usual dose is 5 ml containing 250 mcg fluprostenol (1 ml contains 50 mcg fluprostenol).
Warnings: Not for use in horses intended for food.
Women of child-bearing age, asthmatics and persons with bronchial and other respiratory problems should exercise extreme caution when handling this product. In the early stage, women may be unaware of their pregnancies, Equimate® is readily absorbed through the skin and can cause abortion and/or bronchospasms. Direct contact with the skin should therefore be avoided. Accidental spillage on the skin should be washed off immediately with soap and water.
How Supplied:
Code: 0121 (5 ml)—10 per drum
Precautions: Protect from light. After opening ampule, discard any unused product.

ESTRUMATE®
(cloprostenol sodium)
Equivalent to 250 mcg. Cloprostenol/ml.
Prostaglandin Analogue for Cattle

Composition: Estrumate® cloprostenol is a synthetic prostaglandin analogue structurally related to prostaglandin $F_2\alpha$ ($PGF_2\alpha$). Each ml. of the colorless aqueous solution contains 263 mcg of cloprostenol sodium (equivalent to 250 mcg. of cloprostenol) in a sodium citrate, anhydrous citric acid and sodium chloride buffer containing 0.1% w/v chlorocresol B.P. as a bactericide.
Action: Estrumate causes functional and morphological regression of the *corpus luteum* (luteolysis) in cattle. In normal, non-pregnant cycling animals this effect on the life span of the corpus luteum usually results in estrus two to five days after treatment. In animals with prolonged luteal function (mummified fetus and luteal cysts) the induced luteolysis usually results in resolution of the condition and return to cyclicity. Pregnant animals may abort depending on the stage of gestation.

Indications: For intramuscular use to induce luteolysis in beef and dairy cattle. The luteolytic action of Estrumate can be utilized to manipulate the estrous cycle to better fit certain management practices and to terminate pregnancies resulting from mismatings and to treat certain conditions associated with prolonged luteal function.

Recommended Uses:

Unobserved or non-detected estrus

Cows which are not detected in estrus although ovarian cyclicity continues can be treated with ESTRUMATE if a mature corpus luteum is present. Estrus is expected to occur two to five days following injection, at which time animals may be inseminated. Treated cattle should be inseminated at the usal time following detection of estrus. If estrous detection is not desirable or possible, treated animals may be inseminated twice at about 72 and 96 hours post injection.

Mummified fetus

Death of the conceptus during gestation may be followed by its degeneration and dehydration. Induction of luteolysis with ESTRUMATE usually results in expulsion of the mummified fetus from the uterus. (Manual assistance may be necessary to remove the fetus from the vagina.) Normal cyclical activity usually follows.

Luteal Cysts

A cow may be non-cyclic due to the presence of a luteal cyst (a single, anovulatory follicle with a thickened wall which is accompanied by no external signs and by no changes in palpable consistency of the uterus). Treatment with ESTRUMATE can restore normal ovarian activity by causing regression of the luteal cyst.

Pregnancies from mismating: Unwanted pregnancies can be safely and efficiently terminated from one week after mating until about five months of gestation. The induced abortion is normally uncomplicated and the fetus and placenta are usually expelled about four to five days after the injection with the reproductive tract returning to normal soon after the abortion. The ability of Estrumate to induce abortion decreases beyond the fifth month of gestation while the risk of dystocia and its consequences increases. Estrumate has not been sufficiently tested under feedlot conditions therefore recommendations cannot be made for its use in heifers placed in feedlots.

Controlled Breeding: The luteolytic action of Estrumate can be utilized to schedule estrus and ovulation for an individual cycling animal or a group of animals. This allows control of the time at which cycling cows or heifers can be bred. Estrumate can be incorporated into a controlled breeding program by the following methods:

1. Single Estrumate injection: Only animals with a mature *corpus luteum* should be treated to obtain maximum response to the single injection. However, not all cycling cattle should be treated since a mature *corpus luteum* is present for only 11-12 days of the 21-day cycle.

Prior to treatment, cattle should be examined rectally and found to be anatomically normal, be non-pregnant and have a mature *corpus luteum.* If these criteria are met, estrus is expected to occur two to five days following injection, at which time animals may be inseminated. Treated cattle should be inseminated the usual time following detection of estrus. If estrus detection is not desirable or possible, treated animals may be inseminated either once at about 72 hours post injection or twice at about 72 and 96 hours post injection.

With a single injection program it may be desirable to assess the cyclicity status of the herd before Estrumate treatment. This can be accomplished by heat detecting and breeding at the usual time following detection of estrus for a six-day period, all prior to injection. If by the sixth day the cyclicity status appears normal (approximately 25-30% detected in estrus) all cattle not already inseminated should be palpated for normality, non-pregnacy, and cyclicity, then injected with Estrumate. Breeding should then be continued at the usual time following signs of estrus on the seventh and eighth day. On the ninth and tenth day breeding may continue at the usual time following detection of estrus or all cattle not already inseminated may be bred either once on the ninth day (at about 72 hours post injection) or on both the ninth and tenth day (at about 72 and 96 hours post injection).

2. Double Estrumate injections.

Prior to treatment, cattle should be examined rectally and found to be anatomically normal, non-pregnant and cycling (the presence of a mature *corpus luteum* is not necessary when the first injection of a double injection regimen is given). A second injection would be given 11 days after the first injection. In normal cycling cattle estrus is expected two to five days following the second injection. Treated cattle should be inseminated at the usual time following detection of estrus. If estrus detection is not desirable or possible, treated animals may be inseminated either once at about 72 hours post injection or twice at about 72 and 96 hours following the second Estrumate injection.

Many animals will come into estrus following the first injection. These animals can be inseminated at the usual time following detected estrus. Animals not inseminated should receive a second injection 11 days after the first injection. Animals receiving both injections may be inseminated either once at about 72 hours or twice at about 72 and 96 hours post second injection.

Any controlled breeding program recommended should be completed by either: observing animals (especially during the third week after injection) and inseminating or hand mating any animals returning to estrus, or turning in clean-up bull(s) five to seven days after the last injection of Estrumate to cover any animals returning to estrus.

Requirements for Controlled Breeding Programs: A variety of programs can be designed to best meet the needs of individual management systems. A controlled breeding program should be selected which is appropriate for the existing circumstances and management practices.

Before a controlled breeding program is planned the producers objectives must be examined and he must be made aware of the projected results and limitations. The producer and his consulting veterinarian should review the operations breeding history, herd health and nutritional status and agree that a controlled breeding program is practical in the producers specific situation. For any successful controlled breeding program:

Cows and heifers must be normal, nonpregnant, and cycling, (rectal palpation should be performed).

Cattle must be in a fit and thrifty breeding condition and on an adequate or increasing plane of nutrition.

Proper program planning and record keeping are essential.

If artificial insemination is used it must be performed by competent inseminators using high quality semen.

It is important to understand that Estrumate is effective only in animals with a mature *corpus luteum* (ovulation must have occurred at least five days prior to treatment). This must be considered when breeding is intended following a single Estrumate injection.

Adverse Reactions: At 50 and 100 times the recommended dose, mild side effects may be detected in some cattle. These include increased uneasiness, slight frothing, and milk let-down.

Contraindications: Estrumate should not be administered to a pregnant animal whose calf is not to be aborted.

Dosage and Administration: 2 ml. of Estrumate (500 mcg. of cloprostenol) should be administered by **Intramuscular Injection** for all indications in both beef and dairy catle.

Precautions: There is no effect on fertility following the single or double dosage regimen when breeding occurs at induced estrus or at 72 and 96 hours post treatment. Conception rates may be lower than expected in those fixed time breeding programs which omit the second insemination (i.e., the insemination at or near 96 hours). This is especially true if a fixed time insemination is used following a single Estrumate injection. As with all parenteral products, careful aseptic techniques should be employed to decrease the possibility of post injection bacterial infection. Antibiotic therapy should be employed at the first sign of infection.

Warning: Women of child-bearing age, asthmatics and persons with bronchial and other respiratory problems should exercise extreme caution when handling this product. In the early stages, women may be unaware of their pregnancies. Estrumate is readily absorbed through the skin and may cause abortion and/or bronchospasms. Direct contact with the skin should therefore be avoided. Acci-

Continued on next page

Haver—Cont.

dental spillage on the skin should be washed off immediately with soap and water.

Storage Conditions:
Protect from light.
Store in container.
Store at controlled room temperature (15°-30°C, 59°-86°F).

Caution: Federal (U.S.A.) law restricts this drug to use by or on the order of a licensed veterinarian.

How Supplied:

Code 0122	5 Doses (10 ml)
Code 0123	10 Doses (20 ml)

FLEA ANTIGEN

Description: A phenolized glycerine buffered saline extract of fleas
Indications: For desensitizing dogs and cats against flea bite irritation.
Dosage and Administration: Give 3 intradermal injections of 0.5 ml. at 5 to 7 day intervals. Repeat course of treatment as indicated.
How Supplied:
Code 4900—5 ml vial

FLEATOL™ SHAMPOO

Composition: Active Ingredients: Ammonium lauryl sulfate 18.60% w/w Piperonyl butoxide, technical* 0.50% w/w, Pyrethrins 0.05% w/w, Petroleum oils 0.2%. Inert Ingredients: 80.65%.
Indications: Combines an insecticide and bluing in a shampoo to remove dirt; kill fleas, lice and ticks and whiten white coats and markings.
Dosage and Administration: Wet animal thoroughly, apply shampoo and work up a good lather. Let lather remain a few minutes; then rinse, dry thoroughly and comb.
How Supplied:
Code: 0740—8 oz
0665—1 gal.

H

HAVA-CIDE™ LIQUID

Composition: Contains: Squalane (Hexamethyltetracosane) 25.00%, Pyrethrins, 0.05%; Technical Piperonyl Butoxide, 0.50%, Inert ingredients, 74.45%.
Indications: For treatment of ear mites in dogs and cats.
Dosage and Administration: After cleansing ears thoroughly, administer in each ear daily for 7 to 10 days according to the following schedule: 5-15 lbs, 4-5 drops; 15-30 lbs, 5-10 drops; 30 lbs or over, 10-15 drops.
How Supplied:
Code: 0282—½ ounce dropper bottle

HAVA-SPAN™
(sulfamethazine)
Prolonged Release Bolus

Composition: Each bolus contains 22.5 grams of sulfamethazine in a prolonged release base.
Description: Hava-Span (Sulfamethazine) Prolonged Release Bolus is a controlled release broad spectrum antibacterial formulation containing sulfamethazine. Sulfamethazine is a well established drug for the treatment of bovine shipping fever and other bacterial diseases of cattle. In Hava-Span (Sulfamethazine) Prolonged Release boluses, the sulfamethazine is formulated with a unique Servospa™ base that slowly releases the sulfamethazine for absorption into the blood stream to achieve minimum effective blood levels of 5 mg/100 ml of blood for prolonged periods.
Sulfamethazine is n^1-(4,6-dimethyl-2-pyrimidinyl) sulfanilamide.
Indications: Hava-Span (Sulfamethazine) Prolonged Release Bolus is indicated for the sustained treatment of shipping fever pneumonia caused or complicated by *Pasteurella multocida* in beef and nonlactating dairy cattle. It is also indicated as an aid in the treatment of foot rot, mastitis, pneumonia, metritis, bacterial enteritis, calf diphtheria and septicemia in beef and nonlactating dairy cattle when caused or complicated by bacteria susceptible to sulfamethazine.
Contraindications: Hava-Span (Sulfamethazine) Prolonged Release Bolus should not be administered to cattle with a known sensitivity to sulfonamides or with known renal impairment. Do not administer to cattle too small to swallow boluses (usually less than 200 lb body weight).
Dosage and Administration: Cattle which are acutely ill should be treated parenterally with a suitable antibacterial product to obtain immediate therapeutic blood levels. Hava-Span Sulfamethazine) Prolonged Release Boluses, which provide effective blood levels starting 14 to 18 hours following administration, should be administered concurrently to provide long lasting therapy. The duration of therapeutic levels (5 mg/100 ml or greater) in acutely ill animals is related to the dosage of Hava-Span (Sulfamethazine) Prolonged Release Bolus administered.
Depending on the duration of therapeutic blood level desired, administer Hava-Span (sulfamethazine) Prolonged Release Bolus as follows:

Hava-Span dosage	*Duration of Therapeutic Blood Levels* (5 mg/100 ml or greater)*
1 bolus/200 lb body wt	3½ days
1 bolus/100 lb body wt	5 days

*Duration of blood levels are based on studies on acutely ill animals with elevated body temperatures. Therapeutic blood levels following treatment with Hava-Span (Sulfamethazine) Prolonged Release Bolus rise quicker and are of a shorter duration in non-feverish animals (see section on blood levels).
Administration: Administer Hava-Span. (Sulfamethazine) Prolonged Release Bolus orally with a balling gun. Allow sufficient time between the administration of each bolus for the swallowing reflex to occur. Regurgitation may be a possibility with any bolus if not administered properly.
Safety: Two groups of four cattle weighing 490 to 665 lb were administered respectively four and six times the usual clinical dose of Hava-Span (Sulfamethazine) Prolonged Release Bolus. None of the animals revealed any visible signs of toxicity during a two week observation period. A profile of blood chemistry tests was also performed during this period and the only abnormality noticed was that one animal in the group which received four times the usual dose had a rise in blood urea nitrogen five days after dosing and a persistent low blood level of sulfamethazine for 16 days after medication.
Warning: Do not use in lactating dairy cattle. Do not administer within 16 days of slaughter.
Precautions: Do not limit drinking water to cattle being medicated. Estimated body weights carefully to assure accurate dosing. Observe animals following dosing to insure that boluses are not regurgitated. If treated animals do not respond within 2 to 3 days, the diagnosis should be redetermined and appropriate supplemental medication administered. Use only intact bolus, do not break or crush!
Adverse Reactions: Sulfonamides may infrequently cause allergic or toxic reactions such as skin rashes, drug fever, leukopenia, granulocytopenia, agranulocytosis, aplastic or hemolytic anemia, hepatotoxicity, jaundice, cyanosis, toxic nephrosis or serum sickness. However, none of these symptoms has been recorded during preclinical or clinical studies involving Hava-Span (Sulfamethazine) Prolonged Release Bolus.
Caution: Federal law restricts this drug to use by or on the order of a licensed veterinarian.
How Supplied:
Code 1407—Box of 50

HAVIDOTE
(calcium disodium edetate injection)

Composition: Calcium disodium edetate (anhydrous) 6.6% in Purified Water. Sodium Hydroxide added to adjust pH.
Indications: An aid in the treatment of acute lead poisoning in horses.
Dosage and Administration: Administer by slow intravenous injection at the rate of 1 ml per 2 lb of body weight daily. Is best administered in divided doses 2 to 3 times daily and continued for three to five days. If additional treatment is indicated, a two-day rest period is recommended, which may be followed by another 3 to 5 day period of therapy.
Warning: The recommended dose should not be exceeded. Overdosage may cause necrosis of the kidney. Avoid concomitant administration of barbiturates or sulfonamides. Watch heart rate and administer carefully to avoid tachycardia, dyspnea and body tremors. Do not use in horses intended for food purposes. This product does not contain a preservative. Do not save fractional contents for later use.
Side effects: Adverse reactions with some deaths may follow therapy with

Calcium disodium edetate in animals carrying a high blood lead burden.
Caution: Federal (U.S.A.) law restricts this drug to use by or on the order of a licensed veterinarian.
How Supplied:
Code: 0221—50 ml bottles

HAVO-LEP™-5
Leptospira Canicola-Grippotyphosa-Hardjo-Icterohaemorrhagiae-Pomona Bacterin

Composition: Chemically inactivated, aluminum hydroxide adsorbed cultures of the organisms listed above.
Indications: For the immunization of healthy cattle and swine against *Leptospira canicola-grippotyphosa-hardjo-icterohaemorrhagiae-pomona.*
Dosage and Administration: 2 ml injected subcutaneously or intramuscularly. Annual revaccination is recommended for breeding stock.
Precautions: Shake well before using. Store at 35° to 45°F (2° to 7°C). Use entire contents when first opened. Do not vaccinate within 21 days of slaughter. Anaphylactoid reactions may occur. *Antidote:* Epinephrine. Contains thimerosal as a preservative.
How Supplied:
Code 4705—20 ml (10 doses)
4706—100 ml (50 doses)

HEIFEX®
Prostaglandin Analogue for Pregnant Feedlot Heifers

Description: HEIFEX® cloprostenol is a synthetic prostaglandin analogue structurally related to prostaglandin $F_2a(PGF_2a)$. Each ml. of the colorless solution contains 131.5 mcg. of cloprostenol sodium (equivalent to 125 mcg. of cloprostenol) in a sodium citrate, anhyrdous citric acid and sodium chloride buffer containing 0.1% w/v chorocresol B.P. as a bactericide.

Action: HEIFEX® causes functional and morphological regression of the corpus luteum (luteolysis) in cattle. In non-pregnant animals, this effect on the life span of the corpus luteum normally results in estrus two to five days after treatment. The regression of the corpus luteum in pregnant animals usually results in abortion depending upon the state of gestation.
Indications: For intramuscular use to induce abortion in pregnant feedlot heifers. Unwanted pregnancies can be safely and efficiently terminated from one week after mating until about 4-½ months of gestation.
Administration and Dosage: 3 ml. of HEIFEX® (375 mcg. of cloprostenol) should be administered by INTRAMUSCULAR INJECTION.
Safety and Toxicity: The induced abortion is normally uncomplicated. The fetus and placenta are usually expelled about four or five days after the injection with the reproductive tract returning to normal soon after the abortion.
In pregnant animals, no adverse reactions associated with HEIFEX® treatment and no unusual side effects associated with the induced abortion have been observed at three times the recommended dose. At 67 and 133 times the recommended dose, mild side effects have been detected in some non-pregnant cattle. These include increased uneasiness, slight frothing and milk letdown.
Contraindications: HEIFEX® should not be administered to a pregnant animal whose calf is not be be aborted.
Precautions: The ability of HEIFEX® to induce abortion decreases beyond 4-½ months of gestation while the risk of dystocia and its consequences increases. Therefore, animals over 4-½ months gestation should not be treated. Factors causing stress may reduce efficacy and increase risks for treated animals. Animals should be observed following treatment.
Cattle administered a progestogen may be expected to have a reduced response to HEIFEX® (cloprostenol). As with all parenteral products, careful aseptic techniques should be employed to decrease the possibility of post injection bacterial infection. Antibiotic therapy should be employed at the first sign of injection.
Caution: Federal (U.S.A.) law restricts this drug to use by or on the order of a licensed veterinarian.
Warning: For Veterinary Use Only.
Women of child-bearing age, asthmatics and persons with bronchial and other respiratory problems should exercise exteme caution when handling this product. In the early stages, women may be unaware of their pregnancies. HEIFEX® is readily absorbed throught the skin and may cause abortion and/or bronchospasms. Direct contact with the skin should therefore be avoided. Accidental spillage on the skin should be washed off immediately with soap and water.
Storage Conditions: Protect from light. Store in carton.
Code: 323-00—30 ml vial

H-L BI-PEN™
(sterile penicillin G benzathine and penicillin G procaine in aqueous suspension) For veterinary use in beef cattle, horses and dogs

Composition: Each ml of suspension contains: 150,000 units penicillin G benzathine; 150,000 units penicillin G procaine; 3.0 mg sodium formaldehyde sulfoxylate; 14.0 mg lecithin; 1.20 mg methylparaben (as preservative); 0.14 mg propylparaben (as preservative); 0.25% Phenol (as preservative); 7.0 mg between 40; 10.0 mg span 40; 10.0 mg sodium citrate; 20.0 mg procaine hydrochloride; 1.5 mg sodium carboxymethylcellulose; 3.5 mg povidone; 0.15 ml sorbitol solution; and water for injection q.s.
Indications: H-L Bi-Pen™ is indicated for treatment of the following bacterial infections in dogs, horses and beef cattle due to penicillin G susceptible micro-organisms that are susceptible to the serum levels common to this particular dosage form, such as:
1. Bacterial Pneumonia (shipping Fever complex) (*Streptococcus spp., Corynebacterium pyogenes, Staphylococcus aureus*)
2. Upper Respiratory Infections such as Rhinitis or Pharyngitis (*Corynebacterium pyogenes*)
3. Equine Strangles (*Streptococcus equi*)
4. Blackleg (*Clostridium Chauvoei*)
5. Anthrax (*Bacillus anthracis*)

Contraindications: H-L Bi-Pen™ is contraindicated in patients which have shown hypersensitivity to penicillin.
Adverse Reactions: Anaphylactic reactions have been reported in cattle given penicillin. Treated animals should be closely observed and if allergic or anaphylactic reactions occur, administer epinephrine or antihistamines immediately.
Administration: H-L Bi-Pen™should be given by intramuscular injection to horses. In beef cattle the recommended dosage should be administered by subcutaneous injection only. Dogs may be injected by either the intramuscular or subcutaneous route.
Dosage: *Horses:* 2 ml per 150 lb body weight given intramuscularly (2,000 units penicillin G procaine and 2,000 units penicillin G benzathine per lb body weight). Treatment should be repeated in 48 hours.
Beef cattle: 2 ml per 150 lb body weight given subcutaneously only (2,000 units penicillin G procaine and 2,000 units penicillin G benzathine per lb body weight). Treatment should be repeated in 48 hours.
Important: Treatment in beef cattle should be limited to two (2) doses of H-L Bi-Pen™ given by subcutaneous injection only.
Dogs: 1 ml per 10 to 25 lb body weight given intramuscularly or subcutaneously (6,000 to 15,000 units penicillin G procaine and 6,000 to 15,000 units penicillin G benzathine per body weight). Treatment should be repeated in 48 hours. Keep in a cool place —store below 15°C (59°F).
Warning: Beef cattle should be withheld from slaughter for food use for 30 days following last treatment. Treatment in beef caltle must be limited to two (2) doses. Not to be used in horses intended for food purposes.
Caution: Federal law restricts this drug to use by or on the order of a licensed veterinarian.
How Supplied:
Code: 3152—100 ml vial
3154—250 ml vial

Continued on next page

Haver—Cont.

H-L DEX™
Dexamethasone Injection
2 mg/ml

Composition: H-L Dex™ is intended for intravenous or intramuscular administration. Each milliliter contains 2 mg dexamethasone, 500 mg polyethylene glycol 400, 9 mg benzyl alcohol, 1.8 mg methylparaben and 0.2 mg propylparaben as preservatives, 0.05 ml alcohol, water for injection q.s.
Dosage: *Canine* —0.25 to 1 mg intravenously or intramuscularly. The dose may be repeated if necessary.
Feline —0.125 to 0.5 mg intravenously or intramuscularly. The dose may be repeated if necessary.
Equine —2.5 to 5 mg intravenousiy or intramuscularly.
Note: When using dexamethasone as supportive therapy in horses, dogs and cats, the doses suggested above may be used. It should be kept in mind that the use of this product in these cases does not preclude the necessity for employing standard therapy to combat the primary condition.
Doses of H-L Dex™ above 5 mg may produce transient drowsiness or lethargy in some horses. The lethargy usually abates in 24 hours.
Not for use in horses intended for food.
Caution: Federal law restricts this drug to use by or on the order of a licensed veterinarian.
How Supplied:
Code: 3150—100 ml vials

HY-GUARD™ with HAVLOGEN

H

Composition: A formaldehyde inactivited and adjuvanted whole culture of Treponema hyodysenteriae.
Indications: Recommended for use in healthy swine as an aid in the prevention of swine dysentery caused by Treponema hyodysenteriae.
Dose: Inject 5 ml. intramuscularly. Repeat in 3–4 weeks and at any time epidemic conditions exist or are reported and exposure is imminent. Pigs vaccinated prior to weaning should be revaccinated 3 weeks after weaning.
Shake well before using. Store at 35° to 45°F (2° to 7°C). Do not vaccinate within 21 days of slaughter. Use entire contents when first opened. Anaphylactoid reactions may occur. Antidote: Epinephrine. Contains thimerosal as preservative.
How Supplied:
Code: 4738—50 ml.—10 doses
4740—250 ml.—50 doses

HYPODERMIN™ INJECTION
(Counter irritant)

Composition: Iodine 1.9% in Peanut Oil base containing approximately 9% ether.
Note: Variation in ether content is unavoidable.
Indications: A counterirritant for subcutaneous use in horses.
Dosage and Administration: Inject subcutaneously over the periosteum of exostoses from ½to 1 ml totaling no more than 6 ml and rub the skin firmly to distribute the solution evenly over and around the entire enlargement.
Repeat at intervals of ten days, if necessary.
Store at room temperature 50° to 86°F.
How Supplied:
Code: 0230—50 ml bottle

INTRANASAL BOVINE RHINOTRACHEITIS-PARAINFLUENZA$_3$ VACCINE
Modified Live Virus
IBR-PI$_3$ (Cutter label)

Indications: For the active immunization of healthy cattle against infectious bovine rhinotracheitis and parainfluenza$_3$ virus.
Caution: Store at not over 45°F or 7°C. Use entire contents when first opened. Do not use chemical disinfectants to sterilize syringes, needles or cannulas. Burn container and all unused contents. Do not vaccinate within 21 days before slaughter. Contains penicillin and streptomycin as added preservatives. Anaphylactoid reactions, although rare, may occur. **Antidote:** Epinephrine.
Administration and Dosage: For Intranasal Use Only. For use in healthy cattle. Slowly transfer contents of diluent vial to vaccine vial, using aseptic technique and boiled or autoclaved syringes and needles. Administer 2 ml intranasally—1 ml in each nostril. Use a separate disposable cannula for each animal. Calves vaccinated under 6 months of age should be revaccinated at 6 months or weaning.
How Supplied:
Code: 240-95—20 ml—10 doses
240-96—50 ml—25 doses
240-97—100 ml—50 doses

KIT-TONNE™ LAXATIVE

Composition: Benzoic acid 0.2% (preservative) in Lecithin —Malt Extract —Petrolatum —Heavy Mineral oil base.
Indications: A laxative paste for dogs and cats which is also used as an aid in removing hairballs.
Directions: If animal at first refuses to take Kit-Tonne from the tube, place a small amount on its nose or on cats paws; afterward animal usually licks Kit-Tonne from the tube.
Dosage and Administration: ***Cats*** ⅛–¼ tube. ***Dogs:*** small, ¼; average, ½; large, up to 1 tube. May be repeated as necessary.
Do not store above 80°F.
How Supplied:
Code: 1094—2¼ oz. tubes

KRS® Spray Foam (Cutter label)

Active Ingredient: Coumaphos
Indications: For treatment and prevention of screw worms and fly maggots on livestock. For control of ear ticks on beef and dairy cattle.
Contains:
ACTIVE INGREDIENT
O,O-Diethyl O-(3-chloro-4-methyl -2-oxo-2H-1-benzopyran-7-yl) phosphorothioate.......................... 3.0%
INERT INGREDIENTS.................97.0%
100.0%
Storage: Store in a cool place. Do not expose to freezing or heat above 130°F.
Directions: Shake well before using. SCREW WORMS AND FLY MAGGOTS ON BEEF AND DAIRY CATTLE, SHEEP, GOATS, SWINE AND HORSES: Hold spray nozzle 3–10 inches from the wound area to be treated and apply a protective coating on and around the wound. For the **treatment** of wounds infested with fly maggots and screw worms on beef and dairy cattle, sheep, goats, swine and horses, spray wounds until complete coverage is obtained. Repeat as necessary. For **prevention,** spray a protective coating on new wounds from dehorning, castration, docking, injury, etc. as soon as possible to avoid infestation. Repeat as necessary. EAR TICKS ON BEEF AND DAIRY CATTLE: For **control** spray directly into each ear canal until complete coverage is obtained (approximately 5 seconds). Repeat as necessary.
Use Restrictions: For external insecticidal use only on above-specified animals. Do not contaminate feed, troughs, water or water utensils. Provide thorough ventilation while spraying. Use caution when spraying in area of face to avoid exposure to eyes.
Packaging:
Code: 336-80—16 oz. spray foam

LEG TONE™ EQUINE LEG PAINT

Composition: Each pint contains

Iodine Tincture Strong	20.0% w/v
Camphor	1.0%
Propylene glycol	15.0%
Methyl salicyate	5.0%
Turpentine	1.0%
Ammonium iodide	1.0%
Oil of Origanum Red	1.0%
Oil of Pennyroyal	1.0%
Isopropyl Alcohol	45.0%
Alcohol, U.S.P.	10.0%
	100.0%

Indications: A medium strength solution for use when counterirritant-stimulant action falling between stimulating liniment and blistering ointment is desired. To be used as an aid in the temporary relief of minor stiffness and soreness caused by overexertion.
Directions: Paint Leg Tone on the horses leg at undiluted strength daily until desired effect is obtained.
Caution: Do not use tight or heavy air-excluding bandage. Discontinue use if excessive irritation of the skin develops.
Warning: Do not apply to irritated skin. If excessive irritation develops, discontinue treatment and consult your veterinarain. Avoid getting into eyes or on mucous membranes.
For external use only
Keep out of reach of children
How Supplied:
Code: 0742—1 pint

LYSOFF™ INSECTICIDE (Cutter label)

Composition: Contains: Fenthion (0,0-Dimethyl 0-4(methylthio)-m-tolyl

phosphorothioate)*, 7.6%; Petroleum distillate, 56.7%; Xylene, 20.0%; Inert ingredients, 15.7%.
Indications: Easy to mix, convenient and economical control for both biting and sucking lice on beef and non-lactating dairy cattle. Mixes easily to form a creamy emulsion, even in cold water. Provides all the advantages of an easy-touse pour-on product. Concentrated for reduced weight and lower cost. No foul odor. One-half gallon treats up to 57,000 lbs.
Dosage and Administration: Treat when lice become a problem or the existence of lice has been confirmed. Treat every animal in the herd. For 4½ gallons of final pour-on mixture, add ½ gallon of water slowly to ½ gallon Lysoff Insecticide. Stir for one minute, then add remaining 3½ gallons of water. Stir for additional 2 minutes. Pour 1 fl oz of final mixture per 100 lbs body wt uniformly along center line of the animal's back. A second application may be necessary for heavily infested animals or those that become reinfested. For additional final mixture quantities and number of animals treated, see label.
Side Effects: While Lysoff Pour-On is not an effective product for cattle grub control, host-parasite reactions have been reported on rare occasions. In these rare instances (usually 24-72 hours after treatment) animals may exhibit symptoms of stagering or more rarely posterior paralysis, salivation or bloat cause by treating when cattle grubs are in the area of the spinal cord or gullet.
Contraindications: Do not treat lactating dairy cattle, non-lactating dairy cattle within 28 days of freshening, calves less than 3 months old, sick, convalescent or stressed livestock.
Warning: Do not treat for 10 days before or after shipping, weaning, dehorning or after exposure to contagious or infectious diseases. Do not slaughter within 35 days after a single treatment; or within 45 days of a second application.
How Supplied:
Code: 136-65—½ gallon can

NEGUVON POUR-ON
(Cutter label)

Composition:
Contains: Dimethyl (2,2,2-tri chloro-1-hydro-xyethyl) phosphonate, 8%; Inert ingredients, 925.
Indications: Brand of trichlorfon for effective control of grubs and lice on cattle.
Dosage and Administration: Apply at the rate of ½ fluid oz per 100 lbs body weight uniformly
along the back of the animal.
Warning: Do not use milk for human consumption for 7 days after treatment. Do not treat cattle within 21 days of slaughter. Do not apply in conjunction with oral drenches, other internal medications, organic phosphates, or cholinesterase inhibitors.
How Supplied:
Code: 134-41—1 gal can
134-45—5 gal can

NOVIN™ INJECTION
Analgesic-Antipyretic-Antispasmodic

Composition: Dipyrone (Aminopyrine derivative) 50%; Benzyl alcohol, 2%; Distilled water, q.s.
Indications: Aids in the relief of equine colic and similar conditions in dogs and cats, which are caused and accompanied by smooth muscle spasms.
Dosage and Administration: Administer subcutaneously, intravenously or intramuscularly; *Horses*—10 to 20 ccs; *Dogs and cats*—¼ cc per 10 lbs body weight. May be repeated once or twice daily at 8 hour intervals.
Warning: Do not treat food producing animals, those producing milk for human consumption, when there is a history of blood dyscrasia or in conjuction with phenylbutazone and barbiturates. Average or large doses may cause nausea, vomiting, agranulocytosis or leukopenia. See insert.
How Supplied:
Code: 0054—90 ml vial

NOVIN™ TABLETS
Analgesic-Antipyretic-Antispasmodic

Composition: Contains: Dipyrone (Aminopyrine derivative), 5 gr.
Indications: For use in relieving pain, relaxing smooth muscles and reducing fever in dogs and cats.
Dosage and Administration: ***To cats and dogs,*** give 1 grain per each 5 lbs body wt (1 tablet per 25 lbs) 2 or three times daily.
Warning: In exceptional cases, this product may cause agranulocytosis and leukopenia. Do not give in large doses or for prolonged periods of time without frequent complete blood counts.
Not for human use. Keep out of reach of children.
How Supplied:
Code: 1652—bottles of 500

ODOR-BAN DEODORANT

Composition: Active ingredients (Biphenyl and Perfume), 3.7%; Inert ingredients (Ethyl alcohol, 190 proof, denatured), 96.3%.
Indications: A deodorant for use on kennels, instruments, floors. clothing, furniture, rugs, drapes, etc. Chemically neutralizes most odors caused by rancidity, putrefaction, excrement, urine, anal glands, skunk, body odors, tobacco, etc.
Directions: *Spraying*—Use sprayer or atomizer, spray lightly over bedding, cabinets, floors, etc. *Mopping and cleaning*—2 to 3 ounces in 5 gallons of water. *Bathing dogs*—10 cc per gallon of bath water. *Laundry*—3 to 6 ounces per load, household washer. *Shampooing rugs and upholstery*—3 ounces per gallon. *Air conditioners*—spray undiluted solution on air intake and filter.
Precaution: Harmful if taken internally. See label for more complete information.
How Supplied:
Code: 0819—1 gal.

ODOR-TROL™ TABLETS

Composition: Each tablet contains: Methionine, 200 mg.
Indications: For use in preventing fatty infiltration of the liver and kidneys, as a urinary acidifier, in the control of alkaline urinary calculi and the ammoniacal odor of urine.
Dosage and Administration: ***Dogs and cats***—1 tablet per 15 lbs body weight twice daily.
Warning: Do not treat animals with severe liver or kidney damage.
How Supplied:
Code: 1681—1000 tablets

OVINE-ECTHYMA VACCINE
(Cutter Label)

Composition: Live, dried virus vaccine for immunizing sheep and goats against soremouth.
Dosage and Administration: Scratch or scarify the outer layer of skin on the inside of the flank sufficiently to penetrate the skin but not to draw blood. Sheep and goats —rub 1 drop of rehydrated vaccine well into the sacrified area with the supplied brush. Do not use this product within 12 hours of dipping or spraying. Only healthy animals should be vaccinated.
How Supplied:
Code: 316-85 (100 doses)

PARABOCEPTOL® (Cutter label) BOVINE RHINOTRACHEITIS-PARAINFLUENZA-3 VACCINE-LEPTOSPIRA POMONA BACTERIN

Indication: For the immunization of healthy cattle against bovine rhinotracheitis, parainfluenza-3 virus infections and leptospirosis caused by Leptospira pomona.
Procedure: Rehydrate the dried bovine rhinotracheitis-parainfluenza-3 vaccine by aseptically adding the enclosed Leptospira pomona bacterin.
Dosage and Administration:
DOSE: Cattle of all ages - 2 ml. Inject intramuscularly. Only healthy animals should be vaccinated.
It requires 2 to 3 weeks to acquire full immunity after vaccination, therefore, the best time to vaccinate is at least 2 to 3 weeks before exposure. Calves nursing immune cows will acquire passive (temporary) immunity from the mother via the colostrum and be unresponsive to the vaccine until this immunity has expired; therefore, calves vaccinated under 6 months of age should be revaccinated at 6 months of age or at weaning.
Caution: Shake well until dissolved. Use entire contents immediately after bacterin has been added. Protect the rehydrated vaccine from contamination while inoculating cattle by changing to a sterile needle each time the vial is to be entered for withdrawal of vaccine. Sterilize syringe and needles by boiling. Chemical antiseptics should not be used as they might destroy the virus. Store at 35° to 45° F. (2° to 7° C.) Burn this container and all unused contents. Penicillin,

Continued on next page

Haver—Cont.

streptomycin and a fungistat added to the vaccine as preservatives.
Do not vaccinate within 21 days before slaughter. Do not use in pregnant cows or in calves nursing pregnant cows. Anaphylactoid reactions may occur. Antidote: Epinephrine.
How Supplied:
Code: 241–15 - 20ml (10 doses)
241–25 - 100ml (50 doses)

PARABOCINE (Cutter label) Bovine Rhinotracheitis-Parainfluenza-3 Vaccine

Indications: For the immunization of healthy cattle against bovine rhinotracheitis and parainfluenza-3 virus infections. Rehydrate the dried vaccine by aseptically adding dilutent.
Dosage and Administration: Dose: Cattle of all ages, 2 ml. Inject intramuscularly.
Caution: Shake well until dissolved. Use entire contents when first opened. Do not vaccinate within 21 days before slaughter. Do not use in pregnant cows or in calves nursing pregnant cows. Store at 35° to 45°F. (2° to 7°C.) See carton for more complete directions.
How Supplied:
Code: 289–15 - 20 ml (10 doses)
289-23 - 100 ml (50 doses)

PARA-M™-1 PRESSURIZED SPRAY

Composition: Active Ingredients: Pyrethrins, 0.06%; Piperonyl butoxide technical, 0.48%, equivalent to 0.384% of (butylcarbityl) (6-propylpiperonyl) ether and 0.096% related compounds; Malathion (0,0-dimethydithiophos phate of diethyl mercaptosuccinate), 0.50%; 2,3:4,5-Bis (2-butylene) tetrahydro-2-furalde hyde, 0.24%; Petroleum distillate, 23.67%. Inert ingredients, 75.05%.
Indications: An effective insecticide against fleas, lice and ticks on dogs and cats; a repellent for lice, mosquitos, gnats and deodorant against dog odors.
Dosage and Administration: Hold upright 2 to 4 inches from the animal and direct spray over entire coat. For average size dogs, a 30 second application is usually sufficient; for cats, 10 seconds. Most effective when sprayed against the lay of the hair. Spray must hit ticks directly to kill them. Treatment may be repeated at weekly intervals if required. Also useful for spraying kennels and bedding.
Warning: Harmful if swallowed. Avoid contamination of feed and foodstuffs. Skin contact may be harmful, avoid prolonged breathing of spray mist.
How Supplied:
Code: 0573—13 oz aerosol can.

PARA™ MIST WATER BASE PYRETHRIN LIQUID INSECTICIDE

Indications: A liquid insecticide for control of fleas, lice, and ticks on dogs, puppies, cats, and kittens and as a repellent for flies, mosquitoes, and gnats. Controls stable flies, horse flies, deer flies and face flies on horses.
Directions: Dogs and Cats: To kill fleas, lice, and ticks, cover animal's eyes with hand and with a firm, fast stroke, to get a proper spray mist, spray head, ears, and chest until damp. With fingertips rub into face and around mouth, nose and eyes. Then spray neck, middle, and hind quarters, finishing legs last. For best penetration of spray to the skin, direct spray against the natural lay of the hair. On long-haired dogs rub your hand against the lay of the hair, spraying the ruffled hair directly behind the hand. Make sure spray thoroughly wets ticks. Repeat treatment as needed.
Puppies and Kittens: Do not directly spray nursing puppies or kittens, rather spray only along the animal's back or on your fingertips, then rub the spray into the hair.
Pet Sleeping Quarters: Spray around baseboards, windows, door frames, wall cracks, and local area of floors. If mosquitoes, gnats or flies are present, spray lightly into the air. Repeat as needed. Remove and discard old bedding. Spray new bedding for best results.
Cautions: May cause eye injury. Do not get in eyes. Harmful if swallowed or inhaled. Avoid breathing mist. Avoid contamination of food. Wash hands with soap and water after using.
Practical Treatment: If in eyes: Flush with plenty of water. Get medical attention immediately.
If on skin: Wash off with soap and water.
If inhaled: Remove the victim to fresh air.
Get medical attention if victim displays signs of poisoning.
Pesticide Storage: Protect from freezing.
Container Disposal: Do not reuse empty container. Wrap container in newspaper and put into trash.
E.P.A. Reg. No. 7056-100-11556
E.P.A. Est. No. 7056-TX-1
It is a violation of federal law to use this product in a manner inconsistent with its labeling.
How Supplied:
Code: 0579—16 oz spray bottle

PARA™ POWDER

Composition: Active Ingredients: Carbaryl 5.0%. Inert Ingredients, 95.0%.
Indications: Especially designed for the control of resistant, brown dog ticks, fleas and lice. Pleasantly scented to help eliminate "animal odors".
Caution: Harmful if swallowed or inhaled. Avoid treatment of puppies or kittens less than 4 weeks old. Do not use simultaneously or within a few days of treatment with other cholinesterase inhibiting drugs, pesticides or chemicals.
How Supplied:
Code: 2001—4 oz canister

PARA-PREMISE™ RESIDUAL PREMISE INSECTICIDE

Description: Active Ingredients: Resmethrin* cyclopropane carboxylate (0.10% w/w), chlorpyrifos** (Dursban) (0.50% w/w). Inert Ingredients: 99.40% (w/w).
Indications: A premise insecticide for residual kill of:

Fleas	Spiders
Brown dogs ticks	Ants
Lone star ticks	Fire ants
Cockroaches***	Boxelder bugs
Crickets	Scorpions
Silverfish†	Spider beetles
House flies	Bedbugs
Mosquitoes	Clover mites
Gnats	Millipedes
Flying moths	Centipedes
Earwigs	

***Waterbugs
†Firebrats

Directions: To Control Fleas And Ticks: Contact spray: Thoroughly apply as a spot treatment to infested areas such as pets' beds and resting quarters; nearby cracks and crevices; along and behind baseboards, window and door frames, and localized areas of floors and floor coverings where these pests may be present. Old bedding of pets should be removed and replaced with clean fresh bedding after treatment of pet areas. DO NOT TREAT PETS WITH THIS PRODUCT. Treat pets with a product registered for animal application such as PARA™ MIST or PARA™ MIST Water Base to control the source of flea and tick infestation.
Out-of-Doors: For treatment of localized infestations of fleas and ticks in outdoor areas where there are weeds or bushy non-crop areas, spray infested areas thoroughly. Repeat application as infestations warrant and as reinfestations occur. Refer to product label for specific directions to treat for indicated pests other than fleas and ticks.
This product can be used in non-food areas such as corridors, offices, foyers, lavatories, garages, utility rooms, storage rooms, and basements. Also, for use in dogs kennels, and horse stables.
Refer to the label for cautions about use in food preparation areas.
DO NOT SPRAY ON DOGS OR OTHER ANIMALS OR ON THEIR FOOD OR FOOD ITEMS.
For contact and residual sprays, use this product without diluting. For repeat applications, dilute with equal parts of water.
Storage: Do not store this water-based formulation at temperatures below 32F (0C).
Store product in original container in a locked storage area.
Container Disposal: Do not use empty container. Wrap container and put in trash.
Cautions: Harmful if swallowed. Avoid contact with eyes, skin, or clothing. Wash hands after using. Do not allow children or pets to contact treated surfaces until spray has dried. Remove pets and cover fish aquariums before spraying.
Practical Treatment: If swallowed: Get immediate medical attention. If in eyes or on skin: Flush with plenty of wa-

H

ter for at least 15 minutes. For eyes, get medical attention.
To Physician: Chlorpyrifos is a cholinesterase inhibitor. If signs of cholinesterase inhibition appear, atropine only by injection is an antidote.
Environmental Hazards: This product is toxic to fish, birds, and other wildlife. Birds and other wildlife in treated areas may be killed. Do not apply directly to water. Do not apply where runoff is likely to occur. Do not apply when weather conditions favor drift from areas treated. Do not contaminate water by cleaning of equipment or disposal of wastes.
Physical/Chemical Hazards: Do not apply this water-based product in conduits, motor housings, junction and switch boxes, or other electrical equipment because of possible shock hazard. Do not use on surfaces that can be harmed or stained by water.
EPA Reg. No. 432-569-11556
EPA Est. No. 7056-Tx-1
It is violation of federal law to use this product in a manner inconsistent with its labeling.
*Penick's SBP-1382® brand of resmethrin insecticide. U.S. Patent Nos. 3,465,007 and 3,542,928.
**U.S. Patent No. 3,244,586. Dursban is a Trademark of Dow Chemical Co.
Packaging:
Code 2016—32 oz spray bottle
2017—64 oz spray bottle

PARA™ PYRETHRIN MIST
Liquid Insecticide

Composition: Active Ingredients: Pyrethrins 0.150%, Piperonyl butoxide, technical 1.500%, N-Octyl Bicycloheptene dicarboximide 0.333%, 2,3,4,5-Bis (2-butylene) tetrahydro-2-Furaldehyde 0.200%, Inert Ingredients 97.817%.
Indications: A liquid insecticide for fleas, lice and ticks on dogs and cats, and as a repellent for flies, mosquitoes, and gnats.
Directions: It is a violation of federal law to use this product in a manner inconsistant with its labeling.
Dogs and Cats: To kill fleas, lice, and ticks. Cover animal's eyes with hand and with a firm fast stroke to get a proper spray mist, spray head, ears, and chest until damp. With fingertips rub into face around mouth, nose, and eyes. Then spray neck, middle and hind quarters, finishing legs last. For best penetration of spray to the skin, direct spray against the natural lay of the hair. On long-haired dogs rub your hand against the lay of the hair, spraying the ruffled hair directly behind the hand. Make sure spray thoroughly wets ticks. Repeat treatment as needed.
Puppies and kittens: Spray only along animal's back or on your fingertips and rub in animal's fur.
Pet Sleeping Quarters: Spray around baseboards, windows, door frames, wall cracks and local area of floors. If flies, mosquitoes, or gnats are present, spray lightly into the air. Repeat as needed. The bedding can be sprayed. Concurrent treatment of animals is recommended.
Horses: To repel flies, gnats, and mosquitoes. Apply a light mist sufficient to wet the surface of the hair. To control stable flies, horse flies, deer flies, and face flies, apply at the rate of 2 oz per adult horse. Repeat treatment as needed.
Cautions: Keep out of reach of children. Harmful if swallowed or inhaled. Avoid breathing mist. Avoid contact with eyes. In case of contact immediately flush eyes with plenty of water. Get medical attention if irritation persists. Wash hands with soap and water after using. Avoid treatment of nursing kittens and puppies.
Warning: Flammable. Keep away from heat and open flame. Do not use or store near heat or open flame. Do not allow to freeze. Do not contaminate food or feed. Wrap container and put into trash collection.
How Supplied:
Code: 0580—16 oz pump spray plastic bottle;
0581—64 oz refill
0582—16 oz (with sprayer)

PARA S™-1 AEROSOL
Insecticide

Composition: Pyrethrins, 0.06%; Piperonyl butoxide, technical 0.48%; Methoxychlor, technical 0.50%; Carbaryl 0.50%; 2,3:4,5-bis (2 butylene) tetrahydro-2-furaldehyde, 0.24%. Petroleum distillate, 22.84%. Inert ingredients, 75.38%.
Indications: An effective insecticide against fleas, lice and ticks on dogs and cats; a repellent for lice, mosquitos, gnats and deodorant against dog odors.
Dosage and Administration: Hold container 6 to 12 inches from animal and spray lightly over entire body. Do not spray in eyes. For best penetration of spray to the skin, direct spray against the natural lay of the hair. Repeat if necessary but not more often than once weekly.
Warning: Harmful if swallowed. Avoid contamination of feed and foodstuffs. Skin contact may be harmful, avoid prolonged breathing of spray mist.
How Supplied:
Code: 0583—13 oz aerosol can

PARGUARD™ with HAVLOGEN®
Porcine Parvovirus-Killed Virus

Description: An inactivated and adjuvanted suspension of porcine parvovirus.
Indications: Recommended for use in healthy breeding swine for prevention of porcine parvovirus infection considered to be the major cause of SMEDI disease syndrome (Stillbirths, Mummified fetuses, Embryonic Deaths, Infertility).
Administration and Dosage: Inject a single 2 ml. dose intramuscularly 2 to 6 weeks prior to first breeding.
Caution: Shake well before using. Store at 35° to 45° F (2° to 7°C). Do not vaccinate within 21 days of slaughter. Use entire contents when first opened. Anaphylactoid reactions may occur. *Antidote:* Epinephrine. Contains formaldehyde, Neomycin, Polymyxin B and a fungistat as preservatives.
How Supplied:
Code: 4722–20 ml (10 doses)
4723–100 ml (50 doses)

PROBAN®
(Cythioate)
Oral Insecticide

Description: Proban® contains an organic phosphorous drug (cythioate) and is supplied in tablets containing 30 mg. of cythioate and as a liquid containing 1.6% cythioate.
Indications: Proban® (cythioate) is indicated for flea control on dogs of all ages and sizes.
Administration and Dosage: The recommended dosage represents an average effective dose.
Proban® (cythioate) Tablets, 30 mg.—One tablet orally for each 20 lbs. of body weight once every third day or twice a week.
Proban® (cythioate) Oral Liquid, 1.6%—1 ml. orally for each 10 lbs. of body weight once every third day or twice a week. The liquid, measured by the supplied dispenser, should be applied to the food and mixed thoroughly.
Duration of treatment—The first week of treatment will usually kill more than 95% of the fleas. Additional treatments for several weeks are necessary to remove the fleas that reinfest dogs from their environment.
Mode of Action: Proban® is a cholinesterase inhibitor. It is rapidly absorbed from the gastrointenstinal tract and distributed throughout the body. Fleas are killed by ingesting the drug from the body fluids. Biological data indicate that Proban® is eliminated rapidly.
Overdosage: Proban® (cythioate) has a good margin of safety. Symptoms at 7 times the recommended dosage are muscular tremors and hyperexcitability. At recommended doses there have been few side effects.
The symptoms of toxicity are similar to those described for organic phosphate drugs, namely; vomition, muscular tremors, hyperexcitability, salivation, and diarrhea. When toxic signs occur, treatment with Proban® should be discontinued. Atropine is antidotal.
Contraindications: Do not use in greyhounds. Available data are not adequate to recommend for this breed, which is more sensitive than other breeds to organic phosphate insecticides.
Proban® is a cholinesterase inhibitor. Do not use in animals that are pregnant, sick, under stress, or recovering from surgery.
Do not use this product simultaneously with other drugs, insecticides, pesticides, or chemicals having cholinesterase inhibiting activity, nor within a few days before or after treatment with any other cholinesterase inhibitors.
Warning: Keep out of reach of children.
If swallowed by a human, immediately call a physician, poison control center or hospital emergency room.

Continued on next page

H

Haver—Cont.

How Supplied:
Code: 2264—(100's)—30 mg. Tablets
2273—(1000's)—30 mg. Tablets in 2×5 foil strips
2270—(25 ml.)—1.6% Liquid
2272—(120 ml.)—1.6% Liquid

PRO-KILL™
Insecticide Dip for Dogs

Composition:
ACTIVE INGREDIENTS:
Rotenone 1.1% w/w
Other Cube Extractives 2.2%
Pyrethrins 0.8%
Petroleum Distillate 3.2%
Aromatic Petroleum Solvent 84.7%
INERT INGREDIENTS: 8.0%
To Kill Fleas, Ticks And Lice On Dogs And Premises: (KEEP DILUTED SPRAY AWAY FROM LIGHT).
ON DOGS: DO NOT USE MORE THAN 1 FLUID OUNCE (2 Tbsp.) (30 ml) PER GALLON (3.79 L) *ON PUPPIES:* For fleas and lice, dilute Pro-Kill Insecticide at the rate of 1 fluid ounce (2 Tbsp.) (30 ml) per 1 gallon (3.79 L) of water. [For young animals, use 1/2 fluid ounce (1 Tbsp.) (15 ml) per 1 gallon (3.79 L) of water.] Apply directly to animal as a spray, sponge-on or a wash. Dip until animal's skin is wet. Do not rinse. For ticks, dilute Pro-Kill Insecticide at the rate of 2 fluid ounces (4 Tbsp.) (60 ml) per 1 gallon (3.79 L) of water. [For young animals, use 1 fluid ounce (2 Tbsp.) (30 ml) per 1 gallon (3.79 L) of water.] Apply directly to animal as a spray, sponge-on or a wash. Dip until animal's skin is wet. Do not rinse. Avoid contact with eyes, nose or mouth of animal. To prevent reinfestation, thoroughly spray the animal's living quarters with Pro-Kill Insecticide.
How Supplied:
Code: 2093—8 oz.
2095—1 gal
Refer to label for detailed information.

H

PRO-POWDER™
INSECTICIDAL DUST FOR DOGS AND CATS

Description: Active Ingredients: pyrethrins 1.0%, piperonyl butoxide technical 10.0%, amorphous silica gel 40.0%, petroleum distillate 49.0%.
Indications: A desiccant dust for control of fleas, lice, ticks, ants, cockroaches, silverfish, and spiders. Use directly on dogs and cats and in their surroundings.
Directions: Fleas: Dogs and Cats: Liberally apply powder to the animal, rubbing thoroughly to the skin. Begin with the neck and include the underbody, legs, feet, and the base of the tail. Repeat as necessary.
Surfaces of kennels should be dusted at the rate of one ounce per 50 square feet. Heavily infested lawns, basements, and crawl spaces should be dusted at the rate of one ounce per 60 square feet. Repeat as necessary.
Caution: Keep out of the reach of children. Avoid inhalation.
Disposal: Do not reuse container. Destroy when empty.
Packaging:
Code: 2006—1 oz container

PRO-SPOT™
(Fenthion)

Description: Pro-Spot (fenthion) Solution is a topically applied organophosphate flea-control product combining effective systemic action with convenience of use. Pro-Spot Solution is available as 5.6% and 13.8% concentrations of fenthion in a glycol ether base. Each concentration is available in two sizes, each for a different weight range of dog (See PACKAGING below).
Action: Pro-Spot Solution contains an organophosphate with systemic activity. It will control fleas on the dog at the time of treatment and has good residual activity against many of the fleas that may reinfest the dog after treatment.
Special Note: As with all the flea-control products for dogs, treatment with Pro-Spot Solution must be used with a control program aimed at reducing flea populations and flea breeding areas in the dog's environment (bedding, carpets, yard, etc.).
Indication: Pro-Spot (fenthion) Solution is indicated for the control of fleas on dogs only.
Caution: Federal law restricts this drug to use by or on the order of licensed veterinarian.
Dosage and Administration: Dogs should be weighed prior to selection and use of Pro-Spot Solution to ensure the recommended dose of 4 to 8 mg/kg bodyweight is applied.
Young, growing dogs should be reweighed periodically to ensure the proper size of Pro-Spot Solution is used for repeat treatments. The frequency of repeat treatments depends upon the rate of flea reinfestation. This will vary greatly with season and location. Treatments should not be repeated more often than once every two weeks.
How To Apply:
1. To avoid contact with human skin, gloves may be worn.
2. Cut as indicated to remove one tube from card.
3. Hold applicator tube in an upright position and twist cap to break seal, then remove cap from tube.
4. Invert the tube and use it to part the hair on the dog's back between the shoulder blades.
5. Squeeze the tube firmly twice to apply all the solution *in one spot* directly on the skin. While applying the liquid, the tube should remain in contact with the dog's skin to ensure that the total dose is properly applied Do *not* apply on top of hair as this will result in reduced flea control. Care should be taken to avoid contact of solution with human skin.
6. Wrap empty tube in paper and discard in trash.

Overdosage: Signs of overdosage are neurotoxicity (muscular tremors), weakness, salivation, vomition, and diarrhea.
Client Reminder: Consult veterinarian at first sign of adverse effects.
Precautions: Repeated or prolonged use may cause marked cholinesterase depression. Fenthion is a cholinesterase inhibitor. Do not use this product on dogs at the same time or within 14 days before or after treatment with other cholinesterase inhibiting pesticides, drugs, or chemicals. Do not use with flea or tick collars. Toxicologic interactions between cholinesterase inhibitors and various muscle relaxants and central nervous system depressants have been reported. The use of Pro-Spot with these drugs is not recommended. The following drugs may enhance fenthion toxicity: succinylcholine, procaine, aminoglycosides, and various neuromuscular blocking agents. Do not use more often than once every two weeks.
Treatment with Pro-Spot Solution at two-week intervals should not exceed six months as controlled safety studies of longer duration have not been conducted.
Contraindications: Do not use on puppies under 10 weeks of age. Do not use on sick, stressed, or convalescing dogs.
The safe use of fenthion in breeding males has not been established.
Adverse Reactions: Adverse reactions reported from the use of fenthion in clinical field trials included occasional incidences of vomiting, loose stool, diarrhea, anorexia, and intermittent coughing.
Animal Toxicology: Multiple treatments with Pro-Spot Solution at two-week intervals with 60 mg/kg (7.5X) have induced toxicosis.
Pro-Spot has been applied to female dogs at rates of 18 mg/kg during all stages of reproduction without adverse effects.
Tests indicate no effect on circulating microfilariae or adult *Dirofilaria immitis* with three applications of 40 mg/kg (5X). However, it is reported in the literature that fenthion has been used clinically to reduce numbers of microfilariae.[1]
Concurrent use of diethylcarbamazine formulations and Pro-Spot Solution has been tested with no adverse effects observed.
Anemic, parasitized, young puppies showed an increased incidence of diarrhea following multiple treatments with 10 or 50 mg/kg.
Warning: Keep out of reach of children. *This material contains a cholinesterase inhibitor.* If swallowed by a human being, ***immediately*** *call a physician, poison control center, or hospital emergency room.* Upon medical advice induce vomiting with ipecac syrup. If ipecac is not available, have person drink water then *gently* try to induce vomiting with finger—be extremely careful not to damage throat. May be harmful if absorbed through the skin. Do not get in eyes, on skin, or on clothing. Avoid breathing vapors. Wash thoroughly with soap and warm water after handling. Wash contaminated clothing. Do not contaminate feed or food. If spilled on skin, wash immediately with soap and warm water. If in eyes, rinse immediately with large

amounts of water and obtain medical aid. Skin swab tests on dogs treated with Pro-Spot Solution at greater than label rate revealed that the amount of active ingredient at the treatment site declined rapidly with only 51% of the dose remaining at 15 minutes, 22% at two hours, and less than 3% at eight hours post-treatment. Avoid grooming, direct contact, or unventilated confinement with dog(s) for eight hours after administration of Pro-Spot.

To Physician: Pro-Spot (fenthion) is a cholinesterase inhibitor. If necessary, establish an airway and support respiration. Atropine is antidotal. 2-PAM is also antidotal, but must be administered in conjunction with atropine.

Storage and Disposal: Do not store above 25C (77F).

Keep single dose applicators stored in their original container until use. Do not store near heat or open flame. Wrap empty tubes in paper and discard in trash.

How Supplied: Pro-Spot Solution is supplied in four sizes containing different concentrations and volumes of drug. Single-dose applicator tubes are packaged six per card.

[See table above right.]

NAME	Dog Weight	Concentration	Net Contents	Code No.
Pro-Spot 10 Solution	5–10 lb	5.6%	0.34 ml	2096
Pro-Spot 20 Solution	11–20 lb	5.6%	0.74 ml	2097
Pro-Spot 40 Solution	21–40 lb	13.8%	0.56 ml	2098
Pro-Spot 80 Solution	41–80 lb	13.8%	1.09 ml	2099

(Over 80 lb use two Pro-Spot 80 applicators)

Reference

[1] Kirk-*Current Veterinary Therapy VIII, Small Animal Practice,* p 357; 1983.

REDWOL® with Spur Clostridium Haemolyticum Bacterin (Cutter Label)

Composition: Formalin inactivated whole culture Clostridium haemolyticium bacteria with Spur, which extends the absorption of the vaccine and increases immunity for cattle and sheep.

Dosage and Administration:

Cattle and Sheep: Inject 2 ml intramuscularly. Repeat dose every 5 to 6 months in animal subject to reexposure. Grazing calves may become reinfected. Vaccinate after 3 months of age.

How Supplied:

Code 213—10—20 ml (10 doses)
213—15—100 ml (50 doses)

RINTAL® PASTE (febantel) Equine Anthelmintic

Description: Rintal® Paste can be used as low volume oral paste or a palatable feed additive. Contains: febantel.

Indications: Rintal® (febantel) is indicated for the removal of Large Strongyles *(Strongylus vulgaris, Strongylus edentatus, Strongylus equinus);* Ascarids *(Parascaris equorum*—adult and sexually immature forms); Pinworms *(Oxyuris equi* adult and 4th stage larva) and the various Small Strongyles, in horses, breeding stallions and mares, pregnant mares, foals and ponies.

Dosage: Recommended dosage for febantel in horses is 6 mg/kg (2.73 mg/lb) of body weight. To obtain this dosage, administer Rintal® Paste at the rate of one mark on plunger for each 250 lbs of body weight.

Partially Used Syringes—A partially used syringe, if recapped, may be stored up to 1 year for future use provided the expiration date on the product is not exceeded.

Breeding Stallions and Mares: Rintal® Paste has been tested at multiple and elevated dosages and shown not to produce any adverse effects on fertility, conception, fetal development or pregnancy. Rintal® Paste can be administered safely to either breeding stallions or mares. In addition, pregnant mares may be treated during any stage of pregnancy.

Precaution: For horses maintained on premises where reinfection is likely to occur, retreatment may be necessary. For most effective results, retreat these horses in 6 to 8 weeks.

Note to Veterinarian: Symptoms of Overdosing: Single overdoses of up to 40 times the therapeutic dose have not produced any adverse reactions in test animals. Repeat doses of 8 times the therapeutic dose produced a self-limiting diarrhea after 3 consecutive daily doses. The diarrhea ceased 4 days after the drug was withdrawn. As with any drug, anaphylactic reactions could occur and should be treated symptomatically.

Warning: Keep out of reach of children. Not for human use. Not for use in horses intended for food.

How Supplied:

Code: 0161—6 gm syringe
0162—36 gm multi-dose syringe

Combotel Paste (trichlorfon and febantel) is also available from HAVER.

RINTAL® Suspension (febantel)* Equine Anthelmintic

Indications: Rintal® (febantel) is indicated for the removal of Ascarids (*Parascaris equorum*-adult and sexually immature forms), Pinworms (*Oxyuris equi* adult and 4th stage larvae), Large Strongyles *(Strongyles vulgaris, Strongylus edentatus, Strongylus equinus)* and the various Small Stronglyles in horses, breeding stallions and mares, pregnant mares, foals and ponies.

Contraindications: There are no known contrain dications to the use of this drug.

Dosage: Recommended dosage for febantel in the horse is 6 mg/kg, body weight. Rintal® Suspension may be administered at the rate of 3 ml of suspension for each 100 lbs of body weight (1 oz per 1,000 lbs). This rate will provide a dosage of 6 mg/kg of body weight.

Shake Well Before Using.

Directions for Use: *Stomach Tube*—Rintal® Suspension may be adminstered by stomach tube. Because of the small volume of RintalSuspen sion required when using the suspension alone, care should be taken to flush the stomach tube with enough water after dosing to remove all drug from the tube. For use directions with Combot (brand of trichlorfon) Liquid, see Combinations for Bot Control.

Drench—Rintal® Suspension may be administered as a drench with conventional dose syringes or similar dosing equipment.

Feed—Rintal® Suspension is palatable and readily accepted when administered on the grain ration. The appropriate dose should be poured on a portion of the normal grain ration and mixed well. After consumption of the medicated feed, the remainder of the grain may be fed.

Overdosing—Single overdoses of febantel of up to 40 times the therapeutic dose have not pro duced any adverse reactions in test animals. Three consecutive daily doses of 8 times the therapeutic dose produced self-limiting diarrhea. The diarrhea ceased four days after the drug was withdrawn. As with any drug, anaphylactic reactions could occur and should be treated symptomatically.

Breeding Stallions and Mares—Febantel Suspension has been tested at multiple and elevated dosages and shown not to produce any adverse effects on fertility, conception, fetal development or pregnancy. Febantle Suspension can be administered safely to either breeding stallions or mares. In additon, pregnant mares may be treated during any stage of pregnancy.

Combinations for Bot Control—For broad spectrum control, Rintal® Suspension may be combined with Combot® Liquid** in the ration of 1 part Rintal® to 5 parts Combot and the mixture administered by stomach tube at the rate of 18 ml per 100 lbs of body weight. This will provide a dosage of 6 mg febantel/kg body weight and 40 mg trichlorfon/kg body weight. Note: Always administer the mixture of febantel and trichlorfon following at least a protion of the daily grain ration. Mixtures containing Combot® (trichlorfon) should not be administered on an empty stomach, nor should they be administered as a drench or feed additive. Normal precautions and contraindications for Combot® Liquid as well as Rintal® Suspension must be followed when using the mixture.

Overdoses of febantel and trichlorfon mixtures will produce signs compatible with trichlorfon overdosage.

Continued on next page

Haver—Cont.

Storage of Rintal®/Combot® mixtures—The mixture of Rintal® Suspension and Combot® Liquid may be stored in a tightly closed container at room temperature (below 86F) for 6 days. If not used within 6 days, the mixture stored at room temperature loses its potency and should be discarded. If it is desirable to keep the mixture longer than 6 days, the mixture must be refrigerated in a tightly closed container. When refrigerated within 24 hours of mixing and maintained at 40°F (or below), the mixture will remain stable for 2 months. If after refrigeration the mixture is brought to room temperature, the content should be used within 24 hours or discarded. Stored mixtures should be mixed well by shaking before use.
Precaution: For horses maintained on premises where reinfection in likely to occur, retreatment may be necessary. For most effective results, retreat horses in 6 to 8 weeks.
Caution: Federal Law restricts this drug to use by or on the order of a licensed veterinarian.
Warning: Keep out of the reach of children. Not for human use. Not for use in horses intended for food.
**Combot® (brand of trichlorfon) Equine Anthelmintic (Boticide) is available from Haver Laboratories.
How Supplied:
Code: 0159—26 fl. oz. bottle

ROMPUN® 20 mg/ml INJECTABLE (xylazine)

Composition: Xylazine 2.3%. Inert ingredients: 97.7%.
Indications: For use in dogs and cats for restraint facilitation of minor procedures and preanesthesia.
Dosage and Administration: Inject intravenously 0.5 mg per lb of body weight; intramuscularly or subcutaneously 0.5 to 1 mg per lb of body weight.
Precautions: Do not use in conjunction with tranquilizers. Use with caution when used in addition to barbiturate compounds.
Caution: Federal law restricts this drug to use by or on the order of a licensed veterinarian.
How Supplied:
Code: 6899—20 ml

ROMPUN® 100 mg/ml INJECTABLE (xylazine)

Composition: Xylazine 11.4%. Inert ingredients: 88.6%
Indications: In horses when it is desirable to produce a state of sedation accompanied by a shorter period of analgesia.
Dosage and Administration: Inject intravenously 0.5 ml per 100 lbs body weight (0.5 mg per lb); intramuscularly 1.0 ml per 100 lbs body weight (1 mg per lb) Following injection the animal should be allowed to rest quietly until the full effect has been reached. These dosages produce sedation which is usually maintained for one or two hours, and analgesia which lasts for 15 to 30 minutes.
Precautions: Do not use in conjunction with tranquilizers. Use caution when administering in addition to barbiturate compounds. Avoid intracarotid arterial injection.
Warning: Not for use in food-producing animals.
Caution: Federal law restricts this drug to use by or on the order of a licensed veterinarian.
How Supplied:
Code: 6900—50 ml

SENDRAN® CAT COLLAR

Composition: Active Ingredients: o-Isopropoxy phenyl methylcarbamate + 9.4%, Inert Ingredients: 90.6%.
Indications: For cats of all sizes. Kills fleas and ticks for up to 4 months. Do not use on cats less than 6 weeks of age. Consult product insert for detailed information.
How Supplied:
Code: 2392—1 collar

SENDRAN® FLEA AND TICK SPRAY

Composition: Contents: Active ingredients: o-Isopropoxyphenyl methylcarbamate*, 0.25%; Inert ingredients, 99.75%.
Indications: Provides rapid kill of fleas on dogs and cats and ticks on dogs.
Dosage and Administration: Hold container 6 to 10 inches from the animal and spray lightly over the entire body. Do not spray in eyes. For best penetration of spray to the skin, direct spray against the natural lay of the hair to cause fluffing of the coat. Repeat as necessary but not more often than once weekly. For more prolonged insect control, the animal's bedding should also be treated to help prevent reinfestation.
Caution: Harmful if swallowed, inhaled or absorbed through the skin. Avoid breathing of spray mist and provide adequate ventilation of treatment area. If swallowed, induce vomiting. Contact with skin, eyes or clothing should be avoided. See label for more complete information.
How Supplied:
Code: 0567—13 oz. aerosol can

SENDRAN® INSECTICIDE SHAMPOO

Composition: Active Ingredients: o-Isopropoxy phenyl methylcarbamate, 0.125%. Inert Ingredients, 99.875%.
Indications: For control of fleas on dogs and cats.
Dosage and Administration: Use enough shampoo to form a lather adequate to cover the entire body. Rub the lather into the haircoat and allow it to remain in contact with the skin for a minimum of 5 minutes; then rinse well with warm water. Care should be taken to avoid contact of the shampoo with the animal's eyes. The treatment may be administered twice a week if necessary due to reinfestation.
Caution: Harmful if swallowed, inhaled or absorbed through the skin. Do not get in eyes. Excessive or prolonged contact of the product with the skin should be avoided. Wash thoroughly with soap and warm water after bathing animals. Wash contaminated clothing with soap and hot water before reuse. Avoid contamination of foodstuffs.
Keep out of reach of children.
0-Isopropoxyphenyl methylcabamate is a cholinesterase inhibitor—Atropine sulfate is antidotal. Do not reuse container. Destroy when empty.
How Supplied:
Code: 2086—8 oz. bottle
2087—1 gallon bottle

SENDRAN® Liquid Tick and Flea Dip For Dogs and Cats

Composition: Active Ingredients: o-Isopropoxy phenyl methylcarbamate 8%, Inert Ingredients: 92%.
Caution: Do not treat nursing animals or animals under one month of age. Avoid submerging the mouth, nose and eyes. Do not use diluted dip solution that has been stored for more than 30 days.
Directions: To Kill Ticks and Fleas on Dogs and Cats: Mix two (2) ounces (4 tablespoons) of Sendran® Liquid to one gallon of warm tap water. Measure accurately and stir well. Dip animal in the solution or pour solution on animal until the hair coat is thoroughly wet to the skin. Initial kill of fleas and nonengorged ticks is rapid, but 24 to 48 hours may be required for complete kill of engorged ticks. For residual activity, do not rinse—allow solution to dry on the animal. Apply as needed, but not more often than weekly. To help prevent reinfestation, the animal's bedding and kennel should be treated with a suitable product effective against fleas and ticks. Although ticks are generally not a problem on cats, this product may be used to kill ticks on cats should they become a problem.
Caution: Harmful if swallowed, inhaled or absorbed through the skin.
KEEP OUT OF REACH OF CHILDREN.
o-Isopropoxyphenyl methylcarbamate is a cholinesterase inhibitor. Atropine sulfate is antidotal.
How Supplied:
Code: 2083—8 oz bottle
2089—1 gal bottle

SENDRAN® TICK AND FLEA COLLAR

Composition: Contains: 0-Iosopropoxyphenyl methylcarbamate*.
Indications: Kills ticks and fleas rapidly and controls them any place on the dog's body. Proven effective for many weeks following application.
Dosage and Administration: When either ticks or fleas are a problem the collar should be worn constantly. Replace when effectiveness diminishes. A separate flea collar should not be used.
How Supplied:
Code: 2391—22″ collars
2393—30″ collars

H

SPOTTON® 20% SOLUTION
(Cutter Label)

Composition: Fenthion (phosphorothioate) 20%; Inert ingredients, 80%.
Indications: Ready to use Fenthion for effective control of grubs and as an aid in controlling lice on cattle. Provides systemic kill of grubs before they can cause damage to meat and hides.
Dosage and Administration: Apply 4 cc for each 300 lbs body weight in one spot on the back of the animal. For maximum effectiveness use as soon as possible after heel fly activity has ceased.
Warning: Do not use in conjunction with, or within a few days of, treatment with cholinesterase inhibitors. Do not slaughter cattle within 45 days of treatment.
How Supplied:
Code: 136-62—1 pint bottle
136-60—6 pint bulk pack

STREPGUARD™ with HAVLOGEN

Composition: An adjuvanted, concentrated, enzyme extract of Streptococcus equi, U.S. Patent pending.
Indications: Recommended for use in healthy equines as an aid in the prevention of strangles disease due to Streptococcus equi infection.
Dose: Horses and foals—Inject 2 ml. intramuscularly using aseptic techniques. Repeat in 3–4 weeks. Foals vaccinated when less than 3 months of age should receive an additional 2 ml. dose at 6 months of age or at time of weaning. A 2 ml. booster should be administered annually or prior to expected exposure.
Shake well before using. Store at 35° to 45°F (2° to 7°C). Use entire contents when first opened. Do not vaccinate within 21 days before slaughter. Certain hypersensitive individuals may demonstrate local or generalized reactions, sometimes severe, following exposure to streptococcal proteins. To minimize reactions, free exercise is recommended after injection. Do not use in pregnant mares as safety in pregnant mares has not been established. Anaphylactoid reactions may occur. Antidote: Epinephrine. Contains thimerosal as preservative.
How Supplied:
Code: 4661—2 ml.—1 dose
4662—20 ml.—10 doses

STYQUIN®
Butamisole Hydrochloride Parenteral

Composition: Styquin® (butamisole hydrochloride) Parenteral 1.1% contains 11 mg of butamisole per milliliter. Inactive ingredients: propylene glycol 70.0% and benzyl alcohol 4.0%. The liquid formulation allows for the accurate measurement of the required dosage in a syringe.
Indications: Butamisole hydrochloride is indicated for the treatment of dogs infected with whipworms *(Trichuris vulpis)* and the hookworm *(Ancylostoma caninum)*.
Contraindication: Do not administer this product concurrently with bunamidine hydrochloride. Adverse reactions, sometimes fatal, have been reported when animals are concurrently treated with Styquin® and bunamidine hydrochloride.
Do not administer this product to heartworm positive dogs. Adverse reactions, sometimes fatal, have been reported when Styquin® is administered to heartworm positive dogs.
Do not use in breeding females prior to the third week of pregnancy. The safety of butamisole in pregnant females the first three weeks of gestation has not been determined.
Do not use in puppies less than 8 weeks of age. The safety of butamisole in puppies less than 8 weeks of age has not been established.
Toxicology: Styquin® (butamisole) is well tolerated at the effective therapeutic level. In several laboratory studies, no clinical symptoms of toxicity were noted in dogs that received butamisole injectable at a dose that was three times the recommended dosage (7.2 mg per kg or 3.3 mg/lb body weight), with the exception of one study where death occurred in one of eight dogs in which hepatic and renal lesions were noted. Incoordination, emesis, tremors, convulsions, lateral recumbency, and death occurred in dogs that receive a four-fold overdose in the laboratory.
Dosage and Administration: All animals should be accurately weighed prior to receiving butamisole injectable. The dosage should be calculated on the basis of 0.1 (1/10) ml per pound of body weight. It is recommended that a tuberculin syringe be used for animals weighing less than 5 pounds body weight. Administer subcutaneously, with no more than 3 ml injected at one site. Intramuscular use is not recommended, since pain may be produced at the injection site.
Retreatment: In problem cases, retreatment of whipworms may be necessary in approximately 3 months. For hookworms, a second injection should be given 21 days after initial treatment. Since butamisole is primarily effective against adult hookworms, the initial injection will not affect the larvae. Twenty-one days after the initial injection of butamisole, the larvae will be developed sufficiently to be eliminated by a second injection. To determine the effect of treatment, conduct a fecal examination three days after injection. Periodic fecal examinations should also be conducted because of the possibility of reinfection. Severe hookworm infestation, particularly in puppies, can result in marked anemia and death. Supportive therapy, such as blood transfusions, or injection of iron compounds, may be advisable prior to butamisole therapy.
Adverse Reactions: Occasional swelling, stinging, and irritation have been observed at the injection site. Field reports have indicated adverse reactions and some deaths following treatment of dogs with established *Dirofilaria immitis* infection with butamisole.
Caution: As in the care with other anthelmintics, butamisole injectable should be administered with caution to severely diseased or debilitated animals or to animals with a history of renal or hepatic ailments.
Caution: Federal law restricts this drug to use by or on the order of a licensed veterinarian.
How Supplied:
Code: 2288—50 ml vial

STYRID® CARICIDE®
Oral Liquid, Film Coated Tablets, Edible Tablets

Composition: Styrid® Caricide® Oral Liquid: Each ml contains 50 mg styrylpyridinium chloride and 30 mg of diethylcarbamazine (as base) when administered at the recommended dose. Base is equivalent to citrate.
Styrid® Caricide® Film Coated Tablets: Each tablet will provide 3 mg of diethylcarbamazine citrate and 2.5 mg of styrylpyridinium chloride per pound of body weight when administered at the recommended dose.
Styrid® Caricide® Edible Tablets: Each tablet will provide 3 mg of diethylcarbamazine citrate equivalent and 2.5 mg of styrylpyridinium chloride equivalent per pound body weight when administered at the recommended rate. Active ingredients are absorbed on an inert resin in a palatable matrix.
Indications: Styrid® Caricide® is recommended as an aid in the control of the ascarid, *Toxocara canis,* the hookworm, *Ancylostoma caninum,* aand for the prevention of heartworm disease *(Dirofilaria immitis)* in dogs.
Dosage and Administration: Styrid® Caricide® Oral Liquid-1 ml per 20 lb body weight, administered daily in the food. When given with dry food, add the dose to the water used to moisten the food. When given with canned food, the dose is added and mixed thoroughly.
Styrid® Caricide® Film Coated Tablets-available in four sizes: No. 20 (Peach), No. 35 (yellow), No. 50 (Green), and No. 65 (Purple). Follow the respective dosage on the chart below.
[See table on next page].
Styrid® Caricide® Edible Tablets - available in two sizes: Dosage: No. 20 - One tablet per 20 lbs. body weight, administered daily as a treat or crumbled in food. Dosage: No. 50-One tablet per 50 lbs body weight, administered daily as a treat or crumbled in food.
The first seven days of medication will eliminate intestinal hookworm and large roundworm burdens from most dogs. Continue medication at low daily dosage levels during periods of exposure to hookworm, roundworm and heartworm.
Styrid® Caricide® may be given to dogs of all ages including bitches throughout the reproductive period and following whelping.
Under kennel conditions, place all dogs (including breeding dogs) on treatment. Medication may be started at any time; however, it is best to begin before bitches are bred and then continue through the growing period of the puppies.

Continued on next page

Haver—Cont.

Administration of Styrid® Caricide® in heartworm endemic areas should start one month prior to the beginning of mosquito season, continue daily throughout the season, and for approximately two months therafter. This regimen prevents heartworm disease from arresting the development of the infective larvae of *Dirofilaria immitis.*
Styrid® is active against the adult hookworm *Ancylostoma caninum.* Caricide® is active against the adult roundworm *Toxocara canis* and the infective larval stages of the heartworm *Dirofilaria immitus.*
Residual anthelmintic efficacy following discontinuation of medication is negligible and treatment must be continued for as long as medicinal activity is indicated in light of the potential for extended exposure to, and the life cycles of, *Toxocara canis, Ancylostoma caninum,* or *Dirofilara immitus.*
Overdosage: Styrid® Caricide® has a high margin of safety. This product may cause emesis when inadvertently given at a rate that is five times greater than the recommended dosage.
Precautions: Styrid® Caricide® will not affect hookworm or roundworm encystyed larvae in tissues.
Pups of treated bitches may require individual worming in the first four weeks of life.
Dogs on prophylactic therapy should be examined for the presence of microfilaria every six weekls.
Contraindications: Do not use in dogs that may be harboring adult heartworms. Dogs with established heartworm infections should not receive Styrid® Caricide® until they have been converted to a negative status. Inadvertant administration to heartworm-infected dogs may cause adverse reactions.
Warning: Federal law restricts this drug to use by or on the order of a licensed veterinarian.
Caution: Keep out of reach of children.
Precautions: Indications, Contraindications and Directions May be Abbreviated. Consult Label and Package Information Before Use.
How Supplied: Styrid® Caricide® Oral Liquid Code:
2282 - 8 oz
2284 - 1 gal
2283 - 55 gal
Styrid® Caricide® Film Coated Code:
2276 - (200's) - No. 20 (Peach)
2275 - (200's) - No. 35 (Yellow)
2278 - (100's) - No. 50 (Green)
2277 - (100's) - No. 65 (Purple)
Styrid® Caricide® Edibles Code:
2279 - (100's) - No. 20
2280 - (50's) - No. 50

Tablet	*Daily Dose*	*Body Weight*
No. 20 (Peach)	¼ tablet	5 lbs
No. 20	½ tablet	10 lbs
No. 20	1 Tablet	20 lbs
No. 35 (Yellow)	¼ tablet	17 lbs
No. 35	1 tablet	35 lbs
No. 50 (Green)	½ tablet	25 lbs
No. 50	1 tablet	50 lbs
No. 65 (Purple)	½ tablet	32 lbs
No. 65	1 tablet	65 lbs
No. 65	1½ tablet	97 lbs

SUPER-TET®
Tetanus Toxoid with Havlogen®

Composition: Tetanus toxoid which is highly purified and highly concentrated to yield a finished product high in antigenicity but low in tissue reactivity. Havlogen adjuvant is then added to facilitate production of superior immune titers.
Dosage and Administration: For initial immunization: ***Horses*** —1 ml.; ***Sheep*** —½ ml. Inject intramuscularly and repeat in 3 to 4 weeks. A booster dose should be administered annually. Mature ewes should be vaccinated at least one month before lambing.
How Supplied:
Code: 4786—1 dose (1 ml)
4791—10 doses (10 ml)

TETANUS ANTITOXIN
(Bayvet Label)
Equine Origin

Indication: For use in the prevention and treatment of tetanus. Tetanus Antitoxin is derived from the blood of horses hyperimmunized with the toxin of Clostridum tetani.
Precautions: Keep refrigerated at 35° to 45°F. Avoid freezing. Entire contents of a vial should be used at time when first opened. Do not inject in food producing animals within 21 days before slaughter. In case of anaphylactoid reactions, administer epinephrine or equivalent.
Equine serum hepatitis (Theiler's disease), an acute hepatic disease of the horse, has been reported sporadically with prior administration of biological products of equine serum origin in horses. The cause of this disease is unknown. Until more scientific knowledge is available as to the true cause of the equine serum hepatitis, Tetanus Antitoxin, as well as all other products of equine serum origin, when administered to horses must be used with the full awareness that there may be some risk of this disease within 30 to 90 days following injection.
Dosage & Administration: The recommended prophylactic dose for horses and other large animals is 1500 units administered intramuscularly or subcutaneously. For therapeutic dose administer 10,000 to 50,000 units intramuscularly or intravenously, and repeat as indicated.
Contains Phenol and Thimerosal as preservatives.
Packaging: Code: 320-40 (1500 units)

THRAXOL®-2
(Cutter Label)
anthrax spore vaccine

Description: A suspension of live anthrax spores (from a nonencapsulated strain) in a diluent containing saponin.
Indication: Recommended for prevention of anthrax in cattle, horses, sheep, goats and swine.
Dosage and Administration DOSE: Cattle and horses - 2 ml.; Sheep, goats and swine - 1 ml. Inject subcutaneously.
Caution: Shake well before using. Store at 35° to 45° F. (2° to 7° C.). Do not freeze. Do not vaccinate within 6 weeks before slaughter. Use entire contents when first opened. Burn this container and all unused contents. Anaphylactoid reactions may occur. Antidote: Epinephrine. See insert for complete directions.
How Supplied:
Code: 235-16 20 ml (10 doses)
235-23 100 ml (50 doses)

TIGUVON® POUR-ON
(Cutter Label)
Cattle Insecticide (3%)

Composition: Contains: Fenthion phosphorothioate, 3%: Inert ingredients, 97%.
Indications: For effective control of grubs and lice on cattle. No dilutions or mixing required.
Dosage and Administration: Apply ½ ounce per 100 lbs body weight along the back line of the animal. For maximum effectiveness use as soon as possible after heel fly activity has ceased.
Caution: Do not use milk for human consumption for 28 days after treatment. Do not slaughter cattle within 35 days following a single treatment or if a second application is made for louse control within 45 days of the second treatment. Do not slaughter swine within 14 days of treatment. Do not use in conjunction with, or within a few days of treatment of cholinesterase inhibitors.
How Supplied:
Code: 136-51—1 gal cans
Dippers—Supplied with Pour-Ons.

TIGUVON® POUR-ON
(Cutter Label)
Swine Insecticide

Active Ingredient:
fenthion 3%
Inert Ingredients: 97%
100%
Directions For Use: A single application placed on the backline of swine.
Indication: Controls lice.
Dosage and Administration: Apply Tiguvon Pour-On at the rate of ½ fluid ounce (15cc) per 100 pounds of body weight.
Contraindications and Restrictions: Do not treat sick, convalescent or stressed animals.

Warning: DO NOT SLAUGHTER SWINE WITHIN 14 DAYS OF TREATMENT.
Tiguvon (Brand of fenthion) is a cholinesterase inhibitor. Do not use this product on animals simultaneously or within a few days before or after treatment with or exposure to cholinesterase inhibiting drugs, pesticides or chemicals.
Warning: May be poisonous if swallowed. Harmful if absorbed through the skin. Do not get in eyes or on skin. Wash thoroughly with soap and warm water after handling. Wash contaminated clothing with soap and hot water before reuse.
Caution: Do not contaminate feed or food. Keep out of reach of children.
This material contains a cholinesterase inhibitor. If poisoning should occur, obtain prompt medical aid.
To Physician and Veterinarian—Atropine is antidotal. 2-PAM is also antidotal and may be administered in conjunction with atropine.
How Supplied:
Code: 137-05-1 qt.
137-10-gal.

VELTRIM®
(clotrimazole)
Dermatologic Cream

Composition: Veltrim® (clotrimazole) Cream is a topical preparation for the treatment of fungus infections in dogs and cats.
Each gram contains 10 gm of clotrimazole in a base containing sorbitan monostearate, polysorbate 60, spermaceti, cetostearyl alcohol, octyldodecanol, benzyl alcohol and purified water.
Indications: Veltrim® (clotrimazole) Dermatologic Cream is indicated for the treatment of fungal infections of dogs and cats caused by *Microsporum canis* and *Trichophyton mentagrophytes.*
Dosage and Administrations:
Apply ¼" ribbon per square inch of lesion once daily for 2 to 4 weeks.
Precaution: Because of the nature of the inert ingredients, this cream is not intended for use in the eye.
How Supplied:
Code: 1996—15 g tube (boxes of 12)

VERCOM™ PASTE
Broad Spectrum* Anthelmintic Paste for Dogs and Cats

Contains: 3.4% febantel and 0.34% praziquantel.
Description: Vercom Broad Spectrum Anthelmintic Paste contains 34 mg febantel and 3.4 mg praziquantel per gram (ml) formulated for oral administration to dogs, puppies, cats, and kittens for removal of nematode and cestode intestinal parasites.
Action: Febantel is primarily active against nematode parasites. It is rapidly absorbed and metabolized in the animal. Current evidence suggests that the parasite's energy metabolism is blocked, leading to energy exchange breakdown and inhibited glucose uptake.
Praziquantel is also rapidly absorbed, metabolized in the liver, and rapidly eliminated from the body. With cestodes, it produces a rapid alteration of the permeability of cell membranes, resulting in a contraction of the tapeworm musculature and detachment. It alters the integrity of the integument making it susceptible to damage by the host's defense mechanisms. Additionally, praziquantel inhibits glucose uptake and promotes glycogen breakdown. Following treatment, only partially digested fragments of the cestode may be seen.
Indications: Vercom (Febantel and Praziquantel) Paste is indicated for the removal of the following nematode and cestode parasites. Dogs and Puppies —*Ancylostoma caninum, Trichuris vulpis, Toxocara canis, Dipylidium caninum, and Taenia pisiformis.*
Cats and Kittens—*Ancylostoma tubaeforme, Toxocara cati, Dipylidium caninum, and Taenia taeniaeformis.*

Directions:

Dosage: The animal to be treated should be accurately weighed prior to calculating the amount of paste to be given. The dosage is based on a daily rate of one gram of paste for each 7.5 lb body weight for mature dogs and cats (10 mg febantel and 1 mg praziquantel per kg) and one gram of paste for each 5 lb body weight for puppies and kittens (15 mg febantel and 1.5 mg. praziquantel per kg). The same dose is to be given once daily for three days.
Note: One gram is equivalent to one ml of paste.
Filling Syringes for Dispensing:
The use of clean disposable syringes provides an accurate and convenient means of paste dosing. Use a clean disposable syringe for each animal.
The paste may be transferred for daily dosing from the 36-g Vercom (Febantel and Praziquantel) Paste syringe into an appropriate size disposable syringe. One syringe for each of the three daily doses is recommended. Dispensing labels for the disposable syringes are provided.
Begin by removing the cap to the 36-g syringe, backing the rowel nut away from the barrel and pushing the plunger until paste begins to emerge.
Next, insert the tip of the selected disposable syringe into the tip of the 36-g syringe and withdraw the correct amount of paste into the disposable syringe. One gram of paste is equivalent to 1 ml. Exercise care to avoid letting air pockets interfere with the accuracy of the fill.
Administration: Vercom Paste has been developed for administration directly by mouth or by mixing in food. For administration directly *by mouth,* insert the disposable syringe containing the correct daily dose into the side of the mouth between the teeth. Administer the entire daily dose on the base of the tongue. For administration *in the food,* mix the proper daily dose of paste into a small portion of food immediately prior to routine feeding.
Mature dogs and cats may be dosed either directly by mouth or in the food with equal effect upon parasites. Fasting or feeding is not necessary for mature dogs and cats. Puppies and kittens less than six months old ***must be dosed on a full stomach*** and thus should be dosed by mouth only.
Precaution: Clients should be instructed in the measures to be taken to prevent reinfection. If preventive steps are not taken, reinfection is likely to occur such as with *Dipylidium caninum* where fleas, the intermediate host, must be removed from the animal and its environment.
Contraindications: DO NOT USE IN PREGNANT ANIMALS. Elevated treatments (six consecutive days with three times the labeled dosage rate) to dogs and cats in early pregnancy induced an increased incidence of abortion and fetal abnormalities.
Safety and Toxicity: Controlled safety evaluations have been conducted with Vercom Paste. Two series of treatments at a 14-day interval, with each series consisting of six consecutive daily doses of 150 mg febantel and 15 mg praziquantel/kg did not produce drug-induced deaths in either dogs or cats. Clinical signs observed at this excessive rate (15X for mature dogs and cats, 10X for puppies and kittens) included transient salivation, vomition, diarrhea, and loss of appetite. No significant clinical chemistry, hematologic or histopathologic changes occurred. There was no effect on cholinesterase values.
Vercom Paste can cause adverse effects when administered at elevated doses during pregnancy in dogs and cats. No effect was observed on spermatogenesis or libido.
Testicular and prostatic hypoplasia was observed in dogs when febantel was administered at dosage rates of 5 and 10 mg/kg for 90 consecutive days.
Twelve of 514 dogs (2.3%) and nine of 125 cats (7.2%) exhibited side effects during clinical trials. In dogs, these consisted of four cases of salivation, four cases of emesis or gagging, two cases of diarrhea or soft stool, and two cases of reduced appetite. In cats, the effects consisted of six cases of salivation, and one case each of vomition, depression, and paste rejection. All the drug related effects seen were mild and self-limiting.
Caution: Federal (U.S.A.) law restricts this drug to use by or on the order of a licensed veterinarian.
Warning: Keep out of the reach of children. Wash hands thoroughly with soap and warm water immediately after handling.
How Supplied:
Code 1836—36 gm Syringes (6 per box)
Code 1842—HAVER Syringe Kit
Code 1845—Cartons of 4.8 gm Syringes (12 per box)

VIBRIO-BAC™
Vibrio Fetus Bacterin

Composition: Inactivated Havlogen® adjuvanted whole culture of Vibrio fetus venerealis to be used in the prevention of bovine infertility caused by infection with Vibrio fetus venerealis.

Continued on next page

H

Haver—Cont.

Dosage and Administration: Cattle —2 ml. Inject intramuscularly using strict aseptic techniques. Vaccinate at least 30 days before breeding —repeat annually. A second dose at 2 to 4 weeks is advised for infected herds and in endemic areas.
How Supplied:
Code: 4826—20 ml (10 doses)
4827—100 ml (50 doses)

VIBRIO-BAC™ -H-L5 with HAVLOGEN®

Description: A chemically inactivated, HAVLOGEN® adjuvanted suspension of *Vibrio fetus, Leptospira-canicola-grippotyphosa-hardjo-icterohaemorrhagie-pomona* and *Clostridium haemolvticum.* Contains formaldehyde as preservative.
Indications: For use in healthy cattle as an aid in preventing Vibriosis, Leptospirosis and Bacillary Hemaglobinuria (Red Water).
Administration And Dosage: Inject 5 ml. intramuscularly using strict aseptic techniques. Vaccinate at least 30 days before breeding and repeat annually. Revaccination against Vibriosis and Leptospirosis is recommended at 2 to 4 weeks for infected herds and in endemic areas. Revaccinate for Bacillary hemoglobinuria (Red Water) every 5 to 6 months in animals subject to re-exposure.
Caution: Shake well before using Store at 35° to 45° F (2° to 7° C). Use entire contents when first opened. Do not vaccinate within 21 days before slaughter. Anaphylactoid reactions may occur. *ANTIDOTE:* Epinephrine.
Packaging:
Code: 4838 - 50 ml (10 doses)
4840 - 250 ml (50 doses)

VIBRIO-BAC™-L with Havlogen® Vibrio Fetus-Leptospira Pomona Bacterin

Composition: A chemically inactivated, detoxified and Havlogen adjuvanted bivalent bacterin containing Vibrio (campylobacter) fetus and Leptospira pomona. One 2 ml. IM dose is recommended as an aid in the prevention of infertility, abortions, prolonged conceptions and economic cattle losses caused by these diseases.
Dosage and Administration: 2 ml. injected intramuscularly. Vaccinate at least 30 days before breeding and repeat annually. A second dose at 2 to 4 weeks is advised for infected herds and in endemic areas.
How Supplied:
Code: 4831—20 ml (10 doses)
4832—100 ml (50 doses)

VIBRIO-BAC™ L5 with HAVLOGEN®

Vibrio fetus and *leptospria canicola-grippotyphosa - harjo icterohaemorrhagiae-pomona bacterin*
Description: A chemically inactivated and adjuvanted suspension of *Vibrio fetus* and *Leptospira canicola, grippotyphosa, hardjo, icterohaemorrhagiae* and *pomona.*
Indications: For use in healthy cattle as an aid in the prevention of disease caused by *Vibrio fetus venerealis* and *Leptospira canicola, grippotyphosa, hardjo, icterohaemorrhagiae* and *pomona.*
Dosage and Administration: Inject 5 ml intramuscularly using strict aseptic techniques. Vaccinate at least 30 days before breeding and repeat annually. A second dose at two to four weeks is advised for infected herds and in endemic areas.
Caution: Shake well before using. Store at 35 to 40F (2 to 7C). Use entire contents when first opened. Do not vaccinate within 21 days before slaughter. Anaphylactoid reactions may occur. *Antidote:* Epinephrine.
How Supplied:
Code: 4836—50 ml—(10 doses)
4837—250 ml—(50 doses)

WART VACCINE

Composition: Formalin-inactivated bovine wart tissue suspension as an aid in prophylactic treatment of warts in cattle.
Dosage and Administration: Inject subcutaneously in two or more sites and repeat 3 to 5 weeks. **Calves** —10 to 15 ml.; **Cattle** —15 to 25 ml.
How Supplied:
Code: 4830—50 ml.

Hoechst-Roussel Agri-Vet Company
SOMERVILLE, NJ 08876

LASIX®
(furosemide)
A diuretic-saluretic for prompt relief of edema.
For Veterinary Use Only

Caution: Federal law restricts this drug to use by or on the order of a licensed veterinarian.
Description: Lasix® (furosemide) is a chemically distinct diuretic and saluretic pharmacodynamically characterized by the following:
1) A high degree of efficacy, low-inherent toxicity and a high therapeutic index.
2) A rapid onset of action and of comparatively short duration.[1,2]
3) A pharmacological action in the functional area of the nephron, i.e., proximal and distal tubules and the ascending limb of the loop of Henle.[2–4]
4) A dose-response relationship and a ratio of minimum to maximum effective dose range greater than tenfold.[1,2]
5) It may be administered orally or parenterally. It is readily absorbed from the intestinal tract and well tolerated. The intravenous route produces the most rapid diuretic response.

Lasix® (furosemide), a diuretic, is an anthranilic acid derivative with the following structural formula: Generic name: Furosemide (except in United Kingdom - frusemide). Chemical name: 4-chloro-N-furfuryl-5-sulfamoylanthranilic acid).
Actions: The therapeutic efficacy of Lasix® (furosemide) is from the activity of the intact and unaltered molecule throughout the nephron, inhibiting the reabsorption of sodium not only in the proximal and distal tubule but also in the ascending limb of the loop of Henle. The prompt onset of action is a result of the drug's rapid absorption and a poor lipid solubility. The low lipid solubility and a rapid renal excretion minimize the posibility of its accumulation in tissues and organs of crystalluria. Lasix® (furosemide) has no inhibitory effect on carbonic anhydrase or aldosterone activity either in presence of acidosis or alkalosis.[1–7]
Indications:
Dogs, Cats, & Horses: Lasix® (furosemide) is an effective diuretic possessing a wide therapeutic range. Pharmacologically it promotes the rapid removal of abnormally retained extracellular fluids. The rationale for the efficacious use of diuretic therapy is determined by the clinical pathology producing the edema.
Lasix® (furosemide) is indicated for the treatment of edema (pulmonary congestion, ascites) associated with cardiac insufficiency and acute noninflammatory tissue edema.
The continued use of heart stimulants, such as digitalis or its gylcosides is indicated in cases of edema involving cardiac insufficiency.
Cattle: Lasix® (furosemide) is indicated for the treatment of physiological parturient edema of the mammary gland and associated structures.
Contraindications—Precautions:
Lasix® (furosemide) is a highly effective diuretic-saluretic which if given in excessive amounts may result in dehydration and electrolyte imbalance. Therefore, the dosage and schedule may have to be adjusted to the patient's needs. The animal should be observed for early signs of electrolyte imbalance, and corrective measures administered. Early signs of electrolyte imbalance are: increased thirst, lethargy, drowsiness or restlessness, fatigue, oliguria, gastro-intestinal disturbances and tachycardia. Special attention should be given to potassium levels. Lasix® (furosemide) may lower serum calcium levels and cause tetany in rare cases of animals having an existing hypocalcemic tendency.[10–14]
Although diabetes mellitus is a rarely reported disease in animals, active or latent diabetes mellitus may on rare occasions be exacerbated by Lasix® (furosemide). While it has not been reported in animals the use of high doses of salicyl-

ates, as in rheumatic diseases, in conjunction with Lasix® (furosemide) may result in salicylate toxicity because of competition for renal excretory sites.

Transient loss of auditory capacity has been experimentally produced in cats following intravenous injection of excessive doses of Lasix® (furosemide) at a very rapid rate.[15–17]

Electrolyte balance should be monitored prior to surgery in patients receiving Lasix® (furosemide). Imbalances must be corrected by administration of suitable fluid therapy.

Lasix® (furosemide) is contraindicated in anuria. Therapy should be discontinued in cases of progressive renal disease if increasing azotemia and oliguria occur during the treatment. Sudden alterations of fluid and electrolyte imbalance in an animal with cirrhosis may precipitate hepatic coma, therefore observation during period of therapy is necessary. In hepatic coma and in states of electrolyte depletion, therapy should not be instituted until the basic condition is improved or corrected. Potassium supplementation may be necessary in cases routinely treated with potassium-depleting steroids.

Warnings: Lasix® (furosemide) is a highly effective diuretic and if given in excessive amounts as with any diuretic may lead to excessive diuresis which could result in electrolyte imbalance, dehydration and reduction of plasma volume enhancing the risk of circulatory collapse, thrombosis, and embolism. Therefore, the animal should be observed for early signs of fluid depletion with electrolyte imbalance, and corrective measures administered. Excessive loss of potassium in patients receiving digitalis or its glycosides may precipitate digitalis toxicity. Caution should be exercised in animals administered potassium-depleting steroids.

It is important to correct potassium deficiency with dietary supplementation. Caution should be exercised in prescribing enteric-coated potassium tablets.

There have been several reports in human literature, published and unpublished, concerning nonspecific small-bowel lesions consisting of stenosis, with or without ulceration, associated with the administration of enteric-coated potassium tablets alone or when they are used with nonenteric-coated thiazides, or certain other oral diuretics. These small-bowel lesions may have caused obstruction, hemorrhage, and perforation. Surgery was frequently required, and deaths have occurred. Available information tends to implicate enteric-coated potassium salts, although lesions of this type also occur spontaneously. Therefore, coated potassium-containing formulations should be discontinued immediately if abdominal pain, distention, nausea, vomiting, or gastrointestinal bleeding occurs.

Human patients with known sulfonamide sensitivity may show allergic reactions to Lasix® (furosemide); however, these reactions have not been reported in animals.

Sulfonamide diuretics have been reported to decrease arterial responsiveness to pressor amines and to enhance the effect of tubocurarine. Caution should be exercised in administering curare or its derivatives to patients undergoing therapy with Lasix® (furosemide) and it is advisable to discontinue Lasix® (furosemide) for one day prior to any elective surgery.

Warning:

Cattle: Milk taken from animals during treatment and for 48 hours (four milkings) after the last treatment must not be used for food. Cattle must not be slaughtered for food within 48 hours following last treatment.

Horses: Do not use in horses intended for food.

Dosage and Administration: The usual dosage of Lasix® (furosemide) is 1 to 2 mg/lb. body weight (approximately 2.5 to 5 mg/kg). The lower dosage is suggested for cats. Administer once or twice daily at 6 to 8-hour intervals either orally, intravenously, or intramuscularly. A prompt diuresis usually ensues from the initial treatment. Diuresis may be initiated by the parenteral administration of Lasix® (furosemide) injection and then maintained by oral administration.

The dosage should be adjusted to the individual's response. In severe edematous or refractory cases the dose may be doubled or increased by increments of 1 mg per pound body weight. The established effective dose should be administered once or twice daily. The daily schedule of administration can be timed to control the period of micturition for the convenience of the client or veterinarian. Mobilization of the edema may be most efficiently and safely accomplished by utilizing an intermittent daily dosage schedule, i.e., every other day or 2 to 4 consecutive days weekly.

Diuretic therapy should be discontinued after reduction of the edema, or maintained after determining a carefully programmed dosage schedule to prevent recurrence of edema. For long-term treatment, the dose can generally be lowered after the edema has once been reduced. Re-examination and consultations with client will enhance the establishment of a satisfactorily programmed dosage schedule. Clinical examination and serum BUN, CO and electrolyte determinations should be performed during the early period of therapy and periodically thereafter, especially in refractory cases. Abnormalities should be corrected or the drug temporarily withdrawn.

Dosage: Oral Tablet Dog and Cat

One-half to one 50 mg scored tablet per 25 pounds body weight.

One 12.5 mg tablet per 5 to 10 pounds body weight.

Administer once or twice daily, permitting a 6- to 8-hour interval between treatments. In refractory or severe edematous cases, the dosage may be doubled or increased by increments of 1 mg per pound body weight as recommended in preceding paragraphs, "Dosage and Administration."

Oral Bolus Cattle

One bolus (2g) per cow daily. Treatment not to exceed 48 hours postparturition.

Oral Syrup Dog Only

One to two ml (10 to 20 mg furosemide) per 10 lb body weight (approximately 2.5 to 5 mg/kg).

Parenteral Dog and Cat

Administer intramuscularly or intravenously ¼ to ½ ml per 10 pounds body weight. Administer once or twice daily, permitting a 6- 8-hour interval between treatments. In refractory or severe edematous cases, the dosage may be doubled or increased by increments of 1 mg per pound body weight as recommended in preceding paragraphs, "Dosage and Administration."

Horse

The individual dose is 250 to 500 mg (5 to 10 ml) administered intramuscularly or intravenously once or twice daily at 6-8-hours intervals until desired results are achieved. The veterinarian should evaluate the degree of edema present and adjust dosage schedule accordingly. Do not use in horses intended for food.

Cattle

The individual dose administered intramuscularly or intravenously is 500 mg (10 ml) once daily or 250 mg (5 ml) twice daily at 12-hour intervals. Treatment not to exceed 48 hours postparturition. Milk taken from animals during treatment and for 48 hours (four milkings) after the last treatment must not be used for food. Cattle must not be slaughtered for food within 48 hours following last treatment.

How Supplied Parenteral:

Lasix® (furosemide) Injection 5% (50 mg/ml)

Each ml contains: 50 mg furosemide as a diethanolamine salt preserved and stabilized with myristylgammapicolinium chloride 0.02%, EDTA sodium 0.1%, sodium sulfite 0.1% with sodium chloride 0.2 in distilled water, pH adjusted with sodium hydroxide. Available in 50 ml multidose vials.

Tablets: 50 mg (scored) tablets

Each tablet contains 50.0 milligrams of furosemide.

12.5 mg tablets

Each tablet contains 12.5 milligrams of furosemide. Available in bottles of 100 and 500 tablets.

Bolus:

Lasix® (furosemide) 2g. Bol-O-Tabs®

Each bolus contains 2g. of furosemide. Available in boxes with 12 Bol-O-Tabs® each.

Syrup:

Lasix® (furosemide) Syrup 1% (10 mg/ml).

Available in 60 ml bottles with calibrated pipette.

Toxicology Acute Toxicity:

The following table illustrates low acute toxicity of Lasix® (furosemide) in three different species. (Two values indicate two different studies.)

LD_{50} of Lasix® (furosemide) in mg/kg body weight

Species	Oral	Intra-venous

Continued on next page

H

Hoechst-Roussel—Cont.

Mouse	1050-1500	308
Rat	2650-4600*	680
Dog	>1000 and >4640	>300 and >464

*NOTE: The lower value for the rat oral LD was obtained in a group of fasted animals; the higher figure is from a study performed in fed rats.

Toxic doses lead to convulsions, ataxia, paralysis and collapse. Animals surviving toxic dosages may become dehydrated and depleted of electrolytes due to the massive diuresis and saluresis.

Chronic Toxicity: Chronic toxicity studies with Lasix® (furosemide) were done in a one-year study in rats and dogs. In a one-year study in rats, renal tubular degeneration occurred with all doses higher than 50 mg/kg. A six-month study in dogs revealed calcification and scarring of the renal parenchyma at all doses above 10 mg/kg.

Reproductive Studies: Reproductive studies were conducted in mice, rats and rabbits. Only in rabbits administered high doses (equivalent to 10 to 25 times the recommended average dose of 2 mg/kg for dogs, cats, horses, and cattle) of furosemide during the second trimester period did unexplained maternal deaths and abortions occur. The administration of Lasix® (furosemide) is not recommended during the second trimester of pregnancy.

References:

1. Timmerman, R.J., Springman, F.R., and Thoms, R.K. Evaluation of Furosemide, a New Diuretic Agent. *Current Therapeutic Research* 6(2):88–94, February 1964
2. Muschaweck, R., and Hajdu, P.: Die salidiuretische Wirksamkeit der Chlor-N-(2-furylmethyl)-5-sulfamyl-anthranilsaure. *Arzneimittel-Forschung* 14:44–47, 1964. (The Saluretic Action of 4-Chloro-N-(2-furylmethyl)-5-sulfamyl-anthranilic acid).
3. Suki, W.; Rector, Jr., F.C., and Seldin, D.W.: The Site of Action of Furosemide and Other Sulfonamide Diuretics in the Dog. *Journal of Clinical Investigation* 44(9):1458–1469, 1965
4. Deetjen, P.: Mikropunktionsuntersuchungen zur Wirkung von Furosemid. *Pflugers Archiv fuer die Gesamte Physiologie* 284:184–190, 1965 (Micropuncture Studies of the Action of Furosemide)
5. Berman, L.B. and Ebrahimi, A.: Experiences with Furosemide in Renal Disease. *Proceedings of the Society for Experimental Biology and Medicine* 118:333–336, February 1965.
6. Schmidt, H.A.E.: "Animal Experiments with S35 Tagged Lasix in Canine and Bovine." Radio-chemical Pharmacological Laboratory. Farbwerke Hoechst, Frankfurt, West Germany.
7. Haussler, A., and Hajdu, P.: "Methods Biological Identification and Results of Studies on Absorption, Elimination and Metabolism." Research Laboratories, Farbwerke Hoechst, Frankfurt, West Germany.
8. Wilson, A.F., and Simmons, D.H. Diuretic Action in Hypochloremic Dogs. *Clinical Research* 14(1):158, January 1966.
9. Hook, J.B., and Williamson, H.E.: Influence of Probenecid and Alterations in Acid-Base Balance of the Saluretic Activity of Furosemide. *Journal of Pharmacology and Experimental Therapeutics* 149(3):404–408, 1965.
10. Antoniou, L.D.; Eisner, G.M.; Slotkoff, L.M., and Lilienfield, L.S.: Sodium and Calcium Transport in the Kidney. *Clincial Research* 15(4):476, December 1967.
11. Duarte, C.G.: Effects of Furosemide (F) and Ethacrynic Acid (ETA) on the Renal Clearance of Phosphate (Cp) Ultrafilterable Calcium (CUfCA) and Magnesium (CUfMg). *Clincial Research* 15(2):357, April 1967.
12. Duarte, C.G.: Effects of Ethacrynic Acid and Furosemide on Urinary Calcium, Phosphate and Magnesium. *Metabolism* 17:867–876, October 1968.
13. Nielsen, S.P., Anderson, O., and Steven, K.E.: Magnesium and Calcium Metabolism during Prolonged Furosemide (Lasix) Administration to Normal Rats. *Acta Pharmacol. et Toxicol.* 1969, 27:469–479.
14. Reimold, E.W.: The Effect of Furosemide on Hypercalcemia Due to Dihydrotachysterol. *Metabolism* 21(7), July 1972.
15. Brown, R.D., and McElwee, Jr., T.W.: Effects of Intra-Arterially and Intravenously Administered Ethacrynic Acid and Furosemide on Cochlear N, in Cats. *Toxicology and Applied Pharmacology* 22:589–594, 1972.
16. Mathog, R.H., Thomas, W.G., and Hudson, W.R.: Ototoxicity of New and Potent Diuretics. *Archives of Otolaryngology* 92(1):7–13, July 1970.
17. Mathog, R.H. and Matz, G.J.: Ototoxic Effects of Ethacrynic Acid. *Annals of Otolaryngology* Vol. 81, 1972.

Lasix® (furosemide)
Tablets 12.5 mg and 50.0 mg
Manufactured by:
Hoechst-Roussel Pharmaceuticals Inc.
Somerville, N.J. 08876

Lasix® (furosemide)
Injection 5%
Manufactured by:
Taylor Pharmacal Co.
Decatur, Illinois
62525

Lasix® (furosemide)
Bol-O-Tabs®
Manufactured by:
Hoechst-Roussel Pharmaceuticals Inc.
Somerville, N.J. 08876

Lasix® (furosemide)
Syrup 1%
Manufactured by:
Hoechst-Roussel
Pharmaceuticals Inc.
Somerville, N.J. 08876
Hoechst-Roussel Agri-Vet Company
Somerville, N.J. 08876

PANACUR®
(fenbendazole) For Use In Horses
Panacur® (fenbendazole) Granules 22.2% (222 mg/g)
Panacur® (fenbendazole) Suspension 10% (100 mg/ml)
Panacur® (fenbendazole) Paste 10% (100 mg/g)

Indications: Equine dewormer for control of large strongyles, small strongyles, pinworms and ascarids.

Dosage: 5 mg/kg (2.3 mg/lb) for the control of large strongyles (*Strongylus edentatus, S. equinus, S. vulgaris*), small strongyles (*Cyathostomum* spp., *Cylicocylus* spp., *Cylicostephanus* spp., *Tridontophorus* spp.) and pinworms (*Oxyuris equi*).

Example: Suspension - 2.3 ml/100 lb; 23 ml/1000 lb
Granules - One 5g pkg/450-480 lbs

10 mg/kg (4.6 mg/lb) for the control of ascarids (*Parascaris equorum*).

Example: Suspension - 2.3 ml/50 lb; 23 ml/500 lb
Granules - One 5g pkg/225-240 lb

Directions for use: Panacur® (fenbendazole) Granules 22.2% (222 mg/g). Sprinkle the appropriate amount of drug on a small amount of the usual grain ration. Prepare for each horse individually. Withholding of feed or water not necessary.

Panacur® (fenbendazole) Suspension 10% is approved for use concomitantly with an approved form of trichlorfon for the treatment of stomach bots (*Gasterophilus* spp.). Refer to the manufacturer's label for directions for use and cautions for trichlorfon.

Panacur® (fenbendazole) Paste 10% (100 mg/g) The contents of one syringe will deworm a 1,100 lb horse. Each syringe contains 2.5g of fenbendazole. Panacur® (fenbendazole) given at the rate of 2.3 mg/lb controls the listed parasites. For foals and weanlings (less than 18 months of age) where ascarids are a common problem, one syringe for each 550 lb body weight is recommended. Regular deworming at intervals of six to eight weeks may be required. Consult your veterinarian for assistance in the diagnosis, treatment, and control of parasitism.

Caution: Keep this and all medication out of the reach of children.

Warning: Do not use in horses intended for food.

How Supplied:
Suspension- Bottles of 1000 ml
Granules- Packages of 5g
Paste- 25g Syringe

PANACUR®
(fenbendazole) Granules 22.2% (222 mg/g)
For Dogs

Dosage: 50 mg/kg (22.7 mg/lb) daily for 3 consecutive days for the removal of ascarids (*Toxocara canis, Toxascaris leon-*

ina), Hookworms (*Ancylostoma caninum, Uncinaria stenocephala*), Whipworms (*Trichuris vulpis*) and Tapeworms (*Taenia pisiformis*).
Directions: The daily dosage of 50 mg/kg (22.7 mg/lb) can be achieved as follows:
1. Using a gram scale, weigh out 1 gram of Panacur® (fenbendazole) Granules 22.2% for each 4.44 kg or 10 pounds of body weight;
OR
2. Using standard measuring devices,
   measure 1/4 level teaspoon (1.25cc) of Granules for 2.73 kg or 6 lbs. body weight.
   measure 1 level teaspoon (5.0cc) of Granules for 11.36 kg or 25 lbs. body weight.

Daily dosage must be repeated for 3 consecutive days.
Mix the appropriate amount of drug with a small amount of the usual food: dry dog food may require slight moistening to facilitate mixing with the drug.
Contraindications: None known.
Toxicology Data: Panacur® (fenbendazole) Granules 22.2% did not cause toxicity when administered to weaned pups at doses equal to 5 times the recommended daily dose and for 2 times the duration of treatment.
Adverse Reactions: Another benzimidazole has been reported to cause hepatotoxicity clinically in canines. However, this effect has not been reported during the clinical use of fenbendazole. In U.S. clinical studies, 3 of 240 dogs vomited which may have been drug related.
Drug Interactions: Panacur® (fenbendazole) Granules 22.2% has been administered to dogs in clinical trials along with a wide variety of other drugs including antibiotics, steroids, anesthetics, tranquilizers, vitamins, and minerals. No incompatibilities with other drugs are known at this time.
Precautions: Medicated food must be fully consumed to be effective.
Store at controlled room temperature (59-86°F).
Keep this and all medications out of the reach of children.
Caution: Federal law restricts this drug to use by or on the order of a licensed veterinarian.
How Supplied: 1 lb. Plastic container.

PANACUR®
(fenbendazole) Paste 10% (100 mg/g) Cattle Dewormer

Dosage: Panacur® (fenbendazole) Paste is given orally for the removal and control of:
Lungworm: (*Dictyocaulus viviparus*); Stomach worms; (*Haemonchus contortus, Ostertagia ostertagi, Trichostrongylus axei*) Intestinal worms: (*Bunostomum phlebotomum, Nematodirus helvetianus, Cooperia punctata* & *C. oncophora, Trichostrongylus colubriformis, Oesophagostomum radiatum*). The dose is 5 mg fenbendazole/kg (2.3 mg/lb.) or 5 g Panacur® (fenbendazole) Paste per 220 lb. body weight (100 kg).
Each full depression of the dispensing gun trigger delivers approximately 5 g Panacur® (fenbendazole) Paste. Administer according to the following table:

Cattle Weight	Number of Depressions	One Tube Will Treat
220 lbs	1	58 head
440 lbs	2	29 head
660 lbs	3	19 head
880 lbs	4	14 head
1,100 lbs	5	11 head

DO NOT UNDERDOSE.
Under conditions of continued exposure to parasites, retreatment may be needed after 4–6 weeks. There are no known contraindications to the use of the drug in cattle.
Warning: Cattle must not be slaughtered within 8 days following last treatment. Because a withdrawal time in milk has not been established, do not use in dairy cattle of breeding age. Sales to licensed veterinarians only. Consult your veterinarian for assistance in the diagnosis, treatment and control of parasitism.
Keep this and all medications out of the reach of children.
Store at room temperature.
How Supplied: 10.2 oz cartridge.
92 g syringe

PANACUR®
(fenbendazole)-Suspension 10% (100 mg/ml) Cattle Dewormer

Directions: Determine the proper dose according to estimated body weight. Administer orally.
Dosage: 5 mg/kg (2.3 mg/lb) for the removal and control of - Lungworm: (*Dictyocaulus viviparus*); Stomach worms: Barberpole worm (*Haemonchus contortus*), Brown stomach worm (*Ostertagia ostertagi*), Small stomach worm (*Trichostrongylus axei*); intestinal worms: Hookworm (*Bunostomum phlebotomum*), Thread-necked intestinal worm (*Nematodirus helvetianus*), Small intestinal worms, (*Cooperia punctata* & *C. oncophora*), Bankrupt worm (*Trichostrongylus colubriformis*), Nodular worm (*Oesophagostomum radiatum*).
The recommended dose of 5 mg/kg is achieved when 2.3 mL of the drug is given for each 100 lb. body weight.

EXAMPLES:	Dose	Cattle Weight
	2.5 mL	109 lb.
	5.0 mL	217 lb.
	10.0 mL	435 lb.
	15.0 mL	652 lb.
	23.0 mL	1,000 lb.

Under conditions of continued exposure to parasites, retreatment may be needed after 4–6 weeks. There are no known contraindications to the use of the drug in cattle.
Warning: Cattle must not be slaughtered within 8 days following last treatment. Because a withdrawal time in milk has not been established, do not use in dairy cattle of breeding age.
Caution: Consult your veterinarian for assistance in the diagnosis, treatment and control of parasitism.
Sales to licensed veterinarians only.
Keep this and all medications out of the reach of children.
How Supplied: Bottles of 1000 ml.

REGU-MATE® (altrenogest) Solution
0.22% (2.2 mg/ml)
Oral Progestin for mares only.

Caution: Federal law restricts this drug to use by or on the order of a licensed veterinarian.
Description: REGU-MATE® (altrenogest) Solution 0.22% contains the active synthetic progestin, altrenogest. The chemical name is 17α-Allyl-17β-hydroxyestra-4,9,11-trien-3-one.
Each mL of REGU-MATE® (altrenogest) Solution 0.22% contains 2.2 mg of altrenogest in an oil solution.
Actions: REGU-MATE® (altrenogest) Solution 0.22% produces a progestational effect in mares.
Indications: REGU-MATE® (altrenogest) Solution 0.22% is indicated to suppress estrus in mares.
Suppression of estrus allows for a predictable occurrence of estrus following drug withdrawal. This facilitates the attainment of regular cyclicity during the transition from winter anestrus to the physiological breeding season. Suppression of estrus will also facilitate management of prolonged estrus conditions. Suppression of estrus may be used to facilitate scheduled breeding during the physiological breeding season.
Contraindications: REGU-MATE® (altrenogest) Solution 0.22% is contraindicated in pregnant mares. The safety of the drug in pregnant mares has not been established. Various synthetic progestins, including altrenogest, when administered to rats during the embryogenic stage of pregnancy at doses manyfold greater than the recommended equine dose caused fetal anomalies, specifically masculinization of the female genitalia.
Warning: Do not use in horses intended for food. Pregnant women and others of childbearing age should exercise extreme caution when handling this product. Accidental absorption could lead to a disruption of the menstrual cycle or prolongation of pregnancy. Direct contact with the skin should therefore be avoided. Accidental spillage on the skin should be washed off immediately with soap and water.
Caution: For oral use in horses only.
Dosage & Administration: Administer orally at the rate of 1 mL per 110 pounds body weight (0.44 mg/kg) to be given one dose daily for 15 consecutive days. Administer directly on the posterio-dorsal surface of the mare's tongue using a dose syringe or suitable plastic syringe. The drug may also be administered on the usual grain ration.

Dosage Chart

Approximate Weight in lbs.	Dose in mL

Continued on next page

H

Hoechst-Roussel—Cont.

770	7
880	8
990	9
1100	10
1210	11
1320	12

Which Mares Will Respond to REGU-MATE® (altrenogest) Solution 0.22%: Extensive clinical trials have demonstrated that estrus will be suppressed in appoximately 95% of the mares within three days; however, the post-treatment response depended on the level of ovarian activity when treatment was initiated. Estrus in mares exhibiting regular estrus cycles during the breeding season will be suppressed during treatment; these mares return to estrus four to five days following treatment and continue to cycle normally. Mares in winter anestrus with small follicles continued in anestrus and failed to exhibit normal estrus following withdrawal.

Response in mares in the transition phase between winter anestrus and the summer breeding season depended on the degree of follicular activity. Mares with inactive ovaries and small follicles failed to respond with normal cycles post-treatment, whereas a higher proportion of mares with ovarian follicles 20 mm or greater in diameter exhibited normal estrus cycles post-treatment.

REGU-MATE® (altrenogest) Solution 0.22% was very effective for suppressing the prolonged estrus behavior frequently observed in mares during the transition period (February, March, and April). In addition, a high proportion of these mares responded with regular estrus cycles post-treatment.

Specific Uses For REGU-MATE® (altrenogest Solution 0.22%:

Suppression of Estrus to:

1. Facilitate attainment of regular cycles during the transition period from winter anestrus to the physiological breeding season.
   To facilitate attainment of regular cycles during the transition phase, mares should be examined to determine the degree of ovarian activity. Estrus in mares with inactive ovaries (no follicles greater than 20 mm in diameter) will be suppressed but these mares may not begin regular cycles following treatment. However, mares with active ovaries (follicles greater than 20 mm in diameter) frequently respond with regular post-treatment estrus cycles.
2. Facilitate management of the mare exhibiting prolonged estrus during the transition period.
   Estrus will be suppressed in mares exhibiting prolonged behavioral estrus either early or late during the transition period. Again, the post-treatment response depends on the level of ovarian activity. The mares with greater ovarian activity initiate regular cycles and conceive sooner than the inactive mares. REGU-MATE® (altrenogest) Solution 0.22% may be administered early in the transition period to suppress estrus in mares with inactive ovaries to aid in the management of these mares or to mares later in the transition period with active ovaries to prepare and schedule the mare for breeding.
3. Permit scheduled breeding of mares during the physiological breeding season.
   To permit scheduled breeding, mares which are regularly cycling or which have active ovarian function should be given REGU-MATE® (altrenogest) Solution 0.22% daily for 15 consecutive days beginning 20 days before the date of the planned estrus. Ovulation will occur 5 to 7 days following the onset of estrus as expected for non-treated mares. Breeding should follow usual procedures for mares in estrus. Mares may be regulated and scheduled either individually or in groups.

Store At Room Temperature.

How Supplied: REGU-MATE® (altrenogest) Solution 0.22% (2.2mg/mL). Each mL contains 2.2 mg altrenogest in an oil solution.

Available in 1000 mL plastic bottles.

T-61® EUTHANASIA SOLUTION*

***Not subject to the regulations of the 1970 Controlled Substances Act.**

Composition: Each ml contains:
200 mg N-[2-(m-methoxy-phenyl)-2-ethyl-butyl-(1)]-gamma-hydroxybutyramide;
50 mg 4.4′-methylene-bis(cyclohexyl-trimethyl-amonium iodide);
5 mg tetracaine hydrochloride; with 0.6 ml dimethylformamide in distilled water.

Actions: T-61® contains three chemically and pharmacologically different substances to provide a combination of general anesthetic, strong muscle relaxant, and local anesthetic actions fulfilling the requirements for a professional euthanasia solution. Euthanasia is due to cerebral death in conjunction with respiratory arrest and circulatory collapse. T-61® is painless, humane, rapidly effective, and easy to administer.

N-[2-(m-methoxy-phenyl)-2-ethyl-butyl-(1)]gamma—hydroxybutyramide has a general anesthetic action inducing a rapid and deep anesthesia, followed by respiratory arrest, cerebral death and circulatory collapse.

4,4′-methylene-bis (cyclohexyl-trimethyl-ammonium iodide) has a neuromuscular blocking action inducing skeletal muscular relaxation by blocking the transfer of stimuli from nerve endings to muscle fibers.

Tetracaine hydrochloride has a local anesthetic effect to permit completion of the injection without local pain or struggling.

Pharmacodynamic Activity: The sequence of neurologic effects of T-61®, when properly administered, produces a general anesthesia including first an analgesic stage, followed by deep anesthesia with suppression of consciousness, respiratory paralysis, cerebral death and circulatory collapse. The stage of involuntary excitation that normally occurs between the analgesic and deep anesthesia stages is omitted when the recommended dose of T-61® is properly injected. (Please refer to section on "Dosage and Administration.") The cortical encephalographic changes are typical of the anesthetic component alone. They occur almost immediately following proper administration and advance rapidly to cerebral death. The second component exerts its effect during the deep anesthesia stage, augmenting skeletal muscle relaxation and respiratory paralysis. Cerebral death occurs prior to circulatory collapse.

Animals euthanized with T-61®, when it is properly administered, do not experience anoxic pain, since the neuropharmacologic action of the anesthetic component is evident prior to apneusis.

Indications: T-61® is exclusively intended for the humane euthanasia of animals without excitation or pain. T-61® is indicated for use in dogs, cats, horses, as well as in mink, small laboratory animals, and birds.

Warnings: T-61® must not be used for therapeutic purposes. Do not use in animals intended for food.

The euthanasia effect may sometimes be delayed in animals with severe cardiac or circulatory deficiencies. This may be explained in such cases by the impaired movement of the drug to its site of action.

Caution: Caution should be exercised to avoid contact of the drug with open wounds or accidental self-inflicted injections. The following procedures should be taken in case of accidental exposure. The wound should be thoroughly washed with tap water and compression applied laterally to the site of puncture. Antidotes include central analeptic agents to combat the anesthetic components and physostigmine to counteract the curariform component. For euthanasia only.

Dosage and Administration: Intravenous injection is the preferred route of administration of T-61®; however, intrapulmonary or intracardiac injections may be made where the intravenous injection is impractical, as in the very small dog and cat, or in the comatose animal with depressed vascular function.

Injection Technique: Two thirds (⅔) of the total dose should be administered without interruption at a moderate rate (1 ml/5 sec). The remaining one third (⅓) may be administered rapidly. The correct injection technique is a prerequisite to effect euthanasia without excitation or pain.

Dog:

Intravenous Injection—The onset of effect is rapid and occurs during injection. Cardiac activity may continue for several seconds or, in some cases, for 1 to 3 minutes following cerebral death.

Dosage: 0.3 ml/kg (0.14 ml/lb) (Weight in pounds × 0.14 ml = ml required for dosage).

Example: 25 lb dog × 0.14 ml = 3.5 ml.

Intracardiac Injection has the same effect as intravenous administration. Good injection skill is necessary; the dosage is the same as for intravenous administration.

Intrapulmonary Injection: This technique is less desirable for the dog due to variations in individual dosage response, which may result in the delayed action of the drug.

Dosage: Dogs weighing up to 10 kg are given 7 to 10 ml. In larger dogs the initial administration of 10 ml is followed by another 3 to 10 ml by intrapulmonary or intracardiac route after initial anesthesia has occurred.

Proper technique is particularly important for intrapulmonary injection.

Horse:

Intravenous Injection—The recommended dosage is 4 to 6 ml/50 kg (110 lb body weight). Usually, 50 ml T-61® solution is effective for 1000 lb animal.

Cat:

Intravenous Injection—The onset of effect is rapid and occurs during injection. Cardiac activity may continue for several seconds or, in some cases, for 1 to 3 minutes following the cerebral death.

Dosage: 0.3 ml/kg (0.14 ml/lb) (Weight in pounds × 0.14 ml = ml required for dosage).

Example: 10 lb cat × 0.14 = 1.4 ml

Intrapulmonary Injection:

Dosage:

kittens a few days old	1 ml
kittens up to six months of age	3 ml
cats over six months of age	5 ml
cats weighing more than 5 kg (11 lb)	10 ml

The injection is best carried out with the animal held in a prone position. A sharp needle of the appropriate size for the animal is inserted about 2 to 3 cm (approximately 1 in) below the vertebral column in the center of the chest, directed toward the opposite elbow.

Mink:

Intraperitoneal Injection: 0.5 to 1 ml

Birds (Pigeons and Parakeets) and ***Small Laboratory Animals*** (Mice, Rats, Guinea Pigs and Rabbits.)

Intrapulmonary Injection of 0.5 to 2 ml, according to size.

Caution: Federal law restricts this drug to use by or on the order of a licensed veterinarian.

How Supplied: Available in 50 ml and 250 ml multidose vials. This product is not subject to regulations under the 1970 controlled substances act.

References:

Eikmeier H; Experiences with a new preparation for painless destruction of small animals.

(Erfahrungen mit einem neuen Praeparat zur schmerzlosen Toetung von Kleintieren.) *(Tieraerztl Umsch* 16:397–399, 1961.

Kuepper G: T-61® used in large animals, in *The Blue Book for the Veterinary Profession,* Frankfurt, West Germany, Hoechst AG, No. 8:32–33, 1964.

Quinn AH; Observations of a new euthanasia agent for small animals. *Vet Med* June 1963, pp 494–495.

International Minerals And Chemical Corp.

Animal Health & Nutrition Division
P.O. BOX 207
TERRE HAUTE, IN 47808

RALGRO®

Composition: Zeranol, the active drug in RALGRO is a chemical derivative of resorcylic acid lactone which is a fermentation product. The RALGRO implant is a new concept in producing increased rate of gain and greater feed efficiency in all classes of beef cattle.

Zeranol is an anabolic agent and has a positive influence on the dynamic state of protein metabolism in the animal. Studies indicate that one mode of action of zeranol is stimulation of the pituitary gland to produce increased amounts of somatotrophin, the true growth hormone. Implanted animals can be expected to gain 10 percent faster and improve feed conversion 8 percent better than nonimplanted animals.

Indications: For use in beef cattle to increase weight gains and improve feed conversion. Animals may be reimplanted every 90–100 days.

Dosage and Administration: RALGRO is implanted subcutaneously on the back side of the ear, 1 inch from the base of the head. The dose for all classes of beef cattle is 36 mg. (three 12-mg. pellets).

Precautions: Not recommended for breeding animals. Do not implant beef cattle 65 days before slaughter.

How Supplied: RALGRO is available in cylindrical pellets. The cylindrical pellets are in a plastic cartridge disc for use with a RALOGUN® implant gun. Each cartridge disc has 24 chambers, each chamber containing three 12-mg. pellets (one dose) positioned for delivery with one pull of the trigger. Ten cartridges are packed in one carton (240 doses). Two cartons are packed in one shipper unit (480 doses).

International Multifoods

See OSBORN

Luitpold Pharmaceuticals, Inc.

ANIMAL HEALTH DIVISION
ONE LUITPOLD DRIVE
SHIRLEY, NY 11967

ADEQUAN®

Brand Of
Polysulfated Glycosaminoglycan (PSGAG)
Solution 250 mg/ml
For intraarticular use in horses

Description: Each milliliter of Adequan® contains 250 mg of Polysulfated Glycosaminoglycan and water for injection q.s. Sodium Hydroxide or Hydrochloric Acid added when necessary to adjust pH.

Pharmacology: Polysulfated Glycosaminoglycan is chemically similar to the mucopolysaccharides of cartilagenous tissue. It is a potent proteolytic enzyme inhibitor and diminshes or reverses the processes which result in the loss of cartilagenous mucopolysaccharides. PSGAG improves joint function by stimulating synovial membrane activity, reducing synovial protein levels and increasing synovial fluid viscosity in traumatized equine carpal joints.

Toxicity: Toxicity studies were conducted in horses. Doses as high as 1,250 mg were administered intracarpally to 6 horses once a week for 18 weeks. This dosage is 5 times the recommended dosage and 3.6 times the recommended therapeutic regimen. Clinical observations revealed a soreness and swelling in 1.8% (2 of 109 animals) at the injection site which was mild, self limiting and lasted less than one day. There was a dose related elevation on partial thromboplastin time, creatinine and glucose. No animal had any clinical illness during the trial and none showed clinical evidence of toxicity except for transient swelling at the injection site, possibly due to mechanical invasion of the joint.

Indication: Adequan® is recommended for the treatment of non-infectious degenerative and/or traumatic joint dysfunction and associated lameness of the carpal joint in horses.

Contraindications: Do not use in horses showing hypersensitivity to Polysulfated Glycosaminoglycan.

Warning: Not for use in horses intended for food.

Dosage and Administration: The recommended dosage of Adequan® in horses is 250 mg (1 ampule) once a week for five weeks, intraarticularly. The joint area must be shaved, cleansed and sterilized as in a surgical procedure prior to injection. Do not mix Adequan® with other drugs or solvents.

Precautions: After intraarticular treatment, reactions in the joint may occur within 48 hours post-injection. If the joint reacts with excessive inflammation, cease therapy with Adequan®. Serious reactions of this type may indicate the presence of joint infection. Appropriate antibacterial therapy should be initiated if joint infection is suspected or confirmed. Excessive joint inflammation may be manifested by tenderness, swelling and warmth at the inflammed site.

Impairment of Fertility: Fertility impairment studies in mares and stallions have not been conducted. Do not use in horses intended for breeding.

Caution: Federal law restricts this drug to use by or on the order of a licensed veterinarian.

How Supplied: Adequan® solution, 250 mg/ml is available in 1 ml glass ampules, boxes of six.

Storage Conditions: Store in a cool place.

Molecular Genetics Inc.

10320 BREN ROAD EAST
MINNETONKA, MINNESOTA
55343

GENECOL® 99 brand Escherichia coli Monoclonal Antibody Murine Hybridoma Cell Line, Mouse Origin

For veterinary use only.

As an aid in the reduction of fatal calf scours due to infection with enteropathogenic *E. coli* organisms.

Product Description: Genecol® 99 consists of a specific monoclonal K99-*E. coli* antibody derived from a secreting hybridoma cell line using the ascitic fluid of the mouse for the production of the monoclonal antibody. The cell line has been specifically selected for its high antibody producing capacity. Monoclonal antibodies are a recent scientific development which offer an alternative means of delivering protection to the small intestine of newborn animals. K99 antigen is one of the main attributes of virulence found on enterotoxigenic strains of *E. coli* (ETEC) isolated from calves, sheep and pigs (1,2,3,4). This pilus has been shown to be one of the main attachment mechanisms which allow the ETEC to colonize the small intestine (5). Since colonization is an essential step in the pathogenesis of diarrhea, interference with attachment will prevent the disease. Several vaccine trials have been conducted to show that the passive antibody against the K99 antigen within the lumen of the small intestine will prevent severe, fatal enterotoxigenic colibacillosis (6,7,8,9,10). In these previous studies passive antibody has been "delivered" to the intestine of suckling calves through the colostrum of dams vaccinated prior to parturition.

Mode of Action: The first 12 hours post partum are the most critical in terms of preventing pathogenic *E. coli* with the K99 antigen from adhering to the intestinal villi. Genecol 99 contains the antibody against this pilus antigen and consequently must be present in the intestines during this critical period to reduce mortality which could result.

Dosage and Administration: The entire contents of one 10 ml syringe are to be administered ORALLY to the newborn calf within 12 hours after birth.

Safety: The safety of Genecol 99 has been demonstrated by the administration to calves of 30 times the recommended dose with no adverse effects. Genecol 99 may also be administered to calves regardless of other agents that may already have been given to the calf or its dam.

Precautions: 1. Store the product at 2°-7°C (35° to 45°F). DO NOT FREEZE.
2. Syringes must be kept sealed until the time of use.
3. Contains thimerosal as a preservative.

It should be appreciated that calf scours in general is a complex disorder with many possible contributing factors. These factors may be of nutritional parasitic or management origin as well as viral and bacterial organisms which could be implicated.

How Supplied: Unit Size. Package of 5 and 10 single doses.

References:

1. Orskov I, Orskov F, Smith HW, et al: The establishment of K99, of thermolabile transmissible *Escherichia coli* K antigen, previously called "Kco" possessed by calf and lamb enteropathogenic strains. Acta Pathol Microbiol Scand (B) 83:31–36, 1975.
2. Moon HW, Whip SC, Skartvedt SN: Etiologic diagnosis of diarrheal diseases of calves: Frequency and methods for detecting enterotoxin and K99 antigen production by *Escherichia coli.* AM J Vet Res 37:1025–1029, 1976.
3. Guinee PAM, Jansen WH: Detection of enterotoxigenicity and attachment factors in *Escherichia coli* strains of human, porcine and bovine origin; The comparative study. Zentralbl Bakteriol(A) 243:245–257, 1979.
4. Moon HW, Nagy B, Isaacson RE, et al: Occurrence of K99 antigen on *Escherichia coli* isolated from pigs and colonization of pig ileum by K99+ enterotoxigenic *E. coli* from calves and pigs. Infect Immun 15:614–620, 1977.
5. Smith HW, Huggins MB: The influence of plasmid-determined and other characteristics of enteropathogenic *Escherichia coli* on their ability to proliferate in the alimentary tract of piglets, calves and lambs. J Med Microbiol 11:471–492, 1978.
6. Acres SD, Isaacson RE, Babiuk LA, et al: Immunization of calves against enterotoxigenic colibacillosis by vaccinating dams with purified K99 antigen and whole cell bacterins. Infect Immun 25:121–126, 1979.
7. Contrepoi SM, Girardeau JP, Dubourguier HC, et al: Specific protection by colostrum from cows vaccinated with the K99 antigen in newborn calves experimentally infected with i E. coli+ and K99+. Ann Res Vet 9:385–388, 1978.
8. Morris JA, Wray C, Sojka WJ: Passive protection of lambs against enteropathogenic *Escherichia coli:* Role of antibodies and serum in colostrum of dams vaccinated with K99 antigen. J Med Microbiol 13:265–271, 1980.
9. Nagy B: Vaccination of cows with K99 extract to protect newborn calves against experimental enterotoxigenic colibacillosis. Infect Immun 27:21–24, 1980.
10. Sojka WJ, Wray C, Morris JA: Passive protection of lambs against experimental enteric colibacillosis by colostral transfer of antibodies from K99 vaccinated ewes. J Med Microbiol 11:493–499, 1978.

U.S. Patent #4,443,549

Genecol® 99 is a Registered Trademark of Molecular Genetics, Inc.

U.S. Veterinary License No. 284

Manufactured by
Molecular Genetics, Inc.
10320 Bren Road East
Minnetonka, MN 55343

MSD AGVET

Division of Merck & Co., Inc.
P.O. BOX 2000
RAHWAY, NJ 07065

CORID® 1.25% Crumbles (amprolium) Medicated

Composition: Active drug ingredient
Amprolium....................................1.25%

Ingredients: Dehydrated Alfalfa Meal, Corn Gluten Feed, Animal Fat preserved with BHA and citric acid, Citric Acid, and Soybean Oil

Indications: An aid in the prevention and treatment of coccidiosis caused by *Eimeria bovis* and *E. zurnii* in calves.

Caution: For a satisfactory diagnosis, a microscopic examination of the feces should be done before treatment. When treating outbreaks, the drug should be administered promptly after diagnosis is determined.

Mixing Directions: Corid 1.25% Crumbles should be thoroughly and evenly mixed in the feed in accordance with good manufacturing practice.

Dosage and Administration: Prevention: Corid 1.25% Crumbles should be fed at the rate of 1 lb. (453.6 g) for each 2500 lb (1134 kg) body weight, or approximately 1/10 lb (1.6 oz) (45.4 g) for each 250 lb (113.4 kg) calf. This amount will supply 226.8 mg amprolium/100 lb (5 mg/kg) body weight. It should be fed daily for 21 days during periods of exposure or when experience indicates that coccidiosis is likely to be a hazard.

Treatment: Feed 2/10 lb (3.2 oz) (90.8 g) Corid 1.25% Crumbles per 250 lb.(10 mg/kg) body weight daily for 5 days. Use on a herd basis only; when one or more calves show signs of coccidiosis, it is likely that the rest of the group have been exposed, and all calves in the group should be treated.

The proper amount of Corid 1.25% Crumbles is mixed with the ration consumed each day. If preferred, it may be top-dressed on the feed. The tables below give suggested directions for feeding the Corid 1.25% Crumbles.

[See table on next page].

Warning: Withdraw 24 hours before slaughter.

How Supplied: Corid 1.25% Crumbles for top-dressing is supplied in 50-lb bags. Product No. 23111.

For Veterinary Use only.

CORID 9.6% SOLUTION (amprolium)

Composition: Corid Solution contains 9.6% amprolium.

Indication: An aid in the treatment and prevention of coccidiosis caused by *Eimeria bovis* and *E. zurnii* in calves.

Caution: For a satisfactory diagnosis a microscopic examination of the feces should be done before treatment. When treating outbreaks, drug should be administered promptly after diagnosis is determined.

Dosage and Administration: 1 fl. oz. = 2 measuring tablespoonfuls; 16 fl. oz. = 1 pint.

In Drinking Water: Treatment—Add Corid Solution to drinking water at the rate of 16 fl. oz./100 gal. At the usual rate of water consumption this will provide an intake of approximately 10 mg. amprolium/kg. (2.2 lb.) body weight. Offer this solution as the only source of water for 5 days.

Use on a herd basis only; when one or more calves show signs of coccidiosis, it is likely that the rest of the group have been exposed, and all calves in the group should be treated.

Prevention—During periods of exposure or when experience indicates that coccidiosis is likely to be a hazard, add Corid Solution to drinking water at the rate of 8 fl. oz./100 gal. At usual rates of water consumption this will provide an intake of approximately 5 mg. amprolium/kg (2.2 lb.) body weight. Offer this solution as the only source of water for 21 days.

As a Drench: Treatment—Add 3 fl. oz. Corid Solution to 1 pt. of water and, with a dose syringe, give 1 fl. oz. of this solution for each 100 lb. (45 kg.) body weight. This will provide a dose of approximately 10 mg. amprolium/kg. (2.2 lb.) body weight. Give daily for 5 days.

Use on a herd basis only; when one or more calves show signs of coccidiosis, it is likely that the rest of the group have been exposed, and all calves in the group should be treated.

Prevention—During periods of exposure or when experience indicates that coccidiosis is likely to be a hazard, add 1⅔ fl. oz. of Corid Solution to 1 pt. of water and, with a dose syringe, give 1 fl. oz. of this solution for each 100 lbs. (45 kg.) body weight. This will provide a dose of approximately 5 mg. amprolium/kg. (2.2 lb.) body weight. Give daily for 21 days.

Warning: Withdraw 24 hours before slaughter.

Keep above 41°F (5°C).

Benzoic acid 0.1 added as preservative.

How Supplied: Corid 9.6% Solution is supplied in 1-gal plastic jugs, 4 jugs per case. Product No. 23101.

CORID® 20% Soluble Powder (amprolium)

Composition: Corid Soluble Powder contains 20 percent amprolium.

Indications: Corid is highly effective for the prevention and treatment of bovine coccidiosis caused by *Eimeria bovis* and *E. zurnii* in calves. Corid works to control coccidia in a unique way: scientists believe that it actually starves coccidia to death by taking the place of vitamin B_1, a vitamin essential to their growth and reproduction. This operates to retard development of the first-generation schizonts in the cells of the intestinal wall.

An aid in the treatment and prevention of coccidiosis caused by *Eimeria bovis* and *E. zurnii* in calves.

FOR 21-DAY PREVENTION PROGRAM

Animal Weight		Approximate Daily Dose per Head		Amount of CORID 1.25%
		Amprolium	CORID 1.25%	for each 100 Head
lb	kg	mg	g	lb
200	90.8	454	36.3	8
300	136.1	680.5	54.4	12
400	181.5	907.5	72.6	16
500	226.8	1134	90.7	20
600	272.2	1361	108.9	24

FOR 5-DAY TREATMENT PROGRAM

Animal Weight		Approximate Daily Dose per Head		Amount of CORID 1.25%
		Amprolium	CORID 1.25%	for Each 100 Head
lb	kg	mg	g	lb
200	90.8	908	72.6	16
300	136.1	1361	108.8	24
400	181.5	1815	145.2	32
500	226.8	2268	181.4	40
600	272.2	2722	217.8	48

Caution: For a satisfactory diagnosis a microscopic examination of the feces should be done before treatment. When treating outbreaks, drug should be administered promptly after diagnosis is determined.

Dosage and Administration: *In Drinking Water:* Treatment—Add Corid Soluble Powder to drinking water at the rate of 4 oz./50 gal. At the usual rate of water consumption this will provide an intake of approximately 10 mg. amprolium/kg. (2.2 lb.) body weight. Offer this solution as the only source of water for 5 days. Use on a herd basis only; when one or more calves show signs of coccidiosis, it is likely that the rest of the group have been exposed, and all calves in the group should be treated.

Prevention—During periods of exposure or when experience indicates that coccidiosis is likely to be a hazard, add Corid Soluble Powder to drinking water at the rate of 4 oz./100 gal. At usual rates of water consumption this will provide an intake of approximately 5 mg. amprolium/kg. (2.2 lb.) body weight. Offer this solution as the only source of water for 21 days.

As a Drench: Treatment—Add 3 oz. Corid Soluble Powder to 1 qt. of water and, with a dose syringe, give 1 fl. oz. of this solution for each 100 lb. (45 kg.) body weight. This will provide a dose of approximately 10 mg. amprolium/kg. (2.2 lb.) body weight. Give daily for 5 days.

Use on a herd basis only; when one or more calves show signs of coccidiosis, it is likely that the rest of the group have been exposed, and all calves in the group should be treated.

Prevention—During periods of exposure or when experience indicates that coccidiosis is likely to be a hazard, add 1½ oz. of Corid Soluble Powder to 1 qt. of water, and, with a dose syringe, give 1 fl. oz. of this solution for each 100 lb. (45 kg.) body weight. This will provide a dose of approximately 5 mg. amprolium/kg. (2.2 lb.) body weight. Give daily for 21 days.

Warning: Withdraw 24 hours before slaughter.

How Supplied: Corid 20% Soluble Powder is supplied in 4-oz plastic bags, 60 per 15-lb plastic pail, and 10-oz plastic bags, 24 per 15-lb plastic pail.

DIURIL® Boluses (chlorothiazide)

Composition: Diuril (Chlorothiazide) is known chemically as 6-chloro-7-sulfamyl-1, 2, 4-benzothiadiazine-1,1-dioxide and is designated by the generic name of chlorothiazide. Diuril belongs to a class of heterocyclic compounds of which the parent compound is benzo-1,2,4-thiadiazine.

Diuril is a colorless crystalline compound with a molecular weight of 295.7. It has low solubility in water but is readily soluble in dilute aqueous sodium hydroxide. It is soluble in buffer or urine to the extent of about 50 and 150 mg./100 cc. at pH 4 and 7, respectively. Analytic procedures exist for the determination of this compound in plasma and urine.

Indications: For use in cattle as an aid in the reduction of post parturient udder edema.

Dosage and Administration: The usual dose range of Diuril is 2 g. once or twice daily for three or four days.

For optimal therapy the dosage must be adjusted to meet the changing needs of the individual animal. In moderately edematous and moderately responsive animals, 2 g. once a day may be given. Severe conditions may require higher doses.

Continued on next page

M

MSD AGVET—Cont.

Precautions: Diuril is a potent compound in its influence on electrolyte excretion and as a result dosage and administration must be individualized. As with other potent diuretics, the patient should be regularly and carefully observed for the early signs of fluid and electrolyte imbalance and appropriate measures taken to prevent or correct such imbalance if it occurs. The early clinical signs and symptoms of fluid and electrolyte imbalances, whatever the cause, are increased thirst, weakness, lethargy, drowsiness or restlessness, fatigue, oliguria, gastrointestinal disturbances and tachycardia.
Warning: Milk taken from dairy animals during treatment and for 3 days after the latest treatment must not be used for food.
Caution: Federal law restricts this drug to use by or on the order of a licensed veterinarian.
How Supplied: No. 54841—Diuril Boluses Veterinary, 2 g. each, package of 50.

EQUIZOLE®
(thiabendazole)
Suspension

Indications: For the control of gastrointestinal roundworms in cattle*, horses**, sheep and goats***; also active against ova and larvae† passed by sheep from 3 hours to 3 days after treatment.
Directions for Use and Dosage
Shake well before using.
CATTLE
EQUIZOLE is given as a drench. The dose is proportional to body weight and the severity of infection. The routine dose of Thiabendazole for *Trichostrongylus spp., Haemonchus spp., Nematodirus spp., Ostertagia spp.,* and *Oesophagostomum radiatum* is 3 g. (¾ fl. oz. EQUIZOLE) per 100 lb. of body weight. For *Cooperia spp.,* or severe infections of other species, give 5 g. (1¼ fl. oz. EQUIZOLE) per 100 lb.
HORSES
Give EQUIZOLE by stomach tube or as a drench. The routine dose of Thiabendazole is 2 g . (½ fl. oz. EQUIZOLE) per 100 lb. of body weight. A dose of 4 g. (1 fl. oz. EQUIZOLE) per 100 lb. is recommended for use against ascarids.
NOTE: Certain equine parasites may become resistant to anthelmintics.
Thiabendazole is inactive against larvae of the bot fly, *Gasterophilus sp.* However, the drug is compatible with carbon disulfide or piperazine-carbon disulfide complex and these may be given to horses with EQUIZOLE if desired.
Precautions ordinarily observed with carbon disulfide must be observed.
Keep this and all medications out of the reach of children.
0.18% methylparaben, 0.05% ethylparaben, and 0.02% propylparaben added as preservatives.
SHEEP and GOATS
Give EQUIZOLE as a drench. The dose of Thiabendazole is 2 g. (½ fl. oz. EQUIZOLE) per 100 lb. of body weight. Examples of average total doses of EQUIZOLE are:

Lambs and Small Goats (under 50 lb.)	¼ fl. oz.
Ewes and Does (50 to 100 lb.)	½ fl. oz.
Rams and Bucks (100 to 150 lb.)	¾ fl. oz.

Goats with severe infections should be given 3 g. Thiabendazole (¾ fl. oz. EQUIZOLE) per 100 lb. of body weight.
Some strains of the sheep stomach worm, *Haemonchus contortus,* do not respond fully to the usual dose of thiabendazole.

*Cattle—Genera *Trichostrongylus spp., Haemonchus spp., Nematodirus spp., Ostertagia spp., Oesophagostomum radiatum,* and *Cooperia* species.

**Horses—Genera *Strongylus spp., Cyathostomum spp., Cylicobrachytus spp.* and related genera, *Craterostomum spp., Oesophagodontus spp., Poteriostomum spp., Oxyuris spp., Strongyloides spp.,* and *Parascaris* species.

***Sheep and Goats—Genera *Trichostrongylus spp., Haemonchus spp., Ostertagia spp., Cooperia spp., Nematodirus spp., Bunostomum spp., Strongyloides spp., Chabertia spp.,* and *Oesophagostomum* species.

† Good activity against ova and larvae of *T. colubriformis* and *axei, Ostertagia spp., Bunostomum spp., Nematodirus spp.,* and *Strongyloides spp.;* less effective against those of *Haemonchus contortus* and *Oesophagostomum spp.*

NOTE: For most effective results, retreat animals in 3 to 4 weeks; for animals maintained on premises where reinfection is likely to occur, additional treatment may be necessary.
WARNING: *(Cattle, Sheep* and *Goats)* Milk taken from treated animals within 96 hours (8 milkings) after the latest treatment must not be used for food. Do not treat *cattle* within 3 days of slaughter or *sheep* and *goats* within 30 days of slaughter. *(Horses)* Do not use in horses to be slaughtered for human consumption.

EQUIZOLE A®
(thiabendazole-piperazine citrate)
Liquid
Horse Wormer

Composition: Each fluid ounce contains 2 g Thiabendazole and 2.5 g Piperazine (as piperazine citrate).
Indications: For the control of large strongyles, small strongyles, pinworms, *Strongyloides,* and ascarids in horses.*
Dosage: Each fluid ounce of Equizole A (thiabendazole-piperazine citrate) Liquid contains 2 g thiabendazole and 2.5 g piperazine and will treat 100 lb body weight.
Use directions: Equizole A Liquid is designed to be given by stomach tube or as a drench. To promote rapid flow through the stomach tube, Equizole A Liquid should be above 60°F (15°C). *Shake well before using.*
At 1 fl oz per 100 lb it is highly effective against the genera listed below.
Equizole A Liquid is inactive against *Gasterophilus* spp. However, the product is compatible with carbon disulfide and may be given at the same time, if desired. *Cautions ordinarily observed with carbon disulfide should be observed.*
Caution: Do not use in horses to be slaughtered for food purposes.
Keep this and all medications out of the reach of children.
0.18% methylparaben and 0.02% propylparaben added as preservatives.

*Genera *Strongylus* spp., *Cyathostomum* spp., *Cylicobrachytus* spp. and related genera, *Craterostomum* spp., *Oesophagodontus* spp., *Poteriostomum* spp., *Oxyuris* spp., *Strongyloides* spp., and *Parascaris* species.

Caution: Federal law restricts this drug to use by or on the order of a licensed veterinarian.
Protect From Freezing
U.S. Pat. 3,017,415
How Supplied: Equizole A Liquid is available in 1-gal plastic jugs, 4 jugs per case.
Product No. 54803.
For Veterinary Use Only

EQVALAN®
Paste 1.87%
(ivermectin)
Anthelmintic and Boticide
For Oral Use In Horses Only
Removes worms and bots with a single dose.

INDICATIONS: Consult your veterinarian for assistance in the diagnosis, treatment, and control of parasitism. EQVALAN Paste provides effective control of the following parasites in horses: **Large Strongyles** (adults)—*Strongylus vulgaris* (also early forms in blood vessels), *S edentatus* (also tissue stages), *S equinus Triodontophorus* spp; **Small Strongyles** (adults and fourth-stage larvae)—*Cyathostomum* spp, *Cylicocyclus* spp, *Cylicostephanus* spp, *Cylicodontophorus* spp; **Pinworms** (adults and fourth-stage larvae)—*Oxyuris equi;* **Ascarids** (adults)—*Parascaris equorum;* **Hairworms** (adults)—*Trichostrongylus axei;* **Large-mouth Stomach Worms** (adults)—*Habronema muscae;* **Neck Threadworms** (microfilariae)—*Onchocerca* sp; **Bots** (oral and gastric stages)—*Gastrophilus* spp.
Dosage and Administration: This syringe contains sufficient paste to treat one 1250 lb horse at the recommended dose rate of 91 mcg ivermectin per lb (200 mcg/kg) body weight. Each weight marking on the syringe plunger delivers enough paste to treat 250 lb body weight. (1) While holding plunger, turn the knurled ring on the plunger ¼ turn to the left and slide it so the side nearest the barrel is at the prescribed weight marking. (2) Lock the ring in place by making a ¼ turn to the right. (3) Make sure that horse's mouth contains no feed. (4) Remove the cover from the tip of the syringe. (5) Insert the syringe tip into the horse's mouth at the space between the teeth. (6) Depress the plunger as far as it will go, depositing paste on the back of the tongue. (7) Immediately raise the

horse's head for a few seconds after dosing.

Parasite Control Program: All horses should be included in a regular parasite control program. Consult your veterinarian for a control program to meet your specific needs. EQVALAN Paste is highly effective against gastrointestinal nematodesand bots of horses. Regular treatment will reduce the chances of verminous arteritis caused by *S vulgaris.*

Product Advantages: Broad-spectrum Control—EQVALAN Paste kills important internal parasites, including bots and the arterial stages of *Strongylus vulgaris,* with a single dose. EQVALAN Paste is a highly active anti-parasitic agent that is neither a benzimidazole nor an organophosphate. **Safety**—EQVALAN Paste may be used in mares at any stage of pregnancy. Stallions may be treated without adversely affecting their fertility.

Warning: Do not use in horses intended for food purposes.

Caution: Refrain from smoking and eating when handling. Wash hands after use. Avoid contact with eyes. **Keep this and all drugs out of the reach of children.**

Caution: Safety has not been demonstrated in horses under four months old. Do not administer to foals of this age class. Ivermectin may adversely affect aquatic organisms. Do not contaminate ground water. Dispose of container in approved landfill or by incineration.

Note to User: Swelling and itching reactions after treatment with EQVALAN Paste have occurred in horses carrying heavy infections of Neck Threadworms (microfilariae)—*Onchocerca sp.* These reactions were most likely the result of microfilariae dying in large numbers. Symptomatic treatment may be advisable. Consult your veterinarian should any such reactions occur.

How Supplied: Product 25874-EQVALAN (ivermectin) Paste 1.87% is available in 0.21 oz. (6.08 g) individual syringes.

HYDROZIDE® Injection (hydrochlorothiazide)

Composition: Hydrozide is the 3,4-dihydro derivative of chlorothiazide, known chemically as 6-chloro-7-sulfamyl-3, 4-dihydro-1, 2, 4-benzothiadiazine-1, 1-dioxide, and is designated by the generic name of hydrochlorothiazide. Hydrozide belongs to a class of heterocyclic compounds of which the parent compound is benzo-1,2,4-thiadiazine. Hydrozide is a colorless crystalline compound with a molecular weight of 297.73. It has low solubility in water but is readily soluble in dilute aqueous sodium hydroxide. It is soluble in buffer or urine to the extent of about 50 and 150 mg. per 100 cc. at pH 4 and 7, respectively.

Each cc. of Injection Hydrozide contains 25 mg. hydrochlorothiazide, 10.0 mg. benzyl alcohol, 0.45 cc. polyethylene glycol 300, and water for injection, q.s. 1.0 cc.

Indications: For use in cattle as an aid in the treatment of postparturient udder edema.

Usual Dosage: Usual injectable dose is 5 to 10 cc. (125 to 250 mg. hydrochlorothiazide) once or twice a day. Treatment may be continued with Hydrozide (hydrochlorothiazide), if desired, or the patient maintained on Diuril® (chlorothiazide) Boluses.

Clinical Indications: *Udder Edema*—The retention of fluid or secondary congestion of organs or structures of the animal body is often a troublesome problem in veterinary practice.

Perhaps one of the most commonly seen examples of this variety of edema is congestion of the mammary gland in cows, either shortly before or immediately after parturition. This edema is considered physiologic, but can be of such magnitude as to cause the animal much discomfort and reduce milk production, as well as making milking itself difficult and painful. In high-producing first-calf heifers, severe udder edema may delay full milk production, and in older cows the great increase in size and weight of the gland may predispose to the premature breakdown of the udder attachments. Prompt removal of the excess fluid by the use of Hydrozide can be of great advantage in such conditions.

Dosage and Administration: The usual daily dose of Hydrozide in the cow is 5 to 10 cc. (125 to 250 mg.) given either I.V. or I.M. once or twice a day. Treatment with Hydrozide may be continued for several days, if necessary. However, it is often more convenient to use Hydrozide to achieve prompt onset of diuresis and maintain this activity for the desired time with oral administration of Diuril (chlorothiazide) Boluses. These are given at the rate of 2 Gm. once or twice a day for three or four days.

For optimal therapy the dosage must be adjusted to meet the changing needs of the individual animal. In moderately edematous and moderately responsive animals, 125 mg. once a day may be adequate. Severe conditions may require higher doses.

Precautions: Hydrozide is a potent compound in its influence on electrolyte excretion and as a result dosage and administration must be individualized. As with other potent diuretics, the patient should be regularly and carefully observed for the early signs of fluid and electrolyte imbalance and appropriate measures taken to prevent or correct such imbalance if it occurs. The early clinical signs and symptoms of fluid and electrolyte imbalances, whatever the cause, are increased thirst, weakness, lethargy, drowsiness or restlessness, fatigue, oliguria, gastrointestinal disturbances and tachycardia.

Warning: *Milk taken from dairy animals during treatment and for three days after the latest treatment must not be used for food.*

How Supplied: Product 55191—Injection Hydrozide Veterinary, 25 mg. hydrochlorothiazide per cc., in rubber-capped vials of 50 cc.

IVOMEC® (ivermectin)
1% Injection for Cattle
A Parasiticide for the Treatment and Control of Internal and External Parasites of Cattle

Caution: Federal (U.S.A.) law restricts this drug to use by or on the order of a licensed veterinarian.

Introduction: IVOMEC* (ivermectin) is an injectable parasiticide for cattle. One low-volume dose effectively treats and controls many gastrointestinal roundworms (including inhibited *Ostertagia ostertagi*), lungworms, grubs, lice, and mange mites that may impair the health of cattle.

IVOMEC reduces the need for additional handling, dipping, spraying, and many of the other treatments used in the past to control the parasites against which IVOMEC is effective.

Discovered and developed by scientists from Merck Sharp & Dohme Research Laboratories, ivermectin is a novel chemical entity. Its convenience, broad-spectrum efficacy and a wide therapeutic index make IVOMEC Injection a unique product for parasite control of cattle.

Product Description: Ivermectin is derived from the avermectins, a family of highly active, broad-spectrum antiparasitic agents which are isolated from fermentation of *Streptomyces avermitilis.* **IVOMEC** is a clear, ready-to-use, sterile solution containing 1% ivermectin, 40% glycerol formal, and propylene glycol, q.s. ad 100%. It is formulated to deliver the recommended dose level of 200 mcg ivermectin/kilogram of body weight given subcutaneously at the rate of 1ml/110 lb (50 kg).

Product Indications: IVOMEC Injection is indicated for the effective treatment and control of the following harmful species of gastrointestinal roundworms, lungworms, grubs, lice, and mange mites in cattle.

Gastrointestinal roundworms (adults and fourth stage larvae):
Ostertagia ostertagi (including inhibited *O. ostertagi*)
O. lyrata
Haemonchus placei
Trichostrongylus axei
T. colubriformis
Cooperia oncophora
C. punctata
C. pectinata
Oesophagostomum radiatum
Nematodirus helvetianus (adults only)
N. spathiger (adults only)

Lungworms (adults and fourth stage larvae):
Dictyocaulus viviparus

Cattle grubs (parasitic stages):
Hypoderma bovis
H. lineatum

Lice:
Linognathus vituli

Continued on next page

M

MSD AGVET—Cont.

Haematopinus eurysternus
Mites (Scabies)
Psoroptes ovis (syn. *P. communis* var. *bovis*)
Sarcoptes scabiei var. *bovis*
Dosage: IVOMEC should be given only by subcutaneous injection at the recommended dose level of 200 mcg ivermectin per kilogram of body weight. Each ml of IVOMEC contains 10 mg of ivermectin, sufficient to treat 110 lb (50 kg) of body weight.

Body Weight (lb)	Dose (ml)
110–220	2
220–330	3
330–440	4
440–550	5
550–660	6
660–770	7
770–880	8
880–990	9
990–1100	10

Administration: IVOMEC Injection is to be given subcutaneously only. Animals should be appropriately restrained to achieve the proper route of administration. Use of a 16-gauge, ½ to ¾" needle is suggested. Inject under the loose skin in front of or behind the shoulder.
Use sterile equipment and sanitize the injection site by applying a suitable disinfectant. Clean, properly disinfected needles should be used to reduce the potential for injection site infections.
No special handling or protective clothing is necessary.
Mode of Action: Ivermectin inactivates parasitic nematodes, arachnids, and insects. Its action on the nematodes is by inhibiting signal transmission from the ventral cord interneurons to the excitatory motor neurons. It acts by stimulating the release of the inhibitory neurotransmitter gamma-aminobutyric acid (GABA) from presynaptic nerve terminals as well as by potentiating GABA binding to the postsynaptic receptors. The ivermectin-treated nematodes lose central command to move. Ivermectin acts on the anthropods by inhibiting signal transmission at the neuromuscular junctions via the same mechanism of amplifying GABA action. The susceptible parasites become paralyzed and are thereby killed.
Ivermectin has no measurable effect against flukes and tapeworms, presumably because they do not have GABA as a nerve impulse transmitter.
Recommended doses are non-toxic to cattle. The principal peripheral neurotransmitter in mammals, acetylcholine, is unaffected by ivermectin. Ivermectin does not readily penetrate the central nervous system of mammals where GABA functions as a neurotransmitter.
Ivermectin is unrelated structurally to any of the previously available products. Because of this and its unique mode of action not shared by any other antiparasitic agents, cross resistance is unlikely.
Animal Toxicity: Studies have demonstrated a wide therapeutic index for IVOMEC Injection. Toxic signs did not appear until doses exceeded 30 times the recommended use level. In breeding animals (bulls, and cows in early and late pregnancy), the recommended use level had no effect on breeding performance.

Warning: Do not treat cattle within 35 days of slaughter. Because a withdrawal time in milk has not been established, do not use in female dairy cattle of breeding age.

Precautions

- **This product is not for intravenous or intramuscular use.**
- Use sterile equipment and sanitize the injection site by applying a suitable disinfectant. Clean, properly disinfected needles should be used to reduce the potential for injection site infections.
- Instruct clients to observe cattle for injection site reactions. Reactions may be due to clostridial infection and should be aggressively treated with appropriate antibiotics.
- IVOMEC is highly effective against all stages of cattle grubs. However, proper timing of treatment is important. For most effective results, cattle should be treated as soon as possible after the end of the heel fly (warble fly) season.

Destruction of *Hypoderma* larvae (cattle grubs) at the period when these grubs are in vital areas may cause undesirable host-parasite reactions including the possibility of fatalities. Killing *Hypoderma lineatum* when it is in the tissue surrounding the gullet may cause salivation and bloat; killing *H. bovis* when it is in the vertebral canal may cause staggering or paralysis. These reactions are not specific to treatment with IVOMEC, but can occur with any successful treatment of grubs. Cattle should be treated either before or after these stages of grub development.
Cattle treated with IVOMEC after the end of the heel fly season may be retreated with IVOMEC during the winter for internal parasites, mange mites, or lice without danger of grub-related reactions. A planned parasite control program is recommended.

- Transitory discomfort has been observed in some cattle following subcutaneous administration. A low incidence of soft-tissue swelling at the injection site has been observed. These reactions have disappeared without treatment. Divide doses greater than 10 ml between two injection sites to reduce occasional discomfort or site reaction.
- Protect product from light.

Environmental Safety: Studies indicate that when ivermectin comes in contact with the soil, it readily and tightly binds to the soil and becomes inactive over time. Free invermectin may adversely affect fish and certain waterborne organisms on which they feed. Do not permit water runoff from feedlots to enter lakes, streams, or ponds. Do not contaminate water by direct application or by the improper disposal of drug containers.
Package Information: IVOMEC 1% Injection for Cattle is available in three ready-to-use pack sizes:
The 50-ml pack (Product 41262) is a multiple-dose, rubber-capped bottle. Each bottle contains sufficient solution to treat 10 head of 550-lb (250-kg) cattle.
The 200-ml pack (Product 41265) is a soft, collapsible pack designed for use with automatic injection equipment. Each pack contains sufficient solution to treat 40 head of 550-lb (250-kg) cattle.
The 500-ml pack (Product 41266) is a soft, collapsible pack designed for use with automatic injection euipment. Each pack contains sufficient solution to treat 100 head of 550-lb (250-kg) cattle.

NALLINE® Hydrochloride (nalorphine hydrochloride) Injection

Composition: Nalline Hydrochloride (nalorphine hydrochloride) is a specific narcotic antidote. It rapidly overcomes respiratory and circulatory depression resulting from narcotic overdosage due to accident or unusual sensitivity. The effect of Nalline is dramatic and may be life saving. Unlike large doses of some analeptics, doses of Nalline within the therapeutic range do not cause additional depression or convulsions.
Nalline Hydrochloride is a white, odorless, soluble powder. When dissolved in water, it forms a clear, colorless solution that turns yellow on standing. The empirical formula is $C_{19}H_{21}No_3 \cdot HCl$.
Nalline is a congener of morphine formed by substituting an allyl radical for the methyl radical in the parent compound. Though the mechanism of action of Nalline is unknown, it has proved effective in treating poisoning by morphine and certain other narcotics.
Each cc. of Injection Nalline Hydrochloride contains 5 mg. nalorphine hydrochloride, 3 mg. sodium formaldehyde sulfoxylate, 15 mg. sodium citrate, 2.5 mg. phenol as preservative, and water for injection, q.s. 1.0 cc.
Indications: Respiratory and circulatory depression resulting from overdosage or unusual sensitivity to morphine and certain other narcotics. *Not for depression due to any other cause.*
Usual Dosage: DOGS—1 mg./5 lb. but ordinarily no more than 5 mg. in a single dose.
Pharmacology: The pharmacologic effects of nalorphine in animals have been extensively studied. When administered subcutaneously to dogs in doses of 10 to 20 mg./g., it caused no analgesic effect or depression of respiration. When this dose was given 20 to 60 minutes before a dose of 5 to 10 mg./Kg. of morphine, it prevented the usual respiratory depression, drowsiness, incoordination, and vomiting. In rabbits, nalorphine given 30 minutes before morphine, prevented morphine-induced respiratory depression. When it was given 30 minutes after morphine, it stimulated respiration depressed by morphine. Various

investigators have shown that nalorphine protected most of the mice tested against fatal doses of morphine. Nalorphine has been reported to have no analgetic effect in dogs. One group reported a depressant effect on intestinal motility. Generally, nalorphine has a striking effect on respiration but a variable effect on the other manifestations of morphine depression.

Nalorphine has also been shown to antagonize respiratory depression in dogs caused by the fentanyl fraction of Innovar-Vet®, methadone, Metopon®, Dilaudid®, codeine, and Demerol®.

The effect of nalorphine on depth of coma caused by narcotics is ordinarily not as outstanding as its effect on respiratory depression. Peripheral vascular collapse occasionally accompanies severe narcotic intoxication. Nalorphine will often increase blood pressure toward normal in narcotic-induced hypotensive states.

Clinical Use: Nalline may be used in veterinary medicine as a specific antidote to severe respiratory and circulatory depression caused by the fentanyl fraction of Innovar-Vet® (Fentanyl and Droperidol), morphine sulfate, methadone hydrochloride, Dilaudid® Hydrochloride (Hydromorphone Hydrochloride), Dilaudid® Sulfate (Hydromorphone Sulfate), Pantopon® (Hydrochlorides of Opium Alkaloids), Demerol® Hydrochloride (Meperidine Hydrochloride), codeine, and Metopon® Hydrochloride (Methyldihydromorphinone Hydrochloride).

The clinical effectiveness of Nalline (2.5 mg. to 5 mg./dog) was studied in 18 dogs manifesting various degrees of depression following the routine use of morphine as a preanesthetic sedative. The usual response was a prompt return of reflex activity. Often, full consciousness returned within minutes to several hours. Occasionally, though consciousness was regained after the intravenous administration of Nalline, the animal later became depressed. The authors suggest that it may be desirable to inject a smaller dose intravenously for immediate effect and, soon after, another dose intramuscularly or subcutaneously for prolonged effect.

Nalorphine has been used successfully to reverse narcosis induced in the capture of large wild animals. In divided doses, it has been used in the hippopotamus *(Hippopotamus amphibius)* at 1.1 mg./Kg., in the topi *(Damaliscus korrigum)* at 2.2 mg./Kg. and in a rhinocerous at 0.53 mg./Kg. as a single dose. The drug may be useful to improve the safety with which such animals in captivity can be subjected to veterinary treatment, transport or other handling.

TRESADERM®
(thiabendazole—dexamethasone—neomycin sulfate solution)

Composition: Dermatologic Solution Tresaderm (thiabendazole—dexamethasone—neomycin sulfate solution) contains the following active ingredients per cc.: 40 mg. Thiabendazole, 1 mg. Dexamethasone, 3.2 mg. Neomycin (from Neomycin Sulfate). Inactive ingredients: glycerin, propylene glycol, purified water, hypophosphorous acid, calcium hypophosphite; about 8.5 ethyl alcohol and about 0.5 benzyl alcohol.

Indications: Dermatologic Solution Tresaderm is indicated as an aid in the treatment of certain bacterial, mycotic, and inflammatory dermatoses and otitis externa in dogs and cats. Both acute and chronic forms of these skin disorders respond to treatment with Tresaderm. Many forms of dermatosis are caused by bacteria (chiefly *Staphylococcus aureus, Proteus vulgaris* and *Pseudomonas aeruginosa*). Moreover, these organisms often act as opportunistic or concurrent pathogens that may complicate already established mycotic skin disorders, or otacariasis caused by *Otodectes cynotis.* The principal etiologic agents of dermatomycoses in dogs and cats are species of the general *Microsporum* and *Trichophyton.*

The efficacy of neomycin as an antibacterial agent, with activity against both gram-negative and gram-positive pathogens, is well documented. Detailed studies in various laboratories have verified the significant activity thiabendazole displays against the important dermatophytes. Dexamethasone, a synthetic adrenocorticoid steroid, inhibits the reaction of connective tissue to injury and suppresses the classic inflammatory manifestations of skin disease. The Tresaderm formulation combines these several activities in a complementary form for control of the discomfort and direct treatment of dermatitis and otitis externa produced by the above mentioned infectious agents.

Dosage and Administration: Prior to the administration of Dermatologic Solution Tresaderm remove the ceruminous, purulent or foreign material from the ear canal, as well as the crust which may be associated with dermatoses affecting other parts of the body. The design of the container nozzle safely allows partial insertion into the ear canal for ease of administration. The amount to apply and the frequency of treatment are dependent upon the severity and extent of the lesions. Five to 15 drops should be instilled in the ear twice daily. In treating dermatoses affecting other than the ear the surface of the lesions should be well moistened (2 to 4 drops per square inch) with Dermatologic Solution Tresaderm twice daily. The volume required will be dependent upon the size of the lesion.

Tresaderm is limited to 7 days maximum duration of administration.

Cautions: On rare occasions dogs may be sensitive to neomycin. In these animals, application of the drug will result in erythema of the treated area, which may last for 24 to 48 hours. Also, evidence of transient discomfort has been noted in some dogs when the drug was applied to fissured or denuded areas. The expression of pain may last 2 to 5 minutes. Application of Dermatologic Solution Tresaderm should be limited to periods not longer than one week.

While systemic side effects are not likely with topically applied corticosteroids, such a possibility should be considered if use of the solution is extensive and prolonged. If signs of salt and water retention or potassium excretion are noticed (increased thirst, weakness, lethargy, oliguria, gastrointestinal disturbances or tachycardia), treatment should be discontinued and appropriate measures taken to correct the electrolyte and fluid imbalance. Also, it should be remembered that Tresaderm is not a hormonal replacement, hence it will have no effect on the alopecia of hypothyroidism.

For topical use in dogs and cats.

Avoid contact with eyes.

Keep out of the reach of children.

How Supplied: Product 55871—Dermatologic Solution Tresaderm Veterinary is supplied in 15 cc. and 7.5 cc. dropper bottles, each in 12 bottle boxes; also in 4 fl. oz. dropper bottle.

Norden Laboratories, Inc.
601 W. CORNHUSKER
P.O. BOX 80809
LINCOLN, NE 68521

ANTHELCIDE® EQ
(Brand of Oxibendazole)
Paste
Equine Wormer
For Veterinary Use Only

Description: Anthelcide EQ (brand of oxibendazole) Paste is a paste formulation of oxibendazole, a broad spectrum benzimidazole anthelmintic. This formulation has been developed for ease of administration. Each syringe contains 0.85 ounce (24 grams) of paste.

Anthelcide EQ Paste contains:
Oxibendazole....................................22.7%

Indications: Anthelcide EQ (brand of oxibendazole) Paste is indicated for removal and control of: large strongylids *(Strongylus edentatus, S. equinus, S. vulgaris);* small strongylids (species of the genera *Cylicostephanus, Cylicocyclus, Cyathostomum, Triodontophorus, Cylicodontophorus, and Gyalocephalus);* large roundworms *(Parascaris equorum);* pinworms *(Oxyuris equi)* including various larval stages; and threadworms *(Strongyloides westeri).*

Contraindications: Anthelcide EQ is contraindicated in severely debilitated horses or horses suffering from infectious disease, toxemia or colic.

[See table at bottom of next page.]

Dosage and Administration: The dosage of oxibendazole is 10 mg/kg (2.2 lb) of body weight (15 mg/kg for strongyloides). Each mark on the syringe delivers Anthelcide EQ to treat 100 pounds (67 pounds for strongyloides). Horses maintained on premises where reinfection is likely to occur should be retreated in 6 to 8 weeks.

Anthelcide EQ is compatible with carbon disulfide, which can be used concurrently for bot control *(Gasterophilus spp.)*

Continued on next page

Norden—Cont.

when administered by a veterinarian. Routine carbon disulfide cautions must be observed.
Caution: Consult your veterinarian for assistance in the diagnosis, treatment, and control of parasitism.
Use of Syringe: Determine the weight of the horse and dial the correct setting on the plunger, having the side of the wheel nearest the barrel on the desired mark. Remove the cap from the syringe. Insert the tip of the syringe into the side of the animal's mouth between the incisor and molar teeth, and press the plunger down as far as it will go, depositing the paste on the back of the tongue.
Warning:
Keep out of reach of children.
Not for use in horses intended for food.
How Supplied: Anthelcide EQ Paste is supplied in 12-0.85 ounce (24 gram) syringes.

ANTHELCIDE® EQ
(Brand of Oxibendazole)
Suspension
Equine Wormer
For Veterinary Use Only

Composition:
Active Ingredient:
Oxibendazole..10%
Oxibendazole is a broad spectrum benzimidazole anthelmintic.
Indications: Anthelcide EQ (brand of oxibendazole) Suspension is indicated for removal and control of large strongylids *(Strongylus edentatus, S. equinus, S. vulgaris)*; small strongylids (species of the genera *Cylicostephanus, Cylicocyclus, Cyathostomum, Triodontophorus, Cylicodontophorus,* and *Gyalocephalus)*; large roundworms *(Parascaris equorum)*; pinworms *(Oxyuris equi)* including various larval stages; and threadworms *(Strongyloides westeri)*.
Anthelcide EQ is compatible with carbon disulfide, which can be used concurrently for bot control *(Gasterophilus spp.)*. Routine carbon disulfide cautions must be observed.
Dosage and Administration: The dosage of oxibendazole for the horse is 10 mg/kg body weight (15 mg/kg for strongyloides). Each ml of suspension contains 100 mg of oxibendazole. Administer by stomach tube in 3-4 pints of warm water, or if preferred, by top dressing or mixing into a portion of the normal grain ration. Prepare individual doses to assure that each animal receives the correct amount. Horses maintained on premises where reinfection is likely to occur should be retreated in 6 to 8 weeks.

DOSAGE TABLE

Body Weight (lb)	Dosage of 10% Suspension* 10 mg/kg (ml)	15 mg/kg (ml)
220	10	15
440	20	30
660	30	45
880	40	60
1100	50	75
1320	60	90

* Contains 100 mg oxibendazole per ml of suspension
Warning:
Not for use in horses intended for food.
Protect from freezing.
Shake well before using.
Keep out of reach of children.
Caution: U.S. Federal law restricts this drug to use by or on the order of a licensed veterinarian.
How Supplied: 1 Quart (946 ml) & 1 Gallon (3.785 L).

DOSAGE TABLE

10 mg/kg Syringe Mark	10 mg/kg Horse Weight (lb)	15 mg/kg Syringe Mark	15 mg/kg Horse Weight (lb)
100	100	300	200
200	200	600	400
400	400	900	600
600	600	1200	800
800	800		
1000	1000		
1200	1200		

APRALAN®*
Apramycin Sulfate Soluble Powder

Contains apramycin sulfate equivalent to **37.5 g** apramycin activity (medicates 100 gallons or 380 liters of drinking water, 6600 lbs body weight).
An antibiotic for the control of porcine colibacillosis (weanling pig scours).
Indications: For the control of porcine colibacillosis (weanling pig scours) caused by strains of *E. coli* sensitive to apramycin.
Dosage: Treated pigs should consume enough medicated water to receive 12.5 mg of apramycin per kg of body weight per day (5.67 mg/lb/day). **CONTINUE TREATMENT FOR 7 DAYS.**
Mixing Directions: Use the plastic spoon for measuring the amount of powder to be used. Add to the drinking water at the rate of 375 mg of apramycin per gallon according to the following table. Stir on addition, let stand for 15 minutes to allow particles to dissolve. Stir again to disperse medication.
[See table above].

Total Body Weight to be Treated* Lb	Kg	Apralan Soluble Per Day (Plastic spoon leveled full)	Approximate Daily Water Consumption (Gallon)	Apramycin (mg)
264	120	1	4	1,500
1320	600	5	20	7,500
6600	3000	Entire Contents	100	37,500

*Number of pigs × average weight

Water consumption should be monitored closely to determine that the recommended dosage is being consumed. The drug concentration should be adjusted according to water consumption. Water consumption varies considerably with ambient temperature, humidity and other factors. Prepare fresh medicated water daily. Rusty waterers may cause rapid loss of potency.
Actions: Porcine colibacillosis is caused by *E. coli* infection in the intestinal tract. The marked change in the diet and other stresses associated with weaning contribute to the development of the disease. Colibacillosis is characterized by retarded growth, poor feed utilization and diarrhea. Apramycin acts to inhibit *E. coli* in the intestine and results in an increased rate of weight gain and improved feed efficiency in addition to lowering the incidence and severity of diarrhea.
Active Drug Ingredient: Apramycin (as apramycin sulfate) 37.5 g
Warning: Do not slaughter treated swine for 28 days following treatment.
Notice: Organisms vary in their degree of sensitivity to chemotherapeutics. If no improvement is observed after recommended treatment, diagnosis and sensitivity should be reconfirmed.
Storage: Protect from moisture. Keep tightly closed. Store in a cool, dry place.
Warning: Keep out of the reach of children.
*Apralan is a registered trademark of Elanco Products Company, a division of Eli Lilly and Company.

BovEye®
Moraxella Bovis Bacterin

Description: 'BovEye' is for the vaccination of healthy cattle against infectious keratoconjunctivitis ("pink eye") caused by infection with *Moraxella bovis*. 'BovEye' contains a chemically inactivated culture of *M. bovis* combined with a sterile adjuvant to enhance the immune response.
Indications: Infectious bovine keratoconjunctivitis (IBK) is a highly transmissible disease characterized by keratitis, conjunctivitis, and blepharitis. In severe cases, corneal ulceration may occur, leading to scarring and blindness. Clinical signs of IBK include exudative erythema of affected tissues, excessive lacrimation, and photophobia. The disease affects cattle of all ages, but is most severe in young calves.[1] Incidence of IBK is highest during summer months, with morbidity estimated at 20% in calves

and 10% in feedlot cattle.[2] Economic losses caused by IBK primarily are due to decreased weight gain, decreased milk production, and treatment expense.[1,2,3]

Safety and Efficacy: Chemical inactivation renders 'BovEye' incapable of causing infectious disease. 'BovEye' is a gram-negative bacterial product. Like other bacterins of this type, 'BovEye' on occasion can induce anaphylaxis or endotoxic shock and therefore the product should be administered by someone with a thorough knowledge of post-anaphylaxis procedures. Animals should be carefully observed following vaccination, and atropine or epinephrine should be administered at the first sign of anaphylaxis or endotoxic shock, to be followed by supportive therapy as needed, including antihistamines and, when appropriate, steroids.

Efficacy was determined by field studies and challenge-of-immunity tests. Against natural exposure to *M. bovis* in field studies, 'BovEye' protected 92% of vaccinates, whereas 47% of nonvaccinated control calves developed IBK. In rigorous experimental *M. bovis* challenge tests, 93% of nonvaccinated control calves developed IBK, whereas 'BovEye' protected 76% of vaccinates.

Directions:

1. *General Directions:* Vaccination of healthy beef and dairy cattle is recommended. Calves should be at least 21 days or older when vaccinated. Shake well and administer 2 ml. subcutaneously in the neck.
2. *Primary Vaccination:* Primary vaccination with two doses is recommended. Administer one dose at 3 weeks of age or older, and a second dose 3 weeks afterward.
3. *Revaccination:* Annual revaccination is recommended.

Precautions:

1. Anaphylaxis or endotoxic shock may occur following use. Initial antidote of epinephrine or atropine is recommended and should be followed with supportive therapy that would include antihistamines or, when appropriate, steroids.
2. Store at 2°C. to 7°C. Do not freeze.
3. Use entire contents when first opened.
4. Do not vaccinate within 21 days of slaughter.
5. Transient local reactions may occur following administration.
6. Although this product has been shown to be efficacious, some animals may be unable to develop or maintain an adequate immune response following vaccination if they are incubating any disease, are malnourished or parasitized, or stressed due to shipment or adverse environmental conditions.

Supplied: 10-dose and 50-dose vials

References:

1. Blood, D.C., J.A. Henderson, and O.M. Radostits, 1979. Veterinary Medicine. Lea and Febiger, Philadelphia.
2. Gelatt, K. 1981. Textbook of Veterinary Ophthalmology. Lea and Febiger, Philadelphia.
3. Killinger, A.H. *et al.* 1977. Economic impact of infectious bovine keratoconjunctivitis in beef calves. VM/SAC 72:618–620.

For Veterinary Use Only

BRSV™
Bovine Respiratory Syncytial Virus Vaccine
Modified Live Virus

Product Description: BRSV is for the vaccination of healthy cattle against respiratory disease caused by infection with bovine respiratory syncytial virus. BRVS contains an attenuated strain of bovine respiratory syncytial virus propagated on a bovine cell line, and lyophilized to preserve stability.

Disease Description: Bovine respiratory syncytial virus infection is a respiratory disease, and has been reported in cattle of all ages, including nursing calves. The virus causes a discrete disease[1,4] which may predispose cattle to secondary infections,[1,2,3] particularly bacterial pneumonia. Bovine respiratory syncytial virus infection is characterized by rapid breathing, coughing, anorexia, serous nasal and ocular discharge, fever, and subcutaneous edema around the throat and neck. In an acute outbreak, deaths may follow within 48 hours after onset of signs. Pathology typically consists of subpleural and interstitial emphysema with consolidating lesions characteristic of pneumonia. Clinically, bovine respiratory syncytial virus infection may be difficult to distinguish from other viral diseases associated with the bovine respiratory disease complex.

Safety and Efficacy: In controlled studies, no reports of local or systemic reactions were received following use of BRSV. Serologically negative nonvaccinated control animals did not seroconvert when maintained in contact with vaccinates.

Challenge-of-immunity tests were conducted under federally approved protocol. All vaccinated calves remained clinically normal following challenge that produced typical signs of disease in nonvaccinated control calves.

BRSV is not recommended for use in pregnant animals.

Directions:

1. *General Directions:* Vaccination of healthy animals is recommended. Aseptically rehydrate vaccine with sterile diluent supplied. Shake well. Inject 2 ml. intramuscularly.
2. *Primary Vaccination:* Two doses are recommended, 3 to 4 weeks apart. Calves vaccinated before the age of six months should be revaccinated at 6 months of age.
3. *Revaccination:* Annual revaccination with one 2 ml. dose is recommended.

Precautions:

1. Store at 2°C.–7°C.
2. Do not vaccinate within 21 days of slaughter.
3. Vaccination of stressed animals should be delayed.
4. Use only syringes and needles sterilized by boiling. Do not use chemical sterilization.
5. Use entire contents without delay after rehydration.
6. Burn container and all unused contents.
7. If anaphylaxis occurs following use, administer epinephrine or equivalent.
8. Contains penicillin and streptomycin as preservatives.
9. Although this product has been shown to be efficacious, some animals may be unable to develop or maintain an adequate immune response following vaccination if they are incubating any infectious disease, are malnourished or parasitized, or stressed due to shipment or adverse environmental conditions.

Supplied: 10- and 25-dose vials.

References:

1. Bohlender, RE et al. Bovine respiratory syncytial virus infection. Mod. Vet. Prac. 63(8):613–618. 1982.
2. Bryson, DG. Observations on outbreaks of respiratory disease in calves associated with parainfluenza type 3 virus and respiratory syncytial virus infection. Vet. Rec. 104(3):45–49. 1979.
3. Elazhary, MASY et al. Bovine respiratory syncytial virus in Quebec: antibody prevalence and disease outbreak. Can. J. Comp. Med. 44(3):299–303. 1980.
4. Pirie, HM et al. Acute fatal pneumonia in calves due to respiratory syncytial virus. Vet. Rec. 108(19):411–416. 1981.

For Veterinary Use Only

CALF-GUARD®
Bovine Rota-Coronavirus Vaccine
Modified Live Virus

Product Description: Calf-Guard is for the vaccination of healthy newborn calves and pregnant cows against diarrhea (scours) caused by bovine rotavirus and bovine coronavirus. Calf-Guard contains attenuated strains of bovine rotavirus and bovine coronavirus, propagated on the Norden Bovine Cell Line, and lyophilized to preserve stability.

Disease Description: Neonatal calf diarrhea has a complex etiology, but bovine rota- and coronavirus have been found to be two of its most common causative agents.[1-3] Experimental studies have demonstrated that either virus can initiate calf diarrhea.[4-5] Viral diarrhea is often complicated by secondary infection with *Escherichia coli* or other enteric pathogens.

Safety and Efficacy: Immunization must precede natural exposure in order to be effective. Thus, immunization during the first 24 hours of life, the earlier the better, is strongly recommended. Data indicates that the effectiveness of Calf-Guard declines when some animals in a herd are left unprotected.[6] In such cases, infected calves may seed the premises with virus, and expose other calves prior to immunization. All calves should be immunized for best results. Immunization with Calf-Guard may be accom-

Continued on next page

N

Norden—Cont.

plished by oral vaccination of calves at birth, or by intramuscular vaccination of cows during pregnancy; vaccinated cows provide immunity to their calves via protective antibodies transmitted in colostrum and milk.

Calf-Guard was evaluated in field studies where calves in 21 herds and cows in 5 herds were vaccinated and compared with nonvaccinated calves and calves from nonvaccinated cows during corresponding test periods. Incidence of scours was 25.7% among 1,598 vaccinated calves, while incidence among 829 nonvaccinated calves was 52.1%. Death loss from scours was 2.9% among vaccinated calves and 22.9% among nonvaccinated calves. Among 2,927 calves from vaccinated cows, incidence of scours was 11.3%, with 0.9% death loss. In contrast, 21.7% of 2,801 calves from nonvaccinated cows developed scours, and death loss was 4.1%. These results indicate that vaccination with Calf-Guard significantly reduces incidence and death loss from neonatal calf diarrhea. Because the disease has a variety of causes, however, the vaccine should not be expected to entirely eliminate its occurrence.

Experimental calves remained normal following oral administration of Calf-Guard, and adverse reactions in vaccinated calves were not reported during extensive field trials. Similarly, in field trials with vaccinated pregnant cows, abortions or other adverse reactions were not reported.

Directions:

1. *General Directions:* Rehydrate lyophilized vaccine with sterile diluent provided, and administer without delay. Dosage for both calves and cows is 3 ml.
2. *Calf Vaccination:* Remove needle from syringe and administer vaccine into the back of the calf's mouth. Vaccination should occur as soon as possible after birth because susceptible calves are at risk as soon as they are born. Vaccination of calves older than 1 day may not be effective.
3. *Cow Vaccination:* Administer 2 intramucular doses 3 to 6 weeks apart during late pregnancy. Ideally, the second dose should be administered within 30 days prior to calving.
4. *Cow Revaccination:* Cows should be revaccinated with 2 doses during each subsequent pregnancy.

Precautions:

1. Store at 2°C.–7°C.
2. Use entire contents when first opened.
3. Burn container and unused contents.
4. Do not vaccinate within 21 days before slaughter.
5. Contains penicillin and streptomycin as preservatives.
6. If anaphylaxis occurs following use, administer epinephrine or equivalent.
7. Although this product has been shown to be efficacious, some animals may be unable to develop or maintain an adequate immune response following vaccination if they are incubating any infectious disease, are malnourished or parasitized, or stressed due to shipment or adverse environmental conditions.

References:

1. House JA: Economic impact of rotavirus and other neonatal disease agents of animals. JAVMA 173:573-576, 1978.
2. Woods GN: Epizootiology of bovine rotavirus infection. Vet Rec 103:44–46, 1978.
3. White RG, Mebus CA, and Twiehaus MJ: Incidence of herds infected with a neonatal calf diarrhea virus (NCDV). Vet Med 65:487–489, 1970.
4. Mebus CA, Stair EL, Underdahl NR, and Twiehaus MJ: Pathology of neonatal calf diarrhea induced by a reo-like virus. Vet Path 8:490–505, 1971.
5. Mebus CA, Newman LE, and Stair EL: Scanning electron, light, and immunofluorescent microscopy of intestine of gnotobiotic calf infected with calf diarrheal coronavirus. Am J Vet Res 36:1719–1725, 1975.
6. Thurber ET, Bass EP, and Beckenhauer WH: Field trial evaluation of a reo-coronavirus calf diarrhea vaccine. Can J Comp Med 41:131–136, 1977.

For Veterinary Use Only

CALFSPAN™
Sustained-Release Sulfamethazine

Attention Doctor: This product should not be used in those calves slaughtered at an early age due to the extended withdrawal period required for depletion of sulfonamide residues.

It is your responsibility to inform your client that federal law prohibits slaughter of treated animals for food within 18 days after receiving this drug because of residue violations which may be incurred.

For Veterinary Use Only

Composition: Each CalfSpan Tablet contains 8 grams of sulfamethazine in two distinct layers. The white layer provides sulfamethazine in a readily available form while the gray layer provides a slow-release form of the same drug.

Action: It is well established that the action of the sulfonamides as a group is one of bacteriostasis with high concentrations being bactericidal.[1,2,3,4,5] The most commonly accepted theory of this antibacterial action is that the sulfonamide interferes with the normal metabolism of the bacterial cell, more specifically interfering with the utilization of para-aminobenzoic acid (PABA) in the bacterial enzyme system.[1,2,3,4,5]

Successful therapy with the sulfonamides depends heavily upon its proper usage. First, of course, the causative organism must be sensitive to this class of drugs.

Organisms sensitive to sulfonamides include certain gram-positive cocci and diplococci, gram-negative diplococci, and gram-negative bacilli. They are not effective in most viral and rickettsial infections or tuberculosis.[2] Group A *Streptococci*, some strains of *Staphylococci, E. Coli, Bacillus anthracis, Diplococci, Pasteurella, Shigella, Vibrio and Hemophilus* are highly sensitive while *Strep. viridans, Klebsiella, Aerobacter, B. proteus, Pseudomonas, Clostridia, P. tularensis and Brucella* are only moderately sensitive. *Ornithosis, psittacosis* and *actinomycosis* may respond to sulfonamide therapy though most viruses and *fungi* are highly resistant to this group of drugs.[2]

Beyond this, it is extremely important to:

(1) Give the drug early in the course of the disease.
(2) Give adequate dosage.
(3) Continue medication for a short time after the temperature is normal, to give body defenses a chance to eliminate the infecting organism.

Proper case selection and early administration of a sufficient dose are less difficult to achieve in clinical veterinary practice than is the continuation of drug dosage for an adequate length of time. Jones states that "Animals difficult to restrain may receive no more than one or two doses."[4]

Sustained Action: CalfSpan Tablets combine sulfamethazine in a single tablet of two distinct layers. The smaller white layer provides sulfamethazine in a readily available form while the larger gray layer provides a slow-release form of the same drug. Studies with these tablets showed that following a single oral dose at the rate of one tablet per 45 pounds body weight, plasma sulfamethazine levels of 5 mg % were seen consistently within 4 to 6 hours after treatment. Plasma levels of 5 mg % or higher extended to the 3rd or 4th day post treatment. These *in vivo* studies were conducted in calves ranging in weight from approximately 75 pounds to approximately 150 pounds. Bacterial pathogens are thus exposed to sustained levels of sulfamethazine for a period of time sufficient to allow body elimination of those which are sensitive to the drug.

Indications: CalfSpan Tablets are recommended for the treatment of infectious diseases of calves in which the causative organism is sensitive to sulfamethazine. Uses include the following:

1. Colibacillosis (bacterial scours) caused by *Escherichia coli*
2. Bacterial pneumonia caused by *Pasteurella spp.*
3. Calf diphtheria caused by *Fusobacterium necrophorum.*

Dosage: Administer as a single oral dose at the rate of one CalfSpan Tablet for each 45 pounds body weight. If no response is evident within 2-3 days, other therapeutic approaches should be considered. Tablets may be halved if necessary to closely approximate dosage requirement, *but do not crush.*

Administration of CalfSpan Tablets early in the course of the infection is imperative for best results. A single dose will provide adequate blood sulfonamide levels that will be sustained 3 to 4 days.

Warning: Reports of side effects following the use of sulfamethazine in cattle are rare. Renal damage may result from crystallization of the drug in the kidneys. If hematuria develops during CalfSpan Tablet therapy, take measures to increase the fluid intake of the animal. Care should be taken to ascertain that the tablets are swallowed before the animal is released. As with any orally administered tablet, occasional regurgitation will occur in ruminants.

Tissue Residue: Since CalfSpan Tablets provide sustained release of the active ingredient, tissue levels of sulfamethazine remain for a longer period of time than when this drug is administered in conventional forms.

Treated animals must not be slaughtered for food within 18 days after receiving this drug.

Caution: U.S. Federal law restricts this drug to use by or on the order of a licensed veterinarian.

How Supplied: Cartons of 50 tablets.

Bibliography:

1. Davison, F.M., Synopsis of Materia Medica, Toxicology and Pharmacology. The C.V. Mosby Company, Third Edition (1944).
2. Drill's Pharmacology in Medicine, Edited by Joseph R. DiPalma, McGraw-Hill, Third Edition (1965).
3. Goodman, Louis S. and Gilman, Alfred, The Pharmacological Basis of Therapeutics, The MacMillan Company, Third Edition (1969).
4. Jones, L. Meyer, Veterinary Pharmacology and Therapeutics. The Iowa State College Press, Second Edition (1957).
5. Sollman, T.A., Manual of Pharmacology. W.B. Saunders Company, Sixth Edition (1944).

CARMILAX® BOLETS®

For Veterinary Use Only
Antacid and Mild Laxative

Composition: Magnesium hydroxide 27.0 gm.

Directions: 2 to 4 Bolets, depending on size and condition of animal. Carmilax Powder is recommended as the initial dose for prompt action. Carmilax Bolets are excellent as follow-up therapy. Three Carmilax Bolets contain magnesium hydroxide equivalent to one quart of milk of magnesia.

Warning: Milk taken from dairy animals during treatment and within 12 hours (one milking) after the latest treatment must not be used for food.

How Supplied: 50 Bolets.®

For Veterinary Use Only

CARMILAX® POWDER

Antacid and Mild Laxative

Composition: Each one lb. contains: Magnesium hydroxide 361.0 gm.

Directions: Mix one lb. Carmilax into one gallon of water and stir thoroughly. Shake well before administering with a stomach tube. *Cattle*, one gallon of mixture; *Sheep* and *Calves*, one pint to one quart of mixture, depending on size.

Warning: Milk that has been taken from animals during treatment and for 12 hours (1 milking) after the latest treatment must not be used for food.

For Veterinary Use Only

How Supplied: 10 lb. and 25 lb.

CLOSTRIN® 7

Clostridium Chauvoei-Septicum-Novyi-Sordellii-Perfringens Types C and D Bacterin-Toxoid

Product Description: 'Clostrin 7' is for the vaccination of healthy cattle and sheep against clostridial muscle diseases caused by infection with *Clostridium chauvoei, Cl. septicum, Cl. novyi, Cl. sordellii,* and *Cl. perfringens* Types C and D.

Disease Description: Clostridial infections are caused by bacteria called *Clostridia* that live as spores in the soil and are picked up by the cattle as they graze, lie, or stand on contaminated ground. *Clostridia* also become active when introduced into an open wound created by punctures or lacerations. *Clostridium chauvoei,* blackleg, is characterized by lameness, swelling, and a dark red to black discoloration of the heavy, active muscle tissues. *Clostridium septicum,* malignant edema, is characterized by gaseous swelling of the affected muscles, which become gangrenous as the infection kills tissue. *Clostridium novyi,* black disease, is often characterized by black lesions in the brisket and throat upon necropsy. *Clostridium sordellii* is characterized by black lesions in the brisket, throat, and other muscles upon necropsy. Marked yellow gelatinous swelling may be seen between muscle layers. *Clostridium perfringens* Types C and D are characterized by signs ranging from abdominal pain and diarrhea to convulsions and blindness. Many animals die before signs are noticed. In fact, sudden death is a common feature of all these *Clostridia.*

Safety and Efficacy: This product has met all standards required to be federally licensed.

Directions:

1. *General Directions:* Vaccination of healthy beef and dairy cattle and sheep is recommended. Shake well and administer 5 ml, either intramuscularly or subcutaneously.
2. *Primary Vaccination:* Primary vaccination with one dose is recommended, and a second dose 3 to 4 weeks later. Animals vaccinated at less than 3 months of age should be revaccinated at weaning or 4 to 6 months of age.
3. *Revaccination:* Annual revaccination is recommended.

Precautions:

1. Store at not over 45°F or 7°C.
2. Protect from freezing.
3. Use entire contents when first opened.
4. Do not vaccinate within 21 days before slaughter.
5. If anaphylaxis occurs following use, administer epinephrine or equivalent.
6. Although this product has been shown to be efficacious, some animals may be unable to develop or maintain an adequate response following vaccination if they are incubating any infectious disease, are malnourished or parasitized, or stressed due to shipment or adverse environmental conditions.

Supplied: 10- 50- and 200-dose bottles for cattle and sheep.

For Veterinary Use Only

The following Clostrin® products are also available:

- Clostrin M (Cl. chauvoei, Cl. septicum, Cl. sordellii)
- Clostrin MG (Cl. chauvoei, Cl. septicum, Cl. sordellii, Cl. perfringens Types C and D)
- Clostrin MLG (Cl. chauvoei, Cl. septicum, Cl. haemolyticum, Cl. novyi, Cl. sordellii, Cl. perfringens Types C and D)
- Clostrin G (Cl. perfringens Types C and D)
- Clostrin ML (Cl. chauvoei, Cl. septicum, Cl. haemolyticum, Cl. novyi, Cl. sordellii)

COUGHGUARD–B™

Bordetella Bronchiseptica Bacterin

Product Description: 'CoughGuard-B' is for the immunization of healthy dogs against disease caused by *Bordetella bronchiseptica.* The bacterin contains an inactivated culture of this agent.

Disease Description: Although there is no single cause for kennel cough, *B. bronchiseptica* is a primary etiological agent in the kennel cough complex.[1,2] This pathogen predisposes dogs to the influence of other respiratory agents and frequently exists concurrently with them. Kennel cough can be reproduced by challenge with virulent *B. bronchiseptica.* Further, environmental factors such as cold, drafts, and high humidity —often typical conditions in dog kennels—increase susceptibility to the disease.[3] Antibiotics are generally recognized as poor agents to treat the primary disease.[3] In contrast, immunoprophylaxis for *B. bronchiseptica* provides an effective means to aid in the control of disease.

The outstanding sign of *B. bronchiseptica* infection is a harsh, dry cough, which is aggravated by activity or excitement. The coughing occurs in paroxysms, followed by retching or gagging in attempts to clear small amounts of mucus from the throat. Body temperature may be elevated as secondary bacterial invasion takes place.

Because kennel cough is highly contagious, the disease can readily be transmitted to susceptible dogs and produce a severe cough. The most severe signs are noted beginning 2 to 5 days following infection, but can continue for extended periods. Stress, particularly of adverse environmental conditions, may cause relapse during later stages of the disease.

Safety and Efficacy: 'CoughGuard-B' is prepared from a highly antigenic strain of *B. bronchiseptica* which has been inactivated and processed to be nontoxic when administered to dogs. The production method leaves the immunogenic properties of *B. bronchiseptica* intact. Historically, bordetella bacterins have had a tendency toward toxic reactions characterized by lethargy, anorexia, and vomiting 1 to 6 hours following administration. However, 'CoughGuard-B' is safe and effective. In an extensive field trial in which over 1,000

Continued on next page

N **Norden—Cont.**

doses of 'CoughGuard-B' were administered, no reports of these reactions were received.

In tests conducted at Norden Laboratories with normal, susceptible dogs under controlled conditions, experimental infection with the virulent BC strain of *B. bronchiseptica* consistently resulted in coughing and other respiratory signs typical of kennel cough (Table 1).

In the usual research model, palpation of the throat is necessary to produce coughing. Due to severity of the challenge in the Norden test, coughing was spontaneous for extended periods beginning 2 to 5 days following challenge. (Data on file, Norden Laboratories.)

TABLE 1. Protection from Spontaneous Coughing in Challenge of Immunity Tests with BC Strain of *B. bronchiseptica*

Group	Number/ Normal Total Dogs	Percentage
Vaccinated	75/83	90%
Non-Vaccinated Controls	1/34	3%

Directions:

1. *General Directions:* Shake and administer a 1 ml. dose intramuscularly.
2. *Primary Vaccination:* Two doses should be administered 2 to 4 weeks apart. The presence of maternal antibody may interfere with development of an adequate immune response. The age at which maternal antibody drops below interfering levels varies with the amount of antibody absorbed from the colostrum and may persist as late as about 4 months of age. Dogs vaccinated when less than 4 months of age should be revaccinated after reaching the age of 4 months.
3. *Revaccination:* Annual revaccination with a single dose is recomended. Where exposure is likely, such as breeding, boarding, and showing situations, additional boosters are indicated or annual revaccination could be timed 2 to 4 weeks prior to these events.

Precautions:

1. Store at 2°C. to 7°C. Do not freeze.
2. Use entire contents when first opened.
3. If anaphylaxis occurs following use, administer epinephrine or equivalent.
4. Intramuscular vaccination is recommended to avoid petite nodules which may occur if given subcutaneously.
5. Although this product has been shown to be efficacious, some animals may be unable to develop or maintain an adequate immune response following vaccination if they are incubating any disease, malnourished or parasitized, or stressed due to shipment or adverse environmental conditions.

Supplied: 50 × 1 dose vials.

References:

1. Bemis, D.A., H.A. Greisen, and M.J. Appel. 1977. Pathogenesis of Canine Bordetellosis, J. Infect. Dis. *135*:753–762.
2. Thompson, H., I.A.P. McCandlish, and N.G. Wright. 1976. Experimental Respiratory Diseases in Dogs Due to *Bordetella bronchiseptica*. Res. Vet. Sci. *20*:16–23.
3. *The Merck Veterinary Manual*, Fifth Edition. Otto H. Siegmund, ed. Rahway, Merck and Company, 1979, p. 904.

For Veterinary Use Only.

COUGHGUARD–BP™
Canine Parainfluenza Vaccine
Modified Live Virus
Bordetella Bronchiseptica Bacterin

Product Description: 'CoughGuard-BP' is for the immunization of healthy dogs against disease caused by *Bordetella bronchiseptica* and canine parainfluenza virus (CPI). 'CoughGuard-BP' contains an attenuated strain of CPI and an inactivated culture of *B. bronchiseptica* for use as diluent.

Disease Description: Although there is no single cause for kennel cough, both *B. bronchiseptica* and CPI are the primary etiological agents in the kennel cough complex.[1,2,3,5] These pathogens predispose dogs to the influence of other respiratory agents and frequently exist concurrently with them. Kennel cough can be reproduced by challenge with either virulent *B. bronchiseptica* or CPI. Further, environmental factors such as cold, drafts, and high humidity—often typical conditions in dog kennels—increase susceptibility to the disease.[3] Antibiotics are generally recognized as poor agents to treat the primary disease.[3] In contrast, immunoprophylaxis for *B. bronchiseptica* and CPI provides an effective means to aid in the control of the disease.

CPI is a highly contagious respiratory virus which contributes to upper respiratory disease and infectious tracheobronchitis. A characteristic clinical sign of CPI infection is coughing that may be intensified by activity, excitement, or stress. Typically, CPI is self limiting, with a course of 5 to 10 days duration. However, bacterial infections of the respiratory tract, such as *B. bronchiseptica*, may complicate the clinical syndrome.

The outstanding sign of *B. bronchiseptica* infection is a harsh, dry cough, which is aggravated by activity or excitement. The coughing occus in paroxysms, followed by retching or gagging in attempts to clear small amounts of mucus from the throat. Body temperature may be elevated as secondary bacterial invasion takes place.

Because kennel cough is highly contagious, the disease can rapidly be transmitted to susceptible dogs and produce a severe cough. The most severe signs are noted beginning 2 to 5 days following infection, but can continue for extended periods. Stress, particularly of adverse environmental conditions, may cause relapse during later stages of the disease.

Safety and Efficacy: 'CoughGuard-BP' is prepared from an attenuated strain of canine parainfleunza virus propagated on an established canine cell line and a highly antigenic strain of *B. bronchiseptica* which has been inactivated and processed to be non-toxic when administered to dogs. The production method leaves the immunogenic properties of *B. bronchoseptica* intact. Historically, bordetella bacterins have had a tendency toward toxic reactions characterized by lethargy, anorexia, and vomiting 1 to 6 hours following administration. However, 'CoughGuard-BP' is safe and effective. In an extensive field trial in which over 1,000 doses of the *B. bronchiseptica* fraction were administered, no reports of these reactions were received. In more than 16,000 vaccinated dogs where CPI was used no reports of post-vaccination reactions attributable to CPI were received.[4]

In tests conducted at Norden Laboratories with normal, suspectible dogs under controlled conditions, experimental infection with the virulent BC strain of *B. bronchiseptica* consistently resulted in coughing and other respiratory signs typical of kennel cough (Table 1).

TABLE 1. Protection from Spontaneous Coughing in Challenge of Immunity Tests with BC Strain of *B. bronchiseptica*

Group	Number Normal/ Total Dogs	Percentage
Vaccinated	75/83	90%
Non-Vaccinated Controls	1/34	3%

In the usual research model, palpation of the throat is necessary to produce coughing. Due to severity of the challenge in the Norden test, coughing was spontaneous for extended periods beginning 2 to 5 days following challenge. The most severe and extended coughing was observed in non-vaccinated dogs. In contrast, clinical signs in the few vaccinated dogs which coughed were generally mild and of limited duration. (Data on file, Norden Laboratories.)

A test of the CPI immunizing agent showed that hemorrhagic lung lesions characteristic of infection were absent or greatly diminished in vaccinated dogs after challenge.[5] All non-vaccinated control dogs had characteristic lung lesions, in some cases distributed to all lobes (Table 2).

TABLE 2. Lung Lesions in CPI Challenge of Immunity Test

	*Degree of Severity					
Group	0	1	2	3	4	5
Vaccinated	16	3		1		
Non-Vaccinated Controls			2	4	3	1

*0 = Normal
1 = A very few indistinct petechial hemorrhages

2=A few petechial hemorrhages
3=Petechial hemorrhages, all lobes
4=Many petechial hemorrhages, all lobes
5=Widespread and extensive hemorrhages

Directions

1. *General Directions:* Aseptically rehydrate vaccine with bacterin supplied. Shake and administer a 1 ml. dose intramuscularly.
2. *Primary Vaccination:* Two doses should be administered 2–4 weeks apart. The presence of maternal antibody may interfere with development of an adequate immune response. The age at which maternal antibody drops below interfering levels varies with the amount of antibody absorbed from the colostrum and may persist as late as about 4 months of age. Dogs vaccinated when less than 4 months of age should be revaccinated after reaching the age of 4 months.
3. *Revaccination:* Annual revaccination with a single dose is recomended. Where exposure is likely, such as breeding, boarding, and showing situations, additional boosters are indicated or annual revaccination could be timed 2 to 4 weeks prior to these events.

Precautions:

1. Store at 2°C. to 7°C. Do not freeze.
2. Use entire contents when first opened.
3. If anaphylaxis occurs following use, administer epinephrine or equivalent.
4. Contain penicillin and streptomycin as preservatives.
5. Intramuscular vaccination is recommended to avoid petite nodules which may occur if given subcutaneously.
6. Although this product has been shown to be efficacious, some animals may be unable to develop or maintain an adequate immune response following vaccination if they are incubating any disease, malnourished or parasitized, or stressed due to shipment or adverse environmental conditions.

Supplied: 25 × 1 dose vials.

References:

1. Bemis, D.A., H.A. Greisen, and M.J. Appel. 1977. Pathogenesis of Canine Bordetellosis, J. Infect. Dis. *135*:753–762.
2. Thompson, H., I.A.P. McCandlish, and N.G. Wright. 1976. Experimental Respiratory Diseases in Dogs Due to *Bordetella bronchiseptica.* Res. Vet. Sci. *20*:16–23.
3. *The Merck Veterinary Manual,* Fifth Edition. Otto H. Siegmund, ed. Rahway, Merck and Company, 1979, p. 904.
4. Bass, C.P., M.A. Gill, and W.H. Beckenhauer, 1980. Evaluation of a Canine Adenovirus Type 2 Strain as a Replacement for Infectious Canine Hepatitis Vaccine. J. Am. Vet. Med. Assoc. *117*:234–242.
5. Brown, A.L., J.G. Bihr, J.A. Vitamvas, and L. Miers. 1978. An Alternative Method of Evaluating Potency of Modified Live Canine Parainfluenza Virus Vaccine. Jour. Biol. Stand. *6*:271–281.

For Veterinary Use Only.

CYTOBIN® TABLETS ℞
(sodium liothyronine U.S.P.)

Composition: Each tablet contains 60 or 120 micrograms of L-triiodothyronine as the sodium salt.

Description: A unique, effective and rapid acting metabolic regulating agent for treatment of numerous canine disorders resulting from hypothyroid activity.

Indications: Cytobin (brand of liothyronine) is indicated in cases of hypothyroidism in dogs.

Advantages: Because it stimulates metabolism at the cellular level, Cytobin (sodium liothyronine) offers significant advantages:

1. Produces prompt patient response.
2. Facilitates sensitive adjustment of dosage because of its rapid action.
3. Often effective when other thyroid preparations fail.
4. Is valuable as a diagnostic adjunct.
5. Is well tolerated and has no cumulative effect.

Recommended Dosage: Oral administration to dogs is recommended at levels up to, but not exceeding, 12.8 mcg/kg body weight (approximately 6 mcg/lb) per day. Twice daily administration is recommended. Under clinical conditions —in animals having some thyroid function —lesser amounts may be found effective. Dosage should be adjusted according to the severity of the condition and the response of the patient. Dosage at the total replacement level (6 mcg/lb) should then be considered for initiating therapy and then titrated downward for optimum maintenance effect.

Cautions and Side Effects: Symptoms of overdosage would include tachycardia, excitability, nervousness and excessive panting. Some gastric upset has been observed in dogs but is usually controlled by reduction of dosage.

As the onset of action is rapid, symptoms of overdosage are usually seen within 24 to 48 hours. These symptoms will subside in a similar period of time after discontinuance of the drug. Medication may then be resumed in smaller doses.

Caution: U.S. Federal law restricts this drug to use by or on the order of a licensed veterinarian.

How Supplied: 60 mcg. tablets, 500; 120 mcg. tablets, 500.

DARBAZINE® INJECTION
(prochlorperazine and isopropamide)

Composition: A combination of a potent anticholinergic and tranquilizer for subcutaneous injection.

Formula: Each ml. of Darbazine Injection contains 6 mg. prochlorperazine edisylate (equiv. to 4 mg. prochlorperazine), 0.38 mg. isopropamide iodide (equiv. to 0.28 mg. isopropamide), 0.9 mg. sodium saccharin, 5 mg. sodium biphosphate, 12 mg. sodium tartrate, 0.1 mg. benzalkonium chloride, in distilled water.

Indications: Darbazine injection is indicated for dog and cat patients in which gastrointestinal disturbances are associated with emotional stress. Conditions in which Darbazine Injection is indicated are:

Nonspecific gastroenteritis
Drug induced diarrhea, especially following worming.
Infectious diarrhea, in conjunction with other appropriate therapy
Spastic colitis
Motion sickness

Darbazine Injection is of value when used as a routine medication for hospitalized or boarded animals, administered on the day of discharge from the hospital to prevent excitement, excessive salivation, water and food gulping and the vomiting and diarrhea that frequently follows. Darbazine Injection is also indicated in newly hospitalized cases which are highly nervous, salivate excessively, gulp food and water, and have difficulty adjusting to the new environment.

Contraindications: Darbazine Injection is contraindicated in cases of glaucoma, pyloric obstruction or stenosis, and prostatic hypertrophy.

Side Effects: The dry mouth syndrome may occur at recommended dosages. The application of small amounts of water to the tongue at frequent intervals for a period of 10 to 15 minutes will generally relieve this symptom. Animals should be given close supervision for at least one hour after administration of the product.

Dosage and Administration: Administer subcutaneously twice daily to dogs and cats, following last injection in 6 to 8 hours with Darbazine Spansule* Capsules as indicated.

Wt. of Animal	Darbazine Injection
Up to 4 lbs.	0.25 ml
5–14 lbs.	0.5–1 ml
15–30 lbs.	2–3 ml
30–45 lbs.	3–4 ml
45–60 lbs.	4–5 ml
Over 60 lbs.	6 ml

Dosage may be adjusted upward or downward as clinical results indicate.

Overdosage: Isopropamide overdosage produces dryness of mouth, dilated pupils, constipation and urinary retention. Prochlorperazine overdosage may cause nervous depression, rigidity, weakness, tremor, torticollis, salivation, inability to swallow, hypotension and disturbance of gait.

Treatment of overdosage is essentially symptomatic and supportive. Depending on the severity and type of side effects, gastric lavage, purgatives, catheterization and other standard procedures of combating circulatory shock may be employed as indicated.

Note: If it is desirable to administer a vasoconstrictor, norepinephrine is the drug of choice. Other pressor agents, including epinephrine, are not recommended because phenothiazine derivatives may reverse the usual elevating action of these agents and cause a further lowering of blood pressure.

Caution: U.S. Federal law restricts this drug to use by or on the order of a licensed veterinarian.

* Reg. TM of SmithKline Beckman Corporation.

How Supplied: Darbazine Injection —30 ml. multiple dose vial.

Continued on next page

Norden—Cont.

DARBAZINE®
(prochlorperazine and isopropamide) Spansule* Capsules No. 1 and No. 3

Composition: A logical combination of a potent, inherently long-acting anticholinergic with 12-hour effect and a tranquilizer/antiemetic in sustained release form.

Formula: Each Darbazine Spansule capsule No. 1 contains: 3.33 mg. of prochlorperazine, as the dimaleate, in sustained release form; and 1.67 mg. of isopropamide, as the iodide.

Each Darbazine Spansule capsule No. 3 contains: 10 mg. of prochlorperazine, as the dimaleate, in sustained release form; and 5 mg. of isopropamide, as the iodide.

*Registered Trademark of SmithKline Beckman Corporation brand of sustained release capsules.

Indications: Darbazine Spansule capsules are a formulation for those dog patients in which gastrointestinal disturbances are associated with emotional stress. Among the many conditions in which Darbazine Spansule capsules are indicated are:

Nonspecific gastroenteritis
Vomiting
Drug induced diarrhea (especially following worming)
Infectious diarrhea (in conjunction with other appropriate therapy)
Spastic colitis
Nervous stomach
Motion sickness

Contraindications: Darbazine is contraindicated in cases of glaucoma, pyloric obstruction or stenosis, and prostatic hypertrophy.

Do not use with depressants as it will potentiate general anesthesia. Drug should not be used in disease conditions where prolonged activity is not desirable, or where drug may not be properly metabolized or eliminated.

Precautions: Lowest dosages should be used and with care in animals showing debilitation, cardiac disease, sympathetic blockage, hypovolemia, shock, and during general anesthesia.

Epinephrine is contraindicated for the treatment of acute hypotension produced by phenothiazine-derivative tranquilizers since further depression of blood pressure can occur.

Other pressor-amines, such as norepinephrine or neosynephrine are the drugs of choice. Do not use this product in conjunction with organophosphates and/or procaine hydrochloride since Phenothiazine may potentiate the toxicity of organophosphates and the activity of procaine hydrochloride.

Dosage and Administration: Darbazine Spansule capsules are provided in two convenient sizes (No. 1 and No. 3) for adjustment of dosage according to individual needs. (Note: Each Darbazine Spansule capsule No. 3 is equivalent to three Darbazine Spansule capsules No. 1).

Darbazine Spansule capsule No. 1—Dogs: 4 lbs. to 15 lbs., 1 capsule twice daily. 16 lbs. to 30 lbs. 1 or 2 capsules twice daily.

Darbazine Spansule capsule No. 3—Dogs: 30 lbs. and over 1 capsule twice daily.

For animals weighing less than 4 lbs. administer appropriate fraction of the contents of a Darbazine Spansule capsule No. 1. Tolerance of Darbazine is quite good and individual dosage adjustment up to twice the recommended dose may prove beneficial without side effects.

Side Effects: Tranquilizers that are potent central nervous system depressants can produce marked sedation with suppression of the sympathetic nervous system. These drugs may produce prolonged depression or motor restlessness when given in excessive amounts or to sensitive animals.

The dry mouth syndrome occurs at recommended dosages. The application of small amounts of water to the tongue at frequent intervals for a period of 10-15 minutes will generally relieve this condition. Animals should be given close supervision for at least one hour after administration of the product.

Overdosage: Symptoms of overdosage are those of the separate ingredients, isopropamide and prochlorperazine. Isopropamide overdosage produces dilated pupils, constipation and urinary retention. Prochlorperazine overdosage may cause central nervous depression, rigidity, weakness, tremor, torticollis, salivation, inability to swallow, hypotension and disturbance of gait.

Overdosage may be treated as may be indicated, by such means as gastric lavage, purgatives, catheterization and standard procedures of combatting circulatory shock.

How Supplied: Darbazine Spansule capsules No. 1, bottles of 250, 500. Darbazine Spansule capsules No. 3, bottles of 100, 250.

Caution: U.S. Federal law restricts this drug to use by or on the order of a licensed veterinarian.

E COLI BAC™
Escherichia Coli Bacterin For Use in Cattle Only

Description: Neonatal calf diarrhea is a disease of complex etiology. Enterotoxigenic strains of *E. coli* are commonly isolated from scouring calves, often in combination with other bacterial and viral pathogens. Studies have shown that most enterotoxigenic strains isolated from scouring calves have K99 pili, antigenic structures that promote colonization on the mucosal surface of the small intestine.[1,2] Enterotoxins produced by these *E. coli* strains induce secretion of body fluids and electrolytes into the lumen of the gut. Fluid loss into the intestine produces diarrhea resulting in dehydration, electrolyte loss, and in severe cases, metabolic acidosis.

Indications: E Coli Bac is for vaccination of healthy, pregnant cows to protect their calves against calf diarrhea caused by enterotoxigenic strains of *Escherichia coli* having the K99 pili adherence factor. E Coli Bac contains an inactivated *E coli* strain selected because of its high K99 pili content. A sterile adjuvant is used to enhance the immune response.

Safety and Efficacy: Pregnancies in experimental cows were not affected as a result of vaccination with E Coli Bac. Susceptible calves are protected by receiving colostral antibodies from vaccinated cows. In a controlled challenge of immunity study, pregnant cows that received two doses of E Coli Bac provided maternal immunity that fully protected 80% of their calves from virulent challenge. The remaining 20% of the experimental calves had transient diarrhea lasting less than 48 hours. No death loss occurred in vaccinated calves. Following challenge, 100% of the non-vaccinated control calves had severe diarrhea resulting in a 58.8% mortality rate.

Dosage and Administration:

General Directions: Shake well. Administer 2 ml intramuscularly to pregnant cows.

Primary Vaccination: Administer 2 doses, late in pregnancy, at least 2 weeks apart. The last dose should be given at least 3 weeks before calving.

Revaccination: Annual revaccination is recommended.

Precautions:

Store at 2°C.-7°C. Do not freeze.

Use entire contents when first opened. Do not vaccinate within 21 days of slaughter. Anaphylaxis may occur following use (antidote is epinephrine). Although this product has been shown to be efficacious, some animals may be unable to develop or maintain an adequate immune response following vaccination if they are incubating any disease, malnourished or parasitized, or stressed due to shipment or adverse environmental conditions.

How Supplied: 20-dose vials.

For Veterinary Use Only

References;

1. Isaacson R.E., Moon H.W., Schneider, R.A.: Distribution and virulence of Escherichia coli in the small intestine of calves with and without diarrhea. *Am. J. Vet. Res. 39:* 1750-1755, 1978.
2. Moon, W., Whipp, S.C., Skartvedt, S.M.: Etiological diagnosis of diarrheal diseases of calves: Frequency and methods for detecting enterotoxin and K99 antigen production by *Escherichia coli. Am. J. Vet Res. 37:* 1025-1029, 1976.

ENDURALL-K®
Rabies Vaccine Killed Virus

Composition: Endurall-K, consisting of cell culture adapted, inactivated rabies virus, is for the immunization of healthy dogs and cats against rabies. The virus is propagated on a porcine established cell line that has been extensively tested for purity. Endurall-K is chemically inactivated and contains an adjuvant selected for its consistently reaction-free performance.

Indications: For use in the prevention of rabies in healthy dogs and cats only.

Dosage and Administration: Shake and administer a single 1 ml. dose subcutaneously or intramuscularly. Healthy dogs and cats 3 months of age or older should be given a single dose. Annual revaccination is recommended.

Duration of Immunity: A study conducted at Norden Laboratories demonstrated that a single 1.0 ml dose protected dogs and cats satisfactorily following a severe 1 year post-vaccination challenge.

Caution: Store at 2°C–7°C. Do not freeze. Use entire contents when first opened. Contains gentamicin as preservative. Anaphylactoid reactions may follow use of products of this nature. *Antidote:* Epinephrine.

For Use by Graduate Veterinarians Only.

How Supplied: Endurall-K is supplied in 10-dose vials.

For Veterinary Use Only

ENDURALL-R®

Rabies Vaccine, Modified Live Virus, High Egg Passage, Flury Strain
For Use in Dogs and Cats Only!
Not for Use in Any Other Animal!

Composition: Endurall-R® is prepared from the Flury HEP strain of rabies virus grown in tissue culture using the Stable Cell Line (SCL®) process developed at Norden Laboratories. The product is lyophilized for stability and must be rehydrated before use with accompanying diluent.

The Flury HEP strain of rabies virus used in Endurall-R is one of the most highly modified rabies viruses known. At the 227th passage level in embryonated eggs it was adapted to tissue culture by Dr. T. J. Wiktor of the Wistar Institute, Philadelphia, Pennsylvania. It was then further adapted by scientists at Norden to grow in the DK cell line. At this passage level the virus is not pathogenic for dogs and cats when used as directed.

The use of a Stable Cell Line (SCL®) has important advantages. Like our virus strain, Norden Laboratories stable dog kidney (NL-DK-1) cell line, upon which the virus is grown, also has a carefully controlled pedigree. The cells used for vaccine production are maintained under carefully controlled conditions at a uniform passage level. Because these pedigreed cells all have the same genetic background, they all have the same growth rate, the same virus susceptibility, and respond the same way each time they are infected with rabies virus. Therefore, the potency of the vaccine from serial to serial is very uniform. On the basis of all tests conducted, the NL-DK-1 cell line has been found free of adventitious or latent viruses. Their propagation for many generations outside of the host dog virtually eliminates the danger of their transmitting virus infections from the living animal.

Isolated cases of vaccine-induced rabies in cats have been reported following use of modified live virus (MLV) rabies vaccine produced by various manufacturers. Several such cats were positive for feline leukemia, leading to speculation that immunodeficiency may contribute to vaccine-induced rabies in cats.[2-4] Although the cause-and-effect relationship between the HEP-Flury strain and vaccine-induced rabies has been questioned,[5] and reported cases are extremely rare, an overriding public health concern warrants precautions in the product's use. Therefore, use of HEP-Flury strain rabies vaccine is contraindicated in immunosuppressed cats, i.e., those treated with corticosteroids or affected with known immunosuppressive diseases such as feline leukemia and feline panleukopenia.

This vaccine is produced and tested in accordance with a production outline on file with the U.S. Department of Agriculture. It has passed all required tests and been proven to be a safe and efficacious product.

Dosage and Administration: Aseptically rehydrate and administer as follows: Healthy dogs, three months of age or older, a single 1 ml. dose, injected intramuscularly in the thigh. Healthy cats, three months of age, a single 1 ml. dose injected intramuscularly in the thigh. Use sterile disposable syringes and needles which have been sterilized by steam or boiling, not by chemicals. Using syringe, aseptically transfer the entire contents of the diluent vial to the vaccine vial and shake to rehydrate. Use product immediately following rehydration or keep refrigerated and use within one hour.

The entire dose should be given intramuscularly at a single site in the thigh. Aseptic technique should be employed in administering the vaccine.

Protection of Dogs: In a duration of immunity study conducted by veterinarians and scientists at Norden Laboratories it was shown that under the conditions of the experiment, a single intramuscular dose of 'Endurall-R' satisfactorily protected dogs following challenge at 41 months post-vaccination. A table from the complete report published in the American Journal of Veterinary Research[1] summarizes the essential results. A copy of the full report may be obtained from Norden Laboratories upon request.

While laboratory experiments have shown that animals as young as eight weeks often develop satisfactory immunity, in accordance with uniform vaccination regulations, we recommend that vaccine be administered to dogs at 3 months of age or older, with a repeat dose 1 year later. Subsequent vaccinations shall be not less frequently than every 3 years thereafter. 'Endurall-R' inoculation may be combined in any sequence with other vaccination procedures.

Protection of Cats: We recommend that vaccine be administered to cats at 3 months of age or older, with a repeat dose 1 year later. Yearly revaccination is recommended to keep immunity high.

Precautions: Store at 2°C.–7°C. and follow all directions carefully. Although evidence of untoward effects on the fetus has not been observed, vaccination of pregnant animals should be avoided. Contains penicillin and streptomycin as preservatives. If anaphylaxis occurs following use, administer epinephrine or equivalent. Burn containers and all unused contents.

Inadvertent Human Exposure: In event of accidental exposure to the vaccine virus, the possible hazard to human health should be considered and State Public Health Officials should be consulted for specific recommendations.

Caution: For Use By Graduate Veterinarians Only

How Supplied: 25-1 dose, 10 doses, with sterile diluent. Dose is 1 ml.

For Veterinary Use Only

U.S. Patent No. 3,616,203

Canadian Patent 1969 No. 829,277

References:

1. Brown AL, Merry DL, Jr, and Beckenhauer WH: Modified Live-Virus Rabies Vaccine Produced from Flury High Egg-Passage Virus Grown on an Established Canine-Kidney Cell Line: Three-Year Duration-of-Immunity Study in Dogs. Am J Vet Res, 34 (Nov 1973): 1427-1432.
2. Esh JB, Cunningham JG, Wiktor TJ: Vaccine-induced rabies in four cats. J Am Vet Med Assoc 180:1336-1339, 1982.
3. Bellinger DA, Chang J. Bunn TO: Rabies induced in a cat by high-egg passage Flury strain vaccine. J Am Vet Med Assoc 183:997-998, 1983.
4. Eriewein DL: Post-vaccinal rabies in a cat. Feline Pract 11:16-20, March-April, 1981.
5. Beckenhauer WH, Sharpee RL: Vaccine induced rabies. J Am Vet Med Assoc 184:380-382, 1984.

ER BAC®

Erysipelothrix Rhusiopathiae Bacterin

Composition: An inactivated antigenic culture of *Erysipelothrix rhusiopathiae.*

Indications: For the immunization of healthy swine against erysipelas.

Dosage and Administration: Shake well. Using aseptic precautions administer 2 ml. intramuscularly or subcutaneously at weaning age or older. Animals retained for breeding should receive a second dose at selection. Annual revaccination is recommended.

Caution:
Store at 2°C-7°C. Do not freeze. Use entire contents when first opened. Do not vaccinate within 21 days before slaughter. Anaphylaxis may follow use of products of this nature. Antidote: Epinephrine.

How Supplied: 10-, 50- and 250-dose vials

For Veterinary Use Only

ER BAC®/LEPTOFERM-5®

Erysipelothrix Rhusiopathiae-Leptospira Canicola-Grippotyphosa-Hardjo-Icterohaemorrhagiae-Pomona Bacterin
For Use in Swine Only
Aluminum Hydroxide Adsorbed

Composition: An inactivated combination of antigenic cultures of *E. rhusi-*

Continued on next page

Norden—Cont.

opathiae, L. canicola, L. grippotyphosa, L. hardjo, L. icterohaemorrhagiae and *L. pomona.*

Indications: For the immunization of healthy swine against erysipelas and leptospirosis caused by these serotypes

Dosage and Administration: Shake well. Using aseptic precautions administer 5 ml. intramuscularly. A second dose is recommended 3–6 weeks later. Annual revaccination is recommended.

Caution: Store at 2°C–7°C. Do not freeze. Use entire contents when first opened. Do not vaccinate within 21 days befoe slaughter. Anaphylaxis may follow use of products of this nature. Antidote: Epinephrine.

How Supplied: 10- and 50-dose vials.

For Veterinary Use Only

EVA®
Erysipelothrix Rhusiopathiae Vaccine Avirulent Live Culture

Dosage and Administration: Aseptically rehydrate vaccine with diluent supplied. Inject 2 ml. intramuscularly *in pigs of weanling age or older.* Swine held beyond normal marketing period, such as breeding or show animals, should be revaccinated. Vaccination of breeding stock is recommended from 30 days prior to breeding up to the breeding date; however, no adverse reactions have been experienced if vaccinated during the gestation period. If immediate protection is required, administer swine erysipelas antiserum as indicated, using another site of injection.

Caution: Do not vaccinate within 21 days before slaughter. Anaphylaxis may follow the use of products of this nature. Antidote: Epinephrine.

Syringes and needles used in administering this type vaccine should be sterilized by boiling. Do not use chemical sterilization since traces of disinfectant may inactivate the vaccine. Store at 2°C.-7°C. Shake well before using. Do not save fractional contents for later use. Use without delay after rehydration. Burn container after use.

How Supplied: 20 ml (10-dose), 50 ml (25-dose), and 100 ml (50-dose) vials.

EVA®/LEPTOFERM-5®
Erysipelothrix Rhusiopathiae Vaccine Avirulent Live Culture Leptospira Canicola-Grippotyphosa-Hardjo-Icterohaemorrhagiae-Pomona Bacterin

Indications: Eva/Leptoferm-5 is for the vaccination of healthy swine against *Erysipelothrix rhusiopathiae* and *L. canicola, L. grippotyphosa, L. hardjo, L. icterohaemorrhagiae,* and *L. pomona* infections.

Disease Description: Swine erysipelas is an infectious disease of major economic significance throughout the world. Caused by the *Erysipelothrix rhusiopathiae* bacterium, the disease occurs most often in pigs between 3 and 12 months of age. Manifestations include acute septicemia, chronic arthritis, endocarditis, and urticaria (diamond-skin lesions). Abortions may occur in dams infected during pregnancy. Although acute erysipelas can be fatal, the greatest economic loss probably results from a general unthriftiness caused by milder, chronic forms of the disease.

Leptospirosis is a contagious disease caused by several species of *Leptospira* bacteria. Infection in swine is usually subclinical, but may be characterized by mild fever, anorexia and diarrhea over a 1 to 3 day period. Following acute infection, *Leptospira* organisms may localize in the kidneys and be shed in the urine for several months. In pregnant dams, such chronic infection may cause late-term abortions, stillbirths and weak neonatal pigs, resulting in significant economic loss. Swine serve as a reservoir of leptospirosis infection for other animals and man.

Safety and Efficacy: In efficacy studies performed at Norden Laboratories, all of the pigs vaccinated with Eva/Leptoferm-5 were shown to be satisfactorily protected against challenge with a virulent *Erysipelothrix* culture. In contrast, 100% of the controls receiving only the *Leptospira* bacterin exhibited clinical signs of erysipelas, thus demonstrating the severity of the challenge. Comparison of post-vaccination microagglutination (MA) titers in the 2 groups of pigs demonstrated that the *Erysipelothrix* fraction did not significantly interfere with protective seroconversion of the *Leptospira* fractions. In both groups, titers were significantly above protective levels.

No post-vaccination reactions were observed in any of the vaccinated test animals. No adverse reactions attributed to the avirulent *E. rhusiopathiae* fraction have been reported in pregnant swine.

Directions for Use:

1. General Directions: Aseptically rehydrate the *E. rhusiopathiae* vaccine with the *Leptospira* bacterin supplied. Shake well and use without delay after rehydration.
2. Primary Vaccination: Eva/Leptoferm-5 is for use in pigs weighing 50 pounds or more. Administer 2 ml. intramuscularly. Follow in 3-6 weeks with a second 2 ml. dose of Leptoferm-5 bacterin.
3. Revaccination: Breeding stock should be revaccinated with Eva/Leptoferm-5 30 days prior to breeding. Semiannual revaccination is recommended for show animals.

Caution: Store at 2°C.–7°C. Do not save fractional contents of vaccine for later use. Burn containers after use.

Do not use chemical means to sterilize syringes and needles used in administering this type of vaccine.

Do not vaccinate within 21 days before slaughter.

Anaphylaxis may occur following use (antidote is epinephrine).

Although Eva/Leptoferm-5 has been shown to be efficacious, some animals may be unable to develop an adequate immune response following vaccination. Vaccination is an important part of a herd health management program, but does not in itself provide absolute protection. In the case of confined animals, sufficient space, good sanitation, suitable temperature and humidity control, adequate ventilation, and proper nutrition are equally important factors in disease control.

How Supplied: 20 ml (10- dose) and 100 ml (50-dose) vials.

For Veterinary Use Only

FELOCELL CVR®
Feline Rhinotracheitis-Calici-Panleukopenia Vaccine Modified Live Virus

Composition: Felocell CVR is a modified live virus vaccine for protection of healthy cats against feline rhinotracheitis, calicivirus and panleukopenia infections. The viruses are propagated on the Norden Feline Cell Line which has been shown to be free of adventitious agents. The highly antigenic Johnson Snow Leopard Strain of panleukopenia virus is used.

Indications: For the immunization of healthy cats against feline rhinotracheitis, feline calicivirus and panleukopenia infections.

Dosage and Administration: Rehydrate lyophilized vaccine with accompanying sterile diluent to 1 ml. Inoculate entire volume intramuscularly or subcutaneously. Use without delay after rehydration. Cats 9 weeks of age or older should be administered 2 doses 3 to 4 weeks apart. Cats less than 9 weeks of age should be revaccinated every 3 to 4 weeks until at least 12 weeks of age. Annual revaccination is recommended. Vaccination of pregnant queens should be avoided.

Caution: Store at 2°C.-7°C. Use entire contents. Burn container and syringe after use. Contains gentamicin as preservative. Do not use chemically sterilized syringes and needles. If allergic response occurs for any reason, administer epinephrine or equivalent.

How Supplied: Packaged as 25 1-dose vials with sterile diluent.

For Veterinary Use Only.

FELOCINE®
Feline Panleukopenia Vaccine Killed Virus

Composition: Felocine is an inactivated virus antigen for the protection of healthy cats, including pregnant queens, against feline panleukopenia (feline distemper). This vaccine utilizes the highly antigenic snow leopard strain of panleukopenia virus, which is grown on the Norden feline Established Cell Line.

Use of the Norden feline Established Cell Line assures that Felocine is produced under the most advanced conditions known to modern science. These cells all have the same genetic background, growth rate, and virus susceptibility for uniform vaccine antigenicity and potency.

Propagation of the feline Established Cell Line *in vitro* for many generations virtually eliminates the danger of transmitting unrecognized virus diseases originating from the cell culture.
Feline tissue culture virus-laden fluids are harvested at the peak of infection as determined by fluorescent antibody microscopy. The resultant product is highly antigenic and relatively free of extraneous protein. Discomfort is virtually never noted in the patient due to the reduced amount of inactivating agent used in this product.
The potency of each serial of Felocine is determined by protection in susceptible kittens. Every kitten used for vaccination has beeen determined to be free of antibody to the virus prior to its use in protection tests. Sterility, inactivation and safety tests must conform to the requirements of the U.S. Department of Agriculture.
Dosage and Administration: *Dosage:* Inject 1 ml. subcutaneously or intramuscularly using aseptic precautions. Revaccinate annually.
Age: Vaccinate healthy cats of any age with one dose except that if the animal is less than 12 weeks of age, a second dose should be given at 12 to 16 weeks of age. Annual revaccination with a single dose is recommended.
Precautions: Store at 2°C. or 7°C. Sick or malnourished animals are not good subjects for vaccination. If allergic response occurs administer epinephrine or equivalent.
How Supplied: 10-dose vials. Dose is 1 ml.

FELOMUNE CVR®
Feline Rhinotracheitis-Calici Vaccine Modified Live Virus For Intranasal Use

Composition: Felomune CVR® is a modified live virus vaccine for protection of healthy cats against feline rhinotracheitis and calicivirus infections.
It is difficult to differentiate feline rhinotracheitis (FVR) from feline calicivirus (FCV) infections in many cases. Both viral diseases produce respiratory signs characterized by fever varying from 104°–107°F., anorexia, depression and excessive salivation. Violent or paroxysmal sneezing, ocular and nasal discharges, frequently purulent, are most likely to be associated with FVR. Palatine, lingual and nasal septum ulceration is most likely to be associated with FCV. Pneumonia may be a prominent characteristic of FCV.
Indications: For the immunization of healthy cats and kittens against feline rhinotracheitis and feline calicivirus infections.
Dosage and Administration: Rehydrate lyophilized vaccine to 0.5 ml. with accompanying vial of sterile diluent using sterile dropper supplied. Inoculate entire volume into nasal passages; however, one drop may be placed in each eye and remaining vaccine into nasal passages. Use within 30 minutes after rehydration. Vaccinate all healthy cats over 12 weeks of age. If vaccinated at less than 12 weeks of age, administer a second vaccination at 12 weeks or older. Annual revaccination with a single dose is recommended.
Warning: Transient sneezing may be observed 4 to 7 days following inoculation. Oral lesions may be observed postvaccinally but heal without incident. Vaccination of cats incubating or harboring latent infections may result in more pronounced upper respiratory signs, ocular irritation, or febrile response.
Precautions: Store at 2°C.–7°C. Use entire contents immediately after rehydration. Burn container and dropper after use. Contains penicillin and streptomycin as preservatives.
How Supplied: Packaged as 25 1-dose vials with sterile diluent.

Recommended Dosage Schedule for Prevention of Heartworms

Body Weight (lb)	Filaribits Tablets 60 mg.	120 mg.	180 mg.
5	¼ Tablet		
10	½ Tablet		
15			¼ Tablet
20	1 Tablet	½ Tablet	
30			½ Tablet
40		1 Tablet	
60			1 Tablet

FILARIBITS®
(brand of diethylcarbamazine citrate) Chewable Tablets

Composition: Each tablet contains diethylcarbamazine citrate, 60 mg., 120 mg. or 180 mg.
Indications: Filaribits are indicated for use in the prevention of infection with *Dirofilaria immitis* (heartworm disease), and as an aid in the treatment of ascarid *(Toxocara canis* and *Toxascaris leonina)* infections in dogs. Filaribits may be given to dogs of all ages including bitches throughout the reproductive period and following whelping.
Dosage and Administration: Filaribits are chewable tablets that are palatable to most dogs. Tablets may be fed free choice or crumbled and placed on food. Filaribits are scored for convenient adjustment of dosage.
For the Prevention of Heartworm Disease in Dogs: Filaribits are given orally (once a day) at a dosage rate of 3 mg. diethylcarbamazine citrate per pound of body weight. Young dogs may be started on the preventive program at two months of age. Administration of Filaribits in heartworm endemic areas should start 1 month before the beginning of mosquito season and for approximately two months thereafter. Continuous low level administration during the mosquito season effectively prevents the maturation of recently inoculated heartworm larvae into adults *(D. immitis).*
[See table above].
For the Treatment of Ascarid Infection in Dogs: Filaribits are given as a single, oral dose at the dosage rate of 25 to 50 mg. of diethylcarbamazine citrate per pound of body weight (one 180 mg. tablet for each 3.6 to 7.2 pounds of body weight, one 120 mg. tablet for 2.4 to 4.8 pounds of body weight, or one 60 mg. tablet for 1.2 to 2.4 pounds body weight). Fasting or a laxative after treatment is not necessary. To reduce the possibility of vomiting which occasionally occurs, it is preferable to administer Filaribits with food or directly after feeding. Repeat the dose 10 to 20 days later to remove immature worms which may enter the intestine from the lungs after the first treatment.
Precautions and Side Effects: The use of diethylcarbamazine citrate is not recommended in dogs with active *D. immitis* infections. Inadvertent administration to heartworm infected dogs may cause adverse reactions due to pulmonary occlusion. Overdosage may cause emesis. The compound causes no cumulative toxic effects.
Warning: Dogs with established heartworm infections should not receive Filaribits until they have been converted to a negative status by the use of adulticidal and microfilaricidal drugs. A dog on prophylactic therapy should be examined for the presence of microfilaria every six months. Do not use in dogs that may be harboring adult heartworms. Keep out of reach of children.
Caution: U.S. Federal law restricts this drug to use by or on the order of a licensed veterinarian.
How Supplied: Bottles of 100 and 200-60 mg. (quarter scored).
Bottles of 100-120 mg (half scored).
Bottles of 50, 100 and 200-180 mg (quarter scored).
For Veterinary Use Only

FILARIBITS® PLUS
(brand of diethylcarbamazine citrate/oxibendazole) Chewable Tablets For Veterinary Use Only

Composition: Each 60 mg/45 mg 'Filaribits Plus' tablet contains 60 mg diethylcarbamazine citrate and 45.36 mg oxibendazole. Each 180 mg/136 mg 'Filaribits Plus' tablet contains 180 mg diethylcarbamazine citrate and 136.1 mg oxibendazole.
Indications: 'Filaribits Plus' are indicated for use in the prevention of infection with *Dirofilaria immitis* (heartworm

Continued on next page

Norden—Cont.

disease) and *Ancylostoma caninum* (hookworm infection). 'Filaribits Plus' may be given to dogs of all ages including bitches, throughout the reproductive period and following whelping.

Precautions and Side Effects: The use of diethylcarbamazine citrate is not recommended in dogs with active *Dirofilaria immitis* infections. Inadvertent administration to heartworm infected dogs may cause adverse reactions due to pulmonary embolism. Overdosage may cause emesis. The product causes no cumulative toxic effects.

Oxibendazole, the benzimidazole component of 'Filaribits Plus', is safe when administered to dogs under laboratory and clinical conditions. Another benzimidazole has been reported to cause hepatotoxicity clinically in canines. This effect has not been reported during the clinical use of 'Filaribits Plus'. In U.S. clinical studies only 1 of 487 dogs receiving 'Filaribits Plus' exhibited clinical signs of diarrhea, emesis and anorexia.

Warning: Dogs with established heartworm and/or hookworm infection should not receive 'Filaribits Plus' until they have been converted to a negative status by the use of appropriate adulticidal and microfilaricidal heartworm therapy and /or hookworm therapy. A dog on prophylactic therapy should be examined for the presence of heartworm microfilaria every six months.

Dosage and Administration: 'Filaribits Plus' are chewable tablets that are palatable to most dogs. Tablets may be fed free choice or placed on food. 'Filaribits Plus' are scored for convenient adjustment of dosage.

For the Prevention of Heartworm Disease and Hookworm Infection in Dogs.

'Filaribits Plus' are given orally (once a day) at a dosage rate of 3 mg diethylcarbamazine citrate and 2.27 mg oxibendazole per pound of body weight. Young dogs may be started on the preventive program at two months of age. Administration of 'Filaribits Plus' in heartworm or hookworm endemic areas should start prior to hookworm exposure and at least one month before the beginning of the mosquito season. 'Filaribits Plus' administration should continue daily throughout the entire period of exposure to hookworms and two months past the mosquito season since there is little residual effect of the drugs. Continuous low level administration effectively prevents maturation of hookworms *(A. caninum)* and recently inoculated heartworm larvae *(D. immitis)* into adults. In those areas with seasonal heartworm problem, hookworm prevention or therapy should be continued after 'Filaribits Plus' have been discontinued.

Recommended Dosage Schedule

Body Weight (lb.)	'Filaribits Plus' 60 mg/45 mg Tablets
1–5	¼ Tablet
6–10	½ Tablet
11–15	¾ Tablet
16–20	1 Tablet
21–25	1¼ Tablet
26–30	1½ Tablet
31–35	1¾ Tablet
36–40	2 Tablets
41–45	2¼ Tablets
46–50	2½ Tablets

Body Weight (lb.)	'Filaribits Plus' 180 mg/136 mg Tablets
26–30	½ Tablet
31–45	¾ Tablet
46–60	1 Tablet
61–75	1¼ Tablet
76–90	1½ Tablet
91–105	1¾ Tablet
106–120	2 Tablets
121–135	2¼ Tablets
136–150	2½ Tablets

Caution: U.S. Federal law restricts this drug to use by or on the order of a licensed veterinarian.

Do not use in dogs that may be harboring adult heartworms.

KEEP OUT OF REACH OF CHILDREN

Supplied: 'Filaribits Plus' 60 mg/45 mg—Bottles of 100 and 200 tablets
'Filaribits Plus' 180 mg/136 mg—Bottles of 100 and 200 tablets.

U.S. Patent Nos. 3,480,642 and 3,574,845

NORDEN LABORATORIES 75-6423-01
Lincoln, NE 68501, U.S.A. Printed in U.S.A. (May 1985)

FIRSTDOSE CPV™
Parvovirus Vaccine
Modified Live Virus
For Use in Dogs Only

Product Description: 'FirstDose CPV' is for vaccination of healthy dogs against canine parvovirus (CPV) infection. 'FirstDose CPV' contains a strain of CPV attenuated by low passage on an established canine cell line. At that passage level the virus has immunogenic properties capable of overriding maternal antibodies. 'FirstDose CPV' is packaged in liquid form.

Disease Description: Canine parvovirus is generally transmitted through direct contact with infected feces. The virus also can be carried on dogs' hair and feet or other contaminated objects and can remain infective for more than 6 months at room temperature. Incubation period of CPV infection ranges from 4 to 14 days. Infection with CPV results in enteric disease characterized by sudden onset of vomiting and diarrhea, often hemorrhagic. Leukopenia commonly accompanies clinical signs. Course of CPV disease may be aggravated by concurrent parasitism or infection with other enteric pathogens. Susceptible dogs of any age can be affected, but mortality is greatest in puppies. In puppies 4 to 12 weeks of age, CPV may occasionally cause myocarditis that can result in acute heart failure after a brief and inconspicuous illness. Following infection many dogs are refractive to the disease for a year or more. Similarly, seropositive bitches may transfer to their pups CPV antibodies which can interfere with active immunization of the pups through 16 weeks of age.

Safety and Efficacy: 'FirstDose CPV' was subjected to comprehensive safety and efficacy testing at Norden Laboratories. It was shown safe and reaction-free in laboratory tests and in clinical trials under field conditions. Product safety was demonstrated by oral administration of multiple doses of the vaccine strain to susceptible dogs, which remained normal. 'FirstDose CPV' vaccine virus shares a characteristic with other live CPV vaccine strains in that the vaccinal virus may be present in the feces following administration. Although vaccinal virus was found occasionally and in low titers in the feces of vaccinated dogs, testing demonstrated that the vaccine strain did not revert to virulence following 6 consecutive backpassages in susceptible dogs.

Susceptible test dogs all developed CPV antibody titers following vaccination and were protected following oral administration of virulent CPV. Conversely, following challenge exposure, nonvaccinated control dogs all developed clinical signs of CPV infection, including vomiting and diarrhea with blood and mucus in the feces. Challenge virus was isolated from the feces of 1/20 vaccinated dogs, whereas challenge virus was isolated from the feces of 5/5 nonvaccinated control dogs. In addition, all controls developed marked lymphopenia, while no lymphopenia was demonstrated in vaccinates following exposure to virulent CPV.

Research conducted at Norden Laboratories demonstrated a stronger correlation of immunogenicity to number of attenuating virus passages than to antigenic mass; immunogenicity of the vaccinal strain was shown to be in inverse proportion to number of passages. The low-passage vaccinal virus in 'FirstDose CPV', therefore, is highly immunogenic and capable of stimulating active immunity in the presence of maternal antibodies. Procedures to demonstrate that capability involved thirty-nine 6- to 8-week old puppies with a conventional range of maternal CPV antibody titers. By 7 days following 1-dose vaccination with 'FirstDose CPV', more than 92% of those animals exhibited active immunity as shown by rising CPV antibody titers. By 14 days following vaccination, 100% of vaccinates' titers were well above the protective threshold. In contrast, nonvaccinated seropositive sentinel littermate dogs' CPV antibody titers declined, demonstrating that initial antibody titers were indeed of maternal origin and no adventitious exposure occurred during the study.

Directions:

1. *General Directions:* Vaccination of healthy dogs is recommended. Administer 1 ml subcutaneously or intramuscularly.
2. *Primary Vaccination:* A single dose is recommended. Although 'FirstDose CPV' has been specifically designed to

override high levels of maternal antibodies, they may still interfere with active immunization in a low percentage of puppies. Dogs vaccinated at less than 4 months of age, therefore, should be revaccinated after reaching the age of 4 months.

3. *Revaccination:* Annual revaccination is recommended.

Precautions:
1. Store at 2°C. to 7°C. Do not freeze.
2. Use entire contents when first opened.
3. Burn this container and all unused contents.
4. Contains penicillin, streptomycin, and amphotericin B as preservatives.
5. If anaphylaxis occurs following use, administer epinephrine or equivalent.
6. Although this product has been shown to be efficacious, some animals may be unable to develop or maintain an adequate immune response following vaccination if they are incubating any disease, malnourished or parasitized, or stressed due to shipment or adverse environmental conditions.

Supplied: 10-dose vials

References:
1. Pollock RVH: Experimental canine parvovirus infection in dogs. *Cornell Vet* 72:103–119, 1982.
2. Woods CB, Pollock RVH, Carmichael LE: Canine parvoviral enteritis. *J Am An Hosp Assoc* 16:171–179, 1980.
3. Swango LJ: Frequently asked questions about CPV disease. *Norden News* 58:4–10, 1983.

For Veterinary Use Only

FLEA AND TICK POWDER FOR DOGS AND CATS

Active Ingredients:

Carbaryl	3.0%
Inert Ingredients:	97.0%
	100.0%

Claims: Kills fleas.
Kills ticks.
Deodorizes with dichlorophene.

Animal Precautions: Do not use on nursing bitches or queens.
Do not use on puppies or kittens under 4 weeks of age.
Do not use within 30 days before or after treatment with other cholinesterase-inhibiting drugs or chemicals. If signs of cholinesterase inhibition develop, administer atropine.

Human Precautions: Powder is harmful if swallowed or inhaled; avoid contamination of food and foodstuffs, and avoid breathing of dust.
Avoid prolonged contact of powder with skin, and avoid contact of powder with eyes.
If powder contacts eyes, flush with water. Seek medical attention if irritation persists.

How Supplied: 6-ounce shaker top cans.

FLEA, TICK, AND MITE SPRAY FOR DOGS, CATS, AND BIRDS

Formula:

Active Ingredients:

Pyrethrins	0.10%
Piperonyl butoxide, technical	0.20%
N-Octyl bicycloheptene dicarboximide	0.40%
Petroleum distillate	0.60%
Inert Ingredients	98.70%
	100.00%

Indications: Kills fleas and ticks on dogs and cats.
Kills mites on birds.

Precautions:

Animal: Cover fish aquariums before spraying.

Human: Harmful if swallowed.
Avoid breathing vapors.
Wash with soap and water after use.
In the home all food processing surfaces, exposed food and utensils should be covered during treatment, or thoroughly washed before use.
Do not use or store near heat or open flame.

Supplied: 16-ounce cans

FURACIN® DRESSING
Nitrofurazone
Topical Antibacterial

Description: Furacin Dressing Veterinary contains 0.2% Furacin*, brand of nitrofurazone. The ointment-like base is water-soluble. The material becomes less viscous at body temperature and dissolves in wound exudates, but retains sufficient viscosity to resist accidental removal.

*Furacin® is a registered trademark of Norwich Eaton Pharmaceuticals, Inc., Norwich, New York 13815.

Advantages: Furacin Dressing Veterinary has a wide spectrum of antibacterial activity. It is effective against both gram-negative and gram-positive organisms. It remains stable and effective in presence of blood, pus or serum. Development of resistant bacterial strains is infrequent. Toxicity to tissues is low.

Indications: For prevention or treatment of surface bacterial infections of wounds, burns, cutaneous ulcers, eczema, ears, and in the treatment of secondary bacterial infections of cow pox.

Dosage and Administration: Apply directly on the lesion with a spatula or first place on a piece of gauze. Application of a bandage is optional. This preparation should be in contact with the lesion for at least 24 hours. The dressing may be changed several times daily or left on the lesion for a longer period.

Caution: In case of deep or puncture wounds or serious burns use only as recommended by veterinarian. If redness, irritation, or swelling persists or increases, discontinue; reconsult veterinarian.

How Supplied: Furacin Dressing Veterinary is supplied in jars of 135 grams and 1 pound.

FURACIN® SOLUBLE POWDER
(nitrofurazone)
Topical Antibacterial

Composition: Contains 0.2% Furacin*, brand of nitrofurazone, in a water-soluble base.

*Furacin® is a registered trademark of Norwich Eaton Pharmaceuticals, Inc., Norwich, New York 13815.

Advantages: Furacin Soluble Powder Veterinary has a broad spectrum of antibacterial activity. It does not produce local foreign body reactions. It does not delay clotting or healing.

Indications: For the prevention or treatment of surface bacterial infections of wounds, burns, skin ulcers, and abscesses after incision. For use only on dogs, cats, and horses (not for food use).

Dosage and Administration: Apply several times daily to the lesion or affected area from the plastic squeeze bottle.

Caution: In case of deep or puncture wounds or serious burns use only as recommended by veterinarian. If redness, irritation, or swelling persists or increases, discontinue; reconsult veterinarian.

How Supplied: 10 gm. and 50 gm. plastic squeeze bottles.

FURACIN® WATER MIX CONCENTRATE
(nitrofurazone)

Composition: A yellow, fine crystalline material containing 18.35% Furacin*, brand of nitrofurazone, in a stabilizing water-soluble base. It mixes well with water when added with slight agitation and will maintain its stability in metal waterers for a maximum of 7 days.

*Furacin® is a registered trademark of Norwich Eaton Pharmaceuticals, Inc., Norwich, New York 13815.

Advantages: Furacin Water Mix is palatable in water. It is effective against *Salmonella choleraesuis*, the organism causing necrotic enteritis in swine. Infected swine frequently do not eat well but continue to drink normal quantities of water. Development of bacteria resistant to Furacin seldom occurs in animals.

Indications: For treatment of infectious necrotic enteritis of swine caused by *Salmonella choleraesuis*, and for treatment of gray diarrhea in mink.

Dosage and Administration: *For swine:* Provide properly medicated, clean water at all times as the only supply of drinking water. Administer for at least 7 days or longer if needed. *Mixing instructions:* See directions on package label. Use only clean drinking water. Stir until completely dissolved. *NOTE:* Discard solutions in waterers once daily if dirty and provide clean, freshly medicated water. Prepared water solutions of Furacin Water Mix will deteriorate if allowed to remain in continuous contact with metal for over 7 days.

Caution: Remove Furacin Water Mix from drinking water 5 days before slaughter of swine. If no improvement is noted after using this preparation for 2 or 3 days, reconsult your veterinarian.

For Mink: Provide properly medicated fresh feed daily as the only source of feed. Administer for at least 21 days. Depend-

Continued on next page

N **Norden—Cont.**

ing on the severity of the infection and response obtained, treatment may be repeated for an additional period of 21 days if indicated. *Mixing instructions:* See directions on package label. *NOTE:* Discard all unused feed after 24 hours. Prepare fresh feed daily. Mink feed mixes containing Furacin Water Mix tend to deteriorate after 24 hours.
How Supplied: 8 oz. bags, and 25 lb. drums.

FUROXONE® SUSPENSION Veterinary (furazolidone) Intestinal Antibacterial with Automatic Dose Dispenser

Composition: A yellow, uniform, opaque smooth liquid suspension. Each ml. contains 100 mg. of Furoxone*, brand of furazolidone. Supplied with an automatic dose dispenser which, when used as directed, will deliver 100 measured doses.
*Furoxone® is a registered trademark of Norwich Eaton Pharmaceuticals, Inc., Norwich, New York 13815.
Advantages: Furoxone Suspension Veterinary acts rapidly. Improvement may be seen within 24 hours. The drug is safe and nontoxic; it remains stable.
Indications: For the peroral treatment of bacterial enteritis (baby pig scours, colibacillosis or white scours) of pigs under 4 weeks of age.
Dosage and Administration: Shake the bottle thoroughly. Remove cap. Insert the automatic dose dispenser into bottle, and screw on tightly. Prime the pump by depressing plunger until Furoxone Suspension appears from spout. After each dose return the bottle to vertical position before releasing plunger to allow dispenser to refill automatically. When primed, 1 complete depression of the plunger automatically delivers 1 dose. Administer 1 dose by mouth each day to each affected baby pig. Treatment may be continued once a day for a total of 3 days. Since the disease often spreads within a litter, all pigs in the litter should be treated, including those which are not scouring.
Note: If no improvement is noted after 2 or 3 days, reconsult your veterinarian.
How Supplied: In 8 fl. oz. bottles (240 ml.) with automatic dose dispenser.

HEATHCLIFF'S FLEA AND TICK COLLAR FOR CATS

Active Ingredients

Propoxur	9.4%
Inert Ingredients	90.6%
	100.0%

MARMADUKE FLEA AND TICK COLLAR FOR DOGS

Active Ingredients

Propoxur	9.4%
Inert Ingredients	90.6%
	100.0%

Claims: Kills fleas and ticks for up to 5 months.
Effectiveness of the collars is not reduced by temporary wetness.
Animal Precautions: When collar is first worn, observe neck area every few days for irritation. Remove collar at the first sign of irritation or adverse reaction.
Do not use on sick or convalescing animals.
Do not use other pesticides on dog or cat while collar worn.
The dust released by this collar is a cholinesterase inhibitor. If signs of cholinesterase inhibition develop, administer atropine.
Human Precautions: Do not allow children to handle this collar.
Do not open protective pouch until ready to use.
Dust will form on collar during storage. Do not get dust or collar in mouth; it is harmful if swallowed. Do not get dust in eyes; will cause temporary pupillary constriction. In case of contact, flush eyes with water.
Wash hands thoroughly with soap and water after handling collar.
Directions for Use: Buckle collar around pet's neck, and adjust the collar size to allow 2 or 3 fingers to be inserted easily between the collar and neck. Cut off any excess length and throw it away. The collar starts killing fleas as soon as it is placed around pet's neck. Fleas will be killed and new ones which may temporarily appear will also be killed while collar is worn. Use in addition to regular collar. This product has been shown to provide effective flea control for up to 21 weeks. Replace collar when effectiveness diminishes. Ticks are tough and are killed slowly. When the collar is first placed on pet, adult ticks will be killed over entire body in a few days and will fall off or may then be easily removed. Ticks appear in three stages. In the first two stages, ticks are smaller than a match head and are difficult to see. The collar will also control these immature stages. This product has been shown to provide effective tick control up to 5 months. If ticks are a problem, this collar should be worn continuously. Kills ticks that may carry and transmit Rocky Mountain spotted fever and tularemia.
How Supplied: 0.29-ounce collar. And 1.2-ounce collar.

HEATHCLIFF'S FLEA AND TICK SPRAY FOR CATS

Active Ingredients:

Pyrethrins	0.06%
Piperonyl butoxide	0.12%
N-Octyl bicycloheptene dicarboximide	0.20%
Petroleum distillate	0.29%
Inert Ingredients:	99.33%
	100.00%

Claims: Kills fleas and ticks on cats and kittens.
Animal Precautions: Remove pets and birds, and cover fish aquariums before spraying.
Human Precautions: Keep out of reach of children.
Spray is harmful if swallowed, or absorbed through the skin. Avoid inhaling spray mist or vapors. Avoid contact with skin or eyes.
In case of contact, immediately flush eyes or skin with plenty of water.
Seek medical attention if irritation persists.
Directions for Use:
Spray the animal from a distance of 8–12 inches. Start spraying at the tail, moving the dispenser rapidly and making sure that the animal's entire body is covered, including the legs and under the body. As you spray, fluff the hair so the spray will penetrate to the skin. Make sure spray wets ticks thoroughly. Do not spray into the eyes, face or on genitals. Repeat as needed.
For cats apply at the rate of one second per pound of body weight.
Storage and Disposal:
STORAGE: Store in original container in cool, locked storage area away from heat or open flame.
DISPOSAL: Unused insecticide: Securely wrap original container in several layers of newspaper and discard in trash.
Empty Container: Do not reuse bottle or sprayer. Rinse thoroughly before discarding in trash.
How Supplied: 8-ounce, 16-ounce bottles.

HEATHCLIFF'S FLEA, TICK, AND LICE DIP FOR CATS

Formula:
Active Ingredients

Pyrethrins	0.33%
Piperonyl butoxide, technical*	0.66%
N-Octyl bicycloheptene dicarboximide**	1.10%
Petroleum distillates	90.58%
Inert Ingredients	7.33%
	100.00%

Indications: Kills fleas, ticks, and lice on cats and kittens.
Precautions:
Animal: This product is toxic to fish and other aquatic animals. Do not apply directly to water. Do not contaminate water by cleaning of equipment or disposal of wastes.
Avoid contact of material with eyes and mouth of animal.
Do not contaminate food or feedstuffs with concentrate or dip.
Human: Keep out of reach of children.
Concentrate or dip is harmful if swallowed. Avoid inhaling vapors. Avoid contact with eyes.
In case of contact, immediately flush eyes or skin with plenty of water. Obtain medical attention if irritation persists. If swallowed, do not induce vomiting. Call a physician at once.
Store in a cool place away from heat or open flame.
Supplied: 8-ounce and 1-gallon bottles.
Dosage: Dilute 4 ounces of concentrate with 1 gallon of water.
Instructions: Dip animal into solution, making sure hair is thoroughly wet to the skin. The area around the ears should be sponged thoroughly. Avoid contact of material with eyes and mouth of animal. Repeat as necessary for control.

*Equivalent to .53% (butylcarbityl) (6-propylpiperonyl) ether and .13% related compounds.
**MGK 264, Insecticide Synergist

LEPTOFERM-5®
Leptospira-Canicola-Grippotyphosa-Hardjo-Icterohaemorrhagiae-Pomona Bacterin

Composition: An inactivated combination of antigenic cultures of *L. canicola, L. grippotyphosa, L. hardjo, L. icterohaemorrhagiae* and *L. pomona.* For the immunization of healthy cattle and swine against leptospiral infections caused by these serotypes.
Dosage and Administration: Shake well. Inject 2 ml. intramuscularly using aseptic precautions. For swine, a second dose is recommended 3-6 weeks later. Revaccinate annually.
Precautions: Store at 2°C.-7°C. Use entire contents when first opened. Do not vaccinate within 21 days before slaughter. Anaphylaxis may follow use of products of this nature. *Antidote:* Epinephrine.
How Supplied: 10- and 50-dose vials. Dose is 2 ml.

LEPTOFERM-P®
Leptospira Pomona Bacterin

Composition: An inactivated antigenic culture of *L. pomona.* For immunization of healthy cattle and swine against *L. pomona* infection.
Dosage and Administration: Shake well. Inject 2 ml. intramuscularly using aseptic precautions. For swine a second dose is recommended 3-6 weeks later. Revaccinate annually.
Precautions: Store at 2°C.-7°C. Use entire contents when first opened. Do not vaccinate within 21 days before slaughter. Anaphylaxis may follow use of products of this nature. Antidote: Epinephrine.
How Supplied: 10- and 50-dose vials. Dose is 2 ml.

LEUKOCELL®
Feline Leukemia Vaccine Killed Virus

Product Description: 'Leukocell' is for vaccination of healthy cats as an aid in prevention of persistent viremia and lymphoid tumors caused by feline leukemia virus (FeLV) and diseases associated with FeLV infection. 'Leukocell' is prepared by propagating FeLV, subgroups A, B, and C, in feline leukemia virus transformed lymphoid cells. Selection of this production system was a critical factor in developing an immunogenic vaccine (see SAFETY AND EFFICACY). Viral antigens are chemically inactivated, combined with a sterile adjuvant, and packaged in liquid form.
'Leukocell' is prepared from a FeLV transformed lymphoid cell line that releases FeLV viral particles which are soluble in a maintenance medium.[1] The practical benefit of this unique, patented feature is that production of immunosuppressive effects characteristic of fully assembled FeLV antigens, whether live or killed, is reduced or eliminated (see SAFETY AND EFFICACY).[2–4]
Disease Description: Feline leukemia virus is associated with a complex of feline diseases. These include two forms of cancer, (1) lymphosarcoma, characterized by presence of tumors, and (2) leukemia, characterized by presence of malignant cells in the bloodstream. In addition, FeLV is associated with a variety of non-neoplastic diseases, including aplastic anemia, reproductive failure, stomatitis, Fading Kitten Syndrome (thymic atrophy), and upper respiratory infections. Pathogenesis is based on the virus's role as an immunosupressive agent. Following chronic infection, immunosuppression persists until cancer or disease of microbial origin develops, usually after a period of months or years.
The causative agent of FeLV disease is a retrovirus, which was named "feline leukemia virus" after its discovery in 1964. The designation is somewhat inaccurate in view of the variety of clinical conditions that result from FeLV infection, only a minority of which are leukemic. Three FeLV subgroups, designated A, B, and C, have been identified, with subgroup A predominating. Structurally, the FeLV envelope consists of two proteins, gp70 and p15e. The gp70 protein is the more prominent. It is considered to be the immunogenic antigen inasmuch as gp70 antibodies will neutralize FeLV. A variety of other FeLV proteins have been identified (including p10, p12, p15, and p27) although their correlation with FeLV disease has not been established.
Lymphosarcoma is the most common form of cancer caused by FeLV. Tumors resulting from FeLV lymphosarcoma express a non-viral antigen on the surface of the malignant cells. This tumor-specific antigen is designated feline oncornavirus-associated cell membrane antigen (FOCMA). Antibodies to FOCMA have been shown to confer immunity to FeLV-induced lymphosarcoma and are an important factor in successful resistance to tumor development.[5] Studies have shown that cats that develop FeLV malignancies do not have high FOCMA antibody titers,[5] and that inadequate anti-FOCMA response is a cause, rather than an effect, of ensuing FeLV lymphosarcoma.[6]
Safety and Efficacy: 'Leukocell' stimulates antibodies to whole FeLV, the gp70 protein, and the tumor-specific antigen FOCMA (see DISEASE DESCRIPTION). This broad serologic response ensures that 'Leukocell' functions as a comprehensive immunizing agent.
In an immunogenicity study, 25 seronegative cats were vaccinated with a 2-dose primary regimen (given 2 weeks apart) and a booster dose (given 9 weeks after the second dose). Following the initial dose, all vaccinates developed FeLV antibody titers. Following the second dose, the mean FeLV antibody titer increased 2-fold. There was no appreciable increase in mean antibody titer after the third dose, indicating that primary immunization was achieved with 2 doses. (Other tests indicated that while 2 doses produce an optimum serologic response, a third dose will sustain peak antibody levels for a longer period, providing the basis for an initial 3-dose vaccination regimen.) Twenty-three of 25 vaccinates developed FOCMA antibody titers, with the mean value peaking after the second dose.
Following challenge with the Rickard strain of FeLV, 80% of vaccinates were protected against establishment of persistent viremia, and 92% were protected against lymphoid tumor formation. In contrast, following the same challenge, 70% of nonvaccinated control cats developed persistent viremia and died, 60% with lymphoid tumors and the remaining 10% with FeLV-related disease.
In assessing these results, it should be noted that test cats were subjected to a far more rigorous challenge than could be expected under normal conditions. Because FeLV lymphosarcoma usually develops over long periods of time, all test cats (including vaccinates) were artificially immunosuppressed at the time of challenge to enhance susceptibility to FeLV infection and tumor development. Previous testing has indicated that artificially immunosuppressed cats are at considerably greater risk to FeLV pathology than normal cats.[7] Immunosupression was demonstrated in both vaccinates and controls by pronounced reductions in lymphocyte values lasting 6 to 10 weeks after treatment, creating an extended period of vulnerability to FeLV infection and viremia. Challenge inoculum was administered oronasally in droplet form to ensure uniform exposure that conforms to the natural route of infection. To definitively evaluate tumor development, test cats were maintained for a postchallenge obvservation period exceeding two years. The 60% incidence of tumor development in nonvaccinated controls has not been previously described in FeLV immunogenicity testing, and is evidence of a challenge of exceptional severity. In addition, vaccinates and control cats were obtained from individual litters that were evenly divided between the two test groups, minimizing genetic variation in test animals. This feature of the immunogenicity testing precluded assigning to the vaccinated group a disproportionate number of refractory cats that inevitably exist in the feline population.
Demonstrated safety is particularly critical in the case of a FeLV vaccine. Kittens, which are not fully immunocompetent, are particularly prone to progressive effects of live or killed FeLV. Researchers have found that FeLV (live or killed) contains a specific envelope protein designated p15e, that is responsible for host immunosupression.[2–4,8] Rigorous safety tests confirmed that 'Leukocell' is free of FeLV immunosuppressive effects. Kittens vaccinated with 'Leukocell' had normal postvaccination white blood cell (WBC) counts, did not become viremic, remained clinically normal, and developed gp70 and FOCMA antibodies. Adult cats vaccinated with approxi-

Continued on next page

Norden—Cont.

mately 50 times the field dose remained clinically normal, had normal WBC counts, and did not become viremic.

Extensive pre-licensing field trials were conducted with the cooperation of practicing veterinarians. Several types of postvaccination reactions were observed by field trial participants. These included stinging on injection, transient listlessness, depression, and brief temperature elevations. Hypersensitivity evidenced by myxedema and gastrointestinal distress (vomiting and bowel evacuation) was occasionally reported. Satisfactory response followed treatment with steroids, antihistamines or epinephrine.

Though a diagnostic test for FeLV is not required prior to vaccination with 'Leukocell', such a test may be beneficial in evaluating candidates for vaccination. In cases where a FeLV diagnostic test is administered, a positive result indicates the cat may be infected or has been exposed to FeLV. A positive test does not necessarily mean that the cat is immune or will become immune, or that it has disease caused by FeLV. In tests conducted at Norden Laboratories, clinically normal but FeLV-infected cats were vaccinated with 'Leukocell' without inducing frank disease or other adverse effects. However, vaccination is of no known immunologic value in cats with existing FeLV infection, nor will it alter the natural course of disease.

Directions: Vaccination of healthy cats 9 weeks of age or older is recommended. Administer 1 ml. intramuscularly. Primary vaccination with 2 doses should be given, with the second dose administered 2–3 weeks after the first. A third (booster) dose should be given 2 to 4 months later. Annual revaccination with a single dose is recommended.

Precautions:

1. Certain postvaccination reactions may occur (see SAFETY AND EFFICACY).
2. Store at 2°C.–7°C. Do not freeze.
3. Use entire contents when first opened.
4. Contains penicillin, streptomycin, and amphotericin B as preservatives.
5. Anaphylaxis may occur following use (see SAFETY AND EFFICACY). Use epinephrine or equivalent, antihistamine, or steroids.
6. Although this product has been shown to be efficacious, some animals may be unable to develop or maintain an adequate immune response following vaccination if they are incubating any infectious disease, malnourished or parasitized, or stressed due to shipment or environmental conditions.

Supplied: Cartons of 50 1-dose vials.

References:

1. Wolff LH, Mathes LE, Olsen RG: Recovery of soluble feline oncornavirus-associated cell membrane antigen from large volumes of tumor culture fluids. J. Immunol. Methods 26:151, 1979.
2. Schaller JP, Hoover EA, Olsen RG: Active and passive immunization of cats with inactivated feline oncornaviruses. J. Natl. Cancer Inst. 59:144–1450, 1977.
3. Olsen RG, Hoover EA, Schaller JP et al: Abrogation of resistance to feline oncornavirus disease by immunization with killed feline leukemia virus. Cancer Res. 37:2082–2085, 1977.
4. Hoover EA, Olsen RG, Hardy WD Jr et al: Feline leukemia virus infection: Age-related variation in response of cats to experimental infection. J. Natl. Cancer Inst. 57:365–369, 1976.
5. Essex M: Horizontally and vertically transmitted oncornaviruses of cats. Adv. Cancer Res. 21:175, 1975.
6. Essex M, Sliski A, Cotter SM et al: Immunosurveillance of naturally occurring feline leukemia, Science 190:790, 1975.
7. Rojko JL, Hoover EA, Mathes LE et al: Influence of adrenal corticosteroids on the susceptibility of cats to feline leukemia virus infection. Cancer Res. 39:3789–3791, 1979.
8. Olsen RG, Mathes LE, Hebebrand LC et al: Feline leukemia virus disease. Am. J. Path. 98:857–860, 1980.

U.S. Patent No. 4,332,793
For Veterinary Use Only

LIFE-GUARD
Oral Nutrient-Electrolyte Powder

Composition: Dextrose 56.76%; protein concentrate (from hydrolyzed meat by-product) 18.91%; sodium bicarbonate 12.68%; potassium chloride 3.60%; glycine 3.12%; sodium chloride 2.84%; calcium phosphate 1.33%; and magnesium sulfate 0.76%.

Indications: For use as an electrolyte replacement and nutrient supplement. Life-Guard is designed for maximum absorption following oral administration.

Directions for Use:

100 gm size: Mix the contents of one packet with one-half gallon (64 oz) of warm water.

200 gm size: Mix the contents of one packet with one gallon (128 oz) of warm water.

2 Kg size: Mix the contents of one packet with ten (10) gallons (1,280 oz) of warm water.

Administer Life-Guard solution at body temperature. Allow animal to nurse from a nursing bottle or administer via a stomach tube.

Refrigerate if not used immediately.

Shake well before using. Discard solution if not used within 24 hours.

Dosage and Administration: Administer orally 2 to 3 times per day at the following rates:

Calves, Foals, and Sheep: 1 to 2 quarts (32-64 ozs.) per treatment.

Lambs: ½ to 1 pint (8-16 ozs.) per treatment.

Cattle and Horses: 1 to 3 gallons (128-384 ozs.) per treatment.

Dogs, Cats and Pigs: ¼ to ½ pint (4-8 ozs.) per treatment for each 10 pounds of body weight. Use the higher dosages and more frequent administration rates in cases of more severe dehydration and diarheal fluid losses.

Contraindications: Do not use in cases of upper gastrointestinal obstruction or in moribund animals.

Caution: Keep out of the reach of children.

How Supplied: 100 gm, 200 gm, 2 Kg
For Veterinary Use Only

LITTERGUARD®
Escherichia
Coli Bacterin

Description: 'LitterGuard' is for vaccination of healthy, pregnant sows and gilts to protect their pigs against neonatal colibacillosis caused by enterotoxigenic strains of *Escherichia coli* having the K99, K88, 987P, or F41 adherence factors. The addition of F41 now offers broader protection than previously available. The bacterin is prepared from chemically inactivated strains of *E. coli.* A sterile adjuvant is used to enhance the immune response.

Indications: Enterotoxigenic strains of *E. coli* are among the most important etiologic agents of porcine neonatal diarrhea. Studies have shown that enterotoxigenic *E. coli* (ETEC) isolated from diarrheic pigs have two characteristics in common: (1) they have pili, surface antigenic structures which attach the bacteria to cells of the intestinal epithelium; and (2) they express enterotoxins, causing the intestinal cells to secrete body fluids and electrolytes into the gut lumen. The results are diarrhea, dehydration, and in severe cases, death. The four major pili types associated with neonatal enteric colibacillosis in swine are K99, K88, 987P[1], and F41.[2]

Safety and Efficacy: No adverse reactions to 'LitterGuard' were reported in experimental tests conducted at Norden Laboratories, or in clinical trials conducted by private practitioners. Anaphylaxis occasionally has been observed in field use; see precautions. Susceptible pigs are protected by receiving colostral antibodies from vaccinated dams. Thus, adequate and timely consumption of colostrum by the neonatal pig is essential for protection. Controlled challenge of immunity tests were conducted involving 110 gilts and sows and their litters. Components of 'LitterGuard' were tested for effectiveness separately and in combination. Results showed that vaccination of pregnant swine with 2 doses of 'LitterGuard' significantly reduced the incidence and severity of neonatal diarrhea in their litters.

Directions:

1. *General Directions:* Shake well and administer 2 ml. intramuscularly or subcutaneously to pregnant sows and gilts.
2. *Primary Vaccination:* Administer 2 doses at least 3 weeks apart. The last dose should be given at least 2 weeks prior to farrowing.
3. *Revaccination:* A single dose should be administered at least two weeks prior to each subsequent farrowing.

Precautions:

1. Store at 2°C.–7°C. Do not freeze.
2. Use entire contents when first opened.
3. Do not vaccinate within 21 days of slaughter.

4. If anaphylaxis occurs following use, administer epinephrine or equivalent.
5. Although this product has been shown to be efficacious, some animals may be unable to develop or maintain an adequate immune response following vaccination if they are incubating any disease, malnourished or parasitized, or stressed due to shipment or adverse environmental conditions.

Supplied: 10- and 50-dose vials.

References:

1. Moon HW, Isaacson RE, and Pohlenz J: Mechanisms of association of enteropathogenic *Escherichia coli* with intestinal epithelium. Am. J. Clin. Nutr., 32:119–127 (1979).
2. Moon HW, Kohler EM, Schneider RA, and Whipp SC: Prevalence of pilus antigens, enterotoxin types, and enteropathogenicity among K-88 negative enterotoxigenic *Escherichia coli* from neonatal pigs. Infect. Immun., 27:222–230 (1980).

For Veterinary Use Only

LITTERGUARD® LT
Escherichia Coli Bacterin-Toxoid

Description: 'LitterGuard LT' is for vaccination of healthy, pregnant sows and gilts to protect their pigs against neonatal colibacillosis caused by enterotoxigenic strains of *Escherichia coli* producing heat-labile toxin or having the K99, K88, 987P, or F41 adherence factors. The addition of F41 now offers broader protection than previously available. The bacterin is prepared from chemically inactivated strains of *E. coli*. A sterile adjuvant is used to enhance the immune response.

Indications: Enterotoxigenic strains of *E. coli* are among the most important etiologic agents of porcine neonatal diarrhea. Studies have shown that enterotoxigenic *E. coli* (ETEC) isolated from diarrheic pigs have two characteristics in common: (1) they have pili, surface antigenic structures which attach the bacteria to cells of the intestinal epithelium; and (2) they express enterotoxins, causing the intestinal cells to secrete body fluids and electrolytes into the gut lumen. The results are diarrhea, dehydration, and in severe cases, death. The four major pili types associated with neonatal enteric colibacillosis in swine are K99, K88, 987P[1], and F41.[2]

Safety and Efficacy: No adverse reactions to 'LitterGuard LT' were reported in experimental tests conducted at Norden Laboratories, or in clinical trials conducted by private practitioners. Anaphylaxis occasionally has been observed in field use; see precautions. Susceptible pigs are protected by receiving colostral antibodies from vaccinated dams. Thus, adequate and timely consumption of colostrum by the neonatal pig is essential for protection. Controlled challenge of immunity tests were conducted involving 110 gilts and sows and their litters. Components of 'LitterGuard LT' were tested for effectiveness separately and in combination. Results showed that vaccination of pregnant swine with 2 doses of 'LitterGuard LT' significantly reduced the incidence and severity of neonatal diarrhea in their litters.

Directions:
1. *General Directions:* Shake well and administer 2 ml. intramuscularly or subcutaneously to pregnant sows and gilts.
2. *Primary Vaccination:* Administer 2 doses at least 3 weeks apart. The last dose should be given at least 2 weeks prior to farrowing.
3. *Revaccination:* A single dose should be administered at least two weeks prior to each subsequent farrowing.

Precautions:
1. Store at 2°C.–7°C. Do not freeze.
2. Use entire contents when first opened.
3. Do not vaccinate within 21 days of slaughter.
4. If anaphylaxis occurs following use, administer epinephrine or equivalent.
5. Although this product has been shown to be efficacious, some animals may be unable to develop or maintain adequate immune response following vaccination if they are incubating any disease, malnourished or parasitized, or stressed due to shipment or adverse environmental conditions.

Supplied: 10- and 50-dose vials.

References:

1. Moon HW, Isaacson RE, and Pohlenz J: Mechanisms of association of enteropathogenic *Escherichia coli* with intestinal epithelium. Am. J. Clinc. Nutr., 32:119–127 (1979).
2. Moon HW, Kohler EM, Schneider RA, and Whipp SC: Prevalence of pilus antigens, enterotoxin types, and enteropathogenicity among K-88 negative enterotoxigenic *Escherichia coli* from neonatal pigs. Infect. Immun., 27:222–230 (1980).

For Veterinary Use Only

MARMADUKE AUTOMATIC ROOM FOGGER
One Unit Treats Up To 5,000 Cu. Ft.

Kills Fleas and Ticks, Houseflies, Mosquitoes, Cockroaches, Spiders, Centipedes, Wasps, Black Carpet Beetles, Saw-Toothed Grain Beetles, Rice Weevils, Small Flying Moths, Pill Bugs, Crickets and Silverfish.

Active Ingredients:

Chlorpyrifos (0,0,-Diethyl 0-(3,5,6-Trichloro-2-Pyridyl)Phosphorothioate)	1.000%
Pyrethrins	0.050%
*Piperonyl Butoxide, Technical	0.100%
†N-Octyl Bicycloheptene Dicarboximide	0.166%
Petroleum Distillate	0.239%
Inert Ingredients:	98.445%
	100.000%

* Equivalent to 0.08% (Butylcarbityl) (6-Propyl-piperonyl) Ether and 0.02% related compounds
†MGK 264, Insecticide Synergist

For homes, apartments, attics, basements, campers, boats, garages, plants, warehouses, boxcars, trucks, kennels, and pet sleeping areas.

This water-base formula has no strong solvent odor—is non-staining—and won't damage carpets, rugs, drapes or floors.

Directions for Use: It is a violation of Federal Law to use this product in a manner inconsistent with its labeling.

Storage and Disposal: Do not contaminate water, food, or feed by storage or disposal.

Storage: Store in a cool, dry area away from heat or flame.

Disposal: Do not re-use empty container. Replace cap and discard container in trash. Do not incinerate or puncture.

Use one canister for each 5,000 cu. ft. of unobstructed area. Example: 25′ long × 20′ wide × 10′ high = 5,000 cu. ft. Use additional units for remote rooms or where free flow of the mist is not assured. Do not use in an area less than 3000 cu. ft.

Preparation: Cover exposed foods, dishes, and food handling equipment. Cover or remove brass or copper articles (lamps, artifacts, headboards, etc.). Open cabinets and doors to areas to be treated. Shut off fans and air conditioners. Put out all open flames except pilot light. Remove pets and cover fish tanks or fish bowls with paper, or remove from area. Close exterior doors and windows.

To Start Fogging: Place Fogger on table, chair or stand, in center of area, at least six feet from pilot light. Place several thicknesses of newspapers under canister to prevent marring of surface. Hold can at arm's length, with top of can pointing away from face and eyes. Push down on finger pad until it locks—this will start fogging action. Set canister in upright position on table, etc., and leave building at once.

DO NOT RE-ENTER BUILDING FOR TWO HOURS, then open exterior doors and windows and allow to air for one hour before reoccupying area. If additional units are used for remote rooms or where free flow of mist is not assured, increase airing-out time accordingly.

Precautionary Statements: Hazards to Humans and Domestic Animals

Keep Out Of Reach Of Children

Harmful if swallowed. Avoid inhalation of vapors. Avoid contact with skin, eyes, or clothing. Wash contaminated skin promptly with soap and warm water. For eyes, flush with plenty of water. Get medical attention if irritation persists. Avoid contamination of food and foodstuffs. Wash hands with soap and water after using and before eating or smoking. Do not allow children to lie or sleep in treated areas until at least six hours following treatment.

Do not use in commercial food processing preparation, or serving areas or in household storage areas. In home, all food processing surfaces and utensils should be covered during treatment or thoroughly washed before use. Cover or remove exposed food.

Remove pets, birds, and cover fish aquariums before spraying.

Statement of Practical Treatment

If inhaled—Remove victim to fresh air. Apply artificial respiration if indicated.

Continued on next page

Norden—Cont.

If on skin—Remove contaminated clothing and wash affected areas with soap and water.
If in eyes—Flush eyes with plenty of water. Get medical attention, if irritation persists.
Note To Physician: Chlorpyrifos is a cholinesterase inhibitor. Atropine by injection is antidotal only if symptoms of cholinesterase inhibition are present.
Physical Or Chemical Hazards
Contents under pressure. Do not use near heat or open flame. Do not puncture or incinerate container. Exposure to temperatures above 130°F may cause bursting.
How Supplied: 6 oz. canister

MARMADUKE FLEA AND TICK DIP FOR DOGS

Active Ingredients:

Chlorpyrifos	3.84%
Inert Ingredients:	96.16%
	100.00%

Claims: Kills fleas for 28 days.
Controls ticks for 21 days.
Mild Odor.
No Oil Residue
Makes 64 Gallons of Dip
Animal Precautions: Do not use on cats.
Do not use on nursing bitches or puppies under 3 months of age.
Do not use within 30 days before or after treatment with other cholinesterase-inhibiting drugs or chemicals.
Chlopyrifos is a cholinesterase inhibitor. Atropine by injection is antidotal only if symptoms of cholinesterase inhibition are present.
Human Precautions: Keep out of reach of children.
Avoid breathing vapors and spray mist. Keep away from food, feedstuffs, and domestic water supplies.
Keep container closed. Handle concentrate in ventilated area. Wash contaminated clothing before reuse.
Concentrate is harmful if swallowed or absorbed through the skin. May cause eye irritation. Avoid contact with skin, clothing, or eyes. Wash thoroughly with soap and water after handling.
If swallowed... Call a physician or poison control center. Drink a glass of milk or water and induce vomiting by touching finger to back of throat.
If in eyes... Flush with plenty of water. Get medical attention if irritation persists.
If on skin... Wash off with soap and water. Remove contaminated clothing and wash before reuse.
Directions for Use:
It is in violation of federal law to use this product in a manner inconsistent with its labeling.
For use as dip. Shake well before using. Stir four (4) tablespoonfuls (2 fl. oz.) of Marmaduke's Flea & Tick Dip into one (1) gallon of water. Use rubber gloves. Dip, sponge or swab dog with this emulsion until thoroughly wet. Hold hand over dog's nose and mouth to avoid swallowing emulsion. Dipping should not exceed 30 seconds. Allow dog to dry in warm place without rinsing or towelling. Repeat application in 21 day intervals as necessary.
Storage and Disposal:
STORAGE: Store in original container in cool, locked storage area away from heat or open flame.
DISPOSAL: Unused insecticide: Securely wrap original container in several layers of newspaper and discard in trash.
Empty Container: Do not reuse bottle. Rinse thoroughly before discarding in trash.
How Supplied: 8-ounce and 1-gallon containers.

MARMADUKE FLEA AND TICK SPRAY FOR DOGS

Active Ingredients:

Chlorpyrifos	0.225%
Inert Ingredients:	99.775%
	100.000%

Claims:
Kills ticks.
Controls fleas for up to 30 days.
Animal Precautions: Do not use on cats. Do not use on dogs nursing pups or pups under 10 weeks old. Chlopyrifos is a cholinesterase inhibitor. Treat symptomatically. Atropine is an antidote.
Human Precautions:
Keep out of reach of children.
Avoid contact with eyes and inhalation of spray.
If inhaled... Artificial respiration or administration of oxygen may be lifesaving.
If on skin... Wash with water.
If on eyes... Flush with water, get medical treatment.
Directions for Use:
It is in violation of Federal law to use this product in a manner inconsistent with its labeling. Shake well before using.
Place dog on table or bench. Thoroughly spray all over body against lay of the coat. Avoid spraying into the eyes. The hair should be slightly damp down to skin level.
Repeat treatment as necessary. Old bedding of pets should be removed and replaced with clean, fresh bedding after treatment of pet areas.
Free bitches from fleas before they bear pups.
Storage and Disposal:
STORAGE: Store in original container in cool, locked storage area away from heat or open flame.
DISPOSAL: Unused insecticide: Securely wrap original container in several layers of newspapers and discard in trash.
Empty Container: Do not reuse bottle or sprayer. Rinse thoroughly before discarding in trash.
How Supplied: 8-ounce and 24-ounce pump spray bottles.

MITOX LIQUID

Composition: Active Ingredients: Neomycin base (as the sulfate) 0.5%; Sevin 1.0%; Sulfacetamide 9.0%; Tetracaine hydrochloride 0.5%; Mineral oil 88.10%; Inert Ingredients: 0.90%; Total 100.0.%
Indications: An aid in the treatment of bacterial infections of the external ear canal associated with ear mite infestation.
Dosage and Administration: If severe accumulations of ceruminous material are present, clean ear before treatment with a ceruminolytic agent. Follow this cleaning with treatment with Mitox, as directed. Fill lower section with Mitox and massage gently to distribute evenly. For infections, repeat as needed. For ear mites, continue treatments at 10 day intervals until controlled. Do not use on pregnant dogs.
How Supplied: 12-12 ml. squeeze bottles. 12-22 ml. squeeze bottles.

NEO-DARBAZINE®
(prochlorperazine dimaleate and isopropamide iodide with neomycin sulfate)
Spansule* Capsules No. 1 & No. 3

Composition: Neomycin is combined with Darbazine (brand of prochlorperazine and isopropamide) to provide broad spectrum antibiotic therapy for many gastrointestinal infections, especially those associated with emotional stress.
Each No. 1 capsule contains 5.40 mg. of prochlorperazine dimaleate (equivalent to 3.33 mg. prochlorperazine), in *sustained release* form; 2.27 mg. of isopropamide iodide (equivalent to 1.67 mg. isopropamide); and 35.7 mg. of neomycin sulfate (equivalent to 25 mg. neomycin base).
Each No. 3 capsule contains 16.2 mg. of prochlorperazine dimaleate (equivalent to 10 mg. prochlorperazine) in *sustained release* form; 6.8 mg. of isopropamide iodide (equivalent to 5 mg. isopropamide); and 107 mg. of neomycin sulfate (equivalent to 75 mg. neomycin base).
Indications: Neo-Darbazine *Spansule* capsules are indicated for the treatment of infectious gastroenteritis in dogs. It is of special value in those cases in which emotional stress is associated with concurrent bacterial infection.
Note: Systemic disorders giving rise to gastrointestinal symptoms (e.g. uremia; leptospirosis) and enteric infections caused by neomycin resistant organisms would not be expected to respond to therapy with Neo-Darbazine *Spansule** capsules.
Contraindications: Neo-Darbazine *Spansule* capsules are contraindicated in cases of glaucoma, pyloric obstruction or stenosis and prostatic hypertrophy. In view of the possible nephrotoxicity, Neo-Darbazine should not be used in the presence of nephritis.
Possible Side Effects and Precautions: Side effects are most likely to be due to overdosage and are those of the separate ingredients.
Isopropamide overdosage produces dryness of mouth, dilated pupils, constipation and urinary retention.
Prochlorperazine overdosage may cause nervous depression, rigidity, weakness, tremor, torticollis, salivation, inability to

swallow, hypotension and disturbance of gait.
Neomycin is poorly absorbed from the intestinal tract under normal conditions. However, in combination with the above active ingredients, peristalsis is greatly reduced and absorption of neomycin is apparently enhanced. Overdosage or prolonged administration may produce nephrotoxicity as manifested by albuminuria, presence of granular casts and depressed urinary output.
Treatment of overdosage is essentially symptomatic and supportive. Discontinue medication and, depending upon the severity and type of side effects, such means as gastric lavage, purgatives, catheterization and standard procedures of combatting circulatory shock may be employed as indicated.
Note: If it is desirable to administer a vasoconstrictor, norepinephrine is the drug of choice. Other pressor agents, including epinephrine, are not recommended because phenothiazine derivatives may reverse the usual elevating action of these agents and cause a further lowering of blood pressure.
Recommended Dosage: Neo-Darbazine *Spansule* capsules are provided in two convenient sizes (No. 1 and No. 3) for adjustment of dosage according to individual needs. (Note: Each Neo-Darbazine *Spansule* capsule No. 3 is equivalent to three Neo-Darbazine *Spansule* capsules No. 1.)
Neo-Darbazine *Spansule* capsule No. 1

10 lb to 20 lb	1 capsule twice daily
20 lb to 30 lb	2 capsules twice daily
Over 30 lb	3 capsules twice daily

Neo Darbazine *Spansule* capsule No. 3

Over 30 lb	1 capsule twice daily

Dosage may be adjusted up to two No. 3 capsules twice daily for very large dogs (over 60 lb.)
Do not continue medication longer than five days. Most cases show a favorable response within this period of time and a failure to do so warrants a reconsideration of the diagnosis and/or therapy.
Caution: U.S. Federal law restricts this drug to use by or on the order of a licensed veterinarian.
How Supplied: Neo-Darbazine, *Spansule* capsules No. 1 bottles of 500.
Neo-Darbazine *Spansule* capsules. No. 3 in bottles of 100 and 500.
*Reg. Trademark of SmithKline Beckman Corporation

NORCALCIPHOS
Parenteral Solution

Composition:
Contains: Calcium borogluconate, dextrose, magnesium borogluconate, calcium hypophosphite and base.
Total calcium chemically equivalent to calcium borogluconate 26.0%; Dextrose 15.0%; Magnesium borogluconate 6.0%; Total phosphorus in amounts chemically equivalent to elemental phosphorus 0.5%.
Indications: For intravenous use in milk fever, and in calcium, phosphorus, magnesium and glucose deficiency in animals.
Note: Intravenous administration is always preferable. If used subcutaneously, always distribute dose in several places and massage to facilitate absorption.
Dosage:
Cattle: 500 ml. For milk fever prophylaxis, give 200-500 ml. at time of calving.
Horses: 250-500 ml.
Sheep: 50-125 ml. Repeat in 2 to 6 hours if needed.
This product contains no preservatives. Unused portion remaining in bottle must be discarded.
Veterinarians refer to catalog for intravenous injection of small animals.
Warning: Large doses administered intravenously may have toxic action on heart if the blood level of calcium is raised excessively. Doses should be carefully regulated according to severity of hypocalcemia and injected slowly so that administration may be stopped if toxic action becomes evident.
Caution: Federal law restricts this drug to use by or on the order of a licensed veterinarian.
How Supplied: 500 ml.

PARVO-VAC®
Parvovirus Vaccine
Killed Virus
For Use in Swine Only

Description: Porcine parvovirus is a major cause of swine reproductive failure. Infection in susceptible swine is generally subclinical. However, infection of pregnant females may involve the developing fetus. Stillbirths, mummified fetuses, embryonic death, and infertility (SMEDI) are the chief manifestations of the disease. Reproductive failure generally occurs when susceptible females are exposed during the first 70 days of gestation. Thereafter, the fetuses may survive *in utero* infection. The PPV agent is enzootic in the United States[1] and has a worldwide distribution. Thus, a large proportion of adult swine carry antibodies or disseminate the virus.[2] When maternally acquired antibodies decline below protective levels, stock is at risk.
Indications: Parvo-Vac is for the vaccination of healthy swine against porcine parvovirus (PPV) infection. The vaccine is prepared by chemically inactivating a PPV strain grown in a swine cell line, and combining the viral fluids with a sterile adjuvant.
Safety and Efficacy: Post-vaccination reactions were not observed in experimental pigs vaccinated with Parvo-Vac or in swine vaccinated under field conditions in extensive safety trials. In efficacy studies performed at Norden Laboratories, vaccination of seronegative gilts prior to breeding protected 95.7% of developing fetuses from infection and death following challenge with virulent PPV. In contrast, 46.3% of the fetuses from nonvaccinated control gilts became infected and died following the same challenge. Previous studies have shown that PPV vaccination can produce consistent protection despite low hemagglutination inhibition antibody titers.[3]
Dosage and Administration:
1.Shake and administer 2 ml. intramuscularly.
2.For primary immunization, a single dose given 14 to 60 days before breeding is recommended.
3.Semiannual revaccination (before breeding) is recommended for all breeding stock.
Cautions:
1.Store at 2°C–7°C. Do not freeze.
2.Use entire contents when first opened.
3.Do not vaccinate within 21 days of slaughter.
4.Contains penicillin and streptomycin as preservatives.
5.Anaphylaxis may occur following use (antidote is epinephrine).
How Supplied: 10 and 50 dose vials.
References:

1. Mengeling WL: Porcine Parvovirus: Frequency of naturally occuring transplacental infection and viral contamination of fetal porcine kidney cell cultures. Am. J. Vet. Res., 36:41-44, 1975.
2. Johnson RH, Donaldson-Wood CR, Joo HS, and Allender U: Observations on the epidemiology of porcine parvovirus. Austr. Vet. J., 52:80-84, 1976.
3. Mengeling WL, Brown TT, Paul PS, and Gutekunst DE: Efficacy of an inactivated virus vaccine for prevention of porcine parvovirus-induced reproductive failure. Am. J. Vet. Res., 40:204-207,1979.

For Veterinary Use Only

PARVO-VAC®/LEPTOFERM-5®
Parvovirus Vaccine
Killed Virus,
Leptospira Canicola-Grippotyphosa-Hardjo-Icterohaemorrhagiae-Pomona
Bacterin
For Use In Swine Only

Indications: This product is for the vaccination of healthy swine against porcine parvovirus (PPV), *Leptospira canicola, L. grippotyphosa, L. hardjo, L. icterohaemorrhagiae,* and *L. pomona* infections. The parvovirus component is prepared by chemically inactivating a PPV strain grown in a porcine cell line. The *Leptospira* components are prepared from whole cultures of *L. canicola, L. grippotyphosa, L. hardjo, L. icterohaemorrhagiae,* and *L. pomona.*
Description: Porcine parvovirus is a major cause of swine reproductive failure. Infection in swine is generally subclinical. However, infection of pregnant females may involve the developing fetus. Stillbirths, mummified fetuses, embryonic death, and infertility (SMEDI) are the chief manifestations of the disease. The PPV agent is enzootic in the United States[1] and has a worldwide distribution. Thus, a large proportion of adults carry antibodies or disseminate the virus.[2] When maternally acquired antibodies decline below protective levels, stock is at risk.
Swine leptospirosis is characterized by poor production, anemia, and nephritis.

Continued on next page

Norden—Cont.

Late-term abortions are the most important effect of the disease.
Safety and Efficacy: Post-vaccination reactions were not observed in experimental pigs vaccinated with the PPV component, or in swine vaccinated under field conditions in extensive safety trials. In efficacy studies performed at Norden Laboratories, vaccination of seronegative gilts prior to breeding protected 95.7% of developing fetuses from infection and death following challenge with virulent PPV. In contrast, 46.3% of the fetuses from non-vaccinated control gilts became infected and died following the same challenge. Immunogenicity of the *Leptospira* components was confirmed by challenge-of-immunity or serologic tests.
Directions: *General Directions:* Shake vial and administer 5 ml intramuscularly.
Primary Vaccination: A single dose 21 to 60 days before breeding is recommended. For protection against leptospirosis, a second dose is recommended 3 to 6 weeks after the initial dose.
Revaccination: Semi-annual revaccination before breeding is recommended.
Precautions:
Store at 2°C-7°C. Do not freeze.
Use entire contents when first opened.
Do not vaccinate within 21 days of slaughter.
Contains penicillin and streptomycin as preservatives.
Anaphylaxis may occur following use (antidote is epinephrine).
Although this product has been shown to be efficacious, some animals may be unable to develop or maintain an adequate immune response following vaccination if they are incubating any infectious disease, are malnourished or parasitized, or if they are stressed due to shipment or adverse environmental conditions.
How Supplied: 10- and 50-dose vials.
References:
1. Mengeling WL: Porcine Parvovirus: Frequency of Naturally Occurring Transplacental Infection and Viral Contamination of Fetal Porcine Kidney Cell Cultures. Am. J. Vet. Res., 36:41–44; 1975.
2. Johnson RH, Donaldson-Wood CR, Joo HS, Allender U: Observation on the Epidemiology of Porcine Parvovirus. Austr. Vet. J., 52:80–84; 1976.
For Veterinary Use Only

PLEUROGUARD®
Haemophilus Pleuropneumoniae Bacterin
For Use in Swine Only

Description: *Haemophilus pleuropneumoniae* infection is a swine respiratory disease of increasing incidence and commercial importance. Acute and chronic forms are recognized. Acute disease can cause death within 6 hours after onset of signs. Affected pigs may cough, become cyanotic and express a blood-tinged nasal discharge. Extensive pleural hemorrhages occur, with death resulting from pulmonary consolidation and adhesions. Chronic disease may be subclinical and is characterized by deteriorating performance and an extended finishing period. Pathology typically consists of a fibrinopurulent bronchopneumonia and a fibrinous pleuritis. Certain serotypes of *H. pleuropneumoniae* are highly virulent, with serotype 5 being identified in a majority of cases submitted for laboratory diagnosis.[1,2] Serotypes 1, 4, and 5 consistently produce lung lesions following exposure. Until recently, serotype 3 had been isolated from field cases, but had not been shown to produce clinical disease. During the development of PleuroGuard, however, researchers succeeded in reproducing clinical disease using serotype 3.[3]
Indications: PleuroGuard is for the vaccination of healthy swine against respiratory disease caused by *Haemophilus pleuropneumoniae.* PleuroGuard contains chemically inactivated cultures of four serotypes of *H. pleuropneumoniae* (serotypes 1, 3, 4, and 5) combined with a sterile adjuvant to enhance the immune response.
Safety and Efficacy: Chemical inactivation renders PleuroGuard incapable of causing infectious disease. Temporary induration and moderate swelling may be observed at the injection site.
Efficacy of PleuroGuard was established in rigorous challenge-of-immunity tests. Vaccinates received 2 subcutaneous doses administered 2 weeks apart. Respective test groups were challenged with virulent *H. pleuropneumoniae* serotypes 1, 3, 4, and 5 (Table 1). For serotype 1, two tests were conducted. A market weight challenge was administered to one group 120 days following primary vaccination, and a short term challenge was administered to a second group 42 days following primary vaccination. For serotype 3, challenge was administered 38 days following primary vaccination. For serotype 4 and 5, challenge was administered 49 to 28 days following primary vaccination, respectively.In each test, all pigs were necropsied and evaluated for lung disease either following death or termination of the test at 6 to 12 days postchallenge.
[See table below].

Table 1—Results of *H. Pleuropneumoniae* Vaccination and Challenge in Preweaned Pigs

Test No.	Serotype & Procedure	Test Groups	Postvaccination Seroconversion	Percent Protected from Lung Lesions
1	type 1 challenge (market weight)	19 vaccinates	100	74 (14/19)
		5 controls	—	0 (0/5)
2	type 1 challenge	19 vaccinates	100	84 (16/19)
		4 controls	—	25 (1/4)
3	type 3 challenge	25 vaccinates	100	76 (19/25)
		6 controls	—	0 (0/6)
4	type 4 challenge	21 vaccinates	100	95 (20/21)
		5 controls	—	0 (0/5)
5	type 5 challenge, seronegative pigs	20 vaccinates	100	95 (19/20)
		5 controls	—	0 (0/5)
6	type 5 challenge, seropositive pigs*	20 vaccinates	—	90 (18/20)
		5 controls	—	0 (0/5)

* Test animals had maternally derived antibodies

Results are shown in Table 1. All vaccinates seroconverted to each of the four *H. pleuropneumoniae* serotypes tested. Vaccinated pigs demonstrated a high level of protection against a severe challenge that produced lung lesions in 97% of the controls.
The market weight challenge for serotype 1 demonstrated that vaccination provided substantial protection over the course of the feeding period, even against severe challenge.
One of the challenge-of-immunity tests (test 6) was designed to evaluate the effects of vaccination and challenge in pigs with maternal immunity. (Prevaccination geometric mean titers for *H. pleuropneumoniae* were 1:31 in vaccinates and 1:45 in controls.) Postchallenge, all controls developed lung lesions, indicating that passive immunity may be of limited benefit in the face of a severe challenge. Ninety percent of the vaccinates were protected against lung lesions, underscoring the value of active immunization. Following administration of vaccine, pigs developed a 2-fold increase in the geometric mean serologic titer (Table 2), demonstrating that vaccination can produce active immunity in pigs carrying maternal antibodies.
[See table on next page].
Dosage and Administration:
General Directions: Shake well and administer 2 ml. intramuscularly or subcutaneously.
Primary Vaccination: Pigs should receive 1 dose when weaned and a second dose 2 to 3 weeks later. Pregnant swine should receive 2 doses at least 2 weeks apart, with the second dose administered 2 weeks before farrowing.
Revaccination: For sows, revaccination is recommended prior to each subsequent farrowing. Semiannual revaccination is recommended for boars.
Precautions:
Store at 2°C. to 7°C. Do not freeze.
Use entire contents when first opened.
Do not vaccinate within 21 days of slaughter.

Anaphylaxis may occur following use (antidote is epinephrine).
Transient local reactions may occur following administration.
Although this product has been shown to be efficacious, some animals may be unable to develop or maintain an adequate immune response following vaccination if they are incubating any disease, are malnourished or parasitized, or stressed due to shipment or environmental conditions.
How Supplied: 50-dose and 125-dose vials
For Veterinary Use Only
References:

1. Gunnarsson A, Biberstein EL, and Hurvell B: Serologic Studies on Porcine Strains of *Haemophilus parahaemolyticus (pleuropneumoniae)*: Agglutination Reactions. Am. J. Vet. Res. 38:1111–1114 (1977).
2. Schultz RA: Proceedings George A. Young Swine Conference (1980).
3. Norden Laboratories, data on file with USDA.

PLEUROGUARD® 3
Bordetella Bronchiseptica-Erysipelothrix Rhusiopathiae-Haemophilus Pleuropneumoniae Bacterin
For Use in Swine Only

Description: PleuroGuard 3 is for the vaccination of healthy swine against infection caused by *Bordetella bronchiseptica, Erysipelothrix rhusiopathiae,* and respiratory disease caused by *Haemophilus pleuropneumoniae.* PleuroGuard 3 contains chemically inactivated cultures of *B. bronchiseptica, E. rhusiopathiae,* and four serotypes of *H. pleuropneumoniae* (serotypes 1, 3, 4, and 5) combined with a sterile adjuvant to enhance the immune response.
Indications: *Bordetella bronchiseptica* is a principal cause of atrophic rhinitis in swine. Particularly in young pigs, the disease is characterized by acute rhinitis followed by chronic atrophy of the turbinate bones. Impairment of the turbinate filtering system predisposes the animal to respiratory infections, including pneumonia, and is associated with reduced rate of gain and an extended finishing period. *Erysipelothrix rhusiopathiae* infection in swine (swine erysipelas) has a variety of manifestations. These include acute septicemia, skin discoloration characterized by hyperemic or necrotic diamond-shaped lesions, chronic arthritis, and vegetative endocarditis. *Haemophilus pleuropneumoniae* infection is a swine respiratory disease of increasing incidence and commercial importance. Acute and chronic forms are recognized. Acute disease can cause death within 6 hours after onset of signs. Affected pigs may cough, become cyanotic and express a blood-tinged nasal discharge. Extensive pleural hemorrhages occur, with death resulting from pulmonary consolidation and adhesions. Chronic disease may be subclinical and is characterized by deteriorating performance and an extended finishing period. Pathology typically consists of a fibrinopurulent bronchopneumonia and a fibrinous pleuritis. Certain serotypes of *H. pleuropneumoniae* are highly virulent, with serotype 5 being identified in a majority of cases submitted for laboratory diagnosis.[1,2] Serotypes 1, 4, and 5 consistently produce lung lesions following exposure. Until recently, serotype 3 had been isolated from field cases, but had not been shown to produce clinical disease. During the development of PleuroGuard, however, researchers succeeded in reproducing clinical disease using serotype 3.[1]
Safety and Efficacy: Chemical inactivation renders PleuroGuard 3 incapable of causing infectious disease. Temporary induration and moderate swelling may be observed at the injection site.
The *Bordetella bronchiseptica* component has been evaluated in challenge-of-immunity tests in susceptible 12-week old pigs. Results are shown in Table 1, and indicate that the most effective vaccination program requires immunization of both sows and pigs.
[See table below].
Efficacy of the *E. rhusiopathiae* component was demonstrated in a controlled challenge-of-immunity test. A single subcutaneous dose administered to seronegative test pigs protected them from challenge with *E. rhusiopathiae* administered 2 weeks postvaccination. All controls were clinically affected with signs of erysipelas following the same challenge.
Efficacy of the *H. pleuropneumoniae* component in PleuroGuard 3 was established in rigorous challenge-of-immunity tests. Vaccinates received 2 subcutaneous doses administered 2 weeks apart. Respective test groups were challenged with virulent *H. pleuropneumoniae* serotypes 1, 3, 4, and 5. (Table 2). For serotype 1, two tests were conducted. A market weight challenge was administered to one group 120 days following primary vaccination, and a short-term challenge was administered to a second group 42 days following primary vaccination. For serotype 3, challenge was administered 38 days following primary vaccination. For serotypes 4 and 5, challenge was administered 49 and 28 days following primary vaccination, respectively. In each test, all pigs were necropsied and evaluated for lung disease either following death or termination of the test at 6 to 12 days postchallenge.
Results are shown in Table 2. All vaccinates in the challenge studies seroconverted to each of the four *H. pleuropneumoniae* serotypes tested. Vaccinated pigs demonstrated a high level of protection against a severe challenge that produced lung lesions in 97% of the controls.
[See table on next page].
The market weight challenge for serotype 1 demonstrated that vaccination provided substantial protection over the course of the feeding period, even against severe challenge.
One of the challenge-of-immunity tests (test 6) was designed to evaluate the effects of vaccination and challenge in pigs with maternal immunity. (Prevaccination geometric mean titers for *H. pleuropneumoniae* were 1:31 in vaccinates and 1:45 in controls.) Postchallenge, all controls developed lung lesions, indicating that passive immunity may be of limited benefit in the face of a severe challenge. Ninety percent of the vaccinates were protected against lung lesions, underscoring the value of active immunization. Following administration of vaccine, pigs developed a 2-fold increase in the geometric mean serologic titer, (Table 3) demonstrating that vaccination can

Continued on next page

Table 2—Serologic Values in Maternally Immune Pigs Following *H. Pleuropneumoniae* Vaccination and Challenge

No. & Group	*Geometric Mean Serum Agglutination Titers** Pre Vacc.	Post 1st Vacc.	Post 2nd Vacc.	Post Challenge
20 vaccinates	31	69	64	66
5 controls			45	78

* Expressed as the reciprocal of end point dilutions

TABLE 1—Results of Challenge Following Vaccination with *Bordetella Bronchiseptica* Bacterin

No. Animals	Immunization Status	% Incidence of Turbinate Atrophy
25	nonvaccinated pigs from nonvaccinated sows	96
35	nonvaccinated pigs from vaccinated sows	60
23	vaccinated pigs from nonvaccinated sows	39
40	vaccinated pigs from vaccinated sows	20

N **Norden—Cont.**

produce active immunity in pigs carrying maternal antibodies.
[See table at right].

Dosage and Administration:

General Directions: Shake well and administer 2 ml. intramuscularly or subcutaneously.

Primary Vaccination: Pigs should receive 1 dose at 1 week of age and a second dose when weaned. Alternatively, the initial dose may be given at weaning with a second dose 2 to 3 weeks later. Pregnant swine should receive 2 doses at least 2 weeks apart, with the second dose administered 2 weeks before farrowing.

Revaccination: For sows, revaccination is recommended prior to each subsequent farrowing. Semiannual revaccination is recommended for boars.

Precautions:

Store at 2°C. to 7°C. Do not freeze.
Use entire contents when first opened.
Do not vaccinate within 21 days of slaughter.
Anaphylaxis may occur following use (antidote is epinephrine).
Transient local reactions may occur following administration.
Although this product has been shown to be efficacious, some animals may be unable to develop or maintain an adequate immune response following vaccination if they are incubating any disease, are malnourished or parasitized, or stressed due to shipment or environmental conditions.

How Supplied: 50-dose vials
For Veterinary Use Only

References:

1. Gunnarsson A, Biberstein EL, and Hurvell B: Serologic Studies on Porcine Strains of *Haemophilus parahaemolyticus (pleuropneumoniae)*: Agglutination Reactions. Am. J. Vet. Res. 38:1111–1114 (1977).
2. Schultz RA: Proceedings George A. Young Swine Conference (1980).
3. Norden Laboratories, data on file with USDA.

TABLE 3—Serologic Values in Maternally Immune Pigs Following *H. Pleuropneumoniae* Vaccination and Challenge

No. & Group	Geometric Mean Serum Agglutination Titers* Pre Vacc.	Post 1st Vacc.	Post 2nd Vacc.	Post Challenge
20 vaccinates	31	69	64	66
5 controls			45	78

*Expressed as the reciprocal of end point dilutions

TABLE 2—Results of *H. Pleuropneumoniae* Vaccination and Challenge in Preweaned Pigs

Test No.	Serotype & Procedure	Test Groups	Postvaccination Seroconversion	Percent Protected from Lung Lesions
1	type 1 challenge (market weight)	19 vaccinates	100	74 (14/19)
		5 controls	—	0 (0/5)
2	type 1 challenge	19 vaccinates	100	84 (16/19)
		4 controls	—	25 (1/4)
3	type 3 challenge	25 vaccinates	100	76 (19/25)
		6 controls	—	0 (0/6)
4	type 4 challenge	21 vaccinates	100	95 (20/21)
		5 controls	—	0 (0/5)
5	type 5 challenge, seronegative pigs	20 vaccinates	100	95 (19/20)
		5 controls	—	0 (0/5)
6	type 5 challenge, seropositive pigs*	20 vaccinates	—	90 (18/20)
		5 controls	—	0 (0/5)

*Test animals had maternally derived antibodies

PLEUROGUARD® 4
Bordetella Bronchiseptica-Erysipelothrix Rhusiopathiae-Haemophilus Pleuropneumoniae-Pasteurella Multocida Bacterin

For Use in Swine Only

Description: 'PleuroGuard 4' is for the vaccination of healthy swine against infection caused by *Bordetella bronchiseptica, Erysipelothrix rhusiopathiae*, respiratory disease caused by *Haemophilus pleuropneumoniae*, and *Pasteurella multocida* infection. 'PleuroGuard 4' contains chemically inactivated cultures of *B. bronchiseptica, E. rhusiopathiae*, four serotypes of *H. pleuropneumoniae* (serotypes 1, 3, 4, and 5), and *P. multocida* combined with a sterile adjuvant to enhance the immune response.

Indications: *Bordetella bronchiseptica* is a principal cause of atrophic rhinitis in swine. Particularly in young pigs, the disease is characterized by acute rhinitis followed by chronic atrophy of the turbinate bones. Impairment of the turbinate filtering system predisposes the animal to respiratory infections, including pneumonia, and is associated with reduced rate of gain and an extended finishing period. In combined infections, *B. bronchiseptica* and *Pasteurella multocida* have been shown to cause atrophic rhinitis lesions of greater severity than in cases where either agent functions alone.[1,2] *Erysipelothrix rhusiopathiae* infection in swine (swine erysipelas) has a variety of manifestations. These include acute septicemia, skin discoloration characterized by hyperemic or necrotic diamond-shaped lesions, chronic arthritis, and vegetative endocarditis.
Haemophilus pleuropneumoniae infection is a swine respiratory disease of increasing incidence and commercial importance. Acute and chronic forms are recognized. Acute disease can cause death within 6 hours after onset of signs. Affected pigs may cough, become cyanotic and express a blood-tinged nasal discharge. Extensive pleural hemorrhages occur, with death resulting from pulmonary consolidation and adhesions. Chronic disease may be subclinical and is characterized by deteriorating performance and an extended finishing period. Pathology typically consists of a fibrinopurulent bronchopneumonia and a fibrinous pleuritis. Certain serotypes of *H. pleuropneumoniae* are highly virulent, with serotype 5 being identified in a majority of cases submitted for laboratory diagnosis.[3,4] Serotypes 1, 4, and 5 consistently produce lung lesions following exposure. Until recently, serotype 3 had been isolated from field cases, but had not been shown to produce clinical disease. During the development of 'PleuroGuard', however, researchers succeeded in reproducing clinical disease using serotype 3.

Safety and Efficacy: Chemical inactivation renders 'PleuroGuard 4' incapable of causing infectious disease. Temporary induration and moderate swelling may be observed at the injection site.
The *Bordetella bronchiseptica* component has been evaluated in challenge-of-immunity tests in susceptible 12-week old pigs. Results are shown in Table 1, and indicate that the most effective vaccination program requires immunization of both sows and pigs.
[See table on next page].
Efficacy of the *E. rhusiopathiae* component was demonstrated in a controlled challenge-of-immunity test. A single subcutaneous dose administered to seronegative test pigs protected them from challenge with *E. rhusiopathiae* administered 2 weeks postvaccination. All controls were clinically affected with signs of erysipelas following the same challenge.
Efficacy of the *H. pleuropneumoniae* component in 'PleuroGuard 4' was established in rigorous challenge-of-immunity tests. Vaccinates received 2 subcutaneous doses administered 2 weeks apart. Respective test groups were challenged with virulent *H. pleuropneumoniae* serotypes 1, 3, 4, and 5 (Table 2). For serotype 1, two tests were conducted. A market weight challenge was administered to one group 120 days following primary vaccination, and a short-term challenge was administered to a second group 42

days following primary vaccination. For serotype 3, challenge was administered 38 days following primary vaccination. For serotypes 4 and 5, challenge was administered 49 and 28 days following primary vaccination, respectively. In each test, all pigs were necropsied and evaluated for lung disease either following death or termination of the test at 6 to 12 days postchallenge.

Results are shown in Table 2. All vaccinates seroconverted to each of the *H. pleuropneumoniae* serotypes tested. Vaccinated pigs demonstrated a high level of protection against a severe challenge that produced lung lesions in 97% of the controls.

[See table below].

The market weight challenge for serotype 1 demonstrated that vaccination provided substantial protection over the course of the feeding period, even against severe challenge.

One of the challenge-of-immunity tests (test 6) was designed to evaluate the effects of vaccination and challenge in pigs with maternal immunity. (Prevaccination geometric mean titers for *H. pleuropneumoniae* were 1:31 in vaccinates and 1:45 in controls.) Postchallenge, all controls developed lung lesions, indicating that passive immunity may be of limited benefit in the face of a severe challenge. Ninety percent of the vaccinates were protected against lung lesions, underscoring the value of active immunization. Following administration of vaccine, pigs developed a 2-fold increase in the geometric mean serologic titer (Table 3), demonstrating that vaccination can produce active immunity in pigs carrying maternal antibodies.

[See table on next page].

Directions:

1. *General Directions:* Shake well and administer 3 ml. intramuscularly or subcutaneously.
2. *Primary Vaccination:* Pigs should receive 1 dose at 1 week of age and a second dose when weaned. Alternatively, the initial dose may be given at weaning, with the second dose given 2 to 3 weeks later. CAUTION: FIELD TRIALS HAVE SHOWN THAT TRANSIENT LETHARGY, ANOREXIA, AND VOMITING MAY OCCUR IN SOME PIGS IMMEDIATELY AFTER INOCULATION. IF PIGS ARE NOT VACCINATED WITH *B. BRONCHISEPTICA* BY ONE WEEK OF AGE, LOW DOSE NATURAL EXPOSURE MAY PREDISPOSE THEM TO ALLERGIC REACTION. Sows and gilts should receive 2 doses at least 2 weeks apart before farrowing.
3. *Revaccination:* Pregnant swine should receive 2 doses at least 2 weeks apart with the second dose administered 2 weeks before farrowing. For sows, revaccination is recommended prior to each subsequent farrowing. Semiannual revaccination is recommended for boars.

TABLE 1—Results of Challenge Following Vaccination with *Bordetella Bronchiseptica* Bacterin

No. Animals	Immunization Status	% Incidence of Turbinate Atrophy
25	nonvaccinated pigs from nonvaccinated sows	96
35	nonvaccinated pigs from vaccinated sows	60
23	vaccinated pigs from nonvaccinated sows	39
40	vaccinated pigs from vaccinated sows	20

Precautions:

1. Store at 2°C. to 7°C. Do not freeze.
2. Use entire contents when first opened.
3. Do not vaccinate within 21 days of slaughter.
4. If anaphylaxis occurs following use, administer epinephrine or equivalent.
5. Transient local reactions may occur following administration.
6. Although this product has been shown to be efficacious, some animals may be unable to develop or maintain an adequate immune response following administration if they are incubating any disease, are malnourished or parasitized, or stressed due to shipment or environmental conditions.

Supplied: 35-dose vials.

References:

1. Rutter JM and Rojas X: Atrophic Rhinitis in Gnotobiotic Piglets: Differences in the Pathogenicity of *Pasteurella multocida* in Combined Infections with *Bordetella bronchiseptica.* Vet Rec. 110:531–535 (1982).
2. Barfod K and Pedersen KB: Synergism Between *Bordetella bronchiseptica* and a Toxin-Producing Strain of *Pasteurella multocida* in the Causation of Atrophic Rhinitis in SPF Pigs. International Pig Veterinary Congress: 112 (1982).
3. Gunnarsson A, Biberstein EL, and Hurvell B; Serologic Studies on Porcine strains of *Haemophilus parahaemolyticus (pleuropneumoniae):* Agglutination Reactions. Am. J. Vet. Res. 38:1111–1114 (1977).
4. Schultz RA: Proceedings George A. Young Swine Conference (1980).

For Veterinary Use Only

TABLE 2—Results of *H. Pleuropneumoniae* Vaccination and Challenge in Preweaned Pigs

Test No.	Serotype & Procedure	Test Groups	Postvaccination Seroconversion	Percent Protected from Lung Lesions
1	type 1 challenge (market weight)	19 vaccinates	100	74 (14/19)
		5 controls	—	0 (0/5)
2	type 1 challenge	19 vaccinates	100	84 (16/19)
		4 controls	—	25 (1/4)
3	type 3 challenge	25 vaccinates	100	76 (19/25)
		6 controls	—	0 (0/6)
4	type 4 challenge	21 vaccinates	100	95 (20/21)
		5 controls	—	0 (0/5)
5	type 5 challenge, seronegative pigs	20 vaccinates	100	95 (19/20)
		5 controls	—	0 (0/5)
6	type 5 challenge, seropositive pigs*	20 vaccinates	—	90 (18/20)
		5 controls	—	0 (0/5)

*Test animals had maternally derived antibodies

PNEUMO–GUARD H®
Pasteurella Haemolytica Vaccine Avirulent Live Culture

Product Description: 'Pneumo-Guard H' is for use as an aid in the prevention of cattle infections due to *Pasteurella haemolytica.* 'Pneumo-Guard H' contains a lyophilized, avirulent strain of *P. haemolytica.*

Disease Description: Clinical manifestations of *P. haemolytica* infection are commonly associated with bovine respiratory disease (BRD) and are observed as pneumonia. Typically, signs of BRD include fever, coughing, dyspnea, mucopurulent nasal discharge, ocular discharge, depression, anorexia, and death. Upon necropsy, bovine pneumonic pasteurellosis is characterized by inflammation of the airways, fibrinous pneumonia, lobular necrosis, and fibrinous pleuritis. Clinical signs of *Pasteurella* infection include depression; anorexia; nasal discharge; fever; rapid, shallow breathing; and death. Upon necropsy, inflammation and consolidation of the pulmonary lobes has been seen.[1]

Exposure to other pathogens prior to *Pasteurella haemolytica,* such as infectious bovine rhinotracheitis virus,[2] parainfluenza type 3 virus,[3] or bovine respiratory syncytial virus,[4] may increase severity of *P. haemolytica* infection.

Pneumonia is the most common disease of the bovine respiratory tract, and *Pasteurella* are the organisms most often isolated in these cases. With respiratory infection still the most common disease problem affecting the cattle industry,

Continued on next page

Norden—Cont.

economic loss due to *P. haemolytica* infection is substantial.

Safety and Efficacy: Avirulence of the chemically altered vaccine strain was demonstrated by extensive animal testing. During field studies involving approximately 7,000 doses, 'Pneumo-Guard H' was found to be safe and effective. However, stiffness, moderate swelling at the injection site, and transient lameness were observed in some animals following vaccination.

Efficacy of 'Pneumo-Guard H' was demonstrated in challenge-of-immunity studies using susceptible calves. Vaccinates received 2 doses of 'Pneumo-Guard H' intramuscularly 3 weeks apart. Three weeks following revaccination, all test calves were exposed to virulent IBR virus; then five days later they were challenged with virulent *P. haemolytica*. During the 10-day observation period that followed, 'Pneumo-Guard H' vaccinates developed mild signs of respiratory disease, and minor pulmonary involvement was observed upon subsequent necropsy. In contrast, non-vaccinated control calves developed severe, acute respiratory disease and some died. Necropsy revealed extensive pulmonary involvement in all controls.

Directions:

> DO NOT USE in calves weighing less than 400 pounds. Vaccinate intramuscularly in the rear quarter only. Transient swelling, lameness, stiffness, and soreness were observed in 4% and abscesses in less than 1% of the vaccinates in field trials.

1. *General Directions:* Vaccination of healthy animals is recommended. Rehydrate vaccine with diluent supplied, and aseptically administer 2 ml. intramuscularly.
2. *Primary Vaccination:* Administer 2 doses, 3 to 6 weeks apart.
3. *Revaccination:* Annual revaccination is recommended.

Precautions:
1. Store at 2°C. to 7°C.
2. Use only syringes and needles sterilized by boiling. Do not use chemical sterilization.
3. Use entire contents immediately after rehydration.
4. Burn container and all unused contents.
5. Vaccination of stressed animals should be delayed.
6. Do not vaccinate within 21 days before slaughter.
7. Transient local reactions may occur following administration.
8. If anphylaxis occurs following use, administer epinephrine or equivalent.
9. Although this product has been shown to be efficacious, some animals may be unable to develop or maintain an adequate immune response following vaccination if they are incubating any disease, malnourished or parasitized, or stressed due to shipment or adverse environmental conditions.

Supplied: 10- and 25-dose vials.

References:

1. Kucera CJ, Wong JCS, Feldner TJ: Challenge exposure of cattle vaccinated with a chemically altered strain of *Pasteurella haemolytica*. Am J Vet Res 40:1848–1852, 1983.
2. Jericho KWF, Langford EV: Pneumonia in calves produced with aerosols of bovine herpesvirus 1 and *Pasteurella haemolytica*. Can J Comp Med 42:269–277, 1978.
3. Sharp JM, Gilmour NJL, Thompson DA, *et al:* Experimental infection of specific pathogen-free lambs with parainfleunza type 3 and *Pasteurella haemolytica*. J Comp Pathol 88:237–243, 1978.
4. Al-Darraji AM, Cutlip RC, Lehmkuhl HD, *et al:* Experimental infection of lambs with bovine respiratory syncytial virus and *Pasteurella haemolytica:* Clinical and microbiologic studies. Am J. Vet Res 43:236–240, 1982.

For Veterinary Use Only

PRAGMATAR*
Tar-sulfur-salicylic acid Ointment

Composition:

Contains: Cetyl alcohol-coal tar distillate, 4% providing colorless fractions of crude coal tar, 0.35%; special sulfur, 3%; salicylic acid, 3%; base, q.s.

Indications: To aid in the treatment and control of non-specific dermatoses, subacute and chronic eczema, itching lesions of chronic atopic dermatitis and pruritus, and to relieve itching of ringworm and fungus infections of dogs and cats.

Dosage and Administration: Clean area thoroughly. Apply Pragmatar once or twice daily, using small quantities and confining application to affected areas.

Caution: Use with care near the eyes. Do not apply to unusually large areas at one time. Use precautions, when necessary, to prevent animal from ingesting Pragmatar by licking.

TABLE 3—Serologic Values in Maternally Immune Pigs Following *H. Pleuropneumoniae* Vaccination and Challenge

No. & Group	Geometric Mean Serum Agglutination Titers* Pre Vacc.	Post 1st Vacc.	Post 2nd Vacc.	Post Challenge
20 vaccinates	31	69	64	66
5 controls			45	78

*Expressed as the reciprocal of end point dilutions

Warning: Keep out of reach of children.

How Supplied: 1 oz. tubes —400 gm. jars.

PREG-GUARD 9®
Bovine Rhinotracheitis-Virus Diarrhea-Parainfluenza$_3$ Vaccine Modified Live Virus Campylobacter Fetus-Leptospira Canicola-Grippotyphosa-Hardjo-Icterohaemorrhagiae-Pomona Bacterin

Descriptions: Infectious bovine rhinotracheitis is a viral respiratory disease characterized by fever, nasal discharge, conjunctivitis, a hyperemic muzzle ("red nose"), coughing, and increased respiration. *Bovine virus diarrhea* is a viral disease characterized by lesions of the alimentary tract resulting in diarrhea and dehydration. Mucosal disease, a variant of BVD infection, is typified by destruction of lymphoid tissue and ulcerative lesions throughout the alimentary tract. Animals affected with BVD usually become anorectic with loss of weight, condition, and milk production. *Parainfluenza$_3$* is a viral respiratory infection, sometimes mild or inapparent, but often associated with bovine respiratory disease complex. *Vibriosis* is an insidious venereal disease of cattle. The *Campylobacter* organism infects the cow's genital tract causing early embryonic death. The disease is characterized by infertility, repeat breeding, and a prolonged calving season. Leptospirosis caused by *L. canicola, L. grippotyphosa, L. hardjo, L. icterohaemorrhagiae,* and *L. pomona* is clinically indistinguishable. Infection with any of these serovars may cause characteristic hemolysis, anemia, nephritis, reduced milk production, and abortions in pregnant cows.

Indications: Preg-Guard 9 is for the vaccination of healthy cows and heifers against: infectious bovine rhinotracheitis (IBR), bovine virus diarrhea (BVD), parainfluenza$_3$ (PI$_3$), vibriosis, leptospirosis caused by *Leptospira canicola, L. grippotyphosa, L. hardjo, L. icterohaemorrhagiae,* and *L. pomona.*

The IBR and PI$_3$ components are prepared by growing attenuated virus strains on a bovine cell line. The BVD component is prepared by growing an attenuated virus strain on a porcine cell line. The modified live virus components are combined and stabilized by freeze-drying.

The *Campylobacter* bacterin is an inactivated suspension of *Campylobacter fetus venerealis*. It is combined with an inactivated *Leptospira* bacterin prepared from whole cultures of the agents indicated. The *Campylobacter-Leptospira* bacterin is supplied as a diluent for the IBR-BVD-PI$_3$ vaccine.

Safety and Efficacy: The cell lines on which the modified live virus components are produced have been extensively tested to ensure freedom from adventitious agents. In the case of the BVD

component, susceptible calves inoculated intranasally with a field dose, or parenterally with 10 times the field dose remained clinically normal. The immunizing agents in the *Campylobacter-Leptospira* bacterin have been rendered noninfective by means of inactivation.
Separate challenge-of-immunity tests for the modified live virus components were conducted in accordance with federal regulations. All vaccinated calves remained clinically normal following challenge that produced typical signs of disease in nonvaccinated control calves. Immunogenicity of the *Campylobacter* and *Leptospira* components was confirmed by challenge-of-immunity or serologic tests.
Dosage and Administrations:
General Directions: Shake the *Campylobacter-Leptospira* bacterin and use it to aseptically rehydrate the IBR-BVD-PI_3 vaccine. Inject a 5 ml dose intramuscularly.
Primary Vaccination: A single dose should be administered to all breeding cows and heifers 30 to 60 days prior to breeding or being added to the herd. In noninfected herds in endemic areas, a second injection may be desirable with a vaccination interval of at least 2 weeks.
Revaccination: Annual revaccination is recommended.
Precautions:
Do not use in pregnant cows or in calves nursing pregnant cows (abortions can result). Do not vaccinate neonatal calves.
Vaccination of stressed animals should be delayed.
Do not vaccinate within 21 days of slaughter.
Store at 2°C.-7°C. Do not freeze.
Use entire contents without delay after rehydration.
Burn container and unused contents.
Anaphylaxis may occur following use (antidote is epinephrine).
Contains penicillin and streptomycin as preservatives.
Although this product has been shown to be efficacious, some animals may be unable to develop or maintain an adequate immune response following vaccination if they are incubating any infectious disease, are malnourished or parasitized, or stressed due to shipment or environmental conditions.
How Supplied: 10- and 25-dose vials
For Veterinary Use Only

PR–VAC®
Pseudorabies Vaccine
Modified Live Virus
For Use in Swine Only

Composition: PR-Vac® is a modifed live virus vaccine, porcine cell line origin, for the immunization of healthy swine against pseudorabies (Aujeszky's disease, mad itch, infectious bulbar paralysis).
Pseudorabies is an acute infectious disease caused by porcine herpesvirus. The disease affects most mammals, but has historically caused high mortality in newborn and young pigs. In recent years, both the incidence and severity of the infection in pigs and other species has increased. Acute and chronic infections in older pigs, abortions, stillbirths, and mummified fetuses from breeding females are recognized. Clinical signs include vomiting, diarrhea, high temperature, and CNS disturbances progressing from incoordination to paralysis and death.
Laboratory and field evidence to date have indicated no shed or spread of vaccine virus from vaccinated to susceptible contact animals. Developmental studies have shown that vaccination with PR-Vac prevents clinical pseudorabies following exposure to virulent virus. Shedding of virulent virus from swine was reduced by prior vaccination, thus reducing the probability of transmission of virulent virus among swine.
Indications: For the immunization of healthy swine 3 days of age or older against pseudorabies (Aujeszky's disease).
Dosage and Administration: Aseptically rehydrate PR-Vac with diluent supplied. Administer 2 ml. intramuscularly.
1. For Use in Swine Only! Not For Use in Any Other Animal.
2. Pigs nursing non-immune dams may be safely vaccinated at any age after 3 days.
3. Pigs nursing immune sows should be vaccinated when maternal antibody levels have declined, generally when the pigs are 3 to 8 weeks of age.
4. Semiannual revaccination is recommended for animals retained for breeding. Boars may be revaccinated at any time. Revaccinate sows before breeding.
5. In an emergency situation where exposure is imminent, it may be desirable to immediately vaccinate all swine on the premises.
Caution: Vaccination produces an antibody response, thus vaccinated swine become positive to the serum neutralization test. This positive test cannot be differentiated from a positive test caused by infection. Therefore, regulations concerning movement of seropositive swine would apply to both vaccinated swine and to swine that have had previous infections.
Do not vaccinate within 21 days before slaughter. Store at 2°C-7°C. Use entire contents without delay after rehydration. Burn container and all unused contents. Contains penicillin and streptomycin as preservatives. Anaphylaxis may follow use of this product. Antidote: Epinephrine.
How Supplied: 5- and 25-dose vials.
Distribution is limited to authorized recipients designated by proper State Officials, under such conditions as these authorities may require.
For Veterinary Use Only

PR-VAC®—KILLED
Pseudorabies Vaccine
Killed Virus

Composition: Pseudorabies is an acute infectious disease caused by porcine herpesvirus. The clinical signs include fever, vomiting, encephalitis and high mortality in suckling pigs. The signs in older swine may vary from inapparent to anorexia, fever, depression, and occasional death. Pregnant sows may abort or produce stillborn or mummified pigs.
PR-Vac—Killed is not shed from vaccinated pigs and will not transmit to susceptible contact animals. Developmental studies have shown that vaccination of swine with PR-Vac-Killed prevented clinical disease and death losses caused by pseudorabies.
Indications: PR-Vac-Killed is an inactivated, adjuvanted vaccine for use as an aid in the prevention of pseudorabies in healthy swine.
Dosage and Administration: For use in swine only! Not for use in any other animal. Administer a single 2 ml. dose intramuscularly at weaning. If pigs are vaccinated at an earlier age, revaccinate at weaning. Sows may be vaccinated at any stage of pregnancy. Semi-annual revaccination is recommended for animals retained for breeding.
Caution: Vaccination produces an antibody response, thus vaccinated swine become positive to the serum neutralization test. This positive test cannot be differentiated from a positive test caused by infection. Therefore, regulations concerning movement of seropositive swine would apply to vaccinated swine.
Caution: Do not vaccinate within 21 days before slaughter. Store at 2°C.–7°C. Do not freeze the vaccine. Use entire contents when first opened. Contains penicillin and streptomycin as preservatives. In the case of anaphylactoid reaction, administer epinephrine.
How Supplied: 5- and 25-dose vials.
Distribution is limited to authorized recipients designated by proper State Officials, under such conditions as these authorities may require.
For Veterinary Use Only

PR–VAC®/LEPTOFERM-5®
Pseudorabies Vaccine
Modified Live Virus,
Leptospira Canicola-
Grippotyphosa-Hardjo-
Icterohaemorrhagiae-
Pomona Bacterin
For Use in Swine Only

Composition: PR-Vac/Leptoferm-5 is a combined modified live virus vaccine and bacterin for the immunization of healthy swine against pseudorabies (Aujeszky's disease) and Leptospira infections caused by *L. canicola*, *L. grippotyphosa*, *L. hardjo*, *L. icterohaemorrhagiae* and *L. pomona*.
The vaccine is prepared by propagating the attenuated strain of pseudorabies on an established porcine cell line.
The inactivated leptospira fractions are prepared from antigenic cultures of *L. canicola*, *L. grippotyphosa*, *L. hardjo*, *L. icterohaemorrhagiae*, and *L. pomona*.
Pseudorabies is an acute infectious disease caused by porcine herpesvirus. The disease affects most mammals, but has historically caused high mortality in newborn and young pigs. In recent years, both the incidence and severity of the

Continued on next page

Norden—Cont.

infection in pigs and other species has increased. Acute and chronic infections in older pigs, abortions, still-births, and mummified fetuses from breeding females are recognized. Clinical signs include vomiting, diarrhea, high temperature, and CNS disturbances progressing from incoordination to paralysis and death.

Laboratory and field evidence to date have indicated no shed or spread of vaccine virus from vaccinated to susceptible contact animals. Developmental studies have shown that vaccination with PR-Vac/Leptoferm-5 prevents clinical pseudorabies and Leptospiral infections. Shedding of virulent virus from exposed swine was reduced by prior vaccination, thus reducing the probability of transmission of virulent virus among swine.

Dosage and Administration: Aseptically rehydrate with accompanying bacterin. Shake gently. Administer one 5 ml. dose intramuscularly. Revaccination in 3 to 6 weeks with Leptoferm-5 bacterin is recommended. Use only syringes and needles sterilized by boiling or heat rather than chemical sterilization.

1. For Use in Swine Only! Not For Use in Any Other Animal.
2. Pigs nursing non-immune dams may be safely vaccinated at any age after 3 days.
3. Pigs nursing immune sows should be vaccinated when maternal antibody levels have declined, generally when the pigs are 3 to 8 weeks of age.
4. Semiannual revaccination is recommended for animals retained for breeding. Boars may be revaccinated at any time. Revaccinate sows before breeding.
5. In an emergency situation where exposure is imminent, it may be desirable to immediately vaccinate all swine on the premises.

Caution: Vaccination with PR-Vac produces an antibody response to pseudorabies, thus vaccinated swine become positive to the serum neutralization test. The positive test cannot be differentiated from a positive test caused by infection. Therefore, regulations concerning movement of seropositive swine would apply to both vaccinated swine and to swine that have had previous infections.

Do not vaccinate within 21 days before slaughter. Store at 2°C.-7°C. Use entire contents without delay after rehydration. Burn container and all unused contents. Contains penicillin and streptomycin as preservatives. Anaphylaxis may follow use of this product. Antidote: Epinephrine.

How Supplied: 5-dose and 25-dose vials.

Distribution is limited to authorized recipients designated by proper State Officials, under such conditions as these authorities may require.

For Veterinary Use Only

RABGUARD-TC®
Rabies Vaccine
Killed Virus
For Use in Dogs, Cats, Cattle, Horses, and Sheep

Product Description: 'Rabguard-TC' is for the vaccination of healthy dogs, cats, cattle, horses, and sheep against rabies. The vaccine is prepared by growing a cell-culture adapted rabies virus in an established porcine cell line, chemically inactivating the virus, and combining it with an adjuvant. 'Rabguard-TC' is packaged in liquid form for ease of administration.

Disease Description: Rabies is a world-wide, high-mortality disease affecting all mammalian species. Wild animals are common vectors of the disease and a major source of transmission to humans and domestic animals. Despite successful attempts over the years to reduce the incidence of rabies, a recent report indicates that in the U.S. more than 30,000 people undergo treatment every year for possible exposure.[1] Susceptibility varies according to species. Cats, for example, are highly susceptible, humans and dogs somewhat less so.

Historically, dogs have been the major reservoir of rabies. Domestic cats, however, should not be overlooked as a source of the disease. In 1981, for the first time, the reported number of rabid cats in the U.S. outnumbered rabid dogs, by approximately 20%. In one state (Iowa), 42 out of 57 (74%) of known human rabies bite-associated exposures involved cats.[2] The Committee on rabies of the U.S. Animal Health Association has determined that cat rabies is a threat to public health and is not adequately controlled. The Committee has declared that "the incidence of cat rabies is approximately equal to that of dog rabies while efforts to control cat rabies are very limited as compared with those to control dog rabies. The Committee urges that cats be included in rabies immunization programs."[3] The National Academy of Sciences recommends universal rabies vaccination of all domestic dogs and cats as a public health precaution.[4]

Rabies virus infects nervous tissue, but the route of infection can be oral, respiratory, or parenteral. Following infection, a paralytic syndrome ensues, emerging as either the "furious" or "dumb" form. "Furious rabies" is characterized by unusual aggression; "dumb rabies" by lethargy and a desire to avoid contact. Respiratory failure is the immediate cause of death.

Safety and Efficacy: Because 'Rabguard-TC' is produced on an established cell line, it has safety advantages over inactivated rabies vaccines of murine or caprine origin. Tissue origin vaccines contain extraneous protein in addition to rabies antigen. The vaccinated animal is capable of responding to all such proteins. Auto-immune reactions can occur with repeated use, and have in fact been reported following administration of suckling mouse brain rabies vaccine.[5]

The established cell line used in 'Rabguard-TC' has been extensively tested for freedom from contaminating agents. 'Rabguard-TC' proved to be uniformly safe in experimental tests conducted at Norden Laboratories, and adverse reactions were not reported in extensive clinical trials of the vaccine. In addition, use of an established cell line yields a vaccine of consistent potency from serial to serial.

A study conducted in accordance with federal regulations and under U.S. Department of Agriculture direction demonstrated that a single 1 ml. dose protected either dogs or cats satisfactorily. Immunogenicity tests in cattle, horses, and sheep showed that the vaccine provided protection against virulent challenge administered more than a year after vaccination.

Directions:

General Directions: Shake and administer 1 ml. Dogs and cats may be vaccinated subcutaneously or intramuscularly. Vaccination of cattle, horses, and sheep should be by the intramuscular route.

Primary Vaccination: Healthy dogs, cats, cattle, horses, and sheep should be given a single dose at 3 months of age or older. Animals vaccinated when less than 12 months of age should be revaccinated one year later.

Revaccination: For dogs and cats, revaccination every 3 years is recommended. Annual revaccination is recommended for cattle, horses, and sheep.

Precautions:

1. Store at 2°C.–7°C. Do not freeze.
2. Use entire contents when first opened.
3. Contains gentamicin as preservative.
4. If anaphylaxis occurs following use, administer epinephrine or equivalent.
5. Burn container and all unused contents.
6. Although this product has been shown to be efficacious, some animals may be unable to develop or maintain an adequate immune response following vaccination if they are incubating any infectious disease, are malnourished or parasitized, or stressed due to shipment or environmental conditions.
7. FOR USE BY GRADUATE VETERINARIANS ONLY.

How Supplied: 10-dose vials, 25-dose vials, and cartons of 50 1-dose vials.

References:

1. Kaplan, M.M., Koprowski, H.: Rabies. Austr. Vet. Pract., 10:208–215 (1980).
2. Center for Disease Control, Atlanta, GA Morbidity and Mortality Weekly Report, 31:67–68,73 (1982).
3. Proc. 82nd Ann. Meet. U.S. Anim. Health Assn. 7–9 (1978).
4. Control of Rabies. National Academy of Science, Washington DC (1973).
5. Held, J.R., Lopez, Adaros, H.: Neurologic Disease in Man Following Administration of Suckling Mouse Brain Antirabies Vaccine. Bull. Wld. Hlth. Org., 46:321–327 (1972).

For Veterinary Use Only
U.S. Pat. No. 4,347,239

N

RESBO BVD®
Bovine Virus Diarrhea Vaccine
Modified Live Virus

Description: Bovine virus diarrhea is a viral disease characterized by lesions of the alimentary tract resulting in diarrhea and dehydration. Mucosal disease, a variant of BVD infection, is typified by destruction of lymphoid tissue and ulcerative lesions throughout the alimentary tract. Affected animals usually become anorectic with loss of weight, condition, and milk production.
Indications: Resbo BVD is for the vaccination of healthy cattle against bovine virus diarrhea (BVD). The vaccine is prepared by growing an attenuated BVD virus on a porcine cell line. The vaccine is stabilized by freeze-drying.
Safety and Efficacy: The cell line on which the vaccine is produced is an important factor in ensuring product safety. Use of a cell line that has been extensively tested assures virtual freedom from adventitious agents. Susceptible calves inoculated intranasally with a field dose, or parenterally with 10 times the field dose remained clinically normal with no increase in temperature. In challenge-of-immunity tests performed in accordance with federal regulations, all vaccinated calves remained clinically normal following challenge that produced typical signs of disease in all nonvaccinated control calves.
Directions:
General Directions: Aseptically rehydrate vaccine with diluent supplied. Inject 2 ml. intramuscularly.
Primary Vaccination: A single dose is recommended. Calves vaccinated before 6 months of age should be revaccinated at 6 months of age.
Revaccination: Annual revaccination is recommended.
Precautions:
Vaccination of pregnant animals should be avoided (abortions can result).
Do not vaccinate neonatal calves. Vaccination of stressed animals should be delayed.
Do not vaccinate within 21 days of slaughter.
Store at 2°C.-7°C.
Use entire contents without delay after rehydration.
Burn container and unused contents.
Contains penicillin and streptomycin as preservatives.
Anaphylaxis may occur following use (antidote is epinephrine).
Although this product has been shown to be efficacious, some animals may be unable to develop or maintain an adequate immune response following vaccination if they are incubating any infectious disease, are malnourished or parasitized, or stressed due to shipment or adverse environmental conditions.
How Supplied: 25-dose vials.
For Veterinary Use Only

RESBO® IBL5
Bovine Rhinotracheitis-
Virus Diarrhea Vaccine
Modified Live Virus
Leptospira Canicola-
Grippotyphosa-Hardjo-
Icterohaemorrhagiae-
Pomona Bacterin

Description: *Infectious bovine rhinotracheitis* is a viral respiratory disease characterized by fever, nasal discharge, conjunctivitis, a hyperemic muzzle (red nose), coughing, and increased respiration. *Bovine virus diarrhea* is a viral disease characterized by lesions of the alimentary tract resulting in diarrhea and dehydration. Mucosal disease, a variant of BVD infection, is typified by destruction of lymphoid tissue and ulcerative lesions throughout the alimentary tract. Animals affected with BVD usually become anorectic with loss of weight, condition, and milk production. Leptospirosis caused by *L. canicola, L. grippotyphosa, L. hardjo, L. icterohaemorrhagiae,* and *L. pomona* is clinically indistinguishable. Infection with any of these serovars may cause characteristic hemolysis, anemia, nephritis, reduced milk production, and abortions in pregnant cows.
Indications: Resbo IBL5 is for the vaccination of healthy cattle against infectious bovine rhinotracheitis (IBR), bovine virus diarrhea (BVD), and infection caused by *Leptospira canicola, L. grippotyphosa, L. hardjo, L. icterohaemorrhagiae,* and *L. pomona.* The IBR component is prepared by growing an attenuated virus strain on a bovine cell line. The BVD component is prepared by growing an attenuated virus strain on a porcine cell line. The two modified live virus components are combined and stabilized by freeze-drying. The *Leptospira* bacterin is prepared from whole cultures of *L. canicola, L. grippotyphosa, L. hardjo, L. icterohaemorrhagiae,* and *L. pomona* supplied as a diluent.
Safety and Efficacy: The cell lines on which the vaccine components are produced are important factors in ensuring product safety. Use of cell lines that have been extensively tested assures virtual freedom from adventitious agents. In the case of the BVD component, susceptible calves inoculated intranasally with a field dose, or parenterally with 10 times the field dose remained clinically normal with no increase in temperatures. Separate challenge-of-immunity tests for the modified live virus components were conducted in accordance with federal regulations. All vaccinated calves remained clinically normal following challenge that produced typical signs of disease in nonvaccinated control calves. Immunogenicity of the *Leptospira* components was confirmed by challenge-of-immunity or serologic tests.
Directions:
General Directions: Aseptically rehydrate vaccine with Leptospira diluent supplied. Inject 2 ml. intramuscularly.
Primary Vaccination: A single dose is recommended. Calves vaccinated before 6 months of age should be revaccinated at 6 months of age.
Revaccination: Annual revaccination is recommended.
Precautions:
Do not use in pregnant cows or in calves nursing pregnant cows (abortions can result).
Do not vaccinate neonatal calves.
Vaccination of stressed animals should be delayed.
Do not vaccinate within 21 days of slaughter.
Store at 2°C.–7°C.
Use entire contents without delay after rehydration.
Burn container and unused contents.
Contains penicillin and streptomycin as preservatives.
Anaphylaxis may occur following use (antidote is epinephrine).
Although this product has been shown to be efficacious, some animals may be unable to develop or maintain an adequate immune response following vaccination if they are incubating any infectious disease, are malnourished or parasitized, or stressed due to shipment or adverse environmental conditions.
How Supplied: 10-dose and 50-dose vials.
For Veterinary Use Only

RESBO IBR®
Bovine Rhinotracheitis Vaccine
Modified Live Virus

Composition: Resbo IBR is a modified live virus vaccine for the immunization of healthy cattle and calves against *bovine rhinotracheitis* infection.
This vaccine is prepared by propagating an attenuated strain of bovine rhinotracheitis virus on an established cell line developed at Norden Laboratories. This cell line is derived from a normal embryonic bovine kidney cell culture.
Bovine rhinotracheitis is a viral disease of the respiratory tract characterized by high temperature, excessive nasal discharge, increased respiration, coughing and depression.
Affected animals usually go off feed, resulting in a severe loss of weight and condition, and in dairy cattle, a loss in milk production.
For reducing the economic loss associated with this virus, vaccination of healthy animals is recommended before or upon entering the feedlot or dairy herd. Vaccination of stressed animals should be delayed.
Maximum protection, as determined by virus neutralizing antibodies, develops 14 to 21 days after vaccination.
Dosage and Administration: Aseptically rehydrate vaccine with diluent supplied. Inject 2 ml. intramuscularly. Syringes and needles used in administering this type of vaccine should be sterilized by boiling rather than chemical sterilization.
Caution: Do not use in pregnant cows or in calves nursing pregnant cows. (May cause abortion.) Do not vaccinate very young calves. Calves vaccinated before

Continued on next page

N **Norden—Cont.**

the age of 6 months should be revaccinated at six months of age. Do not vaccinate within 21 days before slaughter. Annual revaccination is recommended.
Store at 2°C.-7°C. Use entire contents immediately after rehydration. Burn container and all unused contents. Contains penicillin and streptomycin as preservatives. Anaphylaxis may follow use of products of this nature. Antidote: Epinephrine.
How Supplied: 10- and 50-dose vials. Dose is 2 ml.

RESBO IBR-BVD®
Bovine Rhinotracheitis-Virus Diarrhea Vaccine Modified Live Virus

Description: *Infectious bovine rhinotracheitis* is a viral respiratory disease characterized by fever, nasal discharge, conjunctivitis, a hyperemic muzzle (red nose), coughing, and increased respiration. *Bovine virus diarrhea* is a viral dis ease characterized by lesions of the alimentary tract resulting in diarrhea and dehydration. Mucosal disease, a variant of BVD infection, is typified by destruction of lymphoid tissue and ulcerative lesions throughout the alimentary tract. Animals affected with BVD usually become anorectic with loss of weight, condition and milk production.
Indications: Resbo IBR-BVD is for the vaccination of healthy cattle against infectious bovine rhinotracheitis (IBR) and bovine virus diarrhea (BVD). The IBR component is prepared by growing an attenuated virus strain on a bovine cell line. The BVD component is prepared by growing an attenuated virus strain on a porcine cell line. The vaccine components are combined and stabilized by freeze-drying.
Safety and Efficacy: The cell lines on which the vaccine components are produced are important factors in ensuring product safety. Use of cell lines that have been extensively tested assures virtual freedom from adventitious agents. In the case of the BVD component, susceptible calves inoculated intranasally with a field dose, or parenterally with 10 times the field dose remained clinically normal with no increase in temperature. Separate challenge-of-immunity tests for the IBR, and BVD components have been conducted in accordance with federal regulations. All vaccinated calves remained clinically normal following challenge that produced typical signs of disease in nonvaccinated control calves.
Directions:
General Directions: Aseptically rehydrate vaccine with diluent supplied. Inject 2 ml. intramuscularly.
Primary Vaccination: A single dose is recommended. Calves vaccinated before 6 months of age should be revaccinated at 6 months of age.
Revaccination: Annual revaccination is recommended.
Precautions:
Do not use in pregnant cows or in calves nursing pregnant cows (abortions can result).
Do not vaccinate neonatal calves.
Vaccination of stressed animals should be delayed.
Do not vaccinate within 21 days of slaughter.
Store at 2°C.–7°C.
Use entire contents without delay after rehydration.
Burn container and unused contents.
Contains penicillin and streptomycin as preservatives.
Anaphylaxis may occur following use (antidote is epinephrine).
Although this product has been shown to be efficacious, some animals may be unable to develop or maintain an adequate immune response following vaccination if they are incubating any infectious disease, are malnourished or parasitized, or stressed due to shipment or adverse environmental conditions.
How Supplied: 10-dose and 50-dose vials.

For Veterinary Use Only

RESBO IBR-BVD-LP®
Bovine Rhinotracheitis-Virus Diarrhea Vaccine Modified Live Virus, Leptospira Pomona Bacterin

Description: *Infectious bovine rhinotracheitis* is a viral respiratory disease characterized by fever, nasal discharge, conjunctivitis, a hyperemic muzzle ("red nose"), coughing, and increased respiration. *Bovine virus diarrhea* is a viral disease characterized by lesions of the alimentary tract resulting in diarrhea and dehydration. Mucosal disease, a variant of BVD infection, is typified by destruction of lymphoid tissue and ulcerative lesions throughout the alimentary tract. Animals affected with BVD usually become anorectic with loss of weight, condition, and milk production. *Leptospira pomona* is a common cause of leptospirosis in cattle. Infection may cause hemolysis, anemia, nephritis, reduced milk production, and abortions in pregnant cows.
Indications: Resbo IBR-BVD-LP is for the vaccination of healthy cattle against infectious bovine rhinotracheitis (IBR), bovine virus diarrhea (BVD) and *Leptospira pomona* infection. The IBR component is prepared by growing an attenuated virus strain on a bovine cell line. The BVD component is prepared by growing an attenuated virus strain on a porcine cell line. The modified live virus components are combined and stabilized by freeze-drying. The *Leptospira* bacterin is an inactivated whole culture of *L. pomona* supplied as diluent.
Safety and Efficacy: The cell lines on which the vaccine components are produced are important factors in ensuring product safety. Use of cell lines that have been extensively tested assures virtual freedom from adventitious agents. In the case of the BVD component, susceptible calves inoculated intranasally with a field dose, or parenterally with 10 times the field dose remained clinically normal with no increase in temperature. Separate challenge-of-immunity tests for the IBR, BVD and *Leptospira* components have been conducted in accordance with federal regulations. All vaccinated calves remained clinically normal following challenge that produced typical signs of disease on nonvaccinated control calves.
Directions:
General Directions: Aseptically rehydrate vaccine with *Leptospira pomona* bacterin supplied. Inject 2 ml. intramuscularly.
Primary Vaccination: A single dose is recommended. Calves vaccinated before 6 months of age should be revaccinated at 6 months of age.
Revaccination: Annual revaccination is recommended.
Precautions:
Do not use in pregnant cows or in calves nursing pregnant cows (abortions can result).
Do not vaccinate neonatal calves.
Vaccination of stressed animals should be delayed.
Do not vaccinate within 21 days of slaughter.
Store at 2°C.–7°C.
Use entire contents without delay after rehydration.
Burn container and unused contents.
Contains penicillin and streptomycin as preservatives.
Anaphylaxis may occur following use (antidote is epinephrine).
Although this product has been shown to be efficacious, some animals may be unable to develop or maintain an adequate immune response following vaccination if they are incubating any infectious disease, are malnourished or parasitized, or stressed due to shipment or adverse environmental conditions.
How Supplied: 10-dose and 25-dose, and 50-dose vials.

For Veterinary Use Only

RESBO IBR–LP®
Bovine Rhinotracheitis Vaccine Modified Live Virus Leptospira Pomona Bacterin

Composition: Resbo IBR-LP is a modified live virus vaccine for the immunization of healthy cattle and calves against bovine rhinotracheitis and *Leptospira pomona* infections.
This vaccine is prepared by propagating an attenuated strain of bovine rhinotracheitis virus on an established cell line developed at Norden Laboratories. This cell line is derived from a normal embryonic kidney cell culture.
The leptospira fraction of the vaccine consists of an inactivated antigenic culture of *Leptospira pomona.*
Bovine rhinotracheitis is a viral disease of the respiratory tract characterized by high temperatures, excessive nasal dis-

charge, increased respiration, coughing and depression.
Affected animals usually go off feed, resulting in a severe loss of weight and condition, and in dairy cattle, a loss in milk production.
For reducing the economic loss associated with this virus, vaccination of healthy animals is recommended before or upon entering the feedlot or dairy herd. Vaccination of stressed animals should be delayed.
Maximum protection, as determined by virus neutralizing antibodies, develops 14 to 21 days after vaccination.
Dosage and Administration: Aseptically rehydrate vaccine with Leptospira Pomona Bacterin supplied. Inject 2 ml intramuscularly. Syringes and needles used in administering this type vaccine should be sterilized by boiling rather than chemical sterilization.
Precautions: Do not use in pregnant cows or in calves nursing pregnant cows. (May cause abortion.) Do not vaccinate very young calves. Calves vaccinated before the age of 6 months should be revaccinated at six months of age. Do not vaccinate within 21 days before slaughter. Annual revaccination is recommended.
Store at 2°C–7°C. Use entire contents immediately after rehydration. Burn container and all unused contents. Contains penicillin and streptomycin as preservatives. Anaphylaxis may follow use of products of this nature. *Antidote:* Epinephrine.
How Supplied: 10- and 50-dose vials. Dose is 2 ml.

RESBO IBR–PI$_3$®
Bovine Rhinotracheitis-Parainfluenza$_3$ Vaccine Modified Live Virus

Composition: Resbo IBR-PI$_3$ is a modified live virus vaccine for the immunization of healthy cattle and calves against *rhinotracheitis* and *parainfluenza$_3$* virus infections.
This vaccine is prepared by propagating attenuated strains of these viruses on an established cell line developed at Norden Laboratories. This cell line is derived from a normal embryonic bovine kidney cell culture.
Bovine rhinotracheitis and *parainfluenza$_3$* are viral diseases of the respiratory tract characterized by high temperature, excessive nasal discharge, increased respiration, coughing and depression.
Affected animals usually go off feed, resulting in a severe loss of weight and condition, and in dairy cattle, a loss in milk production.
For reducing the economic loss associated with these viruses, vaccination of healthy animals is recommended before or upon entering the feedlot or dairy herd. Vaccination of stressed animals should be delayed.
Maximum protection, as determined by virus neutralizing antibodies, develops 14 to 21 days after vaccination.
Dosage and Administration: Aseptically rehydrate vaccine with diluent supplied. Inject 2 ml. intramuscularly. Syringes and needles used in administering this type vaccine should be sterilized by boiling rather than chemical sterilization.
Precautions: Do not use in pregnant cows or in calves nursing pregnant cows. (May cause abortion.). Do not vaccinate very young calves. Calves vaccinated before the age of 6 months should be revaccinated at six months of age. Do not vaccinate within 21 days before slaughter.
Store at 2°C.–7°C. Use entire contents immediately after rehydration. Burn container and all unused contents. Contains penicillin and streptomycin as preservatives. Anaphylaxis may follow use of products of this nature. Antidote: Epinephrine.
How Supplied: 10-, 25-and 50-dose vials. Dose is 2 ml.

RESBO 3®
Bovine Rhinotracheitis-Virus Diarrhea-Parainfluenza$_3$ Vaccine Modified Live Virus

Description: *Infectious bovine rhinotracheitis* is a viral respiratory disease characterized by fever, nasal discharge, conjunctivitis, a hyperemic muzzle (red nose), coughing, and increased respiration. *Bovine virus diarrhea* is a viral disease characterized by lesions of the alimentary tract resulting in diarrhea and dehydration. Mucosal disease, a variant of BVD infection, is typified by destruction of lymphoid tissue and ulcerative lesions throughout the alimentary tract. Animals affected with BVD usually become anorectic with loss of weight, condition, and milk production. *Parainfluenza$_3$* is a viral respiratory infection, sometimes mild or inapparent, but often associated with bovine respiratory disease complex.
Indications: Resbo 3 is for the vaccination of healthy cattle against infectious bovine rhinotracheitis (IBR), bovine virus diarrhea (BVD), and parainfluenza$_3$ (PI$_3$). The IBR and PI$_3$ components are prepared by growing attenuated virus strains on a bovine cell line. The BVD component is prepared by growing an attenuated virus strain on a porcine cell line. The vaccine components are combined and stabilized by freeze-drying.
Safety and Efficacy: The cell lines on which the vaccine components are produced are important factors in ensuring product safety. Use of cell lines that have been extensively tested assures virtual freedom from adventitious agents. In the case of the BVD component, susceptible calves inoculated intranasally with a field dose, or parenterally with 10 times the field dose remained clinically normal with no increase in temperatures. Separate challenge-of-immunity tests for the IBR, BVD and PI$_3$ components were conducted in accordance with federal regulations. All vaccinated calves remained clinically normal following challenge that produced typical signs of disease in nonvaccinated control calves.

Directions:
General Directions: Aseptically rehydrate vaccine with diluent supplied. Inject 2 ml. intramuscularly.
Primary Vaccination: A single dose is recommended. Calves vaccinated before 6 months of age should be revaccinated at 6 months of age.
Revaccination: Annual revaccination is recommended.
Precautions:
Do not use in pregnant cows or in calves nursing pregnant cows (abortions can result).
Do not vaccinate neonatal calves.
Vaccination of stressed animals should be delayed.
Do not vaccinate within 21 days of slaughter.
Store at 2°C.–7°C.
Use entire contents without delay after rehydration.
Burn container and unused contents.
Contains penicillin and streptomycin as preservatives.
Anaphylaxis may occur following use (antidote is epinephrine).
Although this product has been shown to be efficacious, some animals may be unable to develop or maintain an adequate immune response following vaccination if they are incubating any infectious disease, are malnourished or parasitized, or stressed due to shipment or adverse environmental conditions.
How Supplied: 5-dose, 10-dose and 25-dose vials.
For Veterinary Use Only

RESBO 4®
Bovine Rhinotracheitis-Virus Diarrhea-Parainfluenza$_3$ Vaccine, Modified Live Virus Leptospira Pomona Bacterin

Description: *Infectious bovine rhinotracheitis* is a viral respiratory disease characterized by fever, nasal discharge, conjunctivitis, a hyperemic muzzle (red nose), coughing, and increased respiration. *Bovine virus diarrhea* is a viral disease characterized by lesions of the alimentary tract resulting in diarrhea and dehydration. Mucosal disease, a variant of BVD infection, is typified by destruction of lymphoid tissue and ulcerative lesions throughout the alimentary tract. Animals affected with BVD usually become anorectic with loss of weight, condition, and milk production. *Parainfluenza$_3$* is a viral respiratory infection, sometimes mild or inapparent, but often associated with bovine respiratory disease complex. *Leptospira pomona* is a common cause of leptospirosis in cattle. Infection may cause hemolysis, anemia, nephritis, reduced milk production, and abortions in pregnant cows.
Indications: Resbo 4 is for the vaccination of healthy cattle against infectious bovine rhinotracheitis (IBR), bovine virus diarrhea (BVD), parainfluenza$_3$ (PI$_3$) and *Leptospira pomona* infection. The IBR and PI$_3$ components are prepared by

Continued on next page

N

Norden—Cont.

growing attenuated virus strains on a bovine cell line. The BVD component is prepared by growing an attenuated virus strain on a porcine cell line. The modified live virus components are combined and stablilized by freeze-drying. The *Leptospira* bacterin is an inactivated whole culture of *L. pomona* supplied as a diluent.

Safety and Efficacy: The cell lines on which the vaccine components are produced are important factors in ensuring product safety. Use of cell lines that have been extensively tested assures virtual freedom from adventitious agents. In the case of the BVD component, susceptible calves inoculated intranasally with a field dose, or parenterally with 10 times the field dose remained clinically normal with no increase in temperature. Separate challenge-of-immunity tests for the IBR, BVD, PI_3 and *Leptospira* components were conducted in accordance with federal regulations. All vaccinated calves remained clinically normal following challenge that produced typical signs of disease in nonvaccinated control calves.

Directions:

General Directions: Aseptically rehydrate vaccine with *Leptospira pomona* bacterin supplied. Inject 2 ml. intramuscularly.

Primary Vaccination: A single dose is recommended. Calves vaccinated before 6 months of age should be revaccinated at 6 months of age.

Revaccination: Annual revaccination is recommended.

Precautions:

Do not use in pregnant cows or in calves nursing pregnant cows (abortions can result).

Do not vaccinate neonatal calves.

Vaccination of stressed animals should be delayed.

Do not vaccinate within 21 days of slaughter.

Store at 2°C.–7°C.

Use entire contents without delay after rehydration.

Burn container and unused contents.

Contains penicillin and streptomycin as preservatives.

Anaphylaxis may occur following use (antidote is epinephrine)

Although this product has been shown to be efficacious, some animals may be unable to develop or maintain an adequate immune response following vaccination if they are incubating any infectious disease, are malnourished or parasitized, or stressed due to shipment or adverse environmental conditions.

How Supplied: 10-dose and 25-dose vials.

For Veterinary Use Only

RESBO 8®
Bovine Rhinotracheitis-Virus Diarrhea-Parainfluenza$_3$ Vaccine Modified Live Virus Leptospira Canicola-Grippotyphosa-Hardjo-Icterohaemorrhagiae-Pomona Bacterin

Description: *Infectious bovine rhinotracheitis* is a viral respiratory disease characterized by fever, nasal discharge, conjunctivitis, a hyperemic muzzle (red nose), coughing, and increased respiration. *Bovine virus diarrhea* is a viral disease characterized by lesions of the alimentary tract resulting in diarrhea and dehydration. Mucosal disease, a variant of BVD infection, is typified by destruction of lymphoid tissue and ulcerative lesions throughout the alimentary tract. Animals affected with BVD usually become anorectic with loss of weight, condition, and milk production. *Parainfluenza$_3$* is a viral respiratory infection, sometimes mild or inapparent, but often associated with bovine respiratory disease complex. Leptospirosis caused by *L. canicola, L. grippotyphosa, L. hardjo, L. icterohaemorrhagiae,* and *L. pomona* is clinically indistinguishable. Infection with any of these serovars may cause characteristic hemolysis, anemia, nephritis, reduced milk production, and abortions in pregnant cows.

Indications: Resbo 8 is for the vaccination of healthy cattle against infectious bovine rhinotracheitis (IBR), bovine virus diarrhea (BVD), parainfluenza$_3$ (PI_3), and infection caused by *Leptospira canicola, L. grippotyhosa, L. hardjo, L. icterohaemorrhagiae,* and *L. pomona.* The IBR and PI_3 components are prepared by growing an attenuated virus strain on a bovine cell line. The BVD component is prepared by growing an attenuated virus strain on a porcine cell line. The modified live virus components are combined and stabilized by freeze-drying. The Leptospira bacterin is prepared from whole cultures of *L. canicola, L. grippotyphosa, L. hardjo, L. icterohaemorrhagiae,* and *L. pomona* supplied as a diluent.

Safety and Efficacy: The cell lines on which the vaccine components are produced are important factors in ensuring product safety. Use of cell lines that have been extensively tested assures virtual freedom from adventitious agents. In the case of the BVD component, susceptible calves inoculated intranasally with a field dose, or parenterally with 10 times the field dose remained clinically normal with no increase in temperature. Separate challenge-of-immunity tests for the modified live virus components were conducted in accordance with federal regulations. All vaccinated calves remained clinically normal following challenge that produced typical signs of disease in nonvaccinated control calves. Immunogenicity of the *Leptospira* components was confirmed by challenge-of-immunity or serologic tests.

Directions:

General Directions: Aseptically rehydrate vaccine with *Leptospira* diluent supplied. Inject 2 ml. intramuscularly.

Primary Vaccination: A single dose is recommended. Calves vaccinated before 6 months of age should be revaccinated at 6 months of age.

Revaccination: Annual revaccination is recommended.

Precautions:

Do not use in pregnant cows or in calves nursing pregnant cows (abortions can result).

Do not vaccinate neonatal calves.

Vaccination of stressed animals should be delayed.

Do not vaccinate within 21 days of slaughter.

Store at 2°C–7°C.

Use entire contents without delay after rehydration.

Burn container and unused contents.

Contains penicillin and streptomycin as preservatives.

Anaphylaxis may occur following use (antidote is epinephrine).

Although this product has been shown to be efficacious, some animals may be unable to develop or maintain an adequate immune response following vaccination if they are incubating any infectious disease, are malnourished or parasitized, or stressed due to shipment or adverse environmental conditions.

How Supplied: 5-dose and 25-dose vials.

For Veterinary Use Only

RHINOBAC™
Bordetella Bronchiseptica Bacterin

Indications: Rhinobac is a chemically inactivated, adjuvanted culture of *Bordetella bronchiseptica.* It is recommended for use in healthy swine as an aid in the prevention of atrophic rhinitis caused by *Bordetella bronchiseptica* infection.

Bordetella bronchiseptica infections in swine are the principal cause of atrophic rhinitis. The disease is characterized by acute rhinitis followed by chronic atrophy of the turbinate bones. Young pigs are primarily affected but older animals may be exposed and become carriers. Bordetella pneumonia may develop as a result of infections. A reduced rate of weight gain leading to an extended finishing period has been associated with atrophic rhinitis.

Dosage and Administration: Shake well. Inject 2 ml intramuscularly or subcutaneously using aseptic technique. For primary immunization of pregnant swine, two doses are recommended at least 2 weeks apart, the second dose to be administered 2 weeks before farrowing. A booster dose is recommended prior to each subsequent farrowing. Semi-annual revaccination is recommended for boars. Primary immunization of piglets should be initiated at one week of age, followed by the second dose at 3 to 5 weeks of age.

Caution: Transient local reaction in vaccinated piglets may be observed following the use of this product. Do not vaccinate within 21 days before slaughter. Store at 2°C–7°C. Do not freeze.

Use entire contents when first opened. Anaphylaxis may follow use of products of this nature. *Antidote:* Epinephrine.
How Supplied: 10 and 50 dose vials.
For Veterinary Use Only

RHINOBAC™-ER
Bordetella Bronchiseptica-Erysipelothrix Rhusiopathiae Bacterin
Aluminum Hydroxide Adsorbed

Description: *Bordetella bronchiseptica* is a principal cause of atrophic rhinitis in swine. In young pigs the disease is characterized by acute rhinitis followed by chronic atrophy of the turbinate bones. Impairment of the turbinate filtering system predisposes the animal to respiratory infections, including *Bordetella*-pneumonia, and is associated with reduced rate of gain and an extended finishing period. *Erysipelothrix rhusiopathiae* infection in swine (swine erysipelas) has a variety of manifestations. These include acute septicemia, skin discoloration characterized by hyperemic or necrotic diamond-shaped lesions, chronic arthritis, and vegetative endocarditis.
Indications: *Bordetella bronchiseptica-Erysipelothrix rhusiopathiae* bacterin is for the vaccination of healthy swine against infection with these organisms. The bacterin contains chemically inactivated cultures of each agent combined with a sterile adjuvant.
Safety and Efficacy: Chemical inactivation renders the bacterin incapable of causing disease. The *Bordetella bronchiseptica* component has been evaluated in challenge-of-immunity tests in susceptible 12-week old pigs. Results indicate that the most effective vaccination program requires immunization of both sows and pigs.
Directions:
General Directions: Shake well. Administer 2 ml. intramuscularly or subcutaneously.
Primary Vaccination: At one week of age, pigs should receive 1 dose of monovalent Bordetella Bronchiseptica Bacterin (Rhinobac). This should be followed at weaning age by vaccination with Bordetella Bronchiseptica-Erysipelothrix Rhusiopathiae Bacterin. Pregnant swine should receive 2 doses at least 2 weeks apart, the second dose to be administered 2 weeks before farrowing.
Revaccination: For sows, a booster dose is recommended prior to each subsequent farrowing. Semiannual revaccination is recommended for boars.
Precautions:
Store at 2°C–7 °C. Do not freeze.
Use entire contents when first opened.
Do not vaccinate within 21 days of slaughter.
Anaphylaxis may occur following use (antidote is epinephrine).
Transient local reactions in vaccinated piglets may occur following administration.
Although this product has been shown to be efficacious, some animals may be unable to develop or maintain an adequate immune response following vaccination if they are incubating any disease or are malnourished, parasitized or stressed due to shipment or environmental conditions.
How Supplied: 10-dose and 50-dose vials.
For Veterinary Use Only

RHINOBAC™-P
Bordetella Bronchiseptica-Pasteurella Multocida Bacterin
For Use in Swine Only

Description: *Bordetella bronchiseptica* is a principal cause of atrophic rhinitis in swine. Particularly in young pigs, the disease is characterized by acute rhinitis followed by chronic atrophy of the turbinate bones. Impairment of the turbinate filtering system predisposes the animal to respiratory infections, including pneumonia, and is associated with reduced rate of gain and an extended finishing period. In combined infections, *B. bronchiseptica* and *P. multocida* have been shown to cause atrophic rhinitis lesions of greater severity than in cases where either agent functions alone.[1,2]
Indications: Rhinobac-P is for the vaccination of healthy swine against infection caused by *Bordetella bronchiseptica* and *Pasteurella multocida*. Rhinobac-P contains chemically inactivated cultures of *B. bronchiseptica* and *P. multocida*, combined with a sterile adjuvant to enhance the immune response.
Safety and Efficacy: Chemical inactivation renders Rhinobac-P incapable of causing infectious disease. Temporary induration and moderate swelling may be observed at the injection site.
The *Bordetella bronchiseptica* component has been evaluated in challenge-of-immunity tests in susceptible 12-week old pigs. The most effective vaccination program requires immunization of both sows and pigs.
Dosage and Administration:
General Directions: Shake well and administer 2 ml intramuscularly or subcutaneously.
Primary Vaccination: Pigs should receive 1 dose at 1 week of age and a second dose when weaned. Pregnant swine should receive 2 doses at least 2 weeks apart, with the second dose administered 2 weeks before farrowing.
Revaccination: For sows, revaccination is recommended prior to each subsequent farrowing. Semiannual revaccination is recommended for boars.
Precautions:
Store at 2°C–7°C. Do not freeze.
Use entire contents when first opened.
Do not vaccinate within 21 days of slaughter.
Anaphylaxis may occur following use (antidote is epinephrine).
Transient local reactions may occur following administration.
Although this product has been shown to be efficacious, some animals may be unable to develop or maintain an adequate immune response following vaccination if they are incubating any disease, malnourished or parasitized, or stressed due to shipment or environmental conditions.
How Supplied: 50-dose and 125-dose vials
For Veterinary Use Only
References

1. Rutter JM and Rojas X: Atrophic Rhinitis in Gnotobiotic Piglets: Differences in the Pathogenicity of *Pasteurella multocida* in Combined Infections with *Bordetella bronchiseptica*. Vet. Rec. 110:531–535 (1982).
2. Barfod K and Pedersen KB: Synergism Between *Bordetella bronchiseptica* and a Toxin-Producing Strain of *Pasteurella multocida* in the Causation of Atrophic Rhinitis in SPF Pigs. International Pig Veterinary Congress: 112 (1982).

RHINOBAC™ 3
Bordetella Bronchiseptica-Erysipelothrix Rhusiopathiae-Pasteurella Multocida Bacterin
For Use in Swine Only

Description: Rhinobac 3 is for the vaccination of healthy swine against infection caused by *Bordetella bronchiseptica, Erysipelothrix rhusiopathiae,* and *Pasteurella multocida*. Rhinobac 3 contains chemically inactivated cultures of *B. bronchiseptica, E. rhusiopathiae,* and *P. multocida* combined with a sterile adjuvant to enhance the immune response.
Indications: *Bordetella bronchiseptica* is a principal cause of atrophic rhinitis in swine. Particularly in young pigs, the disease is characterized by acute rhinitis followed by chronic atrophy of the turbinate bones. Impairment of the turbinate filtering system predisposes the animal to respiratory infections, including pneumonia, and is associated with reduced rate of gain and an extended finishing period. In combined infections, *B. bronchiseptica* and *Pasteurella multocida* have been shown to cause atrophic rhinitis lesions of greater severity than in cases where either agent functions alone.[1,2] *Erysipelothrix rhusiopathiae* infection in swine (swine erysipelas) has a variety of manifestations. These include acute septicemia, skin discoloration characterized by hyperemic or necrotic diamond-shaped lesions, chronic arthritis, and vegetative endocarditis.
Safety and Efficacy: Chemical inactivation renders Rhinobac 3 incapable of causing infectious disease. Temporary induration and moderate swelling may be observed at the injection site.
The *Bordetella bronchiseptica* component has been evaluated in challenge-of-immunity tests in susceptible 12-week old pigs. The most effective vaccination program requires immunization of both sows and pigs.
Efficacy of the *E. rhusiopathiae* component was demonstrated in a controlled challenge-of-immunity test. A single subcutaneous dose administered to seronegative test pigs protected them from challenge with *E. rhusiopathiae* administered 2 weeks postvaccination. All controls were clinically affected with signs of erysipelas following the same challenge.

Continued on next page

Norden—Cont.

Dosage and Administration:
General Directions: Shake well and administer 2 ml intramuscularly or subcutaneously.
Primary Vaccination: Pigs should receive 1 dose at 1 week of age and a second dose when weaned. Pregnant swine should receive 2 doses at least 2 weeks apart, with the second dose administered 2 weeks before farrowing.
Revaccination: For sows, revaccination is recommended prior to each subsequent farrowing. Semiannual revaccination is recommended for boars.
Precautions:
Store at 2°C–7°C. Do not freeze.
Use entire contents when first opened.
Do not vaccinate within 21 days of slaughter.
Anaphylaxis may occur following use (antidote is epinephrine).
Transient local reactions may occur following administration.
Although this product has been shown to be efficacious, some animals may be unable to develop or maintain an adequate immune response following administration if they are incubating any disease, are malnourished or parasitized, or stressed due to shipment or environmental conditions.
How Supplied: 50-dose vials
For Veterinary Use Only
References:
1. Rutter JM and Rojas X: Atrophic Rhinitis in Gnotobiotic Piglets: Differences in the Pathogenicity of *Pasteurella multocida* in Combined Infections with *Bordetella bronchiseptica.* Vet. Rec. 110:531–535 (1982).
2. Barford K and Pedersen KB: Synergism Between *Bordetella bronchiseptica* and a Toxin-Producing Strain of *Pasteurella multocida* in the Causation of Atrophic Rhinitis in SPF Pigs. International Pig Veterinary Congress: 112 (1982).

RHINOMUNE®
Equine Rhinopneumonitis Vaccine Modified Live Virus

Composition: Rhinomune is an attenuated live virus vaccine, equine cell line origin, for use in healthy horses *as an aid in the prevention of respiratory infections* caused by equine herpesvirus Type 1 (EHV-1).
EHV-1 causes acute respiratory disease on primary infection. Annual outbreaks may occur among foals in areas of dense horse population. Asymptomatic reinfection may occur and a latent carrier state is the probable reservoir of infection.
Immunity following natural infection persists 3 to 9 months and is usually augmented by subclinical or mild respiratory reinfection/recrudescence.
Directions: Vaccination of all horses 3 months of age or older on a premise is recommended to enhance herd immunity. For primary immunization administer 2 doses intramuscularly 4–8 weeks apart. Semi-annual revaccination is recommended. Additional boosters may be indicated in an epidemic or prior to exposure anticipated at training stables, races, shows or sales.
Foals younger than 3 months may carry maternal antibodies which interfere with the immune response to vaccination. In circumstances requiring earlier vaccination, foals should receive the 2 dose series after reaching 3 months of age.
Pregnant mares should be vaccinated after the second month of pregnancy.
Rhinomune is not intended for prophylactic or therapeutic use in horses previously exposed, incubating or infected with virulent EHV-1.
Dosage: Aseptically rehydrate with supplied diluent and administer intramuscularly. Appropriate preparation of inoculation site is advised to prevent introduction of bacterial contaminants. Use contents promptly after rehydration.
Precautions:
1. Store at 2°C–7°C.
2. Needles and syringes should not be sterilized with chemicals.
3. Anaphylaxis may occur. Antidote: Epinephrine.
4. Do not vaccinate animals to be slaughtered for human consumption within 21 days before slaughter.
5. Contains penicillin and streptomycin as preservatives.

How Supplied: 25 1-dose vials with diluent; 5 dose vials. Dose is 2 ml.

ROTA-VAC TGE®
Porcine Rotavirus-Transmissible Gastroenteritis Vaccine Modified Live Virus
TGE & 2 Major Rotavirus Serotypes

Introduction: 'Rota-Vac TGE' is a modified live virus vaccine containing three unique virus strains:
1. Rotavirus (2 prevalent serotypes A_1 and A_2)
2. TGE (transmissible gastroenteritis)

All three viruses have been modified so that they do not cause disease in baby pigs, feeder pigs and pregnant swine. The vaccine is recommended as an aid in prevention and control of Rotavirus (2 prevalent serotypes A_1 and A_2) and TGE diseases in swine. Both diseases produce identical clinical signs—occasional vomition and profuse watery diarrhea—in young pigs. Laboratory confirmation of the cause of baby pig diarrhea is recommended since other viral, bacterial and coccidial agents can also cause similar disease signs.
Efficacy of the TGE virus component has been previously reported for pregnant swine and baby pigs, and the importance of oral vaccination emphasized.[1,2] Efficacy of Rotavirus has been demonstrated in both pregnant sows and baby pigs. Pregnant sows, when vaccinated with 'Rota-Vac TGE', subsequently develop high persisting levels of antibody in their milk, thereby aiding in the control of diarrhea in their nursing pigs. Oral vaccination of conventional and gnotobiotic newborn pigs has also been shown to prevent the disease.[2,3] Experimental studies have also shown that two intramuscular doses of 'Rota-Vac TGE' at 5 and 2 weeks before farrowing will also result in good protection of nursing baby pigs and can be used as an alternate vaccination program. This is particularly true for herds in which there has been previous disease exposure.
Dosage and Guidelines: Follow directions carefully. Two vaccination programs may be used:

A. Oral and intramuscular vaccination (*Oral method*):
   1. Each pregnant sow or gilt must receive at least 3 doses of vaccine before farrowing:
      a. 5 weeks before farrowing—one oral dose.
      b. 3 weeks before farrowing—one oral dose.
      c. 1 week before farrowing—one intramuscular dose.
      In subsequent farrowings administer one oral and one intramuscular dose 2–3 weeks before farrowing.
   2. Reconstitute dried vaccine with the sterile diluent provided. Use 2 ml. for the one dose vial and 20 ml. for the 10 dose vial.

B. Two intramuscular vaccinations (*Injection method*):
   1. Each pregnant sow and gilt must receive 2 doses of 'Rota-Vac TGE' before farrowing.
   2. Reconstitute dried vaccine with the sterile diluent provided. Inject 2 ml. intramuscularly.

Oral vaccination—Transfer the desired number of doses to skim milk (prepared by adding one pound dried milk solids to 2½ gallons clean cool water) or to cool pasteurized milk at a ratio of one dose per quart. Add clean ground corn (or other pure ground grain) to vaccine-milk mixture until thickened and immediately feed to sow. Solid feed should be withheld from sows overnight prior to vaccination in order to facilitate vaccine consumption.
Intramuscular vaccination—Inject 2 ml. of the vaccine reconstituted with sterile diluent deep intramuscularly. Do not use chemically sterilized syringes as the chemicals may destroy the vaccine.
Caution: Store vaccine in the dark at temperatures between 35° and 45°F (4°–7°C). Use vaccine immediately after reconstitution; do not save partial contents. Burn this container and all unused contents. Do not use commercial milk replacers or complete rations to prepare oral vaccine mixture as they may adversely affect vaccine potency. Do not pour vaccine-milk mixture on top of ground corn as sows may not receive sufficient vaccine. Use vaccine in healthy animals only. Do not vaccinate within 21 days before slaughter. If allergic reactions follow use of the product treat with epinephrine. Good husbandry and management procedures should always accompany use of a vaccine in a herd. Contains gentamicin as preservative.
References:
1. Welter, C.J. 1980. Experimental and Field Evaluation of a New Oral Vac-

cine for TGE. Vet. Med. Sm. An. Clin. 75:1757–1759.
2. Graham, J.A. 1980. Induction of Active Immunity to TGE in Neonatal Pigs Nursing Seropositive Dams. Vet. Med. Sm. An. Clin. 75:1618–1619.
3. Research data on file, Ambico, Inc.
For Veterinary Use Only

SCOURGUARD 3®
Bovine Rota-Coronavirus Vaccine Modified Live Virus Escherichia Coli Bacterin

Product Description: 'ScourGuard 3' is for vaccination of healthy, pregnant cows to protect their calves against calf diarrhea caused by bovine rotavirus, bovine coronavirus and enterotoxigenic strains of *Escherichia coli* having the K99 pili adherence factor. The rota-coronavirus vaccine is prepared by propagating attenuated strains of virus on an established bovine cell line. It is rehydrated with a bacterin prepared from a chemically inactivated *E. coli* strain selected because of its high K99 pili content. A sterile adjuvant is used to enhance the immune response.
Disease Description: Neonatal calf diarrhea is a disease of complex etiology. The enterotoxigenic *E. coli* and the two viruses used in this product are commonly isolated from scouring calves, often in combination or with other bacterial or viral pathogens. Studies have shown that most enterotoxigenic *E. coli* strains isolated from scouring calves have K99 pili, antigenic structures that promote colonization of the mucosal surface of the small intestine.[1,2] The combination of enterotoxins produced by these strains and the cytopathogenic effects of rotavirus and coronavirus induce secretion of body fluids and electrolytes into the lumen of the gut. Fluid loss into the intestine produces diarrhea resulting in dehydration, electrolyte loss and in severe cases, metabolic acidosis.
Safety and Efficacy: Pregnancies in experimental cows were not affected as a result of vaccination with 'ScourGuard 3'. Susceptible calves are protected by receiving colostral antibodies from vaccinated cows. Thus, adequate and timely consumption of colostrum by the neonatal calf is essential for protection. In dairy herds where calves traditionally are weaned at 1 to 2 days of age, colostrum and first milk should be collected from vaccinated cows, and used for subsequent feedings of their calves.
Efficacy of the rota-coronavirus vaccine was evaluated in field studies in herds where these viral agents were identified by laboratory methods. Incidence of scours was 21.7% in nonvaccinated herds compared with 11.3% in vaccinated herds. Death loss from scours was 4.1% in nonvaccinated herds and 0.9% in vaccinated herds. Serological studies indicate there is a slightly greater antibody response to both viruses following administration of the combination product compared to Bovine Rota-Coronavirus Vaccine alone.
Efficacy of the *E. coli* bacterin was demonstrated in a controlled challenge-of-immunity study. Pregnant cows that received two doses of the bacterin provided maternal immunity that fully protected 80% of their calves from virulent challenge. The remaining 20% of the calves in this group had transient diarrhea lasting less than 48 hours. No death loss occurred in calves from vaccinated cows. Following challenge, 100% of the control calves from non-vaccinated cows had severe diarrhea resulting in a 58.8% mortality rate.
Directions:
1. *General Directions:* Rehydrate vaccine with accompanying bacterin. Shake well. Without delay, using aseptic precautions, administer 2 ml. intramuscularly to healthy pregnant cows.
2. *Primary Vaccination:* Administer 2 doses, late in pregnancy. The second dose may be administered as early as 2 weeks following the first, but not later than 3 weeks before calving.
3. *Revaccination:* Annual revaccination is recommended.
4. *Use in Dairy Cattle:* Calves are protected by receiving colostral antibodies from vaccinated cows. If calves are to be weaned at 1-2 days of age, collect colostrum and first milk from vaccinated cows, and use for subsequent feedings of their calves.
Precautions:
1. Store at 2°C.–7°C. Do not freeze.
2. Use entire contents when first opened.
3. Burn container and all unused contents.
4. Do not vaccinate within 21 days before slaughter.
5. Contains penicillin and streptomycin as preservatives.
6. If anaphylaxis occurs following use, administer epinephrine or equivalent.
7. Although this product has been shown to be efficacious, some animals may be unable to develop or maintain an adequate immune response following vaccination if they are incubating any infectious disease, are malnourished or parasitized, or stressed due to shipment or adverse environmental conditions.
HOW SUPPLIED: 'ScourGuard 3' is supplied in 5 and 20 dose combination packages.
REFERENCES:
1. Isaacson, R.E., Moon, H.W., Schneider, R.A.: Distribution and virulence of *Escherichia coli* in the small intestine of calves with and without diarrhea. *Am. J. Vet Res.* 39:1750-1755, 1978.
2. Moon, H.W., Whipp, S.C., Skartvedt, S.M.: Etiological diagnosis of diarrheal diseases of calves: Frequency and methods fo detecting enterotoxin and K99 antigen production by *Escherichia coli. Am. J. Vet Res.* 37:1025-1029, 1976.
U.S. Patent Nos. 3,838,004; 3,869,547; 3,873,422 and 3,919,412
For Veterinary Use Only

SPANBOLET®II TABLETS
(sustained-release sulfamethazine)

Composition: Each Spanbolet II Tablet contains 27 grams of sulfamethazine in two distinct layers. The smaller white layer provides sulfamethazine in a readily available form while the larger gray layer provides a slow-release form of the same drug.
Action: It is well established that the action of the sulfonamides as a group is one of bacteriostasis with high concentrations being bactericidal.[1,2,3,4,6] The most commonly accepted theory of this antibacterial action is that the sulfonamide interferes with the normal metabolism of the bacterial cell, more specifically interfering with the utilization of paraaminobenzoic acid (PABA) in the bacterial enzyme system.[1,2,3,4,6]
Successful therapy with the sulfonamides depends heavily upon its proper usage. First, of course, the causative organism must be sensitive to this class of drugs.
Organisms sensitive to sulfonamides include certain gram-positive cocci and diplococci, gram-negative diplococci, and gram-negative bacilli. They are not effective in most viral and rickettsial infections or tuberculosis.[2] Group A *Streptococci,* some strains of *Staphylococci, E. coli, Bacillus anthracis, Diplococci, Pasteurella, Shigella, Vibrio* and *Hemophilus* are highly sensitive while *Strep. viridans, Klebsiella, Aerobacter, B. proteus, Pseudomonas, Clostridia, P. tularensis and Brucella* are only moderately sensitive. *Ornithosis, psittacosis* and *actinomycosis* may respond to sulfonamide therapy though most viruses and fungi are highly resistant to this group of drugs.[2]
Beyond this, it is extremely important to: (1) Give the drug early in the course of the disease. (2) Give adequate dosage. (3) Continue medication for a short time after the temperature is normal, to give body defenses a chance to eliminate the infecting organism.
Proper case selection and early administration of a sufficient dose are less difficult to achieve in clinical veterinary practice than is the continuation of drug dosage for an adequate length of time. Jones states that "Animals difficult to restrain may receive no more than one or two doses."[4]
Sustained Action: Sulfamethazine Spanbolet II Tablet combines two forms of sulfamethazine in a single tablet of two distinct layers. The smaller white layer provides sulfamethazine in a readily available form while the larger gray layer provides a slow-release form of the same drug. Studies with these tablets showed that following a single oral dose at the rate of one tablet per 150 pounds body weight, plasma sulfamethazine levels of 5 mg.% were seen as early as 2 hours and consistently within 4 to 6 hours after treatment. A plasma sulfonamide profile was produced which was closely comparable to that produced following 3 doses of non-sustained sulfamethazine (1½ gr/lb + ¾ gr/lb + ¾ gr/lb) at 24-hour intervals. Plasma levels of 5 mg% or higher extended to the 4th or 5th day post treatment.[5] These *in vivo* studies were conducted in beef-type calves ranging in weight from approxi-

Continued on next page

mately 300 pounds to approximately 500 pounds.
Bacterial pathogens are thus exposed to sustained levels of sulfamethazine for a period of time sufficient to allow body elimination of those which are sensitive to the drug.

Indications: Spanbolet II Tablets are recommended for the treatment of infectious diseases of non-lactating cattle in which the causative organism is sensitive to sulfamethazine. Uses include the following:

1. Treatment of bovine respiratory disease complex (shipping fever complex) (*Pasteurella* spp.).
2. An aid in the treatment of necrotic pododermatitis (foot rot) (*Sphaerophorus necrophorus*)
3. Bacterial pneumonia (*Pasteurella* spp.).
4. Colibacillosis (bacterial scours) (*Escherichia coli*).
5. Calf diphtheria (*Sphaerophorus necrophorus*).

Dosage and Administration: (Prophylactic or Therapeutic) Administer as a single oral dose at the rate of one Spanbolet II Tablet for each 150 pounds body weight. If no response is evident within 2–3 days, other therapeutic approaches should be considered. Tablets may be halved if necessary to closely approximate dosage requirement, *but do not crush.*
For best results with Spanbolet II Tablets in reducing the incidence of bacterial infection associated with the shipping of cattle, early administration is imperative. A single dose (2 or 3 Spanbolet II Tablets for most feeder calves) given at the time of arrival at the feedlot will provide sustained blood sulfonamide levels, markedly enhancing his disease resistance while the calf is adjusting to his new environment.

Warning: Reports of side effects following the use of sulfamethazine in cattle are rare. Renal damage may result from crystallization of the drug in the kidneys. If hematuria develops during Spanbolet II Tablet therapy, take measures to increase the fluid intake of the animal.
Care should be taken to ascertain that the tablets are swallowed before the animal is released. As with any orally administered tablet, occasional regurgitation will occur in ruminants.
Because the tablets remain in the rumen-reticulum after administration, many physiologic factors, such as diet, pH and ruminal activity, play a major role in the rate of release of sulfamethazine. If a metal detector is to be used as a diagnostic aid, its use should precede the administration of Spanbolet II Tablets, as these tablets will react the same as a metallic object.

Tissue Residue: Since Spanbolet II Tablets provide sustained release of the active ingredient, tissue levels of sulfamethazine remain for a longer period of time than when this drug is administered in conventional forms. Liver, kidney, muscle and fat tissues from calves were assayed for sulfamethazine at varying intervals following treatment with Spanbolet, II Tablets.
In view of these findings:
Treated animals must not be slaughtered for food within 28 days after receiving this drug. Not for use in lactating dairy animals.

Caution: U.S. Federal law restricts this drug to use by or on the order of a licensed veterinarian.

How Supplied: Available in: Carton of 5 ×10 tablets, bulk 50s.

Bibliography:

1. Davison, F.M., Synopsis of Materia Medica, Toxicology and Pharmacology, The C. V. Mosby Company, Third Edition (1944).
2. Drill's Pharmacology in Medicine, Edited by Joseph R. DiPalma, McGraw-Hill, Third Edition (1965).
3. Goodman, Louis S. and Gilman, Alfred, The Pharmacological Basis of Therapeutics, The MacMillan Company, Second Edition (1956).
4. Jones, L. Meyer, Veterinary Pharmacology and Therapeutics, The Iowa State College Press, Second Edition (1957).
5. Research and Development Files, Norden Laboratories, Inc.
6. Sollman, T. A., Manual of Pharmacology, W. B. Saunders Company, Sixth Edition (1944).

SULKAMYCIN®-S BOLETTES

Composition: Each Sulkamycin-S Bolette contains: Sulfamethazine 2.0 gm.; Neomycin sulfate (Equiv. to neomycin base, 175 mg.) 250.0 mg.; Base, q.s.

Indications: Appropriate for use in respiratory infection-enteritis complex in calves, and enteritis in calves and foals, each caused by bacterial pathogens sensitive to sulfamethazine and neomycin; also, coccidiosis in calves caused by pathogens sensitive to sulfamethazine.

Dosage and Administration: Initial dose is two Bolettes for each 100 lb. body weight. Follow with one Bolette for each 100 lb. body weight every 12 hours. Maintain adequate fluid intake and employ supportive therapy if necessary. If symptoms persist after 2 or 3 days, diagnosis should be reconsidered.

Warning: Treated animals must not be slaughtered for use in food for at least 20 days after the latest treatment with Sulkamycin-S Bolettes. Do not administer Sulkamycin-S Bolettes more than 4 days.

Caution: Keep out of the reach of children.

How Supplied: 50 plastic-pak —100 bulk-pak — dispenser-pak of 25 bolettes with balling gun.

SULKAMYCIN®-S POWDER

Composition: Each 42.8 g packet contains: Sulfamethazine 16 g, neomycin sulfate 2 g (equivalent to 1400 mg. neomycin base) and inert base q.s.

Indications: Appropriate for use in respiratory infection-enteritis complex in calves and enteritis in calves, baby pigs and foals, each caused by bacterial pathogens sensitive to sulfamethazine and neomycin; also coccidiosis in calves caused by pathogens sensitive to sulfamethazine.
For oral treatment of bacterial enteritis (scours and pneumonia in calves, foals and pigs).

Directions for Mixing: To make 8 fl. oz. of finished suspension, measure 8 level teaspoons (21.4 grams) Sulkamycin-S Powder into a container and stir in sufficient cold water to make 8 fl. oz. To make 1 gal. of finished suspension, add contents of 1 jar (350 grams) Sulkamycin-S Powder to a container and stir in sufficient cold water to make 1 gallon. Optimum viscosity will develop in 30 minutes. Finished suspension contains 1 g sulfamethazine and 125 mg neomycin sulfate per fl. oz. Shake suspension well before using. Use suspension within 14 days after mixing.

Dosage for Calves and Foals: *As a Suspension:* Initial dose is 2 fl. oz. finished suspension per 50 lb. body weight, followed with 1 fl. oz. finished suspension per 50 lb. body weight every 12 hours for 2 or 3 days.
As a Powder: Initial dose is two level teaspoons for each 50 lb. body weight followed with one level teaspoon for each 50 lb. body weight every 12 hours for 2 or 3 days.
For severe infections, dosage may be doubled. Powder may be mixed with water, milk or regular animal ration.

Dosage for Baby Pigs: Initial dose is 8 ml. finished suspension per 5 pounds body weight followed with 4 ml. per 5 pounds every 12 hours for 2 or 3 days.

Warning: Animals must not be slaughtered for human consumption within 20 days of last treatment with Sulkamycin-S Powder. If no improvement is noted within 3 days, consult your veterinarian.

Caution: Keep out of the reach of children.

How Supplied: 42.8 and 350 grams.

SUPER SPRAY/REPELLENT FOR DOGS, CATS, AND HORSES

Formula:

Active Ingredients

Pyrethrins	0.15%
*Piperonyl butoxide, technical	0.30%
**N-Octyl bicycloheptene dicarboximide	0.50%
***2,3:4,5-Bis(2-butylene) tetrahydro-2-furaldehyde	0.40%
Inert Ingredients	98.65%
	100.00%

Indications: Kills fleas and ticks on dogs and cats. Effectively repels flies, gnats, and mosquitoes on dogs, cats, and horses.

Precautions:

Animal: Cover fish aquariums before spraying.

Human: Harmful if swallowed.
Avoid breathing vapors.
Wash with soap and water after use.
In the home all food processing surfaces, exposed food and utensils should be covered during treatment, or thoroughly washed before use.
Do not use or store near heat or open flame.
Supplied: 16-ounce cans and ½ gallon containers.

*Equivalent to 0.24% Butycarbityl (6-Propylpiperonyl) ether and 0.06% related compounds.
**MGK 264, Insecticide synergist.
***MGK Repellent II.

TEMARIL-P®
(trimeprazine with prednisolone) Spansule* Capsules No. 1 & No. 2

Composition: Each Temaril-P *Spansule capsule* No. 1 contains: trimeprazine tartrate (equivalent to 3.75 mg. trimeprazine), in sustained release form, and prednisolone, 1 mg.
Each Temaril-P *Spansule* capsule No. 2 contains: trimeprazine tartrate (equivalent to 7.5 mg. trimeprazine), in sustained release form, and prednisolone, 2 mg.
Action: The exclusive Temaril-P formula combines the antipruritic and antitussive actions of trimeprazine with the anti-inflammatory action of prednisolone. Administered as tablets, a therapeutic effect is attained by twice daily dosage. Carefully monitored clinical studies have shown that by sustaining the release of trimeprazine, in combination with non-sustained release prednisolone, a *24-hour therapeutic effect* can be achieved from a Single Daily Dose. In the treatment of either pruritus or coughs, this extended therapeutic effect is equally applicable. *Recommendations for Use Include:*

1. *Antipruritic:* Temaril-P is recommended for the relief of itching regardless of cause. Its usefulness has been demonstrated for the relief of itching and the reduction of inflammation commonly associated with most skin disorders of dogs such as the eczema caused by internal disorders, otitis, and dermatitis (allergic, parasitic, pustular and non-specific). It often relieves pruritus which does not respond to other therapy. With any pruritus treatment, the cause should be determined and corrected; otherwise, signs are likely to recur following discontinuance of therapy.
2. *Antitussive:* Temaril-P has been found to be effective as therapy and adjunctive therapy in various cough conditions of dogs. Therefore, in addition to its antipruritic action, Temaril-P is recommended for the treatment of "kennel cough" or tracheobronchitis, bronchitis including allergic bronchitis, and infections and coughs of non-specific origin. (Coughs due to cardiac insufficiencies would not be expected to respond to Temaril-P therapy.) As with any antitussive treatment, the etiology of the cough should be determined and eliminated if possible. Otherwise, symptoms are likely to recur following discontinuance of therapy.

Precautions and Side Effects: All the precautions applicable to cortisone and to phenothiazine derivatives apply also to Temaril-P. Possible side effects attributable to corticosteroids include: (1) sodium retention and potassium loss, (2) negative nitrogen balance, (3) suppressed adrenal cortical function, (4) delayed wound healing and (5) osteoporosis. Possible increased susceptibility to bacterial invasion and/or the exacerbation of preexisting bacterial infection may occur in patients receiving corticosteroids. As noted above, however, this problem can be avoided by concomitant use of appropriate anti-infective agents. Possible side effects attributable to phenothiazine derivatives include: (1) sedation, (2) protruding nictitating membrane, (3) blood dyscrasias, (4) intensification and prolongation of the action of analgesics, sedatives and general anesthetics and (5) potentiation of organophosphate toxicity and the activity of procaine hydrochloride.
It should be remembered that the premonitory signs of cortisone overdosage, such as sodium retention and edema, may not occur with prednisolone. Therefore, the veterinarian must be alert to detect less obvious side effects, such as blood dyscrasias, polydipsia and polyuria.
The appearance and severity of side effects are dose related and are minimal at the recommended dosage level. If troublesome side effects are encountered, the dosage of Termaril-P should be reduced and discontinued unless the severity of the condition being treated makes its relief paramount.
Prolonged treatment with Termaril-P must be withdrawn gradually.
Warning: Clinical and experimental data have demonstrated that corticosteroids administered orally or parenterally to animals may induce the first stage of parturition when administered during the last trimester of pregnancy and may precipitate premature parturition followed by dystocia, fetal death, retained placenta, and metritis. If a vasoconstrictor is needed, norepinephrine should be used in lieu of epinephrine. Phenothiazine derivatives may reverse the usual elevating action of ephinephrine causing a further lowering of blood pressure.
Recommended Dosage: The same dosage schedule may be followed for both antipruritic and antitussive therapy.
[See table above].

Patient Weight	DOSE No. 1 Capsule	No. 2 Capsule	Frequency
up to 10 lb	1	—	once daily
11 to 20 lb	2	1	once daily
21 to 40 lb	4	2	once daily
over 40 lb	6	3	once daily

After 4 days reduce dosage to one-half of the initial dose or to an amount just sufficient to maintain remission of symptoms. Individual animal response will vary and dosage should be adjusted until proper response is obtained.
If it is necessary to use doses smaller than the No. 1 size, the gelatin capsule can be separated and appropriate fractional portions of the pellets administered. These pellets may be added to a small portion of feed, if desired.
Caution: U.S. Federal law restricts this drug to use by or on the order of a licensed veterinarian.
How Supplied: Temaril-P Spansule capsules, No. 1, bottles of 100, 500.
Temaril-P Spansule capsules, No. 2, bottles of 100, 500.
*Registered trademark of SmithKline Beckman Corporation, brand of sustained release capsules.
*Use Temaril-P Capsule No. 1 for patients weighing 10 lbs. or less.

TEMARIL-P® TABLETS
(trimeprazine with prednisolone)

Composition: Each tablet contains trimeprazine tartrate, U.S.P. 10-[3-(Dimethylamino)-2-methylpropyl] phenothiazine tartrate (2:1)) equivalent to trimeprazine, 5 mg., and prednisolone, 2 mg.
Action: The exclusive Temaril-P formula combines the antipruritic and antitussive action of trimeprazine with the anti-inflammatory action of prednisolone. A therapeutic effect is attained by administering the tablets twice daily.
Usage: *Antipruritic:* Temaril-P is recommended for the relief of itching regardless of cause. Its usefulness has been demonstrated for the relief of itching and the reduction of inflammation commonly associated with most skin disorders of dogs such as the eczema caused by internal disorders, otitis, and dermatitis (allergic, parasitic, pustular and non-specific). It often relieves pruritus which does not respond to other therapy. With any pruritus treatment, the cause should be determined and corrected; otherwise, signs are likely to recur following discontinuance of therapy.
Antitussive: Temaril-P has been found to be effective as therapy and adjunctive therapy in various cough conditions of dogs. Therefore, in addition to its antipruritic action, Temaril-P is recommended for the treatment of "kennel cough" or tracheobronchitis, bronchitis including allergic bronchitis, and infections and coughs of non-specific origin. (Coughs due to cardiac insufficiencies would not be expected to respond to Temaril-P therapy.) As with any antitussive treatment, the etiology of the cough should be determined and eliminated if possible. Otherwise, symptoms are likely

Continued on next page

to recur following discontinuance of therapy.
Note: Temaril-P may be administered to animals suffering from acute or chronic bacterial infections provided the infection is controlled by appropriate antibiotic or chemotherapeutic agents.
Precautions and Side Effects: See Temaril-P® Spansule Capsules
Warning: See Temaril-P® Spansule Capsules
Recommended Dosage: The same dosage schedule may be followed for both antipruritic and antitussive therapy.

Weight of dog	Initiate therapy with
up to 10 lbs	½ tablet, twice daily
11 to 20 lbs	1 tablet, twice daily
21 to 40 lbs	2 tablets, twice daily
over 40 lbs	3 tablets, twice daily

After 4 days reduce dosage to one-half of the initial dose or to an amount just sufficient to maintain remission of symptoms. Individual animal response will vary and dosage should be adjusted until proper response is obtained.
Caution: U.S. Federal law restricts this drug to use by or on the order of a licensed veterinarian.
How Supplied: Bottles of 100 and 1000.

TGE VACCINE
Transmissible Gastroenteritis Vaccine
Modified Live Virus

Introduction: Transmissible gastroenteritis (TGE) vaccine consists of a unique strain of TGE virus which has been modified so that it does not cause disease in newborn pigs, which are most susceptible to the natural disease. The vaccine has also been shown to be safe for feeder pigs, boars, pregnant sows and pregnant gilts. In addition to swine, the vaccine virus has been inoculated into mice, guinea pigs, hamsters, dogs and rabbits which experienced no abnormality after inoculation. Vaccine containing the modified or attenuated virus is in the dried state in order to preserve its potency and it must be reconstituted with the diluent provided immediately prior to use.
Experimental results indicate that sows as well as their baby pigs can be protected from TGE if the sow is fed the vaccine during the later stages of pregnancy. It is well known that feeding virulent TGE virus to pregnant sows a few weeks before farrowing will provide a good immunity to TGE for both the sow and her nursing piglets. It has also been shown that oral immunization provides more effective antibodies associated with the immunoglobulin A fraction in the sow's milk, thus providing more effective passive immunity to TGE for the sow's nursing piglets. Baby pigs, however, will become susceptible to TGE after weaning. Therefore, active immunization of the baby pigs before weaning is recommended. Experimental results have demonstrated that oral administration of TGE vaccine was effective for baby pigs nursing either immune or non-immune sows[1,2]. The virus used in this vaccine has been shown to be safe in both laboratory and field trials in swine[3]. However, due to the nature of TGE immunity in piglets nursing immune sows, any condition in the sow resulting in reduction or cessation of milk flow can seriously impair immunity in her piglets. For this reason, active immunization of baby pigs may also be desirable.
Dosage Guidelines: Follow directions carefully.

A. **Vaccination of Sows:** Two vaccination programs may be used.
   1. **Oral and intramuscular vaccination (Oral method):** Each pregnant sow or gilt must receive at least three doses of vaccine before farrowing:
      a. 5 weeks before farrowing—one oral dose.
      b. 3 weeks before farrowing—one oral dose.
      c. 1 week before farrowing—one intramuscular dose.
      In subsequent farrowings administer one oral and one intramuscular dose, on the same day, about 2–3 weeks before farrowing.
      Reconstitute dried vaccine with the sterile diluent provided, using 2 ml. diluent for the one dose vial and 20 ml. diluent for the 10 dose vial.
   2. **Two intramuscular vaccinations (Injection method):**
      a. Each pregnant sow or gilt must receive two doses of TGE vaccine; 5 and 2 weeks before each farrowing.
      b. Reconstitute dried vaccine with the sterile diluent provided. Inject 2 ml. intramuscularly.

   Oral vaccination—Transfer the desired number of doses to cool skim milk (prepared by adding one lb. dried milk solids to 2½ gal. clean cool water) or to cool pasteurized milk at a ratio of one dose per quart.
   Add clean ground corn to vaccine-milk mixture until thickened and immediately feed to sow. Solid food should be withheld from sows overnight in order to facilitate vaccine consumption and efficacy.
   Intramuscular vaccination—Inject 2 ml. of the vaccine, reconstituted with sterile diluent, deep intramuscularly. Do not use chemically sterilized syringes as the chemicals may destroy the vaccine.

B. **Vaccination of Baby Pigs:** Orally vaccinate each baby pig at 1 to 3 days of age with ⅕ the sow dose. A second dose may be given at 3–7 days of age. Reconstitute the dried vaccine with sterile diluent provided, using 2 ml. diluent for the one dose vial and 20 ml. diluent for the 10 dose vial. Add 0.5 ml. cool milk to the 2 ml. vial and 5 ml. cool milk to the 20 ml. vial.
   Inoculate each pig *per os* with 0.5 ml. of the vaccine-milk mixture using a tuberculin syringe and dropping the inoculum into the pharyngeal region. Do not return the piglets to the sow for at least 30 minutes after oral vaccination. The milk may be prepared from dried milk solids reconstituted with cool clean water, or cool pasteurized milk may be used.

Caution: Store vaccine in the dark at temperatures between 35° and 45°F (4°–7°C). Use vaccine immediately after reconstitution, do not save partial contents, and burn this container and all unused contents. Do not use commercial milk replacers or complete rations to prepare vaccine mixture as they may adversely affect vaccine potency. Do not pour vaccine-milk mixture on top of ground corn as sows may not receive sufficient vaccine. Use vaccine in healthy animals only and do not vaccinate within 21 days of slaughter. If allergic reactions follow use of this product, treat with epinephrine. Conditions which interfere with lactation adversely affect immunity in baby pigs. Good husbandry and management procedures should always accompany use of a vaccine in a herd.
Contain gentamicin as preservative.

References:

1. Welter, C.J. 1980. Experimental and Field Evaluation of a New Oral Vaccine for TGE. Vet. Med. Sm. An. Clin. 75:1757–1759.
2. Graham, J.A. 1980. Induction of Active Immunity to TGE in Neonatal Pigs Nursing Seropositve Dams. Vet. Med. Sm. An. Clin. 75:1618–1619.
3. Research data on file, Ambico, Inc.

For Veterinary Use Only

THERABLOAT®
(brand of poloxalene)
Drench Concentrate

Composition: Each fluid ounce contains poloxalene 25 gm.
Indications: Therabloat Drench Concentrate will relieve legume bloat in cattle within minutes when used as directed. For best results administer at the earliest sign of bloat. If bloat has progressed in its severity to the degree that the animal is down, other means of treatment also are recommended (rumenotomy—rumen puncture). For oral use only—not for injection. May be used in lactating dairy animals.
Directions for Use: Add the proper amount of concentrate to one pint of water. Mix well and administer using a drenching bottle. If a stomach tube is to be used, add concentrate to one gallon of water.
Dosage and Administration: Each fluid ounce (approx. 30 ml.) contains poloxalene 25 gm. For animals up to 500 lb., use one fl. oz. of Drench Concentrate. For animals over 500 lb., use two fl. oz. of Drench Concentrate.
Caution: Keep out of reach of children.
How Supplied: 2 oz. and 30 oz.

TOPAZONE®
AEROSOL POWDER
(furazolidone)
Topical Antibacterial

Composition: Contains Topazone*, brand of furazolidone, as the active ingredient with an inert dispersing agent and propellants, in a metal spray can.

*Topazone® is a registered trademark of SmithKline Beckman Corporation for its brand of furazolidone.

Advantages: Topazone offers all the benefits of a wide-spectrum bactericidal agent plus the benefits of aerosol application. It is effective against both gram-negative and gram-positive bacteria. It is non-irritating. Topazone controls surface bacterial contamination caused by microorganisms susceptible to furazolidone. The aerosol takes only seconds to apply regardless of surface area. Usually no dressing is needed. Little patient restraint is necessary, since wound handling or manipulation of sensitive areas is not required during application. The drug is deposited directly on the lesion and incorporated directly into wound fluids. There is little or no caking, even on moist wounds, when used as directed.

Indications: *In Horses:* Superficial wounds, abrasions, lacerations, and following firing (heat or electrocautery). *In Dogs:* Superficial wounds, abrasions, lacerations, and pyogenic dermatitis. *In Cattle:* Bacterial infections of the eye and infectious bovine keratoconjunctivitis (pinkeye) caused by Moraxella bovis.

Precautions: Use only as recommended by a veterinarian in the treatment of puncture wounds, wounds requiring surgical debridement or suturing, those of a chronic nature involving proud flesh, generalized and chronic infections of the skin, and those skin conditions associated with intense itching. If redness, irritation, or swelling persists or increases, discontinue; reconsult veterinarian.

Conditions other than bacterial infections of the bovine eye and infectious bovine keratoconjunctivitis caused by Moraxella bovis may cause similar signs. Evidence of clinical improvement should be noticeable after 5 treatments; if not, reconsult veterinarian.

Dosage and Administration: Shake Well Before Each Use.

In equine and canine: The affected area should be cleansed thoroughly before application. Holding container about 6 to 12 inches from the affected area, apply only that amount of powder necessary to impart a light yellow color to the affected area. Heavy application may cause caking and retard healing processes. Apply lightly once or twice daily. Repeat treatment as necessary.

In the bovine eye: Holding container 6 to 12 inches from eye, apply Topazone lightly. Treat once daily on each of 3 to 5 consecutive days. In less severe cases recovery may occur with fewer treatments. To reduce the incidence of additional cases of infectious bovine keratoconjunctivitis, also medicate unaffected eyes.

How Supplied: In aerosol containers of 1.2 oz and 2.8 oz.

TRI-SULFA-G
(sulfonamide solution)

Composition: Each ml. contains: Sulfamethazine, 45 mg.; sulfathiazole, 45 mg. and sulfapyridine, 20 mg.; chemically stabilized with dextrose. Ortho-phenylphenol (preservative) 1:10,000 by weight.

Indications: Indicated for the treatment of infections in large animals in which the causative organism is sensitive to sulfonamides.

Dosage and Administration: *Cattle:* For foot rot, shipping fever, bacterial enteritis, upper respiratory infections of bacterial origin, acute mastitis, and acute metritis. Initial dose is 0.7 to 0.9 ml. per lb. body weight for the first day. Subsequent dose is 0.4 to 0.5 ml. per lb. body weight every 12 hours for 2 to 4 additional days. If desired, medication may be administered in drinking water, provided that it is the sole source of water. Add 60 ml. (2 oz.) Tri-Sulfa-G to each gallon of water.

Warnings: Do not administer Tri-Sulfa-G more than 5 days. If symptoms of sulfonamide toxicity should appear, discontinue use and force fluids orally and/or intravenously to facilitate elimination of the drug. If symptoms persist after 2 or 3 days, consult your veterinarian.

Milk taken from animals during treatment and for 84 hours (7 milkings) after the last treatment must not be used for food, and animals must not be slaughtered for human consumption within 10 days of the last treatment with Tri-Sulfa-G.

Caution: Keep out of reach of children.

How Supplied: 1 gallon.

TSV-2®
Bovine Rhinotracheitis-Parainfluenza$_3$ Vaccine
Modified Live Virus

For Intranasal Use

Composition: *Bovine Rhinotracheitis* is a virus disease of the respiratory tract characterized by high temperature, excessive nasal discharge, increased respiration, coughing and depression. Affected animals usually go off feed resulting in a severe loss of weight and condition. In dairy cattle, there is a loss in milk production.

Infection of susceptible cattle with the *Bovine Parainfluenza$_3$* virus sometimes results in the development of a temperature, lacrimation and a moderate nasal discharge in the affected animals. The paramyxovirus infection in cattle is essentially a local infection of the respiratory tract.

Infections with either the IBR or the Parainfluenza$_3$ viruses or the combination of these viruses with other viruses may infect the upper respiratory tract of cattle. These virus infections may establish conditions which may result in secondary bacterial infections of the respiratory tract.

Cattle should be vaccinated before or upon entering the feedlot or dairy herd. The effectiveness of the vaccine will vary depending on the number of animals in the incubative stages of disease due to the IBR or the *Bovine Parainfluenza$_3$* viruses.

Studies of the TSV-2 strains of vaccine viruses indicate the replication to be confined to the cells of the upper respiratory tract of vaccinated animals. The vaccine viruses have been found to be highly effective and remarkably safe in calves and cattle of all ages. Substantial immunity has been shown to develop in healthy cattle within 7 to 14 days in response to the administration of the vaccine viruses.

Safety studies of the TSV-2 strains conducted in bred, IBR-susceptible cattle indicate the IBR fraction of the vaccine will not cause abortion at any stage of gestation. The TSV-2 vaccine may be used in pregnant animals.

Indications: For the immunization of healthy cattle and calves against Bovine Rhinotracheitis and Parainfluenza$_3$ infections.

Dosage and Administration: Aseptically add diluent to the container of vaccine. Shake well. Administer 2 ml. intranasally using a syringe without the needle or with the cannula supplied by Norden Laboratories, Inc. upon request. Place half of the dose (1 ml.) in each nostril.

Caution: Calves vaccinated before the age of six months should be revaccinated at six months of age. Do not vaccinate within 21 days before slaughter. Annual revaccination is recommended. Contains penicillin and streptomycin as preservatives. Should anaphylaxis occur following the use of the product, administer epinephrine.

Use entire contents without delay after rehydration. Syringes, needles, and nasal applicators used in the rehydration and administration of the vaccine should be sterilized by boiling. Do not use chemical sterilization. Store vaccine at 2°C.–7°C. Burn container and all unused contents.

How Supplied: 25 x 1 dose, 5-25-50 dose sizes. Dose is 2 ml.

VANGUARD® CPV (killed)
Parvovirus Vaccine
Killed Virus
For Use in Dogs Only

Composition: The vaccine is prepared by growing a canine parvovirus strain in a canine Stable Cell Line, and chemically inactivating the preparation.

The CPV strain is specially selected for its antigenicity. The CPV antigen contained in Vanguard CPV (killed) consistently provided protection following challenge.

Extensive tests conducted under controlled conditions at Norden Laboratories demonstrated the vaccine was safe and efficacious. No postvaccination reactions were observed.

Extensive field trials performed by practicing veterinarians confirmed vaccine safety.

Indications: Vanguard CPV (killed) is designed for the immunization of healthy dogs against canine parvovirus (CPV) infection.

Dosage and Administration: Administer 1 ml subcutaneously or intramuscularly. Two doses should be administered 3–4 weeks apart. The presence of maternal antibody may interfere with develop-

Continued on next page

ment of an adequate immune response. Scientific evidence indicates that maternal antibody to canine parovirus declines at a constant rate. The age at which maternal antibody drops below interfering levels varies with the amount of antibody absorbed from the colostrum and may persist as late as about 4 months of age. Dogs vaccinated when less than 4 months of age should be revaccinated with two doses 3 to 4 weeks apart after reaching the age of 4 months.
Annual revaccination is recommended.
Precautions: Store at 2°C–7°C. Use entire contents when first opened. Contains penicillin and streptomycin as preservatives. Anaphylaxis may occur.*Antidote:* Epinephrine.
How Supplied: Vanguard CPV (killed) is supplied in 10-dose vials.
For Veterinary Use Only.

VANGUARD® CPV (ML)
Parvovirus Vaccine
Modified Live Virus
For Use in Dogs Only

Description: Canine parvovirus infection results in enteric disease characterized by sudden onset of vomiting and diarrhea, often hemorrhagic. Leukopenia often accompanies clinical signs. Susceptible dogs of any age can be affected, but mortality is greatest in puppies 4 to 12 weeks of age, CPV may occasionally cause myocarditis that can result in acute heart failure after a brief and inconspicuous illness.
Indications: This product is for the vaccination of healthy dogs against canine parvovirus (CPV) infection. The vaccine is prepared by growing an attenuated CPV strain on a canine cell line. An effective stabilizer makes lyophilization unnecessary as a means of preservation. As a result, vaccine is packaged in liquid form for ease of administration.
Safety and Efficacy: The vaccine was subjected to comprehensive safety and efficacy testing at Norden Laboratories. It proved safe and reaction-free in laboratory tests and in clinical trials under field conditions. Susceptible dogs remained normal following oral administration of multiple doses of the vaccine strain. The vaccine strain shares a characteristic with other live CPV strains in that the virus may be present in the feces following administration. Virus was found occasionally and in low titers in the feces of vaccinated dogs, indicating that presence of the vaccine strain in the feces is not a routine occurrence. A test demonstrated that the vaccine strain did not revert to virulence following six consecutive passages in susceptible dogs.
Susceptible test dogs all developed CPV antibody titers following vaccination, and were protected following oral administration of virulent CPV. Challenge virus was not demonstrated in the feces of vaccinated dogs. Following challenge exposure, nonvaccinated control dogs all developed clinical signs of CPV infection, including vomiting and diarrhea with blood and mucous in the feces. Challenge virus was isolated from the feces of all nonvaccinated control dogs, and they all developed marked lymphopenia following exposure to virulent CPV.
Directions for Use:
General Directions: Administer 1 ml. subcutaneously or intramuscularly.
Primary Vaccination: A single dose is recommended. Maternal antibody may interfere with development of an adequate immune response. The age at which maternal antibody drops below interfering levels varies and may persist as late as 4 months of age. Dogs vaccinated less than 4 months of age should be revaccinated after reaching the age of 4 months.
Revaccination: Annual revaccination is recommended.
Precautions:
Store at 2°C–7°C.
Use entire contents when first opened.
Contains penicillin and streptomycin as preservatives.
Anaphylaxis may occur following use (antidote is epinephrine).
Vaccination of pregnant bitches should be avoided.
Burn container and all unused contents.
Although this product has been shown to be efficacious, some animals may be unable to develop or maintain an adequate immune response following vaccination if they are incubating any infectious disease, malnourished or parasitized, or stressed due to shipment or environmental conditions.
How Supplied: 10-dose vials
For Veterinary Use Only

VANGUARD® DA_2L
Canine Distemper-
Adenovirus Type 2 Vaccine
Modified Live Virus,
Leptospira Bacterin

Composition: Canine distemper, adenovirus type 2, modified live virus, and leptospira bacterin is for the immunization of healthy dogs against canine distemper, infectious canine hepatitis (canine adenovirus type 1) infection, respiratory disease caused by canine adenovirus type 2, and *Leptospira canicola* and *icterohaemorrhagiae.*
The bacterin fraction is supplied as diluent for the rehydration of the modified live virus fraction.
Canine adenovirus type 2 (CAV-2) infections are primarily respiratory, evidenced by pneumonia, bronchitis, tonsillitis and pharyngitis. CAV-2 has not been associated with corneal opacity (blue eyes), uveitis or virus localization in the kidneys which may be characteristic of canine adenovirus type 1 (CAV-1) infections.
Infectious canine hepatitis (CAV-1) infections are characterized by fever, leukopenia, enlarged tonsils, hepatitis, nephritis and occasional uveitis with corneal opacity.
Vaccination with modified live canine hepatitis vaccine, although effective in disease prevention, has certain disadvantages. Following vaccination, persistent kidney infections may occur causing vaccine virus shedding in urine. Uveitis and corneal opacity (blue eyes) are occasionally observed 1 to 2 weeks post-vaccination.
It has been reported and demonstrated by evaluations performed at our laboratories that canine adenovirus type 2 vaccine protected against canine hepatitis and respiratory syndromes caused by the canine adenovirus type 2.
Data indicate that the development of corneal opacity is not associated with the use of this product.
The strain of canine adenovirus type 2 used in the vaccine is specially selected to preclude the oncogenic properties characteristic of this group of viruses.
Norden Laboratories developed a combined vaccine, in which the CAV-2 fraction is a replacement for canine hepatitis. This vaccine has significant advantages:
A. This vaccine is designed to protect with a single 1 ml. dose.
B. By using CAV-2, lesions sometimes associated with conventional ICH vaccines are avoided. Tests showed no such lesions following vaccination with the CAV-2 fraction.
C. Dogs vaccinated with CAV-2 vaccine were completely protected against challenge inoculation with virulent infectious canine hepatitis virus while all controls succumbed to challenge.
D. Dogs vaccinated with CAV-2 vaccine were protected against challenge with virulent CAV-2 virus that caused severe respiratory syndromes in the susceptible controls. Challenge virus was not recovered from vaccinated dogs and was not isolated from tissues taken at necropsy.
E. Ocular lesions were not observed in any of the 172 dogs inoculated intravenously with high titer CAV-2 vaccine virus. In comparison, intravenous inoculation of 32 dogs with infectious canine hepatitis vaccine produced ocular lesions in 22. This is one of the critical tests of the ability of a canine adenovirus to produce ocular lesions.
F. The specially selected vaccine strain, $NL\text{-}A_2001$, has been demonstrated to be non-oncogenic.
Dosage and Administration: Aseptically rehydrate with Leptospira diluent supplied. Administer 1 ml. subcutaneously or intramuscularly.
Dogs 3 months of age or older should be administered a single vaccination. If younger dogs are vaccinated, they should be revaccinated upon reaching the age of 3 months. Annual revaccination is recommended. It is generally recommended that vaccination of pregnant females with modified live virus should be avoided.
Caution: Store at 2°C.–7°C. Use without delay after rehydration. Contains penicillin and streptomycin as preservatives. Anaphylaxis may occur. Antidote: Epinephrine. Burn container and all unused contents.
How Supplied: Vanguard DA_2L is supplied in 25 x 1-dose vials.

VANGUARD® DA_2MP
Canine Distemper-Adenovirus Type 2-Measles-Parainfluenza Vaccine Modified Live Virus

Description: *Canine distemper* (CD) is a universal, high-mortality viral infection of dogs. *Infectious canine hepatitis* (ICH) is a worldwide, some times fatal, viral disease of dogs, characterized by hepatic and generalized endothelial lesions. The causative agent is canine adenovirus type 1 (CAV-1). *Canine adenovirus type 2* (CAV-2) respiratory infection is commonly associated with infectious tracheobronchitis ("kennel cough") in dogs of all ages. *Canine parainfluenza* (CPI) is a common viral upper respiratory disease of dogs. Uncomplicated CPI may be mild or subclinical with signs becoming more severe if concurrent infection with other respiratory agents exists.

Indications: Vanguard DA_2MP is for the vaccination of healthy dogs 6 to 12 weeks of age against canine distemper, infectious canine hepatitis, respiratory disease caused by canine adenovirus type 2, and canine parainfluenza. The vaccine is produced by growing attenuated strains of each virus in a canine cell line. The vaccine is freeze-dried to maintain potency.

Safety and Efficacy: Experimental tests demonstrated that Vanguard DA_2MP immunized dogs against CD, ICH, CAV-2 respiratory disease, and CPI, and that no significant immunologic interference existed among the vaccine components. No adverse reactions to vaccination were observed in any of the test dogs. The viral components of the vaccine all have an extensive clinical history of safe and effective use in other Norden vaccines.

Protection against CD is desirable at the earliest possible age. However, successful vaccination may not be possible in puppies with maternal antibodies against CD. By 12 weeks of age, maternal CD antibodies decline in almost all dogs to levels that do not neutralize attenuated vaccine virus. Measles virus stimulates heterotypic protection against canine distemper in puppies regardless of circulating canine distemper antibody levels. The resistance provided by measles virus, however, does not appear to be as effective in very young pups as those six weeks of age or older. Thus, a combined CD and measles virus vaccine increases the probability of protecting pups against CD during the period when they commonly carry maternal antibodies. For example, studies conducted at Norden Laboratories showed that 45 of 76 experimental dogs at 6 weeks of age had maternal antibody levels sufficient to interfere with active immunization. When vaccinated with a combination distemper-measles vaccine at 6 weeks of age, 73 of 76 pups (96%) were protected, 42 of them by the measles virus component.[1]

Use of measles vaccine in adult bitches may produce high levels of measles antibodies that can interfere with successful protection of pups in the next generation. Thus, Vanguard DA_2MP is recommended for use in pups 6 to 12 weeks of age.

It has been demonstrated that CAV-2 vaccine cross-protects against ICH caused by CAV-1. The CAV-2 component in Vanguard vaccines is used as a replacement for CAV-1 because it has significant advantages. Some CAV-1 vaccines, though effective, can produce undesirable reactions, including persistent kidney infections, uveitis, and corneal opacity ("blue eye"), which have not been reported following vaccinations with CAV-2.[2] In addition, the CAV-2 strain used in Vanguard vaccines has been specially selected for freedom from oncogenic properties characteristic of adenoviruses.

Studies conducted at Norden demonstrated that CAV-2 not only protects against ICH, but against CAV-2 respiratory disease as well.[3] Although conventional CAV-1 (ICH) vaccines cross-protect against CAV-2 they may not prevent subclinical infection and spread of the CAV-2 agent. CAV-2 challenge virus was not recovered from CAV-2 vaccinated dogs in tests conducted at Norden Laboratories.

A test of the CPI immunizing agent showed that hemorrhagic lung lesions characteristic of infection were absent or greatly diminished in vaccinated dogs necropsied after challenge. Nonvaccinated control dogs all had characteristic lung lesions, in some cases distributed in all lobes.[4]

Dosage and Administration:

General Directions: Aseptically rehydrate vaccine with diluent supplied. Administer 1 ml. intramuscularly.

Primary Vaccination: Puppies between 6 and 12 weeks of age should be vaccinated with a single dose.

Revaccination: Puppies should be revaccinated at 14 to 16 weeks of age with a canine distemper, canine adenovirus type 2, and canine parainfluenza vaccine. In most cases, a complete immunization program will also include vaccination for canine parvovirus, *Leptospira canicola*, and *L. icterohaemorrhagiae*. At the discretion of the veterinarian, annual revaccination with any or all of these agents is recommended.

Precautions:

Store at 2°C.–7°C.

Use entire contents when first opened.

Contains penicillin and streptomycin as preservatives.

Anaphylaxis may occur following use (antidote is epinephrine).

Vaccination of pregnant bitches should be avoided.

Burn container and all unused contents.

Although this product has been shown to be efficacious, some animals may be unable to develop or maintain an adequate immune response following vaccination if they are incubating any infectious disease, are malnourished or parasitized, or if they are stressed due to shipment or adverse environmental conditions.

How Supplied: 25 × 1-dose vials

For Veterinary Use Only

References:

1. Brown, AL: Vitamvas, JA; Merry, DL; Beckenhauer, WH: Immune Response of Pups to Modified Live-Virus Canine Distemper-Measles Vaccine. Am. J. Vet. Res., 33:1447–1456; 1972.
2. Appel, M; Bistner, SI; Menegus, WH: Pathogenicity of Low Virulence Strains of Two Canine Adenovirus Types. Am. J. Vet. Res., 34:543–550; 1970.
3. Bass, EP; Gill, MA; Beckenhauer, WH: Evaluation of a Canine Adenovirus Type 2 Strain as a Replacement for Infectious Canine Hepatitis Vaccine. J. Am. Vet. Med. Assoc., 177:234–242; 1980.
4. Brown, AL; Bihr, JG; Vitamvas, JA; Miers, L; An Alternative Method of Evaluating Potency of Modified Live Canine Parainfluenza Virus Vaccine. Jour. Biol. Stand., 6:271–281; 1978.

VANGUARD® DA_2P
Canine Distemper-Adenovirus Type 2 Parainfluenza Vaccine Modified Live Virus

Composition: Canine distemper, adenovirus type 2 and parainfluenza vaccine, modified live virus is for the immunization of healthy dogs against canine distemper, infectious canine hepatitis (canine adenovirus type 1) infection, respiratory disease caused by canine adenovirus type 2 and parainfluenza.

Canine adenovirus type 2 (CAV-2) infections are primarily respiratory, evidenced by pneumonia, bronchitis, tonsillitis and pharyngitis. CAV-2 has not been associated with corneal opacity (blue eye), uveitis or virus localization in the kidneys which may be characteristic of canine adenovirus type 1 (CAV-1) infections.

Infectious canine hepatitis (CAV-1) infections are characterized by fever, leukopenia, enlarged tonsils, hepatitis, nephritis and occasional uveitis with corneal opacity.

Vaccination with modified live canine hepatitis vaccine, although effective in disease prevention, has certain disadvantages. Following vaccination, persistent kidney infections may occur causing vaccine virus shedding in urine. Uveitis and corneal opacity (blue eye) are occasionally observed 1 to 2 weeks post-vaccination.

It has been reported and demonstrated by evaluations performed at our laboratories that canine adenovirus type 2 vaccine protected against canine hepatitis and respiratory syndromes caused by the canine adenovirus type 2.

Data indicate that the development of corneal opacity is not associated with the use of this product.

The strain of canine adenovirus type 2 used in the vaccine is specially selected to preclude the oncogenic properties characteristic of this group of viruses.

Norden Laboratories developed a combined vaccine, in which the CAV-2 fraction is a replacement for canine hepati-

Continued on next page

tis. This vaccine has significant advantages:
A. By using CAV-2, lesions sometimes associated with conventional ICH vaccines are avoided. Tests showed no such lesions following vaccination with the CAV-2 fraction.
B. Dogs vaccinated with CAV-2 vaccine were completely protected against challenge inoculation with virulent infectious canine hepatitis virus while all controls succumbed to challenge.
C. Dogs vaccinated with CAV-2 vaccine were protected against challenge with virulent CAV-2 virus that caused severe respiratory syndromes in the susceptible controls. Challenge virus was not recovered from vaccinated dogs and was not isolated from tissues taken at necropsy.
D. Ocular lesions were not observed in any of the 172 dogs inoculated intravenously with high titer CAV-2 vaccine virus. In comparison, intravenous inoculation of 32 dogs with infectious canine hepatitis vaccine produced ocular lesions in 22%. This is one of the critical tests of the ability of a canine adenovirus to produce ocular lesions.
E. The specially selected vaccine strain, NL-$A_2$001, has been demonstrated to be non-oncogenic.

Dosage and Administration: Aseptically rehydrate vaccine with diluent supplied. Administer 1 ml. subcutaneously or intramuscularly.

Dogs 3 months of age or older should be administered a single vaccination. If younger dogs are vaccinated, they should be revaccinated upon reaching the age of 3 months. Annual revaccination is recommended. It is generally recommended that vaccination of pregnant females with a modified live virus should be avoided.

Caution: Store at 2°C–7°C. Use without delay after rehydration. Contains penicillin and streptomycin as preservatives. Anaphylaxis may occur. Antidote: Epinephrine. Burn container and all unused contents.

How Supplied: Vanguard DA_2P is supplied in 25 x 1-dose vials.

VANGUARD® DA_2P+CPV
Canine Distemper-Adenovirus Type 2-Parainfluenza-Parvovirus Vaccine
For Use in Dogs Only

Product Description: 'Vanguard DA_2P+CPV' is for the vaccination of healthy dogs against canine distemper (CD) virus infection, infectious canine hepatitis caused by canine adenovirus type 1 (CAV-1), respiratory disease caused by canine adenovirus type 2 (CAV-2), canine parainfluenza (CPI) virus infection, and canine parvovirus (CPV) infection. 'Vanguard DA_2P+CPV' contains attenuated strains of CD virus, CAV-2, CPI virus, and CPV propagated on an established canine cell line. The CPV component was attenuated by low passage on the canine cell line and at that passage level has immunogenic properties capable of overriding maternal antibodies. 'Vanguard DA_2P+CPV' is packaged in lyophilized form with inert gas in place of vacuum.

Disease Description: *Canine distemper* is a universal, high-mortality viral disease of dogs. Approximately 50% of nonvaccinated, nonimmune dogs infected with CD virus develop clinical signs of disease, and approximately 90% of those dogs die.[1] *Infectious canine hepatitis* (ICH) is a universal, sometimes fatal, viral disease of dogs, characterized by hepatic and generalized endothelial lesions. The causative agent is CAV-1. *Canine adenovirus type 2* infection causes respiratory disease which in severe cases may include pneumonia and bronchopneumonia. *Canine parainfluenza* is a common viral upper respiratory disease of dogs. Uncomplicated CPI may be mild or subclinical, with signs becoming more severe if concurrent infection with other respiratory agents exists. *Canine parvovirus* infection results in enteric disease characterized by sudden onset of vomiting and diarrhea, often hemorrhagic. Leukopenia frequently accompanies clinical signs. Susceptible dogs of any age can be affected, but mortality is greatest in puppies. In puppies 4 to 12 weeks of age CPV may occasionally cause myocarditis that can result in acute heart failure after a brief and inconspicuous illness. Following infection many dogs are refractive to the disease for a year or more. Similarly, seropositive bitches may transfer to their pups CPV antibodies which can interfere with active immunization of the pups through 16 weeks of age.

Safety and Efficacy: Laboratory evaluation demonstrated that 'Vanguard DA_2P+CPV' immunized dogs against CD, ICH, CAV-2 respiratory disease, CPI, and CPV infection and that no immunologic interference existed among the vaccine components.

It has been demonstrated that CAV-2 vaccine cross-protects against ICH caused by CAV-1. The CAV-2 component in 'Vanguard' vaccines is used as a replacement for CAV-1 because it has significant advantages. Some CAV-1 vaccines may produce undesirable reactions, including persistent kidney infections, uveitis, and corneal opacity ("blue eye"), which have not been reported following vaccination with CAV-2.[2] In addition, the CAV-2 strain used in 'Vanguard' vaccines has been specially selected for freedom from oncogenic properties characteristic of adenoviruses.

Studies conducted at Norden Laboratories demonstrated that CAV-2 not only protects against ICH but against CAV-2 respiratory disease as well.[3] Although conventional CAV-1 (ICH) vaccines cross-protect against CAV-2, they may not prevent subclinical infection and spread of the CAV-2 agent. Canine adenovirus type 2 challenge virus was not recovered from CAV-2 vaccinated dogs in tests conducted at Norden.

The CPV component in 'Vanguard DA_2P+CPV' was subjected to comprehensive safety and efficacy testing at Norden. It was shown safe and reaction-free in laboratory tests and in clinical trials under field conditions. Product safety was demonstrated by oral administration of multiple doses of the vaccine strain to susceptible dogs, which remained normal. The CPV virus in 'Vanguard DA_2P+CPV' shares a characteristic with other live CPV vaccine strains in that the vaccinal virus may be present in the feces following administration. Although vaccinal virus was found occasionally and in low titers in the feces of vaccinated dogs, testing demonstrated that the vaccine strain did not revert to virulence following 6 consecutive back-passages in susceptible dogs.

Susceptible test dogs all developed CPV antibody titers following vaccination and were protected following oral administration of virulent CPV. Conversely, following challenge exposure, nonvaccinated control dogs all developed clinical signs of CPV infection, including vomiting and diarrhea with blood and mucus in the feces. Challenge virus was isolated from the feces of 1/20 vaccinated dogs, whereas challenge virus was isolated from the feces of 5/5 nonvaccinated control dogs. In addition, all controls developed marked lymphopenia, while no lymphopenia was demonstrated in vaccinates following exposure to virulent CPV.

Research conducted at Norden demonstrated a stronger correlation of CPV immunogenicity to number of attenuating virus passages than to antigenic mass; immunogenicity of the vaccinal strain was shown to be in inverse proportion to number of passages. The low-passage CPV virus in 'Vanguard DA_2P+CPV', therefore, is highly immunogenic and capable of stimulating active immunity in the presence of maternal antibodies. Procedures to demonstrate that capability involved thirty-nine 6- to 8-week old puppies with a conventional range of maternal CPV antibody titers. By 7 days following 1-dose vaccination with the vaccinal virus, more than 92% of those animals exhibited active immunity as shown by rising CPV antibody titers. By 14 days following vaccination, 100% of vaccinates' titers were well above the protective threshold. In contrast, nonvaccinated seropositive sentinel littermate dogs' CPV antibody titers declined, demonstrating that initial antibody titers were indeed of maternal origin and no adventitious exposure occurred during the study.

Directions:
1. *General Directions:* Aseptically rehydrate vaccine with sterile diluent supplied. Administer 1 ml subcutaneously or intramuscularly.
2. *Primary Vaccination:* Two doses should be administered 3 to 4 weeks apart. Although the CPV virus in 'Vanguard DA_2P+CPV' has been specifically designed to override high levels of maternal antibodies, they may still interfere with active immunization in a low per-

centage of puppies. Dogs vaccinated at less than 4 months of age, therefore, should be revaccinated after reaching the age of 4 months.

3. *Revaccination:* Annual revaccination with a single dose is recommended.

Precautions:

1. Store at 2°C. to 7°C.
2. Use entire contents immediately after rehydration.
3. Burn this container and all unused contents.
4. Vaccination of pregnant bitches should be avoided.
5. Contains penicillin and streptomycin as preservatives.
6. If anaphylaxis occurs following use, administer epinephrine or equivalent.
7. Although this product has been shown to be efficacious, some animals may be unable to develop or maintain an adequate immune response following vaccination if they are incubating any disease, malnourished or parasitized, or stressed due to shipment or adverse environmental conditions.

Supplied: Cartons of 25 1-dose vials

References:

1. Swango LJ: Frequently asked questions about CPV disease. *Norden News* 48:4–10, 1983.
2. Appel M, Bistner SI, Menegus M: Pathogenicity of low-virulence strains of two canine adenovirus types. *Am J Vet Res* 34:543–550, 1970.
3. Bass EP, Gill MA, Beckenhauer WH: Evaluation of a canine adenovirus type 2 strain as a replacement for infectious canine hepatitis vaccine. *J Am Vet Med Assoc* 177:234–242, 1980.

For Veterinary Use Only

VANGUARD® DA_2PL
Canine Distemper-Adenovirus Type 2-Parainfluenza Vaccine Modified Live Virus, Leptospira Bacterin

Composition: Canine distemper, adenovirus type 2, parainfluenza vaccine, modified live virus and leptospira bacterin is for the immunization of healthy dogs against canine distemper, infectious canine hepatitis (canine adenovirus type 1) infection, respiratory disease caused by canine adenovirus type 2, parainfluenza and *Leptospira canicola* and *icterohaemorrhagiae.*

The bacterin fraction is supplied as diluent for the rehydration of the modified live virus fraction.

Canine adenovirus type 2 (CAV-2) infections are primarily respiratory, evidenced by pneumonia, bronchitis, tonsillitis and pharyngitis. CAV-2 has not been associated with corneal opacity (blue eye), uveitis or virus localization in the kidneys which may be characteristic of canine adenovirus type 1 (CAV-1) infections.

Infectious canine hepatitis (CAV-1) infections are characterized by fever, leukopenia, enlarged tonsils, hepatitis, nephritis and occasional uveitis with corneal opacity.

Vaccination with modified live canine hepatitis vaccine, although effective in disease prevention, has certain disadvantages. Following vaccination, persistent kidney infections may occur causing vaccine virus shedding in urine. Uveitis and corneal opacity (blue eyes) are occasionally observed 1 to 2 weeks post vaccination.

It has been reported and demonstrated by evaluations performed at our laboratories that canine adenovirus type 2 vaccine protected against canine hepatitis and respiratory syndromes caused by the canine adenovirus type 2.

Data indicate that the development of corneal opacity is not associated with the use of this product.

The strain of canine adenovirus type 2 used in the vaccine is specially selected to preclude the oncogenic properties characteristic of this group of viruses.

Norden Laboratories developed a combined vaccine, in which the CAV-2 fraction is a replacement for canine hepatitis. This vaccine has significant advantages:

A. By using CAV-2, lesions sometimes associated with conventional ICH vaccines are avoided. Tests showed no such lesions following vaccination with the CAV-2 fraction.

B. Dogs vaccinated with CAV-2 vaccine were completely protected against challenge inoculation with virulent infectious canine hepatitis virus while all controls succumbed to challenge.

C. Dogs vaccinated with CAV-2 vaccine were protected against challenge with virulent CAV-2 virus that caused severe respiratory syndromes in the susceptible controls. Challenge virus was not recovered from vaccinated dogs and was not isolated from tissues taken at necropsy.

D. Ocular lesions were not observed in any of the 172 dogs inoculated intravenously with high titer CAV-2 vaccine virus. In comparison, intravenous inoculation of 32 dogs with infectious canine hepatitis vaccine produced ocular lesions in 22%. This is one of the critical tests of the ability of a canine adenovirus to produce ocular lesions.

E. The specially selected vaccine strain, $NL\text{-}A_2001$, has been demonstrated to be nononcogenic.

Dosage and Administration: Aseptically rehydrate vaccine with Leptospira diluent supplied. Administer 1 ml. subcutaneously or intramuscularly.

Dogs 3 months of age or older should be administered two vaccinations, 3 to 4 weeks apart. If younger dogs are vaccinated, they should be revaccinated upon reaching the age of 3 months. Annual revaccination is recommended. It is generally recommended that vaccination of pregnant females with modified live virus vaccine should be avoided.

Caution: Store at 2°C.–7°C. Use without delay after rehydration. Contains penicillin and streptomycin as preservatives. Anaphylaxis may occur. Antidote: Epinephrine. Burn container and all unused contents.

How Supplied: Vanguard DA_2PL is supplied in 25 x l-dose vials.

VANGUARD® $DA_2PL+CPV$
Canine Distemper-Adenovirus Type 2-Parainfluenza-Parvovirus Vaccine Modified Live Virus Leptospira Bacterin For Use in Dogs Only

Product Description: 'Vanguard $DA_2PL+CPV$' is for the vaccination of healthy dogs against canine distemper (CD) virus infection, infectious canine hepatitis caused by canine adenovirus type 1 (CAV-1), respiratory disease caused by canine adenovirus type 2 (CAV-2), canine parainfluenza (CPI) virus infection, canine parvovirus (CPV) infection, and leptospirosis caused by *Leptospira canicola* and *L. icterohaemorrhagiae.* The vaccine component of 'Vanguard $DA_2PL+CPV$' contains attenuated strains of CD virus, CAV-2, CPI virus, and CPV propagated on an established canine cell line. The CPV antigen was attenuated by low passage on the canine cell line and at that passage level has immunogenic properties capable of overriding maternal antibodies. The vaccine is packaged in lyophilized form with inert gas in place of vacuum. The bacterin component, containing inactivated whole cultures of *L. canicola* and *L. icterohaemorrhagiae,* is supplied as diluent.

Disease Description: *Canine distemper* is a universal, high-mortality viral disease of dogs. Approximately 50% of nonvaccinated, nonimmune dogs infected with CD virus develop clinical signs of disease, and approximately 90% of those dogs die.[1] *Infectious canine hepatitis* (ICH) is a universal, sometimes fatal, viral disease of dogs, characterized by hepatic and generalized endothelial lesions. The causative agent is CAV-1. *Canine adenovirus type 2* infection causes respiratory disease which in severe cases may include pneumonia and bronchopneumonia. *Canine parainfluenza* is a common viral upper respiratory disease of dogs. Uncomplicated CPI may be mild or subclinical, with signs becoming more severe if concurrent infection with other respiratory agents exists. *Canine parvovirus* infection results in enteric disease characterized by sudden onset of vomiting and diarrhea, often hemorrhagic. Leukopenia frequently accompanies clinical signs. Susceptible dogs of any age can be affected, but mortality is greatest in puppies. In puppies 4 to 12 weeks of age CPV may occasionally cause myocarditis that can result in acute heart failure after a brief and inconspicuous illness. Following infection many dogs are refractive to the disease for a year or more. Similarly, seropositive bitches may transfer to their pups CPV antibodies which can interfere with active immunization of the pups through 16 weeks of age. *Leptospirosis* occurs in dogs of all ages, with a wide range of clinical signs and chronic nephritis generally following acute infection. Infection with *L. canicola* and *L. icterohaemorr-*

Continued on next page

N **Norden—Cont.**

hagiae cannot be differentiated clinically.

Safety and Efficacy: Laboratory evaluation demonstrated that 'Vanguard $DA_2PL+CPV$' immunized dogs against CD, ICH, CAV-2 respiratory disease, CPI, CPV infection, and leptospirosis caused by *L. canicola* and *L. icterohaemorrhagiae*, and that no immunologic interference existed among the product antigens.

It has been demonstrated that CAV-2 vaccine cross-protects against ICH caused by CAV-1. The CAV-2 antigen in 'Vanguard' vaccines is used as a replacement for CAV-1 because it has significant advantages. Some CAV-1 vaccines, may produce undesirable reactions, including persistent kidney infections, uveitis, and corneal opacity ("blue eye"), which have not been reported following vaccination with CAV-2.[2] In addition, the CAV-2 strain used in 'Vanguard' vaccines has been specially selected for freedom from oncogenic properties characteristic of adenoviruses.

Studies conducted at Norden demonstrated that CAV-2 not only protects against ICH, but against CAV-2 respiratory disease as well.[3] Although conventional CAV-1 (ICH) vaccines cross-protect against CAV-2, they may not prevent subclinical infection and spread of the CAV-2 agent. Canine adenovirus type 2 challenge virus was not recovered from CAV-2-vaccinated dogs in tests conducted at Norden.

The CPV component in 'Vanguard $DA_2PL+CPV$' was subjected to comprehensive safety and efficacy testing at Norden. It was shown safe and reaction-free in laboratory tests and in clinical trials under field conditions. Product safety was demonstrated by oral administration of multiple doses of the vaccine strain to susceptible dogs, which remained normal. The CPV virus in 'Vanguard $DA_2PL+CPV$' shares a characteristic with other live CPV vaccine strains in that the vaccinal virus may be present in the feces following administration. Although vaccinal virus was found occasionally and in low titers in the feces of vaccinated dogs, testing demonstrated that the vaccine strain did not revert to virulence following 6 consecutive back-passages in susceptible dogs.

Susceptible test dogs all developed CPV antibody titers following vaccination, and were protected following oral administration of virulent CPV. Conversely, following challenge exposure, nonvaccinated control dogs all developed clinical signs of CPV infection, including vomiting and diarrhea with blood and mucus in the feces. Challenge virus was isolated from the feces of 1/20 vaccinated dogs, whereas challenge virus was isolated from the feces of 5/5 nonvaccinated control dogs. In addition, all controls developed marked lymphopenia, while no lymphopenia was demonstrated in vaccinates following exposure to virulent CPV.

Research conducted at Norden demonstrated a stronger correlation of CPV immunogenicity to number of attenuating virus passages than to antigenic mass; immunogenicity of the vaccinal strain was shown to be in inverse proportion to number of passages. The low-passage CPV virus in 'Vanguard $DA_2PL+CPV$', therefore, is highly immunogenic and capable of stimulating active immunity in the presence of maternal antibodies. Procedures to demonstrate that capability involved thirty-nine 6- to 8-week old puppies with a conventional range of maternal CPV antibody titers. By 7 days following 1-dose vaccination with the vaccinal virus, more than 92% of those animals exhibited active immunity as shown by rising CPV antibody titers. By 14 days following vaccination, 100% of vaccinates' titers were well above the protective threshold. In contrast, nonvaccinated seropositive sentinel littermate dogs' CPV antibody titers declined, demonstrating that initial antibody titers were indeed of maternal origin and no adventitious exposure occurred during the study.

Directions:

1. *General Directions:* Aseptically rehydrate vaccine with Leptospira bacterin supplied. Administer 1 ml subcutaneously or intramuscularly.
2. *Primary Vaccination:* Two doses should be administered 3 to 4 weeks apart. Although the CPV virus in 'Vanguard $DA_2PL+CPV$' has been specifically designed to override high levels of maternal antibodies, they may still interfere with active immunization in a low percentage of puppies. Dogs vaccinated at less than 4 months of age, therefore, should be revaccinated after reaching the age of 4 months.
3. *Revaccination:* Annual revaccination with a single dose is recommended.

Precautions:

1. Store at 2°C. to 7°C. Do not freeze.
2. Use entire contents immediately after rehydration.
3. Burn this container and all unused contents.
4. Vaccination of pregnant bitches should be avoided.
5. Contains penicillin and streptomycin as preservatives.
6. If anaphylaxis occurs following use, administer epinephrine or equivalent.
7. Although this product has been shown to be efficacious, some animals may be unable to develop or maintain an adequate immune response following vaccination if they are incubating any disease, malnourished or parasitized, or stressed due to shipment or adverse environmental conditions.

Supplied: Cartons of 25 1-dose vials

References:

1. Swango LJ: Frequently asked questions about CPV disease. *Norden News* 48:4–10, 1983.
2. Appel M, Bistner SI, Menegus M: Pathogenicity of low-virulence strains of two canine adenovirus types. *Am J Vet Res* 34:543–550, 1970.
3. Bass EP, Gill MA, Beckenhauer WH: Evaluation of a canine adenovirus type 2 strain as a replacement for infectious canine hepatitis vaccine. *J Am Vet Med Assoc* 177:234–242, 1980.

For Veterinary Use Only

VANGUARD® D-M
Canine Distemper-Measles Vaccine Modified Live Virus

Composition: Vanguard® D-M is a modified live virus vaccine for the initial vaccination of healthy dogs 6 to 12 weeks of age against canine distemper. The vaccine is prepared by separately growing highly attenuated strains of canine distemper virus and measles virus in tissue culture on the Norden Stable Cell Line (SCL®). The use of this Stable Cell Line has many important advantages. Just as virus strains have pedigrees, so do the cells on which they are grown. Originally derived from a normal dog, the Stable Cell Line used for vaccine production is maintained under carefully controlled conditions at a uniform passage level. Because these pedigreed cells all have the same genetic background, they have the same growth rate and uniform virus susceptibility. Therefore, the vaccine from serial to serial is very uniform. On the basis of all tests that have been conducted, these pedigreed cells have been found free of adventitious or latent virus. Their propagation for many generations outside of the host dog virtually eliminates the possibility of transmitting unrecognized virus infections from the living animal.

Protection against canine distemper is desirable at the earliest possible age. Puppies of any age may be successfully immunized against canine distemper by modified live virus canine distemper vaccine providing they do not have circulating antibody against canine distemper. When passive immunity is present, whether maternal or from inoculation of canine distemper antiserum, vaccination will be unsuccessful until the antibodies decline to a level which will not interfere with the virus. Measles virus stimulates resistance against canine distemper in puppies regardless of circulating canine distemper antibody levels. The resistance provided by measles virus, however, does not appear to be as effective in very young pups as those six weeks of age or older.

Because the immune status and age of a pup presented for vaccination is often unknown, the use of Vanguard D-M provides a solution. Controlled experiments conducted by the Research and Development Division of Norden Laboratories to determine effectiveness of Vanguard D-M at various ages showed that 73 of 76 pups (96%) were protected at six weeks of age. Of these pups, 45 had levels of maternal passive immunity sufficient to interfere with successful protection by canine distemper virus. Forty-two of these pups (93%) were protected by the measles virus component.

The resistance induced by measles virus does not interfere with active immunization against canine distemper. Many authorities believe it may actually stimulate a more rapid serological response and in many cases a higher level of antibody. Heterotypic immunity should not be relied on for protection after 16 weeks of age. Because repeated use of this vaccine may produce high levels of measles antibodies which can interfere with successful protection of pups in the next generation, this vaccine should not be used on female pups over 12 weeks of age or older bitches.

Dosage and Administration: Aseptically rehydrate with diluent supplied and shake well. Inject 1 ml. intramuscularly within one hour after rehydration.

Based on current scientific information, this vaccine is capable of stimulating all the protection which the dog is capable of producing. The following recommendations are for the vaccination of healthy puppies. Vanguard D-M is specifically designed for the temporary protection of young puppies against canine distemper. Puppies between 6 and 12 weeks of age should be inoculated with a single dose of Vanguard D-M, the earlier the better. This should be followed by a dose of canine distemper vaccine at 14 to 16 weeks of age to provide the dog with a high level of distemper protection. In most cases, it will be desirable to combine the canine distemper vaccination with protection against infectious canine hepatitis and *Leptospira canicola* and *L. icterohaemorrhagiae* infections by administering a combination vaccine such as Vanguard DA_2 or Vanguard DA_2L.

Puppies older than 12 weeks of age should respond to a single dose of canine distemper vaccine (rarely, interfering levels of passive maternal antibody may persist longer) and this is the vaccine of choice in these older animals.

Annual revaccination of all dogs with Canine Distemper Vaccine is recommended.

Caution: Store at 2°C.–7°C. Use entire contents within one hour after rehydration. Anaphylactoid reactions are possible following use of any biological product. In this event use epinephrine or its equivalent. Contains penicillin and streptomycin as preservatives. Although it is not anticipated that this vaccine will be used on adult dogs, vaccination of pregnant bitches should be avoided. Burn containers after use.

How Supplied: 25 × 1-dose. Dose is 1 ml.

VANGUARD® DMP

Canine Distemper-Measles-Parainfluenza Vaccine Modified Live Virus

Vanguard DMP is a modified live virus vaccine for the immunization of healthy dogs 6 to 12 weeks of age against canine distemper and canine parainfluenza. The vaccine is prepared by growing highly attenuated strains of canine distemper virus, measles virus and canine parainfluenza virus separately in tissue culture using the Norden Stable Cell Line (SCL®) method.

Protection against canine distemper is desirable at the earliest possible age. Puppies of any age may be successfully immunized against canine distemper by modified live virus canine distemper vaccine providing they do not have circulating antibody against canine distemper.

When passive immunity is present, whether maternal or from inoculation of canine distemper antiserum, vaccination will be unsuccessful until the antibodies decline to a level which will not interfere with the virus. Measles virus stimulates heterotypic protection against canine distemper in puppies regardless of circulating canine distemper antibody levels. The resistance provided by measles virus, however, does not appear to be as effective in very young pups as those six weeks of age or older.

Because the immune status and age of a pup presented for vaccination is often unknown, the use of Vanguard DMP provides a solution. Controlled experiments conducted by the Research and Development Division of Norden Laboratories to determine effectiveness of Vanguard DMP at various ages showed that 75 of 76 pups (96%) were protected at six weeks of age. Of these pups, 45 had levels of maternal passive immunity sufficient to interfere with successful protection by canine distemper virus. Forty-two of these 45 pups (93%) were protected by the measles virus component.

The resistance induced by measles virus does not interfere with active immunization against canine distemper. Many authorities believe it may actually stimulate a more rapid serological response and in many cases a higher level of antibody. Heterotypic immunity should not be relied on for protection after 16 weeks of age. Because repeated use of this vaccine may produce high levels of measles antibodies which may interfere with successful protection of pups in the next generation, this vaccine should not be used on female pups over 12 weeks of age or older bitches.

Canine parainfluenza virus is another disease of dogs which often attacks young pups at the time they are weaned. Since canine parainfluenza may superficially resemble distemper, early protection is desirable.

Directions for Use: Aseptically rehydrate with diluent supplied and shake well. Inject 1 ml. intramuscularly within one hour after rehydration.

Based on current scientific information, this vaccine is capable of stimulating all the protection which the dog is capable of producing. The following recommendations are for the vaccination of healthy puppies. Vanguard DMP is specifically designed for the temporary protection of young pups against canine distemper and as the first dose in a two dose series for canine parainfluenza. Puppies between 6 and 12 weeks of age should be inoculated with a single dose of Vanguard DMP the earlier the better. This should be followed by a dose of canine distemper vaccine and canine parainfluenza vaccine at 14 to 16 weeks of age. In most cases it will be desirable to combine these vaccinations with protection against canine adenovirus type-2, which also serves to protect against infectious canine hepatitis virus, and/or *Leptospira canicola* and *L. icterohaemorrhagiae* infection by administering a combination vaccine such as Vanguard DA_2P or Vanguard DA_2PL.

Puppies older than 12 weeks of age should respond to a single dose of canine distemper vaccine (rarely, interfering levels of passive maternal antibody may persist longer) and this is the vaccine of choice in these older animals.

Annual revaccination of all dogs for canine distemper and canine parainfluenza is recommended.

Caution: Store at 2°C.–7°C. Use entire contents within one hour after rehydration. Anaphylactoid reactions are possible following use of any biological product. In this event use epinephrine or its equivalent. Contains penicillin and streptomycin as preservatives. Although it is not anticipated that this vaccine will be used on adult dogs, vaccination of pregnant bitches should be avoided. Burn container after use.

How Supplied: 25 × 1 dose. Dose is 1 ml.

For Veterinary Use Only

VIBRIN®

Campylobacter Fetus Bacterin

Product Description: 'Vibrin' is for vaccination of healthy cattle against vibriosis. 'Vibrin' is prepared from an inactivated, concentrated suspension of *Campylobacter fetus*, bovine isolate, in a patented repository base.[1]

Disease Description: Vibriosis is a venereal disease of cattle, caused by *Campylobacter fetus*. A worldwide problem for the livestock industry, diagnosis of vibriosis is difficult because the disease is often subclinical. In cows vibriosis causes temporary infertility, irregular estrus cycles, delayed conception, and occasionally, abortion. The disease is transmitted during breeding, either through coitus or artificial insemination with contaminated semen.

Safety and Efficacy: Chemical inactivation renders 'Vibrin' incapable of causing or spreading infectious disease. The special adjuvant base enhances and prolongs antigenic stimulation and may produce a localized vaccine granuloma. These are noninflammatory, however, and usually disappear in several weeks. Field use and extensive, controlled tests in breeding cattle under experimental conditions demonstrated that the serotype of *Campylobacter fetus* used in 'Vibrin' was effective in prevention of vibriosis.[2,3] Pregnancy rates in vaccinated cattle were up to 44% higher than in nonvaccinated control cattle. All research conducted on 'Vibrin' indicated a single dose is effective and there is no advantage in using two injections.[2,4,5]

Directions:

General Directions: Shake well. Administer 2 ml. subcutaneously in the upper part of the neck.

Continued on next page

N **Norden—Cont.**

Primary Vaccination: A single dose of 'Vibrin' should be administered to all breeding cows and heifers between 30 days and seven months prior to breeding. Pregnant animals can be safely vaccinated.[2,4]
Revaccination: Annual revaccination with a single dose is recommended between 30 days and 7 months prior to breeding.
Precautions:
1. Store at 2°C. to 7°C. Do not freeze.
2. Use entire contents when first opened.
3. To avoid vaccination site trim-out, do not vaccinate within 60 days before slaughter.
4. If anaphylaxis occurs following use, administer epinephrine or equivalent.
5. Although this product has been shown to be efficacious, some animals may be unable to develop or maintain an adequate immune response following vaccination. If they are incubating any disease, malnourished or parasitized, or stressed due to shipment or adverse environmental conditions.

Supplied: 10- and 50-dose vials
References:
1. Repository vaccine and method of preparing same. Charles R Kuhns and William H Beckenhauer. U.S. Patent No. 3,435,112. Canadian Patent No. 810,630.
2. Carroll EJ, Hoerlein AB: Current Recommendations for Vibrio Vaccination in Cattle. Presented at 32nd Ann. Conf. Vet. at Coll. Vet. Med. and Bio-Med. Sci., Colorado State University, Fort Collins, Feb. 14–17, 1971.
3. Hoerlein AB, Kramer T: Artificial Stimulation of Resistance to Bovine Vibriosis. Am. J. Vet. Res. 24:951, 1963.
4. Hoerlein AB, Carroll EJ, Kramer T, Beckenhauer WH: Bovine Vibriosis Immunization. JAVMA 146:828–835, 1965.
5. Hoerlein AB, Carroll EJ: Duration of Immunity to Bovine Genital Vibriosis. JAVMA 156:775 (1970).

For Veterinary Use Only
U.S. Patent Nos. 3,329,573 and 3,435,112
Canadian Pat. 1969 No. 818,457
Canadian Pat. 1969 No. 810,630

VIBRIO/LEPTOFERM-P®
Campylobacter Fetus-Leptospira Pomona Bacterin

Product Description: 'Vibrio/Leptoferm-P' is for vaccination of healthy cattle against vibriosis and against leptospirosis caused by *Leptospira pomona.* 'Vibrio/Leptoferm-P' contains an inactivated, adjuvanted suspension of *Vibrio fetus venerealis (Campylobacter fetus venerealis)* combined with an inactivated culture of *L. pomona.*
Disease Description: Vibriosis (campylobacteriosis) is a venereal disease of cattle, caused by *Vibrio fetus venerealis (Campylobacter fetus venerealis).* A worldwide problem for the livestock industry, diagnosis of vibriosis is difficult because the disease is often subclinical. In cows vibriosis causes temporary infertility, irregular estrus cycles, delayed conception, and occasionally, abortion. The disease is transmitted during breeding, either through coitus or artificial insemination with contaminated semen.
Leptospirosis may be caused by several serovars of *Leptospira,* although *L. pomona* is among the most common affecting cattle. *Leptospira* bacteria localize in the kidneys and are shed in the urine. Leptospirosis in calves causes anemia, bloody urine, fever, inappetence, and prostration. Signs are usually subclinical in adult cattle. However, pregnant cows often abort, and dairy cows may exhibit a marked decrease in milk production.
Safety and Efficacy: In product development studies in 20 herds, no adverse reactions were reported. The studies further demonstrated non-interference between the vaccine antigens and higher pregnancy rates in vaccinated cattle than in nonvaccinated control cattle.
Directions:
General Directions: Shake well. Administer 2 ml. intramuscularly.
Primary Vaccination: 'Vibrio/Leptoferm-P' should be administered to all breeding cows and heifers at least 30 to 60 days prior to exposure or being added to the breeding herd. In herds in endemic areas, a second injection may be desirable with a vaccination interval of at least 2 weeks.
Revaccination: Annual revaccination with a single dose is recommended.
Precautions:
1. Store at 2°C. to 7°C. Do not freeze.
2. Use entire contents when first opened.
3. Do not vaccinate within 21 days before slaughter.
4. If anaphylaxis occurs following use, administer epinephrine or equivalent.
5. Although this product has been shown to be efficacious, some animals may be unable to develop or maintain an adequate immune response if they are incubating any disease, malnourished or parasitized, or stressed due to shipment or adverse environmental conditions.

Supplied: 10- and 50-dose vials
For Veterinary Use Only

VIBRIO/LEPTOFERM-5®
Campylobacter Fetus-Leptospira Canicola-Grippotyphosa-Hardjo-Icterohaemorrhagiae-Pomona Bacterin

Bovine Vibriosis: Bovine Vibriosis is an insidious baceterial disease of the genital tract of cattle. The disease is characterized by infertility and occasional abortions. It is a venereal disease spread by breeding and is considered to be an important cause of infertility in cattle.
No clinical symptoms are normally evident in vibriosis infection, therefore, the herd history is very important in diagnosing the disease. A lowered calving rate, prolonged calving season, or a combination of the two point to vibriosis.
'Vibrio/Leptoferm-5' is a chemically inactivated, adjuvanted suspension of *Campylobacter fetus* combined with chemically inactivated Leptospira bacterin prepared from separately grown cultures of *Leptospira canicola, Leptospira grippotyphosa, Leptospira hardjo, Leptospira icterohaemorrhagiae* and *Leptospira pomona.* 'Vibrio/Leptoferm-5' is recommended as an aid in the prevention of infertility or delayed conception due to *Campylobacter fetus* and the prevention of leptospirosis due to *L. canicola, L. grippotyphosa, L. hardjo, L. icterohaemorrhagiae* and *L. pomona.*
Vaccination Recommendations: A single dose of 'Vibrio/Leptoferm-5' should be administered to all breeding cows and heifers at least 30 to 60 days prior to exposure or being added to the breeding herd. In noninfected herds in endemic areas, a second injection may be desirable with a vaccination interval of at least 2 weeks. Annual revaccination is recommended.
Administration: Shake well. Inject 5 ml. intramuscularly using aseptic precautions.
Caution: Store at 2°C.–7°C. Do not freeze. Use entire contents when first opened. Do not vaccinate within 21 days before slaughter.
If anaphylaxis occurs following use, administer epinephrine or equivalent.
For Veterinary Use Only.

WEANGUARD®
Porcine Rotavirus Vaccine Modified Live Virus Two Major Rotavirus Serotypes For Baby Pigs

Introduction: 'WeanGuard' is a modified live virus containing serotypes A_1 and A_2 of porcine Rotavirus which have been modified so that they do not cause disease in baby pigs, feeder pigs or pregnant swine. The vaccine is recommended as an aid in the prevention and control of Rotavirus disease in swine. Rotavirus is one cause of viral gastroenteritis characterized by vomiting, watery diarrhea, dehydration and death in young pigs; therefore, the clinical signs may be identical to those of TGE. The disease is very common in both nursing and weaned pigs, and all swine herds so far examined show serologic evidence of its presence. Efficacy of 'WeanGuard' has been demonstrated in both pregnant sows and baby pigs[1]. Oral and intramuscular vaccination of nursing pigs induces active immunity and will protect them against post-weaning rotavirus-induced scours. Laboratory confirmation of the cause of baby pig diarrhea is recommended since other viral, bacterial and coccidial agents can cause similar disease signs.
It is recommended that pregnant sows and gilts always be vaccinated with 'Rota-Vac TGE' (as directed) prior to farrowing. This should result in increased levels of milk antibody and protection of nursing pigs. Since pigs lose their passive milk protection when they are weaned it is necessary to actively immunize them by oral and intramuscular vaccination prior to weaning.
Dosage Guidelines: Follow directions carefully. Each baby pig should receive, before weaning, at last two doses of vaccine; one oral dose and one intra-

muscular dose about 7–10 days preweaning.
Reconstitute the dried vaccine with sterile diluent provided. Use 50 ml. for the 50 dose size. Reconstitute the 50 dose vaccine vial with 10–15 ml. sterile diluent and then return the liquid vaccine to the remainder of the diluent in the plastic 50 ml. diluent vial. The 50 doses of vaccine can then be administered with either automatic syringes or a plastic oral dosing bottle (holds 50–100 doses and delivers 1 ml. per depression of the dispenser) available through a veterinarian.
Inoculate each pig orally with 1 ml. of the reconstituted vaccine and inject one dose intramuscularly. Do not return the pig to the sow for at least 30 minutes after oral vaccination. Always wash oral vaccine dispensers thoroughly with soap and water and rinse thoroughly with clean water before addition of vaccine.
Caution: Store vaccine in the dark at temperatures between 35° and 45°F (4°–7°C). Use vaccine immediately after reconstitution. Always use clean syringes and dispensers without chemical residues which can destroy the vaccine. Do not save partial contents. Burn this container and all unused contents. Good animal husbandry and management procedures should always accompany use of a vaccine in a herd. Use vaccine in healthy animals only. Do not vaccinate within 21 days of slaughter. If allergic reactions occur following use of this product, treat with epinephrine or atrophine. If diarrhea persists after use of the vaccine additional diagnostic work may be warranted. Contains gentamicin as a preservative.
Reference:
1. Research data on file, Ambico, Inc.
For Veterinary Use Only

Osborn
AN ESSAR CORPORATION
P. O. BOX 1590
FORT DODGE, IOWA 50501

AMCON™
Injectable Amino Acid Concentrate

Indications: For use as a properly balanced nutritional supplement and essential metabolic support in the management of scours, shipping fever or other conditions involving respiratory problems, intestinal disorders, blood loss or nutritional upset.
Composition: Contains pure crystalline amino acid 30 times the concentration, but in the same balance found in blood serum, plus B vitamins, electrolytes and dextrose. Amino Acids: L-Arginine, L-Glutamine, L-Isoleucine, L-Leucine, L-Lycine, L-Methionine, L-Phenylalanine, L-Threonine, L-Tryptophan, L-Valine, L-Histadine, B Vitamins: Thiamine, Riboflavin, Niacinamide, Calcium Pantothenate, Pyridoxine, Vitamin B12. Electrolytes: Calcium, Chloride, Magnesium, Sodium, Potassium.
Side Effects: Dose of 20 ml (cc) per pound body weight have been administered and blood pressure, heart rate, respiratory rate, and urine flow measured. With the exception of transient rise in the blood pressure, a slight increase in respiratory rate, and a slight increase in pulse pressure, these large doses were well tolerated with all values returned to normal within 15 minutes.
Precautions: When used in the management of infectious disease conditions, appropriate concurrent therapeutic measures should be taken.
Dosage and Administration: Product may be administered intraperitoneally, intramuscularly, intravenously or subcutaneously. Intravenous route is recommended for best results.
Small Animals: 1 to 3 ml (cc) per pound body weight, 1 to 3 times daily.
Cattle, Calves, Sheep & Swine: 1 ml (cc) per 10 lbs body weight, 1 to 3 times daily.
Horses: 1 ml (cc) per 10 lbs body weight, 1 to 3 times daily.
Frequency of Administration is indicated by severity of condition. In cattle, calves and horses, doses up to 2 ml (cc) per pound body weight can be used when severity of the condition warrants.
Caution: Store in cool dark place.
How Supplied: 500 ml.

BETA-CON
Water Dispersible Vitamins

Composition: Each pound of Beta-Con contains: Vitamin A, 2,500,000 USP Units; Vitamin D_3 600,000 IC Units; Vitamin E, 1,000 I Units; Vitamin B_{12} 6 mg; Riboflavin 500 mg.; d-Pantothenic Acid, 2,500 mg.; Niacin, 10,000 mg., Choline Bitartrate 45,344 mg.; Vitamin K (MSBC), 2,000 mg.; Folic Acid, 200 mg; Thiamine Mononitrate, 500 mg.; Pyridoxine Hydrochloride, 500 mg.; Ascorbic Acid, 6,000 mg.
Indications: Water dispersible vitamin mix for calves, swine, beef and dairy cattle, horses, turkeys and poultry.
How Supplied: 4 oz.

BOVO-COX™ BOLUSES
(Sulfaquinoxaline)

Composition: Each bolus contains 20 gr. Sulfaquinoxaline; plus inactive ingredients: Colloidal Aluminum Silicate, Ferrous Sulfate, Activated Charcoal, Calcium Carbonate, Copper Sulfate, Activated Attapulgite.
Indications: As an aid in the treatment of Coccidiosis and Dysentery in non-lactating cattle and sheep.
Dosage and Administration: ***Cattle:*** Give one bolus for each 200 lbs of body weight daily for a period of 3 to 5 days. ***Sheep:*** Give one-half bolus daily for each mature sheep for 3 to 5 days.
Notice: Supply adequate quantities of drinking water at all times. Treatment must be accompanied by preventive management practices to avoid unnecessary reinfection. Clean pens daily to hold down concentration of infective oocysts.
Caution: This drug, like all sulfonamides, may cause toxic reactions and irreparable injury unless administered with adequate and continuous supervision.
Warning: Discontinue treatment at least 10 days before animals are marketed for human consumption.
How Supplied: Jars of 50 boluses.

O

BOVO-COX™ CALF BOLUSES
(Sulfaquinoxaline)

Composition: Each bolus contains: *Active Ingredient:* Sulfaquinoxaline 10 gr. *Inactive Ingredients:* Colloidal Aluminum Silicate, Ferrous Sulfate, Activated Charcoal, Calcium Carbonate, Copper Sulfate, Activated Attapulgite.
Indications: As an aid in the treatment of Coccidiosis and Dysentery in calves.
Dosage and Administration: ***Calves:*** Give one bolus for each 100 lbs. of calf weight for a period of 3 to 5 days. ***Lambs:*** Give ½ bolus for each 50 lbs. of body weight for 3 to 5 days.
Notice: Supply adequate quantities of drinking water at all times. Treatment must be accompanied by preventive management practices to avoid unnecessary reinfections. Clean pens daily to hold down concentration of infective oocysts.
Caution: This drug, like all Sulfonamides, may cause toxic reactions and irreparable injury unless administered with adequate and continuous supervision.
Warning: Discontinue treatment at least 10 days before animals are marketed for human consumption.
How Supplied: Jars of 50 boluses.

BOVO-COX™ POWDER
(Sulfaquinoxaline)

Composition: Each ounce contains: Sulfaquinoxaline 900 mg., Colloidal Activated Attapulgite, Ferrous Sulfate, Copper Sulfate, Colloidal Aluminum Silicate (Hydrated), Activated Charcoal, Sugar and Artificial Flavors in a Palatable Cereal Base preserved with Ethoxyquin.
Indications: Indicated in the treatment of Bovine Coccidiosis.
Dosage and Administration: ***Individual Treatment:*** Give one ounce twice daily for each 300 pounds of calf weight for a period of 3 to 5 days.
Herd Treatment: Give one pound twice daily for each 4,800 pounds of calf weight for a period of 3 to 5 days. Thoroughly mix with the total feed consumed to provide accurate dosage.
Notice: Supply adequate quantities of drinking water at all times. Treatment must be accompanied by preventive management practices to avoid unnecessary reinfection. Clean pens daily to hold down the concentration of infective oocysts.
Caution: This drug, like all sulfonamides, may cause toxic reactions and irreparable injury unless administered with adequate and continuous supervision. Not for use in Dairy Cattle.

Continued on next page

Osborn—Cont.

Warning: Discontinue treatment at least 10 days before animals are marketed for human consumption.
How Supplied: 25 lb pails

O

BOVO-LYTE™
For the Correction of Electrolyte Depletion and Dehydration in Cattle and Calves

Composition: Sodium (Na) 140 mEq/Liter; Potassium (K) 10 mEq/Liter; Calcium (Ca) 5 mEq/Liter; Magnesium (Mg) 3 mEq/Liter; Chloride (Cl) 130 mEq/-Liter. Dextrose 5%.
Suggested Dosage: ***Calves***—300–900 ml. ***Cattle***—900–1800 ml.
Administer intravenously avoiding rapid administration. Repeat as indicated by the degree of dehydration.
How Supplied: 900 ml Bottles.

BOVO-LYTE™ CONCENTRATE
A Balanced Concentrated Electrolyte Solution Which Must be Diluted Prior to Use

Composition: Bovo-Lyte™ Concentrate contains: Sodium (Na) 1400 mEq/L; Potassium (K) 100 mEq/L; Calcium (Ca)50 mEq/L; Magnesium (Mg) 30 mEq/L; Chloride (Cl) 1300 mEq/L; Dextrose 200 Cal/Liter.
Indications: For the correction of electrolyte depletion and dehydration of bovines.
Directions: When Bovo-Lyte™ Concentrate is diluted 1 to 10 (1 part Bovo-Lyte™ Concentrate added to 9 parts distilled water) the final solution will have the following approximate Electrolyte Concentration per liter: Sodium (Na) mEq/L 140; Potassium (K) mEq/L 10; Calcium (Ca) mEq/L 5; Magnesium (Mg) mEq/L 3; Chloride (Cl) mEq/L 130; Dextrose 20 Cal/Liter.
Suggested Dosage: ***Calves*** 300 to 900 ml.; ***Cattle*** 900 to 1800 ml.
Administer intravenously avoiding rapid administration. Repeat as indicated by the degree of dehydration.
Caution: This product is highly concentrated and must be diluted prior to use. It is recommended that solutions be diluted just prior to use.
How Supplied: 1 Qt.

BUTATRON™ Oral Gel
Phenylbutazone Oral Gel
FOR USE IN HORSES ONLY

Each 30 grams of gel contain: Phenylbutazone ....4 grams
Indication: Butatron Oral Gel is indicated for the relief of inflammatory conditions associated with the musculoskeletal system of horses.
Dosage: Butatron Oral Gel should be administered at a rate of 0.2 gram to 0.4 grams phenylbutazone per 100 pounds body weight (1 to 2 grams per 500 pounds). Do not exceed 4 grams phenylbutazone daily.
Administration: Calculate dosage to be given and select proper dose on plunger ring. Insert nozzle of syringe through inter-dental space of animal. Gel should be placed on base of tongue.
Precautions: In the treatment of inflammatory conditions associated with infection, specific anti-infection therapy is required.
READ PACKAGE INSERT CAREFULLY FOR COMPLETE INSTRUCTIONS PRIOR TO USE.
WARNING: NOT FOR HORSES INTENDED FOR FOOD
Caution: Federal (U.S.A.) law restricts this drug to use by or on the order of a licensed veterinarian.
CONTENTS: 30 Grams

CAL-PHOS PALATABS®
Calcium, Phosphorus & Vitamin D

Composition: Each tablet contains: Calcium 580 mg, Phosphorus 450 mg., Vitamin D3 400 I.U. in a protein chewable base.
Indications: For preventing calcium and phosphorus deficiences during rapid growth, pregnancy and lactation.
Dosage and Administration: One tablet per 20 pounds body weight daily. Cal-Phos Palatabs® may be given free choice or crumbled and mixed with food.
How Supplied: 50's

CARBAM PALATABS®
(diethylcarbamazine citrate)
Chewable Tablets

Indications: Carbam Palatabs® are indicated in the prevention of heartworm disease *(Dirofilaria immitis)* in dogs.
Carbam Palatabs® are also indicated as an aid in the treatment of ascarid infections in dogs *(Toxocara canis)* and cats *(Toxocara canis* and *Toxascaris leonina)* and as an aid in the control of ascarid infections *(Toxocara canis)* in dogs.
Dosage and Administration: For prevention of heartworm *(Dirofilaria immitis)* infection in dogs, the drug may be added to the daily diet at a dosage rate of 3.0 mg per pound of body weight per day, or given directly by mouth at the same dosage rate. Administration of Carbam Palatabs® (Diethylcarbamazine citrate) should start one month before the mosquito season, continue daily throughout the season and for two months thereafter. Dogs on prophylactic therapy should be examined for the presence of microfilariae every six months.
As an aid in the control of ascarid infections *(Toxocara canis)* in dogs, the drug may be added to the daily diet at a dosage rate of 3.0 mg per pound of body weight, or given directly by mouth at the same dosage rate.
As an aid in the treatment of ascarid infections in dogs *(Toxocara canis)* and cats *(Toxocara canis* and *Toxascaris leonina)* administer 25 mg to 50 mg Carbam Palatabs® (diethylcarbamazine citrate) per pound of body weight as a single dose. A repeat dose may be given in ten to twenty days, to remove immature worms which may enter the intestine from the lung after the first dose.
Carbam Palatabs® should be administered with food or following feeding to reduce the occasional possibility of vomiting.
Warning: Do not use in dogs that have been harboring adult heartworms. Use of diethylcarbamazine citrate is not recommended in dogs with active *Dirofilaria immitis* infection, until they have been converted to a negative status by the use of adulticidal and microfilaricidal drugs. Inadvertent administration to dogs infected with heartworm may cause adverse reactions due to pulmonary occlusion or shock.
Note: Size change as indicated in supplements.
How Supplied:
60 mg tablets: 100's, 200's
120 mg tablets: 100's
180 mg tablets: 50's, 100's, 200's

CARBAM™ TABLETS
(diethylcarbamazine citrate)

Composition: Diethylcarbamazine Citrate Tablets U.S.P.
Indications: For the prevention of heartworm disease *(Dirofilaria immitis)* in dogs, as an aid in the treatment of ascarid infections in dogs *(Toxocara canis)* and cats *(Toxocara canis* and *Toxascaris leonina)* and as an aid in the control of ascarid infections *(Toxocara canis)* in dogs.
Dosage and Administration: For prevention of heartworm *(Dirofilaria immitis)* infection in dogs, the drug may be added to the daily diet at a dosage rate of 3.0 mg. per pound of body weight per day, or given directly by mouth at the same dosage rate. Administration of Carbam Tablets (diethylcarbamazine citrate) should start one month before the mosquito season, continue daily throughout the season and for two months thereafter. Dogs on a prophylactic therapy should be examined for the presence of microfilariae every six months.
As an aid in the control of ascarid infections *(Toxocara canis)* in dogs, the drug may be added to the daily diet at a dosage rate of 3.0 mg. per pound of body weight, or given directly by mouth at the same dosage rate.
As an aid in the treatment of ascarid infections in dogs *(Toxocara canis)* and cats *(Toxocara canis* and *Toxascaris leonia),* administer 25 mg. to 50 mg. Carbam Tablets (diethylcarbamazine citrate) per pound of body weight as a single dose. A repeat dose should be given in ten to twenty days, to remove immature worms which may enter the intestine from the lung after the first dose.
Carbam Tablets should be administered with food or following feeding to reduce the occasional possibility of vomiting.
Warning: Do not use in dogs that have been harboring adult heartworms. Use of diethylcarbamazine citrate is not recommended in dogs with active *Dirofilaria immitis* infection, until they have been converted to a negative status by the use of adulticidal and microfilaricidal drugs. Inadvertent administration to dogs infected with heartworm may cause adverse reactions due to pulmonary occlusion or shock.

Caution: Federal (USA) law restricts this drug to use by or on the order of a licensed veterinarian.

How Supplied:

50 mg	500's
100 mg	300's
200 mg	200's
300 mg	100's
400 mg	100's

CELULASE™
Rumen Inoculant and Media

Composition: Primary Dried Torula Yeast, Active Dry Yeast, Soluble Sugars, Urea, Peptonized Iron, Disodium Phosphate and Artifical Flavor.
Indications: Celulase may be used as media for correcting rumen dysfunction due to deficiency in normal rumen bacterial flora, stimulating and establishing rumen function, improving digestion, and converting cellulose.
How Supplied: 1 lb.

CONVAL™

Composition:
Each Pound Contains:
Vitamins:—Vitamin A, 4480 I.U., Vitamin D_3 3,000 I.U., Vitamin E 56 I.U., Thiamin HCl 0.060 mg., Riboflavin 2.240 mg., Pantothenic Acid 6.670 mg., Niacin 11.280 mg., Pyridoxine HCl 0.060 mg., Folic Acid 0.112 mg., Biotin 0.006 mg., Vitamin B_{12} 0.056 mg., Choline Chloride 0.720 mg., Menadione SBC 1.125 mg.,
Amino Acids:—Lysine 7,450 mg., Methionine 1,950 mg., Cystine 1,095 mg., Threonine 4,975 mg., Valine 6,325 mg., Isoleucine 5,525 mg., Leucine 9,195 mg., Phenylalanine 5,145 mg., Tyrosine 3,625 mg., Histidine 2,740 mg., Arginine 6,070 mg., Aspartic Acid 11,220 mg., Serine 6,325 mg., Glutamic Acid 21,640 mg., Proline 8,605 mg., Glycine 4,595 mg., Alanine 4,680 mg.
In an especially prepared essential fatty acid base containing arachidonic, linoleic and linolenic acids and natural flavors.
Guaranteed Analysis: Protein (Min) . . . 24.00%; Fat (Min) . . . 9.00%; Fiber (Max) . . . 0.75%.
Indications: Conval is indicated particularly during the postsurgical convalescent period and during periods of general hospitalization and confinement. Conval is also indicated for general geriatric debilitation and may be used following periods of chronic disease conditions such as chronic gastritis or enteritis in the dog.
Dosage: *Slight Negative Nitrogen Balance* . . . One tablespoon* for each 30 pounds body weight twice daily mixed in dog food.
Moderate Negative Nitrogen Balance . . . Two tablespoonfuls* for each 15 pounds of body weight twice daily mixed in dog food.
Severe Negative Nitrogen Balance . . . Four tablespoonfuls for each 15 pounds of body weight twice daily mixed in dog food.*
Conval may be used as an adjunct to parenteral therapy.
*NOTE: A special dosage tablespoon is provided which will deliver approximately one ounce.
How Supplied: 2 lb.

DEXAMETHASONE TABLETS
(Dexamethasone U.S.P.)

Composition: Each tablet contains 0.25 mg. Dexamethasone.
Indications: Zonometh™ Tablets are indicated for use as an anti-inflammatory agent.
Actions: Dexamethasone is a synthetic corticosteroid and possesses glucocorticoid activity. Dexamethasone, as with other corticosteroids, is not specific. It differs from other corticosteroids only in its anti-inflammatory potency and ability to manifest mineralocorticoid properties.
Dosage and Administration: Dosage and administration for Zonometh Tablets are as follows:
Dog: 0.25 to 1.25 mg. per day up to 7 days.
Cat: 0.125 to 0.5 mg. per day up to 7 days.
Contraindications: Do not use in viral infections. Except for emergency therapy, do not use in animals with tuberculosis, chronic nephritis, cushingoid syndrome and peptic ulcers. Existance of congestive heart failure, diabetes and osteoporosis are relative contraindications.
Precautions: Because of the anti-inflammatory action of corticosteroids, signs of infection may be hidden and it may be necessary to stop treatment until diagnosis is made. Overdosage of some glucocorticoids may result in sodium retention, fluid retention, potassium loss and weight gain. When therapy with dexamethasone is to be discontinued after long use, the dosage should be reduced gradually. The administration of ACTH during the period of gradual dosage reduction may help to accelerate the return of normal adrenocortical function.
Side Effects: Side reactions such as weight loss, anorexia, diarrhea, polydipsia, and polyuria have been frequently observed during corticosteroid therapy.
Warning: Studies have demonstrated that corticosteroids may cause abortion or premature birth when given in the last trimester of pregnancy and may also lead to difficulty in giving birth, death of fetus, retained afterbirth, and infection of uterus. Therefore, to prevent these side-effects, this preparation should not be given during the last trimester of pregnancy.
Caution: Federal law restricts this drug to use by or on the order of a licensed veterinarian.
How Supplied: Bottles of 1000.

DXT–500
Sterile 50% Dextrose Solution

Composition: Dextrose 500 grams/liter, methyl parahydroxybenzoate (.90 mg/ml) and propyl parahydroxybenzoate (.10 mg/ml) as preservatives.
Indications: Ketosis of dairy cattle and general supportive therapy.
Suggested Dosage: ***Adult cattle*** 50 to 500 ml, ***Calves*** 25 to 150 ml; ***Small animals*** 10 to 50 ml., depending on size and condition. Administer intravenously only. May be diluted with distilled water or normal saline as required.
How Supplied: 500 ml (cc) bottles

O

DYREA–AID PALATABS®

Composition: Each chewable tablet contains: colloidal attapulgite, colloidal aluminum silicate, aluminum hydroxide, kaolin, calcium carbonate, sodium bicarbonate, pectin, and 0.1 mg methyl atropine nitrate in a protein chewable base.
Indications: Dyrea-Aid is used as an aid in the control of non-specific diarrhea in dogs.
Contraindications: Dyrea-Aid should not be used in dogs with glaucoma because of its possible mydriatic effect.
Dosage and Administration: ***Dogs*** —One chewable tablet per 10 pound body weight twice daily. Tablet may be given directly by mouth or crumbled and mixed with food.
Warning: If symptoms persist after using this product for 2 to 3 days, the diagnosis should be redetermined.
How Supplied: Bottles of 50's and 350's.

ELPAK–360™
Balanced Oral Electrolytes for calves and pigs.

Composition: When Elpak-360 is diluted with 2 quarts water, the solution contains:
Sodium (Na) 120 mEq/L; Potassium (K) 10 mEq/L; Bicarbonate (HCO_3) 40 mEq/L; Chloride (Cl) 70 mEq/L; Calcium (Ca) 10 mEq/L; Magnesium (Mg) 5 mEq/L; Sulfate (SO_4) 5 mEq/L; Dextrose 56 mM/L; Glycine 40 mM/L.
Indications: A concentrated electrolyte product fortified with dextrose, glycine and bicarbonate for oral administration.
Directions for Use: Dissolve contents of one packet in 2 quarts of warm water. Administer 2 quarts of solution per calf 2 to 3 times a day. Prepare fresh solution daily.
When mixed as directed, the resulting solution containing electrolytes, dextrose and glycine is approximately 360 mOsm/Liter which is near isotonicity for plasma and at a desirable level for optimal absorption.
Keep in cool dry place.
How Supplied: 60 grams.

ENDOMAGMA™ BOLUSES
Antidiarrhetic, Adsorbent, Demulcent

Composition: Each bolus contains Activated Attapulgite with Roasted Powdered Carob Pulp, Citrus Pectin, Magnesium Trisilicate and Colloidal Aluminum Silicate (Hydrated).

Continued on next page

Osborn—Cont.

Dosage: ***Horses***—½ to 1 bolus. ***Cattle***—1 to 1½ boluses. ***Colts and Calves***—½ bolus. Repeat at 4 hour intervals if indicated.
Endomagma is relatively non-toxic and may be given freely in amounts to effect.
How Supplied: Jars of 50 boluses.

ENDOMAGMA™ POWDER

Description: An adsorbent, anti-diarrhetic, demulcent formula for all animals.
How Supplied: 1 lb.

EQUI-LYTE™ CONCENTRATE

A Concentrated Replacement Electrolyte Solution Especially Formulated for Horses. Must be Diluted Prior to Use.

Composition: Sodium (Na) 1450 mEq/Liter; Potassium (K) 50 mEq/Liter; Calcium (Ca) 60 mEq/Liter; Magnesium (Mg) 30 mEq/Liter; Chloride (Cl) 1040 mEq/Liter; Dextrose 200 Calories/Liter.
Indications: To be used as a replacement electrolyte solution during electrolyte depletion and dehydration in horses.
Directions: Dilute 1 part Equi-Lyte™ Concentrate to 9 parts water (2 quarts to 5 gallons) for injection using aseptic techniques. The diluted solution contains the following electrolytes: Sodium (Na) mEq/L 145; Potassium (K) mEq/L 5; Calcium (Ca) mEq/L 6; Magnesium (Mg) mEq/L 3; Chloride (Cl) mEq/L 104; Dextrose 20 Cal/Liter.
Suggested Diluted Dosage: *Ponies:* 300–900 ml. *Horses:* 900–1800 ml.
Administer intravenously avoiding rapid administration. Repeat as indicated by the degree of dehydration.
Caution: This product is highly concentrated and must be diluted prior to use. It is recommended that solutions be diluted just prior to use.
How Supplied: 1 Qt.

EQUI-LYTE™ SOLUTION

A Replacement Electrolyte Solution Especially Formulated for Horses with 5% Dextrose. Sterile.

Composition: Sodium (Na) 145 mEq/Liter; Potassium (K) 5 mEq/Liter; Calcium (Ca) 6 mEq/Liter; Magnesium (Mg) 3 mEq/Liter; Dextrose 200 Calories/Liter; Chloride (Cl) 104 mEq/Liter.
Suggested Dosage: *Horses*—900–1800 ml. *Ponies*—300–900 ml.
Administer intravenously avoiding rapid administration. Repeat as indicated by the degree of dehydration.
How Supplied: 900 ml. Bottles.

IVS-1830®

Hypertonic Dextrose Buffered with Electrolytes and Fortified with Amino Acids. Sterile.

Composition: Dextrose (grams/liter) 275; Sodium (Na) (mEq/liter) 130; Potassium (K) (mEq/liter) 10; Calcium (Ca) (mEq/liter) 4.5; Magnesium (Mg) (mEq/liter) 2.75; Chloride (mEq/liter) 102; Glutamic Acid (mg./liter) 280; L-Arginine (mg/liter) 225; L-Histidine (mg/liter) 20; L-Leucine (mg/liter) 80; L-Iso-Leucine (mg/liter) 35; L-Lysine (mg/liter) 120; L—Methionine (mg/liter) 20; L-Phenylalnine (mg/liter) 55; L-Threonine (mg/liter) 50; L-Tyrosine (mg/liter) 12; L-Valine (mg/liter) 55; L-Proline (mg/liter) 200.
Indications: Ketosis of dairy animals and general supportive therapy and as an aid in correction of electrolyte depletion.
Ingredients: Dextrose (d-Glucose), Sodium Acetate, Sodium Chloride, Potassium Acetate, Calcium Chloride, Magnesium Chloride, Amino Acids.
Suggested Dosage: *Adult Cattle*—900 ml *Calves*—100-300 ml depending upon size. Administer intravenously only, avoiding rapid administration. May be repeated as indicated.
How Supplied: 900 ml bottles.

KALAMINO™

**Calcium Buffered with Electrolytes and Fortified with Amino Acids and Dextrose.
STERILE.**

Composition: Calcium (mEq./liter) 425; Phosphorus (mEq./liter) 425; Chloride (mEq./liter) 235; Potassium (mEq./-liter) 204; Sodium (mEq./liter) 35; Dextrose (Calories/liter) 1,000; L-Arginine (mg./liter) 225; Glutamic Acid (mg./liter) 280; L-Histidine (mg./liter) 20; L-Leucine (mg./liter) 80; IsoLeucine (mg./liter) 35; L-Lysine (mg./liter) 120; L-Methionine (mg./liter) 20; L-Phenylalanine (mg./liter) 55; L-Threonine (mg./liter) 50; L-Tyrosine (mg./liter) 12; L-Valine (mg./liter) 55; L-Proline (mg./liter) 200.
Ingredients: Calcium Hypophosphite, Potassium Phosphate, Potassium and Sodium Chlorides, Dextrose (d-Glucose), Amino Acids.
Indications: An aid in correction of blood electrolyte levels in hypocalcemic conditions in bovine.
Suggested Dosage: Dairy Cows—450 to 900 ml. Administer intravenously, avoiding rapid administration.
Caution: Federal law restricts this drug to use by or on the order of a veterinarian.
How Supplied: 900 ml Bottles.

KAL-K-DEX®

**Calcium Buffered with Electrolytes and Fortified with Potassium, Phosphorus and Dextrose.
Sterile.**

Composition: Calcium (mEq/liter) 425; Phosphorus (mEq/liter) 425; Chloride (mEq/ liter) 235; Potassium (mEq/-liter) 204; Magnesium (mEq/liter) 3; Sodium (mEq/liter) 35; Dextrose (Calories/-liter) 1,000.
Ingredients: Calcium Hypophosphite, Potassium Phosphate, Magnesium Chloride, Potassium and Sodium Chlorides, Dextrose (d-Glucose).
Indications: As an aid in the correction of blood electrolyte levels in hypocalcemic conditions in dairy cows.
Suggested Dosage: Dairy Cows—450 to 900 ml. Administer intravenously.
How Supplied: 900 ml Bottles.

KETOBAN™

An Oral Glucogenic Formula for the Prevention and Treatment of Ketosis (Acetonemia) in Dairy Cattle

Composition: Choline; Propylene Glycol; Cobalt; Sulfate, Heptahydrate; Saccharin Sodium; Sorbitol; Artificial Flavor and Color.
Directions: Administer orally as drench, in the drinking water, on silage or mixed in the grain ration.
Preventing Relapses: As an aid in preventing relapses and as a follow-up treatment in acetonemia, administer from 3 to 6 fluid ounces once or twice a day for 5 to 7 days.
Preventing Expected Cases: To aid in the prevention of ketosis in dairy cows, begin administering on feed, a few days before calving, and continue for 2 to 6 weeks or as indicated.
Treatment: Depending upon the severity of the case, administer from ½ to 1 pint (8 to 16 fluid ounces) twice daily for the first day; thereafter, give from ¼to ½ pint twice daily for 3 to 5 days.
How Supplied: 1 gal jugs; 55 gallon jugs.

LBA BOLUS

Description: Bolus containing live microbial cultures with Lactobacillus for all animals.
How Supplied: 50's

LBA-GEL

Description: Lactobacillus Gel for all animals
How Supplied: 30 cc dose syringe

LBA POWDER

Description: Water Dispersible microbial culture containing Lactobacillus for all animals.
How Supplied: 1 lb.

MAGNADEX™

**Magnesium Buffered with Electrolytes and Fortified with Calcium, Phosphorus and Dextrose.
Sterile.**

Composition: Magnesium (mEq./liter) 160; Phosphorus (mEq./liter) 185; Potassium (mEq./liter) 5; Calcium (mEq./liter) 200; Sodium (mEq./liter) 140; Dextrose (calories/liter) 400.
Indications: An aid in the correction of blood electrolyte levels in Hypomagnesimic conditions of cattle, such as the the Grass Tetany Syndrome.
Ingredients: Magnesium Chloride, Calcium Hypophosphite, Sodium Chloride, Sodium and Potassium Acetates, Dextrose (d-Glucose).
Suggested Dosage: Cattle 450 to 900 ml. administer intravenously only, avoiding rapid administration. Repeat as indicated.
How Supplied: 900 ml. bottles.

MED-A-SUL™
Soluble Sulfonamide Arsenical Salt, Electrolytes and Vitamin Foritifed.

Composition: Each 8 ounces contains: Active Ingredients: Sodium Sulfathiazole 22.0%, Sodium Arsanilate Anhydrous 24.0% (equiv. to 263.26 gr. elemental arsenic).
Inactive Ingredients: Vitamin A, Vitamin D-3, Menadione Sodium Bisulfite, Calcium Pantothenate, Niacin, Riboflavin, Thiamin, in an electrolyte base composed of Potassium Acetate, Sodium Acetate, Sodium Chloride, Potassium Chloride, Magnesium Sulfate, Calcium Lactate and Flavoring Agents.
Indications: As an aid in the control and treatment of swine dysentery.
Dosage and Administration: Mix contents of container (8 ounces) in sufficient hot water to make one gallon of stock solution.
Treatment: First Day: Mix one pint of stock solution in each 10 gallons of fresh drinking water, allowing free access.
Second and third days: Mix one pint of stock solution in each 20 gallons of fresh drinking water, allowing free access.
Caution: Sulfonamides may cause severe toxic reactions and irreparable damage if blood levels become too high. Constant supervision of animals is essential during treatment. Discontinue treatment if toxic symptoms appear.
Warning: Use as sole source of organic arsenic. Discontinue treatment at least 10 days before animals are marketed for human consumption.
NOTE: Poisonous if swallowed. Induce vomiting. Administer 10% sodium thiosulfate solution by mouth. Avoid breathing dust or spray mist. Avoid contact with skin, eyes and clothing. Wash thoroughly after handling.
How Supplied: 8 oz. (½lb.)

MER-A-LITE® G
Soluble Sulfa Granules

Composition: Each Pound Contains: Sodium Sulfathiazole (NF equivalent)312 grams Electrolytes-Sodium and Potassium Chlorides, Calcium Hypophosphite, Sodium Citrate, Magnesium Sulfate, Solubilizers, Flavoring Agents and Artificial Color.
An instantly soluble granule designed as a water medication for cattle, swine, sheep, poultry and horses. Use as an aid in the treatment of bacterial enteritis, hemorrhagic septicemia and pneumonia in swine. Shipping fever complex, pneumonia foot rot (pododermatitis) of beef cattle, calf diphtheria, pyosepticemia (navel ill) in horses and infectious coryza of poultry.
Dosage and Administration: To prepare stock solution:
Mix contents of package (one pound) in sufficient very hot water (just short of boiling, 200 degrees F) to make one gallon of stock solution. Prepare immediately prior to use and shake well before using. Administer as follows:
[See table above].
Warning: Hazardous —As with all sulfonamides, overdosage may cause toxic

	Pints of Stock Solution	Gallons of Drinking Water First Day	Thereafter
Swine	1	4 to 6	6 gals.
Beef Cattle	1	5 to 10	10 to 20
Sheep*	1	10 to 15	20 to 30
Horses	1	10 to 15	20 to 30
Poultry	1	5 gals.	5 gals.

Maximum treatment period, 4 days

reactions. Discontinue treatment if prolonged depression, blood-tinged urine or cloudy urine are noted. Continuous veterinary supervision is essential.
Not for use in lactating dairy animals since this will result in contamination of the milk.
Discontinue treatment at least 10 days before treated animals are marketed for human consumption.
How Supplied: One Pound, 25 Pound

METHAPYRIN® BOLUSES

Composition: Each Bolus contains;
Active Ingredients: Sulfamethazine 37.5 gr.; Neomycin Base 175.0 mg.; Pyrilamine Maleate 10.0 mg.; Methyl Atropine Nitrate 1.0 mg.
Inactive Ingredients: Vitamin A 10,000 U.S.P. units; Sodium Ascorbate 12.5 mg. and Electrolytes.
Indications: For treatment of enzootic pneumonia, pneumoenteritis, bacterial pneumonia and bacterial enteritis in calves.
Dosage and Administration: *Initial Dose:* Give 2 boluses for each 100 lbs. Repeat dose 12 hours later the first day.
Follow-up Dose: Give 1½ boluses for each 100 lbs. at 12 hour intervals.
Notice: Supply adequate quantities of drinking water at all times. If improvement is not noted within 2 to 3 days of therapy, reconsult a veterinarian. Do not administer over 4 days.
Caution: This drug, like all Sulfonamides, may cause toxic reactions and irreparable injury unless administered with adequate and continuous supervision.
Warning: Discontinue treatment at least 30 days before animals are marketed for human consumption.
How Supplied: Jars of 50 boluses.

METHIONINE PALATABS®

Composition: Each chewable tablet contains, 500 mg D-L Methionine in a protein chewable base.
Indications: For use as an aid to acidify the urine of dogs and cats and to control the ammoniacal odor of urine.
Contraindications: Not for use in animals with severe liver or kidney damage.
Dosage and Administration: Give ½ tablet per 20 pounds of body weight, 2 to 3 times a day.
Methionine Palatabs may be given freely by hand or crumbled and mixed with food.
For optimal results, Methionine Palatabs should be given after food to lessen the chance of stomach upsets.
How Supplied: Bottle of 50's

NITROZONE™ OINTMENT
Topical Antibacterial Ointment

Composition: Contains 0.2% Nitrofurazone in a water soluble base.
Indications: For the prevention or treatment of surface infections of wounds, burns, cutaneous ulcers, by organisms sensitive to nitrofurazone. For use on dogs, cats and horses.
Administration: Apply directly on the lesion with a spatula or on a piece of gauze. This preparation should be in contact with the lesion for at least 24 hours. The dressing may be changed several times daily or left on the lesion for a longer period.
How Supplied: 1 lb.

NRG–PLUS™
Nutritional Concentrate

Composition: Crude Protein, not less than 9%; Crude Fat, not less than 0.25%; Crude Fiber, not more than 1%.
Indications: NRG-Plus provides readily available metabolic sources of amino acids, energy, vitamins, electrolytes and minerals for use in cattle which are convalescent, sick or anorectic. NRG-Plus is also of value as a drench in cattle which have been shipped for substantial distances and are dehydrated.
Dosage and Administration: ***Calves:*** administer 2–4 oz. in 1 gallon of water at the rate of 2 quarts per calf. Repeat 2–3 times daily as indicated. ***Cattle:*** administer 1 lb. for each 1000 lbs. body weight through a stomach tube as a drench. Suspend in at least ½ gal. of warm water.
How Supplied: 4 oz., 1 lb., 20 lb.

PLEXAMINO®
Amino Acids Buffered with Electrolytes and Fortified with B-Complex Vitamins and Dextrose. Sterile.

Composition: Sodium (Na) 140 mEq/L; Potassium (K) 10 mEq/L; Calcium (Ca) 5 mEq/L; Magnesium (Mg)3 mEq/L; Chloride (Cl) 130 mEq/L; Dextrose 200 Calories/L; Thiamine HCl 50 mg./L; Riboflavin 5-Phosphate 10 mg/L; Nicotinamide 10 mg/L; Pyridoxine HCl 20 mg/L; L-Arginine 225 mg/L; Glutamic Acid 280 mg/L; L-Histidine 20 mg/L; L-Leucine 80 mg/L; L-Isoleucine 35 mg/L; L-Lysine 120 mg/L; L-Methionine 20 mg/L; L-Phenylalanine 55 mg/L; L-Threonine 50 mg/L; L-Tyrosine 12 mg/L; L-Valine 55 mg/L; L-Proline 200 mg/L.
Ingredients: Sodium Acetate, Sodium Chloride, Potassium Acetate, Calcium Chloride, Magnesium Chloride, Dextrose (d-Glucose), Amino Acids, Thiamine HCl,

Continued on next page

Osborn—Cont.

Riboflavin 5-Phosphate, Nicotinamide, Pyridoxine HCl.
Indications: As an aid in the correction of electrolyte depletion, dehydration and as an aid in the correction of negative nitrogen balance in the bovine.
Dosage and Administration: ***Calves*** —200-300 ml. ***Cattle*** —900-1800 ml. Administer intravenously avoiding rapid administration. Repeat as indicated by the degree of dehydration.
How Supplied: 900 ml Bottles

PLEXAMINO BOLUS™
Balanced Amino Acid Formula

Composition: Each bolus contains: Enzymatic Protein Hydrolysate 11.00g., Vitamin A Acetate, d-Activated Animal Sterol, dl-Alpha Tocopheryl Acetate, Vitamin B_{12}, Riboflavin, d-Calcium Pantothenate, Choline Bitartrate, Niacin, Menadione Sodium Bisulfite Complex, Folic Acid, Thiamin Mononitrate, Pyridoxine Hydrochloride, Ascorbic Acid, Dextrose, Sucrose, Ethylenediamine dihydriodide chelates of Iron (Fe), Manganese (Mn), Copper (Cu), Cobalt (Co) and Zinc (Zn) with the electrolytes Sodium (Na) and Potassium (K).
Indications: Plexamino has been formulated to provide a readily available source of amino acids, carbohydrates, vitamins and trace minerals as an aid in nutritional support for cattle. Plexamino Bolus is of value to aid in rehabilitation following specific therapy.
Directions: *Cattle, Calves:* Administer orally 1 to 2 boluses for each 200 pounds of body weight, depending upon the severity of the condition and the animal's daily nutritional intake. Dosage may be doubled where severe nutritional upset indicates increased fortification. The bolus may be given by means of a balling gun, or crushed and mixed with other feed or crushed and mixed with milk. Store boluses in a dry place avoiding excess humidity. Keep box closed when not in use.
How Supplied: 50's

SG-SEVEN®
Sulfonamide Solution for Oral Veterinary Use

Composition: Each ml contains: Sulfamerazine 20 mg, Sulfathiazole 45 mg and Sulfamethazine 45 mg as a complex of dextrose with methyl, propyl and butyl-p-hydroxybenzoates (calculated as derivatives of methyl parahydroxy benzoate) as preservatives 0.25%. The total sulfonamide content of this product is approximately equivalent to a solution of 12.5% of sodium sulfonamides.
Indications: SG-Seven is indicated for large animal therapy and treatment of infections in which the causative agent is sensitive to sulfonamides.
Dosage and Administration: ***Swine:*** For treatment of bacterial enteritis, pneumonia and other respiratory infections of bacterial origin and sensitive to sulfonamide therapy. Add 60 ml (2 fl oz) of SG-Seven to each gallon of drinking water and use as sole source of drinking water for 3 to 5 days.
Cattle: For treatment of shipping fever, foot rot, bacterial enteritis and upper respiratory infections of bacterial origin and sensitive to sulfonamide therapy. The initial loading dosage is 0.9 ml per lb body weight for the first day followed by subsequent dosage of 0.45 ml per lb body weight every 12 hours for the next 4 days. SG-Seven may be administered in the drinking water as the sole source of drinking water at a level of 60 ml (2 fl oz) SG-Seven per gallon of drinking water.
Note: 1 ml of SG-Seven contains the equivalent of approximately 1.69 grains of total Sodium Sulfonamides.
Warning: Do not administer SG-Seven more than 5 consecutive days. If symptoms of sulfonamide toxicity appear, discontinue use and force fluids to facilitate elimination of the drug.
Warning: Milk taken from treated animals within 96 hours (8 milkings) after the latest treatment, must not be used for food. Do not market treated swine for food within 15 days of the last treatment. Do not market other treated animals for food within 10 days of the last treatment.
How Supplied: 1 gal jugs.

SUSTAIN III
Sulfamethazine Sustained Release Bolus

Composition: Each bolus contains: Sulfamethazine (Formulated in a sustained release base) 495 grains (32.1 grams)
Indications: Sustain III Boluses (Sulfamethazine Sustained Release Boluses) are intended for oral administration to beef cattle and non-lactating dairy cattle. Sustain III boluses are indicated for the treatment of the following diseases when caused by one or more of the following pathogenic organisms sensitive to sulfamethazine: Bacterial Pneumonia and Bovine Respiratory Disease Complex (Shipping Fever Complex) *(Pasteurella spp),* Colibacillosis (Bacterial Scours) *(E. coli),* Necrotic pododermatitis (Foot rot) *(Fusobacterium necrophorum)* Calf Diphtheria *(Fusobacterium necrophorum),* Acute Mastitis *(Streptococcus spp.)* Acute Metritis *(Streptococcus spp).*
Dosage and Administration: Sustain III boluses are designed to be administered orally to beef cattle and non-lactating dairy cattle. Sustain III boluses should be given at a rate of one bolus per 200 lbs. body weight.
The bolus may be divided for better approximation of correct dose, however, care should be taken not to crush the bolus. Care should also be taken to insure the entire dose has been swallowed by the animal. Observe animals following administration to insure boluses are not regurgitated. Lubricate Sustain III before dosing animals.
Sustain III boluses are designed to provide a therapeutic sulfamethazine level in approximately 6 hours, and persist in providing this level for 72 hours (3 days). After 72 hours, all animals should be re-examined for persistence of observable disease signs. If signs are present, re-consult your veterinarian. It is strongly recommended that a second dose be given to provide for an additional 72 hours of therapy, particularly in those more severe cases. The above dose schedule should be used at each 72 hour interval.
Animals should not receive more than 2 doses of Sustain III boluses because of the possibility of incurring residue violations.
Caution: This drug, like all sulfonamides, may cause toxic reactions and irreparable injury unless administered with adequate and continuous supervision, follow recommended dosages carefully.
Fluid intake must be adquate at all times throughout the three day therapy provided by the sustained release bolus.
Warning: Do not use in lactating dairy cattle. Animals intended for human consumption should not be slaughtered for food for at least 12 days after the last dose.
How Supplied: Box of 5-10 Paks (50 Boluses)
Box of 50 Boluses and
Box of 100 Boluses

SUSTAIN III™ CALF BOLUS
Sulfamethazine Sustained Release

Composition: Each bolus contains 8.02 grams sulfamethazine in a sustained release base.
Indications: Sustain III™ Calf Boluses are intended for oral administration only to ruminating replacement calves (calves over one month old that are not on a milk diet). Sustain III™ Calf Boluses are indicated for the treatment of the following diseases when caused by one or more of the following pathogenic organisms sensitive to sulfamethazine: Bacterial Pneumonia *(Pasteurella spp),* *Colibacillosis* (Bacterial Scours) *(E.Coli),* and Calf Diphtheria *(Fusobacterium Necrophorum).*
Dosage and Administration: Sustain III™ Calf Boluses are to be given at a rate of two boluses per 100 lbs. body weight. This bolus may be divided for better approximation of correct dose, however, care should be taken not to crush the bolus. Care should be taken to insure the entire dose has been swallowed by the animal. Observe animals following administration to insure boluses are not regurgitated. Lubricate bolus before dosing animals. Sustain III™ Calf Boluses are designed to provide a therapeutic sulfamethazine level in approximately 6 hours, and persist in providing this level for 72 hours (3 days). After 72 hours, all animals should be re-examined for persistence of observable disease signs. If signs are present, consult a veterinarian. It is strongly recommended that a second dose be given to provide for an additional 72 hours of therapy, particularly in those more severe cases. The above schedule should be used at each 72 hour interval.
Caution: This drug, like all sulfonamides, may cause toxic reactions and irreparable injury unless administered

with adequate and continuous supervision: follow recommended dosage carefully.
Fluid intake must be adequate at all times throughout the three day therapy provided by the sustained release bolus. This product has not been shown to be effective for non-ruminating calves.
Warning: Treated animals must not be slaughtered for food for at least 12 days after the last dose. Exceeding two consecutive doses may cause violative tissue residue to remain beyond the withdrawal time. Do not use in calves under one month of age or calves fed an all milk diet. Use in these classes of calves may cause violative tissue residue to remain beyond the withdrawal time.
How Supplied: Bottles of 25's.
Box of 50's.

TRIPLE SULFA-699™ BOLUSES

Composition: Each bolus contains: Sulfamethazine 60 gr.; Sulfathiazole 90 gr.; Sulfanilamide 90 gr.
Indications: For oral administration to non-lactating cattle as an aid in treatment of shipping fever (hemorrhagic septicemia), foot rot, calf diphtheria, acute metritis, bacterial enteritis, peritonitis, nephritis, calf scours and other bacterial infections caused by organisms susceptible to the bacteriostatic action of these sulfonamides.
Dosage and Administration: Give 1½ boluses for each 240 lbs. of body weight as initial dose. Thereafter, give ½ bolus for each 240 lbs. of body weight, every 8 to 12 hours, until the temperature has been normal for at least 48 hours.
Notice: Supply adequate quantities of drinking water at all times.
Caution: This drug, like all Sulfonamides, may cause toxic reactions and irreparable injury unless administered with adequate and continuous supervision.
Warning: Discontinue treatment at least 10 days before animals are marketed for human consumption.
How Supplied: Jars of 50 boluses.

TS-543™
Triple Sulfa Oral Solution

Composition: Sulfamethazine Sodium 4.0% w/v; Sulfathiazole Sodium 5.0% w/v; Sulfamerazine Sodium 3.0% w/v.
Indications: For oral administration as an aid in the treatment of bacterial pneumonia of cattle, foot-rot, acute metritis, calf diphtheria and secondary infections in calf scours; bacterial pneumonia of swine and secondary infections associated with respiratory infections; shipping fever of sheep; strangles and secondary bacterial infections associated with respiratory infections in horses; coccidiosis of chickens and turkeys (E. tenella, E. necatrix, E. Acervulina, E. meleagrimitis, E. gallopavonis).
Dosage and Administration: *Cattle, Calves, Sheep and Horses —Dosage:-*
Administer orally 80 ml (approx. 3 fluid ounces) for each 100 pounds of body weight as the initial dose. Follow with 25 to 27 ml (approx. 1 fluid ounce) for each 100 pounds of body weight, every 12 hours, until the temperature has been normal for 48 hours. Give animals, up to one week of age, two-thirds the above dosage schedules. Discontinue treatment after 4 days. Calculated dosage may be given as a drench, or in drinking water.
Caution: This preparation, like all sulfonamides, may cause toxic reactions. It should be administered under adequate supervision and sufficient drinking water should be provided at all times. If any signs of toxicity appear, discontinue the drug.
Warning: Milk taken from treated animals within 96 hours (8 milkings) after the latest treatment, must not be used for food. Do not market treated swine for food within 15 days of the last treatment. Do not market other treated animals for food within 10 days of the last treatment.
How Supplied: 1 gal.

VICETON™ TABLETS
(chloramphenicol)

Description: Chloramphenicol is a broad- spectrum antibiotic shown to have specific therapeutic activity against a wide variety of organisms.
Actions: At low concentrations, chloramphenicol exerts a bacteriostatic effect on a wide range of pathogenic organisms, including many Gram-positive and Gram-negative bacteria, spirochetes, several rickettsiae and certain large viruses and Mycoplasma (PPLO). At high concentrations, it inhibits growth of animal and plant cells.
Chloramphenicol exerts its bacteriostatic action by inhibiting protein synthesis in susceptible organisms. Complete suppression of the assimilation of ammonia and of the incorporation of amino acids, particularly glutamic acid, together with an increased formation of ribonucleic acid (RNA), lead to an inhibition of bacterial growth.
Chloramphenicol antagonizes the action of such antibiotics as penicillin and streptomycin, which act only on growing cells, but is synergistic to tetracycline, which also acts by inhibiting protein synthesis. It is possible the chloramphenicol would produce similar synergism with other antibiotics which act by inhibiting protein synthesis.
In this respect, the experimentally demonstrated synergistic action between chloramphenicol and gamma-globulin should be mentioned. Clinical observations in man and corresponding investigations in laboratory animals experimentally infected with various pathogenic bacteria have shown that a combination of chloramphenicol with gamma-globulin or specific antisera has a greater therapeutic effect than would be expected from a mere addition of the individual effects.
Many experiments have revealed that the development of resistance to chloramphenicol is rare compared with that occurring with other important antibiotics. Bacterial resistance may develop in some strains against chloramphenicol but has been encountered only in-frequently in clinical usage.
Chloramphenicol achieves maximum serum levels very rapidly following, oral, intravenous and intraperitoneal administration. Intramuscular injection with chloramphenicol, except certain soluble forms, results in a somewhat delayed absorption and lower serum levels than when given by the oral, intravenous or intraperitoneal route.
Chloramphenicol diffuses readily into all body tissues, but at different concentrations. Highest concentrations are found in the liver and kidney of dogs indicating that these organs are the main route of inactivation and excretion for the metabolites. The lungs, spleen, heart and skeletal muscles contain concentrations similar to that of the blood.
Chloramphenicol reaches significant concentration in the acqueous and vitreous humors of the eye from the blood.
A significant difference from other antibiotics is its marked ability to diffuse into the cerebrospinal fluid. Within three to four hours after administration, the concentration in the cerebrospinal fluid has reached, on the average, 50% of the concentration in the serum. If the meninges are inflamed, the percentage may be even higher.
Chloramphenicol diffuses readily into milk, pleural and ascitic fluids and crosses the placenta attaining concentrations of about 75% of that of the maternal blood.
Chloramphenicol is rather rapidly metabolized, mainly in the liver, by conjugation with glucuronic acid.
Approximately 55% of a single daily dose can be recovered from the urine of a treated dog. A small fraction of this is in the form of unchanged chloramphenicol.
A single intravenous dose of 150 mg/kg (approximately 68 mg/lb) in propylene glycol is the maximum dose tolerated by the dog. No toxic effect was observed when dogs were administered orally, 200 mg/kg (approximately 91 mg/lb) daily for over four months. In the mouse, the $LD_{50}$is 150-250 mg/kg (68 to 114 mg/lb) body wt by intravenous injection and 1,500 mg/kg (approximately 681 mg/lb) by the oral administration.
Indications: Viceton (Chloramphenicol) tablets are indicated for treatment of the following conditions in dogs caused by susceptible microorganisms:
Bacterial gastro-enteritis associated with bacterial diahrrea, bacterial infections of the urinary tract and bacterial pulmonary infections.
Additional adjunctive therapy should be used when indicated. Most susceptible infectious disease organisms will respond to chloramphenicol therapy in three to five days when the recommended dosage regime is followed.
Laboratory tests should be conducted including in vitro culturing and susceptibility tests on samples collected prior to treatment.
If no response to chloramphenicol therapy is obtained in three to five days, dis-

Continued on next page

Osborn—Cont.

continue its use and review the diagnosis. Also, change of therapy should be considered.

Contraindications: Because of potential antagonism, chloramphenicol should not be administered simultaneously with penicillin or streptomycin.

Warning: Not for use in animals which are raised for food production. Chloramphenicol products should not be administered in conjunction with or 2 hours prior to the induction of general anesthesia with pentobarbital because of prolonged recovery.

Chloramphenicol should not be administered to dogs maintained for breeding purposes.

Hazards and precautions:

1. This antibiotic contains a chemical structure (nitrobenzene group) that is characteristic of a group of drugs long known to depress hematopoietic activity of the bone marrow.
2. *In vitro* tissue culture studies using canine bone marrow cells have demonstrated that extremely high concentration of chloramphenicol inhibit both uptake of iron by the nucleated red cells and incorporation of iron into heme.
3. Chloramphenical products should not be administered in conjunction with or two hours prior to the induction of general anesthesia with pentobarbital because of prolonged recovery time.
4. Chloramphenicol products should not be administered to dogs maintained for breeding purposes. Some experiments indicate that chloramphenicol causes, in experimental animals, particularly females, significant disorders in morphology as well as in function of the gonads.

Adverse Reactions: Certain individual dogs may exhibit transient vomiting or diarrhea after an oral dose of 25 mg/lb body wt.

Dosage and Administration:
Dogs —25 mg/lb body wt every 6 hours for oral administration.

Caution: Federal law restricts this drug to use by or on the order of a licensed veterinarian. Keep out of reach of children.

How Supplied:
500 mg tablets: 100's, 500's
250 mg tablets: 500's, 1000's
100 mg tablets: 500's

IDENTIFICATION PROBLEM?
Consult the
Product Identification Section
where you'll find
products pictured
in full color.

Pfizer Inc.

Agricultural Division
235 EAST 42ND STREET
NEW YORK, NY 10017

COMBIOTIC®
(penicillin and dihydrostreptomycin in aqueous suspension)
For Intramuscular Use Only

Composition: Combiotic is a highly effective antimicrobial preparation containing procaine penicillin and dihydrostreptomycin as the sulfate. Each ml of this suspension contains 200,000 units of procaine penicillin G and dihydrostreptomycin sulfate equivalent to 250 mg dihydrostreptomycin base. Penicillin is a potent antibiotic possessing a high degree of activity chiefly against organisms in the gram-positive category. Dihydrostreptomycin is a potent antibiotic possessing a high degree of activity chiefly against organisms in the gram-negative category. The combination permits treatment of many mixed bacterial infections with the convenience of a single dosage form.

Indications: *Cattle:* Actinomycosis; bronchitis; calf diphtheria; foot rot; joint infections; leptospirosis; mastitis; metritis; navel infections; pleurisy; pneumonia; shipping fever; systemic bacterial complications associated with scours; tracheitis; wound infections, and other infections caused by or associated with penicillin- and dihydrostreptomycin-susceptible organisms.

Swine: Bronchitis, leptospirosis; mastitis; metritis; pleurisy; pneumonia; systemic bacterial complications associated with scours; tracheitis; wound infections, and other infections caused by or associated with penicillin- and dihydrostreptomycin-susceptible organisms.

Sheep: Joint infections; leptospirosis; mastitis; metritis; navel infections; shipping fever; pneumonia; systemic bacterial complications associated with scours; tularemia; wound infections, and other infections caused by or associated with penicillin- and dihydrostreptomycin-susceptible organisms.

Horses: Bacterial complications associated with influenza; bronchitis; joint infections; metritis; navel infections; pleurisy; pneumonia; shipping fever; systemic bacterial complications associated with scours; wound infections, and other infections caused by or associated with penicillin- and dihydrostreptomycin-susceptible organisms.

Small Animals (dogs, cats, rabbits, foxes): Bacterial complications associated with viral diseases, such as those in distemper; bronchitis; middle ear infections; leptospirosis; metritis; pleurisy; pneumonia; snuffles; sore hocks; systemic bacterial complications associated with enteritis; tracheitis; tularemia; wound infections, and other infections caused by or associated with penicillin-and dihydrostreptomycin-susceptible organisms.

RECOMMENDED DAILY DOSAGE

Continue treatment for 1 to 2 days after symptoms disappear.

CATTLE	
Body Weight	Dosage
Up to 100 lbs.	2 ml
100 to 300 lbs.	2 to 6 ml
300 to 700 lbs.	6 to 10 ml
700 lbs. or over	10 to 15 ml
SWINE	
Body Weight	Dosage
8 to 10 lbs.	¼ to ½ ml
10 to 20 lbs.	½ to 1 ml
20 to 40 lbs.	1 to 2 ml
40 to 100 lbs.	2 to 4 ml
100 to 200 lbs.	4 to 6 ml
200 lbs. or over	6 to 10 ml
SHEEP	
Body Weight	Dosage
8 to 10 lbs.	¼ to ½ ml
10 to 20 lbs.	½ to 1 ml
20 to 50 lbs.	1 to 2 ml
50 lbs. or over	2 to 6 ml
HORSES	
Body Weight	Dosage
Up to 300 lbs.	4 to 8 ml
300 to 600 lbs.	8 to 10 ml
600 lbs. or over	10 to 15 ml
SMALL ANIMALS (dogs, cats, rabbits, foxes)	
Body Weight	Dosage
3 to 5 lbs.	1/8 to ¼ ml
5 to 10 lbs.	¼ to ½ ml
10 to 15 lbs.	½ to ¾ ml
15 to 20 lbs.	¾ to 1 ml
20 to 25 lbs.	1 to 1¼ ml
25 to 50 lbs.	1¼ to 2 ml
50 to 75 lbs.	2 to 3 ml
75 lbs. or over	3 to 4 ml

Caution: 1. Combiotic Aqueous Suspension should be injected deep within the fleshy muscles of the hip, rump, round or thigh. Do *not* inject this material subcutaneously, into a blood vessel, or near a major nerve.

2. When properly used in the treatment of diseases caused by susceptible organisms, most sick animals that have been treated with antibiotics show a noticeable improvement within 48 hours. If improvement does not occur within that period of time, the diagnosis should be reconsidered and appropriate treatment initiated.
3. Procaine penicillin G is a substance of low toxicity. However, side effects, or so-called allergic or anaphylactic reactions—sometimes fatal, have been known to occur in animals hypersensitive to penicillin and procaine. The use of this product is therefore contraindicated in animals that are hypersensitive to either penicillin or procaine. Animals treated with Combiotic Aqueous Suspension should be kept under close observation for at least one-half hour. Should allergic or anaphylatic reactions occur, discontinue use of this product and administer epinephrine and antihistamines immediately.
4. Dihydrostreptomycin is eliminated to a large extent through the kidneys. The use of this product is therefore contraindicated in animals suffering from conditions in which there is impairment of kidney function or obstruction to the free flow of urine.
5. Combiotic Aqueous Suspension must be stored between 2° to 8°C. (36° to 46°F.) Warm to room temperature and

shake well before using. Keep under refrigeration when not in use. If product is not kept at recommended storage temperatures, degradation may occur with subsequent loss of penicillin activity. If product fails to resuspend to a uniform consistency or has a strong objectionable odor, it should not be used.

Warning: Milk that has been taken from animals during treatment and for 72 hours (6 milkings) after the latest treatment must not be used for food. The use of this drug must be discontinued for 30 days before treated animals are slaughtered for food. In lactating dairy animals, do not inject more than 2,000 units of penicillin or 2.5 mg. of dihydrostreptomycin per pound of body weight per day. Exceeding the highest recommended dosage level may result in antibiotic residues in meat or milk beyond the withdrawal time.

How Supplied: Combiotic Aqueous Suspension is available in vials of 100 ml. and 250 ml. with a potency of 200,000 units of procaine penicillin G and 250 mg. of dihydrostreptomycin base per ml.

LIQUAMAST®
(oxytetracycline HCl)
For Mastitis

Composition: Liquamast (oxytetracycline HCl), a broad-spectrum antibiotic is derived from the metabolic activity of the actinomycete, *Streptomyces rimosus.* Oxytetracycline is yellow in color and crystalline in nature. It is amphoteric, being soluble in both acid and basic solutions. Solutions of oxytetracycline possess a high order of stability.

In the animal, oxytetracycline is very stable and its activity does not diminish in the presence of body fluids, serums or exudates. It is effective in the treatment of mastitis caused by a variety of gram-positive and gram-negative bacteria.

Liquamast contains oxytetracycline hydrochloride in a water-soluble base. Each gram contains 30 mg of oxytetracycline hydrochloride. Each ½ ounce tube contains 426 mg of oxytetracycline hydrochloride.

Indications: Liquamast is indicated in the treatment of acute chronic mastitis in lactating cows caused by organisms susceptible to oxytetracycline therapy.

Symptoms of Mastitis: Mastitis may be acute or chronic and may occur in one or more quarters of the animal at one time.

The acute form may show painful swelling of the udder, abnormal milk (clumps of milk, blood, straw-colored liquid), sharp drop in milk flow and an increase in body temperature.

The affected animal often refuses to eat or drink and, if fresh, may not allow her calf to nurse.

The chronic form may show abnormal milk (lumpy, off-color, flaky, stringy). Hard cheesy lumps may be felt up in the udder.

Dosage and Administration: Treatment is most effective when the solution is injected into the udder immediately after milking. If weather is cold, warm solution to body temperature (leave cap on while warming).

1. Milk the cow out, but do not strip.
2. Wash hands thoroughly and use clean towel to dry.
3. Carefully wash the teats and udder with soap and warm water; rinse and dry udder with a clean towel.
4. Wipe off end of teat with cotton and alcohol.
5. Just before insertion into the teat, screw plastic collar tight to break seal. Remove clear plastic tip cover. Do not touch tip of tube with fingers.
6. Insert tip of tube into teat and squirt entire contents of tube into the quarter.

Remove the tip of tube from udder. Hold the end of the teat with the fingers of the left hand, and with the thumb and first finger of the right hand, force the contents of the teat canal into the quarter. Then with both hands, massage upward to distribute the solution throughout the quarter.

Treatment of lactating cows should be limited to three (3) infusions at 12 to 24 hour intervals.

Mastitis usually responds to treatment with Liquamast within 48 hours. Infected quarter should be treated following each milking.

Milk the treated quarter at 12 or 24 hour intervals as indicated.

In cases of acute mastitis, nursing care is essential and should accompany the treatment with Liquamast. Apply clean, warm, moist cloths every three or four hours until swelling is reduced.

No case of mastitis may be considered cure unless bacteriological examination of the milk from infected quarters no longer shows the presence of the causative organisms, approximately three weeks after last treatment.

Sanitation: Sanitation is essential for controlling mastitis. Barns and gutters should be clean; lime or superphosphate should be spread on the floor and gutters daily. Supply ample clean, dry bedding; rid the barn of flies, since they can spread mastitis. Before milking, wash the udder with an antiseptic solution and dry with disposable paper towels. Keep milking machines clean. After milking each cow, dip the teat cups in water and then in an antiseptic solution. Milk clean and fast and remove machine as soon as the milk flow stops. Follow the manufacturer's instructions on the use of milking machines. In hand milking, milk with clean hands. Milk infected cows last and disinfect hands after each cow. The feeding of mastitis milk to calves and swine may cause scours in these animals.

Caution: *Warning:* Milk taken from animals during treatment and for 96 hours (8 milkings) after the latest treatment for mastitis must not be used for food.

Animals infused with this product must not be slaughtered for food within 96 hours of latest treatment.

1. When properly used as indicated, most sick animals that have been treated with antibiotics show a noticeable improvement within 36 to 48 hours. If improvement is not noted in that time, the diagnosis should be re-examined.
2. Rarely do side reactions or so-called allergic manifestations occur in animals treated with antibiotics. If any undesirable reactions are noted, discontinue use of the drug immediately.
3. For a rapid response to treatment and the correct use of a drug in a treated animal, a prompt accurate diagnosis should be made. Professional investigation and laboratory assistance are often requisites to the correct diagnosis of complicated animal diseases.

How Supplied: Liquamast is available in ½ oz. tubes.

LIQUAMYCIN® INJECTABLE
(oxytetracycline hydrochloride injection)
50 mg/ml

Composition: Liquamycin Injectable is a sterile, preconstituted solution of the broad-spectrum antibiotic oxytetracycline hydrochloride (Terramycin®). Each ml contains 50 mg oxytetracycline hydrochloride and on a w/v basis 1.9% magnesium chloride hexahydrate; 73.5% propylene glycol; 0.5% sodium formaldehyde sulfoxylate (as a preservative); 2-aminoethanol to adjust pH; water for injection, q.s.

Oxytetracycline is derived from the metabolic activity of the actinomycete, *Streptomyces rimosus.* Discovered and developed in the research laboratories of Pfizer Inc., oxytetracycline is an antimicrobial agent that is effective in the treatment of a wide range of diseases caused by susceptible gram-positive and gram-negative bacteria.

Liquamycin Injectable is a stable product requiring no refrigeration; and, although the viscosity increases at extremely low temperatures, it does not freeze under normal use conditions. It is recommended that Liquamycin Injectable be stored below 77°F (25°C). The antibiotic activity of oxytetracycline is not appreciably diminished in the presence of body fluids, serum, or exudates.

Liquamycin Injectable is rapidly absorbed from the injection site and in a relatively short period of time can be found in the blood and in most body fluids and tissues. Oxytetracycline diffuses readily through the placenta and is present in the fetal circulation. It diffuses into the pleural fluid and in some circumstances into the cerebrospinal fluid. Oxytetracycline appears to be concentrated in the hepatic system and is excreted in the bile. It appears in the feces, milk, and urine in relatively high concentrations and in a biologically active form.

Precautions: Exceeding the highest recommended dosage level of 5 mg per pound of body weight, administering at recommended levels for more than 4 consecutive days, and/or exceeding 10 ml intra-muscularly per injection site, may result in antibiotic residues beyond the withdrawal time.

Continued on next page

Pfizer—Cont.

Use of this product may result in some local tissue irritation manifested by temporary swelling and discoloration. When administered intramuscularly to animals within 30 days of slaughter, muscle discoloration may necessitate trimming of the injection site(s) and surrounding tissues during the dressing procedure.
Reactions of an allergic or anaphylactic nature, sometimes fatal, have been known to occur in hypersensitive animals following administration of Liquamycin Injectable, but such reactions are rare. Should such reactions occur, discontinue treatment with Liquamycin Injectable and consider the administration of epinephrine, antihistamines, and corticosteroids, as the condition may warrant.
Shock is occasionally observed following intravenous administration, especially where large volumes are involved. To minimize this occurrence, dilution with sterile water, physiological saline, or 5 percent dextrose is recommended.
Shortly after injection, treated animals may have transient hemoglobinuria resulting in darkened urine.
Chicks and poults may exhibit some drowsiness for a short period following handling and injection.
As with all antibiotic preparations, use of this drug may result in overgrowth of nonsusceptible organisms, including fungi. A lack of response by the treated animal, or the development of new signs or symptoms suggest that an overgrowth of nonsusceptible organisms has occurred. If superinfections occur, the use of this product should be discontinued and appropriate specific therapy should be instituted.
Since bacteriostatic drugs may interfere with the bactericidal action of penicillin, it is advisable to avoid giving Liquamycin in conjunction with penicillin.
Indications: Liquamycin Injectable is intended for use in the treatment of diseases due to oxytetracycline-susceptible organisms in beef cattle, nonlactating dairy cattle, swine, and poultry (broilers, turkeys and breeding chickens).
Cattle: In cattle, Liquamycin Injectable indicated in the treatment of pneumonia and shipping fever complex associated with *Pasteurella* spp. and *Hemophilus* spp.; foot-rot and diptheria caused by *Spherophorus necrophorus;* bacterial enteritis (scours) caused by *Escherichia coli;* wooden tongue caused by *Actinobacillus lignieresi;* leptospirosis caused by *Leptospira pomona;* anaplasmosis caused by *Anaplasma marginale;* anthrax caused by *Bacillus anthracis;* wound infections and acute metritis caused by staphylococcal and streptococcal organisms.
Swine: In swine, Liquamycin Injectable is indicated in the treatment of bacterial enteritis (scours, colibacillosis) caused by *Escherichia coli;* pneumonia caused by *Pasteurella multocida;* and leptospirosis caused by *Leptospira pomona.*
In sows, Liquamycin Injectable is indicated as an aid in control of infectious enteritis (baby pig scours, colibacillosis) in suckling pigs caused by *Escherichia coli.*
Poultry: In poultry (broilers, turkeys and breeding chickens), Liquamycin Injectable is indicated in the treatment of air sacculitis (air sac disease, chronic respiratory disease) caused by *Mycoplasma gallisepticum* and *Escherichia coli;* fowl cholera caused by *Pasteurella multocida;* infectious sinusitis caused by *Mycoplasma gallisepticum;* and infectious synovitis caused by *Mycoplasma synoviae.*
Dosage Levels: Liquamycin Injectable is to be administered to beef cattle and nonlactating dairy cattle at a level of 3 to 5 milligrams of oxytetracycline per pound of body weight per day. In treatment of anaplasmosis, severe foot-rot and severe forms of the indicated diseases, a dosage level of 5 milligrams per pound of body weight is recommended.
In swine, Liquamycin Injectable is to be administered at a level of 3 to 5 milligrams of oxytetracycline per pound of body weight per day.
For sows, administer 3 milligrams of oxytetracycline per pound of body weight approximately 8 hours before farrowing or immediately after completion of farrowing.
When the intramuscular route is used, no more than 10 ml. should be injected at any one site in adult livestock. The volume administered per injection site should be reduced according to age and body size so that 1 to 2 ml. is injected in the case of smaller animals such as small calves and young pigs.

Chickens

Age	Dilution	Amount
1 day- 2 weeks	1:3	½ ml. diluted product* (6.25 mg)
2 weeks- 4 weeks	1:3	1 ml diluted product* (12.5 mg)
4 weeks- 8 weeks	None	½ ml. undiluted product (25 mg)
8 weeks- broilers & light pullets	None	1 ml. undiluted product (50 mg)
Adult chickens	None	2 ml. undiluted product (100 mg)

*To prepare 1:3 dilution, add one part Liquamycin Injectable (oxytetracycline hydrochloride injection) to three parts sterile water.
Do not attempt to store diluted solutions for later use.

Turkeys

Age	Dilution	Amount
1 day- 2 weeks	1:3	½ ml. diluted product* (6.25 mg)
2 weeks- 4 weeks	1:3	1 ml. diluted product* (12.5 mg)
4 weeks- 6 weeks	None	1 ml. undiluted product (50 mg)
6 weeks- 9 weeks	None	2 ml. undiluted product (100 mg)
9 weeks- 12 weeks	None	3 ml. undiluted product (150 mg)
12 weeks and older	None	4 ml. undiluted product (200 mg)

Caution: In light turkey breeds, do not inject more than 25 mg per pound of body weight.
* To prepare 1:3 dilution, add one part Liquamycin Injectable to three parts sterile water.

Do not attempt to store diluted solutions for later use.
For the treatment of infectious sinusitis in turkeys, inject ¼ to ½ ml. of Liquamycin Injectable (oxytetracycline hydrochloride) directly into each swollen sinus depending on the age of the bird and the severity of the condition. At the time that the sinuses are treated, Liquamycin Injectable should also be injected subcutaneously into the birds according to the dosage indicated in the above table. If refilling of the sinuses occurs, the treatment may be repeated in 5 to 7 days.
Treatment for all diseases should be instituted early. Treatment should continue for 24 to 48 hours beyond the remission of disease signs, but the total number of consecutive days on medication should not exceed four. If improvement is not noted within 24 to 48 hours of the beginning of treatment, diagnosis and course of therapy should be re-evaluated.
Administration: Liquamycin Injectable should be administered subcutaneously in poultry, and by the intravenous and intramuscular routes in beef cattle and nonlactating dairy cattle, and intramuscularly in swine.
Intravenous administration is recommended in cattle when daily dosage exceeds 50 ml. As with all highly concentrated materials, Liquamycin Injectable must be administered slowly by the intravenous route. Dilution with sterile water, physiological saline, or 5 percent dextrose is satisfactory if the resulting solution is used within a few hours. Do not attempt to store diluted Liquamycin Injectable for later use.
Intramuscular injections should be made well within the fleshy part of heavy muscles, such as are found in the gluteal region of livestock. Proper anatomical selection of injection sites should be observed as a precaution against inadvertent injection into or near a major nerve. No more than 10 ml should be injected at any one site in adult livestock; rotate injection sites for each succeeding treatment.
Subcutaneous administration injections in poultry should be made under the loose skin on top of the neck, halfway between the head and the base of the neck.
Warning: Discontinue treatment at least 5 days prior to slaughter for chickens and turkeys, and at least 22 days prior to slaughter for cattle and swine.
Not for use in lactating dairy animals.
Do not administer Liquamycin Injectable to laying hens unless the eggs are used for hatching only.
How Supplied: Liquamycin Injectable is available in 500 ml multidose vials containing 50 mg of oxytetracycline hydrochloride per milliliter.

LIQUAMYCIN® 100
Oxytetracycline Hydrochloride Injection
100 mg Oxytetracycline Base (as Oxytetracycline hydrochloride) per ml

Composition: Liquamycin 100 is a sterile, preconstituted solution of the broad-spectrum antibiotic oxytetracycline hydrochloride. Each ml contains 100 mg oxytetracycline base as oxytetracycline hydrochloride and on a w/v basis, 0.96% magnesium oxide; 0.43% magnesium formaldehyde sulfoxylate (as a preservative); 19% povidone; monoethanolamine to adjust pH; up to 0.05% simethicone emulsion; water for injection, q.s.
Oxytetracycline is derived from the metabolic activity of the actinomycete, *Streptomyces rimosus.* Discovered and developed in the research laboratories of Pfizer Inc., oxytetracycline is an antimicrobial agent that is effective in the treatment of a wide range of diseases caused by susceptible gram-positive and gram-negative bacteria.
The antibiotic activity of oxytetracycline is not appreciably diminished in the presence of body fluids, serum or exudates.
Liquamycin 100 is rapidly absorbed from the injection site and in a relatively short period of time can be found in the blood and in most body fluids and tissues. Oxytetracycline diffuses readily through the placenta and is present in the fetal circulation. It diffuses into the pleural fluid and in some circumstances into the cerebrospinal fluid. Oxytetracycline appears to be concentrated in the hepatic system and is excreted in the bile. It appears in the feces, milk and urine in relatively high concentrations and in a biologically active form.
Indications: Liquamycin 100 (oxytetracycline HCl injection) is intended for use in the treatment of the following diseases in beef cattle, nonlactating dairy cattle and swine when due to oxytetracycline-susceptible organisms:
Cattle: In cattle, Liquamycin 100 is indicated in the treatment of pneumonia and shipping fever complex associated with *Pasteurella* spp. and *Hemophilus* spp.; foot-rot and diphtheria caused by *Fusobacterium necrophorum;* bacterial enteritis (scours) caused by *Escherichia coli;* wooden tongue caused by *Actinobacillus lignieresi;* leptospirosis caused by *Leptospira pomona;* anaplasmosis caused by *Anaplasma marginale;* anthrax caused by *Bacillus anthrasis;* wound infections and acute metritis caused by strains of staphylococci and streptococci organisms sensitive to oxytetracycline.
Swine: In swine, Liquamycin 100 is indicated in the treatment of bacterial enteritis (scours, colibacillosis) caused by *Escherichia coli;* pneumonia caused by *Pasteurella multiocida;* and leptospirosis caused by *Leptospira pomona.*
In sows, Liquamycin 100 in indicated as an aid in control of infectious enteritis (baby pig scours, colibacillosis) in suckling pigs caused by *Escherichia coli.*
Dosage: *Cattle:* Liquamycin 100 is to be administered by intramuscular injection to beef cattle and nonlactating dairy cattle at a level of 3 to 5 milligrams of oxytetracycline per pound of body weight per day. In treatment of anaplasmosis, severe foot-rot and advanced cases of other indicated diseases, a dosage level of 5 milligrams per pound of body weight is recommended. Treatment should be continued 24 to 48 hours following remission of disease signs, however, not to exceed a total of four consecutive days. If improvement is not noted within 24 to 48 hours of the beginning of treatment, diagnosis and therapy should be re-evaluated.
Swine: In swine, Liquamycin 100 is to be administered by intramuscular injection at a level of 3 to 5 milligrams of oxytetracycline per pound of body weight per day. Treatment should be continued 24 to 48 hours following remission of disease signs, however, not to exceed a total of four consecutive days. If improvement is not noted within 24 to 48 hours of the beginning of treatment, diagnosis and therapy should be re-evaluated.
For sows, administer once intramuscularly 3 milligrams of oxytetracycline per pound of body weight approximately 8 hours before farrowing or immediately after completion of farrowing.
Administration: Liquamycin 100 should be administered by the intramuscular route in beef cattle and nonlactating dairy cattle.
Intramuscular injections should be made well within the fleshy part of heavy muscles, such as are found in the gluteal region of beef cattle and nonlactating dairy cattle. Proper anatomical selection of injection sites should be observed as a precaution against inadvertent injection into or near a major nerve. No more than 10 ml should be injected at any one site in adult livestock: rotate injection sites for each succeeding treatment.
Precautions: Exceeding the highest recommended level of 5 mg per pound of body weight per day, administering at recommended levels for more than 4 consecutive days and/or exceeding 10 ml intramuscularly per injection site, may result in antibiotic residues beyond the withdrawal period.
Reactions of an allergic or anaphylactic nature, sometimes fatal, have been known to occur in hypersensitive animals following administration of Liquamycin 100, but such reactions are rare. Should such reactions occur, discontinue treatment with Liquamycin 100 and consider the administration of epinephrine, antihistamines and/or corticosteroids as the condition may warrant.
As with all antibiotic preparations, use of this drug may result in overgrowth of nonsusceptible organisms, including fungi. The absence of a favorable response following treatment, or the development of new signs or symptoms, may suggest an overgrowth of nonsusceptible organisms. If superinfections occur, the use of this product should be discontinued and appropriate specific therapy should be instituted.
Since bacteriostatic drugs may interfere with the bactericidal action of penicillin, it is advisable to avoid giving Liquamycin 100 in conjunction with penicillin.
Caution: Do not store above 86°F (30°C). Keep from freezing.
Warning: Discontinue treatment at least 15 days prior to slaughter of cattle, and 22 days prior to slaughter of swine. Not for use in lactating dairy animals.
How Supplied: Liquamycin 100 is available in 500 ml multidose vials containing 100 mg of oxytetracycline base (as oxytetracycline hydrochloride) per ml.

P

LIQUAMYCIN® LA-200®
(oxytetracycline)

Composition: Liquamycin® LA-200® (oxytetracycline injection) is a sterile preconstituted solution of the broad-spectrum antibiotic oxytetracycline. Each ml contains 200 mg of oxytetracycline base as amphoteric oxytetracycline and on a w/v basis, 40.0% 2-pyrrolidone, 5.0% povidone, 1.8% magnesium oxide, 0.2% sodium, formaldehyde sulfoxylate (as a preservative), monoethanolamine and/or hydrocholoric acid as required to adjust pH.
Oxytetracycline is derived from the metabolic activity of the actinomycete, *Streptomyces rimosus.* Discovered and developed in the research laboratories of Pfizer Inc., oxytetracycline is an antimicrobial agent that is effective in the treatment of a wide range of diseases caused by susceptible gram-positive and gram-negative bacteria.
The antibiotic activity of oxytetracycline is not appreciably diminished in the presence of body fluids, serum, or exudates.
Indications: Liquamycin® LA-200® is intended for use in treatment of the following diseases in beef cattle, nonlactating dairy cattle and swine when due to oxytetracycline-susceptible organisms:
Cattle—In cattle, Liquamycin® LA-200® is indicated in the treatment of pneumonia and shipping fever complex associated with *Pasteurella* spp. and *Hemophilus* spp.; foot-rot and diphtheria caused by *Fusobacterium necrophorum;* bacterial enteritis (scours) caused by *Escherichia coli;* wooden tongue caused by *Actinobacillus lignieresii;* leptospirosis caused by *Leptospira pomona;* wound infections and acute metritis caused by strains of staphylococci and streptococci organisms sensitive to oxytetracycline.
Swine—In swine, Liquamycin® LA-200® is indicated in the treatment of bacterial enteritis (scours, colibacillosis) caused by *Escherichia coli;* pneumonia caused by *Pasteurella multocida;* and leptospirosis caused by *Leptospira pomona.*
In sows, Liquamycin® LA-200® is indicated as an aid in control of infectious enteritis (baby pig scours, colibacillosis) in suckling pigs caused by *Escherichia coli.*
Dosage: *Cattle:* Liquamycin® LA-200® (oxytetracycline injection) is to be administered by intramuscular or intravenous injection to beef cattle and nonlactating dairy cattle at a level of 3 to 5 milligrams of oxytetracycline per pound of body weight per day. In treatment of severe foot-rot and advanced cases of

Continued on next page

Pfizer—Cont.

other indicated diseases, a dosage level of 5 milligrams per pound of body weight is recommended. Treatment should be continued 24 to 48 hours following remission of disease signs; however, not to exceed a total of four consecutive days. If improvement is not noted within 24 to 48 hours of the beginning of treatment, diagnosis and therapy should be re-evaluated.

A single dosage of 9 milligrams of oxytetracycline per pound of body weight administered *intramuscularly* is recommended in the treatment of bacterial pneumonia caused by *Pasteurella spp.* (shipping fever) in calves and yearlings where re-treatment is impractical due to husbandry conditions, such as animals on range, or where repeated restraint is inadvisable.

Swine: In swine, Liquamycin® LA-200® is to be administered by intramuscular injection at a level of 3 to 5 milligrams of oxytetracycline per pound of body weight per day. Treatment should be continued 24 to 48 hours following remission of disease signs; however, not to exceed a total of four consecutive days. If improvement is not noted within 24 to 48 hours of the beginning of treatment, diagnosis and therapy should be reevaluated.

A single dosage of 9 milligrams of oxytetracycline per pound of body weight administered *intramuscularly* is recommended in the treatment of bacterial pneumonia caused by *Pasteurella multocida* in swine, where re-treatment is impractical due to husbandry conditions or where repeated restraint is inadvisable.

For sows, administer once intramuscularly 3 milligrams of oxytetracycline per pound of body weight approximately 8 hours before farrowing or immediately after completion of farrowing.

For swine weighing 25 lb of body weight and under, Liquamycin® LA-200® should be administered *undiluted* for treatment at 9 mg/lb but should be administered *diluted* for treatment at 3 or 5 mg/lb.

	9 MG/LB DOSAGE Volume of UNDILUTED Liquamycin LA-200	3 OR 5 MG/LB DOSAGE Volume of DILUTED Liquamycin LA-200		
Body Weight	9 mg/lb	3 mg/lb	Dilution*	5 mg/lb
5 lb	0.2 ml	0.6 ml	1:7	1.0 ml
10 lb	0.5 ml	0.9 ml	1:5	1.5 ml
25 lb	1.1 ml	1.5 ml	1:3	2.5 ml

*To prepare dilutions, add one part Liquamycin® LA-200® to three, five or seven parts of sterile water, or 5 percent dextrose solution as indicated; the diluted product should be used immediately.

Administration: When the intramuscular route is used, no more than 10 ml should be injected at any one site in adult beef cattle and nonlactating dairy cattle, and not more than 5 ml per site in adult swine. The volume administered per injection site should be reduced according to age and body size so that 1 to 2 ml per site is injected in small calves. Intramuscular injections should be made well within the fleshy part of heavy muscles, such as are found in the gluteal region of beef cattle, nonlactating dairy cattle, and swine. Injections should be made into properly selected anatomical locations as a precaution against inadvertent injection into or near a major nerve; rotating injection sites for each succeeding treatment is recommended.

As with all highly concentrated materials, Liquamycin® LA-200® should be administered *slowly* when used by the intravenous route.

Animal Pharmacology: Using blood concentrations of oxytetracycline following injection (a measure of the total amount of drug available in the animal's circulatory system) as the criterion, Liquamycin® LA-200® has been shown to be bioequivalent with that of Liquamycin® Injectable—50 mg/ml when administered intramuscularly or intravenously at 3 to 5 mg oxytetracycline per pound of body weight. When administered intramuscularly at these dose levels, blood oxytetracycline concentrations for Liquamycin® LA-200® do not peak as high as those of Liquamycin® Injectable—50 mg/ml, but persist for a longer duration. The half-life of oxytetracycline in blood following intramuscular treatment with Liquamycin® LA-200® at 5 mg per pound of body weight has been observed to be approximately 23 hours in cattle and 18 hours in swine versus approximately 12 hours for these species with Liquamycin® Injectable—50 mg/ml.

When Liquamycin® LA-200® is administered to cattle at an intramuscular dosage of 9 mg per pound of body weight, blood oxytetracycline concentrations (≥0.2 mcg/ml) have been observed for 3–4 days. Clinical trials (cattle, swine) evaluating the treatment of bacterial pneumonia have shown that a single intramuscular treatment of Liquamycin® LA-200® at 9 mg per pound of body weight is as effective as two or three repeated, daily treatments of Liquamycin® Injectable at 3–5 mg per pound of body weight.

Warning: Discontinue treatment at least 28 days prior to slaughter of cattle and swine. Not for use in lactating dairy animals.

Precautions: Exceeding the highest recommended level of drug per pound of body weight per day, administering more than the recommended number of treatments, and/or exceeding 10 ml intramuscularly per injection site in adult beef cattle and nonlactating dairy cattle, and 5 ml intramuscularly per injection site in adult swine, may result in antibiotic residues beyond the withdrawal period.

Reactions of an allergic or anaphylactic nature, sometimes fatal, have been known to occur in hypersensitive animals following injection of oxytetracycline. Should such reactions occur, discontinue treatment with Liquamycin® LA-200® and consider the administration of epinephrine, antihistamines, and/or corticosteroids, as the conditions may warrant.

Shortly after injection, treated animals may have transient hemoglobinuria resulting in darkened urine.

As with all antibiotic preparations, use of this drug may result in overgrowth of nonsusceptible organisms, including fungi. The absence of a favorable response following treatment, or the development of new signs may suggest an overgrowth of nonsusceptible organisms. If any of these conditions occur, the use of this product should be discontinued and appropriate specific therapy should be instituted.

Since bacteriostatic drugs may interfere with the bactericidal action of penicillin, it is advisable to avoid giving Liquamycin® LA-200® in conjunction with penicillin.

Storage: Store at room temperature, 15°–30°C (59°–86°F). Keep from freezing.

How Supplied: Liquamycin® LA-200® is available in vials containing 100, 250, or 500 ml.

NEMEX™
(pyrantel pamoate)
Canine anthelmintic suspension

Composition: Nemex is a suspension of pyrantel pamoate in a palatable caramel-flavored vehicle. Each ml contains 2.27 mg of pyrantel base as pyrantel pamoate.

Pyrantel pamoate is a compound belonging to a family classified chemically as tetrahydropyrimidines. It is a yellow, water-insoluble crystalline salt of the tetrahydropyrimidine base and pamoic acid containing 34.6% base activity.

Indications: Nemex suspension is a highly palatable formulation intended as a single treatment for the removal and control of ascarids (*Toxocara canis* and *Toxascaris leonina*) and hookworms (*Ancylostoma caninum* and *Uncinaria stenocephala*) in dogs and puppies.

Consult your veterinarian for assistance in the diagnosis, treatment, and control of parasitism.

Dosage and Administration: Administer one full teaspoon (5 ml) for each 5 pounds of body weight (2.27 mg base per lb of body weight). Although most dogs have been observed to find this formulation very palatable and willingly consume it undiluted, it may be necessary to mix a small quantity of formulation in the dog's normal ration to encourage consumption. Fasting prior to or after treatment is not necessary.

Caution: This product is a suspension and as such will separate. To insure uniform re-suspension and to achieve proper dosage, it is extremely important that the product be shaken thoroughly before every use.

How Supplied: Nemex is available in 60 ml bottles.

NEMEX™ TABS
(pyrantel pamoate)
Canine Anthelmintic Tablets

Composition: Pyrantel pamoate is a compound belonging to a family classified chemically as tetrahydropyrimidines. It is a yellow, water-insoluble crystalline salt of the tetrahydropyrimidine base and pamoic acid contained 34.7% base activity.
Indications: For removal of ascarids (*Toxocara canis; Toxascaris leonina*) and hookworms (*Ancylostoma caninum; Uncinaria stenocephala*) in dogs.
Dosage:
Large Dogs: For the removal of large roundworms (Ascarids) and hookworms, give 1 tablet for each 50 lb of body weight (2.27 mg pyrantel per pound of body weight). Tablets may be broken in half to provide ½ tablet for 25 lb of body weight.
Small Dogs: For the removal of large roundworms (Ascarids) and hookworms, give 1 tablet for each 10 lb of body weight (dosage is designed to provide at least 2.27 mg per pound body weight for dogs weighing over 5 lb and at least 4.54 mg per pound of body weight for dogs weighing less than 5 lb). For dogs weighing more than 10 lb, tablets may be broken in half to provide ½ tablet for each additional 5 lb of body weight.
Administration: Place tablet directly into back of mouth or conceal tablet in a small amount of food. A follow-up fecal examination should be conducted in 2 to 4 weeks after the first treatment to determine the need for re-treatment.
Consult your veterinarian for assistance in the diagnosis, treatment, and control of parasitism. The presence of these parasites should be confirmed by laboratory fecal examination. Do not withhold food from dog prior to or after treatment.
Caution: If dog looks or acts sick, do not treat with the product. Keep out of reach of children. For use only as directed on label. Not for human use. Restricted drug, use only as directed.
Recommended Storage: Store below 30°C (86°F).
How Supplied: For small Dogs and Puppies: bottle of 100 tablets; For Large Dogs: bottle of 50 tablets.

NEMEX™-2
(pyrantel pamoate)
Canine Anthelmintic Suspension

Composition: Nemex-2 is a suspension of pyrantel pamoate in palatable caramel-flavored vehicle. Each ml contains 4.54 mg of pyrantel base as pyrantel pamoate.
Pyrantel pamoate is a compound belonging to a family classified chemically as tetrahydropyrimidines. It is a yellow, water-insoluble crystalline salt of tetrahydropyrimidine base and pamoic acid containing 34.7% base activity.
Indications: Nemex-2 suspension is a highly palatable formulation intended as a single treatment for the removal and control of ascarids (*Toxocara canis and Toxascaris leonina*) and hookworms (*Ancylostoma caninum* and *Uncinaria stenocephala*) in dogs and puppies.
Consult your veterinarian for assistance in the diagnosis, treatment, and control of parasitism.
Dosage and Administration: Administer one full teaspoon (5 ml) for each 10 pounds of body weight (2.27 mg base per lb of body weight). Although most dogs have been observed to find this formulation very palatable and willingly consume it undiluted, it may be necessary to mix a small quantity of formulation in the dog's normal ration to encourage consumption. Fasting prior to or after treatment is not necessary.
Caution: This product is a suspension and as such will separate. To insure uniform resuspension and to achieve proper dosage, it is extremely important that the product be shaken thoroughly before every use.
How Supplied: Nemex-2 is available in 60 ml and 1 pint bottles.

PARATECT®
(morantel tartrate)*
Sustained Release Cartridge

Each cartridge contains 22.7 grams of morantel tartrate equivalent to 13.5 grams of morantel base.

READ ENTIRE BROCHURE CAREFULLY BEFORE USING THIS PRODUCT.

Composition: The **Paratect** cartridge contains a pale yellow to buff paste containing 55% w/w morantel tartrate in an inert vehicle. Morantel tartrate is a compound belonging to a family classified chemically as tetrahydropyrimidines. It is a yellow, water-soluble crystalline salt of the tetrahydropyrimidine base and tartaric acid containing 59.5% base activity. The chemical structure and name are given below:

Chemical Name: Trans-1,4,5,6-tetrahydro-1-methyl-2-[2(3-methyl-2-thienyl) vinyl] pyrimidine tartrate (1:1).
Dosage Form: The **Paratect** cartridge consists of a stainless steel cylinder containing 22.7 grams of morantel tartrate (13.5 grams of morantel base activity) in a polyethylene glycol vehicle. It is administered orally to cattle by means of a special dosing gun and is of a weight sufficient to prevent regurgitation. The **Paratect** cartridge with its special polyethylene diffusing discs at each end is designed to provide for the continuous release of morantel into the reticulum/rumen fluid of the animal for at least ninety days after administration.
Indications for Use: The **Paratect** cartridge is indicated for control of the adult stage of the following gastrointestinal nematode infections in weaned calves and yearling cattle: *Ostertagia* spp., *Trichostrongylus axei*, *Cooperia* spp., *Oesophagostomum radiatum*. Efficacy of the PARATECT cartridge is dependent upon continuous control of the gastrointestinal parasites for approximately 90 days following administration.
Dosage Recommendations: The **Paratect** cartridge should always be administered orally with a specially designed dosing gun.
Cattle turned out to pasture:
Administer one **Paratect** cartridge to each weaned calf and yearling weighing at least 200 pounds.
Cattle that remained on pasture:
The cartridge should be administered to all animals at the start of the grazing season. Criteria for predicting periods of greatest exposure to parasites are described in the "Concepts of the Sustained Release Cartridge" section, but for optimum efficacy, follow the husbandry guidelines in the "Precautions" section.
Dosing Instructions: Insert the **Paratect** cartridge through the rubber sleeve of the dosing gun as far as possible into the metal holder. Restrain the animal with its head in the forward extended position. Take care to keep the neck straight or the animal will have difficulty in swallowing. Open the mouth and hold the dosing gun by its shaft, with the apex of the curve pointing upwards towards the roof of the mouth (the V-notch in the finger guard should be at the top) as shown in Diagram 1. Insert the dosing gun from the front (not the sides) of the mouth and over the back of the tongue (Diagram 2). Gentle firm pressure (not force) is all that is required.

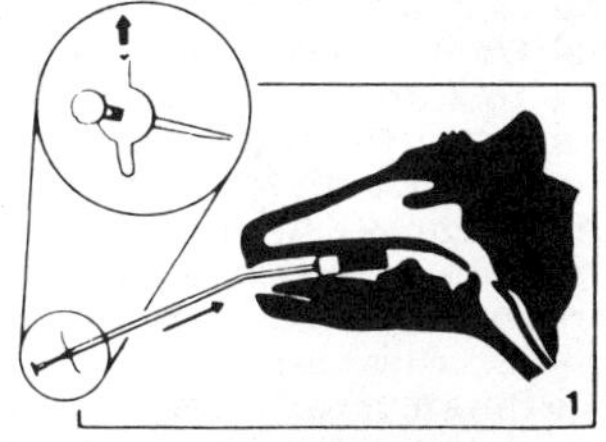

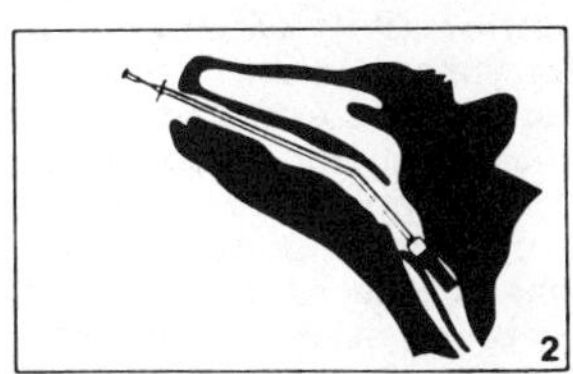

Easy passage of the **Paratect** cartridge and dosing gun in the throat indicates that the animal has swallowed. When this occurs, depress the plunger to eject the cartridge (Diagram 3). If there is resistance to depressing the plunger, the end of the dosing gun is not in the correct position and should be gently reintroduced until swallowing does take place. The resistance will then disappear and the plunger can be easily depressed. Then, carefully withdraw the dosing gun (Diagram 4).
Excessive force should be avoided when dosing cattle.

Continued on next page

Pfizer—Cont.

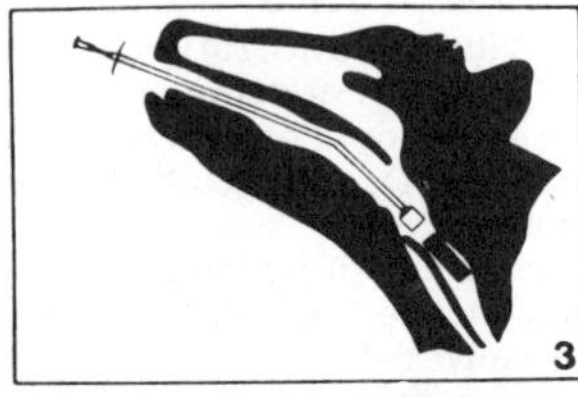

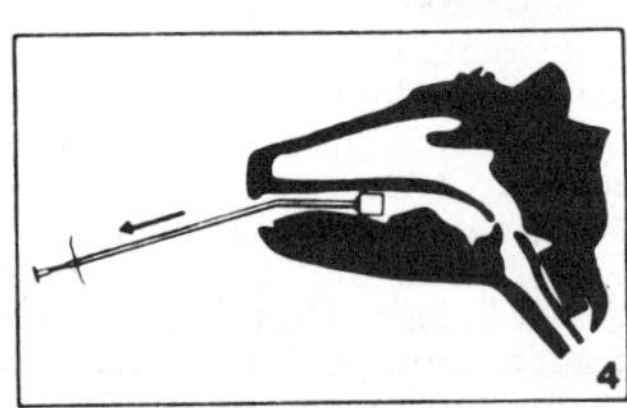

Concept of the Sustained Release Cartridge: The **Paratect** cartridge is indicated for control of the adult stage of gastrointestinal nematode infections in weaned calves and yearling cattle. Under normal management conditions when a pasture is grazed by cattle in successive years, the concentration of infective parasite larvae on the pasture normally follows a predictable pattern with highest larval populations generally occurring during relatively warm, moist environmental conditions. These are the same conditions which promote pasture herbage growth. Animals, when turned out, become infected by ingesting larvae from the previous grazing season. These larvae develop into adults in the gastrointestinal tract of the animal and produce eggs that are deposited back onto the pasture that the cattle are grazing. These eggs develop into infective larvae and may accumulate to very high levels on the pasture. Ingestion of these high concentrations of larvae may result in severe parasitic disease.

When the **Paratect** cartridge is administered as directed, the broad-spectrum anthelmintic activity of morantel in the reticulum/rumen fluid averts the development of ingested overwintered larvae into adult egg-laying parasites. Therefore, worm egg production remains very low, pasture contamination with infective larvae is reduced, and the cycle of parasite propagation is interrupted. Thus, the cartridge protects cattle from gastrointestinal parasites and reduces populations of infective larvae on pastures.

Precautions

All cattle that will be grazing in the same pasture must be treated with the **Paratect** *cartridge. As the effect of the* **Paratect** *cartridge is dependent upon continous control of the gastrointestinal parasites for approximately 90 days following administration, cattle treated with the* **Paratect** *cartridge should not be moved to pastures grazed in the same season/calendar year by cattle not treated with the* **Paratect** *cartridge. Consult veterinarian before using in severely debilitated animals.*

WARNING: DO NOT ADMINISTER TO CATTLE WITHIN 160 DAYS OF SLAUGHTER. KEEP OUT OF REACH OF CHILDREN.

CAUTION: Consult your Veterinarian for assistance in the diagnosis, treatment and control of parasitism.

RECOMMENDED STORAGE: STORE AT ROOM TEMPERATURE, 15°–30°C (59°–86°F)

PEN BP-48®
penicillin G benzathine and penicillin G procaine Aqueous Suspension Veterinary Injection for Use in Beef Cattle

FOR SUBCUTANEOUS USE ONLY

Read entire insert carefully before using this product.

Description: Each ml contains 150,000 units penicillin G benzathine; 150,000 units penicillin G procaine and, approximately: 0.08% sodium carboxymethylcellulose; 0.40% sodium citrate dihydrate; 1.17% lecithin; 0.31% povidone; 0.04% polysorbate 40; 0.06% sorbitan monopalmitate 40; 0.01% propylparaben and 0.12% methylparaben, and 0.25% phenol, as preservatives; trisodium phosphate, as required to adjust pH; water for injection q.s.

Action: Penicillin G is an antibiotic which shows a marked bactericidal effect against certain organisms during their growth phase. It is relatively specific in its action against gram-positive bacteria but is usually ineffective against gram-negative organisms.

It is normally recommended that any bacterial infection be treated as early as possible and with a dosage which will give effective blood levels. Although the recommended dosage of Pen BP-48 Aqueous Suspension will give longer detectable penicillin blood levels than penicillin G procaine alone, it is recommended that a second dose be administered at 48 hours when treating a penicillin-susceptible bacterial infection.

The use of antibiotics in the management of disease is based on an accurate diagnosis and an adequate course of treatment. When properly used in the treatment of diseases caused by penicillin-susceptible organisms, most animals treated with Pen BP-48 Aqueous Suspension show a noticeable improvement within 24 to 48 hours. If improvement does not occur within this period of time, the diagnosis and course of treatment should be re-evaluated. It is recommended that the diagnosis and treatment of animal diseases be carried out by a veterinarian. Since many diseases look alike but require different types of treatment, the use of professional veterinary and laboratory services can reduce treatment time, costs, and needless losses. Good housing, sanitation, and nutrition are important in the maintenance of healthy animals and are essential in the treatment of disease.

Warning: Beef cattle should be withheld from slaughter for food use for 30 days following last treatment. Treatment of beef cattle must be limited to two (2) doses. BY SUBCUTANEOUS INJECTION ONLY. Do not inject intramuscularly.

Indications: Pen BP-48 Aqueous Suspension is indicated for treatment of the following bacterial infections in beef cattle due to penicillin-susceptible microorganisms that are susceptible to the serum levels common to this particular dosage form, such as:

1. Bacterial Pneumonia (shipping fever complex) (*Streptococcus* spp., *Corynebacterium pyogenes, Staphylococcus aureus*)
2. Upper Respiratory Infections such as Rhinitis or Pharyngitis (*Corynebacterium pyogenes*)
3. Blackleg (*Clostridium chauvoei*)

Precautions: Exceeding the recommended doses and dosage levels may result in antibiotic residues beyond the withdrawal time. Do not inject this material intramuscularly.

Penicillin G is a substance of low toxicity. However, side effects, or so-called allergic or anaphylactic reactions—sometimes fatal, have been known to occur in animals hypersensitive to penicillin and procaine. Such reactions can occur unpredictably, with varying intensity. Animals administered penicillin G should be kept under close observation for at least one-half hour. Should allergic or anaphylactic reactions occur, discontinue use of the product and immediately administer epinephrine following manufacturer's recommendations; call a veterinarian.

As with all antibiotic preparations, use of this drug may result in overgrowth of nonsusceptible organisms, including fungi. A lack of response by the treated animal, or the development of new signs or symptoms suggest that an overgrowth of nonsusceptible organisms has occurred. In such instances, consult your veterinarian.

Since bactericidal drugs may interfere with the bacteriostatic action of tetracyclines, it is advisable to avoid giving penicillin in conjunction with tetracyclines.

Pen BP-48 Aqueous Suspension should be stored under refrigeration below 59°F (15°C). Avoid freezing. Warm to room temperature, and shake well before using.

Administration: The recommended dosage for beef cattle should be administered by SUBCUTANEOUS INJECTION ONLY. Failure to use the subcutaneous route of administration may result in antibiotic residues in meat beyond the withdrawal time.

Dosage: Beef Cattle: 2 ml per 150 lb body weight GIVEN SUBCUTANEOUSLY ONLY (2,000 units penicillin G procaine and 2,000 units penicillin G benzathine per lb body weight). Treatment should be repeated in 48 hours.

IMPORTANT: Treatment in beef cattle should be limited to two (2) doses given by subcutaneous injection only.

Directions for Use: A thoroughly cleaned, sterile needle and syringe should be used for each injection (needles and syringes may be sterilized by boiling in water for 15 minutes). Before withdrawing the solution from the bottle, disinfect the rubber cap on the bottle with a suitable disinfectant, such as 70 per cent alcohol. The injection site should be similarly cleaned with the disinfectant. Needles of 14 to 16 gauge and not more than 1 inch long are adequate for injections.
A subcutaneous injection should be made by pinching up a fold of the skin between the thumb and forefinger. The mid-neck region is the preferred injection site. Insert the needle under the fold in a direction approximately parallel to the surface of the body. When the needle is inserted in this manner the medication will be delivered underneath the skin between the skin and the muscles. Proper restraint, such as the use of a chute and nose lead, is needed for proper administration of the product.
How Supplied: Pen BP-48 is available in vials containing 100 or 250 ml.

SHAKE WELL BEFORE USING
LIVESTOCK DRUG, NOT FOR HUMAN USE.
RESTRICTED DRUG. USE ONLY AS DIRECTED.

PROCAINE PENICILLIN G
IN AQUEOUS SUSPENSION
For Intramuscular Use Only

General Information: Procaine Penicillin G is a potent antibacterial agent which is effective against a variety of pathogenic organisms, chiefly in the gram-positive category. Procaine Penicillin G Suspension is a free-flowing product prepared by combining penicillin G and procaine, molecule for molecule, with dispersing agents.
Indications: Procaine Penicillin G Suspension is recommended for treatment of bacterial pneumonia (shipping fever) caused by *Pasteurella multocida* in cattle and sheep, erysipelas caused by *Erysipelothrix insidiosa* in swine, and strangles caused by *Streptococcus equi* in horses.
Dosage Levels: The recommended daily dosage of penicillin is 3,000 units per pound of body weight (one ml per 100 lbs body weight).
Continue daily treatment until recovery is apparent and for at least 1 day after symptoms disappear, usually in 2 or 3 days. Treatment should not exceed 4 consecutive days.
Directions for Use: Procaine Penicillin G Suspension should be administered by the intramuscular route.
A thoroughly cleaned sterile needle and syringe should be used for each injection (needles and syringes may be sterilized by boiling in water for 15 minutes). Before withdrawing the solution from the bottle, disinfect the rubber cap on the bottle with a suitable disinfectant, such as 70 percent alcohol. The injection site should be similarly cleaned with the disinfectant. Needles of 16 to 18 gauge and 1 to 1½ inches long are adequate for intramuscular injections.
Warning: Milk that has been taken from animals during treatment and for 72 hours (6 milkings) after the latest treatment must not be used for food.
Discontinue use of this drug for the following time periods before treated animals are slaughtered for food: *Cattle*—10 days, *Sheep*—9 days, *Swine*—7 days.
Not for use in horses intended for food.
Precautions: Exceeding the recommended daily dosage of 3,000 units per pound of body weight, administering at the recommended level for more than 4 consecutive days, and/or exceeding 10 ml intramuscularly per injection site, may result in antibiotic residues beyond the withdrawal time.
Procaine Penicillin G Suspension should be injected deep within the fleshy muscles of the hip, rump, round, or thigh. Do not inject this material subcutaneously, into a blood vessel, or near a major nerve.
Procaine Penicillin G is a substance of low toxicity. However, allergic or anaphylactic reactions—sometimes fatal, have been known to occur in animals hypersensitive to penicillin and procaine. Such reactions can occur unpredictably with varying intensity. Animals administered Procaine Penicillin G should be kept under close observation for at least one-half hour. Should allergic or anaphylactic reactions occur, discontinue use of the product and immediately administer epinephrine following manufacturers recommendations.
As with all antibiotic preparations, use of this drug may result in overgrowth of nonsusceptible organisms, including fungi. A lack of response by the treated animal or the development of new signs or symptoms suggest that an overgrowth of nonsusceptible organisms has occurred.
Since bactericidal drugs may interfere with the bacteriostatic action of tetracyclines, it is advisable to avoid giving penicillin in conjunction with tetracyclines.
Procaine Penicillin G Suspension should be stored between 2-8°C (36-46°F). Warm to room temperature and shake before using.
How Supplied: Procaine Penicillin G Suspension is available in 100 ml, 250 ml, and 500 ml vials with a potency of 300,000 units per ml.

STRONGID® Paste
(pyrantel pamoate)
Equine Anthelmintic

Description: Strongid Paste is a pale yellow to buff paste containing 43.9% w/pyrantel pamoate in an inert vehicle. Each syringe contains 3.6 grams pyrantel base in 23.6 grams (20 ml) paste. Each milliter contains 180 milligrams pyrantel base as pyrantel pamoate.
Composition: Pyrantel pamoate is a compound belonging to a family classified chemically as tetrahydropyrimidines. It is a yellow, water-insoluble crystalline salt of the tetrahydropyrimidine base and pamoic acid containing 34.7% base activity.
Indications: For the removal and control of mature infections of large strongyles (*Strongylus vulgaris, S. edentatus, S. equinus*); small strongyles; pinworms (*Oxyuris equi*); and large roundworms (*Parascaris equorum*) in horses and ponies.
Consult your veterinarian for assistance in the diagnosis, treatment, and control of parasitism.
Dosage and Administration: Strongid Paste is to be administered as a single dose of 3 milligrams pyrantel base per pound of body weight. The syringe has four weight mark increments. Each weight mark indicates the recommended dose for 300 pounds of body weight.

Dosage

Body Weight Range	*Volume*	*mg Pyrantel Base*
up to 300 lb	¼ syringe (5 ml)	900 mg
301 to 600 lb	½ syringe (10 ml)	1800 mg
601 to 900 lb	¾ syringe (15 ml)	2700 mg
901 to 1200 lb	1 full syringe (20 ml)	3600 mg

Note: Position screw-gauge over appropriate mark on plunger. Each milliliter contains 180 milligrams pyrantel base as pyrantel pamoate.
For maximum control of parasitism, it is recommended that foals (2-8 months of age) be dosed every 4 weeks. To minimize the potential source of infection that the mare may pose to the foal, the mare should be treated 1 month prior to anticipated foaling date followed by re-treatment 10 days to 2 weeks after birth of foal. Horses and ponies over 8 months of age should be routinely doses every 6 weeks.
Warning: Not for use in horses intended for food. Keep out of reach of children.
It is recommended that severly debilitated animals not be treated with this preparation.
Recommended Storage: Store at room temperature, 15°–30°C (59–86°F).
How Supplied: Available in 20 ml syringes.

STRONGID® T
(pyrantel pamoate)
Equine Anthelmintic Suspension

Description: Strongid T is a suspension of pyrantel pamoate in a palatable caramel-flavored vehicle. Each ml contains 50 mg of pyrantel base as pyrantel pamoate.
Pyrantel pamoate is a compound belonging to a family classified chemically as tetrahydropyrimidines. It is a yellow, water-insoluble crystalline salt of the tetrahydropyrimidine base and pamoic acid containing 34.7% base activity.
[See Chemical Formula]

Continued on next page

Pfizer—Cont.

(E)-1.4.5.6-Tetrahydro-1-methyl-2-[2-(2-thienyl) vinyl] pyrimidine 4.4′ methylenebis[3-hydroxy-2-naphthoate] (1:1)

Indications: For the removal and control of mature infections of large strongyles *(Strongylus vulgaris, S. edentatus, S. equinus);* small strongyles *(Trichonema,* sp., *Triodontophorus):* pinworms *(Oxyuris);* and large roundworms *(Parascaris)* in horses and ponies.

Dosage and Treatment: Administer 3 mg pyrantel base per pound of body weight (6 ml Strongid T per 100 lbs. body weight).

For maximum control of parasitism, it is recommended that foals (2–8 months of age) be dosed every 4 weeks. To minimize potential hazard that the mare may pose to the foal, she should be treated 1 month prior to anticipated foaling date followed by retreatment 10 days to 2 weeks after birth of foal. Horses over 8 months of age should be routinely dosed every 6 weeks.

Directions For Use: Strongid T may be administered by means of a stomach tube, dose syringe or by mixing into the feed.

Stomach Tube—Measure the appropriate dosage of Strongid T and mix in the desired quantity of water. Protect drench from direct sunlight and administer to the animal immediately following mixing. Do not attempt to store diluted suspension.

Strongid T is inactive against the common horse bot (*Gastrophilus* sp.). However, Strongid T may be administered concurrently with carbon disulfide observing the usual precautions with carbon disulfide.

Dose Syringe—Draw the appropriate dosage of Strongid T into a dose syringe and administer to the animal. Do not expose Strongid T to direct sunlight.

Feed—Mix the appropriate dosage of Strongid T in the normal grain ration. Fasting of animals prior to or following treatment is not required.

Caution: THIS PRODUCT IS A SUSPENSION AND AS SUCH WILL SEPARATE. TO INSURE UNIFORM RE-SUSPENSION AND TO ACHIEVE PROPER DOSAGE, IT IS EXTREMELY IMPORTANT THAT THE PRODUCT BE SHAKEN THOROUGHLY BEFORE EVERY USE.

Efficacy: Critical (worm count) studies in horses demonstrated that Strongid T administered at the recommended dosage was efficacious against mature infections of *Strongylus vulgaris* ($>$90%), *S. edentatus* (69%), *S. equinus* ($>$90%), *Triodontophorus* ($>$90%), *Trichonema* sp. ($>$90%), *Oxyuris* (81%), and *Parascaris* ($>$90%).

Safety: Strongid T (pyrantel pamoate) is well tolerated by horses and ponies of all ages. No adverse drug response was observed when dose rates up to 60 mg pyrantel base per pound of body weight were administered by stomach tube nor when 3 mg base per pound was given by intratracheal injection. The reproductive performance of pregnant mares and stud horses dosed with Strongid T has not been affected.

Warning: NOT FOR HORSES OR PONIES INTENDED FOR FOOD. KEEP OUT OF REACH OF CHILDREN.

Caution: FEDERAL LAW RESTRICTS THIS DRUG TO USE BY OR ON THE ORDER OF A LICENSED VETERINARIAN.

It is recommended that severely debilitated animals not be treated with this preparation.

Recommended Storage: Store below 86°F.(30°C.).

How Supplied: Strongid T is available in 60 ml or 1-quart bottles.

TERRA-CORTRIL®
(oxytetracycline hydrochloride and hydrocortisone)
Spray
For Dogs and Cats

Composition: Terra-Cortril Spray unites the potent anti-inflammatory action of hydrocortisone with the broad-spectrum antibacterial activity of Terramycin® (oxytetracycline HCl) for rapid relief of symptoms and resolution of lesions in many types of allergic infectious and traumatic skin conditions. This product affords the convenient aerosol spray method of application.

Each unit contains 300 mg of Terramycin (oxytetracycline HCl) and 100 mg of hydrocortisone with an inert non-chlorofluorocarbon propellant.

Pharmacology: Hydrocortisone has been shown to exert a potent anti-inflammatory action by direct hormonal effect at the cellular level. Prompt relief from the physical signs of inflammation can be anticipated due to a reduction in hyperemia, swelling, cellular exudation, and pain. No sensitization due to hydrocortisone has been reported, and since it is not ordinarily absorbed through the skin, it can be used without expectation of systemic side reactions. The addition of the broad-spectrum antibiotic, oxytetracycline, helps prevent infections of initially noninfected lesions, or controls infections due to oxytetracycline-susceptible organisms, if already established.

Indications: Terra-Cortril Spray is indicated for prompt relief of discomfort and continued treatment of many allergic, infectious, and traumatic skin conditions. The anti-inflammatory action of hydrocortisone provides prompt symptomatic relief while Terramycin helps protect against bacterial invasion, or acts against susceptible organisms that may already be present. Terra-Cortril Spray is thus useful as therapy for skin conditions in which anti-inflammatory and antibacterial effects are desired. Indications include: prevention of bacterial infections in superficial wounds, cuts, and abrasions; treatment of allergic dermatoses, including urticaria, eczemas, insect bites and cutaneous drug reactions, infections associated with minor burns and wounds, and nonspecific pruritus.

In the management of allergic dermatoses, the inciting agents in the food or environment should be determined and avoided. Supplemental therapy with oral or parenteral Terramycin is advisable in the treatment of severe infections, or those which may become systemic.

Administration: *Terra-Cortril Spray is not for ophthalmic use; do not spray into or near the eyes.* Shake the container gently once or twice before use, pull off the cap, and depress the nozzle gently with the tip of the forefinger or thumb. A small quantity should be sprayed onto the affected surface by holding the container about six inches from the area to be treated and depressing the nozzle. Only sufficient spray to coat the skin thinly is necessary. The application of small amounts at frequent intervals will give best results. Before treating animals with long or matted hair, it may be necessary to carefully clip the affected area or at least spread the hairs apart to allow the medication to come into contact with the skin surface. Relief will usually be noted following the first or second treatment; however, do not discontinue therapy too soon after the initial favorable response has been obtained.

Tolerance: Hydrocortisone is nonirritating when applied topically and no instances of hypersensitivity have been reported. Terramycin (oxytetracycline HCl) is also well tolerated by the epithelial tissues and only rarely have untoward reactions of an allergic nature occurred. Should any adverse reactions develop, the use of Terra-Cortril Spray should be discontinued immediately.

Precautions: The pleasant, cooling effect of Terra-Cortril Spray is quite desirable for the symptomatic relief of dermatitis. However, it should be anticipated that some highly excitable animals may become alarmed by this mild cooling sensation and by the sound of the spray leaving the container.

Do not use where pyogenic infection is present since the drug may allow this infection to spread. The use of Terramycin and other antibiotics may result in an overgrowth of resistant organisms—particularly Monilia and staphylococci. If new infections due to nonsusceptible bacteria or fungi appear during therapy, appropriate measures should be taken.

Danger: EXTREMELY FLAMMABLE Spray may ignite near an open flame or operating electrical equipment. Do not use when smoking.

Caution: KEEP AWAY FROM EYES OR OTHER MUCOUS MEMBRANES. Use with adequate ventilation. Avoid inhaling. Use only as directed. Intentional misuse by deliberately concentrating and inhaling the contents can be harmful or fatal. Keep out or reach of children.

Warning: CONTENTS UNDER PRESSURE
Do not puncture or incinerate container. Do not expose to heat or store at temperatures above 120°F.
How Supplied: Terra-Cortril Spray is available in a can containing 1.27 ounces.

TERRAMYCIN®
(ophthalmic ointment with polymyxin B sulfate)
Veterinary
For Topical Use Only

Composition: Terramycin (oxytetracycline HCl) is an antibiotic, bright yellow in color, possessing potent antimicrobial activity. It is one of the most versatile of the broad-spectrum antibiotics, and is effective in the treatment of infections due to gram-positive and gram-negative bacteria, both aerobic and anaerobic, the spirochetes, the rickettsiae, and certain of the larger viruses.
Polymyxin B sulfate is one of a group of related antibiotics derived from *Bacillus polymyxa.* The polymyxins are rapidly bactericidal, this action being exclusively against gram-negative bacteria.
The broad-spectrum effectiveness of Terramycin against both gram-positive and gram-negative organisms is enhanced by the particular effectiveness of polymyxin B against infections associated with gram-negative organisms, especially those due to *Pseudomonas aeruginosa,* where polymyxin B is the antibiotic of choice. In addition, there is evidence to indicate that polymyxin B sulfate possesses some antifungal activity. The combined antibacterial effect of Terramycin plus polymyxin is at least additive and, in many instances, an actual synergistic action is obtained.
Terramycin Ophthalmic Ointment with Polymyxin B Sulfate is a suspension of oxytetracycline hydrochloride and polymyxin B sulfate in a special petrolatum base. Each gram of ointment contains oxytetracycline HCl equivalent to 5 mg oxytetracycline, and 10,000 units of polymyxin B as the sulfate.
Indications: Terramycin Ophthalmic Ointment with Polymyxin B Sulfate is indicated for the prophylaxis and local treatment of superficial ocular infections due to oxytetracycline-and polymyxin-sensitive organisms, including infections due to streptococci, rickettsiae, *E. coli,* and *A. aerogenes,* such as conjunctivitis, keratitis, pink eye, corneal ulcer, blepharitis in dogs, cats, cattle, sheep, and horses; ocular infections due to secondary bacterial complications of distemper in dogs, and bacterial inflammatory conditions which may occur secondary to other infectious diseases in the above species.
Dosage and Administration: Terramycin Ophthalmic Ointment with Polymyxin B Sulfate should be administered topically to the eye 2 to 4 times daily.
Recommended Storage: Store below 25°C (77°F).
Precautions: Allergic reactions may occasionally occur. Treatment should be discontinued if reactions are severe.
Note: The use of oxytetracycline and other antibiotics may result in an overgrowth of resistant organisms such as Monilia, staphylococci and other species of bacteria. If new infections due to nonsensitive bacteria or fungi appear during therapy, appropriate measures should be taken.
How Supplied: Terramycin Ophthalmic Ointment with Polymyxin B Sulfate (Veterinary): 1/8 oz. tubes.

Pharmaderm
a division of Altana Inc.
60 BAYLIS ROAD
MELVILLE, NY 11747

CAT LAX®
Feline Laxative

Composition: Contains: Cod Liver Oil, Caramel, Lecithin, Malt Syrup, White Petrolatum, 0.1% Sodium Benzoate (preservative), 0.036 I.U./g Vitamin E (dl-alphatocopheryl acetate) (antioxidant), Purified Water.
Indications: A palatable formula for the elimination and prevention of hair balls in cats.
Dosage and Administration: Many cats will accept Cat Lax readily. For finicky animals place a small amount on paw—cat will lick its paw and become accustomed to the pleasant taste.
For hairball removal: For average weight adult cats, administer once daily. Squeeze approximately one inch of Cat Lax from tube. For smaller cats, vary amount accordingly.
For hairball prevention: Administer two or three times per week.
Warning: For veterinary use only. Keep out of reach of children.
How Supplied: 2 oz. tubes cellowrapped in sixes. NDC #0462-0084-28.
Other veterinary products available from Pharmaderm are:
[See table below].

NDC #0462-00	Product	Size
28–38	Bacitracin-Neomycin-Polymyxin Veterinary Ophthalmic Ointment	⅛ oz. tube
30–38	Bacitracin-Neomycin-Polymyxin Hydrocortisone Acetate 1% Veterinary Ophthalmic Ointment	⅛ oz. tube
93–38	Chloramphenicol 1% Veterinary Ophthalmic Ointment	⅛ oz. tube

Pioneer Brand Microbial Products

Pioneer Hi-Bred Intl., Inc.
P.O. BOX 258
JOHNSTON, IOWA 50131

The following biologicals manufactured by:
DIAMOND SCIENTIFIC CO.
DES MOINES, IOWA

P

BRSV VAC™ BOVINE RESPIRATORY SYNCYTIAL VIRUS VACCINE
Modified Live Virus

BRSV VAC™ is a modified live vaccine for the prevention of bovine respiratory syncytial virus (BRSV) infection in cattle. The virus antigen is stabilized and desiccated.

Serologic surveys indicate the virus is widespread in the cattle population. The virus is considered a contributor to the respiratory disease complex of cattle. Multiple infections do occur, and secondary bacterial infections may exacerbate the disease signs.

BRSV infections generally affect weaned calves although susceptible cattle of any age may become infected. BRSV signs follow an incubation of 5 to 7 days and may include fever; cough; nasal discharge; ocular discharge; anorexia; hyperpnea; pulmonary edema and emphysema; and denuding of the ciliated epithelium, leading to secondary bacterial pneumonia and associated sequela. BRSV signs vary in severity but may rapidly progress to a crisis phase.

Safety of combined vaccine was demonstrated experimentally in serologically negative calves inoculated repeatedly with multiple doses of vaccine.

Vaccine antigenicity and lack of antigenic interference were determined by measuring antibody responses of serologically negative calves to vaccination.

Vaccine efficacy was demonstrated by resistance of vaccinated calves to challenge with virulent BRSV in comparison to nonvaccinated controls and by measuring antibody levels before and after vaccination.

Potency Standards: Virus titrations are performed on each serial of BRSV VAC™. Each serial must have the stated minimum amount of viable virus (expressed as Tissue Culture infective $Doses_{50}$; i.e., $TCID_{50}$) per dose at the time of release for sale and must remain at or above government established requirements throughout dating.

The viruses of this product were extensively tested both at master seed virus and vaccine virus cell culture passages. These tests provide evidence of satisfactory virus identity, safety, and freedom from bacteria, fungi, mycoplasma and extraneous viruses. Antigenic and immunogenic capabilities of the vaccine were demonstrated in susceptible animals.

Serologic responses and resistance to challenge with virulent virus showed the high value of the product in eliciting protection in susceptible animals under the test conditions.

Bovine Respiratory Syncytial Virus

The vaccine must have the high virus release titer stated in the Outline of Production at the time of release for sale and must remain at or above the approved titer limit throughout its dating period.

Indications: For the immunization of healthy cattle against bovine respiratory syncytial virus infections.

Directions: Aseptically add the accompanying bottle of diluent to the vaccine. Agitate until dissolved and use entire contents immediately.

Dosage: Inject 2 ml intramuscularly for cattle of all ages, using aseptic techniques. Immunization against bovine respiratory syncytial virus requires a second dose of bovine respiratory syncytial virus vaccine given approximately three weeks after the first dose.

Calves vaccinated less than 6 months of age should be revaccinated at 6 months.

Caution:
1. Protect from light and hold at temperatures from 35° to 45°F. (2° to 7°C).
2. Allergic reactions may follow the use of products of this nature; antidote, epinephrine.
3. Burn this container and all unused contents.
4. Use entire contents when first opened.
5. Do not vaccinate within 21 days before slaughter.
6. Administer only to healthy animals. Animals infected by disease agents may suffer adverse reactions after vaccination.

Contains penicillin, streptomycin and mycostatin as preservatives.

BRSV VAC™ is supplied in:
10 dose (20 ml) vials
50 dose (100 ml) vials

U.S. Veterinary License No. 213
For Veterinary Use Only

BRSV VAC™ 2 BOVINE PARAINFLUENZA$_3$ RESPIRATORY SYNCYTIAL VIRUS VACCINE
Modified Live Virus

BRSV VAC™ 2 is a multiantigenic modified live vaccine for the prevention of bovine parainfluenza$_3$ (PI_3) and respiratory syncytial virus (BRSV) infection in cattle. The two viral antigens are combined in the proper ratio, stabilized and dessicated.

Serologic surveys indicate the viruses are widespread in the cattle population. The viruses are considered contributors to the respiratory disease complex of cattle. Multiple infections may exacerbate the disease signs.

BRSV infections generally affect weaned calves although susceptible cattle of any age may become infected. BRSV signs follow an incubation of 5 to 7 days and may include fever; cough; nasal discharge; ocular discharge; anorexia; hyperpnea; pulmonary edema and emphysema; and denuding of the ciliated epithelium, leading to secondary bacterial pneumonia and associated sequela. BRSV signs vary in severity but may rapidly progress to a crisis phase.

Disease signs caused by PI_3 virus generally appear within 14 days after shipment and arrival of calves at their destination. Signs are weakness, depression, watery to mucopurulent nasal discharge, fever, coughing and weight loss.

Safety of the combined vaccine was demonstrated experimentally in serologically negative calves inoculated repeatedly with multiple doses of vaccine.

Vaccine antigenicity and lack of antigenic interference were determined by measuring antibody responses of serologically negative calves to vaccination.

Vaccine efficacy was demonstrated by resistance of vaccinated calves to challenge with virulent BRSV or PI_3 in comparison to nonvaccinated controls and by measuring antibody levels before and after vaccination.

Potency Standards: Virus titrations are performed on each serial of BRSV VAC™ 2. Each serial must have the stated minimum amount of viable virus (expressed as Tissue Culture Infective $Doses_{50}$; i.e., $TCID_{50}$) per dose at the time of release for sale and must remain at or above government established requirements throughout dating.

The viruses of this product were extensively tested both at master seed virus and vaccine virus cell culture passages. These tests provide evidence of satisfactory virus identity, safety, and freedom from bacteria, fungi, mycoplasma, and extraneous viruses. Antigenic and immunogenic capabilities of the vaccine were demonstrated in susceptible animals.

Serologic responses and resistance to challenge with virulent virus showed the high value of the product in eliciting protection in susceptible animals under the test conditions.

Bovine Respiratory Syncytial Virus

The vaccine must have the high virus release titer stated in the Outline of Production at the time of release for sale and must remain at or above the approved titer limit throughout its dating period.

Parainfluenza$_3$

The vaccine must contain at least 160,000 $TCID_{50}$ (log $10^{5.2}$) per dose at time of release for sale and must remain at or above government established requirement at 16,000 $TCID_{50}$ (log $10^{4.2}$) throughout its dating period.

Indications: For the immunization of healthy cattle against bovine parainfluenza$_3$ and respiratory syncytial virus infections.

Directions: Aseptically add the accompanying bottle of diluent to the vaccine. Agitate until dissolved and use entire contents imediately.

Dosage: Inject 2 ml intramuscularly for cattle of all ages, using aseptic techniques. Immunization against bovine respiratory syncytial virus requires a second dose of bovine respiratory syncytial virus vaccine given approximately three weeks after the first dose.

Calves vaccinated less than 6 months of age should be revaccinated at 6 months.

Caution:
1. Protect from light and hold at temperatures from 35° to 45°F. (2° to 7° C).

2. Allergic reactions may follow the use of products of this nature; antidote, epinephrine.
3. Burn this container and all unused contents.
4. Use entire contents when first opened.
5. Do not vaccinate within 21 days before slaughter.
6. Administer only to healthy animals. Animals infected by disease agents may suffer adverse reactions after vaccination.

Contains penicillin, streptomycin and mycostatin as preservatives.
BRSV VAC™ 2 is supplied in:
10 dose (20 ml) vials
50 dose (100 ml) vials
U.S. Veterinary License No. 213
For Veterinary Use Only

BRSV VAC™ 3
BOVINE RHINOTRACHEITIS-PARAINFLUENZA$_3$-RESPIRATORY SYNCYTIAL VIRUS VACCINE
Modified Live Virus

BRSV VAC™ 3 is a multiantigenic modified live vaccine for the prevention of bovine rhinotracheitis (IBR), parainfluenza$_3$ (PI$_3$) and respiratory syncytial virus (BRSV) infection in cattle. The three viral antigens are combined in the proper ratio, stabilized and desiccated.
Serologic surveys indicate the three viruses are widespread in the cattle population. The viruses are considered contributors to the respiratory disease complex of cattle. Mutiple infections do occur, and secondary bacterial infections may exacerbate the disease signs.
Signs of IBR may include higher fever, hyperpnea, dyspnea and severe inflammation of the nasal mucosa with formation of mucoid plaques.
Disease signs caused by PI$_3$ virus generally appear within 14 days after shipment and arrival of calves at their destination. Signs are weakness, depression, watery to mucopurulent nasal discharge, fever, coughing and weight loss.
BRSV infections generally affect weaned calves although susceptible cattle of any age may become infected. BRSV signs follow an incubation of 5 to 7 days and may include fever; cough; nasal discharge; ocular discharge; anorexia; hyperpnea; pulmonary edema and emphysema; and denuding of the ciliated epithelium, leading to secondary bacterial pneumonia and associated sequela. BRSV signs vary in severity but may rapidly progress to a crisis phase.
Safety of the combined vaccine was demonstrated experimentally in serologically negative calves inoculated repeatedly with multiple doses of vaccine.
Vaccine antigenicity and lack of antigenic interference were determined by measuring antibody responses of serologically negative calves to vaccination.
Vaccine efficacy was demonstrated by resistance of vaccinated calves to challenge with virulent IBR, PI$_3$ or BRSV in comparison to nonvaccinated controls and by measuring antibody levels before and after vaccination.

Potency Standards: Virus titrations are performed on each serial of BRSV VAC™ 3. Each serial must have the stated minimum amount of viable virus (expressed as Tissue Culture Infective Doses$_{50}$; i.e., TCID$_{50}$) per dose at the time of release for sale and must remain at or above government established requirements throughout dating.
The viruses of this product were extensively tested both at master seed virus and vaccine virus cell culture passages. These tests provide evidence of satisfactory virus identity, safety and freedom from bacteria, fungi, mycoplasma and extraneous viruses. Antigenic and immunogenic capabilities of the vaccine were demonstrated in susceptible animals.
Serologic responses and resistance to challenge with virulent virus showed the high value of the product in eliciting protection in susceptible animals under the test conditions.

Bovine Rhinotracheitis
The vaccine must have at least 200,000 TCID$_{50}$ (log $10^{5.3}$) per dose at time of release and must remain at or above government established standard requirement of 16,000 TCID$_{50}$ (log $10^{4.2}$) throughout its dating period.

Parainfluenza$_3$
The vaccine must contain at least 160,000 TCID$_{50}$ (log $10^{5.2}$) per dose at time of release for sale and must remain at or above government established requirement of 16,000 TCID$_{50}$ (log $10^{4.2}$) throughout its dating period.

Bovine Respiratory Syncytial Virus
The vaccine must have the high virus release titer stated in the Outline of Production at the time of release for sale and must remain at or above the approved titer limit throughout its dating period.

Indications: For the immunization of healthy cattle against bovine rhinotracheitis, parainfluenza$_3$ and bovine respiratory syncytial virus infections.
Directions: Aseptically add the accompanying bottle of diluent to the vaccine. Agitate until dissolved and use entire contents immediately.
Dosage: Inject 2 ml intramuscularly for cattle of all ages, using aseptic techniques. Immunization against bovine respiratory syncytial virus requires a second dose of bovine respiratory syncytial virus vaccine given approximately three weeks after the first dose.
Calves vaccinated less than 6 months of age should be revaccinated at 6 months.
Caution:
1. Protect from light and hold at temperatures from 35° to 45°F. (2° to 7°C).
2. Allergic reactions may follow the use of products of this nature; antidote, epinephrine.
3. Burn this container and all unused contents.
4. Use entire contents when first opened.
5. Do not use in pregnant animals or in calves nursing pregnant animals; abortion may follow use of this vaccine in pregnant animals.
6. Do not vaccinate within 21 days before slaughter.
7. Administer only to healthy animals. Animals infected by disease agents may suffer adverse reactions after vaccination.

Contains penicillin, streptomycin and mycostatin as preservatives.
BRSV VAC™ 3 is supplied in:
10 dose (20 ml) vials
50 dose (100 ml) vials
U.S. Veterinary License No. 213
For Veterinary Use Only

P

BRSV VAC™ 4
BOVINE RHINOTRACHEITIS-VIRUS DIARRHEA-PARAINFLUENZA$_3$-RESPIRATORY SYNCYTIAL VIRUS VACCINE
Modified Live Virus

BRSV VAC™ 4 is a multiantigenic modified live vaccine for the prevention of bovine rhinotracheitis (IBR), virus diarrhea (BVD), parainfluenza$_3$ (PI$_3$), and respiratory syncytial virus (BRSV) infection in cattle. The four viral antigens are combined in the proper ratio, stabilized and desiccated.
Serologic surveys indicate the four viruses are widespread in the cattle population. The viruses are considered contributors to the respiratory disease complex of cattle. Multiple infections do occur, and secondary bacterial infections may exacerbate the disease signs.
Signs of IBR may include high fever, hyperpnea, dyspnea and severe inflammation of the nasal mucosa with formation of mucoid plaques. BVD manifests itself in many ways making diagnosis difficult. Since diarrhea may be one of the lesser signs seen, it is unfortunate the word diarrhea is associated with the name of the disease. A transient diarrhea may be unnoticed until more severe signs are observed in the herd. Respiratory signs, rough hair coat, laminitis and decreased weight gains are also seen. Generally, morbidity is high and mortality is low; however, complications with other conditions are common and will increase the severity and mortality.
BVD is often obscured or confused with other conditions of the respiratory disease complex. BVD in pregnant animals may cause abortions or malformed and weak calves at birth. Chronic disease with erosions in the alimentary tract is referred to as "Mucosal Disease" and is usually fatal.
Disease signs caused by PI$_3$ virus generally appear within 14 days after shipment and arrival of calves at their destination. Signs are weakness, depression, watery to mucopurulent nasal discharge, fever, coughing and weight loss.
BRSV infections generally affect weaned calves although susceptible cattle of any age may become infected. BRSV signs follow an incubation of 5 to 7 days and may include fever; cough; nasal discharge; ocular discharge; anorexia; hyperpnea; pulmonary edema and emphysema; and denuding of the ciliated epithelium, leading to secondary bacterial pneumonia and associated sequela.

Continued on next page

Pioneer—Cont.

BRSV signs vary in severity but may rapidly progress to a crisis phase.
Safety of the combined vaccine was demonstrated experimentally in serologically negative calves inoculated repeatedly with multiple doses of vaccine.
Vaccine antigenicity and lack of antigenic interference were determined by measuring antibody responses of serologically negative calves to vaccination.
Vaccine efficacy was demonstrated by resistance of vaccinated calves to challenge with virulent IBR, PI_3 or BRSV in comparison to nonvaccinated controls and by measuring antibody levels before and after vaccination.
Potency Standards: Virus titrations are performed on each serial of BRSV VAC™ 4. Each serial must have the stated minimum amount of viable virus (expresed as Tissue Culture Infective $Doses_{50}$; i.e., $TCID_{50}$) per dose at the time of release for sale and must remain at or above government established requirements throughout dating.
The viruses of this product were extensively tested both at master seed virus and vaccine virus cell culture passages. These tests provide evidence of satisfactory virus identity, safety, and freedom from bacteria, fungi, mycoplasma and extraneous viruses. Antigenic and immunogenic capabilities of the vaccine were demonstrated in susceptible animals.
Serologic responses and resistance to challenge with virulent virus showed the high value of the product in eliciting protection in susceptible animals under the test conditions.

Bovine Rhinotracheitis
The vaccine must have at least 200,000 $TCID_{50}$ (log $10^{5.3}$) per dose at time of release and must remain at or above government established standard requirement of 16,000 $TCID_{50}$ (log $10^{4.2}$) throughout its dating.

Bovine Virus Diarrhea
The vaccine must have at least 50,000 $TCID_{50}$ (log $10^{4.7}$) per dose at time of release and must remain at or above government established standard requirement of 10,000 $TCID_{50}$ (log $10^{4.0}$) throughout its dating.

$Parainfluenza_3$
The vaccine must contain at least 160,000 $TCID_{50}$ (log $10^{5.2}$) per dose at time of release for sale and must remain at or above government established standard requirement of 25,000 $TCID_{50}$ (log $10^{4.4}$) throughout its dating.

Bovine Respiratory Syncytial Virus
The vaccine must have the high virus release titer stated in the Outline of Production at the time of release for sale and must remain at or above the approved titer limit throughout its dating period.
Indications: For the immunization of healthy cattle against bovine rhinotracheitis, bovine virus diarrhea, $parainfluenza_3$ and bovine respiratory syncytial virus infections.
Directions: Aseptically add the accompanying bottle of diluent to the vaccine. Agitate until dissolved and use entire contents immediately.
Dosage: Inject 2 ml intramuscularly for cattle of all ages, using aseptic techniques. Immunization against bovine respiratory syncytial virus requires a second dose of bovine respiratory syncytial virus vaccine given approximately three weeks after the first dose.
Calves vaccinated less than 6 months of age should be revaccinated at 6 months.
Caution:
1. Protect from light and hold at temperatures from 35° to 45°F. (2° to 7°C).
2. Allergic reactions may follow the use of products of this nature; antidote, epinephrine.
3. Burn this container and all unused contents.
4. Use entire contents when first opened.
5. Do not use in pregnant animals or in calves nursing pregnant animals; abortion may follow use of this vaccine in pregnant animals.
6. Scientific evidence demonstrates the inability of some animals of an occasional herd to develop antibodies to bovine virus diarrhea after vaccination. This affected animal may exhibit symptoms similar to mucosal disease.
7. Do not vaccinate within 21 days before slaughter.
8. Administer only to healthy animals. Animals infected by disease agents may suffer adverse reactions after vaccination.

Contains penicillin, streptomycin and mycostatin as preservatives.
BRSV VAC™ 4 is supplied in:
10 dose (20 ml) vials
50 dose (100 ml) vials

U.S. Veterinary License No. 213
For Veterinary Use Only

BRSV VAC™ 9
BOVINE RHINOTRACHEITIS-VIRUS DIARRHEA-PARAINFLUENZA$_3$-RESPIRATORY SYNCYTIAL VIRUS VACCINE
Modified Live Virus
LEPTOSPIRA CANICOLA GRIPPOTYPHOSA-HARDJO-ICTEROHAEMORRHAGIAE-POMONA BACTERIN

BRSV VAC™ 9 is a multiantigenic modified live vaccine for the prevention of bovine rhinotracheitis (IBR), virus diarrhea (BVD), $parainfluenza_3$ (PI_3), and respiratory syncytial virus (BRSV) infection and a bacterin to aid in the prevention of *Leptospira canicola, Leptospira grippotyphosa, Leptospira hardjo, Leptospira grippotyphosa* and *Leptospira pomona* infection in susceptible cattle.
The four viral antigens are combined in proper ratio, stabilized, and desiccated into one cake. The desiccated viral fractions are rehydrated for use with specially procesed liquid *Leptospira Canicola-Grippotyphosa-Hardjo-Icterohaemorrhagiae-Pomona Bacterin.*
Safety of the viral fraction has been demonstrated in young serologically negative calves inoculated with multiple doses of vaccine. Safety of the *Leptospira Canicola-Grippotyphosa-Hardjo-Icterohaemorrhagiae-Pomona* Bacterin and the rehydrated combination has been demonstrated in calves.
Efficacy of the viral fractions was demonstrated by resistance of vaccinated calves to challenge with virulent IBR, BVD, PI_3, or BRSV in comparison to nonvaccinated calves. The *Leptospira canicola, Leptospira grippotyphosa* and *Leptospira icterohaemorrhagiae, Leptospira pomona* efficacy has been demonstrated by antibody response in cattle. These cattle efficacy studies have been further confirmed by the laboratory animal potency test described.
The Diseases: Serologic surveys indicate the four viruses are widespread in the cattle population. The viruses are considered contributors to the respiratory disease complex of cattle. Multiple infections do occur, and secondary bacterial infections may exacerbate the disease signs.
Signs of IBR may include high fever, hyperpnea, dyspnea and severe inflammation of the nasal mucosa with formation of mucoid plaques. BVD manifests itself in many ways making diagnosis difficult. Since diarrhea may be one of the lesser signs, it is unfortunate the word diarrhea is associated with the name of the disease. A transient diarrhea may be unnoticed until more severe signs are observed in the herd. Respiratory signs, rough hair coat, laminitis and decreased weight gains are also seen. Generally morbidity is high and mortality is low; however, complications with other conditions are common and will increase the severity and mortality.
BVD is often obscured or confused with other conditions of the respiratory disease complex. BVD in pregnant animals may cause abortions or malformed and weak calves at birth. Chronic disease with erosions in the alimentary tract is referred to as "Mucosal Disease" and is usually fatal.
Disease signs caused by PI_3 virus generally appear within 14 days after shipment and arrival of calves at their destination. Signs are weakness, depression, watery to mucopurulent nasal discharge, fever, coughing and weight loss.
BRSV infections generally affect weaned calves although susceptible cattle of any age may become infected. BRSV signs follow an incubation of 5 to 7 days and may include fever; cough; nasal discharge; ocular discharge; anorexia; hyperpnea; pulmonary edema and emphysema; and denuding of the ciliated epithelium, leading to secondary bacterial pneumonia and associated sequela. BRSV signs vary in severity but may rapidly progress to a crisis phase.
Leptospirosis is widespread in the animal population of the United States and is considered one of the most infectious diseases of farm animals.
Man can become infected either from animals with the disease or from an infective environmental source. In animals, the disease is known to cause reproductive disorders, loss of weight, decreased milk production and sometimes death. The economic losses suffered are

very large. The disease can be caused by several specific leptospires.

Five important serovars have been identified and are included in this product. Because specific serovar diagnosis is very difficult, and also due to the widespread nature of potential infection, it is recommended that all animals be vaccinated before introduction into the concentrated holding areas currently utilized on many premises. When infection is diagnosed, it is advisable to separate those animals showing disease signs and to vaccinate the remainder of the herd. The apparent effectiveness of vaccination will depend upon the number of animals exposed and incubating the disease at the time of vaccination. Vaccination cannot be expected to protect animals already in the incubating stages of the disease.

Serologic studies indicate widespread distribution of all these causative agents.

Potency Standards: Virus titrations are performed on each serial of BRSV VAC™ 9. Each serial must have the stated minimum amount of viable virus (expressed as Tissue Culture Infective $Doses_{50}$; i.e., $TCID_{50}$) per dose at the time of release for sale and must remain at or above government established requirements throughout dating.

The viruses of this product were extensively tested both at master seed virus and vaccine virus cell culture passages. These tests provide evidence of satisfactory virus identity, safety and freedom from bacteria, fungi, mycoplasma and extraneous viruses. Antigenic and immunogenic capabilities of the vaccine were demonstrated in susceptible animals.

Serologic responses and resistance to challenge with virulent virus showed the high value of the product in eliciting protection in susceptible animals under the test conditions.

Bovine Rhinotracheitis

The vaccine must have at least 200,000 $TCID_{50}$ (log $10^{5.3}$) per dose at time of release and must remain at or above government established standard requirement of 16,000 $TCID_{50}$ (log $10^{4.2}$) throughout its dating.

Bovine Virus Diarrhea

The vaccine must have at least 50,000 $TCID_{50}$ (log $10^{4.7}$) per dose at time of release and must remain at or above government established standard requirement of 10,000 $TCID_{50}$ ($log^{4.0}$) throughout its dating.

$Parainfluenza_3$

The vaccine must contain at least 160,000 $TCID_{50}$ (log $10^{5.2}$) per dose at time of release for sale and must remain at or above government established standard requirement of 25,000 $TCID_{50}$ (log $10^{4.4}$) throughout its dating.

Bovine Respiratory Syncytial Virus

The vaccine must have the high virus release titer stated in the Outline of Production at the time of release for sale and must remain at or above the approved titer limit throughout its dating period.

Leptospira canicola. Leptospira grippotyphosa, Leptospira hardjo, Leptospira icterohaemorrhagiae, Leptospira pomona. The *Leptospira canicola, grippotyphosa, icterohaemorrhagiae* and *pomona* antigen fractions are tested by sensitive hamster protection evaluation that has been related to host animal response. This test allows each serial of the product to be critically evaluated against these 4 serovars of Leptospira. Each serial must show satisfactory hamster protection with 1/800th of the field dose in USDA established testing for potency of each serovar. Each component is tested against a hamster challenge dose of at least 10–10,000 LD_{50}'s. The *Leptospira hardjo* fraction is tested by a serologic evaluation in rabbits that has been related to host animal response.

Indications: For the immunization of healthy cattle against bovine rhinotracheitis, bovine virus diarrhea, $parainfluenza_3$, bovine respiratory syncytial virus and *Leptospira canicola, Leptospira grippotyphosa, Leptospira hardjo, Leptospira icterohaemorrhagiae, Leptospira pomona* infections.

Directions: Aseptically add the accompanying bottle of *Leptospira Canicola Grippotyphosa-Hardjo-Icterohaemorrhagiae-Pomona* Bacterin (diluent) to the vaccine. Agitate until dissolved and use entire contents immediately.

Dosage: Inject 2 ml intramuscularly for cattle of all ages, using aseptic techniques. Immunization against bovine respiratory syncytial virus requires a second dose of bovine respiratory syncytial virus vaccine given approximately three weeks after the first dose.

Calves vaccinated less than 6 months of age should be revaccinated at 6 months.

Caution:

1. Protect from light and hold at temperatures from 35° to 45°F (2° to 7°C).
2. Allergic reactions may follow the use of products of this nature; antidote, epinephrine.
3. Burn this container and all unused contents.
4. Use entire contents when first opened.
5. Do not use in pregnant animals or in calves nursing pregnant animals; abortion may follow use of this vaccine in pregnant animals.
6. Scientific evidence demonstrates the inability of some animals of an occasional herd to develop antibodies to bovine virus diarrhea after vaccination. This affected animal may exhibit symptoms similar to mucosal disease.
7. Do not vaccinate within 21 days before slaughter.
8. Administer only to healthy animals. Animals infected by disease agents may suffer adverse reactions after vaccination.

The virus vaccine contains penicillin, streptomycin and mycostatin as preservatives. The bacterin contains thimerosal as preservative.

BRSV VAC™ 9 is supplied in:
10 dose (20 ml) vials
50 dose (100 ml) vials

U.S. Veterinary License No. 213
For Veterinary Use Only

HORIZON™ I
BOVINE VIRUS DIARRHEA VACCINE, KILLED VIRUS

Horizon™ I is recommended for the immunization of healthy cattle against bovine virus diarrhea virus. The disease manifests itself in many ways making diagnosis difficult. Since diarrhea may be one of the lesser symptoms seen, it is unfortunate that the word diarrhea became associated with the name of the disease. A transient diarrhea may be unnoticed until more severe symptoms are observed in the herd. Respiratory distress, rough hair coat, laminitis, and decreased weight gains are also seen.

The Disease: The disease, bovine virus diarrhea, is commonly referred to as virus diarrhea or BVD. Generally, morbidity is high and mortality is low; however complications with other conditions are common and will increase the severity and mortality. It is often obscured or confused with other conditions, as the bovine respiratory disease complex. The disease in pregnant animals may cause abortions or malformed and weak calves at birth. Chronic disease with erosions in the alimentary tract is referred to as "Mucosal Disease" and is usually fatal.

The Vaccine: Virus-laden diploid bovine kidney tissue culture fluids are harvested, chemically inactivated, neutralized, suitably concentrated as may be required, and preserved.

Each serial of Horizon™ I is evaluated for purity, safety and potency before it is released for sale.

Indications: For the vaccination of healthy dairy and beef cattle of all ages against bovine virus diarrhea (BVD).

Directions: This product may be used alone or as a diluent for accompanying desiccated product.

Dosage: Inject 2 ml subcutaneously or intramuscularly into cattle of all ages, using aseptic technique. Repeat in 21 to 28 days. Calves vaccinated before weaning should be revaccinated after weaning. Annual revaccination is recommended.

Caution:

1. Store protected from light and hold at temperatures from 35° to 45° F (2° to 7° C).
2. DO NOT FREEZE.
3. Allergic reactions may follow use of products of this nature; antidote, epinephrine.
4. Use entire contents when first opened.
5. Do not vaccinate within 21 days before slaughter.
6. Administer only to healthy animals. Animals infected by disease agents may suffer adverse reactions after vaccination.

Contains penicillin and streptomycin as preservatives.

Horizon™ I is supplied as follows:
10 dose (20 ml) vials
50 dose (100 ml) vials

For Veterinary Use Only

Continued on next page

Pioneer—Cont.

NEO–VAC® 7

Neo-Vac® 7 is recommended for the prevention and reduction of morbidity and mortality in baby pigs of atrophic rhinitis caused by *Bordetella bronchiseptica,* of enterotoxemia caused by *Clostridium perfringens* Type C and of colibacillosis caused by K88, K99, 987p positive *E. coli* serotypes.

The antigens are prepared from specially selected porcine origin bacterial cultures. The cultures are grown separately in modern mass culture propagation equipment. Careful control of the growth conditions and subsequent production processing for purification and concentration provide consistent high quality to each serial of product. The production method allows the reduced 2 ml final product to contain a full dose of these antigens. Special *in vitro* laboratory tests provide a means to quantify product antigen during product preparation. These procedures ensure uniform high product quality with assurance of safety.

Indications: This product is for the prevention and reduction of morbidity and mortality losses in neonatal swine due to atrophic rhinitis caused by *Bordetella bronchiseptica,* enterotoxemia caused by *Clostridium perfringins* Type C and enteric colibacillosis due to enterotoxigenic *Escherichia coli* which have serotype classifications with K88ab, K88ac, K99 or 987p antigens. The protective effect for the baby pigs is passively transferred in the colostrum and /or milk from the previously vaccinated sow according to recommendations.

Recommendations: Shake well before using. Administer 3 ml intramuscularly using aseptic techniques. Two doses of this product should be given. The first dose should be given five to eight weeks before farrowing; the repeat dose, four weeks after the first dose, approximately seven to 30 days before farrowing.

Caution: Protect from light and hold at temperatures from 35 to 45 degrees F. (2 to 7 degrees C.). Do not freeze. Allergic reactions may follow the use of products of this nature. Antidote: epinephrine. On rare occasions, adverse reactions may be observed within an hour or so of inoculation. Affected animals may exhibit varying degrees of distress observed as transitory temperature rise and anorexia. Other signs of adverse reactions to the antigens occur in very sensitive animals. Transient swelling at the injection site may occur following injection of *Bordetella bronchiseptica* products. Do not vaccinate within 21 days before slaughter. Use entire vaccine contents when first opened. Burn container and all unused contents.

Neo-Vac® 7 is available as follows:
10 dose (1 × 30 ml) vial
25 dose (1 × 75 ml) vial

U.S. Veterinary License No. 213
For Veterinary Use Only

TGE/ECOLI–VAC 4–C

TGE/ECOLI-Vac 4-C Vaccine is recommended for use as an aid in the prevention of losses in baby pigs due to transmissible gastroenteritis, to enterotoxemia caused by *Clostridium perfringens* Type C and colibacillosis in neonatal swine caused by K88, K99 and 987p positive *E. coli* serotypes.

Indications: The protective effect for the baby pigs is passively transferred in the colostrum and/or milk from the sow previously vaccinated with the TGE/ECOLI-Vac 4-C Vaccine according to recommendations.

Recommendations: Shake well before using. Administer 2 ml intramuscularly using aseptic techniques. Two doses of bacterin should be given. The first dose should be given five to eight weeks before farrowing; the repeat dose should be given four weeks after the first dose, or seven to 30 days before farrowing. In order to further enhance the level of protection through antibody concentration in colostrum and milk, sows should be given a repeat treatment during each pregnancy.

Caution: Protect from light and hold at temperatures from 35 to 45 degrees F (2 to 7 degrees C.). Do not freeze. Allergic reactions may follow the use of products of this nature. Antidote: epinephrine. Use entire vaccine contents when first opened. Burn container and all unused contents. On rare occasions, adverse reactions may be observed within an hour or so of inoculation. Affected animals may exhibit varying degrees of distress observed as transitory temperature rise and anorexia. Other signs of adverse reactions to the antigens may occur in very sensitive animals. Do not vaccinate within 21 days before slaughter.

TGE/ECOLI-Vac 4-C Vaccine is available as follows:
1 dose (5 × 2 ml) vials
10 dose (1 × 20 ml) vials

TGE-VAC is protected under U.S. Pat. No. 3,479,430, 3,585,108 and 4,070,053.

U.S. Veterinary License No. 213
For Veterinary Use Only

TGE/NEO–VAC® 7

TGE/Neo-Vac® 7 is recommended for use as an aid in the prevention of losses in baby pigs due to transmissible gastroenteritis, and for prevention and reduction of morbidity and mortality in baby pigs of atrophic rhinitis caused by *Bordetella bronchiseptica,* enterotoxemia caused by *Clostridium perfringens* Type C and of colibacillosis caused by K88, K99 and 987p positive *E. coli* serotypes.

The combination vaccine is achieved by using the liquid Neo-Vac® 7 to rehydrate the desiccated TGE Vaccine.

Recommendations: Shake well before using. Administer 3 ml intramuscularly using aseptic techniques. Two doses of this product should be given. First dose administered five to eight weeks before farrowing; repeat dose given four weeks after the first dose, approximately seven to 30 days before farrowing. Rehydrate the desiccated TGE-Vac with the liquid Neo-Vac® 7 Bacterin-toxoid and use entire contents immediately. Do not save unused amounts for later use. In order to further enhance the level of protection through antibody concentration in colostrum and milk, sows should be given a repeat treatment during each pregnancy.

Caution: Protect from light and hold at temperatures from 35 to 45 degrees F. (2 to 7 degrees C.). Do not freeze. Allergic reactions may follow the use of products of this nature. Antidote: epinephrine. On rare occasions, adverse reactions may be observed within an hour or so of inoculation. Affected animals may exhibit varying degrees of distress observed as transitory temperature rise and anorexia. Other signs of adverse reactions to the antigens may occur in very sensitive animals. Transient swellings at the injection site may ocur following injection of *Bordetella bronchiseptica* products. Do not vaccinate within 21 days before slaughter. Maintain the best possible sanitary conditions and protect all pigs from virulent TGE exposure. The degree of protection afforded by the sow's milk is passive, limited and may be overcome by severe exposure. Use entire vaccine contents when first opened. Burn container and all unused contents.

TGE/Neo-Vac® 7 is available as follows:
5 × 1 dose vials with rehydrating bacterin-toxoid, 3 ml each
1 × 10 dose vials with rehydrating bacterin-toxoid, 30 ml each

TGE Vaccine is protected under U.S. Pat. Nos. 3,479,430, 3,585,108 and 4,070,053.
U.S. Veterinary License No. 213
For Veterinary Use Only

TGE–VAC

TGE-Vac is a modified live virus vaccine produced from porcine tissue culture for vaccination of pregnant sows which usually transfer antibodies through their milk to suckling pigs.

Indications: TGE-Vac is recommended for use as an aid in the prevention of losses of baby pigs due to transmissible gastroenteritis.

Directions: Rehydrate the desiccated vaccine with the accompanying diluent and use entire contents immediately.

Recommendations: Two doses of vaccine should be given with a 30-day interval between vaccinations. The second dose is recommended to be given to sows one month after the first vaccination and seven to 30 days before farrowing. In order to further increase level of immunity (antibody concentration in serum and milk), sows should be revaccinated with two doses of vaccine during each pregnancy. Inject 2 ml intramuscularly using aseptic techniques.

Caution: Protect from light and hold at temperatures from 35 to 45 degrees F. (2 to 7 degrees C.). Allergic reactions may follow the use of products of this nature. Antidote: epinephrine or atropine. Use entire vaccine contents when first opened. Burn container and all unused contents. Do not vaccinate within 21 days before slaughter.

Inject vaccine-diluent combination intramuscularly to assure full potency. Maintain the best possible sanitary conditions and protect all pigs from virulent virus exposure. The degree of protection afforded by the sow's milk is passive, limited and may be overcome by severe exposure. Administer only to healthy animals. Animals infected by disease agents may suffer adverse reactions after vaccinations.

Contains penicillin, streptomycin and mycostatin as preservatives.

TGE-Vac is available as follows:
1 dose (5 × 2 ml) vials
10 dose (1 × 20 ml) vials

U.S. Veterinary License No. 213
For Veterinary Use Only

The following Probiocin® brand microbial products manufactured and distributed by:

PIONEER HI-BRED INTL., INC.
MICROBIAL GENETICS DIVISION
JOHNSTON, IOWA

PROBIOCIN® brand Microbial Products

History: Domestic animals frequently respond to sudden changes in diet, environment and weather by developing a change in the normal gut flora. Clinical therapy has also been shown to upset the gut ecosystem. PROBIOCIN® brand Microbial Products can help maintain effective levels of viable Lactobacilli under conditions which tend to diminish the normal flora. PROBIOCIN microbial products are especially useful as first-day-of-life application, to assist the newborn in establishing beneficial bacterial defenses.

Product Description: PROBIOCIN products contain blended combinations of naturally occurring Lactobacillus and *Streptococcus faecium* species selected for bile tolerance and the ability to produce a beneficial effect in a specific test animal. PROBIOCIN Microbial Products are dehydrated and stabilized to insure extended viability and shelf life in the finished product.

Safety: PROBIOCIN products can be administered to both newborn and mature animals. PROBIOCIN products are not classified as drugs: there are no residues and no withdrawal requirements.

Contraindications: Research indicates that beneficial Lactobacilli are the gut organisms most susceptible when the animal experiences digestive upset. Therefore, little or no activity can be expected from PROBIOCIN products when adverse conditions are *absent* in treated animals. In such instances, resident populations of intestinal microflora will be in a stable condition.

Summary: All warm-blooded animals are dependent upon populations of identified strains of select intestinal bacteria, especially Lactobacilli. When fed at established use levels, PROBIOCIN products can provide positive performance responses where conditions are less than ideal. The influences of lactic acid bacteria preparation have been demonstrated. They include:

- Increase in beneficial intestinal bacteria.
- Association with the gut wall to effectively compete with potential enteric pathogens during normal gut microflora development.
- Reduction of intestinal pH by the production of lactic acid.
- Reduction of the intestinal oxidation-reduction potential, creating a more positive anaerobic atmosphere and thereby inhibiting many pathogens.
- Possible reduction of undesirable metabolic by-product synthesis.
- Under certain situations, increases the rates of gain and feed efficiency.

Mortality and morbidity may be decreased.

Product Stability: Stability data for PROBIOCIN® brand Microbial Products have been developed with a variety of products stored under controlled conditions. These studies demonstrate the tolerance of these viable microorganisms to varying environmental conditions. There is a definite, measurable effect of long periods of high temperature on culture viability. Storage at recommended temperatures of 70°F. or less, however, results in excellent extended product shelf life.

Bile Tolerance: One criteria for selecting strains of beneficial intestinal bacteria used in the formulation of PROBIOCIN® brand Microbial Products is bile tolerance. Bile tolerance is essential for the survival of the living culture as it passes from the stomach into the upper small intestine, where concentrations are the highest.

The chart below shows the results of testing the tolerance of PROBIOCIN® brand Dispersible powder in the presence of bile. These tests were conducted in the laboratory and not in the animal, and therefore are actually more severe than would be experienced in the intestinal tract. It is believed that the organisms rarely are exposed to concentrations of bile exceeding 2% in the intestinal tract.

PROBIOCIN® brand BOLUS Microbial Product

An ingestible live microbiotic bolus to inoculate the gastro-intestinal tract of ruminants of all ages.

Benefits: Each bolus contains concentrations of select strains of beneficial micro-organisms.

Provides important vitamins.

Can also be crushed and added to milk replacer, or used as a top dressing on feed.

Not classified as a drug; no withdrawal necessary.

Directions For Use: Administer with balling gun, or by hand. **Newborn calves,** pre-shipment **cattle,** incoming **feeder lambs, sheep** showing persistent appetite loss, during periods of clinical therapy: one ¼-oz. bolus. Incoming **cattle/calves** on arrival, freshening **dairy cows** immediately after calving, adult **sheep and cattle** showing persistent appetite loss, during periods of clinical therapy: 2 ¼-oz. boluses, or 1 ½-oz. bolus. KEEP COOL, DRY.

Technical Specifications
PROBIOCIN® BRAND BOLUS MICROBIAL PRODUCT

Guaranteed Analysis	**(%)**
Protein, minimum	0
Fat, minimum	1
Fiber, maximum	6
Physical Character	
Body	Compressed bolus
Color	Tan
Moisture	Approximately 3%
pH	6.4
Taste	Bland
Odor	None

Contents & Standards Ingredients: Dried *Lactobacillus acidophilus* fermentation product, dried *Lactobacillus plantarum* fermentation product, dried *Streptococcus faecium* fermentation product, dried *Lactobacillus casei* fermentation product, yeast culture, lactose, dicalcium phosphate, vitamin B_{12}, vitamin E, magnesium stearate, TBHQ a preservative.

Microbial Standard: 5×10^6 cfu/gm.

Storage recommendations: Store at 70°F. or below.

Packaging:	
Jars:	¼ oz., 100 count
	½ oz., 50 count
Blister paks:	¼ oz., 12 count
	½ oz., 12 count

PROBIOCIN® brand DISPERSIBLE Microbial Product

An ingestible live microbiotic dispersible powder to help establish and maintain gastro-intestinal well-being in ruminants of all ages.

Benefits: A means to provide continuous introduction of beneficial bacteria to the digestive tract of milk-fed calves.

Can be prepared as a drench in combination with electrolytes and amino acids.

Especially useful at evidence of persistent appetite loss/common intestinal distress.

Mixes easily with milk replacer; poor-eating calves will readily ingest the powder in dry form from the bottom of the pail.

Not classified as a drug; no withdrawal necessary, meat or milk.

Directions For Use: Add to finished milk replacer just before feeding. For maximum results, wait until milk replacer has cooled to 120°F or below before adding powder. **Dairy and veal calves:** feed at rate of 4 grams/hd/day, or 1 pound per 100 calves for 28–30 days. **Lambs:** 2 grams/hd/day, feed continuously for maximum results. As a drench, add 10 grams/hd/day for period of use. Store at 70°F. or below.

Technical Specifications
PROBIOCIN® BRAND DISPERSIBLE

Pioneer—Cont.

MICROBIAL PRODUCT

Guaranteed Analysis	**(%)**
Protein, minimum	2
Fat, minimum	2
Fiber, maximum	5
Physical Character	
Body	Free-flowing powder
Color	Sandy brown
Bulk Density	47 lb/cu ft.
Solubility in Water	Dispersible only
Moisture	Approximately 1%
pH (in 10% solution)	5.60
Angle of repose	34 degrees
Taste	Sweet
Odor	Faint, malt-like

Typical Sieve Size Analysis (Tyler)	**(%)**
Through 20 mesh	99
Through 80 mesh	12

Contents & Standards Ingredients: Dried *Lactobacillus acidophilus* fermentation product, dried *Lactobacillus plantarum* fermentation product, dried *Streptococcus faecium* fermentation product, dried *Lactobacillus casei* fermentation product, yeast culture, sucrose, vegetable oil, Polysorbate 80, TBHQ and ethoxyquin preservatives.
Microbial Standard: 1×10^7 cfu/gm.
Storage recommendations: Storage temperature below 70°F (21°C) recommended. Keep plastic liners sealed when not in use.
Packaging: 2 lb. jars.

PROBIOCIN® brand EQUINE ONE GEL
Microbial Product

An ingestible live microbiotic gel to help establish and maintain gastro-intestinal well-being in newborn foals and adult horses.
Benefits: Especially important as first day-of-life application.
Also useful as first evidence of common intestinal upset in foals.
Helps restore depleted intestinal microflora in horses subjected to rigorous training, transporting, racing and clinical therapy.
No-drip gel formula assures positive oral delivery.
Not classified as a drug.
Directions For Use: Administer orally on back of tongue.
Foals: one dose (15gm) on day of birth; repeat on day four and at weaning.
General: one dose (colts), two doses (adult horses) indicated for lack of food or water, severe environmental temperature change and related conditions leading to physical strain. Store at 70°F or below.
Technical Specifications
PROBIOCIN® BRAND
EQUINE ONE GEL
MICROBIAL PRODUCT

Guaranteed Analysis	**(%)**
Protein, minimum	0
Fat, minimum	40
Fiber, maximum	6
Physical Character	
Body	Gel
Color	Brown/yellow
Bulk Density	1,100 gms/liter
Solubility in Water	None
Moisture	Approximately 1%
pH	4.7
Viscosity (cps at 70°F.)	Approximately 2×10^6
Taste	Sweet
Odor	None

Contents & Standards Ingredients: Dried *Lactobacillus acidophilus* fermentation product, dried *Lactobacillus plantarum* fermentation product, dried *Streptococcus faecium* fermentation product, dried *Lactobacillus casei* fermentation product, yeast culture, vegetable oils, sucrose, silicon dioxide, titanium dioxide, vitamin A, vitamin D_3, vitamin B_{12}, pantothenic acid, riboflavin, thiamine, FD&C Yellow No. 6 Lake, Polysorbate 80, TBHQ a preservative.
Microbial Standard: 1×10^7 cfu/gm.
Storage recommendations: Store at 70°F or below.
Packaging: 30gm syringe

PROBIOCIN® brand GRANULES
Microbial Product

An ingestible live microbiotic in granular form to help establish and maintain gastrointestinal well-being in maturing ruminants, swine and horses.
Benefits:
Helps maintain levels of beneficial bacterial to the intestinal tract.
Feed grade formulation blends with starter or grower rations for beef and dairy cattle, swine, horses and sheep.
Not classified as a drug; no withdrawal necessary.
Especially useful as an aid in overcoming adjustment problems during conditioning to a new environment.
Directions For Use: Blend with ration or top dress. **Incoming feeder cattle:** Total intake should approximate 150 grams in the receiving ration, i.e., 10 grams per/hd/day for 14–15 days, or optionally 20 grams per/hd/day for 7–8 days. Specific daily dosage rate will depend on length of receiving period. **Stale cattle:** add to ration at rate of 15–30 grams per/hd/day for 4–7 days. **Dairy cows, horses:** top dress 5 grams/hd/day during periods of clinical therapy, pre/post-parturition, severe environmental temperatures, ration change or any other adverse condition which might affect animal performance. **Swine:** growing pigs, 2 pounds per ton of feed to 40 pounds. BW. **Sows:** 2 pounds per ton in pre/post-farrowing ration. **Sheep:** feeder lambs, 2–4 grams per/hd/day for 7–14 days, breeding ewes 1–2 grams per/hd/day for 15–30 days in dry lot. Store at 70°F or below.
Technical Specifications
PROBIOCIN® BRAND
MICROBIAL PRODUCTS

Guaranteed Analysis	**(%)**
Protein, minimum	1
Fat, minimum	1
Fiber, maximum	20
Physical Character	
Body	Free-flowing granules
Color	Brown-Grey
Bulk Density	46 lbs/cu ft.
Solubility in Water	Not Soluble
Moisture	Approximately 2%
pH	6.0
Angle of repose	37 degrees
Taste	Bland
Odor	Faint, malt-like

Typical Sieve Size Analysis (Tyler)	**(%)**
Through 20 mesh	94
Through 80 mesh	1

Contents & Standards Ingredients: Dried *Lactobacillus acidophilus* fermentation product, dried *Lactobacillus plantarum* fermentation product, dried *Streptococcus faecium* fermentation product, dried *Lactobacillus casei* fermentation product, yeast culture, calcium carbonate, corn cob fractions, vegetable oil, TBHQ and ethoxyquin preservatives.
Microbial Standard: 1×10^7 cfu/gm.
Storage recommendations: Store at 70°F or below.
Packaging: 5 lb. jars
25 lb jars

PROBIOCIN® brand PET GEL
Microbial Product

An ingestible live microbiotic gel to help establish a balanced intestinal microbial flora in dogs and cats of all ages.
Benefits: Especially important as first-day-of-life application, or at first handling.
Also useful at first evidence of upset.
Each dose contains important vitamins.
No-drip gel formula assures positive oral delivery.
Not classified as a drug.
Directions For Use: Administer orally on back of tongue, or on food.
Newborn pups, kittens: ½gm at birth, 4 days and 7 days of age, and at weaning.
Post-weaning and older: to 10 pounds, 1gm. Over 10 pounds, 1gm each additional 10 pounds (repeated in 3 days) prior to or following periods of marked environmental change such as clinical therapy, simple digestive upsets, grooming, worming, training, shows and pre/post-parturition. Store at 70°F or below.
Technical Specifications:
PROBIOCIN® BRAND
PET GEL
MICROBIAL PRODUCT

Guaranteed Analysis	**(%)**
Protein, minimum	0
Fat, minimum	40
Fiber, maximum	6
Physical Character	
Body	Gel
Color	Rust brown
Bulk Density	1,100 gms/liter
Solubility in water	None
Moisture	Approximately 1%

pH	4.8
Viscosity (cps at 70°F.)	Approximately 2×10^6
Taste	Sweet
Odor	None

Contents & Standards Ingredients:
Dried *Lactobacillus acidophilus* fermentation product,
dried *Lactobacillus plantarum* fermentation product,
dried *Streptococcus faecium* fermentation product,
dried *Lactobacillus casei* fermentation product, yeast culture, vegetable oils, sucrose, silicon dioxide, vitamin A, vitamin D_3, vitamin E, vitamin B_{12}, riboflavin, niacin, pantothenic acid, folic acid, pyridoxine, thiamine, FD&C Yellow No. 6 Lake, Polysorbate 80, TBHQ a preservative.
Microbial Standard: 1×10^7 cfu/gm.
Storage recommendations: Store at 70°or below.
Packaging: 10gm Syringe

PROBIOCIN® brand RUMINANT GEL
Microbial Product

An ingestible live microbiotic gel to inoculate the gastro-intestinal tract of ruminants of all ages.
Benefits: Aids in rapidly populating the intestinal tract of newborn calves.
Helps restore depleted intestinal microflora in cattle subject to transporting, sudden diet/temperature change, calving, worming and clinical therapy.
Not classified as a drug. No withdrawal necessary, meat or milk.
No-drip gel formula assures positive oral delivery.
Directions For Use: Administer orally on back of tongue. **Newborn dairy calves, vealers, beef cattle** under 400 pounds, 10gm; over 400 pounds, 15gm. **Feeder lambs,** 5gm. **Adult sheep,** 10gm. **Dairy cows** post-calving, 15gm. Persistent appetite loss all cattle weights, 10–15gm. During periods of clinical therapy, 15gm. Store at 70°F or below.
Technical Specifications:
PROBIOCIN® BRAND
RUMINANT GEL
MICROBIAL PRODUCT

Guaranteed Analysis	**(%)**
Protein, minimum	0
Fat, minimum	40
Fiber, maximum	6
Physical Character	
Body	Gel
Color	Sandy brown
Bulk Density	1,100 gms/liter
Solubility in Water	None
Moisture	Approximately 1%
pH	4.8
Viscosity (cps at 70°F.)	Approximately 2×10^6
Taste	Sweet
Odor	None

Contents & Standards Ingredients:
Dried *Lactobacillus acidophilus* fermentation product,
dried *Lactobacillus plantarum* fermentation product,
dried *Streptococcus faecium* fermentation product,
dried *Lactobacillus casei* fermentation product, yeast culture, vegetable oils, sucrose, silicon dioxide, titanium dioxide, vitamin A, vitamin D_3, vitamin B_{12}, pantothenic acid, riboflavin, thiamine, Polysorbate 80, TBHQ a preservative.
Microbial Standard: 2.3×10^7 cfu/gm.
Storage recommendations: Store at 70°F or below.
Packaging: 300 gm cartridge
30 gm syringe

PROBIOCIN® brand SWINE GEL
Microbial Product

An ingestible live microbiotic gel to help establish and maintain gastro-intestinal well-being in the newborn and weanling pig.
Benefits: Especially important as first-day-of-life application, or at first handling.
Also useful at first evidence of common upset.
Each dose provides important vitamins.
No-drip gel formula assures positive oral delivery.
Not classified as a drug.
Directions For Use: Administer orally on back of tongue. **Newborn pigs:** at birth or first handling, 1gm. An additonal 2gm's should be given at weaning and whenever common upset or persistent appetite loss occurs. Store at 70°F or below.
Technical Specifications:
PROBIOCIN® BRAND
SWINE GEL
MICROBIAL PRODUCT

Guaranteed Analysis	**(%)**
Protein, minimum	0
Fat, minimum	40
Fiber, maximum	6
Physical Character	
Body	Gel
Color	Light sandy brown
Bulk Density	1,100 gms/liter
Solubility in Water	None
Moisture	Approximately 1%
pH	4.5
Viscosity (cps at 70°F.)	Approximately 2×10^6
Taste	Sweet
Odor	None

Contents & Standards Ingredients:
Dried *Lactobacillus acidophilus* fermentation product,
dried *Lactobacillus plantarum* fermentation product,
dried *Streptococcus faecium* fermentation product,
dried *Lactobacillus casei* fermentation product, yeast culture, vegetable oils, sucrose, silicon dioxide, titanium dioxide, vitamin A, vitamin D_3, vitamin E, vitamin B_{12}, FD&C Yellow No. 6 Lake, Polysorbate 80, TBHQ a preservative.
Microbial Standard: 1×10^7 cfu/gm.
Storage recommendations: Store at 70°F or below.
Packaging: 30gm syringe

Pitman-Moore, Inc.
P.O. BOX 344
WASHINGTON CROSSING, NJ 08560

BACTROVET*
(sulfadimethoxine)
Oral Suspension, 12.5%

Composition: Each ml contains: sulfadimethoxine 125 mg.
Action: Bactrovet (sulfadimethoxine) Oral Suspension in low doses at 24 hour intervals provides therapeutic results against a wide range of bacterial infections, including those due to both gram-negative and gram-positive pathogens such as streptococci, staphylococci, salmonella, *Klebsiella spp.* and *Escherichia coli.* Respiratory, urinary tract, and soft tissue infections due to susceptible organisms have responded well to Bactrovet.
There is little likelihood that Bactrovet will cause crystalluria or kidney damage because the drug is primarily excreted as a highly soluble glucuronide which is even more soluble than the parent compound.
Indications: Bactrovet (sulfadimethoxine) Oral Suspension is indicated for the treatment of a wide variety of bacterial infections in dogs and cats. Bactrovet is appropriate for use in the following specific disease conditions when they are caused by pathogens sensitive to sulfadimethoxine:

tonsillitis	abcesses
pharyngitis	cellulitis
pneumonia	cystitis
sinusitis	bacterial enteritis
urethritis	wound infections
bronchitis	

Contraindications: No specific contraindications are known.
Precautions: Although drug induced toxicity has not been reported following the use of Bactrovet (sulfadimethoxine) Oral Suspension, patients with impaired hepatic or renal function or with urinary obstruction should be closely evaluated before and during therapy.
The usual precautions used in sulfonamide therapy should be observed, including the maintenance of adequate fluid intake. Discontinue if toxic reactions occur.
As with any antibacterial agent, there may be occasional failures due to resistant microorganisms. If a satisfactory clinical response is not obtained after three or four days of Bactrovet therapy, the diagnosis and use of Bactrovet should be re-evaluated. Bactrovet is not effective in virus and rickettsial infections.
Dosage and Administration: The recommended dose of Bactrovet (sulfadimethoxine) Oral Suspension is 1 ml per 5 pounds body weight (25 mg per pound) the first day followed by one-half (12.5 mg per pound) the initial dose every

Continued on next page

24 hours thereafter. Administer directly into patient's mouth. In most cases, treatment for three to six days is adequate. Treatment should be continued until the patient is free of symptoms for 48 hours.
Shake well before using.
Caution: Federal law restricts this drug to use by or on the order of a licensed veterinarian.
How Supplied: Bactrovet (sulfadimethoxine) Oral Suspension 12.5%—12 × 1 fl oz and 16 fl oz (pint) bottles.
*Trademark

BACTROVET*
(sulfadimethoxine)
Tablets

Description: Bactrovet (sulfadimethoxine) Tablets are available in two sizes containing 125 mg or 250 mg of sulfadimethoxine.
Action: Bactrovet (sulfadimethoxine) in low doses at 24 hour intervals provides therapeutic results against a wide range of bacterial infections, including those due to both gram-negative and gram-positive pathogens such as streptococci, staphylococci, salmonellae, *Klebsiella spp.* and *Escherichia coli.* Respiratory, urinary tract, and soft tissue infections due to susceptible organisms have responded well to Bactrovet.
There is little likelihood that Bactrovet will cause crystalluria or kidney damage because the drug is primarily excreted as a highly soluble glucuronide, which is even more soluble than the parent compound.
Indications: Bactrovet (sulfadimethoxine) Tablets are indicated for the treatment of a wide variety of bacterial infections in dogs and cats.
BACTROVET is appropriate for use in the following disease conditions when caused by pathogens sensitive to sulfadimethoxine.

tonsillitis	urethritis	cellulitis
pharyngitis	bronchitis	wound infections
pneumonia	bacterial enteritis	cystitis
sinusitis	abscesses	

Contraindications: No specific contraindications are known.
Precautions: Although drug induced toxicity has not been reported following the use of Bactrovet (sulfadimethoxine), patients with impaired hepatic or renal function or with urinary obstruction should be closely evaluated before and during therapy.
The usual precautions used in sulfonamide therapy should be observed, including the maintenance of an adequate fluid intake.
As with any antibacterial agent, there may be occasional failures due to resistant microorganisms. If a satisfactory clinical response is not obtained after three or four days of Bactrovet (sulfadimethoxine) therapy, the diagnosis and use of Bactrovet should be reevaluated. Bactrovet is not effective in virus and rickettsial infections.
Dosage and Administration: The usual dose of Bactrovet (sulfadimethoxine) is 25.0 mg per pound body weight the first day followed by one-half (12.5 mg) the initial dose every 24 hours thereafter. Length of treatment will depend upon clinical response. In most cases, treatment for three to six days is adequate. Treatment should be continued until the patient is free of symptoms for 48 hours.
Dogs and Cats:
Initial dose—25.0 mg per pound body weight.
Maintenance dose—12.5 mg per pound body weight.
How Supplied:
Bactrovet (sulfadimethoxine) Tablets
125 mg (double scored) Bottles of 500 Tablets
250 mg (double scored) Bottles of 500 Tablets
SOLD TO VETERINARIANS ONLY

BORDEGEN*
Bordetella Bronchiseptica Bacterin

Description: Bordegen is an inactivated Bordetella Bronchiseptica Bacterin that has been adjuvanted to ensure high levels of protection.
Indications: For the immunization of healthy, pregnant swine and piglets against atropic rhinitis caused by *Bordetella bronchiseptica.*
Dosage and Administration: Shake well before using—Aseptically vaccinate healthy sows and piglets intramuscularly or subcutaneously according to the following schedule:
Sows:
2ml 4–5 weeks before farrowing.
2ml 1–2 weeks before farrowing.
2ml 2 weeks prior to each subsequent farrowing.
Piglets:
2ml 3 days of age or older.
2ml at weaning. The interval between the first and second vaccination must be at least 14 days.
Boars:
2ml annual revaccination
Precautions: Store at 2–7°C (35–45°F). Do not vaccinate within 21 days before slaughter. Use entire contents when first opened. Local reactions may occur at the site of injection. In case of anaphylactoid reaction, administer epinephrine. For Veterinary Use Only.
How Supplied: Bordegen is supplied in plastic vials containing 100ml (50 doses).
*Trademark

CANEX* SOLUTION
Oil Solution of Rotenone
EPA Reg. No. 773-4
EPA Est. No. 773-NJ-1

Composition:
Active Ingredients:

Rotenone	0.12% w/w
Other ether extractives of cube	0.2% w/w
Inert ingredients:	99.68% w/w

Indications: For the treatment of demodectic mange. Also used for ear mites.
Directions for Use: It is a violation of Federal law to use this product in a manner inconsistent with its labeling.
Directions for Demodectic Mange: Dogs should be clipped and bathed if necessary, and thoroughly dried. Apply petrolatum or other bland ointment to eyes to prevent conjunctival irritation. Thoroughly massage CANEX Solution into and around infested areas. If animal is in poor physical condition, correct before applying CANEX. Apply to a small area to determine tolerance. Discontinue if gastrointestinal or other systemic complications occur. Demodectic mange is difficult to accurately diagnose and often requires prolonged treatment and attention to other factors such as diet. Apply daily for 7–10 days; if no improvement is noted after 10 days, consult veterinarian.
Direction for Ear Mites: Dilute 1 part CANEX Solution with 3 parts of mineral oil. Shake well before using. Apply several drops in ear canal, massage to distribute over external ear structure. Repeat every 5 to 7 days for several applications, then as indicated.
Storage and Disposal
Keep product in original container. Store in a cool, dry place preferably in a locked storage area out of reach of children or pets. Do not reuse empty container. Rinse thoroughly before discarding. Securely wrap original container in several layers of newspaper and discard in trash.
Caution
Harmful if swallowed. Avoid contact with the eyes. Wash hands thoroughly after using.
How Supplied: 1 gallon.
*Trademark

CERBINOL* SOLUTION
Antiseptic and Keratolytic

Composition: Neutral salicylic and benzoic esters of propylene glycol, 0.07% w/w; Acid ester calculated as propylene glycol monomalic ester, 3.77% w/w; Malic acid 2.77% w/w; Salicylic acid, 1.07% w/w; Benzoic acid, 0.72% w/w.
Indications: For use on domestic animals as an aid in the treatment of minor wounds, lacerations and abrasions. Also soothes irritation and assists healing by softening and facilitating the removal of necrotic (dead) tissue.
Direction For Use: Thoroughly clean the affected area, clipping hair if necessary. Apply full-strength CERBINOL Solution with a cotton swab or gauze pad and bandage if needed. Repeat as required. If condition fails to improve within a reasonable amount of time, a veterinarian should be consulted.
For External Use Only
Warning: Keep out of reach of children.
How Supplied: 1 gallon
*Trademark

CONOFITE* CREAM, 2%
(miconazole nitrate)

Composition: Conofite (miconazole nitrate) Cream is a new, highly effective synthetic antifungal agent for use in dogs and cats. Each gram contains 23 mg

of miconazole nitrate (equivalent to 20 mg miconazole base) in a base containing: cetyl alcohol, stearyl alcohol, butylated hydroxytoluene, white petrolatum, mineral oil, polyoxyl 40 stearate, butylparaben and purified water.
Indications: Conofite (miconazole nitrate) Cream is indicated for the treatment of fungal infections in dogs and cats caused by *Microsporum canis*, *Microsporum gypseum* and *Trichophyton mentagrophytes*.
Precautions: Avoid contact with eyes, since irritation may result.
Wash hands thoroughly after administration to avoid spread of fungal infection.
Dosage and Administration: Accurate diagnosis of the infecting organism is essential. Identification should be made either by direct microscopic examination of a mounting of infected tissue in a solution of potassium hydroxide, or by culture on an appropriate medium.
Apply a ¼-inch ribbon of Conofite (miconazole nitrate) Cream once daily per square inch of lesion for 2 to 4 weeks. Rub into infected site and immediate surrounding vicinity. Application is best accomplished using a finger cot or cotton swab. Medication must be continued until the infecting organism is completely eradicated as indicated by appropriate clinical or laboratory examinations. If no improvement is noticed within 2 weeks, diagnosis should be reevaluated. Difficult cases may require treatment for 6 weeks.
General measures in regard to hygiene should be observed to control sources of infection or reinfection. Clipping of hair around and over the sites of infection should be done at the start of treatment and again as necessary.
Caution: Federal law restricts this drug to use by or on the order of a licensed veterinarian.
How Supplied: 12 × 15 g tubes.
*Trademark

CONOFITE* LOTION, 1%
(miconazole nitrate)

Composition: Conofite (miconazole nitrate) Lotion is a new, highly effective synthetic antifungal agent for use in dogs and cats. It contains: 1.15% miconazole nitrate (equivalent to 1 miconazole base by weight), polyethylene glycol 400%, and ethyl alcohol 55%.
Indications: Conofite (miconazole nitrate) Lotion is indicated for the treatment of fungal infections in dogs and cats caused by *Microsporum canis*, *Microsporum gypseum* and *Trichophyton mentagrophytes*.
Precautions: In the event of sensitization or irritation due to Conofite Lotion, treatment should be discontinued. Avoid contact with eyes, since irritation may result.
Wash hands thoroughly after administration to avoid spread of fungal infection.
Dosage and Administration: Accurate diagnosis of the infecting organism is essential. Identification should be made either by direct microscopic examination of a mounting of infected tissue in a solution of potassium hydroxide, or by culture on an appropriate medium.
Apply a light covering of Conofite (miconazole nitrate) Lotion to affected areas, once daily, for 2 to 4 weeks. Application is best accomplished using a gauze pad or cotton swab. Medication must be continued until the infecting organism is completely eradicated as indicated by appropriate clinical or laboratory examination. If no improvement is noticed within 2 weeks, diagnosis should be reevaluated. Difficult cases may require treatment for 6 weeks.
General measures in regard to hygiene should be observed to control sources of infection or reinfection. Clipping of hair around and over the sites of infection should be done at the start of treatment and again as necessary.
Caution: Federal law restricts this drug to use by or on the order of a licensed veterinarian.
How Supplied: 12 × 30 ml containers.
*Trademark

DIRYL*
Insecticidal Powder
EPA Reg. No. 773-16
EPA Est. No. 773-NJ-1

Composition:
Active Ingredients:
Carbaryl (1-naphthyl N-methylcarbamate†...............5.0% w/w
Pyrethrins...............0.1% w/w
Technical piperonyl butoxide‡...............1.0% w/w
Inert Ingredients...............93.9% w/w
†SEVIN®—Trademark of Union Carbide Corporation.
‡Equivalent to 0.8% (butylcarbityl) (6-propyl-piperonyl) ether and 0.2% of related compounds.
Indications: For control of fleas, ticks and lice on dogs and cats.
Directions for Use: It is a violation of Federal law to use this product in a manner inconsistent with its labeling.
Sprinkle DIRYL Insecticide Powder freely over animal, working well into the hair. To prevent reinfestation, application should be made to the animal and its quarters, especially crevices, at weekly intervals, as needed. Do not use on pregnant dogs.
Storage and Disposal
Keep product in original container. Store in a cool, dry place preferably in a locked storage area out of reach of children or pets. Do not reuse empty container. Securely wrap original container in several layers of newspaper and discard in trash.
Precautionary Statements
Hazards to Humans and Domestic Animals
Caution
HUMAN—Harmful if swallowed or inhaled. Avoid breathing of dust. Avoid contact with eyes. Avoid repeated contact with skin. Wash thoroughly after using. Avoid contamination of food. Do not use this product in commercial food areas of food handling establishments, restaurants, or other places where food is prepared or processed.
ANIMAL—Avoid contact with animal's eyes. Avoid treatment of kittens less than 4 weeks of age and nursing puppies. Repeated applications may produce skin or nasal irritation in sensitive animals—if this occurs, DIRYL Insecticide Powder should be discontinued.
Statement of Practical Treatment
If swallowed: induce vomiting by drinking 1 or 2 glasses of water and touching finger to back of throat. Contact physician immediately.
If in eyes: flush with plenty of water.
If on skin: wash with soap and water.
How Supplied: Twelve 3.5 oz containers.
*Trademark

DISPOSAJECT*
(dioctyl sodium sulfosuccinate)
Enema for dogs and cats

Composition: Each syringe contains 250 mg dioctyl sodium sulfosuccinate in 12 ml of glycerine U.S.P.
Action: Lubricates and softens the stool.
Indications: As an aid in the relief of all forms of constipation, for preoperative preparations and for restoration of bowel habits in postoperative patients.
Dosage and Administration: Gently insert flexible nozzle into rectum and press plunger to express contents. In resistant cases, treatment may be repeated in one hour.
How Supplied: 24 x 12 ml syringes.
*Trademark

ECTORAL* Emulsifiable Concentrate
(ronnel)

Description: Ectoral (ronnel) Emulsifiable Concentrate contains ronnel 33.34%, petroleum derivatives 56.32%, inert ingredients 10.34%.
Indications: The use of the topical product, is effective against certain ectoparasites of dogs and cats. Repeated therapy may be necessary to prevent reinfestation.
In dogs, demodectic and sarcoptic mange, and ear mite, tick, flea and louse infestations have responded to therapy.
In cats, therapeutic indications for the topical solution include infestation with ear mites and fleas.
Dosage and Administration: Although the topical application has an immediate killing effect on the parasites, reinfestation may be expected in heavily infested areas and continued treatment is necessary to maintain adequate control. Clinical experience indicates that failures are due, in most cases, to inadequate dosages or early discontinuance of therapy.
The dosage recommendations that follow have been widely used by veterinarians and may be used as a guide to establishing effective therapy.
Preparation of topical solutions: A freshly prepared topical solution should be used for each patient. To prepare a 1%

Continued on next page

P

Pitman-Moore—Cont.

solution add 1 oz. (2 tablespoonfuls) to 1 qt. of water, or add ½ oz. (tablespoonful) to 1 pt. of water. To prepare a 0.25% solution add ¼ oz. (1½ teaspoonfuls) to 1 qt. of water.

Demodectic mange in dogs: Apply a 1% solution of ronnel over entire body every 4 days. In very severe infections, dose may be increased to 35 mg per lb. per day. Treatment should be based on appearance of the mange mite upon periodic microscopic examination of skin scrapings from the affected area. Continue treatment for 3 weeks after all mites on skin scrapings are apparently dead.

Sarcoptic mange in dogs: Treat 3 times, at 7 to 10 day intervals, by sponging entire body with a 1% solution of ronnel.

Ticks on dogs: Apply a 1% solution of ronnel over entire body following a bath, while hair coat is still damp. Improvement is usually noted in 7 to 10 days in moderate infestations, but in severe infestations, 2 to 3 weeks of high dosage therapy may be required.

Ear mites in dogs and cats: Apply a 1% solution of ronnel to ears as needed.

Fleas and lice on dogs or fleas on cats: Apply a 0.25% solution of ronnel over entire body by sponging or dipping when necessary.

WARNING: *Human*—Ectoral (ronnel) is harmful if swallowed by humans. Call a physician, hospital, poison control center or rescue unit immediately. Avoid prolonged contact of the solution with the skin: rubber gloves should be used to protect the hands of the operator (avoid plastic gloves). Wash after handling. Avoid contact with eyes. Avoid contamination of foods.

Note to Physician: Ectoral (ronnel) is a cholinesterase inhibitor. The emulsifiable concentrate formulation contains petroleum derivatives which can cause chemical pneumonitis if aspirated. Remove from stomach if amount ingested is large enough to be considered systemically dangerous. Give supporting therapy. Atropine is an antidote; give after cyanosis is overcome and to effect. 2-PAM is a supplemental treatment.

WARNING: *Animal*—Ectoral (ronnel) is a cholinesterase inhibitor. Do not use this product on animals simultaneously or within a few days before or after treatment or exposure to cholinesterase inhibiting drugs, pesticides or chemicals.

Do not use Ectoral (ronnel) in conjunction with phenothiazine derived tranquilizers since phenothiazines may potentiate the toxicity of organophosphates.

Precautions: Ronnel is a cholinesterase inhibitor. Vomiting is the principal side-effect.

As with most insecticide dips, rubber gloves should be used to protect the hands of the operator.

Adverse Reactions: In dogs, doses exceeding 500 mg of ronnel per kg of body weight cause emesis. Lower doses cause only transient emesis or no effect. Dogs have received 10 mg/kg per day for 90 days without incidence of adverse effects. One dog was fed 25 mg/kg per day for 11 months without evidencing toxicity.

Adverse reactions may occur, however, due to drug sensitivity or improper dosing. Vomiting is the principal side effect of ronnel therapy. Excessive salivation, constriction of the pupil, purgation, pronounced muscle tremors and extreme muscular weakness with eventual collapse may also occur.

Overdosing: Atropine is an antidote. 2-PAM in conjunction with atropine is beneficial. Give supportive treatment. Avoid the use of tranquilizers, sedatives, narcotics, aminophylline, theophylline and neuromuscular blocking agents. In addition, animals that show toxic symptoms as a result of being overtreated topically should be thoroughly bathed with a detergent to prevent further absorption of the compound.

How Supplied: Ectoral (ronnel) Emulsifiable Concentrate: 33.34% in 4 fluid ounce bottles.

**Trademark*

ENTROMYCIN* POWDER
(bacitracin methylene disalicylate and streptomycin sulfate oral veterinary with carob powder)

Composition: Each gram contains: Bacitracin methylene disalicylate 200 units; streptomycin sulfate equivalent to 20 mg streptomycin; roasted, powdered carob pulp 850 mg and diluent, chocolate flavor q.s.

Indications: For treatment of bacterial enteritis caused by pathogens susceptible to bacitracin and streptomycin, such as *Escherichia coli, Proteus spp., Staphylococcus spp., Streptococcus spp.*, and for the symptomatic treatment of associated diarrhea in dogs.

Dosage and Administration: Administer one level teaspoonful for 10 pounds of body weight three times daily, as indicated.

Mix with a quantity of liquid or food small enough to assure total consumption.

For Oral Veterinary Use Only

Caution: Federal law restricts this drug to use by or on the order of a licensed veterinarian.

How Supplied: 1 lb containers.

*Trademark

FVR*-C-P
Feline Rhinotracheitis-Calici-Panleukopenia Vaccine Modified Live and Killed Virus

Composition: FVR*-C-P is a combination of antigens for convenient use in cats of any age for the prevention of disease caused by feline rhinotracheitis, feline calici and feline panleukopenia viruses. The feline rhinotracheitis-calici component is a lyophilized suspension of modified live viruses propagated in a stable cell line of feline origin and backfilled with an inert gas. The panleukopenia vaccine is propagated in a stable cell line of feline origin, and has been chemically inactivated and processed to be nonviricidal when used as a diluent to rehydrate feline rhinotracheitis—calici vaccine. Safety and immunogenicity of each virus strain have been demonstrated by vaccination and challenge tests in healthy susceptible cats.

Indications: For the immunization of healthy cats of any age against disease caused by feline rhinotracheitis, feline calici and feline panleukopenia viruses.

Dosage and Administration: Aseptically rehydrate vaccine with accompanying diluent (feline panleukopenia vaccine) and vaccinate cat intramuscularly or subcutaneously. Administer two 1 ml doses three to four weeks apart to healthy cats of any age except if the animal is less than 12 weeks of age it should be revaccinated at three to four week intervals until it is 12 to 16 weeks of age. Annual revaccination with a single dose is recommended.

Precautions: Store at 2° to 7° C (35° to 45° F). Use entire contents when first opened. Do not use chemicals to sterilize syringes and needles. Burn this container and all unused contents. Contains neomycin, polymyxin B and a fungistat as preservatives. It is generally recommended to avoid vaccination of pregnant cats. In case of anaphylactoid reaction, administer epinephrine.

This product was tested before release for sale and meets all tests required by the United States Government as well as our own laboratories.

Sold to Veterinarians Only.

U.S. Patent Nos. 3944469, 3937812 and patent pending.

For Veterinary Use Only

*Trademark

FVR*-C-P (MLV)
Feline Rhinotracheitis-Calici-Panleukopenia Vaccine Modified Live Virus

Composition: FVR*-C-P (MLV) is a lyophilized suspension of modified live feline rhinotracheitis and feline calici viruses propagated in a cell line of feline origin, and backfilled with an inert gas, and a liquid suspension of modified live feline panleukopenia virus propagated in a cell line of feline origin. The vaccine is a combination of antigens for convenient use in cats of all ages for the prevention of disease caused by feline rhinotracheitis, feline calici, and feline panleukopenia viruses. The safety and immunogenicity of this vaccine has been demonstrated by vaccination and challenge tests in susceptible cats.

Indications: For the immunization of healthy cats of any age against disease caused by feline rhinotracheitis, feline calici and feline panleukopenia viruses.

Dosage and Administration: Aseptically rehydrate vaccine with accompanying diluent and vaccinate cat intramuscularly or subcutaneously. Administer two 1 ml doses 3 to 4 weeks apart to healthy cats of any age, except that if the animal is less than 12 weeks of age, it should be revaccinated at 3 to 4 week intervals until it is 12 to 16 weeks of age.

Annual revaccination with a single dose is recommended.
Precautions: Store at 2° to 7°C (35° to 45°F). Use entire contents when first opened. Do not use chemicals to sterilize syringes and needles. Burn this container and all unused contents. Contains neomycin, polymyxin B and a fungistat as preservatives. Do not vaccinate pregnant cats. In case of anaphylactoid reaction, administer epinephrine.
This product was tested before release for sale and meets all tests required by the United States Government as well as our own laboratories.
Sold to Veterinarians Only.
U.S. Patent Nos. 3944469, 3937812, and patent pending.
For Veterinary Use Only
*Trademark

IMRAB™
Rabies Vaccine, Killed Virus

Dosage and Administration: Using aseptic technique inject 1 ml subcutaneously or intramuscularly in healthy cats, dogs, sheep and 2 ml in healthy cattle and horses when 3 months old or older. Revaccinate cattle and horses annually; cats, dogs and sheep one year later, and then every three years.
Cautions: Store in the dark at 2–7°C (35–45°F). DO NOT FREEZE. SHAKE WELL BEFORE USING. Use entire contents when first opened. Do not vaccinate food producing animals within 21 days of slaughter. Contains penicillin, streptomycin, and a fungistat as preservatives. A local reaction may occur at the injection site following subcutaneous administration. In case of anaphylactoid reaction, administer epinephrine. For Veterinary Use Only.
RESTRICTED TO USE BY A VETERINARIAN
T.M.—Trademark Institut Merieux
Made in U.S.A. PM7

IMRAB–1™
Rabies Vaccine, Killed Virus

Dosage and Administration: Using aseptic technique inject 1 ml subcutaneously or intramuscularly in healthy dogs and cats, when 3 months old or older. Revaccinate annually.
Cautions: Store in the dark at 2–7°C (35–45°F). DO NOT FREEZE. SHAKE WELL BEFORE USING. Use entire contents when first opened. Contains penicillin, streptomycin, and a fungistat as preservatives. A local reaction may occur at the injection site following subcutaneous administration. In case of anaphylactoid reaction, administer epinephrine. For Veterinary Use Only.
RESTRICTED TO USE BY A VETERINARIAN
T.M.—Trademark Institut Merieux
Made in U.S.A. PM3

INFLOGEN®
Equine Influenza Vaccine Killed Virus

Description: Inflogen is a bivalent vaccine derived from the allantoic fluid of embryonated chicken eggs infected with Types A/1 and A/2 equine influenza strains. The vaccine virus strains have been carefully selected and tested for antigenicity. The virus-laden fluids are clarified and concentrated by sucrose gradient centrifugation. This process insures that the final product is virtually free of unwanted protein and insures maximum antigenicity of each strain in a 1 ml dose. The virus is then chemically treated and irradiated to insure complete inactivation. Safety and immunogenicity of this vaccine have been demonstrated by vaccination in susceptible horses. Being an inactivated virus vaccine, it will not cause the disease in vaccinated animals.
Indications: For the immunization of healthy horses against equine influenza infection. Influenza is a disease complex caused by two subtypes of related viruses. All equine influenza virus substrains isolated to date have been classified as Type A. Two subtypes of influenza Type A virus have been identified as the cause of equine influenza; these are A/Equi-1 and A/Equi-2. Inflogen, which contains strains from both subtypes of equine influenza virus has undergone extensive field evaluation.
Dosage and Administration: SHAKE WELL before using. Using aseptic technique, vaccinate healthy horses with 1 ml intramuscularly. Administer a second dose 2 to 4 weeks later. Vaccination should be timed to achieve peak antibody response prior to possible exposure. Annual revaccination or revaccination in the event of a threatened epizootic is recommended. To minimize local tissue reaction, ensure that injection is administered in deep muscle tissue.
Precautions: Store at 2–7°C (35–45°F). Do not freeze. Use entire contents when first opened. Do not use chemicals to sterilize syringes and needles. In case of an anaphylactoid reaction, administer epinephrine.
How Supplied: Inflogen is supplied in packages containing ten 1 ml doses and one 10 ml (10 dose) vial
For Veterinary Use Only
® Connaught Laboratories

INFLOGEN®–T
Equine Influenza Vaccine-Tetanus Toxoid Killed Virus

Description: Inflogen-T is a bivalent equine influenza vaccine combined with tetanus toxoid. The equine influenza viral antigens are derived from the allantoic fluid of embryonated chicken eggs infected with Types A/1 and A/2 equine influenza strains. The virus laden fluids are clarified and concentrated by sucrose gradient centrifugation. This process insures that the final product is virtually free of unwanted protein and insures the maximum antigenicity of each strain in a 1 ml dose. The virus is then chemically treated and irradiated to insure complete inactivation. Safety and immunogenicity of this vaccine have been demonstrated by vaccination in suspectible horses. Being an inactivated virus vaccine, it will not cause disease in vaccinated animals.
The tetanus toxoid component is alum precipitated and highly purified prior to combining with the equine influenza antigens.
Indications: For active immunization of healthy horses against equine influenza infection and tetanus. Influenza is a disease complex caused by two subtypes of related viruses. All equine influenza virus substrains isolated to date have been classified as Type A. Two subtypes of influenza Type A virus have been identified as the cause of equine influenza; these are A/Equi-1 and A/Equi-2. Inflogen-T which contains strains from both subtypes, has undergone extensive field evaluation.
Dosage and Administration: SHAKE WELL before using. Using aseptic technique, vaccinate healthy horses with 1 ml intramuscularly. Administer a second dose 2 to 4 weeks later. Vaccination should be timed to achieve peak antibody response prior to possible exposure. Annual revaccination or revaccination in the event of a threatened epizootic is recommended. To minimize local tissue reaction, ensure that injection is administered in deep muscle tissue.
Precautions: Do not freeze. Store at 2–7°C (35–45°F). Use entire contents when first opened. Do not use chemicals to sterilize syringes and needles. In case of anaphylactoid reaction, administer epinephrine.
How Supplied: Inflogen-T is supplied in packages containing ten 1 ml doses and one 10 ml (10 dose) vial.
For Veterinary Use Only
® Connaught Laboratories

INNOVAR*–VET INJECTION ©II
Analgesic/Tranquilizer for Intramuscular or Intravenous Use in Dogs Only

Composition: Each ml contains 0.4 mg Sublimaze* [fentanyl] (as citrate salt) and 20 mg Inapsine* [droperidol], with 1.8 mg methylparaben and 0.2 mg propylparaben as preservatives, and lactic acid for pH adjustment to 3.1 ± 0.4.
Indications: The analgesic-tranquilizing effects of Innovar-Vet Injection given intravenously are qualitatively similar to those noted following intramuscular injection. However, the effects are produced quicker and for a shorter duration by the intravenous route. Thus Innovar-Vet intravenously is generally recommended for use in dogs when it is desirable to produce a quicker tranquilization with pain relief for a short period; intramuscular injection is indicated when prolonged analgesia is desired (about 30 to 40 minutes) and when quiescence and relative unresponsiveness to disturbing stimuli is needed for several hours.
Innovar-Vet has been used safely and effectively in a wide variety of procedures.
This experience indicates it to be useful for:

1. *Diagnostic manipulations,* such as vaginal examination, abdominal pal-

Continued on next page

Pitman-Moore—Cont.

pation, rectal palpation, examination of mouth and ears, spinal tap, bronchoscopy, proctoscopy, catheterization of the bladder, and radiographic examinations.
2. *Orthopedic procedures,* such as setting and casting of fractures.
3. *Dental procedures,* such as removal of teeth and scaling.
4. *Minor surgical procedures* of relatively short duration, such as debridement, removal of cutaneous neoplasms, biopsy of tumors and lymph nodes, cropping of ears, suturing of lacerations, tail amputation, and removal of superficially embedded foreign objects.

NOTE: For cropping of ears, best results are obtained by using Innovar-Vet in conjunction with barbiturates or other general anesthetics. (See Dosage and Administration)

5. *Therapeutic manipulations,* such as irrigation and packing of anal sacs, cleaning of ears, treatment of ears and eyes, and application and changing of dressings.
6. *Endotracheal intubation.*
7. *Grooming.*
8. *Pre-* and *postoperative* medication for sedation and relief of pain.
9. *Restraint* of vicious, hyperactive animals.
10. Major surgical procedures
    a. Used in conjunction with barbiturates or other general anesthetics;
    b. Used alone or with infiltration of local anesthetics, as in caesarean section, traumatic injury, or procedures in older dogs.

Note: For caesarian section, it is not recommended that Innovar-Vet be used with parenteral general anesthetics, since the latter may be hazardous to the neonate.

Dosage and Administration:

1. *FOR ANALGESIA AND TRANQUILIZATION:* The recommended intramuscular dose of Innovar-Vet Injection is 1 ml per 15 to 20 pounds. Intravenously, 1 ml per 25 to 60 pounds body weight is recommended, although the dose should be administered according to the response desired. For brief analgesia-tranquilization and rapid recovery, 1 ml per 60 pounds body weight given over 2 to 4 seconds is recommended, while for deeper more prolonged effects 1 ml per 25 pounds body weight should be given. A standard dose of atropine (0.02 mg per pound) should be administered prior to or in conjunction with Innovar-Vet to minimize bradycardia and salivation.

The recommended procedure is as follows:

A. *Intramuscular*
1. Administer a standard dose of atropine sulfate (0.02 mg/lb).
2. Inject Innovar-Vet intramuscularly 1 ml per 15 to 20 lbs.
3. In 10 to 15 minutes the operant procedure may be started.

This schedule produces marked analgesia for 30-40 minutes; tranquilization lasts for several hours. In most cases animals will be ambulatory in 2 hours; however, there is a tendency for the animals to remain quiet for several hours unless disturbed.

B. *Intravenous*
1. Administer a standard dose of atropine sulfate (0.02 mg/lb)
2. Inject Innovar-Vet intravenously 1 ml per 25 to 60 lbs.
3. After 3 minutes the operant procedure may be started.

This procedure produces quick tranquilization with pain relief of short duration; most animals recover from all effects by 90 minutes.

Innovar-Vet can also be used with infiltration of local anesthetics, such as procaine or lidocaine. *If supplemental analgesia is required for longer procedures:* With the exception of caesarean section, for a procedure extending beyond the period of surgical analgesia (30 to 40 minutes), a subsequent dose of Innovar-Vet, from ½ to full recommended dose may be given.

2. *FOR GENERAL ANESTHESIA* Innovar-Vet potentiates or is additive with central nervous system depressants such as sodium pentobarbital, thiopental and thiamylal. Thus it is necessary to reduce the dose of such products to the desired effect, and to reduce the intramuscular dose of Innovar-Vet by approximately one half. For example, when Innovar-Vet is used in conjunction with sodium pentobarbital, the recommended procedure is as follows:

A. *Intramuscular*
1. Administer a standard dose of atropine sulfate (0.02 mg/lb).
2. Inject Innovar-Vet intramuscularly 1 ml per 40 lbs.
3. In 10 minutes inject sodium pentobarbital intravenously, approximately 3 mg/lb.

B. *Intravenous*
1. Administer a standard dose of atropine sulfate (0.02 mg/lb).
2. Inject Innovar-Vet intravenously 1 ml per 25 to 60 lbs.
3. Within 15 seconds administer sodium pentobarbital intravenously at approximately 3 mg/lb.

The combined effect is a general anesthetic state of relatively short duration with no emergence excitement.

Innovar-Vet can be used successfully with sodium pentobarbital, sodium thiopental, sodium thiamylal, amobarbital, nitrous oxide, ether, halothane and methoxyflurane.

Warning: This drug is for use in dogs only and is not for use in food producing animals. Sublimaze (fentanyl) may be habit forming. Although studies indicate that Innovar-Vet Injection has a sedative-analgesic effect in some animals other than dogs, an undesirable central nervous stimulant effect has been noted in cattle, sheep, cats and horses.

Precautions: There are no known contraindications to the use of Innovar-Vet Injection in dogs. However, it is possible that its use may be undesirable in dogs in which respiration is significantly depressed or advanced kidney or liver disease is present.

Brachycephalic breeds, because of their inherent susceptibility to respiratory problems, should be observed frequently during the operative period and postoperatively until ambulatory.

Because Innovar-Vet has been shown to potentiate or be additive with sodium pentobarbital, it should be used with caution with central nervous system depressants, particularly anesthetics. Products known to produce respiratory depression or apnea, such as thiopental, should be given at reduced dosage and when injected intravenously, should be administered slowly; apnea has been noted when thiopental is rapidly injected following Innovar-Vet. Laboratory data have indicated that following a therapeutic intramuscular dose of Innovar-Vet, it is not safe to administer a full anesthetic dose of pentobarbital for four hours. Tranquilizers, analgesics and antitussives should not be given in conjunction with or for at least eight hours following the intramuscular administration of Innovar-Vet.

As with any injectable agent, care should be taken to avoid injection near the sciatic nerve. Care should also be exercised when giving the intravenous injection since perivascular injection may be irritating to the tissue.

Since parenteral general anesthetics may be hazardous to the neonate, these agents should not be used in conjunction with Innovar-Vet for caesarean section. For this procedure, Innovar-Vet may be used with or without infiltraton of local anesthetics.

Bradycardia may occur due to a vagal effect caused by Sublimaze [fentanyl] and can be antagonized or prevented by a standard dose of atropine. A desirable degree of analgesia and tranquility may not be obtained in an occasional dog after a recommended dose of the drug. This is especially true of Australian terriers. (See Dosage and Administration.)

Antidote: Naloxone hydrochloride (also available under the trademark P/M* Naloxone HCl Injection) reverses the respiratory depression which may be produced by the drug as a result of the action of fentanyl. Naloxone hydrochloride may be given intravenously, intramuscularly or subcutaneously. A dose of 0.4 mg naloxone hydrochloride counteracts 0.4 mg of fentanyl. The animal should be kept under continued surveillance and repeat doses of naloxone hydrochloride should be given if significant narcosis recurs. For full prescribing information, please refer to package insert accompanying P/M Naloxone HCl Injection.

Side Effects: A therapeutic intramuscular dose of Innovar-Vet Injection may cause defecation and flatulence; anal sphincter relaxation is not an uncommon occurrence. Salivation and bradycardia may be observed in dogs not pretreated with atropine. Respiratory depression or panting may occur. Oscillation of the eyes may be noted. In some instances spontaneous movements, or movement

in response to sharp auditory stimuli, may be seen. As may be expected, minor local discomfort of short duration may follow intramuscular injection. These effects, in addition to whining, also have been noted following intravenous administration, although they may occur less frequently. On rare occasions dogs receiving Innovar-Vet have exhibited transient personality changes. Animals exhibiting aggressive traits should be confined and handled carefully until normal behavior returns. Head bobbing, thought to occur spontaneously in Doberman Pinschers, has also been observed on rare occasion during 2 days to 2 weeks following Innovar-Vet usage in this breed; however, no long-term effects have been observed.
Overdosage: Innovar-Vet Injection is well tolerated in dogs at three to four times the recommended dose. Doses of six to eight times the recommended dose, given intramuscularly, may produce a relatively high incidence of spontaneous movements or even transient, mild to moderate tonic-clonic convulsions and long-lasting extension and rigidity of the neck. These effects can be antagonized by a small intravenous dose of sodium pentobarbital (3 mg/lb).
Caution: Federal law restricts this drug to use by or on the order of a licensed veterinarian.
How Supplied: 20 ml multiple dose vials.
*Trademark

KAT–A–LAX*
Feline Laxative

Composition: Contains: Cod liver oil, caramel, lecithin, malt syrup, white petrolatum, sodium benzoate 0.1% (as a preservative), vitamin E (dl-alpha-tocopheryl acetate,) 0.036 IU/g (as an antioxidant), and purified water.
Indications: A palatable formula for the elimination and prevention of hair balls in cats.
Dosage and Administration: Many cats will accept Kat-A-Lax Feline Laxative readily. For finicky animals, place a small amount on paw—cat will lick its paw and become accustomed to the pleasant taste.
For Hairball Prevention: Administer two or three times per week.
For Hairball Removal: For average weight adult cats: administer once daily. Squeeze approximately one inch of Kat-A-Lax from tube. For smaller cats, vary amount accordingly.
Warning: Keep out of reach of children.
How Supplied: 12 × 2 oz tube.
For Veterinary Use Only.
*Trademark

K.F.L.*
Insecticide Shampoo
EPA Reg. No. 773-46
EPA Est. No. 773-NJ-1

Composition:
Active Ingredients (w/w basis):

Pyrethrins	0.05%
Piperonyl Butoxide,	0.50%
Technical‡	
Inert Ingredients:	99.45%

‡ Equivalent to 0.4% (butylcarbityl) (6-propyl-piperonyl) ether and 0.1% of related compounds.
Indications: A foaming detergent shampoo with flea and louse killer for routine use on dogs and cats.
Directions for Use: It is a violation of Federal law to use this product in a manner inconsistent with its labeling. Apply liquid petrolatum to eyes prior to shampooing and avoid contact of eyes with K.F.L. Insecticide Shampoo. Wet the hair coat with warm water. Apply K.F.L. Insecticide Shampoo along the back of the animal. Add additional water to aid in dispersing the shampoo over the entire body. After 5 minutes, rinse the hair coat thoroughly and dry the animal in the customary manner.
Storage and Disposal: Keep product in original container. Store in a cool, dry place preferably in a locked storage area out of reach of children or pets. Do not reuse empty container. Rinse thoroughly before discarding. Securely wrap original container in several layers of newspaper and discard container in trash.
Caution: Harmful if swallowed. Avoid contact with eyes. Wash hands thoroughly after using.
How Supplied: Twelve 6 fl oz bottles; 1 Gallon bottles.
*Trademark

LEVASOLE*
(levamisole hydrochloride)
Cattle Wormer Boluses
Anthelmintic for Oral Use in Cattle

Composition: Each bolus contains 2.19 grams of levamisole hydrochloride activity.
Indications: Levasole (levamisole hydrochloride) is a broad-spectrum anthelmintic and is effective against the following nematode infections:
Stomach Worms: (*Haemonchus, Trichostrongylus, Ostertagia*)
Intestinal Worms: (*Trichostrongylus, Cooperia, Nematodirus, Bunostomum, Oesophagostomum*)
Lungworms: (*Dictyocaulus*)
Dosage and Administration:

Single Oral Dosage	No. Boluses
Cattle 250 to 450 lb	½
Cattle 450 to 750 lb	1
Cattle 750 to 1050 lb	1½

Consult your veterinarian for a routine worming program.
Warning: Do not administer within 48 hours of slaughter for food. Do not administer to dairy animals of breeding age.
Caution: Muzzle foam may be observed. However, this reaction will disappear within a few hours. If this condition persists, a veterinarian should be consulted. Follow recommended dosage carefully.
Cattle maintained under conditions of constant helminth exposure may require treatment within two to four weeks after the first treatment.
Consult veterinarian before using in severely debilitated animals.
Consult your veterinarian for assistance in the diagnosis, treatment and control of parasitism.
How Supplied: Box of 50 Boluses.
*Trademark

LEVASOLE* GEL
(levamisole hydrochloride 11.5%)
Cattle Anthelmintic

Description: This cartridge will deliver 27.3 g of levamisole hydrochloride activity and will treat 15 cattle weighing 500 lb each, 18 cattle weighing 400 lb each, 25 cattle weighing 300 lb each, or 37 cattle weighing 200 lb each.
Store at Room Temperature
Indications: Levasole (levamisole hydrochloride) is a broad spectrum anthelmintic and is effective at a dose of 8 mg/kg of body weight (3.6 mg lb) against the following nematode infections in cattle:
Stomach Worms: *(Haemonchus, Trichostrongylus, Ostertagia)*
Intestinal Worms: *(Trichostrongylus, Cooperia, Nematodirus, Bunostomum, Oesophagostomum)*
Lungworms: *(Dictyocaulus)* Use this cartridge with dosing guns designed for anthelmintic cattle paste products.
Dosage and Administration: To administer Levasole Gel follow these steps:
Gel gun and cartridge preparation: To fuction properly, the contents of the cartridge must be above 5°F.

1. Turn plunger rod so that notches face up, and retract plunger fully.
2. Insert large end of cartridge into the gun handle, and turn the cartridge a quarter turn clockwise to secure the cartridge to the gun.
3. Remove small cap from nozzle end of cartridge.
4. Turn plunger rod so that notches face down.
5. Depress trigger until plunger is seeded in cartridge against contents.
6. Continue to depress the trigger until the Gel completely fills the nozzle (two to three clicks). Discard the ejected Gel. This is to insure a full initial dose.

Administration: Set weight selector to desired position. Insert the nozzle of the cartridge in the interdental space, and direct it over the tongue and toward the throat. Depress trigger completely. When set properly, each full depression delivers 0.36 g of levamisole hydrochloride per 100 lb of body weight.
Cattle maintained under condition of constant helminth exposure may require retreatment within two to four weeks after the first treatment.
Warning: Keep this and all drugs out of reach of children.
Do not administer to cattle within 6 days of slaughter for food. To prevent residues in milk, do not administer to dairy animals of breeding age.
Caution: Muzzle foam may be observed. However, this reaction will disappear within a few hours. If this condition persists, a veterinarian should be consulted. Follow recommended dose care-

Continued on next page

Pitman-Moore—Cont.

fully. Consult veterinarian before using in severely debilitated animals.
Consult your veterinarian for assistance in the diagnosis, treatment and control of parasitism.
How Supplied: 237.4 g cartridge.
*Trademark

P

LEVASOLE* (levamisole phosphate) Injectable Solution 13.65% Sterile Anthelmintic

Composition: Each ml of solution contains levamisole phosphate equivalent to 136.5 mg of levamisole hydrochloride.
Indications: For subcutaneous injection in cattle. Levasole (levamisole phosphate) is a broad-spectrum anthelmintic and is effective against the following nematode infections in cattle:
Stomach Worms: (*Haemonchus, Trichostrongylus, Ostertagia*).
Intestinal Worms: (*Trichostrongylus, Cooperia, Nematodirus, Bunostomum, Oesophagostomum, Chabertia*).
Lungworms: (*Dictyocaulus*).
Dosage and Administration: Inject 2 ml per 100 lb body weight, subcutaneously. It is recommended that no more than 10 ml be injected at one site.
Cattle maintained under conditions of constant helminth exposure may require re-treatment with in two to four weeks after the first treatment.
Consult your veterinarian for assistance in the diagnosis, treatment and control of parasitism.
Warnings: Do not administer to cattle within 7 days of slaughter for food to avoid tissue residues. To prevent residues in milk, do not administer to dairy animals of breeding age.
Caution: Careful cattle weight estimates are essential for proper performance of the product. It is recommended that Levasole Injectable Solution, 13.65% be injected only in cattle in stocker or feeder condition. Cattle nearing slaughter weight and condition may show objectionable reactions at the site of injection. An occasional animal in stocker or feeder flesh may show swel ling at the injection site. The swelling will subside in 7 to 14 days and is no more severe than that observed from commonly used vaccines and bacterins.
The mid-neck region is the preferred injection site. Always use sterile needles and syringes. Nonsterile equipment may cause abscesses at the site of injection. Care should be used in maintaining the sterility of the solution. Contents should be used as soon as possible after the seal has been broken. It is recommended that the cap be wiped with alcohol prior to withdrawing solution. Also, skin at injection site should be swabbed with alcohol to avoid infection.
Experience under field conditions indicates that stressful procedures such as vaccination, castration, dehorning, concurrent exposure to cholinesterase-inhibiting drugs, pesticides, or chemicals, may increase the risk associated with the use of the product. Such concurrent stresses should be avoided when using the product.
Consult veterinarian before using in severely debilitated animals.
Muzzle foam may be observed; however, this reaction will disappear within a few hours. If this condition persists, a veterinarian should be consulted. Follow recommended dosage carefully.
How Supplied: 100 ml and 500 ml vials.
*Trademark

LEVASOLE* (levamisole hydrochloride) Sheep Wormer Boluses Anthelmintic for Oral Use in Sheep

Composition: Each bolus contains 0.184 grams of levamisole hydrochloride activity.
Indications: Levasole (levamisole hydrochloride) is a broad-spectrum anthelmintic and is effective against the following nematode infections:
Stomach Worms: (*Haemonchus, Trichostrongylus, Ostertagia*).
Intestinal Worms: (*Trichostrongylus, Cooperia, Nematodirus, Bunostomum, Oesophagostomum, Chabertia*).
Lungworms: (*Dictyocaulus*).
Dosage and Administration: *Single Oral Dosage*

	No. Boluses
Sheep 25 lb	½
Sheep 50 lb	1
Sheep 75 lb	1½
Sheep 100 lb	2
Sheep 150 lb	3

Sheep maintained under conditions of constant helminth exposure may require retreatment within two to four weeks after the first treatment. *Consult your veterinarian for assistance in the diagnosis, treatment and control of parasitism.*
Warning: Do not administer within 72 hours of slaughter for food.
Caution: Consult veterinarian before using in severely debilitated animals. Follow recommended dosage carefully.
How Supplied: 100 Boluses.
*Trademark

LEVASOLE* (levamisole hydrochloride) Soluble Drench Powder Anthelmintic for Oral Use in Cattle and Sheep

Composition: Each packet contains 46.8 grams of levamisole hydrochloride activity.
Indications: Levasole (levamisole hydrochloride) is a broad-spectrum anthelmintic and is effective against the following nematode infections in cattle and sheep:
Stomach Worms: (*Haemonchus, Trichostrongylus, Ostertagia*)
Intestinal Worms: (*Trichostrongylus, Cooperia, Nematodirus, Bunostomum, Oesophagostomum*) [*Chabertia*—Sheep only]
Lungworms: (*Dictyocaulus*)
Dosage and Administration: *Cattle: Standard Drench Solution:* Place the contents of the packet in a 1 quart (32 fl oz) container, fill with water; swirl until dissolved. Administer as a single drench dose according to the following table:

Weight	Drench Dosage	Package Will Treat
200 lb	½ fl oz	64 head
400 lb	1 fl oz	32 head
600 lb	1½ fl oz	21 head
800 lb	2 fl oz	16 head

Concentrated Drench Solution: For use with Cooper 20 ml Automatic Mark II Syringe. Place the contents of the packet in a standard household measuring container and add water to the 8¾ fl oz level; or use the measuring container available from your supplier and add water to the mark. Swirl until dissolved. Give 2 ml (milliliter) per 100 lb body weight. Refer to the table above for the number of cattle each packet will treat.
Sheep: Standard Drench Solution: Place the contents of the packet in a 1 gallon (128 fl oz) container, fill with water; swirl until dissolved. Administer as a single drench dose according to the following table:

Weight	Drench Dosage	Packet Will Treat
50 lb	½ fl oz	256 head
100 lb	1 fl oz	128 head
150 lb	1½ fl oz	84 head
200 lb	2 fl oz	64 head

Concentrated Drench Solution: For use with Cooper 20 ml Automatic Mark II Syringe. Place the contents of the packet in a standard household measuring container and add water to the 17½ fl oz level. Swirl until dissolved. Give 2 ml per 50 lb body weight. Refer to the table above for the number of sheep each packet will treat.
NOTE: Careful weight estimates are essential for proper performance of the product. Prepare solutions as needed. However, excess solutions may be stored in clean closed containers up to 90 days without loss of anthelmintic activity.
Consult your veterinarian for assistance in the diagnosis, treatment and control of parasitism.
Cattle and Sheep maintained under conditions of constant helminth exposure may require retreatment within two to four weeks after the first treatment.
Warnings: Do not administer to cattle within 48 hours of slaughter for food. Do not administer to sheep within 72 hours of slaughter for food. To prevent residues in milk, do not administer to dairy animals of breeding age.
Cautions: Muzzle foam may be observed. However, this reaction will disappear within a few hours. If this condition persists, a veterinarian should be consulted. Follow recommended dosage carefully.
Consult veterinarian before using in severely debilitated animals.

How Supplied: 30 × 52 g packets and 52 g individual packets.
*Trademark

LEVASOLE*
(levamisole hydrochloride) Soluble Drench Powder Anthelmintic for Oral Use in Sheep

Composition: Each packet contains 11.7 grams levamisole hydrochloride activity.
Indications: Levasole (levamisole hydrochloride) is a broad-spectrum anthelmintic and is effective against the following nematode infections in sheep:
Stomach Worms: (*Haemonchus, Trichostrongylus, Ostertagia*).
Intestinal Worms: (*Trichostrongylus, Cooperia, Nematodirus, Bunostomum, Oesophagostomum, Chabertia*).
Lungworms: (*Dictyocaulus*).
Dosage and Administration: Administer as a standard drench with standard drench syringe or administer as a concentrated drench solution with an automatic drenching syringe.
Preparation of Standard Drench Solution: For use with standard drench syringe. Place the contents of this packet in a 1 quart (32 fl oz) container. Fill with water and swirl briefly until dissolved. Administer as a single drench dose according to the following table:

Weight	Drench Dosage	Package Will Treat
50 lb	½ fl oz	64 head
100 lb	1 fl oz	32 head
150 lb	1½ fl oz	21 head
200 lb	2 fl oz	16 head

Preparation of Concentrated Drench Solution: For use with Cooper 20 ml Automatic Mark II Syringe: Place the contents of this packet in a household measuring container add water to the 10.9 fl oz level. Swirl briefly to dissolve and then administer at the rate of 1 ml per 10 lb body weight. Refer to the table above for the number of sheep each packet will treat.
Note: Careful sheep weight estimates are essential for proper performance of this product. Prepare solutions as needed. However, excess solutions may be stored in clean closed containers up to 90 days without loss of anthelmintic activity.
Sheep maintained under conditions of constant helminth exposure may require re-treatment within two to four weeks after the first treatment.
Consult your veterinarian for assistance in the diagnosis, treatment and control of parasitism.
Warning: Do not administer within 72 hours of slaughter for food.
Consult veterinarian before using in severely debilitated animals.
Follow recommended dosage carefully.
How Supplied: Twelve 13 g packets.
*Trademark

LEVASOLE*
(levamisole hydrochloride) Soluble Pig Wormer Anthelmintic For Use in Drinking Water

Composition: Each bottle contains 18.15 grams of levamisole hydrochloride activity which will treat the following:
200—25 lb pigs, or
100—50 lb pigs, or
50—100 lb pigs, or
25—200 lb pigs
Indications: Levasole (levamisole hydrochloride) is a broad spectrum anthelmintic, and is effective against the following nematode infections in swine:
Large Roundworms: (*Ascaris suum*)
Nodular Worms: (*Oesophagostomum spp.*)
Lung worms: (*Metastrongylus spp.*)
Intestinal Threadworms: (*Strongyloides ransomi*)
Dosage and Administration: Withholding water from pigs prior to treatment is not necessary for optimum anthelmintic efficacy and is not recommended during hot weather. Add 10 ml (2 teaspoons) of the solution from the bottle to 1 gallon of water; mix thoroughly. Allow one gallon of medicated water for each 100 pounds body weight of pigs to be treated. No other source of water should be offered. As soon as pigs have consumed all the medicated water resume use of regular water.
Note: Careful estimates of pig weights are essential for proper performance of this product. Pigs maintained under conditions of constant worm exposure may require retreatment within 4–5 weeks after the first treatment due to reinfection.
Warning: Do not administer within 72 hours of slaughter for food.
Caution: Consult veterinarian before administering Levasole to sick swine.
Consult your veterinarian for assistance in the diagnosis, treatment and control of parasitism.
Salivation or muzzle foam may be observed. This reaction is occasionally seen and will disappear in a short time after medication.
If pigs are infected with mature lungworms, coughing and vomiting may be observed soon after medicated water is consumed. This reaction is due to the expulsion of worms from the lungs and will be over in several hours. Follow recommended dosage carefully to assure removal of worms and avoid an overdose of Levasole.
How Supplied: 20.17 g bottles.
*Trademark

LUBRIVET* CONCENTRATE
Veterinary Lubricant

Indications: Lubrivet is a concentrate and must be diluted with water to produce its lubricating properties. Especially indicated for obstetrical and rectal use and all other procedures in which a lubricant is needed, as for lubricating stomach tubes and catheters, and capsules prior to administration. Its use in obstetrical cases keeps the arms free of offensive odors. It can be used in any dilution suited to the convenience of the veterinarian.
Dosage and Administration: For arm lubrication, apply a small portion to the wet skin. Additional water may be supplied until the desired viscosity is achieved. To prepare larger amounts of lubricant, stir Lubrivet into approximately an equal volume of water. Then stir in more water until the desired thickness is attained.
Note: Mixtures of Lubrivet and water, while stable, should not be stirred after standing.
In obstetrical cases, the more fetid the condition, the thicker the mixture should be. The drier the fetus, the more liquid the dilution should be.
How Supplied: 15 oz jar.
*Trademark

METOFANE*
(methoxyflurane) Inhalation Anesthetic

Composition: Metofane (methoxyflurane) is a halogenated ethyl methyl ether with the chemical name, 2,2-dichloro-1, 1-difluoroethyl methyl ether. It contains 0.01% w/w B.H.T. (butylated hydroxytoluene) as the antioxidant.
Metofane (methoxyflurane) is a non-explosive type of inhalation anesthetic at ordinary temperature and use conditions. It exhibits low toxicity, maintains anesthesia with ease, possesses marked muscle relaxing and analgesic properties, demonstrates a remarkable resistance to overdose and respiratory failure, and possesses light analgesic properties for several hours postoperatively. It has a wide margin of safety between surgical anesthetic levels and toxic levels. Recovery is smooth and of short duration. It is compatible with commonly used preanesthetic and other anesthetic agents.
Indications: Metofane (methoxyflurane) can be used for induction and maintenance of general anesthesia for all types of surgery in a wide variety of animal species.
Contraindications: Although no specific contraindications or incompatibilities for the use of Metofane (methoxyflurane) have been discovered, the veterinarian should observe his usual criteria for surgery under any anesthetic agent.
Precautions: Metofane (methoxyflurane) should be cautiously used in animals with liver disease and toxemia. Clinical-pathological tests with methoxyflurane have shown that minimal hepatic damage occurs only on gross over-dosing. As with other anesthetic agents, it is imperative that the patient receives an adequate supply of oxygen to sustain vital functions. Hypoxia at deep levels of anesthesia increases the possibility of hepatic damage occurring. Methoxyflurane has been used extensively in patients with renal, hepatic, cardiac, and pulmonary pathology and in patients suffering from traumatic, hypovolemic, vascular and toxic shock. No con-

Continued on next page

Pitman-Moore—Cont.

traindications to the use of methoxyflurane in these cases has been demonstrated.
Preanesthetic agents and narcotics should be used conservatively since they may accentuate respiratory depression and prolong recovery. The veterinarian should use his judgment based on experience and knowledge of their effects in his choice and use of these agents.
Investigations demonstrate that large doses of epinephrine could produce atrioventricular block and arrhythmias. However, based on clinical studies, the use of usual doses of epinephrine during methoxyflurane anesthesia appears to be tolerated without undue difficulties when used with caution.
NOTE TO VETERINARIANS: Caution should be taken to minimize exposure of hospital personnel to anesthetic gases and vapors. Evacuation systems and adequate ventilation should be used to remove waste gases.
Side Effects: Vomiting is infrequent and mild when it does occur. Metofane (methoxyflurane) will cross the placental barrier and, like other general anesthetics, cause depression of the newborn. To minimize the amount of depression, the patient should be induced with the minimal amount of ultra short-acting barbiturate necessary for intubation, maintained with methoxyflurane in as light a plane of anesthesia as possible, and surgery should be completed as rapidly as possible. If depression of the newborn does occur, the administration of oxygen will usually bring about prompt recovery.
Dosage and Administration: Metofane (methoxyflurane) can be administered by open drop or vaporizer in semiclosed or closed systems. It is preferably used at room temperatures.
Small Animals
The amount of Metofane (methoxyflurane) used will depend on the weight of the patient, the depth of anesthesia and the type of equipment used. In an efficient closed system, 2 or 3 ml are adequate for 2 hours surgery on a 11.3 kg (25 lb) dog. Open drop methods require more.
Preanesthetic Medication: The need, selection and dosage of an appropriate preanesthetic is best left to the judgment and experience of the clinician.
The combined effects of a preanesthetic agent and Metofane (methoxyflurane) will be different from those of Metofane alone. For example: a patient in pronounced depression as the result of premedication with a tranquilizer or sedative will not tolerate the same amount of Metofane that it would unmedicated. Similarily, depression of pulmonary ventilation to the point of hypopnea as a result of premedication requires that extra precautions be taken to assure an adequate supply of oxygen and to assure the effective elimination of carbon dioxide.
Induction: Anesthesia may be induced with Metofane alone, by the intravenous administration of a short-acting general anesthetic or by inhalation of another anesthetic agent.
Because induction time with Metofane (methoxyflurane) alone is relatively slow (requiring 5 to 10 minutes), an ultra short-acting intravenous anesthetic is generally used for induction. Dosage of these anesthetics should be only sufficient to cause collapse of the animal with sufficient relaxation to allow easy insertion of an endotracheal tube and is best determined by experience and judgment of the veterinarian.
Maintenance of Anesthesia: The clinical signs of anesthesia with methoxyflurane are not as well defined as those produced by some other inhalation agents. Since the pedal and palpebral reflexes are abolished relatively early, they are not reliable signs of anesthesia. The depth of anesthesia is best judged by the degree of muscle relaxation, the presence or absence of the swallowing reflex and, if breathing is not controlled, by the rate and character of the respiration.
Loss of muscular tension of the limbs, operative site, and jaws are reliable signs of adequate surgical anesthesia. The swallowing reflex is lost under surgical anesthesia and its return, as manifested by attempts to swallow the endotracheal catheter, is an indication of light anesthesia.
In cats, the "ear flick" reflex returns before the jaw and swallowing reflexes. This reflex is elicited by lightly touching the hairs on the inside surface of the pina or by gently blowing in the ear canal.
The concentration of vapor necessary to maintain surgical anesthesia is much less than that required to induce it.
Large Animals
As with small animals, the semi-closed and the closed circle or closed system machines are the most efficient and economical. Pigs are exceptionally responsive to Metofane (methoxyflurane) and may also be anesthetized by the open method. Information concerning preanesthetics, induction, maintenance of anesthesia and recovery described under Small Animals also apply to large animals.
Birds
Methods of administration have varied with the ingenuity of the veterinarian. The two most common methods have been to place the bird in a closed container (e.g. fruit jar) containing a pledget wet with Metofane (methoxyflurane), or holding the head of the bird in the vapor stream delivered from an anesthetic machine.
Birds respond very rapidly to Metofane (methoxyflurane) and induction is accomplished very quickly. Once induced, very little vapor is required to maintain anesthesia. Recovery from anesthesia is rapid and smooth.
Caution: Federal law restricts this drug to use by or on the order of a licensed veterinarian.
How Supplied: Metofane (methoxyflurane) is available in glass bottles containing 118 ml (4 fl oz) methoxyflurane.
*Trademark

PALADIN*
Insecticide Spray with Repellent for Horses, Dogs and Cats

Composition:
Active Ingredients:

Pyrethrins	0.06%
Technical Piperonyl Butoxide	0.48%
2,3:4,5-bis (2-butylene) tetrahydro-2-furaldehyde	0.24%
Malathion [s-(1, 2-dicarbethoxyethyl) O,O-dimethyldithiophosphate]	0.50%
Petroleum Distillate	0.97%
Inert Ingredients	97.75%
	100.00%

Indications: Paladin is recommended for horses, dogs and cats to kill fleas, ticks and lice and as a repellent to gnats, mosquitoes and flies.
Directions: Remove safety cap and insert sprayer. Hold container upright. Adjust nozzle to either stream or mist as indicated on nozzle. To close, turn nozzle to off position.
Horses: Kills and repels horse flies, stable flies, face flies, house flies, gnats and mosquitoes.
Before application, brush animal to remove loose dirt, dust and debris.
Spray animal from a distance of about 12 inches with special attention to shanks, legs, neck and facial area. Avoid spraying eyes and nostrils. The hair should be slightly dampened. Apply once a day, perferably in the morning.
Dogs and Cats: Apply Paladin from a distance of about 12 inches, protecting animal's eyes from spray. Direct spray over the animal beginning from the back of the neck to the tail. The entire coat should be slightly dampened. Ticks that are attached should be sprayed directly.
NOTE: Do not treat or cause exposure of puppies or kittens less than four weeks old.
In kennels or other sleeping quarters, to control these insects and to deodorize the quarters, spray the animal regularly as above and spray bedding, walls, cracks, crevices and flooring as often as necessary.
Precautionary Statements: Hazards to Humans and Domestic Animals
Caution: Harmful if swallowed or inhaled. Avoid breathing of spray mist. Avoid contact with skin; wash thoroughly after use. Avoid contamination of feed, and foodstuffs. Do not treat or cause exposure of puppies or kittens less than four weeks old.
Physical and Chemical Hazards: Keep away from heat and open flame.
Directions for Use: It is a violation of Federal law to use this product in a manner inconsistent with its labeling.
Storage and Disposal: Store in a cool, dry area away from heat or open flame. Do not reuse empty container. Wrap container and put in trash collection.
How Supplied: 12 x 16 fluid ounce container with trigger sprayer.
EPA Reg. No. 9688-65-773
EPA Est. No. 9688-MO-1
*Trademark

PELLITOL* OINTMENT
Antiseptic—Protective

Composition; Resorcinol 5%; bismuth subgallate 1%; bismuth subnitrate 9%; zinc oxide 17%; calamine 10%; juniper tar 1%
Indications: For use on domestic animals as an aid in the treatment of minor wounds, abrasions, and inflammation of the external ear canal. Pellitol Ointment forms a protective coating and helps reduce pain, irritation and itching.
Dosage and Administration: Apply a layer of Pellitol Ointment, approximately one-eighth inch thick, over the affected area. Treat once or twice daily. Cover with a bandage if possible.
Ears should be checked for the presence of foreign bodies and/or parasites and treated as necessary before application of Pellitol Ointment. Attach applicator to tube and gently insert into the ear canal. Continually apply pressure to the tube as applicator is withdrawn from the ear canal. Apply a layer of Pellitol Ointment over any existing lesions on the outer surface of the ear. Repeat application once or twice daily.
Caution: Do not use in eyes.
How Supplied: 12 x 20 g tubes.
*Trademark

PESTISOL*-R
Flea and Tick Spray with Repellent

Composition:
Active Ingredients:

Ingredient	%
Propoxur (o-Isopropoxyphenyl methyl-carbamate)	0.50%
Pyrethrins	0.15%
Technical Piperonyl Butoxide	1.50%
N-Octyl bicycloheptene dicarboximide	0.50%
2,3:4, 5-bis (2-butylene) tetrahydro-2-furaldehyde	0.50%
Petroleum Distillate	0.60%
Inert Ingredients	96.25%
	100.00%

Indications: Pestisol-R is recommended for use on dogs to kill fleas, ticks and lice and as a repellent against gnats, mosquitoes and flies. It is also recommended for residential use to kill ants, roaches, waterbugs, silverfish, crickets and spiders.
Directions for Fleas and Ticks on Dogs: Remove safety cap and insert sprayer. Hold container upright. Adjust nozzle to either stream or mist as indicated on nozzle. To close, turn nozzle to off position. Apply Pestisol-R from a distance of about 12 inches, protecting animal's eyes from spray. Direct spray over the animal beginning from the back of the neck to the tail. The entire coat should be slightly dampened. Ticks that are attached should be sprayed directly.
NOTE: Do not treat or cause exposure of puppies less than four weeks old.
In kennels or other sleeping quarters, to control these insects and to deodorize the quarters, spray the animal regularly as above and spray bedding, walls, cracks, crevices and flooring as often as necessary.
Directions for Residential Use: Apply to surface only. Do not spray up into air. Point nozzle toward surface to be sprayed and squeeze handle firmly. Hold about 12 inches from the surface being sprayed. Spray until surfaces are wet. Avoid excessive wetting of asphalt tile, rubber and plastics.
Ants: Apply to ant trails, around doors, windows and wherever ants enter the house. Repeat as necessary.
Roaches and Waterbugs: Apply to baseboards, window frames, the undersides of shelves and drawers, under sinks and stoves and to other places insects may hide. Also, spray cracks and crevices and surfaces where insects may crawl when they come out of hiding. Repeat as necessary.
Silverfish, Crickets, Spiders: Spray areas infested by these pests. Repeat as necessary.
Precautionary Statements: Hazards to Humans ***Caution:*** Harmful if swallowed, inhaled or absorbed through the skin. Avoid breathing spray mist and provide adequate ventilation of area being treated. Avoid contact with eyes, skin or clothing. Wash thoroughly after handling. Avoid contamination of foods, utensils, or food preparation areas. Do not use in food areas of food processing plants, restaurants or other areas where food is commercially prepared or processed. Cover fish aquariums before spraying. Do not allow children to contact treated surfaces until spray is dried.
Note to Physician: Atropine sulfate is antidotal only if symptoms of cholinesterase inhibition appear.
Physical or Chemical Hazards: Flammable. Keep away from heat and open flame.
Statement of Practical Treatment: If swallowed, drink 1 or 2 glasses of water and induce vomiting by touching finger to back of throat. Contact physician immediately.
If on skin: wash with soap and water.
If in eyes: flush with plenty of water.
Directions for Use: It is a violation of Federal law to use this product in a manner inconsistent with its labeling.
Storage and Disposal: Store in a cool, dry area away from heat or open flame. Do not reuse empty container except to refill with Pestisol-R Spray. Wrap container and put in trash collection.
How Supplied: 12 x 16 ounce container with trigger sprayer and one gallon container.
EPA Reg. No. 9688-64-773
EPA Est. No. 9688-MO-1
*Trademark

P/M* NALOXONE HCl INJECTION
A Specific, Rapid-Acting, Narcotic Antagonist
For use in dogs

Composition: P/M Naloxone HCl Injection, a narcotic antagonist, is a synthetic cogener of oxymorphone. In structure it differs from oxymorphone in that the methyl group on the nitrogen atom is replaced by an allyl group.
Each ml of the injectable aqueous solution contains: Naloxone hydrochloride, 0.4 mg; Sodium chloride, U.S.P., 8.6 mg; Methylparaben and Propylparaben in a ratio of 9 to 1, 2.0 mg; Water for injection q.s. ad 1.0 ml; pH is adjusted with hydrochloric acid.
Naloxone hydrochloride occurs as a white to slightly off-white powder, and is soluble in water, in dilute acids, and in strong alkali; slightly soluble in alcohol; practically insoluble in ether and in chloroform.
Actions: P/M Naloxone HCl Injection is a selective narcotic antagonist. It is unique in that it is a pure antagonist and does not possess the agonistic, or morphine-like, properties characteristic of other narcotic antagonists. Unlike other narcotic antagonists P/M Naloxone HCl Injection does not produce respiratory depression or psychotomimetic effects, even after successive doses, nor will tachyphylaxis occur.
P/M Naloxone HCl Injection will prevent and promptly reverse the depressant effects of narcotics as well as the agonistic or depressant effects of other narcotic antagonists. P/M Naloxone HCl Injection has also been shown to be an effective antagonist in protecting mice and rats from convulsive and lethal effects of propoxyphene.
Its onset of action is very rapid; administered intravenously its effects are usually noticeable within 2 to 3 minutes; administered subcutaneously or intramuscularly its onset of action is slightly longer. The duration of action is approximately 2 to 3 hours.
Aside from counteracting the depressant effects of narcotics and other narcotic antagonists naloxone produces essentially no pharmacodynamic effects of its own in the absence of these agents. This selectivity of action provides a wide margin of safety.
P/M Naloxone HCl Injection is not effective against respiratory depression due to barbiturates, tranquilizers or other non-narcotic agents or pathologic causes.
Indications: For the treatment, prevention or control of narcotic depression, including respiratory depression induced by morphine and its derivatives including meperidine, oxymorphone, fentanyl and the narcotic antagonist analgesic pentazocine. In addition to its obvious application in frank narcotic overdosage P/M Naloxone HCl Injection is of therapeutic and practical value in poor risk or critically ill animals who have received narcotics for surgical or diagnostic procedures, and in whom the veterinarian desires to safely and promptly reverse all or part of the usual or subclinical narcotic-depressant effects.
P/M Naloxone HCl Injection may be safely administered to animals who have received both narcotic and non-narcotic drugs. Unlike other narcotic antagonists it will not aggravate respiratory depression due to non-narcotic causes.
To Terminate Postoperative Central Nervous System Narcotic Effects: As premedication or adjunctive medication to surgery or other manipulative proce-

Continued on next page

Pitman-Moore—Cont.

dures, narcotics are used alone or in combination with barbiturates or tranquilizers to sedate the animal. When the diagnostic or surgical procedure is completed, P/M Naloxone HCl Injection produces a safe, simple, and rapid recovery from narcosis, yet permitting advantages of continued action of the bariturate or tranquilizer.

Administration of P/M Naloxone HCl Injection reduces postoperative waiting time and promotes early ambulation thereby reducing postoperative complication.

P/M Naloxone HCl Injection, a safe, effective, fast acting, selective narcotic antagonist makes the use of narcotic anesthesia/analgesia a safer and more easily controlled procedure than at any previous time.

Pregnancy and the Newborn: When narcotics are employed to ease labor, i.e., difficult deliveries, caesarean section, etc., P/M Naloxone HCl Injection can be administered to the mother just prior to delivery and/or to the newborn pups after delivery to terminate depressant effects of the narcotic. P/M Naloxone HCl Injection will promptly reverse any narcotic depressant effects.

Narcotic Overdosage: Studies conducted by various investigators confirm that P/M Naloxone HCl Injection safely and promptly counteracted the depressant effects of narcotic overdosage. In addition to its indication in frank narcotic overdosage P/M Naloxone HCl Injection is useful for the diagnosis of suspected opiate overdosage or hypersensitivity. P/M Naloxone HCl Injection unlike other narcotic antagonists, will not add to the depressant effects of barbiturates or tranquilizers.

Contraindications: There are no known contraindications to P/M Naloxone HCl Injection.

Warnings: P/M Naloxone HCl Injection should be administered cautiously to animals who have received exceedingly large doses of narcotics. In such cases, the usual recommended dosage of P/M Naloxone HCl Injection may produce an acute withdrawal syndrome and smaller doses should be employed.

A dog which has satisfactorily responded to P/M Naloxone HCl Injection can occasionally show signs of a relapse because the duration of action of some narcotics may exceed that of P/M Naloxone HCl Injection. Therefore, the dog should be closely observed for several hours, and repeat doses of P/M Naloxone HCl Injection administered if necessary.

Precautions: Other resuscitative measures such as maintenance of a free airway, artificial ventilation, cardiac massage and vasopressor agents should be available and employed when necessary to counteract acute narcotic poisoning.

Adverse Reactions: There are no known side effects to P/M Naloxone HCl Injection counteracts the following narcotic dosages:

Oxymorphone hydrochloride	1.5 mg
Morphine sulfate	15.0 mg
Meperidine	100.0 mg
Fentanyl	0.4 mg

In the event that the quantity of narcotic to be reversed is not known, a very simple and effective rule of thumb is to administer an initial dose of 0.04 mg/kg subcutaneously, intramuscularly, or intravenously. The most rapid onset of action is achieved by intravenous administration. Administered intravenously its onset of action is usually within 2 to 3 minutes, and may be repeated at 2 to 3 minute intervals if necessary. The onset of action following intramuscular and subcutaneous administration is slightly longer.

Administration of small doses, such as may be used in pups, requires the dilution of P/M Naloxone HCl Injection with STERILE WATER or SODIUM CHLORIDE INJECTION. For example, add 4.5 ml of diluent to 0.5 ml P/M Naloxone HCl Injection, which results in a concentration of 0.04 mg per ml.

Caution: Federal law restricts this drug to use by or on the order of a licensed veterinarian.

How Supplied: 0.4 mg/ml of P/M Naloxone HCl Injection for intravenous, intramuscular and subcutaneous administration in dogs.

Available in 1 ml ampuls in boxes of 10.

*Trademark

PORCIMUNE*
Escherichia Coli Bacterin

Description: Porcimune is an inactivated quadrivalent liquid bacterin containing the four antigens found in over 90% of the virulent enterotoxigenic *E. coli* strains isolated from neonatal swine.

Indications: For the prevention of neonatal enteric colibacillosis caused by *E. coli* of pilus types K88ab, K88ac, K99, 987P, and F41 through immunization of pregnant sows and gilts.

Dosage and Administration: Shake well. Using asceptic technique, vaccinate healthy pregnant sows and gilts with 2 ml (1 dose) subcutaneously or intramuscularly according to the following schedule:

Sows and Gilts

- 2ml 35 to 150 days before farrowing
- 2ml 7 to 21 days before farrowing
- 2ml Booster 7 to 21 days prior to subsequent farrowings. If the interval between farrowings exceeds 8 months, the 2 dose immunization should be followed.

E. coli protection for the newborn piglet is provided by the maternal antibodies contained in the colostrum. The piglet should, therefore, receive the colostrum as soon as possible after birth.

Precautions: Do not freeze. Store at 2–7°C (35–45°F). Do not vaccinate within 21 days before slaughter. Use entire contents when first opened. Burn this container and all unused contents. Do not use chemicals to sterilize syringes and needles. In case of anaphylactoid reaction, administer epinephrine. For Veterinary Use Only.

How Supplied: Porcimune is supplied in plastic vials containing 20ml (10 doses) and 40ml (20 doses).

This product was tested before release for sale and meets all tests required by the United States Government as well as our own laboratories.

PORCIMUNE* B
Bordetella Bronchiseptica-Escherichia Coli Bacterin

Description: Porcimune B is a combination inactivated liquid bacterin containing the four antigens found in over 90% of the virulent enterotoxigenic *E. coli* strains isolated from neonatal swine combined with a Bordetella Bronchiseptica Bacterin.

Indications: For the prevention of neonatal enteric colibacillosis caused by *E. coli* of pilus types K88ab, K88ac, K99, 987P, F41 and atropic rhinitis caused by *B. bronchiseptica* through immunization of pregnant sows and gilts.

Dosage and Administration: Shake well. Using aseptic technique, vaccinate healthy pregnant sows and gilts with 2ml (1 dose) subcutaneously or intramuscularly according to the following schedule.

Sows and Gilts:

- 2ml 35 to 150 days before farrowing
- 2ml 7 to 21 days before farrowing
- 2ml Booster 7 to 21 days prior to subsequent farrowings. If the interval between farrowings exceeds 8 months, the 2 dose immunization should be followed.

E. coli protection for the newborn piglet is provided by the maternal antibodies contained in the colostrum. The piglet should, therefore, receive the colostrum as soon as possible after birth. For active immunization against atrophic rhinitis, vaccinate each pig with a Bordetella Bronchiseptica Bacterin.

Precautions: Do not freeze. Store at 2–7°C (35–45°F). Do not vaccinate within 21 days before slaughter. Use entire contents when first opened. In case of anaphylactoid reaction, administer epinephrine. For Veterinary Use Only.

How Supplied: Porcimune B is supplied in plastic vials containing 20ml (10 doses) and 40ml (20 doses).

*Trademark

PSEUDOVAX*
Pseudorabies Vaccine Modified Live Virus

Description: Pseudorabies Vaccine, Modified Live Virus is prepared by growing a highly antigenic strain of pseudorabies virus in an established bovine cell line. Laboratory studies have demonstrated this vaccine to be safe and effective for the protection of susceptible swine as young as three days of age against challenge with virulent pseudorabies virus.

Indications: For active immunization of healthy swine older than 2 days of age against pseudorabies.

Dosage and Administration: For use in swine only! Not for use in any other animal. Aseptically rehydrate with ac-

companying diluent. Vaccinate healthy swine three days of age or older intramuscularly with 2 ml (1 dose). Because maternal antibody may interfere with vaccination until pigs are 8 to 10 weeks old, vaccination of young pigs in endemically infected swine herds at 3 to 4 week intervals until the pigs are 10 to 12 weeks of age is recommended. Semiannual revaccination of sows and gilts before breeding is recommended.
Precautions: Store at 2–7°C (35–45°F). Use entire contents when first opened. Burn this container and all unused contents. Do not vaccinate within 21 days of slaughter. In case of anaphylactoid reaction administer epinephrine. Contains neomycin, polymyxin B and a fungistat as preservatives. Do not use chemical disinfectants to sterilized syringes and needles. Do not use if vacuum is lost. It is generally recommended to avoid vaccination of pregnant females.
Distribution in each state shall be limited to authorized recipients designated by proper state officials—under such conditions as these authorities may require.
Caution: Vaccination results in an antibody response indistinguishable from that induced by infection. State and federal regulations restricting the movement of seropositive swine apply to vaccinated animals.
How Supplied: Pseudorabies Vaccine is supplied in packages containing 5 doses, 10 doses and 50 doses.
This product was tested before release for sale and meets all tests required by the United States Government as well as our own laboratories.

For Veterinary Use Only
*Trademark

QUANTUM*
Parvovirus Vaccine
Modified Live Virus
For Use in Dogs
Canine Isolate Parvovirus
Liquid

Description: Quantum* is a modified live canine isolate parvovirus vaccine propagated in a stable cell line of feline origin. Safety and immunogenicity of this vaccine have been demonstrated by vaccination and challenge tests in dogs.
Indications: For active immunization of healthy susceptible dogs against parvovirus infection.
Dosage and Administration: Using aseptic technique vaccinate healthy dogs with 1 ml (1 dose) subcutaneously or intramuscularly. One dose of this vaccine is required to immunize susceptible puppies and dogs. However, the age at which maternal antibody no longer interferes with development of active immunity varies according to the bitch's titer and quantity of colostral antibodies absorbed by the puppy. In some instances, interference may last as long as four months. Therefore, dogs vaccinated when younger than 16 weeks of age should receive one dose every 2 to 4 weeks until reaching this age. An annual booster dose is recommended for all dogs.
Precautions: Store at 2–7°C (35–45°F). Use entire contents when first opened. Do not use chemicals to sterilize syringes and needles. Burn this container and all unused contents. Contains neomycin, polymyxin B, and a fungistat as preservatives. It is generally recommended to avoid vaccination of pregnant dogs. In case of anaphylactoid reaction administer epinephrine.

For Veterinary Use Only
*Trademark

QUANTUM* 4
Canine Distemper-Hepatitis-Parainfluenza-Parvovirus Vaccine
Modified Live Virus
For Use in Dogs
Canine Isolate Parvovirus

Description: Quantum* 4 is a combination of a lyophilized suspension of canine distemper, hepatitis, and parainfluenza modified live viruses propagated in a stable cell line of canine origin and backfilled with an inert gas; and a modified live canine isolate parvovirus propagated in a stable cell line of feline origin. Production by the stable cell line process ensures maximum uniformity with regard to safety and immunogenicity. The safety and immunogenicity of the virus strains have been demonstrated by vaccination and challenge tests in healthy dogs. Data indicates that the development of corneal opacity is not associated with the use of this product.
Indications: For active immunization of healthy dogs against canine distemper, canine hepatitis, canine adenovirus type 2, canine parainfluenza and canine parvovirus-induced disease.
Dosage and Administration: Aseptically rehydrate lyophilized vaccine with accompanying diluent (Parvovirus Vaccine). Using aseptic technique, inject 1 ml (1 dose) subcutaneously or intramuscularly. Susceptible puppies and dogs should receive two doses 2 to 4 weeks apart. Two doses of this vaccine are required in the initial immunization in order to develop a higher level of immunity against canine parainfluenza. The age at which maternal antibody no longer interferes with development of active immunity varies according to the bitch's titer and quantity of colostral antibodies absorbed by the puppy. In some instances, interference may last as long as four months. Therefore, dogs vaccinated when younger than 16 weeks of age should receive one dose every 2 to 4 weeks until reaching this age. An annual booster dose is recommended for all dogs.
Precautions: Store at 2–7°C (34–45°F). Use entire contents when first opened. Do not use chemicals to sterilize syringes and needles. Burn this container and all unused contents. In case of anaphylactoid reaction, administer epinephrine. Contains neomycin, polymyxin B, and a fungistat as preservatives. It is generally recommmended to avoid vaccination of pregnant dogs. Central nervous system reactions have been temporally associated with the administration of modified live canine distemper vaccines. Clinical experience indicates that the incidence of such reactions is extremely low.

For Veterinary Use Only
*Trademark

QUANTUM* 6
Canine Distemper-Hepatitis-Parainfluenza-Parvovirus Vaccine
Modified Live Virus
Leptospira Bacterin
For Use in Dogs
Canine Isolate Parvovirus

Description: Quantum* 6 is a combination product. The lyophilized suspension of canine distemper, hepatitis, and parainfluenza modified live viruses is back-filled with an inert gas. The liquid modfied live canine isolate parvovirus is combined with inactivated cultures of *Leptospira canicola* and *Leptospira icterohaemorrhagiae* which have been processed to be non-viricidal. Production of the viral components by the stable cell line process ensures maximum uniformity with regard to safety and immunogenicity. The lepto fractions have been prepared by a unique and improved process that provides a highly purified bacterin. The immunogenicity and safety of the product have been demonstrated by vaccination and challenge tests in healthy susceptible dogs. Data indicate that the development of corneal opacity is not associated with the use of this product.
Indications: For the immunization of healthy unexposed puppies and dogs against canine distemper, canine hepatitis, canine parvovirus-induced disease, respiratory disease induced by canine adenovirus type 2 and canine parainfluenza, as well as leptospirosis caused by *L. canicola and L. icterohaemorrhagiae.*
Dosage and Administration: Aseptically rehydrate vaccine with accompanying diluent. Using aseptic technique, inject 1 ml (1 dose) either subcutaneously or intramuscularly. Two doses of this vaccine are required in the initial immunization. Susceptible puppies and dogs should receive two doses, 2 to 4 weeks apart. The age at which maternal antibody no longer interferes with development of active immunity varies according to the bitch's titer and quantity of colostral antibodies absorbed by the puppy. In some instances, interference may last as long as four months. Therefore, dogs vaccinated when younger than 16 weeks of age should receive one dose every 2 to 4 weeks until reaching this age. An annual booster dose is recommended for all dogs.
Precautions: Store at 2–7°C (35–45°F). Use entire contents when first opened. Do not use chemicals to sterilize syringes and needles. Burn this container and all unused contents. Contains neomycin, polymyxin B and a fungistat as preservatives. It is generally recommended to avoid vaccination of pregnant dogs. In case of anaphylactoid reaction administer epinephrine. Central nervous system reactions have been temporally associated with the administration of modified live canine distemper vaccines. Clinical experience indicates that the

Continued on next page

Pitman-Moore—Cont.

incidence of such reactions is extremly low.
How Supplied: Quantum* 6 is supplied in packages of 10 x 1 dose vials.
U.S. Pat. No. 3,950,512
For Veterinary Use Only
*Trademark

RHIVIN*
Bovine Rhinotracheitis-Parainfluenza 3 Vaccine Modified Live Virus Intranasal

Composition: Bovine Rhinotracheitis-Parainfluenza 3 Vaccine, is a lyophilized suspension of bovine rhinotracheitis and bovine parainfluenza 3 viruses propagated in bovine tissue culture. Both viruses have been modified to the point where they are nonpathogenic but have retained their capacity for stimulating immunity for the respective diseases.
Indications: For the immunization of healthy beef and dairy cattle against bovine rhinotracheitis and bovine parainfluenza 3 infections.
General Information: Bovine Rhinotracheitis-Parainfluenza 3 Vaccine is a combination of antigens for convenient use in healthy beef and dairy cattle, which produces specific immunity against bovine rhinotracheitis and bovine parainfluenza 3 infections. The safety and immunogenicity of both virus strains have been demonstrated by vaccination and challenge tests in susceptible cattle. One intranasal dose of 2 ml administered 1 ml per nostril, is required to produce specific and durable protection. Calves vaccinated under six months of age should be revaccinated at six months or older since specific maternal antibody, if present, may interfere with successful vaccination.
Intranasal inoculation of Bovine Rhinotracheitis-Parainfluenza 3 Vaccine has been shown to induce levels of interferon in the nasal secretions within 40 to 72 hours after vaccination. Infections may be diminished depending on the sensitivity of specific viruses to interferon.
Cattle studies with Rhivin* indicate it will not cause abortions when used in IBR susceptible cattle at various stages of gestation.
Vaccinating cattle after exposure during shipment or at the time of arrival at the feed-lot may have merit if one understands that some animals may be in the incubation stage of the disease without any signs evident. Those in the incubation stage may come down with active disease after vaccination.
Dosage and Administration: For Intranasal Use Only. Aseptically rehydrate vaccine with accompanying diluent. Mix thoroughly. Using the syringe applicator provided administer 2 ml, 1 ml in each nostril.
Precautions: Store at 2°–7°C (35°–45°F). Do not vaccinate within 21 days before slaughter. Vaccinate all animals in the group. Use entire contents when first opened. Do not use chemical disinfectants to sterilize syringes, needles and applicators. Burn the container and all unused contents. Do not use if vacuum is lost. Contains penicillin, streptomycin and amphotericin B as preservatives. In case of anaphylactoid reaction use epinephrine or atropine sulfate.
How Supplied: Bovine Rhinotracheitis-Parainfluenza 3 Vaccine Intranasal is distributed in packages containing 5 doses and 25 doses.
For Veterinary Use Only
*Trademark

RHUSIGEN*
Erysipelothrix Rhusiopathiae Bacterin

Indications: For the immunization of healthy swine and turkeys against erysipelas.
Dosage and Administration: Shake Well. Using aseptic technique, vaccinate healthy swine and turkeys according to the following schedule:
Swine:
2ml 8 weeks of age or older subcutaneously or intramuscularly. For breeding animals, revaccinate 21 days later and annually.
Turkeys:
0.5 ml 8 weeks of age or older subcutaneously preferably on the neck near the head.
0.5 ml Repeat dose every 3 months.
Precautions: Store at 2–7°C (35–45°F). Do not freeze. Do not vaccinate within 21 days before slaughter. Use entire contents when first opened. In case of anaphylactoid reaction, administer epinephrine. For Veterinary Use Only.
Warning: Do not use as diluent for live vaccines.
For Veterinary Use Only
*Trademark

SIRLENE®
Feed Grade Propylene Glycol†

Indications: For the prevention and treatment of acetonemia (ketosis) in dairy cattle.
A humectant and conditioner for animal feeds.
Dosage and Administration: As an aid in the prevention of acetonemia (ketosis) in dairy cattle. Feed at the rate of 0.25 lb to 0.50 lb of Sirlene® per head per day, starting 2 weeks prior to calving and continuing for 6 weeks after calving. Mix with feed or use as a drench.
As a treatment for acetonemia (ketosis) in dairy cattle, feed at the rate of 0.25 lb (approximately 4 fl oz) to 1 pound (approximately 1 pint) of Sirlene® per head per day for 10 days. Mix with feed or use as a drench.
Note: Some cows may not respond to treatment as a result of complicating factors, such as milk fever, hardware, etc. These conditions must be treated in conjunction with the acetonemia. Consult your veterinarian if in doubt.
Use up to 5 per cent in animal feeds as a humectant and conditioner of feeds. Prevents drying out of feeds.
†U.S.P. grade—the distilling range of this product is 185°–190°C.
How Supplied: One Gallon.
Sirlene® is a U.S. Registered Trademark of the Dow Chemical Company.

SPRECTO*
with Repellent Insecticide-Repellent
EPA Reg. No. 773-36
EPA Est. No. 9688-MO-1

Composition:
Active Ingredients:
Pyrethrins .... 0.05% w/w
Technical piperonyl butoxide† .... 0.1% w/w
Carbaryl (1-naphthyl N-methylcarbamate)‡ .... 0.5% w/w
2, 3:4, 5-bis (2-butylene) tetrahydro-2-furaldehyde... 0.2% w/w
N-octyl bicycloheptene dicarboximide .... 0.4% w/w
Petroleum distillate .... 3.35% w/w
Inert Ingredients:.................. 95.4%
†Equivalent to 0.08% (butylcarbityl) (6-propyl-piperonyl) ether and 0.02% of related compounds.
‡SEVIN®—Trademark of Union Carbide Corporation.
Indications: For control of fleas, lice and ticks on dogs and cats; also temporarily repels annoying mosquitoes and flies.
Directions for Use: It is a violation of Federal law to use this product in a manner inconsistent with its labeling.
SHAKE WELL BEFORE USING
Apply SPRECTO with Repellent from a distance of 4 to 6 inches, protecting animal's eyes from spray.
Adult dogs—spray along the back from head to tail for light infestation. For heavy infestation, entire hair coat should be slightly dampened. Ticks that are attached should be sprayed more heavily. Do not use on pregnant dogs.
Adult cats—spray lightly on hair coat along the back from head to base of tail. To prevent reinfestation, apply at weekly intervals, as needed, and spray living quarters thoroughly. Operates best at room temperature.
Storage and Disposal
Store in a cool, dry area away from heat or open flame preferably in a locked storage area out of reach of children or pets. Securely wrap original container in several layers of newspaper and discard container in trash. Do not puncture or incinerate container.
Precautionary Statements
Hazards to Humans and Domestic Animals
CAUTION
HUMAN—Harmful if swallowed or inhaled. Avoid breathing mist. Avoid contact with eyes and skin. Wash hands after applying. Avoid contamination of food. Do not use this product in commercial food areas of food handling establishments, restaurants, or other places where food is prepared or processed.
ANIMAL—Avoid contact with animal's eyes. Avoid treatment of kittens less than 4 weeks of age and nursing puppies.

Overtreatment may cause toxic reactions.

Statement of Practical Treatment
If swallowed: do not induce vomiting. Contact physician immediately.
If inhaled: remove victim to fresh air. Apply artifical respiration, if indicated.
If in eyes: flush with plenty of water.
If on skin: wash with soap and water.

Physical and Chemical Hazards: Flammable!
Contents under pressure. Do not use near fire, sparks or flame. Do not puncture or incinerate container. Exposure to temperatures above 130°F may cause bursting.

How Supplied: Twelve 14 oz spray cans.

*Trademark

SPRECTO*-F
Total Release Fogger

Composition:
Active Ingredients:
d-trans. Allethrin........................0.3000%
(allyl homolog of Cinerin 1)
Related compounds........................0.023%
†3-Phenoxybenzyl d-cis and.........0.191%
trans†† 2,2-dimethyl-3-(2-methlpropenyl) cyclopropanecarboxylate
Other isomers................................0.009%
N-octyl bicycloheptene dicarboximide 2.500%
Petroleum distillate 11.954%
Inert Ingredients 85.023%
† d-(cis, trans) phenothrin
†† cis/trans isomer ratio; max 25% (+ or −) cis; min 75% or (+ or −) trans

Indications: For apartments, homes or buildings up to 10,000 cubic feet.
Kills Fleas, Ticks and Mosquitoes
One unit treats an entire room (up to 10,000 cu. ft.) with an effective bug killing fog that leaves no unpleasant residual odor.
This easy-to-use exclusive water-based formula DOES NOT CONTAIN CHLORINATED SOLVENTS. When used as directed, it will not harm drapes, upholstery, fabrics, carpeting, bedspreads, clothing, linens, furniture, walls, floor tiles, ceilings, shades or blinds.

Directions: For use in rooms, apartments, homes, attics, basements, campers, boats, garages, pet sleeping areas, household storage areas, cabins.
This product will kill fleas, ticks, flies, mosquitoes, cockroaches, black carpet beetles, sawtoothed grain beetles, rice weevils, small flying moths, spiders, centipedes, wasps, pill bugs, crickets and silverfish.
Cover exposed food, dishes and food-handling equipment. Open cabinets and doors to areas to be treated. Shut off fans and air conditioners. Put out all flames. Close doors and windows.
Shake Well Before Using
To operate valve: Point valve opening away from face and eyes when releasing. To lock valve in open position for automatic discharge press valve button all the way down, hooking the catch. Then place fogger on stand or table in center of room with valve locked open, place several layers of newspaper or pad under fogger. Do not remain in the area during treatment. Leave building at once and keep building closed for two hours before airing out. Ventilate thoroughly before reentry. Open all windows and allow to air for 30 minutes. Repeat spraying in two weeks or when necessary. Use one unit for each 10,000 cubic feet of unobstructed area. Use additional units for remote rooms or where free flow of mist is not assured.
To kill fleas, or ticks: Remove and destroy pet's old bedding. Apply this product as for other insects. Put fresh bedding in pet's quarters after treatment. Treat dogs and cats with a registered tick control product before allowing them to enter treated area.

Precautions Statements: Hazards to Humans and Domestic Animals
Caution: Harmful if swallowed. If swallowed, do not induce vomiting. Call a physician immediately. Avoid inhalation of vapors. Avoid contact with skin, eyes or clothing. Wash contaminated skin promptly with soap and warm water. For eyes, flush with plenty of water and get medical attention if irritation persists. Avoid contamination of food and feedstuffs.
Do not use in commerical food processing, preparation, storage or serving areas. In the home, all food processing surfaces and utensils should be covered during treatment or thoroughly washed before use. Cover exposed food.
Remove pets, birds, and cover fish aquariums before spraying.

Physical and Chemical Hazards: Contents under pressure. Do not use or store near heat or open flame. Do not puncture or incinerate container. Exposure to temperatures above 130°F may cause bursting.

Directions for Use: It is a violation of Federal law to use this product in a manner inconsistent with its labeling.

Storage and Disposal: Store in a cool, dry area away from heat or open flame. Do not reuse empty container. Wrap container and put in trash collection.

How Supplied: 12 x 10 ounce spray can.

*Trademark

SPRECTO-CCR*
Complete Carpet & Room Spray with lemon-scented, non-staining formula to kill fleas and ticks on contact. (Does not contain chlorinated solvents.)

Active Ingredients: **By Weight**
Chlorpyrifos [0,0-diethyl 0-(3,5,6-trichloro-2-pyridyl) phosphorothioate]........................0.5000%
Xylene range aromatic solvent...0.3300%
d-trans Allethrin (allyl homolog of Cinerin 1)................................0.0500%
Related Compounds.....................0.0036%
Petroleum distillate 4.0000%
Inert Ingredients 95.1164%

Directions for use: It is a violation of Federal law to use this product in a manner inconsistent with its labeling.

For Control of Fleas and Brown Dog Ticks: Controls adult fleas and larvae for up to 4 weeks. Thoroughly spray for spot treatment to infested areas such as pet beds and resting quarters; nearby cracks and crevices; along and behind baseboards, windows and door frames and localized areas of floor and floor covering where these pests may be present. TEST INCONSPICUOUS SAMPLE OF FABRIC OR RUG FOR STAINING BEFORE USE. Old bedding of pet should be removed and replaced with clean, fresh bedding after treatment of pet area. DO NOT TREAT PETS WITH THIS PRODUCT. To control the source of flea infestation, pets inhabiting the treated premises should be treated with a product registered for application to animals.

For Cockroaches, Ants, Clover Mites, Crickets, Firebrats, Silverfish and Spiders: Spray localized areas where these pests are found or normally occur including dark corners of rooms and closets; cracks and crevices in walls; along and behind sinks, stoves, refrigerators and cabinets; around plumbing and other utility installations. For ants, apply to ant trails, also around doors and windows and wherever else these pests may find entrance. NOTE: a period of 4 to 7 days is normally required for maximum effect on cockroaches.

For Control of Carpet Beetles: Thoroughly spray for spot treatment along baseboards and edges of carpeting, under carpeting, rugs and furniture, in closets and shelving, and wherever else these insects are seen or suspected.

Storage and Disposal: Store in cool dry area away from heat or open flame. Do not reuse empty container. Wrap container and put in trash collection.

Precautionary Statements—Hazards to Humans:
CAUTION: Avoid contact with eyes, skin and clothing. Avoid breathing vapors or spray mist. Keep away from food, feedstuffs and domestic water supplies. Wash thoroughly after handling. Do not use in edible product areas of food processing plants, restaurants or other areas where food is commercially prepared or processed. Do not use in serving areas while food is exposed.

Statement of Practical Treatment: If swallowed: Call a physician or Poison Control Center. Drink 1 or 2 glasses of water and induce vomiting by touching back of throat with finger. Do not induce vomiting or give anything by mouth to an unconscious person.
If on skin: In case of contact, remove contaminated clothing and immediately wash skin with plenty of water.
If in eyes: Flush eyes with plenty of water.

Note to Physician: Chlorpyrifos is a cholinesterase inhibitor. Treat symptomatically. Atropine only by injection is an antidote.

Environmental Hazards: This product is toxic to fish, birds and other wildlife. Do not apply directly to water. Do not contaminate water by cleaning of equipment or disposal of wastes. Apply this product only as specified on this label.

Continued on next page

Pitman-Moore—Cont.

This product is highly toxic to bees exposed to direct treatment or residues on plants. Protective information may be obtained from your Cooperative Agricutural Extension Service.
Physical and Chemical Hazards: Contents under pressure. Do not use or store near heat or flame. Do not puncture or incinerate container. Exposure to temperatures above 130°F may cause bursting.
How Supplied: 12 × 12 oz.
**Trademark*

SPRECTO*

Dog Insecticide Collar
Kills ticks & fleas up to 7 months
Aids in the prevention of Sarcoptic Mange for up to 7 months

Active Ingredient:
N-(Mercaptomethyl) phthalimide *S*-(*O,O*-dimethylphosphorodithioate) 15.0%
Inert Ingredients 85.0%

Keep Out of Reach of Children
Precautionary Statements
Hazards to Humans and Domestic Animals

Caution: Dust will form on this collar during storage. Do not get dust or collar in mouth, or allow dust in eyes. Do not open protective pouch until ready to use. Do not allow children to handle collar.
Statement of Practical Treatment: If dust is on skin—wash promptly with soap and water. Rinse thoroughly. If dust is in eyes—rinse eyes with plenty of water. Get medical attention if irritation persists.
Note to Physician: The dust released by this collar is a cholinesterase inhibitor. If signs of cholinesterase inhibition appear atropine is antidotal.
Directions for use: It is a violation of Federal law to use this product in a manner inconsistent with its labeling.
Buckle collar around dog's neck. Collar should be worn loosely to prevent irritation. Attach collar so two or three fingers may be inserted easily between collar and dog's neck. Cut off any excess length and dispose of it. When collar is first worn, observe neck area every few days for irritation. Remove collar at first sign of irritation or adverse reaction. Collar is intended for use only as an insecticide generator and is not to be taken internally by man or animals. Use in addition to regular collar. Do not use on sick or convalescing dogs. Do not use other pesticides on dogs while collar is worn. *Product not to be used on puppies under 12 weeks of age.* Remove collar when bathing.
The collar starts killing fleas as soon as it is placed around dog's neck. Fleas on the dog will be killed and new ones, which may temporarily appear on the dog, will also be killed while collar is worn. This product has been shown to provide effective flea kill up to 7 months plus aiding in kill for an additional 3 months. Replace collar when effectiveness diminishes.
Ticks are tough and are killed slowly. When the collar is first placed on dog, adult ticks will be killed over entire body in a few days and will fall off, or may then be easily removed. Ticks appear on dogs in three stages. In the first two stages, ticks are smaller than a match head and are difficult to see. The collar will also kill these immature stages. This product has been shown to provide effective tick kill up to 7 months plus aiding in kill for an additional 3 months. If ticks are a problem, this collar should be worn continuously. Kills ticks that may carry and transmit Rocky Mountain spotted fever and tularemia. Replace when effectiveness diminishes.
The collar will also aid in the prevention of Sarcoptic Mange for up to 7 months.
Storage and Disposal: Store in original unopened container, away from children. Do not reuse container or used collar. Wrap and put in trash.
How Supplied: One collar per box, two sizes—20″ & 26″.
*Trademark

SPRECTO*

Cat Insecticide Collar
For Cats of All Sizes
Kills ticks & fleas up to 5 months

Active Ingredient:
o-Isopropoxyphenyl methylcarbamate 9.4%
Inert Ingredients 90.6%

Directions: Remove collar from package and place around cat's neck. Adjust for proper fit and buckle in place. Collar must be worn loosely but securely enough to prevent easy removal and loss. Cut off any excess length of collar, leaving ample length for expansion as the cat grows, and dispose of by discarding in trash. Check and adjust collar periodically to assure a proper fit.
Do not use on kittens under 6 weeks of age.
Results Expected: The flea and tick collar starts killing fleas and ticks when it is placed around the cat's neck. Fleas will be killed and new ones which may temporarily appear on the cat will also be killed during the five months. Ticks are tough occasional pests of cats and will be killed within a few days. For continuous protection, replace collar when effectiveness diminishes.
Storage and Disposal: Store in original unopened container, away from children. Do not reuse container or used collar. Wrap and put in trash.
Caution: Do not open inner envelope until ready to use. Do not allow children to play with this collar. Dust will form on this collar during storage. Do not get dust or collar in mouth, harmful if swallowed. Do not get dust in eyes, will cause temporary pupillary constriction.† In case of contact, flush eyes with water. Wash hands thoroughly with soap and water after handling collar. The dust released by this collar is a cholinesterase inhibitor.
Note to Physician: Atropine and †homatropine are antidotal.
When collar is first worn, observe neck area every few days for irritation. Any collar, when fastened too tightly, may cause skin irritation. Remove collar at the first sign of irritation or adverse reaction. Collar is intended for use as an insecticide generator and is not to be taken internally by man or animal. Do not use on sick or convalescing animals. Do not use any other pesticide on cat while collar is worn.
How Supplied: One collar per box (one size fits all).
*Trademark

SPRECTO*-D

Triple Action Dip
Sponge-on or dip for dogs & cats
An insecticide for the control of sarcoptic mange on dogs, and for fleas and ticks on dogs and cats

Active Ingredients:
Phosmet [*N*-(Mercaptomethyl) phthalimide *S*-(*O,O*-dimethyl phosphorodithioate)] 11.60%
Aromatic petroleum solvent 72.90%
Inert Ingredients 15.50%
Protect from temperatures below 20°F.

Gives control of sarcoptic mange on dogs with one dip treatment
Gives 16 day residual control of fleas and Brown Dog ticks on dogs
Gives 9 day residual control of fleas on cats
Gives 16 day residual control of ticks on cats

Directions for Use: Sarcoptic mange on dogs is characterized by loss of hair; thickened skin and intense itching, caused by the mite *Sarcoptes scabiei var canis.* Mix 1 oz (2 tbs.) Sprecto D with 1 gal. water. Dip dog until skin is wet and allow to shake dry. Do not rinse. If no improvement is seen within 14 days, consult your veterinarian. If mange mites reinfest your dog, retreatment may be necessary.
Fleas and Ticks on Dogs: Mix 1 oz (2 tbs.) Sprecto D with 1 gal. water. Dip or sponge on solution until skin is wet. For maximum residual control, allow to dry on animal.
Occasionally, cats get ticks.
Fleas and Ticks on Cats: Mix ½ oz. (1 tbs.) Sprecto D with 1 gal. water. Dip or sponge on solution until skin is wet. For maximum residual control, allow to dry on animal.
Retreat as necessary but not more often than every 7 days. Do not treat dogs or cats under 8 weeks of age. The Sprecto D solution may be stored or used for 30 days.
Warning: Sprecto D is a cholinesterase inhibitor. Do not use this product on animals simultaneously or within a few days before or after treatment with or exposure to cholinesterase inhibiting drugs, pesticides, or chemicals. Do not treat sick or debilitated animals.
May be harmful if swallowed, inhaled or absorbed through skin. If swallowed, do not induce vomiting. Immediately give large quantities of water or milk. If vomiting does occur, give fluids again. Never give anything by mouth to an unconscious person. Call a physician or Poison Control Center immediately.

Do not get in eyes, on skin or clothing. Do not breathe spray mist. Use only in well ventilated areas. Wear rubber gloves, goggles and protective clothing. In case of skin contact, wash immediately with soap and water; for eyes, flush with water. Wash all contaminated clothing with soap and hot water before re-use. Do not store near heat or open flame. Do not contaminate food or feed.
This product is toxic to fish and wildlife. Keep out of lakes, streams or ponds. Do not apply where runoff is likely to occur. Do not contaminate water by cleaning of equipment or disposal of wastes. Apply this product only as specified on this label.
Storage and Disposal: Store in original container, away from children. Do not reuse container. Wrap and put in trash.
Note to Physician and Veterinarian: Sprecto D is an organophosphorous insecticide. Atropine is antidotal. Usual symptoms of organophosphorous poisoning in man include: headache, blurred vision, weakness, nausea, discomfort in the chest, vomiting, abdominal cramps, diarrhea, salivation, sweating, and pinpoint pupils. Usual symptoms of organophosphorous poisoning in animals include salivation and labored breathing.
How Supplied: Available in 4 fl. oz. & 1 gal. containers.
*Trademark

SPRECTO*–CF
Complete
Insecticide Fogger

Kills Fleas, Ticks and Mosquitoes
Controls Adult Fleas and Larvae for up to Four Weeks
For apartments, homes or buildings.
This easy-to-use exclusive water based formula DOES NOT CONTAIN CHLORINATED SOLVENTS. When used as directed, it will not harm drapes, upholstery, fabrics, carpeting, bedspreads, clothing, linen, furniture, walls, floor tiles, ceilings, shades or blinds.

Active Ingredients:	**By Weight**
Chlorpyrifos [0,0-diethyl 0-(3,5,6-trichloro-2-pyridyl) phosphorothioate]	0.5000%
Xylene range aromatic solvent	0.3300%
d-trans Allethrin (allyl homolog of Cinerin I)	0.0500%
Related compounds	0.0036%
Petroleum Distillate	4.0000%
Inert Ingredients	95.1164%

Keep Out of Reach of Children
Directions for use: It is a violation of Federal law to use this product in a manner inconsistent with its labeling.
For use in rooms, apartments, homes, attics, basements, campers, boats, garages, pet sleeping areas, household storage areas, cabins.
This product will kill fleas, cockroaches, flies, mosquitoes, black carpet beetles, sawtoothed grain beetles, rice weevils, wasps, ticks, spiders, small flying moths, pillbugs, crickets and silverfish.
Cover exposed food, dishes and food handling equipment. Open cabinets and doors to areas to be treated: Shut off fans and air conditioners. Put out all flames except pilot lights. Close doors and windows.
SHAKE WELL BEFORE USING
To Operate Valve: Remove cap and point valve opening away from face and eyes when releasing. To lock valve in open position for automatic discharge, invert cap and place actuator hole over nozzle. Press cap all the way down, locking cap into place. Then place fogger on stand or table in center of room with valve locked open, placing several layers of newspaper or pad under fogger. Do not remain in area during treatment. Leave building at once and keep building closed for two hours before airing out. Ventilate thoroughly before re-entry. Open all doors and windows and allow to air for 30 minutes. Repeat spraying in two to four weeks if necessary.
Use one unit for each 8,000 cubic feet of unobstructed area. Do not use this unit in an area less than 100 cubic feet. Use additional units for remote rooms or where free flow of mist is not assured.
To kill fleas or ticks: Remove and destroy pets old bedding. Apply this product as for other insects. Put fresh beeding in pet's quarters after treatment. Treat dogs and cats with a registered flea or tick control product before allowing them to enter treated areas.
Storage and Disposal: Store in cool, dry area away from heat or open flame. Discard container in trash. Do not incinerate or puncture container.

PRECAUTIONARY STATEMENTS
Hazards to Humans
Caution: May be harmful if swallowed. Avoid contact with eyes, skin or clothing. Avoid breathing vapors or spray mist. Wash thoroughly after handling. Do not allow children to lie or sleep in treated areas until at least six hours following treatment. Avoid contamination of food, feedstuffs and domestic water supplies. Do not use in commercial food processing, preparation, storage or serving areas. In the home, all food processing surfaces and utensils should be covered during treatment or thoroughly washed before use.
Remove pets, birds and cover fish aquariums before spraying.

STATEMENT OF PRACTICAL TREATMENT
If swallowed: call a physician or Poison Control Center. Drink 1 or 2 glasses of water and induce vomiting by touching back of throat with finger. Do not induce vomiting or give anything by mouth to an unconscious person.
If on skin: In case of contact, remove contaminated clothing and immediately wash skin with plenty of water.
If in eyes: flush eyes with plenty of water. Get medical attention if irritation persists.
If inhaled: remove victim to fresh air. Apply artificial respiration if indicated.
NOTE TO PHYSICIAN: Chlorpyrifos is a cholinesterase inhibitor. Treat symptomatically. Atropine only by injection is an antidote.

PHYSICAL OR CHEMICAL HAZARDS:
Contents under pressure. Do not use or store near heat or open flame. Do not puncture or incinerate container. Exposure to temperatures above 130°F may cause bursting.
How Supplied: 4 oz. and 8 oz. cans

*Trademark

STIGLYN* 1:500
(neostigmine methylsulfate) Injection

Composition: Each ml contains: Neostigmine methylsulfate 2.0 mg, phenol (as a preservative) 4.5 mg, sodium hydroxide (to adjust pH).
Actions: Stiglyn produces marked vagotonic effects similar to those of physostigmine (eserine), but in therapeutic doses, its use is not likely to be attended by disturbing side reactions. It inhibits the destruction of acetylcholine by cholinesterase, thus facilitating transmission of nerve impulses across the myoneural junction and enhancing cholinergic action.
Indications: For treating rumen atony; initiating peristalsis which causes evacuation of the bowel; emptying the urinary bladder; and stimulating skeletal muscle contractions. It is a curare antagonist.
Contraindications: Stiglyn 1:500 (neostigmine methylsulfate) Injection is contraindicated in mechanical intestinal or urinary tract obstructions, late pregnancy, and in animals treated with other cholinesterase inhibitors. When large doses are administered, muscle twitching may occur, but animals will usually recover if atropine sulfate is administered to overcome cardiovascular effects. For this reason, atropine is sometimes administered simultaneously with Stiglyn. The standard dose of atropine is 0.02 mg per pound of body weight.
Warning: Not for use in animals producing milk, since this use will result in contamination of the milk.
Precautions: Neostigmine exerts a parasympathomimetic activity by inhibiting cholinesterase. In addition to the stimulating effect upon the smooth muscle of the digestive and urinary tracts, it stimulates skeletal muscles, causes pupillary constriction, and excessive doses cause dyspnea, muscular weakness, vomiting and diarrhea.
Dosage and Administration: Cattle and horses, 0.5 ml per 100 lbs of body weight—subcutaneously; sheep, 0.5 to 0.75 ml per 100 lbs of body weight—subcutaneously; swine, 1.0 to 1.5 ml per 100 lbs of body weight—intramuscularly. These doses may be repeated as indicated.
Caution: Federal law restricts this drug to use by or on the order of a licensed veterinarian.
How Supplied: Stiglyn 1:500 (neostigmine methylsulfate) Injection is supplied in 20 ml multiple dose vials.
*Trademark

Continued on next page

Pitman-Moore—Cont.

STRESNIL* INJECTION
(azaperone)
40 mg/ml

Description: Azaperone, the active ingredient of STRESNIL (azaperone) Injection, is a neuroleptic of the butyrophenone series. Chemically, it is 4′-fluoro-4-[4-(2-pyridyl)-1-piperazinyl] butyrophenone. Each ml of STRESNIL Injection contains: azaperone 40 mg; tartaric acid 14 mg; sodium bisulfite 2 mg; methylparaben 0.5 mg; propylparaben 0.05 mg; sodium hydroxide (to adjust pH).

Actions: STRESNIL (azaperone) Injection is a potent neuroleptic which produces a predictable and consistent response in pigs. The drug is fast-acting; the onset of action is approximately 5–10 minutes after intramuscular injection. The peak effect is reached in approximately 30 minutes and generally lasts for one to several hours. The animal remains conscious but is quiet and indifferent to the environment.

Indications: STRESNIL (azaperone) Injection is indicated for the control of aggressiveness when mixing or regrouping weanling or feeder pigs weighing up to 80 lbs. of body weight.

The drug is recommended for use when pigs from different litters or pens are brought together, since they often fight in an attempt to establish a social order. Following a single dose of STRESNIL, pigs may be mixed; fighting is eliminated or greatly reduced.

Contraindications: There are no known contraindications to the use of STRESNIL (azaperone) Injection when used as directed.

Adverse Effects: STRESNIL (azaperone) Injection is generally well-tolerated. In clinical trials, salivation, piling and shivering have been observed; these reactions were of short duration and left no lasting effects.

Dosage and Administration: Accurate dosing is essential. The recommended dose of azaperone for the feeder pig is 2.2 mg/kg (1 mg/lb) of body weight. One ml of STRESNIL (azaperone) Injection will treat 40 lbs. of body weight. STRESNIL must be given by **deep intramuscular injection** either behind the ear and perpendicularly to the skin or in the back of the ham.

All animals must be treated. Retreatment is necessary each time mixing or regrouping occurs.

The onset of action of STRESNIL Injection is five to ten minutes after dosing. Administer immediately prior to mixing and do not disturb the animals during the period of drug action (approximately one to several hours).

How Supplied: STRESNIL (azaperone) Injection, 40 mg/ml, is available in cartons of six 20-ml vials.

Storage: Store at controlled room temperature: 59°–86°F (15°–30°C).

Caution: Federal law restricts this drug to use by or on the order of a licensed veterinarian.

*Trademark

SWIVAX*6
Parvovirus Vaccine, Killed Virus Leptospira Canicola—Grippotyphosa—Hardjo—Icterohaemorrhagiae—Pomona Bacterin

Description: SWIVAX 6 is an inactivated porcine parvovirus vaccine combined with an inactivated leptospira bacterin.

The parvovirus component is prepared by chemically inactivating a porcine parvovirus strain grown on an established bovine cell line.

The leptospira components are prepared from whole cultures of *L. canicola, L. grippotyphosa, L. hardjo, L. icterohaemorrhagiae,* and *L. pomona.*

Indications: For the immunization of healthy swine against leptospirosis caused by L. canicola, L. grippotyphosa, L. hardjo, L. icterohaemorrhagiae, L. pomona, and parvovirus-induced reproductive disease.

Dosage and Administration: Use alone or as diluent to rehydrate accompanying vaccine. Using aseptic technique, administer 2ml intramuscularly or subcutaneously according to the following schedule:

Sows and Gilts:
- 2 ml 4–8 weeks prior to breeding
- 2ml 2–4 weeks prior to breeding. The interval between first and second vaccinations must be at least 14 days.
- 2ml Booster 3–4 weeks prior to subsequent breedings. If the interval between breedings exceeds 8 months, the two dose immunization schedule should be followed.

Boars, 8 weeks of age or older:
- Two 2ml doses 2–4 weeks apart
- 2ml annual booster

Precautions: Do not freeze. Store at 2–7°C (35–45°F). Use entire contents when first opened. Do not vaccinate within 21 days before slaughter. Do not use chemicals to sterilize syringes and needles. Contains neomycin, polymyxin B, and a fungistat as preservatives. In case of anaphylactoid reaction, administer epinephrine. For Veterinary Use Only.

How Supplied: SWIVAX 6 is supplied in plastic vials containing 20ml (10 doses) and 40ml (20 doses).

*Trademark

SWIVAX*6 + PRV
Parvovirus—Pseudorabies Vaccine, Modified Live and Killed Virus Leptospira Canicola—Grippotyphosa—Hardjo—Icterohaemorrhagiae—Pomona Bacterin

Description: Swivax 6 + PRV is a combination of a lyophilized, modified live virus pseudorabies vaccine, an inactivated porcine parvovirus vaccine, and an inactivated leptospira bacterin.

The pseudorabies component is prepared by growing a highly antigenic strain of pseudorabies virus in an established bovine cell line.

The parvovirus component is prepared by chemically inactivating a porcine parvovirus strain grown on an established bovine cell line.

The leptospira components are prepared from whole cultures of *L. canicola, L. grippotyphosa, L. hardjo, L. icterohaemorrhagiae,* and *L. pomona.*

Indications: For the immunization of healthy swine against leptospirosis caused by *L. canicola, L. grippotyphosa, L. hardjo, L. icterohaemorrhagiae, L. pomona,* and parvovirus-induced reproductive disease and pseudorabies.

Dosage and Administration: For use in swine only! Not for use in any other animal. Aseptically rehydrate with accompanying diluent. Vaccinate healthy pigs with 2ml (1 dose) intramuscularly or subcutaneously according to the following schedule:

Sows and Gilts:
- 2ml 4–8 weeks prior to breeding
- 2ml 2–4 weeks prior to breeding. The interval between first and second vaccinations must be at least 14 days.
- 2ml Booster 3–4 weeks prior to subsequent breedings. If the interval between breedings exceeds 8 months, the two dose immunization schedule should be followed.

Boars, 8 weeks of age or older:
- Two 2ml doses 2–4 weeks apart
- 2ml annual booster

Precautions: Do not freeze. Store at 2–7°C (35–45°F). Use entire contents when first opened. Burn containers and all unused contents. Do not vaccinate within 21 days before slaughter. Do not use chemicals to sterilize syringes and needles. Contains neomycin, polymyxin B, and a fungistat as preservatives. Do not use if vacuum is lost. It is generally recommended to avoid vaccination of pregnant swine. In case of anaphylactoid reaction, administer epinephrine. For Veterinary use Only.

Distribution in each state shall be limited to authorized recipients designated by proper state officials—under such conditions as these authorities may require.

Caution: Vaccination results in an antibody response indistinguishable from that induced by infection. State and federal regulations restricting the movement of seropositive swine apply to vaccinated animals.

How Supplied: Swivax 6 + PRV is supplied in packages of 10 doses and 20 doses.

*Trademark

SWIVAX*8
Parvovirus Vaccine, Killed Virus Erysipelothrix Rhusiopathiae-Leptospira Canicola-Grippotyphosa-Hardjo-Icterohaemorrhagiae-Pomona-Pasteurella Multocida Bacterin

Description: Swivax 8 is a combination of an inactivated porcine parvovirus vaccine, an inactivated erysipelothrix rhusiopathiae bacterin, an inactivated leptospira bacterin, and an inactivated pasteurella multocida bacterin.

The parvovirus component is prepared by chemically inactivating a porcine par-

vovirus strain grown on an established bovine cell line.
The leptospira components are prepared from whole cultures of *L. canicola, L. grippotyphosa, L. hardjo, L. icterohaemorrhagiae,* and *L. pomona.*
The pasteurella multocida and erysipelothrix rhusiopathiae components are lysed, and the total bacterin is adjuvanted.
Indications: For the immunization of healthy swine against disease produced by *Erysipelothrix rhusiopathiae* and *Pasteurella multocida;* leptospirosis caused by *L. canicola, L. grippotyphosa, L. hardjo, L. icterohaemorrhagiae* and *L. pomona,* and parvovirus-induced reproductive disease.
Dosage and Administration: Using aseptic technique, administer 2ml intramuscularly or subcutaneously according to the following schedule:
Sows and Gilts:
- 2ml 4–8 weeks prior to breeding
- 2ml 2–4 weeks prior to breeding. The interval between first and second vaccinations must be at least 14 days.
- 2ml Booster 3–4 weeks prior to subsequent breedings. If the interval between breedings exceeds 8 months, the two dose immunization schedule should be followed.

Boars, 8 weeks of age or older:
- Two 2ml doses 2–4 weeks apart
- 2ml annual booster

Precautions: Do not freeze. Store at 2–7°C (35–45°F). Use entire contents when first opened. Burn containers and all unused contents. Do not vaccinate within 21 days before slaughter. Do not use chemical to sterilize syringes and needles. Contains neomycin, polymyxin B, and a fungistat as preservatives. In case of anaphylactoid reaction, administer epinephrine. For Veterinary Use Only.
Caution: Do not use as diluent for live vaccines.
How Supplied: Swivax 8 is supplied in plastic vials containing 20ml (10 doses) and 40ml (20 doses).
*Trademark

TELMIN*
(mebendazole)
Equine Wormer

Composition: Each g contains 166.7 mg mebendazole.
Indications: Telmin (mebendazole) Equine Wormer is indicated for infections of: large roundworms (*Parascaris equorum*); large strongyles (*Strongylus edentatus, S. equinus, S. vulgaris*); small strongyles (*Cyclicocyclus spp., Gyalocephalus spp., Poteriostomum spp., Trichonema spp., Triodontophorus spp.,*) and pinworms (*Oxyuris equi*), including many larval stages.
Dosage and Administration: The recommended dose of mebendazole for the horse is 8.8 mg/kg body weight. Each 384 g bottle will treat sixteen 1,000 lb horses. Administer by sprinkling directly on the grain portion of the ration, or by stomach tube in 2–4 pints of water. Prepare individual doses. Withholding feed or water is not necessary.
Telmin is compatible with carbon disulfide, which can be used concurrently for bot control (*Gastrophilus spp.*). Routine carbon disulfide cautions must be observed.
Warning: Not for use in horses intended for food.
Caution: Federal law restricts this drug to use by or on the order of a licensed veterinarian.
How Supplied: 384 g bottle.
*Trademark

TELMIN* B
(mebendazole-trichlorfon)
Equine Wormer

Composition: Each gram of Telmin B Equine Wormer contains 83.3 mg mebendazole and 375.0 mg trichlorfon.
Indications: Telmin B Equine Wormer is indicated for infections of bots (*Gastrophilus intestinalis* and *G. nasalis*), large roundworms (*Parascaris equorum*), large strongyles (*Strongylus edentatus, S. equinus, S. vulgaris*), small strongyles, and pinworms (*Oxyuris equi*).
Dosage and Administration: Packet: Each 24 g packet of Telmin B Equine Wormer will treat 500 pounds of body weight at the recommended dose. Prepare individual doses and administer by stomach tube, or thoroughly mix with the ground grain portion of the ration to be consumed in one feeding. Remove any treated grain not consumed by the next feeding.
Bulk Bottle: Use one level scoop (12 g) for each 250 lbs. of body weight. Prepare individual doses and administer as described above for packets.
Precautions: Use only as directed. Do not administer more than once every 30 days. Do not treat sick or debilitated animals, foals under 4 months of age or mares in the last month of pregnancy. Symptoms of overdosage are ataxia and colic.
Trichlorfon is a cholinesterase inhibitor. Do not administer Telmin B Equine Wormer to animals simultaneously or within a few days before or after treatment with or exposure to cholinesterase-inhibiting drugs, pesticides or chemicals. Do not administer intravenous anesthetics, especially muscle relaxants, concurrently with Telmin B. Do not allow poultry access to medicated feed or feces of treated animals as consumption of trichlorfon by poultry can be fatal.
Notice to Physicians and Veterinarians: Trichlorfon is a cholinesterase inhibitor. Atropine is an antidote; give after cyanosis is overcome and to effect. 2-PAM is a supplemental treatment. Do not walk patient or give morphine.
Warnings:
Not for use in horses intended for food.
Not for human use.
If swallowed by a human, immediately call physician, poison control center or hospital emergency room.
Upon medical advice, induce vomiting with ipecac syrup.
If ipecac is not available, give milk or water and induce vomiting by touching the back of the throat with finger or blunt object.
Avoid prolonged or repeated contact with the skin.
Wash hands after use. Keep out of reach of children.
Caution: Federal law restricts this drug to use by or on the order of a licensed veterinarian.
How Supplied: 24 g packets, cartons of ten
768 g bottle
*Trademark

P

TELMIN* SUSPENSION
(mebendazole)
Equine Wormer

Composition: Each ml contains 33.3 mg mebendazole.
Indications: Telmin (mebendazole) Suspension Equine Wormer is indicated for infections of: large roundworms (*Parascaris equorum*); large strongyles (*Strongylus edentatus, S. equinus, S. vulgaris*); small strongyles and pinworms (*Oxyuris equi*), including many larval stages.
Dosage and Administration: The recommended dose of mebendazole for the horse is 8.8 mg/kg body weight. To provide this, administer one fluid ounce (30 ml) of Telmin Suspension per 250 pounds of body weight, via stomach tube. Following administration, flush the stomach tube with water to insure complete delivery of the dose. Each gallon will treat thirty-two 1000 pound horses. Withholding feed or water is not necessary.
Telmin Suspension should be warmed to approximately 60°F (15°C) for ease of administration.
Warning:
Not for use in horses intended for food.
Shake well before using.
Caution: Federal law restricts this drug to use by or on the order of a licensed veterinarian.
How Supplied: One gallon bottles.
For Oral Veterinary Use Only
*Trademark

TELMIN*
(mebendazole)
Syringe Formula
Equine Wormer

Composition: Each g contains 200 mg mebendazole.
Indications: Telmin (mebendazole) Syringe Formula Equine Wormer is indicated for infections of common equine gastrointestinal nematodes: large roundworms (*Parascaris equorum*); large strongyles (*Strongylus edentatus, S. equinus, S. vulgaris*); small strongyles; and mature and immature (4th larval stage) pinworms (*Oxyuris equi*). See below.
Dosage and Administration: The recommended dose of mebendazole is 8.8 mg per kg of body weight. The Telmin (mebendazole) Syringe Formula Equine Wormer syringe, calibrated in 250 pound weight increments, provides this dosage by delivering 1 g of mebendazole for each 250 pounds (see dosage table). Use one syringe per 1,250 pound horse.

Continued on next page

Pitman-Moore—Cont.

Consult your veterinarian for assistance in the diagnosis, treatment and control of parasitism and before using in severely debilitated animals.
[See table below].
Warning: Not for use in horses intended for food.
How Supplied: 12 x 25 g syringes.
*Trademark

Dosage Table

Syringe† Mark	Horse Wt. (lbs.)	Telmin SF delivered	g mebendazole delivered
0	—	—	—
250	250	5 g	1 g
500	500	10 g	2 g
750	750	15 g	3 g
1,000	1,000	20 g	4 g
1,250	1,250	25 g	5 g

†Use dial edge nearest syringe barrel to mark dose.

TELMINTIC* POWDER
(mebendazole)
Anthelmintic for Dogs

Composition: Telmintic (mebendazole) Powder is an off-white granular powder containing mebendazole, a broad-spectrum benzimidazole anthelmintic, as the active ingredient. Each gram of Telmintic Powder contains 40 mg of mebendazole.
Actions: Mebendazole exerts nematocidal activity by inhibiting glucose uptake by the parasite, thereby reducing the energy level necessary for survival. Mebendazole is not a cholinesterase inhibitor.
Indications: Telmintic (mebendazole) Powder is recommended for infections of roundworms (*Toxocara canis*), hookworms (*Ancylostoma caninum, Uncinaria stenocephala*), whipworms (*Trichuris vulpis*), and tapeworms (*Taenia pisiformis*) in dogs.
The anthelmintic effectiveness of Telmintic was first determined in three controlled-critical trials using 201 naturally parasitized dogs and was confirmed in 502 clinical cases. In these studies, Telmintic was administered at the recommended dose of 22 mg/kg (10 mg/lb) once daily for five consecutive days in a small quantity of food. Results of these studies showed Telmintic to be effective against infections of *T. canis, A. caninum, T. vulpis* and *T. pisiformis* when given at the recommended dose for five consecutive days.
Subsequently, two additional critical studies using 114 naturally or experimentally infected dogs have shown that Telmintic is effective against *T. canis, A. caninum, U. stenocephala, T. vulpis* and *T. pisiformis* when given at the recommended dose for three consecutive days (Table I).
The efficacy obtained in the critical studies was confirmed in a clinical trial using 223 dogs. The animals were given Telmintic Powder at the recommended dose of 22 mg/kg for three or five consecutive days on a blind basis. Results of this study showed that the efficacy obtained with the 3-day dosage regimen was no different from that obtained with the 5-day regimen (Table II).

Table I: Percent Efficacy of Telmintic in Critical Trials

Parasite	*Trial 1* Telmintic (3 days)	*Trial 1* Untreated Control	*Trial 2* Telmintic (3 days)	*Trial 2* Telmintic (5 days)	*Trial 2* Placebo Control	Overall Efficacy (3 days)
T. canis	100	16	100	100	1.2	100
A. caninum	97.8	0.2	99.4	100	0.3	98.6
U. stenocephala	100	0	100	100	0	100
T. vulpis	100	0	100	100	0.6	100
T. pisiformis	100	—	93.9	100	0	96.9
No. of Dogs	27	14	26	23	24	114

Table II: Percent Efficacy of Telmintic in Clinical Trials

Parasite	3-Day Treatment	5-Day Treatment
T. canis	99.4	96.8
A. caninum	99.4	99.9
U. stenocephala	100	100
T. vulpis	100	100
T. pisiformis	100	100
No. of Dogs	109	114

Dosage and Administration: Telmintic (mebendazole) Powder is available in three packet sizes, containing 2.5, 5.0, and 10.0 grams, respectively. Each packet bears a number—either 10, 20 or 40—which corresponds to the size (weight) of a dog the packet will treat as follows:

No. on Packet	Lbs Body Wt Packet Will Treat	Packet Size
10	10 lbs	2.5 g
20	20 lbs	5.0 g
40	40 lbs	10.0 g

Dose to the nearest 10 lbs of body weight using a single packet size or a combination of packets which provides a dose appropriate to the weight of the dog. Administer once daily for 3 consecutive days by mixing with a small quantity of food, preferably prior to the regular meal.
Contraindications: No specific contraindications are known at this time.
Adverse Reactions: Occasionally in dogs, hepatic dysfunction, sometimes fatal, especially following retreatment, has been reported with the use of Telmintic Powder.
Vomiting and diarrhea/soft stools are the most frequently reported side effects. In clinical trials, these effects appeared in approximately 2–6% of the dogs treated.
Animal Toxicology: The safety of mebendazole in dogs has been well established. In acute toxicity studies, the highest single oral dose given, 640 mg/kg, elicited no significant side effects. Similarly, the oral administration of mebendazole at doses up to 40 mg/kg once daily for 90 days and also for 24 months did not produce any significant abnormality. In reproductive studies, mebendazole was not embryotoxic or teratogenic when administered in an oral dose of 20 mg/kg/day beginning on the first day of pregnancy and continuing for 56 consecutive days.
The market formulation of Telmintic (mebendazole) Powder when given to dogs at five times the recommended daily dose for 10 days produced no side effects other than occasional vomiting and diarrhea. In a second study, when dogs were given up to five times the recommended daily dose for 15 days, the only side effects noted were a moderate increase in the incidence of diarrhea or soft stools and vomiting, when compared to untreated and placebo controls. No drug-related clinicopathological or histopathological alterations were noted in the test animals. In another study Telmintic has been shown to be compatible with organophosphate, carbamate and chlori nated hydrocarbon compounds commonly used in flea collars, shampoos and dipping solutions. Also Telmintic has been proven safe for use in heartworm-infected dogs which were also infected with intestinal parasites.
Caution: Federal law restricts this drug to use by or on the order of a licensed veterinarian.
How Supplied: Telmintic (mebendazole) Powder is supplied in 2.5 and 5.0 g packets, cartons of 100; and 10.0 g packets, cartons of 50.
*Trademark

TETNOGEN®
Tetanus Toxoid
Alum Precipitated Purified

For Use in Horses, Cattle, Swine, and Sheep
Dosage and Administration: Shake well before using. Acceptically vaccinate

horses, cattle, and swine with 1 ml; sheep, 0.5. ml intramuscularly or subcutaneously. A second dose should be given 30 days later. Annual revaccination with a single dose is recommended.
Precautions: Store at 2–7°C (35–45°F). Do not freeze. Use entire contents immediately after opening. Do not vaccinate within 21 days before slaughter. In case of anaphylactoid reaction, administer epinephrine.
How Supplied: Tetnogen is supplied in packages containing ten 1 ml and one 10 ml vials.

For Veterinary Use Only
® Connaught Laboratories

TISSUVAX* 5
Canine Distemper-Hepatitis-Parainfluenza Vaccine
Modified Live Virus
Leptospira Bacterin

Description: Tissuvax* 5 is a combination of lyophilized suspension of canine distemper, canine hepatitis, and parainfluenza modified live viruses and leptospira bacterin. The lyophilized suspension of canine distemper, hepatitis, and parainfluenza modified live viruses is propagated in a stable cell line of canine origin and backfilled with an inert gas. The bacterin, inactivated cultures of *Leptospira canicola* and *Leptospira icterohaemorrhagiae*, has been processed to be non-viricidal when used as diluent to rehydrate the Canine Distemper-Hepatitis-Parainfluenza Vaccine. Production of the viral components by the stable cell line process ensures maximum uniformity with regard to safety an immunogenicity. The immunogenicity and safety of the product have been demonstrated by vaccination and challenge tests in healthy susceptible dogs. Data indicate that the development of corneal opacity is not associated with the use of this product.
Indications: For the immunization of healthy unexposed puppies and dogs against canine distemper, canine hepatitis, canine adenovirus type 2, canine parainfluenza and leptospirosis caused by *L. canicola* and *L. icterohaemorrhagiae.*
Dosage and Administration: Aseptically rehydrate vaccine with accompanying diluent. Using aseptic technique, inject 1 ml either subcutaneously or intramuscularly. Two doses of this vaccine are required in the initial immunization in order to develop a higher level of immunity against canine parainfluenza. Susceptible puppies and dogs should receive two doses, 2 to 4 weeks apart. The age at which maternal antibody no longer interferes with development of active immunity varies according to the bitch's titer and quantity of colostral antibodies absorbed by the puppy. In some instances, interference may last as long as three months. Therefore, dogs vaccinated when younger than 12 weeks of age should receive one dose every 2 to 4 weeks until reaching this age. An annual booster is recommended for all dogs.
Precautions: Store at 2–7°C (35–45°F). Use entire contents when first opened. Do not use chemicals to sterilize syringes and needles. Burn this container and all unused contents. In case of anaphylactoid reaction, administer epinephrine. Contains neomycin, polymyxin B, and a fungistat as preservatives. It is generally recommended to avoid vaccination of pregnant dogs. Central nervous system reactions have been temporally associated with the administration of modified live canine distemper vaccines. Clinical experience indicates that the incidence of such reactions is extremely low. For Veterinary Use Only.
This product was tested before release for sale and meets all tests required by the United States Government as well as our own laboratories.
U.S. Pat. No. 3,950,512
*Trademark

TISSUVAX* 6
Canine Distemper-Hepatitis-Parainfluenza-Parvovirus Vaccine
Modified Live Virus
Leptospira Bacterin
For Use in Dogs

Description: Tissuvax* 6 is a combination of a lyophilized suspension of canine distemper, hepatitis, and parainfluenza modified live virus, and a liquid diluent composed of a parvovirus (feline isolate) and Leptospira bacterin. The lyophilized suspension of canine distemper, hepatitis, and parainfluenza modified live viruses is propagated in a stable cell line of canine origin and backfilled with an inert gas. The liquid modified live parvovirus is propagated in a stable cell line of feline origin, and combined with inactivated cultures of *Leptospira canicola* and *Leptospira icterohaemorrhagiae* which have been processed to be non-viricidal when used as diluent to rehydrate the Canine Distemper-Hepatitis-Parainfluenza Vaccine. Production of the viral components by the stable cell line process ensures maximum uniformity with regard to safety and immunogenicity. The immunogenicity and safety of the product has been demonstrated by vaccination and challenge tests in healthy susceptible dogs. Data indicate that the development of corneal opacity is not associated with the use of this product.
Indications: For the immunization of healthy unexposed puppies and dogs against canine distemper, canine hepatitis, canine parvovirus-induced disease, respiratory disease induced by canine adenovirus type 2, and canine parainfluenza, as well as leptospirosis caused by *L. canicola* and *L. icterohaemorrhagiae.*
Dosage and Administration: Aseptically rehydrate vaccine with accompanying diluent. Using aseptic technique, inject 1 ml either subcutaneously or intramuscularly. Two doses of this vaccine are required in the initial immunization in order to develop a higher level of immunity against canine parainfluenza and parvovirus. Susceptible puppies and dogs should receive two doses 2 to 4 weeks apart. The age at which maternal antibody no longer interferes with development of active immunity varies according to the bitch's titer and quantity of colostral antibodies absorbed by the puppy. In some instances, interference may last as long as four months. Therefore, dogs vaccinated when younger than 16 weeks of age should receive one dose every 2 to 4 weeks until reaching this age. An annual booster dose is recommended for all dogs.
Precautions: Store at 2–7°C (35–45°F). Use entire contents when first opened. Do not use chemicals to sterilize syringes and needles. Burn this container and all unused contents. In case of anaphylactoid reaction, administer epinephrine. Contains neomycin, polymyxin B, and a fungistat as preservatives. It is generally recommended to avoid vaccination of pregnant dogs. Central nervous system reactions have been temporally associated with the administration of modified live canine distemper vaccines. Clinical experience indicates that the incidence of such reactions is extremely low. For Veterinary Use Only.
This product was tested before release for sale and meets all tests required by the United States Government, as well as our laboratories.

For Veterinary Use Only
U.S. Pat. No. 3,950,512
*Trademark

TITAN*3
Bordetella Bronchiseptica-Erysipelothrix Rhusiopathiae-Pasteurella Multocida Bacterin

Description: Titan 3 is a trivalent bacterin composed of inactivated Bordetella Bronchiseptica, Pasteurella Multocida, and Erysipelothrix Rhusiopathiae Bacterins.
The *Pasteurella multocida* and *Erysipelothrix rhusiopathiae* components are lysed, and the total bacterin is adjuvanted.
Indications: For use in healthy unexposed swine for the prevention of atrophic rhinitis caused by *Bordetella bronchiseptica* and against disease produced by *Erysipelothrix rhusiopathiae* and *Pasteurella multocida.*
Dosage and Administration: Shake well. Using aseptic technique, vaccinate healthy swine with 2 ml (1 dose) intramuscularly or subcutaneously according to the following schedule:
Sows and Gilts:
- 2ml 4–5 weeks before farrowing
- 2ml 1–2 weeks before farrowing
- 2ml Booster 2 weeks prior to each subsequent farrowing

Pigs:
- 2ml at 3 days of age or older
- 2ml at weaning. The interval between the first and second vaccination must be at least 14 days.

Boars:
- 2ml annual revaccination

Precautions: Do not freeze. Store at 2–7°C (35–45°F). Use entire contents when first opened. Local reactions may occur at injection site. Do not vaccinate within 21 days before slaughter. In case of anaphylactoid reaction, administer epinephrine. For Veterinary Use Only.

Continued on next page

Pitman-Moore—Cont.

Caution: Do not use as a diluent for live vaccines.
How Supplied: TITAN 3 is supplied in plastic vials containing 100ml (50 doses) and 200ml (100 doses).
*Trademark

P

TRIPLE-E™
Encephalomyelitis Vaccine
Eastern, Western, and Venezuelan, Killed Virus

Description: Triple-E is a trivalent inactivated virus vaccine grown in cell cultures infected with the Eastern, Western, and Venezuelan strains of encephalomyelitis. It is formalin inactivated and adjuvanted with aluminum hydroxide.
Indications: For active immunization of healthy horses against Eastern, Western, and Venezuelan Encephalomyelitis.
Dosage and Administration: SHAKE WELL before using. Using aseptic technique, vaccinate healthy horses with a 1 ml dose intramuscularly followed by a second 1 ml dosee 2 to 4 weeks later. A booster is recommended annually, or in the event of a threatened epizootic.
Precautions: Local reactions following vaccination are rare. To minimize such reactions, ensure that injections are administered in deep muscle tissue. Thimerosal added as a preservative. Contains residual neomycin and streptomycin remaining from cell cultures. Store at 2–7°C (35–45°F). Do not freeze. Use entire contents when first opened. Do not use chemicals to sterilize syringes and needles. In case of anaphylactoid reaction, administer epinephrine. For Veterinary Use Only.
How Supplied: Triple-E is supplied in packages containing ten 1ml dose syringes (10 doses) and one 10ml tank vial (10 doses).
™ Trademark Connaught Laboratories

TRIPLE-E™FT
Encephalomyelitis-Influenza Vaccine-Tetanus Toxoid
Eastern, Western, and Venezuelan, Killed Virus

Description: Triple-E FT is a trivalent equine encephalomyelitis vaccine combined with a bivalent equine influenza vaccine and tetanus toxoid. The encephalomyelitis portion is an inactivated virus vaccine grown in cell cultures infected with the Eastern, Western, and Venezuelan strains of encephalomyelitis. The influenza portion is derived from the allantoic fluid of embryonated chicken eggs infected with types A/1 and A/2 equine infleunza strains. The vaccine virus laden fluids are clarified and concentrated to provide maximum antigenicity. The vaccine is formalin inactivated and adjuvanted with aluminum hydroxide. The tetanus toxoid component is alum precipitated and highly purified prior to combining with the encephalomyelitis and influenza antigens.
Indications: For active immunization of healthy horses against Eastern, Western, and Venezuelan Encephalomyelitis and Tetanus and as an aid in the prevention of equine influenza due to types A_1 and A_2.
Dosage and Administration: SHAKE WELL before using. Using aseptic technique, vaccinate healthy horses with a 1 ml dose intramuscularly followed by a second 1 ml dose 2 to 4 weeks later. A booster is recommended annually, or in the event of a threatened epizootic.
Precautions: Local reactions following vaccination are rare. To minimize such reactions, ensure that injections are administered in deep muscle tissue. Thimerosal added as a preservative. Contains residual neomycin and streptomycin remaining from cell cultures. Store at 2–7°C (35–45°F). Do not freeze. Use entire contents when first opened. Do not use chemicals to sterilize syringes and needles. In case of anaphylactoid reaction, administer epinephrine. For Veterinary Use Only.
How Supplied: Triple-E FT is supplied in packages containing ten 1ml dose syringes (10 doses) and one 10ml tank vial (10 doses).
™ Trademark Connaught Laboratories

TRIPLE-E™T
Encephalomyelitis Vaccine—Tetanus Toxoid
Eastern, Western, and Venezuelan, Killed Virus

Description: TRIPLE-ET is a trivalent equine encephalomyelitis vaccine combined with tetanus toxoid. The encephalomyelitis portion is an inactivated virus vaccine grown in cell cultures infected with the Eastern, Western, and Venezuelan strains of encephalomyelitis. This vaccine is formalin inactivated and adjuvanted with aluminum hydroxide.
The tetanus toxoid component is alum precipitated and highly purified prior to combining with the equine encephalomyelitis antigens.
Indications: For active immunization of healthy horses against Eastern, Western, and Venezuelan Encephalomyelitis and Tetanus.
Dosage and Administration: SHAKE WELL before using. Using aseptic technique, vaccinate healthy horses with a 1 ml dose intramuscularly followed by a second 1 ml dose 2 to 4 weeks later. A booster is recommended annually, or in the event of a threatened epizootic.
Precautions: Local reactions followng vaccination are rare. To minimize such reactions, ensure that injections are administered in deep muscle tissue. Thimerosal added as a preservative. Contains residual neomycin and streptomycin remaining from cell cultures. Store at 2–7°C (35–45°F). Do not freeze. Use entire contents when first opened. Do not use chemicals to sterilize syringes and needles. In case of anaphylactoid reaction, administer epinephrine. For Veterinary Use Only.
How Supplied: TRIPLE-ET is supplied in packages containing ten 1ml dose syringes (10 doses) and one 10 ml tank vial (10 doses).
™ Trademark Connaught Laboratories

VERMIPLEX* CAPSULES
Anthelmintic for Dogs & Cats

Composition:

Each No. 000-Orange capsule contains:	
Dichlorophene	50 mg
Toluene	60 mg
Each No. 00-Blue capsule contains:	
Dichlorophene	125 mg
Toluene	150 mg
Each No. 0-Yellow capsule contains:	
Dichlorophene	250 mg
Toluene	300 mg
Each No. 1-Green capsule contains:	
Dichlorophene	500 mg
Toluene	600 mg
Each No. 2-Red capsule contains:	
Dichlorophene	1.0 g
Toluene	1.2 g
Each No. 3-Brown capsule contains:	
Dichlorophene	2.0 g
Toluene	2.4 g
Each No. 4-Maroon capsule contains:	
Dichlorophene	4.0 g
Toluene	4.8 g

Indications: For removal of ascarids (*Toxocara canis* and *Toxascaris leonina*) and hookworms (*Ancylostoma caninum* and *Uncinaria stenocephala*) and as an aid in the removal of tapeworms (*Taenia pisiformis, Dipylidium caninum* and *Echinococcus granulosus*) from dogs and cats.
Dosage and Administration: Withhold solid food and milk (broth may be given) for at least 12 hours prior to medication and for 4 hours afterward.
Single Dose Method: Administer one:
No. 000 capsule per ½ lb body weight.
No. 00 capsule per 1¼ lbs body weight.
No. 0 capsule per 2½ lbs body weight.
No. 1 capsule per 5 lbs body weight.
No. 2 capsule per 10 lbs body weight.
No. 3 capsule per 20 lbs body weight.
No. 4 capsule per 40 lbs body weight.
Divided dose method: Divide the total body weight by 5 and administer the appropriate sized Vermiplex capsule daily for 6 days.
Repeat treatment in 2 to 4 weeks in dogs subject to reinfection.
Side effects: May cause severe salivation if animal bites capsule; discontinue administration until symptoms subside.
Caution: Consult your veterinarian for assistance in the diagnosis, treatment and control of parasitism, and before administering to weak or debilitated animals.
How Supplied:
No. 000 (orange) capsules, bottles of 100
No. 00 (blue) capsules, bottles of 100.
No. 0 (yellow) capsules, bottles of 100.
No. 1 (green) capsules, bottles of 100.
No. 2 (red) capsules, bottles of 100.
No. 3 (brown) capsules, bottles of 25.
No. 4 (maroon) capsules, bottles of 25.
*Trademark

VETRACHLORACIN*
(chloramphenicol)
Veterinary Ophthalmic Ointment 1%
Sterile

Composition: Each gram contains: Chloramphenicol U.S.P. 10 mg, in a Light Mineral Oil N.F., White Petrolatum U.S.P., Polyoxyethylene Sorbitan Monostearate base.

Action: Chloramphenicol is a broad spectrum antibiotic providing rapid clinical response and having therapeutic activity against susceptible strains of a number of gram-positive and gram-negative organisms including *Escherichia coli, Staphylococcus aureus* and *Streptococcus hemolyticus.*

Indications: Vetrachloracin (chloramphenicol) Veterinary Ophthalmic Ointment 1% is appropriate for use in dogs and cats for the topical treatment of bacterial conjunctivitis caused by pathogens susceptible to chloramphenicol.

Contraindications: Chloramphenicol products must not be used in meat, egg, or milk-producing animals. The length of time that residues persist in milk or tissues has not been determined.

Warning: Not for use in animals which are raised for food production. Prolonged use in cats may produce blood dyscrasias.

Precautions: Most susceptible bacteria will respond to chloramphenicol therapy in a few days. If improvement is not noted in this period of time, a change of therapy should be considered.

When infection is suspected as the cause of a disease process, especially in purulent or catarrhal conjunctivitis, attempts should be made to determine, through susceptibility testing, which antibiotics will be effective prior to applying ophthalmic preparations.

Dosage and Administration: Application of Vetrachloracin (chloramphenicol) Veterinary Ophthalmic Ointment 1% should be preceded by cleansing to remove discharge and crusts. The ointment is applied every three hours around the clock for 48 hours, after which night instillations may be omitted. A small amount of ointment should be placed in the lower conjunctival sac. Treatment should be continued for two days after the eye appears normal. Therapy for cats should not exceed seven days.

Caution: Federal law restricts this drug to use by or on the order of a licensed veterinarian.

How Supplied: 12 × ⅛ oz (3.5 g) sterile tamper-proof tubes.

*Trademark

VETROPOLYCIN*
(bacitracin-neomycin-polymyxin) Veterinary Ophthalmic Ointment Antibacterial

Composition: Each gram contains: Bacitracin zinc U.S.P., 400 units; Neomycin sulfate U.S.P. (equivalent to 3.5 mg/g neomycin base) 0.5%; Polymyxin B sulfate U.S.P. 10,000 units. In a base of white petrolatum U.S.P. and mineral oil U.S.P.

Action: The three antibiotics present in Vetropolycin (bacitracin-neomycin-polymyxin) Ophthalmic Ointment provide a broad spectrum of activity against the gram-positive and gram-negative bacteria commonly involved in superficial infections of the eyelid and conjunctiva. Polymyxin B is bactericidal to gram-negative bacteria especially Pseudomonas. No resistant strains have been found to develop *in vivo.* Bacitracin is effective against gram-positive bacteria including hemolytic and non-hemolytic streptococci and staphylococci. Resistant strains rarely develop. Neomycin is effective against both gram-positive and gram-negative bacteria including staphylococci, *Escherichia coli, Haemophilus influenzae* and many strains of Proteus and Pseudomonas.

Indications: Vetropolycin (bacitracin-neomycin-polymyxin) Ophthalmic Ointment is indicated for the treatment of superficial bacterial infections of the eyelid and conjunctiva in dogs and cats when due to organisms susceptible to the antibiotics contained in the ointment. Laboratory tests should be conducted including *in vitro* culturing and susceptibility tests on samples collected prior to treatment.

Precautions: Sensitivity to this ophthalmic ointment is rare; however, if a reaction occurs, discontinue use of the preparation. As with any antibiotic preparation, prolonged use may result in the overgrowth of nonsusceptible organisms including fungi. Appropriate measures should be taken if this occurs. If infection does not respond to treatment in two or three days, the diagnosis and therapy should be reevaluated.

Care should be taken not to contaminate the applicator tip of the tube during application of the preparation. Do not allow the applicator tip to come in contact with any tissue.

Adverse Reactions: Itching, burning or inflammation may occur in animals sensitive to the product. Discontinue use in such cases.

Dosage and Administration: Apply a thin film over the cornea three or four times daily in dogs and cats. The area should be properly cleansed prior to the use of Vetropolycin (bacitracin-neomycin-polymyxin) Ophthalmic Ointment. Foreign bodies, crusted exudates and debris should be carefully removed.

Caution: Federal law restricts this drug to use by or on the order of a licensed veterinarian.

How Supplied: 12 × ⅛ ounce tubes.

*Trademark

VETROPOLYCIN* HC
(bacitracin-neomycin-polymyxin with hydrocortisone acetate 1%) Veterinary Ophthalmic Ointment Antibacterial Sterile

Composition: Each gram contains Bacitracin zinc U.S.P. 400 units; Neomycin sulfate U.S.P. (equivalent to 3.5 mg/g of neomycin base) 0.5%; Polymyxin B sulfate U.S.P. 10,000 units; Hydrocortisone acetate U.S.P. 1.0%. In a base of white petrolatum U.S.P. and mineral oil U.S.P.

Actions: The overlapping spectra of the three antibiotics present in Vetropolycin HC (bacitracin-neomycin-polymyxin with hydrocortisone acetate 1%) provide effective bactericidal action against most commonly occurring gram-positive and gram-negative bacteria associated with infections of the eyes. The range of bactericidal activity encompasses many bacteria which are, or have become, resistant to other antibiotics, notably Pseudomonas and Staphylococcus. In susceptible organisms, resistance rarely develops, even on repeated or prolonged usage. Hydrocortisone acetate exerts a marked anti-inflammatory action at the tissue level and effectively suppresses inflammation in many disorders of the anterior segment of the eye. Local application to the eye often gives rapid relief of pain and photophobia, particularly in lesions of the cornea.

The combined anti-inflammatory and antimicrobial activity of Vetropolycin HC permits effective management of many disorders of the anterior segment of the eye in which combined activity is needed.

Indications: Vetropolycin HC (bacitracin-neomycin-polymyxin with hydrocortisone acetate 1%) may be used in acute or chronic conjunctivitis, when due to organisms susceptible to the antibiotics contained in this ointment. Laboratory tests should be conducted including *in vitro* culturing and susceptibility tests on samples collected prior to treatment.

Contraindications: Ophthalmic preparations containing corticosteroids are contraindicated in the treatment of those deep, ulcerative lesions of the cornea where the inner layer (endothelium) is involved, in fungal infections and in the presence of viral infections.

Warning: All topical ophthalmic preparations containing corticosteroids with or without an antimicrobial agent, are contraindicated in the initial treatment of corneal ulcers. They should not be used until the infection is under control and corneal regeneration is well under way.

Clinical and experimental data have demonstrated that corticosteroids administered orally or by injection to animals may induce the first stage of parturition if used during the last trimester of pregnancy and may precipitate premature parturition followed by dystocia, fetal death, retained placenta, and metritis.

Additionally, corticosteroids administered to dogs, rabbits, and rodents during pregnancy have resulted in cleft palate in offspring. Corticosteroids administered to dogs during pregnancy have also resulted in other congenital anomalies, including deformed forelegs, phocomelia, and anasarca.

Precautions: Sensitivity to this ophthalmic ointment is rare; however, if reactions occur, discontinue use of the preparation.

The prolonged use of antibiotic-containing preparations may result in overgrowth of nonsusceptible organisms including fungi. Appropriate measures should be taken if this occurs. If infection does not respond to treatment in two or three days, the diagnosis and therapy should be reevaluated.

Continued on next page

Pitman-Moore—Cont.

Animals under treatment with this product should be observed for usual signs of corticosteroid overdose which include polydipsia, polyuria and occasionally an increase in weight.
Care should be taken not to contaminate the applicator tip during administration of the preparation.
Adverse Reactions: Itching, burning or inflammation may occur in animals sensitive to the product.
Dosage and Administration: Apply a thin film over the cornea three or four times daily. The area to be treated should be properly cleansed prior to use. Foreign bodies, crusted exudates and debris should be carefully removed. Insert the tip of the tube beneath the lower lid and express a small quantity of the ointment into the conjunctival sac in dogs and cats.
Caution: Federal law restricts this drug to use by or on the order of a licensed veterinarian.
How Supplied: 12 × 1/8 oz tubes.
*Trademark

V–TERGENT* 8X
Detergent—Deodorant

Composition: Contains: Benzethonium chloride 1.6%; Isopropyl alcohol 13.5%.
Indications: Widely useful detergent and deodorant. Liquefies pus and fatty exudates.
General cleaner and deodorizer for equipment, premises and animals.
May be used on hands and arms
Not germicidal in these applications.
Directions for Use: *Undiluted:* As a deodorant shampoo, wet the hair coat of the animal before applying and rinse thoroughly after completing the shampoo. As a presurgical preparation, rinse the area thoroughly with water after application.
Diluted: 1–3 teaspoonfuls per gallon of water (hard or soft) as a cleanser and deodorizer for operating tables, utensils, cages, floors; to clean syringes, slides and other glassware. Especially indicated for cleaning ears and removing secretions from arms, hands, gloves and utensils used in odorous veterinary obstetrical procedures.
Do not use with common laundry detergents or soap.
Caution: Avoid getting the concentrate in eyes. In case of eye contact, wash thoroughly with water. If irritation persists (human), get medical attention.
How Supplied: 16 fl. oz.
*Trademark

WELADOL*
Antiseptic Shampoo
Antibacterial—Antiseptic

Composition:
Contains: Polyalkyleneglycol-Iodine Complex in a shampoo base. Available Iodine—1%.
Indications: Weladol Antiseptic Shampoo is indicated as an aid in the control of bacterial skin infections in dogs and cats.
Dosage and Administration: Wet the hair coat with warm water. Apply liquid petrolatum to eyes before shampooing. Avoid contact with eyes. Apply Weladol Antiseptic Shampoo over the entire body using additional warm water to aid in application. Rinse the hair coat thoroughly and repeat procedure. Use as indicated.
Shake well before using.
Note: This product tends to discolor metal. Do not allow it to come in contact with jewelry.
Warning: For external use only.
How Supplied: 3⅞ oz (110 g) and 31 oz (900 g) bottles.
*Trademark

WELADOL* DISINFECTANT
General Purpose Iodine Disinfectant for Veteninary Use
Bactericidal, Fungicidal (pathogenic fungi) and Virucidal (Canine parainfluenza virus and Canine reovirus)
EPA Reg. No. 773-52
EPA Est. No. 773-NJ-1

Composition: Active Ingredients: Polyethoxy polypropoxy polyethoxy ethanol-iodine Complex 7.8%; Nonyl phenoxy polyethoxy ethanol-iodine Complex 7.5%.
Inert Ingredients: 84.7%. (Provides 1.6% titratable iodine).
Indications: For veterinary use as a sanitizer, cleaner and disinfectant.
Directions for Use: Weladol Disinfectant is a concentrate and must be diluted before using. Solutions should be freshly prepared and not used in combination with other cleaners or sanitizers.

1. *As a Sanitizer:* 1 fluid ounce Weladol Disinfectant to 5 gallons water (25 ppm. of Iodine); for previously cleaned floors, walls, cages, glassware, utensils, dishes, etc.
2. *As a Cleanser and Disinfectant:* 3 fluid ounces Weladol Disinfectant to 5 gallons water (75 ppm. of Iodine), for cleaning and disinfecting in one operation. Scrub or mop thoroughly. Recommended for use in operating room, animal rooms, animal cages, lavatories, laboratories and refuse areas. For surfaces difficult to clean, use 6 fluid ounces Weladol Disinfectant to 5 gallons water.
3. *As a Disinfectant:* 3 fluid ounces Weladol Disinfectant to 5 gallons water; for thermometers, tubing, surgical and hospital instruments, rubber gloves, etc. Preclean, removing all foreign matter.

Dilutions for 18 cc. Dispensing Pump; 18 cc. to 1 gallon gives 75 ppm. of Iodine; 18 cc. to 3 gallons gives 25 ppm. of Iodine.
Diluted Weladol Disinfectant is a self indicator of germicidal activity. Activity persists as long as amber color is evident.
Storage and Disposal: Do not reuse empty container. Rinse thoroughly before discarding. Securely wrap original container in several layers of newspaper and discard in trash.
Precautions: Avoid contact with eyes and skin. In case of contact, flush with plenty of water. If eye irritation persists, get medical attention. Harmful if swallowed. Avoid contamination of food.
Note: This concentrate and its dilutions will discolor jewelry.
How Supplied: 1 gallon.
*Trademark

The Purdue Frederick Company
100 CONNECTICUT AVENUE
NORWALK CT 06856

BETADINE® Aerosol Spray
Topical Antiseptic Germicide

Composition: Betadine Aerosol Spray is a germicidal solution of povidone-iodine in a pressurized spray form. Povidone-iodine, a uniquely complexed form of elemental iodine with polyvinylpyrrolidone, essentially retains the broad microbicidal spectrum of iodine in a form that is virtually free of iodine's undesirable features. It is virtually non-stinging and nonirritating to skin, wounds, and mucous membranes, and may be used even on denuded areas. Virtually nontoxic and noncorrosive to skin and mucosa, Betadine Aerosol Spray may be applied with or without bandages. It is nonstaining to skin, hair or natural fabrics. Betadine Aerosol Spray penetrates into skin crevices and creases.
Action: Betadine Aerosol Spray kills both gram-positive and gram-negative bacteria (including antibiotic-resistant organisms). The action of Betadine Aerosol Spray is bactericidal—not merely bacteriostatic—and is more prolonged than that of iodine tincture. It maintains microbicidal action in the presence of blood, pus, serum and necrotic tissue.
Directions: Hold container about 10 inches from the animal; press valve firmly to cover desired area. Keep spray away from animal's eyes. Allow to dry. Improved actuator permits use from any angle. Not for use on food-producing animals. As with all medication, keep out of reach of children.
How Supplied: Available in 3 oz. bottles.

BETADINE® OINTMENT
Topical Antiseptic Germicide

Composition: Povidone-iodine (titratable iodine, 1%).
Indications: Kills germs—helps prevent bacterial infections in minor burns, superficial cuts and abrasions—virtually nonirritating, nonstaining to skin, hair and natural fabrics.
Dosage and Administration: Apply directly to affected area once or twice daily until healed. May be bandaged.
Caution: In case of deep or puncture wounds or serious burns, consult veterinarian. If redness, irritation or swelling persists or increases, discontinue use and consult veterinarian. Not for use on food-producing animals. As with all medication, keep out of reach of children.
How Supplied: 1 oz tubes, 1 lb, and 5 lb jars.

BETADINE® SOLUTION
Topical Antiseptic Germicide

Composition: Povidone-iodine (available iodine 1%)
Dosage and Administration: Apply Betadine Solution, full strength once or twice daily until healed, as a paint, wet soak, or spray. May be covered with gauze or adhesive bandage. Not for use on food-producing animals. As with all medication, keep out of reach of children.
How Supplied: 8 oz, 16 oz, 32 oz and 1 gal. plastic bottles.

BETADINE® Surgical Scrub
Topical Antiseptic Germicide

Composition: Povidone-iodine (titratable iodine, 0.75%).
Indications: Antiseptic, germicidal sudsing skin cleanser. A microbicidal cleanser for the preoperative and postoperative scrubbing or washing by the veterinarian and preoperative and postoperative prepping of the animal.
Directions: *A. For Preoperative Washing by Veterinarian and Operating Personnel* —1. Wet hands with water. Pour about 5 cc (1 teaspoonful) of Betadine Surgical Scrub on the palm of the hand and spread over both hands. Without adding more water, scrub in the usual manner. Use a brush if desired. Clean thoroughly under fingernails. Add a little water and develop copious suds. Rinse thoroughly under running water. 2. Complete the wash by scrubbing with another 5 cc of Betadine Surgical Scrub in the same way.
B. For Preoperative and Postoperative Prepping on Animals —After the surgical area is shaved, wet with water. Apply Betadine Surgical Scrub. (1 cc is sufficient to cover an area of 20 to 30 square inches). Develop lather and scrub thoroughly. Rinse off by aid of a sterile gauze saturated with water. The area may then be painted with Betadine Solution Veterinary, or sprayed with Betadine Aerosol Spray and allowed to dry. Not for use on food-producing animals. As with all medication, keep out of reach of children.
Note: Blue stains on starched linen will wash off with soap and water.
How Supplied: 16 oz. with and without pump dispenser; 32 fl oz (1 qt) and 1 gal plastic bottles.

Products are cross-indexed by generic and chemical names in the
Active Ingredients Section

lbs. DECCOX Per Ton of Supplement	Decoquinate Levels Gms/Ton	%	Mgs./Lb.	Daily Feeding Rate Per Head
16.7	454	0.05%	227	1/10 lb./100 lbs. body wt.
33.4	908	0.1%	454	1/10 lb./200 lbs. body wt.
41.75	1136	0.125%	568	1/10 lb./250 lbs. body wt.
167.0	4542	0.5%	2271	*(See footnote)

*This supplement must be mixed with grain at the rate of 1 part supplement with 9 parts grain. Th resulting mixture contains 0.05% decoquinate and is then to be fed at the rate of 1/10 lb. per 100 lbs. body weight daily.

Rhone-Poulenc Inc.
FEED ADDITIVES DIVISION
500 NORTHRIDGE ROAD
SUITE 620
ATLANTA, GA 30338
404-256-2889
(outside of Georgia) 800-554-1059

DECCOX®
(decoquinate)
Coccidiostat for cattle, poultry
Medicated premix for feed manufacturing

Composition: Deccox contains 6% decoquinate (ethyl 6-(declyoxy)-7-ethoxy-4-hydroxy-3-quinoline-carboxylate). This is 27.2 grams of active drug per pound of Deccox. A cream to pale buff, microcrystalline powder with a slight odor, decoquinate is blended with degerminated corn meal, soybean oil, lecithin and silicon dioxide to produce Deccox. Deccox is practically insoluble in water and has been found to be stable for four years or more when stored in a cool, dry area with the bag kept tightly closed.
Indications: As an aid in the prevention of coccidiosis in ruminating calves and cattle—caused by *E. bovis* and *E. zurnii.*
As an aid in the prevention of coccidiosis in broiler chickens—caused by *E. tenella, E. necatrix, E. acervulina, E. mivati, E. maxima,* and *E. brunetti.*
Background: Coccidia are most commonly parasites of intestinal epithelial cells, though some species attack the liver and other organs. The species which cause important infections in domestic animals belong to 2 genera, *Eimeria* and *Isospora.* Members of the genus *Eimeria* have a marked host specificity and are the most economically important in animal husbandry. Chickens harbor as many as 9 species; cattle harbor up to 21. In cattle, a low level of oocyst ingestion may result in a subclinical infection that would not be diagnosed as coccidiosis but could have subtle adverse effects on the animal. Clinical signs are often not demonstrated until 3–8 weeks following initial infection. In severe clinical cases, marked diarrhea occurs, with feces containing stringy masses of mucus and clotted blood. This is often accompanied by a loss of appetite, dehydration, general weakness and loss of vigor. The pathology produced by coccidia in cattle is either the direct or indirect result of the tremendous multiplication of coccidia in the epithelial lining of the lower small intestine, cecum, colon or rectum. Gross lesions include loss of surface epithelium, mucosal thickening, diffuse hemorrhage, catarrhal interitis, and destruction of intestinal glands. In this weakened state the animal is subject to secondary disease such as pneumonia, bacterial enteritis and viral infections.
In poultry, signs of coccidiosis show considerable variation. They range from decreased rates of growth to a significant number of obviously sick birds with severe diarrhea and a high mortality rate. Water and feed consumption are usually decreased. Clinical infections result in weight loss, the development of culls, reduced egg production by hens, and increased mortality.
Dosage and Administration: For cattle, thoroughly mix Deccox into the ration at a rate to provide decoquinate at a daily dose of 22.7 mg/100 lb. (0.5 mg/kg) of body weight. Feed for at least 28 days during periods of coccidiosis exposure or when experience indicates that coccidiosis is likely to be a hazard.
Mixing & Feeding Directions
1. *For Supplements*
The table below shows the amounts of DECCOX required per ton of supplement to provide the proper decoquinate levels per head daily.
[See table above]
2. *For Complete Rations*
The table below shows the amounts of DECCOX required per ton of complete feed to provide the proper decoquinate levels daily for animals weighing an average of 600 pounds.
[See table below]

Lbs. DECCOX Per Ton of Feed	Decoquinate Levels Gms/Ton	%	Mgs/Lb.	Daily Feeding Rate Per Head
5	13.6	0.00149%	6.8	20 lbs.
7	19	0.00209%	9.5	14.5 lbs.
1.0	27.2	0.00299%	13.6	10 lbs.

Note: Mix the DECCOX with several pounds of ground grain before adding it to the mixer.
For cattle of other weights calculate the amount of DECCOX needed from the daily dosage of 22.7 mg. decoquinate per 100 lbs. of body weight.
For poultry, thoroughly mix one (1) pound of Deccox in each ton of complete ration and feed continuously.
Warning: Do not feed to laying chickens, breeding cattle, or cows producing milk for food.
Precautions: Restricted drug—use only as directed. Must be mixed with other ingredients before feeding. Mixing and conveying equipment should be properly grounded.
How Supplied: Packed in 50-pound and 4×10-pound multiwall bags with a coated inner liner.
NO FDA 1800 REQUIRED

A.H. Robins Company
1407 CUMMINGS DRIVE
RICHMOND, VA 23220

BOVICON–PM™ PASTEURELLA MULTOCIDA VACCINE
Live Culture, Lyophilized

Description: BOVICON-PM™ is a live *Pasteurella multocida* vaccine for the immunization of healthy cattle as an aid in the prevention of infection due to *Pasteurella multocida.*

Application of Vaccine: This vaccine is recommended for the immunization of healthy cattle a minimum of 7 to 10 days prior to weaning, shipping, or exposure to stress or infectious conditions.

Directions for Use:
1. Rehydrate the lyophilized vaccine with sterile diluent. Shake well before using.
2. Use immediately.
3. Vaccinate only healthy cattle a minimum of 7 to 10 days prior to weaning, shipping, or exposure to stress or infectious conditions.
4. DOSAGE: INJECT 0.5 ml INTRADERMALLY. The use of a short (3/16–1/4") 22–24 gauge needle is recommended for the intradermal injection. Vaccination site should be palpated to ascertain the injection has been made intradermally.

Precautions:
1. Use entire contents of vial immediately after mixing.
2. Store the vaccine at not over 7°C (45°F).
3. Do not spill or spatter the vaccine. Burn used vials and all unused contents (see special caution).
4. If a vial of reconstituted vaccine or the vial containing the lyophilized powder is broken, pour concentrated Clorox® or a similar hypochlorite bleach onto the vial and the adjacent contaminated area and allow to stand for several hours prior to disposal.
5. Do not vaccinate within 21 days of slaughter.
6. Do not use chemicals to sterilize syringes and needles.
7. Although rare, anaphylactoid reactions may occur with this or any biological. If such a reaction occurs, administer epinephrine or equivalent and supportive treatment, as required.
8. Since BOVICON-PM™ is a live vaccine, the concurrent use of parenteral antibiotics may interfere with the production of immunity.
9. A swelling up to 5 cm in diameter may occur at the injection site in from 5–50% of vaccinated animals. These swellings should not be treated and will usually resolve within a 2- to 3-week period.

Special Caution: *Pasteurella multocida* can cause local, pulmonary and systemic infections in man. This infection can be serious and life-threatening in special populations which include diabetics and those with cirrhosis, cancer patients, individuals with various forms of immunosuppression and those who have surgical prostheses. The lyophilized powder constitutes a greater risk than the reconstituted vaccine, both because of the increased concentration of the bacteria per unit weight and the possibility of inhalation. Should the operator inoculate or otherwise contaminate himself, he should seek immediate medical advice (see note below).

Note to Physician: The strain of *Pasteurella multocida* used in BOVICON-PM™ has been shown to be sensitive to the following antibiotics *in vitro:* ampicillin, carbenicillin, cephalosporins. chloramphenicol, tobramycin, gentamicin, cefoxitin, cefamandole, amikacin, trimethoprim/sulfamethoxazole and tetracycline.

Package Sizes: Live *Pasteurella multocida* vaccine is available in boxes of one 5 dose vial and boxes of one 20 dose vial with corresponding diluent.

Warranty: This vaccine is thoroughly tested before sale and meets the requirements of the U. S. Department of Agriculture.

CARPET CONTROL™ POWDER
Carpet Insecticide and Freshener

EPA Reg. No. 778-75
EPA Est. No. 773-VA-1

Purpose: CARPET CONTROL™ is a quick-acting flea and tick killing rug deodorizer. This dry, fresh-scented powder works on all types of floors, floor coverings, and upholstered furniture to kill fleas, pre-adult fleas, ticks, lice, ants, silverfish and roaches. At the same time, it overcomes household odors, leaving a clean, fresh smell. CARPET CONTROL is perfect for periodic treatments of any carpet exposed to your pet.

Directions: It is a violation of federal law to use this product in a manner inconsistent with its labeling. Shake before using as some settling may occur during shipment. Sprinkle CARPET CONTROL evenly and lightly over carpet and adjacent floors by shaking container from side to side. Wait 30 minutes, then vacuum. Sprinkle only over areas that can be vacuumed. If ticks are present, leave powder on surface for two hours. Avoid use on wet spots. If product adheres to spot, rub with stiff brush and vacuum.

Storage and Disposal: Store in cool, dry place. Dispose empty container in trash. Do not re-use container.

Precautionary Statements
Hazards to Humans and Domestic Animals

Caution: Harmful if swallowed. Avoid breathing of dust and contact with eyes, skin, or clothing. Wash hands with soap and warm water after handling. If in eyes, flush with plenty of water. If irritation persists, get medical attention. Do not contaminate feed, water, or food stuffs. Cover fish aquariums before use. Keep children and pets off carpet during treatment.

Active Ingredients:
*3-Phenoxybenzyl d-cis and trans**2,2-dimethyl-3-(2-methylpropenyl) cyclopropanecarboxylate 0.23%
*Other isomers 0.01%
d-trans Allethrin (allyl homolog of Cinerin 1) 0.16%
Piperonyl butoxide, technical*** 1.67%
*d-(cis, trans) phenothrin
**cis/trans isomer ratio:
Max. 25% (+ or −) cis
Min. 75% (+ or −) trans
***equivalent to 1.34% of (butylcarbityl) (6-propylpiperonyl) ether and 0.33% related compounds.

Inert Ingredients 97.93%

How Supplied: 14 oz. (396 grams) shaker cannister.

DOPRAM®-V INJECTABLE
(doxapram hydrochloride)

Composition: Each 1 ml contains: doxapram hydrochloride 20 mg; water for injection, USP q.s.; chlorobutanol (as preservative) 0.5%.

Dopram-V® (doxapram hydrochloride), a product of Robins' research, is a potent respiratory stimulant. It is unique in its ability to stimulate respiration at dosages considerably below those required to evoke cerebral cortical stimulation. In non-anesthetized animals the dose required to produce convulsions is some 70 to 75 times the dose required to produce respiratory stimulation. In anesthetized subjects, doxapram also exerts a marked arousal effect. Thus, by promoting the restoration of normal ventilation and producing early arousal following general anesthesia, doxapram minimizes or prevents the undesirable effects of post-anesthetic respiratory depression or hypoventilation and hastens recovery.

Chemistry: The chemical name of doxapram hydrochloride is 1-ethyl-4-(2-morpholinoethyl)-3,3-diphenyl-2-pyrrolidinone hydrochloride hydrate.
The material is prepared as a clear, colorless, 2% aqueous solution with a pH of 3.5 to 5.0 and is stable at room temperature. Stability studies of 24 months' duration have shown doxapram to have excellent stability characteristics. The preservative is chlorobutanol, 0.5% and sterilization is accomplished by aseptic filtration technique. Doxapram is compatible with 5% and 10% dextrose in water or normal saline, but is physically incompatible with alkaline solutions, such as 2.5% thiopental sodium.

Indications: For Dogs, Cats and Horses:
1. To stimulate respiration during and after general anesthesia.
2. To speed awakening and return of reflexes after anesthesia.

For Neonate Dogs and Cats:
1. Initiate respirations following dystocia or cesarean section.
2. To stimulate respirations following dystocia or cesarean section.

Caution: For intravenous use only in dogs, cats and horses. May be administered subcutaneously, sublingually (topically) or via umbilical vein in neonatal puppies and either subcutaneously or sublingually (topically) in neonatal kittens. Do not mix with alkaline solutions. Dopram-V is neither an antagonist of muscle relaxant drugs nor a specific nar-

cotic antagonist.
Doses of Dopram-V should be adjusted to meet the requirements of the situation. Excessive doses may produce hyperventilation which may lead to respiratory alkalosis. A patent air passageway is essential. Adequate, but not excessive, doses should be used and the blood pressure and reflexes should be checked periodically.
[See table at right]

Dosage of Dopram-V For Neonate Use: *Neonate Canine:* Doxapram may be administered either subcutaneously, sublingually (topically) or via the umbilical vein in doses of 1–5 drops (1–5 mg) depending on size of neonate and degree of respiratory crises.

Technique for Umbilical Vein Administration: When the neonate is presented through the incision of the uterus, placental membrane and fluid are removed from mouth and nose. A clamp is placed across the umbilical cord approximately 1–2 inches from abdomen of neonate. The umbilical vein is isolated and the selected dose of doxapram injected directly into the umbilical vein.

Neonate Feline: Doxapram may be administered either subcutaneously or sublingually (topically) in a dose of 1–2 drops (1–2 mg) depending on severity of respiratory crisis.

Dosage and Administration: The action of Dopram-V is rapid, usually beginning in a few seconds. The duration and intensity of response depends upon the dose, the condition of the animal at the time the drug is administered, and depth of anesthesia. Repeated doses should not be given until the effects of the first dose have passed and the condition of the patient requires it.
Dosage should be adjusted for depth of anesthesia, respiratory volume and rate. Dosage can be repeated in 15 to 20 minutes, if necessary.

How Supplied: Dopram-V (doxapram hydrochloride) is available in 20 ml multiple dose vials of the sterile solution.

Dosage of Dopram-V for Intravenous Injection:
Dogs and Cats

Weight of Animal (lb)	Barbiturate Anesthesia Use 1/8 ml (2.5 mg) to 1/4 ml (5.0 mg) per pound body weight	Gas Anesthesia Use 1/40 ml (0.5 mg) per pound body weight
10	1¼ ml (25 mg) to 2¼ ml (50 mg)	¼ ml (5 mg)
20	2½ ml (50 mg) to 5 ml (100 mg)	½ ml (10 mg)
30	3¾ ml (75 mg) to 7½ ml (150 mg)	¾ ml (15 mg)
50	6¼ ml (125 mg) to 12½ ml (250 mg)	1¼ ml (25 mg)

Dosage should be adjusted for depth of anesthesia, respiratory volume and rate. Dosage can be repeated in 15 to 20 minutes, if necessary.

Horses

Weight of Animal (lb)	Chloral hydrate, chloral hydrate and magnesium sulfate barbiturates, use .0125 ml (0.25 mg) per pound body weight	Inhalation anesthesia halothane, methoxflurane use 0.01 ml (0.02 mg) per pound body weight
100	1¼ ml (25 mg)	1 ml (20 mg)
200	2½ ml (50 mg)	2 ml (40 mg)
500	6¼ ml (125 mg)	5 ml (100 mg)
1000	12½ ml (250 mg)	10 ml (200 mg)

ELANONE®–V
(brand of lenperone hydrochloride)
Tranquilizer for Dogs and Cats
Tablets 10 mg and 25 mg
Injectable 5 mg/mL in 50 mL vials

Description: Lenperone (butyrophenone[1]) posesses potent tranquilizing activity in various mammalian species. It has a depressant effect on the central nervous system[2] and therefore causes sedation, muscular relaxation, and a reduction in spontaneous activity. The need for manual or physical restraint is reduced to a minimum. It has a low order of toxicity and has an added advantage of rapid action and lack of hypnotic effect, as well as antiemetic activity. These properties are similar to those demonstrated by other major tranquilizing drugs[3]. Lenperone is a butyrophenone with the chemical name: 4'fluro-4-[p-flourobenzoyl) piperidino] butyrophenone hydrochloride.

Pharmacology: Controlled laboratory[4] and clinical studies have demonstrated the effectiveness of lenperone as a tranquilizer. It is a centrally acting drug with a low order of toxicity. Intravenous administration to dogs and cats at doses of 0.10 to 0.40 mg per pound resulted in tranquilization varying from slight to pronounced. Intramuscular administration to dogs and cats at doses of 0.20 to 0.40 mg per pound resulted in tranquilization varying from slight to pronounced.
The principal pharmacological activities develop within 3 to 5 minutes following intravenous administration and 10 to 15 minutes following intramuscular administration. The maintenance of tranquilization is dose related with disappearance in 1 to 2 hours at low doses and 5 to 6 hours at high doses.
Following oral administration drug effect is evident within 30 minutes, with peak effect occuring between 1 and 2 hours. The maintenance of tranquilization is dose related with disappearance in 3 to 4 hours at low doses and 5 to 8 hours at high doses.
Lenperone blocks aggressive behavior and amphetamine toxicity in mice. Conditioned avoidance behavior is blocked by lenperone in mice and rats. Lenperone protects against apomorphine-induced emesis in the dog. In comparison to chlorpromazine, lenperone showed greater antiemetic potency and a reduced incidence of sedative-like side effects.
Lenperone resulted in a slowing of cortical waves and a reduced cortical desynchronization produced by stimulation of the ascending activating systems, abolished cortical and hippocampal afterdischarges, and produced biphasic effects on thalamic recruitment.
Arterial blood pressure was usually lowered with lenperone and the nictitating membrane relaxed. In the anesthetized dog lenperone has no effect on blood chemistry, hemogram, or blood clotting time.

Toxicology: Acute and chronic toxicity studies have shown lenperone to have a low order of toxicity. The LD_{50} in cats by either intravenous or intramuscular injections was greater than 16 mg/kg. In dogs the LD_{50} by intravenous, intramuscular, and oral administration was greater than 24, 32, and 128 mg/kg, respectively.
Chronic toxicity studies in dogs, cats, and rats indicate no adverse effects on physical condition, pharmacological signs, electrocardiogram, heart rate, blood pressure, hemogram or blood chemistry.
A teratological study in rats showed lenperone to have no teratological effect.

Indications: Elanone®-V injectable is indicated for use in dogs and cats. Elanone-V Tablets are restricted to use in dogs. Elanone-V can be used in dogs and cats as an aid in controlling intractable animals during examination, treatment, grooming, radiology, dental procedures, minor surgery procedures; to alleviate self-mutilation due to itching as a result of skin irratation; as an antiemetic to control vomiting associated with motion sickness; pre- and postoperative medications; and in other conditions where a tranquilizer is indicated.

Continued on next page

R

Robins—Cont.

Precautions: There are no known contraindications to the use of lenperone in dogs and cats. Generally, this class of drug should not be given if some central nervous system depression or hypotension is unwanted. Following a full therapeutic dose of lenperone a full anesthetic dose may not be required. Although rat studies have indicated no adverse effects on the pregnant female, fetus, or neonate, Elanone-V should not be used during pregnancy unless in the judgment of the veterinarian the potential benefits outweigh the possible hazards.

Dosage and Administration: ***Dogs and Cats***

Parenteral: Elanone-V Injectable may be given intravenously or intramuscularly. The dosage should be individualized and will depend on the clinical procedure and degree of tranquilization required. Drug effects develop within 3–5 minutes following intravenous administration and 10–15 minutes following intramuscular administration. The maintenance of tranquilization disappears in 1–2 hours at low doses and 5–6 hours at high doses.

The recommended intravenous dose is 0.10 to 0 .40 mg/lb and the intramuscular dose is 0.20 to 0.80 mg/lb. Do not exceed 4 mL per injection site when administering intramuscularly.

Oral - Dogs Only: The dosage should be individualized and will depend on clinical procedure and degree of tranquilization desired. Drug effect will be evident within 30 minutes with peak effect occurring between 1 and 2 hours. The maintenance of tranquilization is dose related with disappearance in 3–4 hours at low doses and 5–8 hours at high doses. The dose may be repeated at 5–8 hour intervals. The recommended oral dose is 0.25 to 1.0 mg/lb.

Caution: Federal law restricts this drug to use by or on the order of a licensed veterinarian.

How Supplied: Elanone-V Injectable (lenperone hydrocloride) is supplied in 50 ml vials (5 mg/ml) (00031-4905-90).

Elanone-V (lenperone hydrochloride) 10 mg tablets in bottles of 100 (0031-4911-63) and 500 (0031-4911-70), and 25 mg tablets in bottles of 100 (0031-4921-63) and 500 (0031-4921-70).

References:

1. Duncan, R.L., Jr., *et al.*:Aroylpiperidines and Pyrrolidines. A new Class of Potent Central Nervous System Depressants. J. Med. Chem 13:1, 1970.
2. Johnson, D. N.; Funderburk, W. H.; Ward, J.W.: Neuropharmacologic Analysis of AHR-2277, A New Psychotherapeutic Agent. Arch. Int. Pharmacodyn. 194:197, 1971.
3. Monograph on AHR-2277, Pharmacology and Acute Toxicity, A. H. Robins Co., Inc. Spetember 4, 1970
4. Cloyd, Grover D.; Gilbert Donald L.: Dose Calibration Studies of lenperone, A New Tranquilizer for Dogs, Cats, and Swine. Veterinary Medicine/ Small Animal Clinician 68(4):344-8., 1973.

GUAILAXIN®
brand of
Guaifenesin Sterile Powder
FOR USE IN HORSES

Description: Guailaxin® (guaifenesin) is 3-(0-methoxyphenoxy)-1,2-propanediol, an intravenous muscle relaxant for horses.

Action and Uses: Guaifenesin (formerly termed glyceryl guaiacolate) is an intravenous, central-acting skeletal muscle relaxant of the myanesin group that selectively depresses or blocks nerve impulse transmission at the internuncial neuron level of the spinal cord, brainstem, and subcortical areas of the brain.[1]

In therapeutic amounts guaifenesin produces relaxation of skeletal muscles but the diaphragm continues to function unaffected so that no respiratory paralysis occurs and respiratory activity usually remains normal. Relaxation of the pharyngeal and laryngeal muscles is sufficient to faciliate intubation.[2] These muscle relaxing properties make it an excellent drug for use in induction of general anesthesia with both injectable and inhalant anesthetics.

In addition to its muscle relaxant properties, guaifenesin appears to produce some analgesia and sedation due to its action on the brainstem and subcortical areas of the brain.[3]

Inductions are usually smooth and quiet with duration of action lasting from 10-20 minutes.[2,3] In a study in ponies a significant sex difference in the duration of action was observed with guaifenesin use, the stallions requiring a longer period to recover.[7] Changes in ventilation are small with the usual effect being an increase in respiratory rate associated with a decrease in tidal volume.[4] At increased doses (160 mg/kg) guaifenesin produced only minor changes in heart and respiratory rates and a slight fall in mean arterial blood pressure and in arterial blood PO_2 values.[4] Administration of guaifenesin at 134 mg/kg caused insignificant changes in heart rate, respiratory rate, right atrial pressure, pulmonary arterial pressure, and cardiac output.[5] At recommended doses liver and kidney function are unimpaired while gastrointestinal activity is slightly increased.[2] The activity of guaifenesin can be shortened by conventional central analeptic agents.[6]

The liver is the main site of degradation of guaifenesin, where it undergoes dealkylation to form catechol that is then conjugated to more polar substances.[7] Following degradation and conjugation in the liver the metabolites are excreted largely in the urine.[6,8] The drug has been administered to pregnant mares without ill effects.[3]

In a toxicity study using Guailaxin (guaifenesin) the margin of safety was determined to be at least 2 times the recommended dose. Clinical signs of toxiciy observed included extensor rigidity in 4 horses, apnea in 1 horse, and nystagmus in 1 horse all of which occurred at 100 mg per pound of body weight or 2 times the recommended dose of Guailaxin (guaifenesin).

Indications: Guailaxin (guaifenesin) is indicated for intravenous administration for muscle relaxation in horses.

Contraindications: Administration of physostigmine is contraindicated in horses receiving Guailaxin (guaifenesin).

Warning: Not to be used in horses intended for food.

Precautions: Perivascular leakage should be avoided as this may result in irritation to surrounding tissues. Hemolysis may be induced when guaifenesin is used in concentrations in excess of 5%. This effect is related to concentration of guaifenesin rather than to total dosage administered.[1] As is true with use of any drugs incorporated in anesthetic regimens, care should be taken when anesthetizing anemic or hypovolemic animals with cardiac or respiratory problems. Oxygen should be available when guaifenesin is used in conjunction with barbiturates and/or tranquilizers.

Caution: Guailaxin (guaifenesin) is supplied as a sterile powder but contains no bacteriostatic agent and therefore Guailaxin solutions should be prepared aseptically. Sterilization by heating should not be employed. Guailaxin solutions should be used within 24 hours following preparation. If a solution of Guailaxin precipitates slightly within the 24-hour period, it should be warmed (not to exceed 100°F) until in solution once again.

Federal law restricts this drug to use by or on the order of a licensed veterinarian.

Preparation of Guailaxin solutions: The sterile powder contained in the 4-ounce container may be transferred to an empty, sterile 1-liter administration bottle using a pre-sterilized funnel prior to preparing, as described below.

Guailaxin should be prepared as a 5% solution by dissolving 50 g of the sterile powder in warm (not to exceed 100°F) USP sterile water for injection to make 1 liter of solution. This provides 50 mg guaifenesin per 1 ml of solution.

If thiamylal sodium is to be added, 2 g of the barbiturate should be added to the 50 g of Guailaxin sterile powder prior to dissolving in USP sterile water for injection to make 1 liter of solution. This provides 2 mg thiamylal sodium and 50 mg guaifenesin per 1 ml of solution.

Dosage and Administration: Guailaxin (guaifenesin) should be administered only by the intravenous route. If preanesthetic agents are to be used for chemical restraint, the horse should remain quiet for the recommended period of time. The 5% Guailaxin solution should be administered by rapid intravenous infusion through a 12-gauge needle at a dose of 1 ml per pound of body weight. When administered in this way the dose of guaifenesin is 50 mg per pound of body weight. The horse will fall gently, usually after receiving 1/3 to 1/2 the dose, however the entire dose should be given unless adverse respiratory or cardiovascular effects are observed. The duration of action of a single dose is usually from 10-20 minutes.

Recovery from Guailaxin (guaifenesin) effects is normally smooth with very little incoordination or struggling observed. The horse will usually rest quietly until adequate muscle tonus returns and it can assume a standing position.[3] After standing, some weakness occurs initially, but maximum stability is regained in a short period of time with slow exercise.[3,9]

When thiamylal sodium is added to the guaifenesin as described, the resulting solution should also be administered by rapid intravenous infusion through a 12-gauge needle at a dose of 1 ml per pound of body weight. This provides a dose of 50 mg per pound of guaifenesin and 2 mg per pound of thiamylal sodium. Anesthesia obtained with this procedure is adequate for short surgical operations and the complete muscle relaxation which results is an aid in performing other procedures. If it becomes necessary to prolong anesthesia additional doses of the solution should be given. Use of additional doses requires the person administering the solution to be familiar with the planes of anesthesia as they relate to ocular reflexes, analgesia, and respiratory and cardiac rates.[3] A longer period of surgical anesthesia generally requires a longer period for recovery.

How Supplied: Guailaxin (guaifenesin) Sterile Powder is supplied 50 g per container in 4-oz containers (0031-5320-12) and 32-oz containers (0031-5320-77).

References

1 Booth, NH; McDonald, LE, eds. 1982. *Veterinary Pharmacology and Therapeutics.* 5th ed. Iowa State University Press.

2 Roberts, D. 1968. The role of glyceryl guaiacolate in a balanced equine anesthetic. VM/SAC *63* (2):157-62.

3 Jackson, LL; Lundvall, RL. 1970. Observations on the use of glyceryl guaiacolate in the horse. JAVMA *157* (8):1093-5.

4 Tavernor, WD. 1970. The influence of guaiacol glycerol ether on cardiovascular and respiratory function in the horse. RES. VET. SCI. *11* :91-3.

5 Hubbell, JA; Muir, WW *et al.* 1980. Guaifenesin: cardiopulmonary effects and plasma concentrations in horses. AM. J. VET. RES. *41* (11):1751-5.

6 Funk, KA. 1970. Glyceryl guaiacolate: a centrally acting muscle relaxant. EQ. VET. J. *2* (4):173-7.

7 Davis, LE; Wolff, WA. 1970. Pharmacokinetics and metabolism of glyceryl guaiacolate in ponies. AM. J. VET. RES. *31* :469-73.

8 Grandy, JL; McDonnell, WN. 1980. Evaluation of concentrated solutions of guaiafenesin for equine anesthesia. JAVMA *176* (4):619-22.

9 Gertsen, KE; Tillotson, PJ. 1968. Clinical use of glyceryl guaiacolate in the horse. VM/SAC *63* (11):1062-6.

PRECON–PH®
PASTEURELLA HAEMOLYTICA VACCINE
Live Culture, Lyophilized

Description: PRECON-PH® is a lyophilized live *Pasteurella haemolytica* vaccine for the immunization of healthy cattle as an aid in the prevention of infection due to *Pasteurella haemolytica.*

Application of Vaccine: This vaccine is recommended for the immunization of healthy cattle a minimum of 7 to 10 days prior to weaning, shipping, or exposure to stress or infectious conditions.

Directions for Use:

1. Rehydrate the lyophilized vaccine with sterile diluent. Shake well before using.
2. Use immediately.
3. Vaccinate only healthy cattle a minimum of 7 to 10 days prior to weaning, shipping, or exposure to stress or infectious conditions.
4. DOSAGE: INJECT 0.5 ml INTRADERMALLY. The use of a short (3/16–1/4") 22–24 gauge needle is recommended for the intradermal injection. Vaccination site should be palpated to ascertain the injection has been made intradermally.

Precautions:

1. Use entire contents of vial immediately after mixing.
2. Store the vaccine at not over 7°C (45°F).
3. Do not spill or spatter the vaccine. Burn used vials and all unused contents.
4. Do not vaccinate within 21 days of slaughter.
5. Do not use chemicals to sterilize syringes and needles.
6. If animal exhibits an anaphylactoid reaction, administer epinephrine or equivalent and supportive treatment.
7. Since PRECON-PH® is a live vaccine, the concurrent use of parenteral antibiotics may interfere with the production of immunity.
8. A swelling up to 5 cm in diameter may occur at the injection site in from 5–50% of vaccinated animals. These swellings should not be treated and will usually resolve within a 2- to 3-week period.

Package Sizes: Live *Pasteurella haemolytica* vaccine is available in boxes of one 5 dose vial and boxes of one 20 dose vial with corresponding diluent.

Warranty: This vaccine is thoroughly tested before sale and meets the requirements of the U. S. Department of Agriculture.

ROBAMOX®–V
brand of amoxicillin
Veterinary Oral Suspension

Description: Robamox®-V (amoxicillin) is a broad spectrum, semisynthetic antibiotic which provides bactericidal activity against a wide range of common gram-positive and gram-negative pathogens. Amoxicillin chemically is D-(-)a-amino-p-hydroxybenzyl penicillin trihydrate.

Action: Amoxicillin has bactericidal activity against susceptible organisms similar to that of ampicillin. It acts by inhibiting the biosynthesis of bacterial cell wall mucopeptide. Most strains of the following gram-positive and gram-negative bacteria have demonstrated susceptibility to amoxicillin, both *in vitro* and *in vivo:* non-pencillinase-producing staphylococci, alpha- and beta-hemolytic streptococci, *Streptococcus faecalis, Escherichi coli,* and *Proteus mirabilis.* Amoxicillin does not resist destruction by penicillinase; therefore, it is not effective against penicillinase-producing bacteria, particularly resistant staphylococci. Most strains of Enterobacter and Klebsiella and all strains of Pseudomonas are resistant.

Amoxicillin may be given without regard to meals because it is stable in gastric acid. It is rapidly absorbed following oral administration and diffuses readily into most body fluids and tissues. It diffuses poorly into the brain and spinal fluid except when the meninges are inflamed. Most of amoxicillin is excreted in the urine unchanged.

R

Indications: Robamox-V (amoxicillin) oral suspension is indicated in the treatment of the following infections in dogs when caused by susceptible strains of organisms:

BACTERIAL DERMATITIS due to *Staphylococcus aureus, Streptococcus spp., Staphylococcus spp.,* and *E. coli*

SOFT TISSUE INFECTIONS (abscesses, wounds, lacerations) due to *Staphylococcus aureus, Streptococcus spp., E. coli, Proteus mirabilis,* and *Staphylococcus spp.*

As is true with all antibiotic therapy, appropriate *in vitro* cultures and sensitivities should be conducted prior to treatment.

Contraindications: Use of amoxicillin is contraindicted in animals with a history of an allergic reaction to penicillin.

Adverse Reactions: Amoxicillin is a semisynthetic penicillin and, therefore, has the potential for producing allergic reactions. Epinephrine and/or steroids should be administered if an allergic reaction occurs.

Warnings: For use in dogs only.

Precautions: Until adequate reproductive studies are accomplished, Robamox-V (amoxicillin) oral suspension should not be used in pregnant or breeding animals.

Caution: Federal law restricts this drug to use by or on the order of a licensed veterinarian.

Dosage and Administration: The recommended dosage is 5 mg per pound of body weight administered twice daily for 5 to 7 days or 48 hours after all symptoms have subsided. If no improvement is noted in 5 days, the diagnosis should be reconsidered and therapy changed.

Directions for Mixing Oral Suspension: Add sufficient water to the bottle as indicated in the table below and shake vigorously. Each ml of suspension will contain 50 mg of amoxicillin as the trihydrate.

Continued on next page

Robins—Cont.

Bottle Size	Amount of Water to Add for Reconstitution
15 ml	11 ml
30 ml	21 ml

NOTE: When stored at room temperature or in refrigerator, discard unused portion of reconstituted suspension after 14 days.

Supply: Robamox-V (amoxicillin) oral suspension is supplied in bottles containing 0.75 g or 1.5 g of amoxicillin activity. After reconstitution with the required amount of water, each ml will contain 50 mg of amoxicillin as the trihydrate.

15 ml Bottles	0.75 g	NDC 0031-7180-78
30 ml Bottles	1.5 g	NDC 0031-7180-85

ROBAMOX®–V
(brand of amoxicillin)
Veterinary Tablets

R

Description: Robamox®-V (amoxicillin) is a broad spectrum, semisynthetic antibiotic which provides bactericidal activity against a wide range of common gram-positive and gram -negative pathogens. Amoxicillin chemically is D-(-)a-amino-p-hydroxybenzyl penicillin trihydrate.

Action: Amoxicillin has bactericidal activity against susceptible organisms similar to that of ampicillin. It acts by inhibiting the biosynthesis of bacterial cell wall mucopeptide. Most strains of the following gram-positive and gram-negative bacteria have demonstrated susceptibility to amoxicillin, both *in vitro* and *in vivo:* non-penicillinase-producing staphylococci, alpha- and beta-hemolytic streptococci, *Streptococcus faecalis, Escherichia coli,* and *Proteus mirabilis.* Amoxicillin does not resist destruction by penicillinase; therefore, it is not effective against penicillinase-producing bacteria, particularly resistant staphylococci. Most strains of Enterobacter and Klebsiella and all strains of Pseudomonas are resistant.

Amoxicillin may be given without regard to meals because it is stable in gastric acid. It is rapidly absorbed following oral administration and diffuses readily into most body fluids and tissues. It diffuses poorly into the brain and spinal fluid except when the meninges are inflamed. Most of amoxicillin is excreted in the urine unchanged.

Indications: Robamox-V (amoxicillin) tablets are indicated in the treatment of the following infections in dogs when caused by susceptible strains of organisms:

BACTERIAL DERMATITIS due to *Staphococcus aureus, Streptococcus spp., Staphylococcus spp.,* and *E. coli.*

SOFT TISSUE INFECTIONS (abscesses, wounds, lacerations) due to *Staphylococcus aureus, Streptococcus spp., E. coli, Proteus mirabilis,* and *Staphylococcus spp.*

As is true with all antibiotic therapy, appropriate in vitro cultures and sensitivities should be conducted prior to treatment.

Contraindications: Use of amoxicillin is contraindicated in animals with a history of an allergic reaction to pencillin.

Adverse Reactions: Amoxicillin is a semisynthetic pencillin and, therefore, has the potential for producing allergic reactions. Epinephrine and/or steroids should be administered if an allergic reaction occurs.

Dosage and Administration: The recommended dosage is 5 mg per pound of body weight administered twice daily for 5 to 7 days or 48 hours after all symptoms have subsided. If no improvement is noted in 5 days, the diagnosis should be reconsidered and therapy changed.

Warnings: For use in dogs only.

Precautions: Until adequate reproductive studies are accomplished, Robamox-V (amoxicillin) tablets should not be used in pregnant or breeding animals.

Caution: Federal law restricts this drug to use by or on the order of a licensed veterinarian.

Supply: Robamox-V (amoxicillin) tablets are supplied in 50 mg, 100 mg, and 200 mg concentrations in bottles of 500 and 1,000 tablets; and 400 mg concentration in bottles of 250 and 500 tablets. [See table below].

ROBAMOX-V TABLETS

Tablet Concentration	NDC Numbers Bottles of 500	Bottles of 1000
50 mg	0031-7131-70	0031-7131-74
100 mg	0031-7141-70	0031-7141-74
200 mg	0031-7151-70	0031-7151-74
Tablet Concentration	**Bottles of 250**	**Bottles of 500**
400 mg	0031-7171-67	0031-7171-70

ROBAXIN®-V INJECTABLE
(methocarbamol)
Injectable 100 mg/ml in 20 ml. vial and 100 ml. vial

ROBAXIN®-V TABLETS
(methocarbamol)
Tablets 500 mg.
Skeletal Muscle Relaxant
For Dogs, Cats, and Horses

Description: Robaxin-V® (methocarbamol, Robins) is a potent skeletal muscle relaxant which has an unusually selective action on the central nervous system, specifically on the internuncial neurons of the spinal cord. This specific action results in a diminution of skeletal muscle hyperactivity without concomitant alteration in normal muscle tone. It is long-acting and essentially nontoxic, and has proved effective in a wide range of disorders involving acute muscle spasm.

Pharmacology: Animal studies have shown that methocarbamol acts primarily on the internuncial neurons of the spinal cord. It exerts a prolonged blocking effect on polysynaptic reflex pathways at dosages which do not significantly alter transmission through monosynaptic reflex arcs and interrupts abnormal impulses from areas of disturbed muscle. It has no direct action on the contractile mechanism of striated muscle, the motor endplate, or the nerve fiber.

Methocarbamol affords a marked protective action against the effects of strychnine in rats, cats, and dogs. It prevents both convulsions and death when administered prior to strychnine in the rodent. In dogs and cats, it promptly controls the classical and severe symptoms of strychnine poisoning. Methocarbamol is more potent than mephenesin or mephenesin carbamate in blocking convulsions induced with pentylenetetrazol or electroshock.

Signs of central nervous system depression are produced by large doses of methocarbamol. Included are loss of righting reflex, prostration and ataxia. Also indicative of CNS depression is the finding that methocarbamol potentiates barbiturate hypnosis in mice.

The results of acute and subchronic studies emphasize that methocarbamol is relatively non-toxic. It does not significantly alter hematologic or biochemical values. Similarly, gross and microscopic tissue examinations revealed no significant findings attributable to it.

Indications: *Dogs and Cats. Oral and Intravenous.* Robaxin-V is indicated as an adjunct to therapy of acute inflammatory and traumatic conditions of the skeletal muscle and to reduce muscular spasms. The efficacy of both tablets and injectable in the treatment of acute skeletal muscle hyperactivity secondary to the following conditions has been demonstrated:

1. Intervertebral disc syndrome, compressive myelitis, spinal cord injury where cord remains intact.
2. Traumatism causing muscular and ligamentous sprains and strains.
3. Myositis, fibrositis, bursitis, synovitis.
4. Muscular spasm prior to or following surgical procedures.
5. Miscellaneous conditions: Tablets—To maintain therapeutic benefits of the injectable form in strychnine poisoning and tetanus.

Horses. Intravenous. As an adjunct to therapy of acute inflammatory and traumatic conditions of the skeletal muscle to reduce muscular spasms, and effect striated muscle relaxation. The efficacy in the treatment of acute skeletal muscle hyperactivity secondary to the following conditions has been demonstrated:

1. Trauma, muscular and ligamentous sprains and strains.
2. Myositis, fibrositis, bursitis and synovitis.
3. Tying up syndrome.
4. Muscular spasm prior to, or following, surgical procedures.
5. Maintenance of muscle relaxation in tetanus.

Robaxin-V can be used concurrently with adrenal corticosteroids and other

medications usually employed in these cases without untoward effects.
Contraindications: Although rat studies have indicated no adverse effects on the pregnant female, fetus or neonate, Robaxin-V should not be used during pregnancy unless in the judgment of the veterinarian the potential benefits outweigh the possible hazards.
Robaxin-V Injectable (methocarbamol) should not be administered to patients with known or suspected renal pathology. This caution is necessary because of the presence of polyethylene glycol 300 in the vehicle. A much larger amount of polyethylene glycol 300 than is present in recommended doses of Robaxin-V Injectable (methocarbamol) is known to have increased pre-existing acidosis and urea retention in humans with renal impairment. Although the amount present in this preparation is well within the limits of safety, caution dictates this contraindication.
Methocarbamol is contraindicated in patients hypersensitive to the ingredients.
Warning: Not to be used in horses intended for food.
Precautions: As with any drug administered intravenously, careful attention must be given to the dose and the rate of injection.
In dogs and cats, the rate should not exceed 2 ml per minute. Since Robaxin-V Injectable (methocarbamol) is hypertonic, vascular extravasation must be avoided. A recumbent position will reduce the likelihood of side reactions.
In the horse, the most effective response is achieved by injecting rapidly through a 15- or 17-gauge needle.
Blood aspirated into the syringe does not mix with the hypertonic solution. This phenomenon occurs with many other intravenous preparations. The blood may be safely injected with the methocarbamol or the injection may be stopped when the plunger reaches the blood.
Adverse Reactions: Side effects following administration of injectable methocarbamol are seldom encountered. Excessive salivation, emesis, muscular weakness and ataxia have been noted in both dogs and cats. These effects were prompt in appearance and were generally of short duration. Their incidence was closely related to administration of large doses and/or to a rapid rate of injection. They may serve, therefore, as indicators of overdosage, particularly when methocarbamol is administered at a slow rate.
Dosage and Administration: *Injectable.* Robaxin-V Injectable (methocarbamol) is supplied in 20 ml vials and in 100 ml vials. Each ml contains 100 mg of drug in sterile 50 percent aqueous solution of polyethylene glycol 300 with 0.1 percent sodium bisulfite as a preservative. This preparation is for intravenous administration and may be given undiluted directly into a vein. Dosage and frequency of injection should be based on the severity of symptoms and on the therapeutic response noted.
Robaxin-V is compatible with general anesthetics, causing no depression of vital body functions or prolongation of anesthesia. However, specific studies using the injectable form have shown that additional muscle relaxation does occur and the anesthetic dosage may be reduced.
Dogs and Cats: For relief of moderate conditions, a dose of 1/5 ml per pound (20 mg per pound) body weight may be adequate.
An initial dose of 1/4 to 1 ml per pound body weight is suggested for controlling the severe effects of strychnine and tetanus. Additional amounts may be neded for relieving residual effects and for preventing the recurrence of symptoms. A daily total cumulative dose of 150 mg per pound body weight should not be exceeded. Administer rapidly half the estimated dose, pause until the animal starts to relax then continue administration to effect. When satisfactory muscular relaxation is achieved, it can usually be maintained with tablets.
Horses. Give drug to effect; moderate conditions, a dose of 2 to 10mg/lb; for severe conditions (tetanus) a dose of 10 to 25 mg/lb.
Tablets. Dogs and Cats. Dosage and frequency of administration should be based on the severity of symptoms and on the therapeutic response noted. The usual canine and feline dose of Robaxin-V is 60 mg per pound body weight in divided doses followed by 30 or 60 mg per pound body weight each following day. The total dose should be divided into two (2) or three (3) equal doses [given at twelve (12) or eight (8) hour intervals respectively].
Due to the nature of the conditions for which Robaxin-V therapy is recommended, it is important that an accurate diagnosis is made. If no response is evident within five (5) days of the initiation of treatment, the diagnosis should be redetermined.
Recommended Dosage Schedule for Tablets: Load dose—1st day, 60 mg/lb. 2nd day and Maintenance dose—60 mg or 30 mg/lb.
[See table above].

ROBAXIN-V TABLETS

Wt. of Dog	1st Day Load Dose	2nd Day and Maintenance Dose
12½ lbs.	½ tablet t.i.d.	¼ to ½ tablet t.i.d.
25 lbs.	1 tablet t.i.d.	½ to 1 tablet t.i.d.
50 lbs.	2 tablets t.i.d.	1 to 2 tablets t.i.d.

Toxicity studies have shown Robaxin-V to be well tolerated at doses of 400 mg/kg divided in two daily doses given 5 days a week for 26 weeks. The usual treatment during clinical trials did not exceed 14 to 21 days.
How Supplied: Robaxin-V (methocarbamol) 500 mg. white, scored tablets in bottles of 100 (0031-7417-63) and 500 (0031-7417-70).
Robaxin-V Injectable (methocarbamol) is supplied in 20 ml vials (0031-7411-83) and 100 ml. vials (0031-7411-09) in cartons of 12.

ROBINUL®-V INJECTABLE
brand of
Glycopyrrolate
Preanesthetic Use for Dogs and Cats

Composition: Each 1 ml contains:
Glycopyrrolate....0.2 mg
Water for Injection, USP....q.s.
Benzyl Alcohol (Preservative)....0.9%
pH adjusted, when necessary with hydrochloric acid and and/or sodium hydroxide.
For intramuscular, intravenous, or subcutaneous use in dogs and intramuscular use in cats.
Robinul®-V (glycopyrrolate) Injectable is a synthetic anticholinergic agent.
Pharmacology: Glycopyrrolate, like other anticholinergic agents, inhibits the action of acetylcholine on structures innervated by postganglionic cholinergic nerves and on smooth muscles that respond to acetylcholine that lack cholinergic innervation. It the dog, it diminishes the volume and free acidity of gastric secretions and reduces intestinal motility. It diminishes and controls excessive pharyngeal, tracheal, and bronchial secretions and has a longer lasting effect than atropine. In the cat, it controls excessive salivation and pharyngeal secretions.
In anesthetized dogs intravenous doses of 0.0023 to 0.0045 mg/lb markedly reduced intestinal tone and moderately inhibited amplitude of intestinal contraction but had essentially no effect on respirations, periodic arterial blood pressure, or cardiac rate. These doses of glycopyrrolate reduced bradycardia, hypertension and the intestinal hyperactivity resulting from peripheral vagal stimulation.
In dog studies, glycopyrrolate antagonized muscarinic symptoms (e.g., bronchorrhea, bronchospasm, bradycardia, and intestinal hypermotility) induced by cholinergic drugs such as the anticholinesterases, affording the same protection as atropine against bradycardia.
The intestinal hyperactivity and copious salivation produced by a subcutaneous dose of methacholine chloride, 0.5 mg/kg, were suppressed by a glycopyrrolate in intravenous doses as low as 0.0045 mg/lb. in the dog.
In a study[1] glycopyrrolate at 0.004 and 0.008 mg/lb had a longer lasting effect and more smooth-muscle relaxation, with little adverse cardiovasculur effect when compared to atropine at 0.02 mg/lb. Glycopyrrolate was effective in preventing aspiration of gastric secretions and the resulting pulmonary complications, not only by producing a higher pH of gastric secretions but in the reduction of intestinal smooth-muscle activity and thus the likelihood of regurgitation.

Continued on next page

Robins—Cont.

The polar ammonium moiety of glycopyrrolate limits its passage across the lipid membranes such as the blood-brain barrier in contrast to the belladonna alkaloids which are non-polar tertiary amines.

In a cat study, ^{14}C-labeled glycopyrrolate was administered intramuscularly at doses ranging from 0.018 to 0.024 mg/kg (0.008 to 0.011 mg/lb). Peak blood levels of radioactivity were detected at 15 minutes following injections. Blood levels of radioactivity declined slowly during a 48-hour period with the drug being excreted approximately equally between urinary and fecal excretion routes.

In dog studies, peak effect occurred approximately 30 to 45 minutes after subcutaneous or intramuscular administration. The vagal-blocking effect persisted for two to three hours and the antisialagogue effect persisted for up to seven hours, periods longer than for atropine. With intravenous injection the onset of action was generally evident within one minute.

Toxicology: Acute and chronic toxicity studies have shown glycopyrrolate to have a low order of toxicity.

In the dog, the LD_{50} for intravenous administration is 25.0 mg/kg and daily intravenous doses of either 0.4 or 2.0 mg/kg five days per week for four consecutive weeks revealed no signs of toxicity. The oral feeding of high levels (27 mg/kg) of glycopyrrolate for seven weeks produced no signs of toxicity in the dog.

In the cat, the LD_{50} for intramuscular administration is 283 mg/kg. In a 10-week study, cats received daily intramuscular doses of 0.01, 0.03, and 0.05 mg/kg. No changes considered to be related to glycopyrrolate were seen in food consumption, hematology, biochemical, urinalysis, or gross pathology. Histopathology showed slight to moderate proliferation of intrahepatic bile ducts at the 0.05 mg/kg/day dose level.

Indications: Robinul-V (glycopyrrolate) Injectable is indicated as a preanesthetic anticholinergic agent in dogs and cats.

In dogs it reduces salivary, tracheobronchial and pharyngeal secretions, reduces the volume and free acidity of gastric secretion, and blocks cardiac vagal inhibitory reflexes during induction of anesthesia and intubation.

In cats, it reduces salivary and pharyngeal secretions.

Precautions: There are no absolute contraindications to the use of Robinul-V Injectable in conjunction with anesthesia except known hypersensitivity to glycopyrrolate. Reproduction studies in rats and rabbits revealed no teratogenic effects from glycopyrrolate; however, the anticholinergic action of this agent resulted in diminished rates of conception and of survival at weaning in rats in a dose-related manner. Reproduction studies have not been conducted on glycopyrrolate in dogs and cats. Therefore, Robinul-V should not be administered to pregnant bitches or queens. The excretion of Robinul-V may be prolonged in animals with impaired renal function or impaired gastrointestinal function.

Side Effects: Mild mydriasis, xerostomia, and tachycardia may be seen with Robinul-V. These are extensions of the fundamental pharmacological action of anticholinergics.

Dosage and Administration: ***Dogs*** —Robinul-V (glycopyrrolate) Injectable may be administered intravenously, intramuscularly or subcutaneously at the rate of 5 micrograms/lb body weight (0.25 ml per 10 pounds body weight).

Cats —Robinul-V (glycopyrrolate) Injectable may be administered intramuscularly at the rate of 5 micrograms/lb body weight (0.25 mL per 10 lb body weight). For maximum anticholinergic effect, administer Robinul-V 15 minutes prior to anesthetic administration in cats.

Federal law restricts this drug to use by or on the order of a licensed veterinarian.

How Supplied: Robinul-V (glycopyrrolate) injectable is supplied in 20-mL vials (0.2 mg/mL) (0031-7895-83).

References

1. Short, Charles E; Paddleford, Robert R.; Cloyd, Grover D. Glycopyrrolate for prevention of pulmonary complications during anesthesia. Modern Veterinary Practice, May, 1974.

VIOKASE®—V

Tablet 425 mg
Powder
Whole pancreas
Not an extract
Not enteric coated

Each 425 mg tablet contains:

Lipase	6,500 USP Units
Protease	32,000 USP Units
Amylase	48,000 USP Units

Each 2.8 grams (1 teaspoonful) of powder contains:

Lipase	56,988 USP Units
Protease	284,938 USP Units
Amylase	427,407 USP Units

Description: Viokase-V is activated whole raw pancreas; a pancreatic enzyme concentrate of porcine origin containing standardized amylase, protease and lipase activities plus esterases, peptidases, nucleases and elastase.

Background Information: A review of the literature over the past 20 years, together with clinical experience, prompts the conclusion that pancreatitis is an important disease in the dog. Evidence of the disease was observed in approximately 3% of a series of dogs necropsied at the Angell Memorial Animal Hospital. Others have classified disease of the pancreas into 4 distinctive categories: acute necrotic pancreatitis; subacute or chronic pancreatitis; pancreatic fibrosis; and collapse or atrophy of the acinar pancreatic tissue. Only acute and chronic pancreatitis is readily recognized clinically.

Dogs that acquire acute pancreatitis usually recover, but are subject to exacerbations of the chronic inflammatory process that may persist. Complete healing of the acute lesion may not occur, and progressive destruction of the gland may take place over a period of months, even in the absence of clinical signs.

Chronic pancreatitis is characterized by acute exacerbations of pancreatic inflammation that occur after the remission of acute pancreatitis. Signs of the disease are similar to those of acute pancreatitis but are usually less severe.

Steatorrhea, diarrhea, weight loss, and increased appetite characterize the digestive impairment caused by failure of pancreatic exocrine secretion. Secretion ceases when the acinar tissue is destroyed in the course of chronic pancreatitis. This sequela does not become evident until virtually total destruction of the acinar pancreas has occurred, because as little as 12 to 20 per cent of the exocrine pancreas can secrete enough pancreatic juice to sustain digestion. Thus, digestive impairment is a relatively late event in the pathogenesis of chronic pancreatitis. Transient episodes of fetid diarrhea may occur at the time of an acute exacerbation, and may be caused by a temporary reduction of pancreatic exocrine secretion. However, food engorgement or the ingestion of fatty food often precipitates an exacerbation of chronic pancreatitis and the character of the food, rather than the absence of pancreatic enzymes, may cause the diarrhea.

The veterinarian should not be too concerned about whether the pancreatic lesion is acute or chronic. His primary concern should be to recognize pancreatic inflammatory disease and begin treatment. The differentiation of acute and chronic pancreatitis is then made on the basis of history, and is of importance in advancing a prognosis.

Vikoase-V will replace pancreatic enzymes secretions after total pancreatectomy.

Indications: As a digestive aid; replacement therapy where digestion of protein, carbohydrate and fat is inadequate due to exocrine pancreatic insufficiency.

Precautions: Discontinue use in animals with symptoms of sensitivity.

Treatment in Acute and Chronic Pancreatitis: The most important aspect of the treatment of *acute* pancreatitis is initiation of vigorous therapy aimed at combating pain and shock, restoring blood volume, blood pressure and renal function, with reducing pancreatic secretions and combating secondary infection of necrotic tissue. Animals surviving an acute attack should be placed on a bland and easily digested diet (such as Prescription Diet®, i/d) and supplemented with Viokase-V.

In *chronic* pancreatitis, replacement therapy must be given for the duration of the animal's life. Three daily feedings of a bland and easily digested diet containing sufficient quantities of good quality proteins and carbohydrates and low levels of fat are recommended (i.e. Prescription Diet®, i/d). Viokase-V is given with each meal at a dosage level sufficient to keep the feces normal.

Dosage and Administration: The Viokase-V tablets are administered before each meal. Viokase-V powder is added to moistened dog food (canned or dry). Thorough mixing is necessary to bring the enzymes into close contact with the food particles. Incubation at room temperature for 15–20 minutes before feeding appears to enhance the digestive process. Frequent feeding, at least 3 times daily, is important.
Usual Dosage: Dogs. Three tablets or 1–1½ teaspoonfuls (2.8 g/teaspoonful) with each meal.
Cats. One tablet or ½–¾ teaspoonful (2.8 g/teaspoonful) with each meal.
Note: No one regimen will be successful for every patient. The above dosage should be adjusted according to the severity of the pancreatic exocrine deficiency and weight of the animal. In cases of chronic insufficiency, the dosage should be increased until desired results are obtained.
How Supplied: Viokase-V Tablets—425 mg each in bottles of 100 (0031-9301-63) and 500 (0031-9301-70).
Viokase-V Powder—Bottles of 4 ounce (0031-9303-12), 8 ounce (0031-9303-25) and 12 ounce (0031-9303-22).

Z-BEC® VETERINARY CHEWABLE TABLETS

Composition:
Each tablet provides:

Zinc (Elemental)	20 mg
Vitamin E	40 I.U.
Vitamin C	150 mg
Vitamin B_1	5 mg
Vitamin B_2	5 mg
Niacin	10 mg
Vitamin B_6	3 mg
Vitamin B_{12}	12 mcg
Pantothenic Acid	10 mg

In a palatable base containing Liver, Brewer's Yeast, Animal Protein, and selected unsaturated Fatty Acids.
Actions and Uses: Z-BEC® Veterinary Chewable Tablets are recommended in conditions where supplemental zinc, B-complex vitamins, vitamin E, and vitamin C are indicated, such as may occur in geriatric dogs or cats with decreased efficiency in nutrient digestive and absorptive processes.
Z-BEC Veterinary Chewable Tablets are also recommended as a dietary supplement for dogs or cats of all sizes and ages to aid in the prevention of deficiencies of zinc, B-complex vitamins, vitamin E and vitamin C.
Suggested Daily Dosage:
Dogs: 1 to 4 tablets
Puppies: ½ to 1 tablet
Cats: ½ to 1 tablet
Tablets may be fed orally or crumbled and mixed with food.
How Supplied: Z-BEC Veterinary Chewable Tablets are available in bottles of 60 (0031-0772-62) and 120 (0031-0772-65).

Roche Animal Health and Nutrition,

Hoffmann-La Roche Inc.
340 KINGSLAND STREET
NUTLEY, NJ 07110
(201) 235-5000

ALBON®
(preparation of sulfadimethoxine) Injection-40%

Composition: Each ml contains 400 mg sulfadimethoxine.
Dogs and Cats—To be used in the treatment of sulfonamide-susceptible bacterial infections in dogs and cats and enteritis associated with coccidiosis in dogs. (See Section I).
Horses —To be used in the treatment of respiratory disease caused by *Streptococcus equi* (strangles) (See Section II).
Cattle —For the treatment of bovine respiratory disease complex (shipping fever complex) and bacterial pneumonia associated with Pasteurella Spp. sensitive to sulfadimethoxine; necrotic pododermatitis (foot rot) and calf diphtheria caused by Fusobacterium necrophorum (Sphaerophorus necrophorus), sensitive to sulfadimethoxine.
Not for human use.
Caution: Federal law restricts this drug to use by or on the order of a licensed veterinarian.
Albon Injection-40% is a low-dosage, rapidly absorbed, long-acting sulfonamide, effective for the treatment of a wide range of bacterial infections commonly encountered in dogs and cats; the treatment of respiratory disease of horses; and the treatment of shipping fever complex, bacterial pneumonia, calf diphtheria, and foot rot in cattle.
Sulfadimethoxine is a white, almost tasteless and odorless compound. Chemically, it is N^1-(2, 6-dimethoxy-4-pyrimidinyl) sulfanilamide.
Section I—Dogs and Cats
Actions: Sulfadimethoxine has been demonstrated clinically or in the laboratory to be effective against a variety of organisms, such as streptococci, klebsiella, proteus, shigella, staphylococci, escherichia, and salmonella.[1,2] These organisms have been demonstrated in respiratory, genitourinary, enteric and soft tissue infections of dogs and cats.
The systemic sulfonamides which include sulfadimethoxine are bacteriostatic agents. Sulfonamides competitively inhibit bacterial synthesis of folic acid (pteroylglutamic acid) from para-aminobenzoic acid. Mammalian cells are capable of utilizing folic acid in the presence of sulfonamides.
The tissue distribution of sulfadimethoxine, as with all sulfonamides, is a function of plasma levels, degree of plasma protein binding, and subsequent passive distribution in the tissues of the lipid soluble un-ionized form. The relative amounts are determined by both its pKa and by the pH of each tissue. Therefore, levels tend to be higher in less acid tissue and body fluids or those diseased tissues having high concentrations of leucocytes.[2]
In the dog sulfadimethoxine is not acetylated as in most other animals, and it is excreted predominantly as the unchanged drug.[3] Sulfadimethoxine has a relatively high solubility at the pH normally occurring in the kidney, precluding the possibility of precipitation and crystalluria. Slow renal excretion results from a high degree of tubular reabsorption,[4] and plasma protein binding is very high, providing a blood reservoir of the drug. Thus, sulfadimethoxine maintains higher blood levels than most other long-acting sulfonamides. Single, comparatively low doses of Albon give rapid and sustained therapeutic blood levels.[1]
To assure successful aulfonamide therapy, (1) the drug must be given early in the course of the disease, and it must produce a high sulfonamide level in the body rapidly after administration; (2) therapeutically effective sulfonamide levels must be maintained in the body throughout the treatment period; (3) treatment should continue for a short period of time after the clinical signs have disappeared; and (4) the causative organisms must be sensitive to this class of drugs.
Toxicity and Safety: Data regarding acute (LD_{50}'s) and chronic toxicities of sulfadimethoxine indicate the drug is very safe. The LD_{50} in mice is greater than 2 g/kg body weight when administered intraperitoneally and greater than 16 g/kg when administered per os. In dogs receiving massive single oral doses of 3.2 g/kg body weight, diarrhea was the only adverse effect observed. Dogs given 160 mg/kg body weight per os daily for 13 weeks showed no signs of toxicity.
Indications: Albon Injection-40% is indicated for the treatment of a wide range of respiratory, genitourinary tract, enteric and soft tissue infections. For example:

tonsillitis	pustular dermatitis
pharyngitis	anal gland infections
bronchitis	abscesses
pneumonia	wound infections
cystitis	canine salmonellosis
metritis	bacterial enteritis
pyometra	associated with coccidiosis in dogs

when caused by streptococci, staphylococci, escherichia, salmonella, klebsiella, proteus or shigella organisms sensitive to sulfadimethoxine.
Limitations: Sulfadimethoxine is not effective in viral or rickettsial infections, and as with any antibacterial agent, occasional failure in the therapy may occur due to resistant microorganisms. The usual precautions in sulfonamide therapy should be observed.
Precautions: During treatment period, make certain that animals maintain adequate water intake.
If animals show no improvement within 2 or 3 days, re-evaluate your diagnosis.
Intramuscular administration is not recommended. Some animals treated by the intramuscular route exhibit signs of pain during and for a few minutes following such injections, and in dogs blood lev-

Continued on next page

Roche—Cont.

els are lower than those obtained by intravenous or subcutaneous treatments.

Dosage and Administration: Albon Injection-40% is recommended for administration by the intravenous or subcutaneous route. Usually the injectable formulation may be used to obtain effective blood levels almost immediately or to facilitate treatment of the fractious animal, and the oral formulations utilized for maintenance therapy. However, the injectable formulation may be used for the entire course of Albon therapy when indicated.

Dogs and cats should receive 1 ml of Albon Injection-40% per 16 pounds of body weight (55 mg/kg) as an initial dose, followed by 0.5 ml per 16 pounds of body weight (27.5 mg/kg) every 24 hours thereafter. Representative weights and doses are indicated in the following table: [See table below].

Each ml contains 400 mg sulfadimethoxine

Animal Weight	Initial Dose 25 mg/lb (55 mg/kg)	Subsequent Daily Dose 12.5 mg/lb (27.5 mg/kg)
8 lb. (3.6 kg)	0.5 ml	0.25 ml
16 lb (7.3 kg)	1 ml	0.5 ml
32 lb (14.5 kg)	2 ml	1 ml
64 lb (29.1 kg)	4 ml	2 ml

Length of treatment depends on the clinical response. In most cases, treatment for 3 to 5 days is adequate. Treatment should be continued until the patient is asymptomatic for 48 hours.

NOTE: Store at room temperature. Should crystallization occur at cold temperatures, crystals will dissolve either by storing at room temperature for several days or by heating the vial in warm water. Crystallization and redissolution do not impair the efficacy of the product.

How Supplied: Albon is available in the following dosage forms for dogs and cats:

Albon Injection-40%—Each ml contains 400 mg sulfadimethoxine compounded with 20% propylene glycol, 1% benzyl alcohol, 0.1 mg disoldium edetate, 1 mg sodium formaldehyde sulfoxylate, and pH adjusted with sodium hydroxide.

100 ml and 250 ml multiple dose vials.

Albon tablets, 0.125, 0.25 or 0.5 g sulfadimethoxine per tablet.

Albon Oral Suspension 5% in 2, 4 and 16 oz. bottles, each tsp. (5 ml) contains 250 mg sulfadimethoxine in a custard-flavored carrier.

Section II—Horses and Cattle

Actions: General principles of sulfonamide treatment, antibacterial spectrum of activity, and the tissue distribution of sulfadimethoxine are discussed in Section I, Dogs and Cats, under Actions.

In the horse the concentration of sulfadimethoxine has been determined to be higher in the wall of the duodenum than in any other part of the intestine. This, together with the high drug concentration in the bile, suggests enterohepatic cycling of the drug. Significat drug concentrations were also present in the cerebrospinal fluid.[5] Single, comparatively low doses of Albon give rapid and sustained therapeutic blood levels.[1]

Toxicity and Safety: No toxic effects were noted in horses receiving up to 3 times the recommended dosage as a single injection or twice the recommended dosage for an entire course of therapy. In cattle sufadimethoxine has been shown to be safe through extensive clinical use with other dosage forms. In addition, studies with intravenous administration of Albon (sulfadimethoxine) Injection-40% have demonstrated that hemolysis of erythrocytes does not occur by this route of administration. Sulfadimethoxine has a high solubility at the pH normally occurring in the kidney, precluding the possibility of precipitation and crystalluria. Toxicity data in laboratory animals is discussed in Section I, Dogs and Cats, under Toxicity and Safety.

Indications: *Horses:* Albon Injection-40% is indicated for the treatment of respiratory disease caused by *Streptococcus equi* (strangles). *Cattle*—Albon Injection-40% is indicated as a treatment for shipping fever complex, bacterial pneumonia, calf diphtheria, and foot rot in cattle caused by strains of organisms susceptible to sufadimethoxine.

Limitations: See Section I, Dogs and Cats, under Limitations.

Warning: Milk taken from the animals during treatment and for 60 hours (5 milkings) after the latest treatment must not be used for food. Do not administer within 5 days of slaughter. Not for use in horses intended for food.

Precautions: During treatment period, make certain that animals maintain adequate water intake.

If animals show no improvement within 2 or 3 days, re-evaluate your diagnosis.

Dosage and Administration: Albon Injection-40% must be administered only by the intravenous route in horses and cattle. Horses and cattle should receive 1 ml of Albon Injection-40% per 16 pounds of body weight (55 mg/kg) as an initial dose, followed by 0.5 ml per 16 pounds of body weight (27.5 mg/kg) every 24 hours thereafter. Albon Boluses may be utilized for maintenance therapy in cattle. Representative weights and doses are indicated in the following table: [See table above].

Each ml contains 400 mg sulfadimethoxine

Animal Weight	Initial Dose 25 mg/lb (55 mg/kg)	Subsequent Daily Doses 12.5 mg/lb (27.5 mg/kg)
250 lb (113.6 kg)	15.6 ml	7.8 ml
500 lb (227.2 kg)	31.2 ml	15.6 ml
750 lb (340.9 kg)	46.9 ml	23.5 ml
1000 lb (454.5 kg)	62.5 ml	31.3 ml

Length of treatment depends on the clinical response. In most cases treatment for 3 to 5 days is adequate. Treatment should be continued until the patient is asymptomatic for 48 hours.

Note: For storage information see NOTE In Section I, Dogs and Cats, under Dosage and Administration.

How Supplied: Albon is available in the following dosage form for horses and cattle.

100 ml and 250 ml multiple dose vials.

For cattle Only:

Albon boluses 2.5 g, 5 g, and 15 g per bolus.

References

1. Data on file from Hoffmann-LaRoche Inc., Nutley, New Jersey.

2. Stowe, C.M., The Sulfonamides, in Jones, L.M. (ed.) *Veterinary Pharmacology and Therapeutics* Ames, Iowa, Iowa State University Press, 1965, chapter 33.

3. Bridges, J.W., Kirby, M.R., Walker, S.R., and Williams, R. T., Species Differences in the Metabolism of Sulfadimethoxine, *Biochem, J.,* 109:851, 1968.

4. Baggot, J.D., Some Aspects of Drug Persistence in Domestic Animals, *Res. Vet. Sci. 11:2,* 130, 1970.

5. Oh-ishi, S., Tissue Distribution of Sulfadimethoxine and Sulfamonomethoxine in Horses after Intravenous Injection, *Jap J. Vet. Sci.,* 30:21, 1968.

This product information issued October 1985.

ALBON®-S.R.
(preparation of sulfadimethoxine) Sustained Release Bolus

Composition: Each bolus contains 12.5 g sulfadimethoxine.

Indications: Albon-S.R. is effective in the treatment of shipping fever complex and bacterial pneumonia associated with organisms such as Pasteurella spp. sensitive to sulfadimethoxine; and calf diphtheria and foot rot associated with *Sphaerophorus necrophorus* sensitive to sulfadimethoxine in beef cattle and nonlactating dairy cattle.

Caution: Not for Human Use.

Federal law restricts this drug to use by or on the order of a licensed veterinarian.

Description: The Albon-S.R. Bolus is a slow release formulation of the low dose, rapidly absorbed, long-acting sulfonamide, sulfadimethoxine.

Actions: Sulfadimethoxine has been demonstrated in laboratory studies to be effective against a wide variety of organisms, such as streptococci, staphylococci, klebsiella, proteus, shigella, and members of the *E. coli*-salmonella group of bacteria.[1,2]

The systemic sulfonamides which include sulfadimethoxine are bacteriostatic agents. Sulfonamides competitively inhibit bacterial synthesis of folic acid (pteroylglutamic acid) from para-aminobenzoic acid. Mammalian cells are capable of utilizing folic acid in the presence of sulfonamides.
The tissue distribution of sulfadimethoxine, as with all sulfonamides, is a function of plasma levels, degree of plasma protein binding, and subsequent passive distribution in the tissues of the lipid-soluble un-ionzied form. The relative amounts are determined by both its pKa and by the pH of each tissue. Therefore, levels tend to be higher in less acid tissue and body fluids or those tissues having high concentrations of leucocytes.[2]
Indications for Use: Albon-S.R. is effective in the treatment of shipping fever complex and bacterial pneumonia associated with organisms such as Pasteurella spp. sensitive to sulfadimethoxine, and calf diphtheria and foot rot associated with *Sphaerophorus necrophorus* sensitive to sulfadimethoxine in beef cattle and non-lactating dairy cattle.
Warning: Do not use in lactating dairy cattle. Do not administer within 21 days of slaughter.
Caution: During treatment period, make certain that animals maintain adequate water intake. Do not repeat treatment for seven days.
Dosage and Administration: Albon-S.R. Boluses are to be orally administered to beef cattle and non-lactating dairy cattle. Care should be taken to make certain the boluses are swallowed before releasing the animal. As with any orally administered bolus, occasional regurgitation will occur in ruminants. To fully maintain the sustained release effect, the boluses must not be divided. Animals should receive one bolus for the nearest 200 pounds of body weight, i.e., 62.5 mg/lb of body weight. Represer tative weights and doses are indicated in the following table:

Animal Weight (lb)	Number of Boluses
200	1
400	2
600	3
800	4
1000	5

To assure successful sulfonamide therapy, (1) drug administration must begin early in the course of the disease, and it must produce a high sulfonamide level in the body rapidly after administration; (2) therapeutically effective sulfonamide levels must be maintained in the body throughout the treatment period; (3) treatment should continue for a short period of time after the clinical signs have disappeared; and (4) the causative organisms must be sensitive to this class of drugs.
Toxicity and Safety: Data regarding acute (LD_{50}'s) and chronic toxicities of sulfadimethoxine indicate the drug is very safe. The LD_{50} in mice is greater than 2 g/kg body weight when administered intraperitoneally and greater than 16 g/kg when administered per os. In dogs receiving massive single oral doses of 3.2 g/kg body weight, diarrhea was the only adverse effect observed. Dogs given 160 mg/kg body weight per os daily for 13 weeks showed no signs of toxicity. Sulfadimethoxine has a relatiely high solubility at the pH normally occurring in the kidney, precluding the possibility of precipitation and crystalluria. Following the administration of Albon (sulfadimethoxine) at the recommended dosage, no undesirable side effects have been observed.
Sustained Action: Use of Albon-S.R. Boluses facilitates treatment and assures effective sulfonamide levels. Since only one treatment is required, both stress due to handling in acutely sick animals and labor costs are reduced. Sulfadimethoxine in itself maintains higher blood levels than most other long-acting sulfonamides.[3] Slow renal excretion results from a high degree of tubular reabsorption and plasma protein binding is very high, providing a blood reservoir of the drug. In addition, the greatly prolonged rumen dissolution rate of Albon-S.R. Boluses assures that the drug will be available for continued absorption over an extended period of time.
Blood Levels: Albon-S.R. given once to cattle at the recommended dose level of sulfadimethoxine of 62.5 mg/lb (137.5 mg/kg) of body weight provides rapid, therapeutically effective plasma sulfonamide levels for a period of 4 days.
How Supplied: Albon-S.R. Bolus is supplied as a 12.5 g sulfadimethoxine bolus.
References:

1. Data on file, Hoffmann-La Roche Inc., Nutley, New Jersey.
2. Stowe, C.M., The Sulfonamides, Jones, L. M. (Ed.), Veterinary Pharmacology and Therapeutic, 1965, Chapter 33.
3. Silvestri, G. *et al.*, Long-acting Sulfonamides in Cattle, a Study of Phamarcologic Properties, *Am. J. Vet. Res.* Vol. 28, No. 127, pp. 1783-1797, November 1967.
4. Baggott, J.D., Some Aspects of Drug Persistence in Domestic Animals, *Res. Vet. Sci.* 11:2, 130, 1970.

This product information issued October 1985.

ALBON®
(sulfadimethoxine)
Boluses 2.5 g, 5 g and 15 g

To be used in the treatment of shipping fever complex, bacterial pneumonia, calf diphtheria and foot rot in cattle. Not for human use.
Albon (sulfadimethoxine) is a low dose, rapidly absorbed, long-acting sulfonamide which is effective in the treatment of bacterial infections which commonly cause shipping fever complex, bacterial pneumonia, calf diphtheria and foot rot in cattle. Sulfadimethoxine has been demonstrated in laboratory studies to be effective against a wide variety of organisms, such as streptococci, staphylococci and members of the E. coli-salmonella group of bacteria.
Albon (sulfadimethoxine) has been shown to be a well-tolerated sulfonamide with relatively high solubility at the pH normally occurring in the kidney and with a low degree of toxicity. Following the administration of Albon (sulfadimethoxine) at the recommended dosage, no undesirable side effects have been observed.
Comparatively low doses of Albon (sulfadimethoxine) give rapid, sustained blood levels required for effective disease therapy.
Indications For Use: Albon (sulfadimethoxine) is indicated in the treatment of the following diseases.
Cattle: Shipping fever complex, bacterial pneumonia, calf diphtheria and foot rot.
Dosage and Administration: Albon (sulfadimethoxine) should be administered to cattle so that the initial dose is equivalent to 25 mg per pound of body weight and each subsequent daily dose is equivalent to 12.5 mg per pound of body weight. Length of treatment will depend on clinical response. In most cases, treatment for 3 to 4 days is adequate. Treatment should not be continued beyond 5 days.
The following tables show the dosage and dosage forms to be used for cattle of different weights.

ALBON (sulfadimethoxine) Boluses, 2.5 Gram

DOSAGE SCHEDULE FOR CATTLE—100 to 300 pounds of body weight

Animal Weight Lbs.	First Day	Daily for the Following 3 to 4 Days
100	1 bolus	½ bolus
200	2 boluses	1 bolus
300	3 boluses	1½ boluses

ALBON (sulfadimethoxine) Boluses, 5 Gram

DOSAGE SCHEDULE FOR CATTLE—200 to 600 pounds of body weight

Animal Weight Lbs.	First Day	Daily for the Following 3 to 4 Days
200	1 bolus	½ bolus
300	1½ boluses	1 bolus
400	2 boluses	1 bolus
500	2½ boluses	1½ boluses
600	3 boluses	1½ boluses

ALBON (sulfadimethoxine) Boluses, 15 Gram

DOSAGE SCHEDULE FOR CATTLE—600 to 1,200 pounds of body weight

Animal Weight Lbs.	First Day	Daily for the Following 3 to 4 Days
600	1 bolus	½ bolus
800	1½ boluses	1 bolus
1,000 to 1,200	2 boluses	1 bolus

Continued on next page

Roche—Cont.

Caution: During treatment period, make certain that animals maintain adequate water intake.
Warning: If animals show no improvement within 2 to 3 days, re-evaluate your diagnosis. Treatment should not be continued beyond 5 days.
Milk that has been taken from animals during treatment and for 60 hours (5 milkings) after the latest treatment should not be used for food.
Do not slaughter animals for food purposes within seven days following the last treatment.
How Supplied: Albon (sulfadimethoxine) is supplied in the following dosage forms:
Single Scored Boluses
2.5 g sulfadimethoxine per bolus
5 g sulfadimethoxine per bolus
15 g sulfadimethoxine per bolus
This product information issued October 1985.

R

ALBON®
(preparation of sulfadimethoxine)
Tablets
125 mg, 250 mg and 500 mg
Oral Suspension 5%

Each teaspoonful (5 ml) contains 250 mg sulfadimethoxine.
To be used in the treatment of sulfonamide-susceptible bacterial infections in dogs and cats and enteritis associated with coccidiosis in dogs.
Not for human use.
Caution: Federal law restricts this drug to use by or on the order of a licensed veterinarian.
Description: Albon is a low-dosage, rapidly absorbed, long-acting sulfonamide, effective for the treatment of a wide range of bacterial infections commonly encountered in dogs and cats.
Sulfadimethoxine is a white, almost tasteless and odorless compound. Chemically, it is N^1-(2,6-dimethoxy-4-pyrimidinyl) sulfanilamide.
Actions: Sulfadimethoxine has been demonstrated clinically or in the laboratory to be effective against a variety of organisms, such as streptococci, klebsiella, proteus, shigella, staphylococci, escherichia and salmonella.[1,2] These organisms have been demonstrated in respiratory, genitourinary, enteric and soft tissue infections of dogs and cats.
The systemic sulfonamides which include sulfadimethoxine are bacteriostatic agents. Sulfonamides competitively inhibit bacterial synthesis of folic acid (pteroylglutamic acid) from para-aminobenzoic acid. Mammalian cells are capable of utilizing folic acid in the presence of sulfonamides.

Tablet Size	Approximate Animal Weight lbs	kg	Initial Dose (55 mg/kg)	Subsequent Daily Dose (27.5 mg/kg)
125 mg	5	2.2	1 tablet	½ tablet
250 mg	10	4.5	1 tablet	½ tablet
500 mg	20	9.1	1 tablet	½ tablet

Animal Weight	Initial Dose (55 mg/kg)	Subsequent Daily Doses (27.5 mg/kg)
5 lbs. (2.2 kg)	½ tsp (2½ ml)	¼ tsp. (¼ml)
10 lbs (4.5 kg)	1 tsp (5 ml)	½ tsp (2½ ml)
20 lbs. (9.1 kg)	2 tsp (10 ml)	1 tsp (5 ml)
40 lbs (18.2 kg)	4 tsp (20 ml)	2 tsp (10 ml)
80 lbs (36.4 kg)	8 tsp (40 ml)	4 tsp (20 ml)

The tissue distribution of sulfadimethoxine, as with all sulfonamides, is a function of plasma levels, degree of plasma protein binding, and subsequent passive distribution in the tissues of the lipid-soluble un-ionized form. The relative amounts are determined by both its pKa and by the pH of each tissue. Therefore, levels tend to be higher in less acid tissue and body fluids or those diseased tissues having high concentrations of leucocytes.[2]
In the dog sulfadimethoxine is not acetylated as in most other animals, and it is excreted predominantly as the unchanged drug.[3] Sulfadimethoxine has a relatively high solubility at the pH normally occurring in the kidney, precluding the possibility of precipitation and crystalluria. Slow renal excretion results from a high degree of tubular reabsorption,[4] and plasma protein binding is very high, providing a blood reservoir of the drug. Thus, sulfadimethoxine maintains higher blood levels than most other long-acting sulfonamides. Single, comparatively low doses of Albon give rapid and sustained therapeutic blood levels.[1]
To assure successful sulfonamide therapy, (1) the drug must be given early in the course of the disease, and it must produce a high sulfonamide level in the body rapidly after administration; (2) therapeutically effective sulfonamide levels must be maintained in the body throughout the treatment period; (3) treatment should continue for a short period of time after the clinical signs have disappeared; and (4) the causative organisms must be sensitive to this class of drugs.
Toxicity and Safety: Data regarding acute (LD_{50}'s) and chronic toxicities of sulfadimethoxine indicate the drug is very safe. The LD_{50} in mice is greater than 2 g/kg body weight when administered intraperitoneally and greater than 16 g/kg when administered per os. In dogs receiving massive single oral doses of 3.2 mg/kg body weight, diarrhea was the only adverse effect observed. Dogs given 160 mg/kg body weight per os daily for 13 weeks showed no signs of toxicity.
Indications: Albon is indicated for the treatment of a wide range of respiratory, genitourinary tract, enteric, and soft tissue infections in dogs and cats. For example:

tonsillitis	pustular dermatitis
pharyngitis	anal gland infections
bronchitis	abscesses
pneumonia	wound infections
cystitis	bacterial enteritis
nephritis	canine salmonellosis
metritis	bacterial enteritis
pyometra	associated with coccidiosis in dogs

when caused by streptococci, staphylocci, escherichia, salmonella, klebsiella, proteus or shigella organisms sensitive to sulfadimethoxine.
Limitations: Sulfadimethoxine is not effective in viral or rickettsial infections, and as with any antibacterial agent, occasional failures in therapy may occur due to resistant microorganisms. The usual precautions in sulfonamide therapy should be observed.
Precautions: During treatment period, make certain that animals maintain adequate water intake.
If animals show no improvement within 2 or 3 days, re-evaluate your diagnosis.
Dosage and Administration: *Initial Dose:* 25 mg/lb (55 mg/kg) of animal body weight.
Subsequent Doses: 12.5 mg/lb (27.5 mg/kg) of animal body weight.
Albon Tablets: For ease of administration in animals of varying weights, 3 tablet sizes are provided. The following table indicates how dosage may be adjusted depending on tablet size and body weight. Subsequent doses should be given at 24 hour intervals.
[See table below].
Albon Oral Suspension 5%: Dogs and cats should receive 1 teaspoonful of Albon Oral Suspension 5% per 10 pounds of body weight (25 mg/lb or 55 mg/kg) as an initial dose, followed by 0.5 teaspoonful per 10 pounds of body weight (12.5 mg/lb or 27.5 mg/kg) every 24 hours thereafter. Representative weights and doses are indicated in the following table:
[See table above].
Treatment may be initiated with Albon Injection-40% to obtain effective blood levels almost immediately or to faciliate treatment of the fractious animal. Length of treatment depends on the clinical response. In most cases, treatment for 3 to 5 days is adequate. Treatment should be continued until the patient is asymptomatic for 48 hours.
How Supplied: Albon is available in the following dosage forms:
Albon Tablets; 125 mg, 250 mg and 500 mg sulfadimethoxine per tablet.
Albon Oral Suspension 5%; each tsp. (5 ml) contains 250 mg sulfadimethoxine in a custard-flavored carrier.
Albon Injection-40%
References
1. Data on file, Hoffmann-La Roche Inc., Nutley, New Jersey.

2. Stowe, C.M., The Sulfonamides, in Jones, L.M. (ed.), *Veterinary Pharmacology and Therapeutics*, Ames, Iowa, Iowa State University Press, 1965, chapter 33.
3. Bridges, J.W., Kirby, M.R., Walker, S.R., and Williams, R.T., Species Differences in the Metabolism of Sulfadimethoxine, *Biochem, J.*, 109:851, 1968.
4. Baggot, J.D., Some Aspects of Drug Persistence in Domestic Animals, *Res. Vet. Sci, 11:2*, 130, 1970.

This product information issued October 1985.

ALBON®
(preparation of sulfadimethoxine) Antibacterial
12.5% Concentrated Solution for Use in Drinking Water

12.5% Concentrated Solution for use in drinking water for oral use in chickens, turkeys and cattle. Protect from light. Each fluid ounce contains 3.75 gm. sulfadimethoxine solubilized with sodium hydroxide.

Dairy Calves, Dairy Heifers and Beef Cattle—Use in the treatment of shipping fever complex, bacterial pneumonia, calf diphtheria, and foot rot.

Broiler and Replacement Chickens—Use for the treatment of disease outbreaks of coccidiosis, fowl cholera and infectious coryza.

Meat-Producing Turkeys—Use for the treatment of disease outbreaks of coccidiosis and fowl cholera.

Dosage and Administration: DAIRY CALVES, DAIRY HEIFERS AND BEEF CATTLE

Dosage: ALBON (sulfadimethoxine) should be administered at 25 mg./lb. first day followed by 12.5 mg./lb./day for 4 days.

	Water Consumption (Summer) 1 gallon/ 100 lbs body weight†	(Winter) 1 gallon/ 150 lbs body weight†
First Day Add:		
1 pt. (16 fl. oz.) to	25 gal.	16 gal.
1 qt. (32 fl. oz.) to	50 gal.	33 gal.
1 gal. (128 fl. oz.) to	200 gal.	127 gal.
Next 4 Days Add:		
1 pt. (16 fl. oz.) to	50 gal.	33 gal.
1 qt. (32 fl. oz.) to	100 gal.	66 gal.
1 gal. (128 fl. oz.) to	400 gal.	266 gal.

†This dosage recommendation is based on a water consumption of 1 gal. per 100 lb. of body weight per day, the expected water consumption rate for summer. Water consumption during cold months (winter) may drop markedly (30–40%). Accordingly, adjustments in drug concentration in drinking water must be made to insure proper drug intake.

For individual treatment of cattle, ALBON (sulfadimethoxine) 12.5% Drinking Water Solution may be given as a drench. Administer using same mg./lb. dosage as outlined above. Four fluid ounces will medicate one 600 lb. animal initially or two 600 lb. animals on maintenance dose.

TREATMENT PERIOD—5 consecutive days

CHICKENS

Dosage: Concentration—0.05%. Add 1 fl. oz.* to 2 gal. of water or 25 fl. oz. to 50 gal. of water.

TURKEYS

Dosage: Concentration—0.025%. Add 1 fl. oz.* to 4 gal. of water or 25 fl. oz. to 100 gal. of water.

TREATMENT PERIOD—6 consecutive days.

Automatic Proportioners Stock Solution**

To make 2 gallons of stock solution use:

CHICKENS: 1 gallon ALBON 12.5% Drinking Water Solution Concentrate plus 1 gallon of water.

TURKEYS: 2 quarts ALBON 12.5% Drinking Water Solution Concentrate plus 6 quarts of water.

TREATMENT PERIOD—6 consecutive days

*1 fl. oz. ALBON 12.5% Drinking Water Solution = 30 ml or 2 tablespoonfuls.

**Set proportioner to a feed rate of 1 fl. oz. ALBON Stock Solution per gallon of water.

Caution: Store at room temperature. If freezing occurs, thaw before using. Protect from light; direct sunlight may cause discoloration. Freezing or discoloration does not affect potency. Prepare a fresh stock solution daily.

Chickens and Turkeys: If birds show no improvement within 5 days, discontinue treatment and re-evaluate diagnosis. Handle the recommended dilutions (chickens 0.05% and turkeys 0.025%) as regular drinking water. Administer as sole source of drinking water and sulfonamide medication. Chickens and turkeys that have survived fowl cholera outbreaks should not be kept for replacements or breeders.

Cattle: During treatment period, make certain that animals maintain adequate water intake. If animals show no improvement within 2 or 3 days, re-evaluate diagnosis. Treatment should not be continued beyond 5 days.

FOR SALE TO VETERINARIANS ONLY
NOT FOR HUMAN USE

WARNING: CHICKENS AND TURKEYS—Withdraw 5 days before slaughter. Do not administer to chickens over 16 weeks (112 days) of age or to turkeys over 24 weeks (168 days) of age.
CATTLE—Withdraw 7 days before slaughter. For dairy calves, dairy heifers and beef cattle only.

How Supplied: Available in 1 gallon bottles.

This product information issued October 1985.

ALBON®
(preparation of sulfadimethoxine) Antibacterial Soluble Powder

Each packet contains 3.34 oz (94.6 gm) sulfadimethoxine in the form of the soluble sodium salt and disodium edetate.

Dairy Calves, Dairy Heifers and Beef Cattle—Use for the treatment of shipping fever complex, bacterial pneumonia, calf diphtheria, and foot rot.

Broiler and Replacement Chickens—Use for the treatment of disease outbreaks of coccidiosis, fowl cholera, and infectious coryza.

Meat-Producing Turkeys—Use for the treatment of disease outbreaks of coccidiosis and fowl cholera.

Dosage and Administration: DAIRY CALVES, DAIRY HEIFERS AND BEEF CATTLE

Dosage: ALBON (sulfadimethoxine) should be administered at 25 mg./lb. first day followed by 12.5 mg./lb./day for 4 days.

Note: Prepare a cattle stock solution by adding 1 packet of ALBON Soluble Powder to 1 gallon of water.

[See table on next page].

TREATMENT PERIOD—5 consecutive days.

CHICKENS

Dosage: Concentration—0.05%. Add contents of packet to 50 gal. of water.

TURKEYS

Dosage: Concentration—0.025%. Add contents of packet to 100 gal. of water.

TREATMENT PERIOD—6 consecutive days

Caution: Chickens and Turkeys—If animals show no improvement within 5 days, discontinue treatment and re-evaluate diagnosis. Prepare a fresh stock solution daily. Handle the recommended dilutions (chickens 0.05% and turkeys 0.025%) as regular drinking water. Administer as sole source of drinking water and sulfonamide medication. Chickens and turkeys that have survived fowl cholera outbreaks should not be kept for replacements or breeders.

Cattle: During treatment period, make certain that animals maintain adequate water intake. If animals show no improvement within 2 or 3 days, re-evaluate diagnosis. Treatment should not be continued beyond 5 days.

FOR SALE TO VETERINARIANS ONLY
NOT FOR HUMAN USE

WARNING: CHICKENS AND TURKEYS—Withdraw 5 days before slaughter. Do not administer to chickens over 16 weeks (112 days) of age or to turkeys over 24 weeks (168 days) of age.
CATTLE: Withdraw 7 days before slaughter. For dairy calves, dairy heifers and beef cattle only.

How Supplied: 107 gm packets.

This product information issued October 1985.

Continued on next page

Roche—Cont.

ALFAVET®
(injectable preparation of alfaprostol)

Product Information: ALFAVET is a clear, sterile solution for injection containing 1 mg of alfaprostol per ml of propylene glycol.

Not for human use.

Caution: Federal law restricts this drug to use by or on the order of a licensed veterinarian.

Description: ALFAVET (alfaprostol) is a synthetic compound — 18,19,20-trinor-17, cyclohexyl-13,14-didehydro $PGF_{2\alpha}$ methyl ester

Chemical Structure:

Alfaprostol is an analog of the naturally-occurring prostaglandin $PGF_{2\alpha}$. It is a synthetic compound with some of the basic characteristics of $PGF_{2\alpha}$, but with the following modifications: the substitution of the double trans bond in the 13 and 14 position with a triple acetylenic bond and the introduction of a cyclohexyl ring instead of three terminal carbons.

Actions: ALFAVET acts primarily as a luteolysin. ALFAVET causes luteolysis in mares with active corpora lutea. Animals belonging to this group may be:

(1) cycling, lactating or non-lactating mares;
(2) lactating mares which have not been bred at the foal heat, or which had no visible foal heat;
(3) anestrous mares which have either persistent corpora lutea or are cycling silently.

Effective treatment with ALFAVET results in a sharp decline of plasma progesterone within 12 to 24 hours. Full luteolysis is achieved in most cases within 24 to 48 hours.

Luteolysis resulting from the use of ALFAVET is followed by follicle growth and estrus, which in most mares will commence 2 to 4 days after treatment and by ovulation, observed in most mares between days 6 and 8 after injection.

In some mares, estrus may not be detected, but palpation of the ovaries will reveal follicular growth followed by ovulation.

At the time of treatment of cycling mares, some mares may either not be in the luteal phase or in the very early luteal phase, when corpora lutea are not yet fully developed (before day 6). Response in these mares may occur within several days or may be delayed up to 10 to 12 days.

Safety Studies: In controlled and open clinical studies with ALFAVET, neither treated mares nor foals suckling treated mares showed any side effects at the recommended dose.

The wide margin of safety of ALFAVET has been shown in cycling mares which received 3 to 5 times the recommended dose daily for 5 consecutive days. There were no clinical or behavioral signs of drug effects, and there were no changes in the blood profile. At 15, 30 and 45 times the recommended dose, a transient period of arrhythmia and tachypnea lasting 120 to 240 minutes was recorded, with no further clinical consequences. At the highest dose, neither sweating nor diarrhea nor intestinal cramping was observed. Body temperature was never elevated.

Indications:

1. *Mares with normal estrous cycle* and having a *fully developed progesterone producing corpus luteum* can be brought into estrus and will ovulate, in most instances, by a single injection of ALFAVET. The conception rate at the induced estrus in healthy, well-managed mares will be normal. This procedure can be used in horse studs to space the heat of brood mares and to manage stallion power accordingly. Groups of mares can be brought into heat simultaneously. This allows the use of artificial insemination more efficiently in horse breeding.
2. *Mares postpartum* which were *not bred at the foal heat* or had *no overt foal heat*. Conception rates from breeding at the foal heat might be normal, but several literature reports indicate lowered fertility rates.

Injecting ALFAVET 8 to 10 days after foal heat — or on days 20 to 22 postpartum — will bring mares back into heat, or will induce heat, and assure renewed ovulations and chances for serving mares 3 to 4 weeks postpartum; breeding at this heat will result in a normal pregnancy rate.

3. *Anestrous Mares* — Anestrus can result from persisting corpora lutea or from covert cycling (silent heat cycles) from ovarian inactivity, or from an early pregnancy loss after PMSG (Pregnant Mare Serum Gonadotropin) production has been established. Mares which have an active corpus luteum (persisting or cycling) will respond to ALFAVET treatment with heat and ovulation. In practice, a certain percentage of mares will be treated which do not have plasma progesterone levels of more than 1 ng/ml. Some of these mares respond also with follicular development and estrus and /or ovulation. This may result from the endogenous gonadotropin release known to occur after ALFAVET treatment in an anestrous mare. Anestrous mares which reacted to treatment and were bred had a normal pregnancy rate.

Before administering ALFAVET, mares should be subjected to a thorough breeding soundness examination, including palpation per rectum.

Warning: Women of childbearing age, asthmatics, and persons with bronchial and other respiratory problems should exercise extreme caution when handling this product. In the early stages, women may be unaware of their pregnancies. Alfaprostol is readily absorbed through the skin and can cause abortion and/or bronchiospasms. Direct contact with the skin should therefore be avoided. Accidental spillage on the skin should be washed off immediately with soap and water.

Not for use in horses intended for food.

Contraindications: ALFAVET can cause abortions or induce premature parturitions; hence it should not be given to pregnant animals.

Non-steroidal anti-inflammatory drugs inhibit the synthesis and release of endogenous prostaglandins. Concurrent use of these drugs and ALFAVET is not advisable.

Dosage And Administration: ALFAVET should be given by intramuscular or subcutaneous injection. An optimal dose of 6 mcg per kg body weight has been established for a mature mare. The recommended dose for a mature 500 kg (1100 lb) mare is a 3 ml injection (3 mg) of ALFAVET.

ALBON (sulfadimethoxine) IN WATER

	Amount of Stock Solution for cattle*	WATER CONSUMPTION (Summer) 1 gallon/ 100 lbs. body weight**	(Winter) 1 gallon/ 150 lbs. body weight**
FIRST DAY ADD:	1 quart	10 gallons	7 gallons
	2 quarts	20 gallons	14 gallons
	1 gallon	40 gallons	28 gallons
NEXT 4 DAYS ADD:	1 quart	20 gallons	14 gallons
	2 quarts	40 gallons	28 gallons
	1 gallon	80 gallons	56 gallons

**This dosage recommendation is based on a water consumption of 1 gallon per 100 lb. of body weight per day, the expected water consumption rate for summer. Water consumption during cold months (winter) may drop markedly (30–40%). Accordingly, adjustments must be made in the dilution rates to compensate for this and insure proper drug intake.

For treatment of individual cattle, ALBON (sulfadimethoxine) Soluble Powder stock solution for cattle may be given as a drench. Administer using same mg./lb. of dosage as outlined above.

*Twenty fluid ounces of cattle stock solution will medicate one 600 lb. animal initially or two 600 lb. animals on maintenance dose. Contents of packet will medicate six 600 lb. animals initially or twelve 600 lb. animals on maintenance dose.

R

How Supplied: ALFAVET is supplied as a sterile solution in 18 ml multiple dose vials.
Store at 59° TO 86°F. (15° TO 30°C.)
This product information issued October 1985.

IPROPRAN®
(preparation of ipronidazole hydrochloride) Antihistomonal Soluble Powder

Description: Each 2.65 oz (75 g) packet of Ipropran Soluble Powder contains 2.15 oz (61 grams) of ipronidazole in the form of ipronidazole hydrochloride. This amount of drug will medicate 128 gallons of drinking water.
Indications: For the treatment of blackhead (histomoniasis) in turkeys, Ipropran Soluble Powder may be used in conjunction with 0.00625% ipronidazole in turkey feeds.
Directions for Use: To provide recommended concentration of 0.0125% ipronidazole:
Prepare fresh solutions daily.
Note: Exposure of galvanized or steel containers to solutions of Ipropran Soluble Powder may accelerate normal corrosion.
(1) Automatic Proportioner—Dissolve contents of packet in 1 gallon of water to prepare concentrate solution using a plastic or glass container. Set metering pump to add 1 fl oz of concentrate per gallon of drinking water.
(2) Complete Solution—Dissolve contents of packet in 128 gallons of drinking water with thorough mixing.
Treatment period: 7 consecutive days.
Warning: Withdraw 5 days before slaughter. Do not use in turkeys producing eggs for food.
Hazardous—Not for human use.
How Supplied: 75 g packets
This product information issued October 1985.

INJACOM®

Composition: Injacom has the following composition: Each ml contains:

Vitamin A	500,000 IU
Vitamin D_3	75,000 IU

Compounded with 5 IU vitamin E per ml; 8% ethyl alcohol; 2% benzyl alcohol, 0.75% BHT and 0.75% BHA as preservatives; in an emulsifiable solution.
Description: Injacom is a water-dispersible solution of vitamins A D_3 for prevention and correction of Vitamin A and D deficiencies in cattle, sheep and swine.
Administration: Injacom is to be given by intramuscular (into the muscle) injection. Intramuscular injection should be made with a 16-18 gauge needle, 1½ or 2 inches long, in a heavily muscled area, preferably high on the rump.
ONLY CLEAN, STERILE NEEDLES AND SYRINGES SHOULD BE USED FOR ADMINISTRATION. INJECTION SITE AND RUBBER CAP OF BOTTLE SHOULD BE CLEANED AND DISINFECTED WITH ALCOHOL OR OTHER SATISFACTORY DISINFECTANT.
Deficiency Symptoms: Vitamin A—Night blindness; watery eyes; retarded growth; staggering gait; edema of the brisket and forelegs; poor hair coat; impaired reproduction and weak or dead offspring.
Vitamin D—Enlarged joints; weakened bones (rickets); curved, abnormal back and legs.
Suggested Dosage

Cattle	
Calves	½ to 1 ml per head
Yearlings	1 to 2 ml per head
Breeding cattle	3 to 6 ml per head
Sheep	
Lambs	¼ to ½ ml per head
Fattening lambs	½ to 1 ml per head
Breeding sheep	1 to 2 ml per head
Swine	
Weanling pigs	¼ to ½ ml per head
Growing pigs	½ to 1 ml per head
Breeding swine	1 to 3 ml per head

Dosage may be repeated after 60 days, if needed.
Caution: For intramuscular injection only. If intended dose in cattle is greater than 4 ml, it should be divided equally and given in two different sites.
Do not exceed recommended dosage.
Occasionally a histamine-like reaction may occur. If so, immediate treatment with epinephrine and/or an antihistamine should be given by injection.
If symptoms of deficiencies persist, diagnosis should be re-evaluated.
Store at 59° to 86°F. Keep partially used vial under refrigeration.
This product is not designed for injection in cats, dogs or horses.
DO NOT INJECT INTO MEAT ANIMALS WITHIN 60 DAYS OF MARKETING
For sale to licensed veterinarians only.
Not for human use.
How Supplied: Available in 100 ml and 250 ml multiple dose vials.
This product information issued October 1985.

INJACOM® 100

Composition: Each ml contains:

Vitamin A	100,000 IU
Vitamin D_3	10,000 IU

Compounded with 20 IU Vitamin E per ml; 16% polyoxyethylated fatty acid derivative, 7.2% glycerin, 0.05% acetate buffer, and 0.01% disodium edetate; with 0.13% BHT, 0.13% BHA and 0.01% thimerosal as preservatives; and water for injection.
Description: Injacom-100 is an aqueous emulsion of vitamins A and D_3 for the prevention and correction of vitamin A and D deficiencies in cats, dogs, horses, calves, lambs, and young pigs.
Deficiency Symptoms: Vitamin A—Night blindness, watery eyes, nasal discharge, retarded growth, staggering gait, edema of brisket and forelegs, poor hair coat, impaired reproduction, and weak or dead offspring.
Vitamin D—Rickets, enlarged joints and weakened bones, lameness, stiff gait, and curved, abnormal back and legs.
Administration: Injacom 100 may be administered by subcutaneous or intramuscular injection. Intramuscular injections should be given in a heavily muscled area such as the gluteal area.
ONLY CLEAN, STERILE NEEDLES AND SYRINGES SHOULD BE USED FOR ADMINISTRATION. INJECTION SITE AND RUBBER CAP OF BOTTLE SHOULD BE CLEANED AND DISINFECTED WITH ALCOHOL OR OTHER SATISFACTORY DISINFECTANT.
Suggested Dosage:

Pets	
Cats	¼ to ½ ml
Dogs (dependent on size)	½ to 2 ml
Horses	
Colts	2½ to 5 ml
Yearlings	5 ml
Breeding horses	5 to 10 ml
Young Livestock	
Calves up to 400 lbs	2½ to 5 ml
Lambs up to 60 lbs	1 to 2½ ml
Pigs up to 100 lbs	1 to 2½ ml

Dosage may be repeated after 60 days, if needed.
Caution: For subcutaneous or intramuscular administration only. If intended dose is greater than 5 ml, it should be divided equally and given in two different sites.
Do not exceed recommended dosage. Occasionally a histamine-like reaction may occur. If so, immediate treatment with epinephrine and/or an antihistamine should be given by injection.
If symptoms of deficiencies persist, diagnosis should be re-evaluated.
DO NOT INJECT INTO MEAT ANIMALS WITHIN 60 DAYS OF MARKETING
Store at 59° to 86°F. Keep partially used vial under refrigeration. This product will solidify at freezing temperatures but returns to its original state and is safe to use when thawed at room temperature.
While Injacom-100 is an essentially stable, opalescent dispersion, a slight separation may occur during storage. This does not, however, affect the potency, safety, or usefulness of the preparation. If separation does occur, gentle agitation will restore the dispersion. Avoid shaking excessively, as this may entrap air in the solution.
For sale to licensed veterinarians only.
Not for human use.
Caution: Federal law restricts this drug to use by or on the order of a licensed veterinarian.
How Supplied: Available in 30 ml multiple dose vials.
This product information issued October 1985.

Continued on next page

R

Roche—Cont.

INJACOM® 100 + B COMPLEX
Injectable Vitamins A, D3 and B Complex

Composition: Each ml contains:

Vitamin A	100,00 IU
Vitamin D_3	10,000 IU
Niacinamide	10 mg
Vitamin B_1 (as thiamine hydrochloride)	5 mg
Vitamin B_6 (pyridoxine hydrochloride)	5 mg
Pantothenic Acid (as dexpanthenol)	5 mg
Vitamin B_2 (as riboflavin 5'-phosphate sodium)	1 mg
d-Biotin	0.05 mg

Compounded with 20 IU vitamin E per ml; 20% polyoxyethylated vegetable oil; 7.2% glycerin; 0.01% disodium edetate; 0.13% BHT, 0.13% BHA and 0.01% thimerosal as preservatives; and water for injection.

R

Description: Injacom 100 + B Complex is an aqueous emulsion of vitamins A, D_3, B_1, (as thiamine HC1), B_2 (as riboflavin 5'-phosphate sodium, B_6 (as pyridoxine HC1), niacin (as niacinamide), pantothenic acid (as dexpanthenol) and d-biotin as an aid in correcting multiple deficiencies of such vitamins in domestic animals including ruminants.

Indications: The administration of Injacom 100 + B Complex containing vitamin A, vitamin D and B complex vitamins, is recommended as an aid in correcting multiple deficiencies of such vitamins in domestic animals.

Vitamin Deficiencies: Vitamin deficiencies are of varied etiology. Such deficiencies may be the result of inadequate diet, but even where the diet is believed to contain adequate quantities of vitamins, many factors such as vitamin instability, disease and/or other stress conditions may result in inadequate intake or in increased vitamin requirements. Adjustment in diet should always be considered, but where, deficiency symptoms exist Injacom 100 + B Complex injection is a rapid, effective and convenient aid in overcoming multiple deficiencies of the essential vitamins contained in this product.

A deficiency of a single vitamin may occur, but often vitamin deficiencies occur in multiple form. Accordingly, symptomatology may vary, but following are the most common symptoms encountered with the vitamins contained in Injacom 100 + Complex.

Vitamin A—Night blindness, watery eyes, retarded growth, staggering gait, edema of the brisket and forelegs, poor hair coat. Breeding animals with a vitamin A deficiency may experience reproduction problems, In the female, retained placenta and impaired ability to become pregnant are two of the milder symptoms. More severe symptoms are weak or blind offspring, abortions or stillborn offspring. In the male, a vitamin A deficiency may result in decreased sperm motility and total sperm count.

Vitamin D_3—Rickets: Enlarged joints and weakened bones, lameness, stiff gait, and curved, abnormal back and legs.

Vitamin B Complex—Ruminants: In young animals, without a fully developed rumen, vitamin B complex supplementation may be needed. Severe inadequacy of protein and other nutrients in the feed may impair rumen fermentation so that sufficient quantities of B vitamins will not be synthesized and would have to be provided by supplementation.

Vitamin B complex would be indicated in animals "off feed"or those with atony of the rumen where bacterial synthesis would be minimal. Polioencephalomalacia appears to be related to thiamine deficiency.

Non-Ruminants: In monogastric animals (dogs, cats, horses and swine) deficiency symptoms are anorexia, nervousness, incoordination, diarrhea and anemic states.

Individual B vitamin deficiency symptoms as reported by the National Academy of Sciences.

Niacin—Calf: Sudden anorexia, severe diarrhea, dehydration and death. Swine: Slow or interrupted growth, reduced feed intake, poor hair and skin condition, lameness, diarrhea, impaired breeding and gestation.

Vitamin B_1—Calf: Polyneuritis with leg weakness and retraction of the head accompanied with anorexia, severe diarrhea, dehydration and death. Swine: Slow or interrupted growth, reduced feed intake, impaired breeding and weakened or dead piglets.

Vitamin B_6—Calf: Anorexia and cessation of growth in the first few weeks of life. Swine: Slow or interrupted growth, reduced feed intake, poor hair and skin condition, lameness and diarrhea.

Pantothenic Acid—Calf: Scaly dermatitis around eyes and muzzle, anorexia, diarrhea, weakness, inability to stand and convulsions. Swine: Slow or interrupted growth, reduced feed intake, lameness, impaired breeding and gestation, weak or dead piglets.

Vitamin B_2—Calf: Hyperemia of the mucosa of the mouth, loss of hair on the abdomen, salivation, lacrimination, anorexia and diarrhea. Swine: Slow or interrupted growth, reduced feed intake, poor hair and skin condition, diarrhea, impaired breeding and gestation, and weak or dead piglets.

Biotin—Calf: Paralysis of hind quarters. Swine: Alopecia, spasticity of hind legs, cracks in the feet and dermatosis.

Administration: Injacom 100 + B Complex may be administered by subcutaneous or intramuscular injection. Intramuscular injections should be given in a heavily muscled area such as the gluteal area.

ONLY CLEAN, STERILE NEEDLES AND SYRINGES SHOULD BE USED. THE INJECTION SITE AND RUBBER CAP OF BOTTLE SHOULD BE CLEANED AND DISINFECTED WITH ALCOHOL OR OTHER SATISFACTORY DISINFECTANT.

Suggested Dosage:

Pets	
Cats	1/4 to 1/2 ml
Dogs (dependent on size)	1/2 to 2 ml
Horses	
Colts	2 1/2 to 5 ml
Yearlings	5 ml
Breeding horses	5 to 10 ml
Other livestock	
Calves up to 400 lbs	2 1/2 to 5 ml
Cattle 400 lbs or more and Breeding Cattle	5 to 10 ml
Pigs up to 100 lbs	1 to 2 1/2 ml
Breeding swine	2 1/2 to 5 ml

Dosage may be repeated after 60 days, if needed.

Caution: For subcutaneous or intramuscular administration only. If the intended dose is greater than 5 ml, it should be divided equally and given in two different sites.

Do not exceed recommended dosage. Occasionally a histamine-like reaction may occur. If so, immediate treatment with epinephrine and/or an antihistamine should be given by injection.

If symptoms of deficiencies persist, the diagnosis should be re-evaluated.

DO NOT INJECT INTO MEAT ANIMALS WITHIN 60 DAYS OF MARKETING

Store at 59° to 86°F. Keep partially used vial under refrigeration.

For sale to licensed veterinarians only. Not for human use.

Caution: Federal law restricts this drug to use by or on the order of a licensed veterinarian.

How Supplied: Available in 100 ml multiple dose vials.

This product information issued October 1985.

Products are cross-indexed

by product classifications

in the

Product Category Section

Solvay Veterinary. Inc.

P.O. BOX 7348
PRINCETON, NJ 08540

CRYSTIBEN®

Sterile Penicillin G Benzathine and Penicillin G Procaine in Aqueous Suspension Veterinary
For Veterinary use in Beef Cattle, Horses and Dogs

Description: Each ml of Crystiben contains 150,000 units penicillin G benzathine, 150,000 units penicillin G procaine, not more than 3 mg sodium formaldehyde sulfoxylate, 14 mg lecithin, 1.2. mg methylparaben and 0.14 mg propylparaben and 0.0025 ml liquefied phenol as preservatives, 7 mg polysorbate 40, 10 mg sorbitan monopalmitate, 10 mg sodium citrate, 20 mg procaine hydrochloride, 1.5 mg carboxymethylcellulose sodium, 3.5 mg povidone, 0.15 ml sorbitol solution and water for injection q.s.

Actions: Penicillin G is an antibiotic which shows a marked bactericidal effect against certain organisms during their growth phase. It is relatively specific in its action against gram-positive bacteria but is usually ineffective against gram-negative organisms.

When treating an animal for a bacterial infection, it is advisable to isolate and identify the causative organism and conduct appropriate *in vitro* susceptibility tests. In cases where organisms other than those susceptible to penicillin are present, reevaluation of treatment should be made. Organisms normally considered susceptible to penicillin include *Clostridium septicum, Corynebacterium pyogenes, Staphylococcus aureus, Streptococcus canis, Streptococcus equi* and *Streptococcus pyogenes.*

It is normally recommended that any bacterial infection be treated as early as possible and with a dosage which will give effective blood levels. Although the recommended dosage of Crystiben will give longer detectable penicillin blood levels than penicillin G procaine alone, it is recommended that a second dose be administered at 48 hours when treating a penicillin-susceptible bacterial infection.

If no definite improvement is noted following the second dose of Crystiben, the diagnosis should be reevaluated and use of another chemotherapeutic agent considered.

Indications: Crystiben is indicated for treatment of the following bacterial infections in dogs, horses and beef cattle due to penicillin G susceptible microorganisms that are susceptible to the serum levels common to this particular dosage form, such as:

1. Bacterial Pneumonia (shipping fever complex) (*Streptococcus spp., Corynebacterium pyogenes, Staphylococcus aureus*).
2. Upper Respiratory Infections such as Rhinitis or Pharyngitis (*Corynebacterium pyogenes*).
3. Equine Strangles (*Streptococcus equi*).
4. Blackleg (*Clostridium chauvoei*).
5. Anthrax (*Bacillus anthracis*).

Contraindications: Crystiben is contraindicated in animals which have shown hypersensitivity to penicillin.

Warnings: Beef cattle must be withheld from slaughter for food use for 30 days following last treatment. Treatment in beef cattle must be limited to two (2) doses. Not to be used in horses intended for food.

Adverse Reactions: Anaphylactic reactions have been reported in animals given penicillin. Treated animals should be closely observed and if allergic or anaphylactic reactions occur, administer epinephrine or antihistamines immediately.

Administration: Crystiben should be given by intramuscular injection to horses. In beef cattle the recommended dosage should be administered by subcutaneous injection only. Dogs may be injected by either the intramuscular or subcutaneous route.

Dosage:

Horses —Two ml per 150 lb body weight given intramuscularly (2,000 units penicillin G procaine and 2,000 units penicillin G benzathine per lb body weight). Treatment should be repeated in 48 hours.

Beef Cattle: —Two ml per 150 lb body weight given subcutaneously only (2,000 units penicillin G procaine and 2,000 units penacillin G benzathine per lb body weight). Treatment should be repeated in 48 hours.

Important: Treatment of beef cattle should be limited to two (2) doses of Crystiben given by subcutaneous injection only.

Dogs: One ml per 10 to 25 lb body weight given intramuscularly or subcutaneously (6,000 to 15,000 units penicillin G procaine and 6,000 to 15,000 units penicillin G benzathine per lb body weight). Treatment should be repeated in 48 hours.

Shake the multiple-dose vial gently to avoid entrapped air bubbles before withdrawing the desired dose.

Caution: Federal law restricts this drug to use by or on the order of a licensed veterinarian.

How Supplied: Crystiben (Sterile Penicillin G Benzathine and Penicillin G Procaine) in Aqueous Suspension Veterinary is supplied in 100 ml multiple-dose vials. Each ml of suspension contains 150,000 units of penicillin G benzathine and 150,000 units of penicillin G procaine.

Storage: Store below 15°C (59°F). Keep from freezing.

CRYSTICILLIN® 300 A.S. VETERINARY

Sterile Penicillin G Procaine Suspension USP
Antibiotic • Injectable

Description: Crysticillin 300 A.S. Veterinary is available as an aqueous suspension in 100 ml and 250 ml multiple dose vials. Each ml provides 300,000 units penicillin G procaine with 0.13% methylparaben, 0.02% propylparaben, and 0.25% phenol as preservatives; 0.5% lecithin; 0.5% povidone; 1% sodium citrate; not more than 0.01% sodium formaldehyde sulfoxylate; and 0.075% carboxymethylcellulose sodium.

Actions: Penicillin G is an effective bactericide in the treatment of infections caused primarily by penicillin-sensitive organisms, such as *Streptococcus equi* and *Erysipelothrix insidiosa,* as well as the gram-negative organism *Pasteurella multocida.*

Indications: Crysticillin 300 A.S. Veterinary is indicated for the treatment of the following bacterial diseases:

1. *Cattle and Sheep* —bacterial pneumonia (shipping fever) caused by *Pasteurella multocida*
2. *Swine* —erysipelas caused by *Erysipelothrix insidiosa*
3. *Horses* —strangles caused by *Streptococcus equi*

Consult your veterinarian about your animals as you would your physician about your family, since effective treatment depends on accurate diagnosis of the infection to be treated.

Directions for Use: Crysticillin 300 A.S. Veterinary should be administered by deep intramuscular injection into the neck or hind leg, changing the site for each injection. Use a 16-gauge, 1½-inch needle. The needle and syringe should be washed thoroughly before use and boiled in water for at least 15 to 20 minutes. The injection site should be washed with soap and water and painted with a germicide such as tincture of iodine or 70% alcohol.

1. Crysticillin 300 A.S. Veterinary is ready for immediate injection after warming the vial to room temperature and shaking to insure uniform suspension.
2. Wipe the rubber stopper in the top of the vial with a piece of absorbent cotton wet with alcohol.
3. Inject air into the vial for easier withdrawal.
4. After filling the syringe, make sure the needle is empty by pulling back the plunger until a small air bubble appears. Then detach the needle from the syringe.
5. Insert the needle deeply into the muscle, attach the syringe and withdraw the plunger slightly. If blood appears, withdraw the needle and insert it in a different location.
6. Inject the dose slowly. 7. Not more than 10 ml should be injected in one location.

Dosage: The dosage for cattle, sheep, swine, and horses is 3,000 units per pound of body weight or 1.0 ml for each 100 pounds of body weight once daily.

Daily treatment should be continued for at least 48 hours after temperature has returned to normal and other signs of infection have subsided. Do not exceed 7 days of treatment in nonlactating dairy and beef cattle, sheep and swine or 5 days in lactating dairy cattle.

Animals treated with Crysticillin 300 A.S. Veterinary (Sterile Penicillin G Pro-

Continued on next page

Solvay—Cont.

caine Suspension USP) should show noticeable improvement within 36 to 48 hours. If improvement is not observed, consult your veterinarian.

Warnings:

1. Not for use in horses intended for food.
2. Milk that has been taken from animals during treatment and for 48 hours (four milkings) after the last treatment must not be used for food. The daily treatment schedule should not exceed 7 days of treatment in nonlactating dairy and beef cattle, sheep and swine or 5 days in lactating dairy cattle.
3. Discontinue use of this drug for the following time periods before treated animals are slaughtered for food: nonruminating cattle (calves)—7 days; all other cattle—4 days; sheep—8 days; swine—6 days.

Precautions: Sensitivity reactions to penicillin and procaine, for example, hives or respiratory distress, may occur in some animals. If such signs of sensitivity occur, stop medication and call your veterinarian. In some instances, particularly if respiratory distress is severe, immediate injection of epinephrine or antihistamine may be necessary.

S

As with any antibiotic preparation, prolonged use may result in overgrowth of nonsusceptible organisms, including fungi. If this condition is suspected, stop medication and consult your veterinarian.

How Supplied: In multiple dose vials of 100 and 250 ml.

Storage: Crysticillin 300 A. S. Veterinary should be stored in a refrigerator at a temperature below 15°C (59°F). Avoid freezing.

DIROCIDE® TABLETS
(diethylcarbamazine citrate tablets U.S.P.)

DIROCIDE® SYRUP
(diethylcarbamazine citrate syrup)

Description: Dirocide Tablets (Diethylcarbamazine Citrate Tablets U.S.P.) are available as Filmlok® tablets containing 50 mg, 100 mg, 200 mg and 300 mg diethycarbamazine citrate. (Filmlok is a Squibb trademark for veneer-coated tablets).

Dirocide Syrup (Diethylcarbamazine Citrate Syrup) is available as a palatable syrup containing 60 mg Diethylcarbamazine Citrate U.S.P. per ml.

Actions: (Diethylcarbamazine citrate is a relatively nontoxic piperazine derivative; no cumulative or toxic effects have been reported in dogs. Daily administration of diethylcarbamazine citrate to dogs has been shown to be effective in both laboratory and field studies in preventing the maturation of *D. immitis*. This preventive regimen has been recommended by participants of the First International Symposium on Canine Heartworm Disease.

Diethylcarbamazine citrate is also effective in the treatment of ascarid infections of *Toxocara canis* and *Toxascaris leonina* in dogs and *Toxocara cati* in cats when administered at therapeutic doses, and for the prevention of *T. canis* and *T. leonina* infections in dogs when administered daily in relatively low dosages.

Indications: Dirocide Tablets (Diethylcarbamazine Citrate Tablets U.S.P.) and Dirocide Syrup (Diethylcarbamazine Citrate Syrup) are indicated for use in dogs for the prevention of infection with *Dirofilaria immitis* (heartworm disease), and *T. canis* and *T. leonina*. They are also used as an aid in the treatment of ascarid infections caused by *T. canis* and *T. leonina* in dogs and *T. cati* in cats.

Warnings: Older dogs should be proven negative for the presence of *D. immitis* infection before starting diethylcarbamazine citrate.

This product should not be used in any dog that has not been determined to be free of heartworm infection.

Dogs with proven infection of *D. immitis* should be rendered negative using adulticidal and microfilaricidal drugs before starting diethylcarbamazine citrate.

Precautions: The use of diethylcarbamazine citrate is NOT RECOMMENDED IN DOGS WITH ACTIVE *D. immitis* INFECTIONS. An infection of *D. immitis* is a serious disease involving vital organs. Once the infection is established, treatment involves a degree of risk in all cases.

NOTE: The activity of diethylcarbamazine citrate against the other most common dog filariae, *Dipetalonema reconditum*, is not known.

Dosage and Administration: Dirocide Tablets (Diethylcarbamazine Citrate Tablets U.S.P.)

Prevention of Heartworm Disease and Ascarid Infection in Dogs: Dirocide Tablets (Diethylcarbamazine Citrate Tablets U.S.P.) are given orally (once a day) at a dosage rate of 3 mg diethylcarbamazine citrate per pound of body weight. Young dogs may be started on the prevention program at two months of age. Heartworm preventive medication should be initiated one month before the mosquito season and continued daily throughout the mosquito season and for two months thereafter.

A recommended dosage schedule for dogs with a body weight of 16 lbs is one 50 mg tablet or ½ of a 100 mg tablet; for 33 lbs, two 50 mg tablets or one 100 mg tablet or ½ of a 200 mg tablet; for 50 lbs, three 50 mg tablets or 1½ 100 mg tablets or ½ of a 300 mg. tablet; for 66 lbs, two 100 mg tablets or one 200 mg tablet; for 85 lbs, 2½ 100 mg tablets; for 100 lbs, 1½ 200 mg tablets or one 300 mg tablet; for 133 lbs, two 200 mg tablets; for 150 lbs, 1½ 300 mg tablets; for 200 lbs, two 300 mg tablets.

Treatment of Ascarid Infection in Dogs and Cats: Dirocide Tablets (Diethylcarbamazine Citrate Tablets U.S.P.) are given orally at a dosage rate of 25 to 50 mg of diethylcarbamazine citrate per pound of body weight. Fasting before treatment or a laxative after treatment is not necessary. To reduce the possibility of vomiting, which occasionally occurs if the animal's stomach is empty, it is preferable to administer the oral dose of Dirocide Tablets (Diethylcarbamazine Citrate Tablets U.S.P.) immediately after feeding. A repeat dose should be given in 10 to 20 days to remove immature worms which may enter the intestine from the lungs after the initial treatment.

Dirocide Syrup (Diethylcarbamazine Citrate Syrup) **Prevention of Heartworm and Ascarid Infections in Dogs:** Dirocide (Diethylcarbamazine Citrate Syrup) may be mixed with either dry or wet feed; it does not require special preparation prior to, or during administration. The drug is added to the daily food ration (once a day) at a dosage rate of 3 mg/lb of body weight. The drug is supplied in a syrup base and has been found to be highly palatable to dogs. Repeated administration over a period exceeding 3 years has shown no rejection of palatability.

Feeding habits have not been observed to be altered upon addition of the drug to feed.

A recommended dosage schedule for prevention of heartworm and ascarid infections in dogs with a body weight of 10 lbs is 0.5 ml of syrup; for 20 lbs, 1.0 ml; for 30 lbs, 1.5 ml; for 40 lbs, 2.0 ml; for 50 lbs, 2.5 ml; for 60 lbs, 3.0 ml; for 70 lbs, 3.5 ml; for 80 lbs, 4.0 ml.

If the dog rejects food, the drug may be given directly by mouth. Young dogs may be started at two months of age. Heartworm preventive medication should be initiated one month before the mosquito season and continued daily throughout the mosquito season and for two months thereafter.

Treatment of Ascarid Infections in Dogs and Cats: Fasting before treatment or giving a laxative after treatment is not necessary. It is preferable to administer the oral dose of Dirocide (Diethylcarbamazine Citrate Syrup) immediately after feeding.

Dosage for treatment of ascarid infections in dogs and cats is 25 mg to 50 mg of diethylcarbamazine citrate per pound of body weight. A recommended dosage schedule for dogs and cats with a body weight of 5 lbs is 2.25 to 4.0 ml; for 10 lbs, 4.5 to 8.0 ml; for 15 lbs, 6.75 to 12.0 ml; for 20 lbs, 9.0 to 16.0 ml; for 25 lbs, 11.25 to 20.0 ml; for 30 lbs, 13.5 to 24.0 ml.

How Supplied: Dirocide Tablets (Diethylcarbamazine Citrate Tablets U.S.P.) are available as scored tablets providing 50 mg diethylcarbamazine citrate per tablet in bottles of 200 and 500 tablets; they are also available as scored tablets providing 100 mg, 200 mg and 300 mg diethylcarbamazine citrate per tablet in bottles of 100 and 200 tablets. The 200 and 300 mg tablets are also available in bottles of 1000 tablets. Dirocide Syrup (Diethylcarbamazine Citrate Syrup) is available in 4 oz and 8 oz plastic bottles and one gallon plastic jugs.

Storage: Store the tablets at room temperature; avoid excessive heat. Store the syrup at room temperature; avoid excessive heat; protect from light.

Caution: Federal law restricts these drugs to use by or on the order of a licensed veterinarian.

DISTRYCILLIN® A.S. VETERINARY
Penicillin G Procaine in Dihydrostreptomycin Sulfate Solution For Intramuscular Use in Animals Only

Description: Distrycillin A.S. Veterinary is a highly effective antimicrobial preparation. Each 2 ml of this sterile, aqueous suspension provides 400,000 units penicillin G procaine and dihydrostreptomycin sulfate equivalent to 0.5 gram dihydrostreptomycin base with 0.015% butylparaben, 0.25% liquefied phenol, and 0.37% sodium formaldehyde sulfoxylate as preservatives, 2% procaine hydrochloride, 1.25% sodium citrate, 2% dibasic sodium phosphite, 0.5% povidone, 0.25% lecithin, 0.21% urea and sodium hydroxide.
Penicillin is a potent antibiotic possessing a high degree of activity chiefly against organisms in the gram-positive category. Dihydrostreptomycin is a potent antibiotic possessing a high degree of activity chiefly against organisms in the gram-negative category. The combination permits treatment of many mixed bacterial infections with the convenience of a single dosage form.
Warnings: Milk that has been taken from animals during treatment and for 48 hours (4 milkings) after the latest treatment must not be used for food. The use of this drug must be discontinued for 30 days before treated animals are slaughtered for food. In lactating dairy animals, do not inject more than 2,000 units of penicillin or 2.5 mg of dihydrostreptomycin per pound of body weight per day. Exceeding the highest recommended dosage level may result in antibiotic residues in meat or milk beyond the withdrawal time.
Indications: *Cattle* — Actinomycosis; bronchitis; calf diphtheria; foot rot; joint infections; leptospirosis; mastitis; metritis; navel infections; pleurisy; pneumonia; shipping fever; systemic bacterial complications associated with scours; tracheitis; wound infections, and other infections caused by or associated with penicillin- and dihydrostreptomycin-susceptible organisms.
Swine —Bronchitis; leptospirosis; mastitis; metritis; pleurisy; pneumonia; systemic bacterial complications associated with scours; tracheitis; wound infections, and other infections caused by or associated with penicillin- and dihydrostreptomycin-susceptible organisms.
Sheep —Joint infections; leptospirosis; mastitis; metritis; navel infections; shipping fever; pneumonia; systemic bacterial complications associated with scours; tularemia; wound infections, and other infections caused by or associated with penicillin- and dihydrostreptomycin-susceptible organisms.
Horses —Bacterial complications associated with influenza; bronchitis; joint infections; metritis; navel infections; pleurisy; pneumonia; shipping fever; systemic bacterial complications associated with scours; wound infections, and other infections caused by or associated with penicillin- and dihydrostreptomycin-susceptible organisms.
Small Animals (dogs, cats, mink, rabbits, foxes) -Bacterial complications associated with viral diseases, such as those in distemper; bronchitis; middle ear infections; leptospirosis; metritis; pleurisy; pneumonia; snuffles; sore hocks; systemic bacterial complications associated with enteritis; tracheitis; tularemia; wound infections, and other infections caused by or associated with penicillin- and dihydrostreptomycin-susceptible organisms.
Recommended Daily Dosage: Continue treatment for one to two days after symptoms disappear.

CATTLE:

Body Weight	Dosage
Up to 100 lbs	2 ml
100 to 300 lbs	2 to 6 ml
300 to 700 lbs	6 to 10 ml
700 lbs or over	10 to 15 ml

For cattle use 16 or 18 gauge, 1 or 1½ inch needle.

SWINE

Body Weight	Dosage
8 to 10 lbs	¼ to ½ ml
10 to 20 lbs	½ to 1 ml
20 to 40 lbs	1 to 2 ml
40 to 100 lbs	2 to 4 ml
100 to 200 lbs	4 to 6 ml
200 lbs or over	6 to 10 ml

For swine use 18 gauge, 1 inch needle.

SHEEP

Body Weight	Dosage
8 to 10 lbs	¼ to ½ ml
10 to 20 lbs	½ to 1 ml
20 to 50 lbs	1 to 2 ml
50 lbs or over	2 to 6 ml

For sheep use 18 gauge, 1 inch needle.

HORSES

Body Weight	Dosage
Up to 300 lbs	4 to 8 ml
300 to 600 lbs	8 to 10 ml
600 lbs or over	10 to 15 ml

For horses use 16 or 18 gauge, 1½ or 2 inch needle.

SMALL ANIMALS (dogs, cats, mink, rabbits, foxes)

Body Weight	Dosage
3 to 5 lbs	⅛ to ¼ ml
5 to 10 lbs	¼ to ½ ml
10 to 15 lbs	½ to ¾ ml
15 to 20 lbs	¾ to 1 ml
20 to 25 lbs	1 to 1¼ ml
25 to 50 lbs.	1¼ to 2 ml
50 to 75 lbs	2 to 3 ml
75 lbs or over	3 to 4 ml

For small animals use 20 gauge, ¾ to 1 inch needle.

Directions for Use:
1. Use sterile equipment only. Syringes and needles should be completely disassembled, scrubbed, rinsed and then boiled in water for 15 minutes (boiling time) before using. Reassemble syringe without touching that portion of plunger that fits into barrel of syringe. When attaching needle to syringe, touch needle at hub only.
2. Shake the vial gently but sufficiently to insure complete mixing of contents, and remove the small round metal seal to expose the rubber cap on the vial.
3. Wipe the rubber cap with a suitable disinfectant, such as 70 percent alcohol; insert the needle through the center of the rubber cap and draw the required dosage into the syringe.
4. Clean the skin of the animal at the site of injection with a suitable disinfectant, such as 70 percent alcohol.
5. Direct the needle into the thick muscles of the rump, hip, or thigh, avoiding blood vessels and major nerves.
6. Pull back on plunger slightly. If blood appears in the syringe, a blood vessel has been entered; withdraw the needle and choose a different injection site.
7. If the above directions have been carefully followed, and if no blood appears in the syringe, complete the injection.

Care of Sick Animals: The diagnosis and treatment of many animal diseases require the professional services of a veterinarian. Proper therapy, good nursing, nutritious diet and good sanitation practices are essential factors in the management of sick animals. Always provide warm, dry quarters, clean bedding, good food and clean water.

Caution:
1. Distrycillin A.S. Veterinary should be injected deep within the fleshy muscles of the hip, rump, round or thigh. Do *not* inject this material subcutaneously (under the skin), into a blood vessel, or near a major nerve.
2. When properly used in the treatment of diseases caused by susceptible organisms, most sick animals that have been treated with antibiotics show a noticeable improvement within 48 hours. If improvement does not occur within that period of time, the diagnosis should be reconsidered and appropriate treatment initiated.
3. Penicillin G procaine is a substance of low toxicity. However, side effects, or so-called allergic or anaphylactic reactions—sometimes fatal—have been known to occur in animals hypersensitive to penicillin and procaine. The use of this product is therefore contraindicated in animals that are hypersensitive to either penicillin or procaine. Animals treated with Districyllin A.S. Veterinary should be kept under close observation for at least one-half hour. Should allergic or anaphylactic reactions occur, discontinue use of this product and call a veterinarian. The immediate injection of epinephrine and antihistamines, following manufacturers recommendations, is considered appropriate emergency therapy.
4. Dihydrostreptomycin is eliminated to a large extent through the kidneys. The use of this product is therefore contraindicated in animals suffering from conditions in which there is impairment of kidney function or obstruction to the free flow of urine.
5. Distrycillin A.S. Veterinary should be stored below 15° C (59° F). Warm to room temperature and shake before using.

Continued on next page

S

Solvay—Cont.

How Supplied: Distrycillin A.S. Veterinary (Penicillin G Procaine in Dihydrostreptomycin Sulfate Solution) is available in 100 ml and 250 ml vials. The 250 ml multiple dose vial is specifically intended for use in treatment of herds of large animals. It may be considered suitable for rabbits, mink and foxes only when an automatic syringe is used to treat large groups of animals at one time.

ECLIPSE™ 1
Feline Panleukopenia Vaccine, Modified Live Virus, Cell Line Origin

Indications: Eclipse 1 is a modified live virus vaccine for immunizing cats against feline panleukopenia. The virus is propagated in feline cell line cultures.
Eclipse 1 produces a rapid prolonged immunity with a 1 ml dose.
Eclipse 1 can be used in cats of all ages (not in pregnant cats.)
Attenuation in cell line eliminates virulence, but maintains a high immune response.
Dosage and Administration: Rehydrate each vaccine vial with 1 ml of vaccine diluent. Inject intramuscularly or subcutaneously into 9–10 week old kittens. Repeat dose in 3–4 weeks until 12 weeks old. Cats 12 weeks of age or older require only one dose of vaccine. Annual revaccination with one dose is recommended. DO NOT VACCINATE PREGNANT CATS. Transfer diluent vial contents to vaccine vial aseptically. Do not chemically sterilize needles and syringes.
Precautions: Use of any biological may produce anaphylactoid reactions:
Antidote: Epinephrine.
The vaccine contains gentamicin and a fungistat as preservatives. Store at 2–7°C. Burn the container and all unused contents.
How Supplied: Unit size: Box of 10 single doses

ECLIPSE™ 1 KP
Feline Panleukopenia Vaccine, Killed Virus Cell Line Origin

Indications: Eclipse 1 KP contains feline panleukopenia virus propagated in feline cell line cultures. The virus is chemically inactivated and is recommended for immunizing cats against feline panleukopenia.
Eclipse 1 KP can be used in cats of all ages and in pregnant queens.
There is no chance of reversion to virulence with a killed product.
Dosage and Administration: Inject intramuscularly or subcutaneously. Vaccinate healthy cats of any age with one dose followed by a second dose 7 to 10 days later. If animals receive both vaccinations prior to 12 weeks of age, a third dose is recommended. Annual revaccination with one dose is recommended.
Precautions: Use of any biological may produce anaphylactoid reactions.
Antidote: Epinephrine.
Store at 2–7°C. Vaccine contains gentamicin, a fungistat, and thimerosal as preservatives; inactivating agent: B-propiolactone.
How Supplied: Unit size: Box of 20 vials each containing 1 ml of Eclipse 1 KP, or one vial, good for 10 injections.

ECLIPSE™ 3
Feline Rhinotracheitis-Calici-Panleukopenia Vaccine, Modified Live Virus—Cell Line Origin

Indications: Eclipse 3 is a modified live vaccine which immunizes cats against feline rhinotracheitis, calici, and panleukopenia viruses. The viruses are propagated in feline cell line cultures.
Modified Live virus insures rapid and prolonged immunization.
Eclipse 3 and Eclipse 4 may be used together to immunize cats against FVR, FCV, and FPL. Give a dose of Eclipse 3, then a dose of Eclipse 4 3–4 weeks later.
Dosage and Administration: Rehydrate each vaccine vial with 1 ml of vaccine diluent. Inject intramuscularly or subcutaneously into 9–10 week old kittens. Repeat dose in 3–4 weeks. Revaccinate those kittens vaccinated before 9 weeks every 3–4 weeks until 12 weeks old. Adult cats require one dose, and another 3–4 weeks later. Annual revaccination with one dose is recommended. DO NOT VACCINATE PREGNANT CATS. Transfer diluent vial contents to vaccine vial aseptically. Do not chemically sterilize needles and syringes.
Eclipse 3 may be used in conjunction with Eclipse 4 (Feline Rhinotracheitis-Calici-Panleukopenia-Pneumonitis Vaccine) for immunization of cats. Kittens 9–10 weeks old may be given one dose of Eclipse 3 followed by a dose of Eclipse 4 3–4 weeks later. Two doses of feline rhinotracheitis and calicivirus are required for a prophylactic dose.
Precautions: Use of any biological may produce anaphylactoid reactions.
Antidote: Epinephrine.
The vaccine contains gentamicin and a fungistat as preservatives. Store at 2–7°C. Burn this container and all unused contents.
How Supplied: Unit size: Box of either 10 or 50 single doses

ECLIPSE™ 3 KP
Feline Rhinotracheitis-Calici-Panleukopenia Vaccine, Modified Live and Killed Virus, Cell Line Origin

Indications: Eclipse 3 KP is a modified live and killed virus vaccine for immunization against feline viral rhinotracheitis, calici, and panleukopenia viruses. Viruses are propagated in feline cell line cultures. Feline panleukopenia virus is chemically inactivated.
Killed feline panleukopenia virus vaccine causes less stress.
Eclipse 3 KP and Fromm's Eclipse 4 KP may be used together to immunize cats against FVR, FCV, and FPL. Give a dose of Eclipse 3 KP, then a dose of Eclipse 4 KP 3–4 weeks later.
Dosage and Administration: Rehydrate each lyophilized vaccine vial with 1 ml of vaccine diluent. Inject intramuscularly or subcutaneously into kittens 9–10 weeks old. Repeat dose in 3–4 weeks. Revaccinate those kittens vaccinated before 9 weeks every 3–4 weeks until 12 weeks old. Adult cats require one dose, and another 3–4 weeks later. Annual revaccination with one dose is recommended. DO NOT VACCINATE PREGNANT CATS. Transfer diluent vial contents to vaccine vial aseptically. Do not chemically sterilize needles and syringes.
Eclipse 3 KP may be used in conjunction with Eclipse 4 KP (Feline Rhinotracheitis-Calici-Panleukopenia-Pneumonitis Vaccine) for immunization of cats. Kittens 9–10 weeks old may be given one dose of Eclipse 3 KP followed by a second dose of Eclipse 4 KP 3–4 weeks later. Two doses of Feline Rhinotracheitis, Calici, and Panleukopenia virus are required for a prophylactic dose.
Precautions: Use of any biological may produce anaphylactoid reactions.
Antidote: Epinephrine.
Vaccines contains gentamicin and a fungistat as preservatives and B-propiolactone as an inactivating agent. Store at 2–7°C. Burn the container and all unused contents.
How Supplied: Unit size: Box of either 10 or 50 single doses

ECLIPSE™ 3 KP-R
Rhinotracheitis-Calici-Panleukopenia-Rabies Vaccine-Modified Live and Killed Virus, Cell Line Origin

Indications: Eclipse 3 KP-R is a modified live and killed virus vaccine for immunization against feline viral rhinotracheitis, calici, panleukopenia and rabies viruses. Viruses are propagated in feline cell line cultures. Feline panleukopenia and rabies viruses are chemically inactivated. Eclipse 3 KP-R consists of a panleukopenia, calici, and rhinotracheitis vaccine with rabies as the diluent.The killed rabies virus, feline cell line origin, provides added safety not found in modified live virus vaccines. Annual revaccination.
Dosage and Administration: Rehydrate each lyophilized vaccine vial with 1 ml of vaccine diluent. ***Inject kittens*** 9-10 weeks old with one dose intramuscularly at one site in the thigh. Repeat dose in 3-4 weeks. ***Adult cats*** require one dose and another dose 3-4 weeks later. Annual revaccination with one dose is recommended. DO NOT VACCINATE PREGNANT CATS. Transfer vaccine diluent vial contents to vaccine vial aseptically. Do not chemically sterilize needles and syringes.
Eclipse 3 KP-R may be used in conjunction with Eclipse 3 or Eclipse 3 KP (Feline Rhinotracheitis-Calici-Panleukopenia Vaccine) or Eclipse 4 or Eclipse 4 KP (Feline Rhinotracheitis-Calici-Panleukopenia-Pneumonitis Vaccine) as the initial dose in kittens 9-10 weeks old fol-

lowed by Eclipse 3 KP-R 3-4 weeks later when cats are 3 months old. Eclipse 3 KP-R must be given intramuscularly at one site in the thigh. Two doses of feline rhinotracheitis and calici vaccines are required for a prophylactic dose. Shake vaccine diluent before use.
Precautions: Store at 2-7°C. Do not freeze. The use of any biological may produce anaphylactoid reactions.
Antidote: Epinephrine.
The vaccine contains gentamicin, a fungistat, and thimerosal as preservatives; and β-propiolactone as an inactivating agent. Burn this container and all unused contents.
How Supplied: Box of either 10 or 50 single doses.

ECLIPSE™ 4
Feline Rhinotracheitis-Calici-Panleukopenia-Chlamydia Vaccine, Cell Line Origin

Description: Eclipse 4 is a modified live virus and chlamydia vaccine which immunizes cats against feline rhinotracheitis, calici, panleukopenia viruses and chlamydia (pneumonitis). The viruses and chlamydia are propagated in approved cell lines.
Dosage and Administration: Rehydrate each lyophilized vaccine vial with 1 ml of sterile diluent. Inject intramuscularly or subcutaneously into 9–10 week old kittens. Revaccinate those kittens vaccinated before 9 weeks every 3–4 weeks until 12 weeks old. Adult cats require one dose, and another 3–4 weeks later (two doses of feline rhinotracheitis and calicivirus are required for a prophylactic dose). Annual revaccination with one dose is recommended. DO NOT VACCINATE PREGNANT CATS. Transfer diluent vial contents to vaccine vial aseptically. Do not chemically sterilize needles and syringes.
Eclipse 3 may be used in conjunction with Eclipse 4 for immunization of cats. Kittens 9–10 weeks old may be given one dose of Eclipse 3 followed by a dose of Eclipse 4, 3–4 weeks later.
Precautions: Use of any biological may produce anaphylactoid reactions.
Antidote: Epinephrine.
The vaccine contains gentamicin and a fungistat as preservatives. Store at 2–7° C. Burn the container and all unused contents.
How Supplied: Unit size: Box of either 10 or 50 single 1 ml doses.

ECLIPSE™ 4 KP
Feline Rhinotracheitis-Calici-Panleukopenia-Pneumonitis Vaccine, Modified Live and Killed Virus and Modified Live Chlamydia, Cell Line Origin

Indications: Eclipse 4 KP is a modified live and killed virus and chlamydia vaccine for immunization against pneumonitis and feline viral rhinotracheitis, calici, and panleukopenia viruses. Viruses and chlamydia are propagated in cell line cultures. Feline panleukopenia virus is chemically inactivated. Killed Feline Panleukopenia Vaccine causes less stress.
Eclipse 4 KP and Eclipse 3 KP may be used together to immunize cats against FVR, FCV, and FPL. Give a dose of Eclipse 3 KP, then a dose of Eclipse 4 KP 3-4 weeks later for complete immunization.
Dosage and Administration: Rehydrate each lyophilized vaccine vial with 1 ml of vaccine diluent. Inject intramuscularly or subcutaneously into kittens 9–10 weeks old. Repeat dose in 3–4 weeks. Revaccinate those kittens vaccinated before 9 weeks every 3–4 weeks until 12 weeks old. Adult cats require one dose, and another 3–4 weeks later. Annual revaccination with one dose is recommended. DO NOT VACCINATE PREGNANT CATS. Transfer diluent vial contents to vaccine vial aseptically. Do not chemically sterilize needles and syringes.
Eclipse 3 KP may be used in conjunction with Eclipse 4 KP (Feline Rhinotracheitis-Calici-Panleukopenia-Pneumonitis Vaccine) for immunization of cats. Kittens 9–10 weeks old may be given one dose of Eclipse 3 KP followed by a second dose of Eclipse 4 KP 3–4 weeks later. Two doses of Feline Rhinotracheitis, Calici, and Panleukopenia virus are required for a prophylactic dose.
Precautions: Use of any biological may produce anaphylactoid reactions.
Antidote: Epinephrine.
Vaccines contain gentamicin and fungistat as preservatives, and B-propiolactone as an inactivating agent. Store at 2–7° C. Burn the container and all unused contents.
How Supplied: Unit size: Box of either 10 or 50 single dose.

ECLIPSE™ 4 KP-R
Feline Rhinotracheitis-Calici-Chlamydia-Panleukopenia-Rabies Vaccine Modified Live and Killed Virus and Modified Live Chlamydia, Cell Line Origin

Indications: Eclipse 4 KP-R is a modified live and killed virus plus chlamydia vaccine for immunization against pneumonitis and feline viral rhinotracheitis, calici, panleukopenia and rabies viruses. Feline panleukopenia is chemically inactivated and desiccated with the attenuated fraction. The rabies vaccine is chemically inactivated.
Dosage and Administration: Rehydrate each lyophilized vaccine vial with 1 ml of vaccine diluent. ***Inject kittens*** 9-10 weeks old with one dose intramuscularly at one site in the thigh. Repeat dose in 3-4 weeks. Annual revaccination with one dose is recommended. Do not vaccinate pregnant cats. Transfer vaccine diluent vial contents to vaccine vial aseptically. Do not chemically sterilize needles and syringes.
Eclipse 4 KP-R may be used in conjunction with Eclipse 3 or Eclipse 3 KP (Feline Rhinotracheitis-Calici-Panleukopenia Vaccine) or Eclipse 4 or Eclipse 4 KP (Feline Rhinotracheitis-Calici-Panleukopenia-Penumonitis Vaccine) as the initial dose in kittens 9-10 weeks old followed by Eclipse 4 KP-R 3-4 weeks later when cats are 3 months old. Eclipse 4 KP-R must be given intramuscularly at one site in the thigh. Two doses of feline rhinotracheitis and calici vaccines are required for a prophylactic dose. Shake vaccine diluent before use.
Precautions: Store at 2-7° C. Do not freeze. The use of any biological may produce anaphylactoid reactions.
Antidote: Epinephrine.
The vaccine contains gentamicin and a fungistat as preservatives; and β-propiolactone as an inactivating agent. Burn this container and all unused contents.
How Supplied: Box of either 10 or 50 single doses

EQUIPOISE®
Boldenone Undecylenate Injection For Intramuscular Use in Horses Only

Description: Equipoise (Boldenone Undecylenate Injection) is a long-acting injectable anabolic agent for horses, supplied in vials providing 25 or 50 mg boldenone undecylenate per ml in sesame oil with 3% (w/v) benzyl alcohol as a preservative. At the time of manufacture, the air in the container is replaced by nitrogen.
Boldenone undecylenate is a steroid ester possessing marked anabolic properties and a minimal amount of androgenic activity.
Anabolic and androgenic agents have come to be used widely in the treatment of certain pathophysiological or catabolic processes in man and animals. In many instances it is desirable to maintain a constant level of effect over a long period of time. Equipoise (Boldenone Undecylenate Injection) is a long-acting injectable agent which has a rapid onset of action; this is advantageous and is preferred over frequent oral dosing or even repeated injections.
Actions: Anabolic agents are related to the sex hormones, but each varies in its anabolic and androgenic effect. Compounds such as methyltestosterone have anabolic activity, but with prolonged use, animals develop marked androgenic activity which makes these compounds unsuitable for prolonged therapy.
Pharmacological studies conducted in laboratory animals to evaluate the pharmacological activity characterized Equipoise (Boldenone Undecylenate Injection) as having distinct anabolic properties together with a certain degree of androgenic activity. It does not have marked antigonadotrophic properties nor does it produce any clear-cut effects on the endometrium, conditions that are commonly observed when similar substances are used.
In clinical trials, at the recommended dosage, Equipoise (Boldenone Undecylenate Injection) has a marked anabolic effect in debilitated horses; appetite improved, vigor increased, and improvement was noted in musculature and haircoat. This would be expected with an anabolic agent such as Equipoise (Boldenone

Continued on next page

Solvay—Cont.

Undecylenate Injection), particularly where there had been marked tissue breakdown associated with disease, prolonged anorexia, or overwork.
Indications: Equipoise (Boldenone Undecylenate Injection) is recommended as an aid for treating debilitated horses when an improvement in weight, haircoat, or general physical condition is desired. Debilitation often follows disease or may occur following overwork and overexertion.
Equipoise (Boldenone Undecylenate Injection) improves the general state of debilitated horses thus aiding in correcting weight losses and improving appetite. It is not a substitute for a well-balanced diet. Optimal results can be expected only when good management and feeding practices are utilized.
Equipoise (Boldenone Undecylenate Injection) should be considered only as adjunctive therapy to other specific and supportive therapy for diseases, surgical cases, and traumatic injuries.
Dosage and Administration: The dosage for horses is 0.5 mg per pound of body weight intramuscularly. Treatment may be repeated at three week intervals. The condition should be assessed by the veterinarian to determine the duration of treatment; however, most horses will respond with one or two treatments.
Adverse Reactions: With Equipoise (Boldenone Undecylenate Injection), androgenic (overaggressiveness) effects may be noted in a few animals. If these effects occur, they may persist for up to 6 to 8 weeks. No additional injections of boldenone undecylenate should be administered.
Warnings: For horses only. Do not administer to horses intended for use as food. In the absence of data on the effect of boldenone undecylenate on stallions, on pregnant mares, and the teratogenicity on the offspring, this drug should not be used in these animals.
How Supplied: Supplied for veterinary use in 10 ml vials providing 25 or 50 boldenone undecylenate per ml and in 50 ml vials providing 50 mg boldenone undecylenate per ml.
Storage: Store at room temperature; avoid freezing.
Caution: Federal law restricts this drug to use by or on the order of a licensed veterinarian.

FLEA COLLAR FOR CATS

Composition:

Active Ingredients:	
2,2-dichlorovinyl dimethyl phosphate	4.8%*
Related compounds	0.2%
Inert ingredients	95.0%
TOTAL	100.00%

*Equivalent to 5% w/w Technical DDVP Insecticide.
Indications: For long-lasting flea control in cats.
Dosage and Administration: Place Flea Collar around cat's neck, adjust for proper fit and snap in place. The collar must be worn loosely and in addition to the regular collar. If collar is worn too tightly, it may produce neck irritation. Cut off and dispose of the excess length. Flea kill begins at once and will continue for 3 months while the collar is worn. For continuous protection, replace collar when effectiveness diminishes. When bathing cat, remove collar until cat is dry.
Caution: Do not open protective pouch until ready to use. Do not allow children to play with this collar. Do not use on Persians. Do not use on sick or convalescing cats. Remove collar at first sign of irritation or adverse reaction. Do not use any other pesticides on cat while collar is worn. Collar is intended for use only as an insecticide generator (US Patent 3,318,769) and is not to be taken internally by man or animals.
How Supplied: Individually packaged, clear collars.

FLEA COLLAR FOR DOGS

Composition:

Active Ingredients:	
2,2-dichlorovinyl dimethyl phosphate	9.6%*
Related compounds	0.4%*
Inert Ingredients:	90.0%
TOTAL	100.0%

*Equivalent to 10% w/w Technical DDVP Insecticide.
Indications: For long-lasting flea control in dogs. Aids in tick control, especially in neck area.
Directions: Place Flea Collar around dog's neck, adjust for proper fit and snap in place. The collar must be worn loosely and in addition to the regular collar. If collar is worn too tightly, it may produce neck irritation. Cut off and dispose of the excess length. Flea kill begins at once and will continue for 3 months while the collar is worn. Ticks are harder to kill but those on the neck area will soon be killed and easily removed. Collar will continue to kill ticks for eight weeks. For continuous protection, replace collar every 3 months.
Flea Collar can be worn with regular collar. Remove collar when washing dog—replace when dry.
Caution: Do not open protective pouch until ready to use. Do not allow children to play with this collar. Do not use on cats, whippets and greyhounds. Some dogs may be sensitive to this collar. Remove collar at first sign of irritation or adverse reaction. Do not use on sick or convalescing dogs. Do not use any other pesticide on dog while collar is worn. Collar is intended for use only as an insecticide generator (US Patent 3,318,769 and Design Patent 214,736) and is not to be taken internally by man or animals.
How Supplied: Individually packaged; available in clear or black.

FOLLUTEIN
Chorionic Gonadotropin for Injection U.S.P.
For veterinary use only

Description: Follutein (Chorionic Gonadotropin for Injection U.S.P.) is a sterile, lyophilized, highly purified powder of the anterior pituitary-like hormone isolated from gravid human urine.
Actions: Cystic ovaries in the cow are primarily due to a derangement of the mechanism of ovulation and corpus luteum formation. In affected cows, the luteinizing hormone from the anterior pituitary is released in inadequate amounts or not at all, so that ovulation does not occur and ovarian cysts develop. The affected cows are nearly always disposed to take the bull, but they rarely conceive.
In an encouragingly high percentage of cases, cows with cystic ovaries respond to therapy with chorionic gonadotropin. The hormone induces luteinization of the cystic follicles and ultimately a normal estrus cycle is reestablished. Within a few days after administration of chorionic gonadotropin, luteinization of the cystic follicles can be ascertained by rectal examination of the ovaries.
Indications: Follutein is intended for parenteral use in cows for the treatment of nymphomania (frequent or constant heat) due to cystic ovaries.
Adverse Reactions: Follutein (Chorionic Gonadotropin for Injection U.S.P.) is highly purified, consequently allergic reactions are extremely rare. If allergic symptoms occur, epinephrine and an antihistamine should be administered promptly.
Dosage and Administration: To reconstitute, draw 10 ml. of the diluent into a sterile syringe and inject it into the vial containing the powder. The resultant mixture provides 1000 U.S.P. Units of chorionic gonadotropin per ml.
The recommended dose is 10,000 U.S.P. Units as a single injection, administered by deep intramuscular injection, or 2500 to 5000 U.S.P. Units administered intravenously. Dosage may be repeated in 14 days if the animals behavior or rectal examination of the ovaries indicates the necessity for retreatment.
One investigator has reported the satisfactory administration of chorionic gonadotropin by injection directly into the ovarian cyst, either through the vaginal wall or by insertion of a long needle through the ischiorectal fossa. He suggests the vaginal route for pluriparous cows and the alternate approach for heifers, young cows, and cows of the smaller breeds. After penetration of the needle into the follicular cyst, some of the cystic fluid is allowed to drain before the hormone is injected. Doses of 500 to 2500 U.S.P. Units are recommended for intrafollicular administration.
Caution: Federal law restricts this drug to use by or on the order of a licensed veterinarian.
How Supplied: Follutein (Chorionic Gonadotropin for Injection U.S.P.) is available in vials providing 10,000 U.S.P. Units with 83 mg. sodium chloride per vial and sodium hydroxide to adjust the pH of the reconstituted solution. When reconstituted with the accompanying 10 ml. sterile aqueous diluent, each ml. provides 1000 U.S.P Units chorionic gonadotropin with 0.5 phenol as a preservative

and sodium hydroxide or hydrochloric acid to adjust the pH to 6.0—8.0. At the time of manufacture, the air in the diluent container is replaced by nitrogen.
Storage: After reconstitution, the preparation should be stored in a refrigerator. When refrigerated, the solution retains its potency for 2 months; thereafter potency slowly diminishes.

FROMM™ D
Canine Distemper Vaccine, Modified Live Virus
Chicken Tissue Culture Origin

Indications: Fromm D is a modified live vaccine for immunization against canine distemper. The canine distemper virus is propagated in chicken cell cultures. Transfer the entire contents of the diluent vial to the vaccine vial aseptically. Needle and syringes must not be sterilized chemically.
Fromm D is totally avirulent, no stress exhibited; has been safely used in ferrets and grey foxes.
It cross immunizes with all known strains of distemper virus for complete protection against distemper.
Dosage and Administration: Rehydrate each vial of vaccine with 1 ml of diluent and inject subcutaneously or intramuscularly. One dose is recommended for dogs 12 weeks or age or older. A dog vaccinated prior to 12 weeks of age should be given a second dose at 12-14 weeks of age. This is necessary because maternally acquired antibodies may interfere with development of active immunity.
Booster immunization is recommended for bitches prior to or after breeding to assure that adequate maternal immunity is conferred to the puppies postwhelping. Annual revaccination of all dogs is recommended for continued immunity.
For best immunization response, the vaccinated dog should be in a good state of health, not heavily parasitized, and on a well-balanced diet.
Precautions: The use of any biological may produce anaphylactoid reactions. In this event, use of epinephrine is recommended. *The vaccine contains gentamicin and a fungistat as preservatives.* Store at 2°–7°C. Burn the container and all unused contents.
How Supplied: Box of 10 single doses

GALAXY® DA$_2$L
Canine Distemper-Adenovirus Type 2-Modified Live Virus-Chicken Tissue Culture and Cell Line Origin, Leptospira Bacterin

Indications: Galaxy DA$_2$L is a modified live vaccine for immunization against canine distemper, adenovirus type 2 and hepatitis viruses combined with inactivated Leptospira canicola and Leptospira icterohaemorrhagiae bacterin (Leptobac) as a diluent. The canine distemper fraction is propagated in chicken embryo cell cultures; canine adenovirus type 2 fraction in canine cell line culture. Data indicate that the development of corneal opacity is not associated with the use of this product. The vaccine strain of adenovirus type 2 has been demonstrated to be nononcogenic.
Corneal opacity ("Blue Eye") does not occur with the use of Galaxy DA$_2$L.
The adenovirus type 2 strain is non-oncogenic.
Anaphylactoid type reactions are minimized because the leptospira components are protein serum free.
Dosage and Administration: Rehydrate each vaccine vial with 1 ml of inactivated bacterin diluent (Leptobac). Inject intramuscularly or subcutaneously. Repeat the dose in 3-4 weeks. Revaccinate those dogs vaccinated before 8 weeks of age when 10-12 weeks old and again 3-4 weeks later. Annual revaccination with one dose is recommended. Vaccinate only healthy, non-parasitized dogs. Transfer the contents of the Leptobac diluent to the vaccine vial aseptically. Do not chemically sterilize needles and syringes.
Precautions: The use of any biological may produce anaphylactoid type reactions.
Antidote: Epinephrine.
The vaccine contains gentamicin and a fungistat as preservatives. The bacterin diluent contains thimerosal as an inactivating agent and a preservative. Store at 2–7°C. Burn this container and all unused contents.
How Supplied: Box of 50 single doses.

GALAXY® DA$_2$PL
Canine Distemper-Adenovirus Type 2-Parainfluenza Vaccine, Modified Live Virus-Chicken Tissue Culture and Cell Line Origin, Leptospira Bacterin

Indications: Galaxy DA$_2$PL is a modified live vaccine for immunization against canine distemper, adenovirus type 2, hepatitis and parainfluenza viruses combined with inactivated Leptospira canicola and Leptospira icterohaemorrhagiae bacterin (Leptobac) as a diluent. The canine distemper fraction is propagated in chicken embryo cell cultures; canine adenovirus type 2 and parainfluenza fractions in canine cell line cultures. Data indicates that the development of corneal opacity is not associated with the use of this product. The vaccine strain of adenovirus type 2 has been demonstrated to be non-oncogenic.
Corneal opacity ("Blue Eye") does not occur with the use of Galaxy DA$_2$PL.
Galaxy DA$_2$PL can be used to vaccinate dogs of any age.
Galaxy DA$_2$PL protects against canine adenovirus type 1 (hepatitis) infections.
Galaxy DA$_2$PL provides excellent protection against canine respiratory disease caused by adenovirus type 1 (hepatitis), adenovirus type 2, and/or parainfluenza virus.
Dosage and Administration: Rehydrate each vaccine vial with 1 ml of inactivated bacterin diluent (Leptobac). Inject intramuscularly or subcutaneously. Repeat the dose in 3–4 weeks. Revaccinate those dogs before 8 weeks of age when 10–12 weeks old and again 3–4 weeks later. Annual revaccination with one dose is recommended. Vaccinate only healthy, non-parasitized dogs. Transfer the contents of the Leptobac diluent to the vaccine vial aseptically. Do not chemically sterilize needles and syringes.
Precautions: The use of any biological may produce anaphylactoid type reactions.
Antidote: Epinephrine.
The vaccine contains gentamicin and a fungistat as preservatives. The bacterin diluent contains thimerosal as an inactivating agent and a preservative. Store at 2–7°C. Burn this container and all unused contents.
How Supplied: Box of 50 single dose.

GALAXY® 6 MHP
Canine Distemper-Adenovirus Type 2-Parainfluenza and Modified Live Canine Origin Parvovirus Vaccine, Modified Live Virus, Chicken Tissue Culture and Cell Line Origin

Indications: Galaxy 6 MHP is a modified live virus vaccine for immunization against canine distemper, adenovirus type 2, adenovirus type 1 (hepatitis), parainfluenza and parvovirus. The canine distemper fraction is propagated in chicken tissue cultures; canine adenovirus type 2, parvovirus (HOMOTYPIC) and parainfluenza fractions in cell line cultures. The parvovirus is of canine origin. Data indicate that the development of corneal opacity is not associated with the use of this product. The adenovirus type 2 vaccine strain has been demonstrated to be non-oncogenic. Galaxy 6 MHP contains a CORNELL STRAIN* of modified live canine origin parvovirus (HOMOTYPIC) which was extensively tested for efficacy, safety and durable immunity against canine parvovirus disease. The parvovirus fraction was further selectively attenuated by Solvay's exclusive high technology cell line system. The Onderstepoort type of distemper virus is used exclusively in Solvay vaccines which is safe in dogs, ferrets, and adult grey foxes. Galaxy 6 MHP contains canine adenovirus type 2 (CAV-2) as a replacement antigen for hepatitis (CAV-1). As such corneal opacity ("Blue Eye") does not occur with the use of Galaxy 6 MHP. Galaxy 6 MHP provides excellent protection against canine respiratory disease associated with adenoviruses and/or parainfluenza virus. Studies have demonstrated no interference between fractions. Annual revaccination recommended.
Dosage and Administration: Rehydrate each vaccine vial with 1 ml. of sterile diluent. Inject intramuscularly or subcutaneously. Repeat the dose in 3–4 weeks.** Puppies should receive an initial vaccination at 8–9 weeks of age; a second dose at 12–13 weeks of age; and a final booster at 16–18 weeks of age. If pups are presented at a younger age, they should receive a first dose at 7–9 weeks of age, a second dose at 10–12 weeks of age, a third dose at 13–15 weeks of age, and a final booster at 16–18 weeks

Continued on next page

S

Solvay—Cont.

of age. **Annual revaccination with one dose is recommended.** Vaccinate only healthy, non-parasitized dogs. Transfer the contents of the sterile diluent to the vaccine vial aseptically. Do not chemically sterilize the needles and syringes.
**Two doses of parainfluenza are required for prophylaxis.
Precautions: The use of any biological may produce anaphylactoid reactions.
Antidote: Epinephrine.
The vaccine contains gentamicin and a fungistat as preservatives. Store at 2–7°C. Burn this container and all unused contents.
How Supplied: Box of 50 single doses of 1 ml.
*Patent No. 4303645

GALAXY® 6 MHP-L
Canine Distemper- Adenovirus Type 2-Parainfluenza and Modified Live Canine Origin Parvovirus Vaccine with Leptospira Bacterin, Modified Live Virus, Chicken Tissue Culture and Cell Line Origin, Leptospira Bacterin

Indications: Galaxy 6 MHP-L is a modified live virus vaccine for immunization against canine distemper, adenovirus type 2, adenovirus type 1 (hepatitis), parainfluenza and parvovirus combined with inactivated Leptospira canicola and Leptospira icterohaemorrhagiae bacterin (Leptobac) as a diluent. The canine distemper fraction is propagated in chicken tissue cultures; canine adenovirus type 2, parvovirus (HOMOTYPIC) and parainfluenza fractions in cell line cultures. The parvovirus is of canine origin. Data indicate that the development of corneal opacity is not associated with the use of this product. The adenovirus type 2 vaccine strain was demonstrated to be nononcogenic.
Galaxy 6 MHP-L contains a CORNELL STRAIN* of modified live canine origin parvovirus (HOMOTYPIC) which was extensively tested for efficacy, safety and durable immunity against canine parvovirus disease.
The parvovirus fraction was further selectively attenuated in Solvay's exclusive high technology cell line system.
The Onderstepoort type of distemper virus is used exclusively in Solvay vaccines which is safe in dogs, ferrets, and adult grey foxes.
Galaxy 6 MHP-L contains canine adenovirus type 2 (CAV-2) as a replacement antigen for hepatitis (CAV-1). As such, corneal opacity ("Blue Eye") does not occur with the use of Galaxy 6 MHP-L.
Galaxy 6 MHP-L protects against canine adenovirus type 1 (hepatitis) infection.
Galaxy 6 MHP-L provides excellent protection against canine respiratory disease associated with adenoviruses and/or parainfluenza virus.
Anaphylactoid reactions are minimized because the leptospirosis components are serum free.
Studies have demonstrated no interference between fractions. Annual revaccination recommended.
Dosage and Administration: Rehydrate each vaccine vial with 1 ml. of LEPTOBAC diluent. Inject intramuscularly or subcutaneously. Repeat the dose in 3–4 weeks.** Puppies should receive an initial vaccination at 8–9 weeks of age; a second dose at 12–13 weeks of age; and a final booster at 16–18 weeks of age. If pups are presented at a younger age, they should receive a first dose at 7–9 weeks of age, a second at 10–12 weeks of age, a third dose at 13–15 weeks of age, and a final booster at 16–18 weeks of age. **Annual revaccination with one dose is recommended.** Vaccinate only healthy, non-parasitized dogs. Transfer the contents of the LEPTOBAC to the vaccine vial aseptically. Do not chemically sterilize the needles and syringes.
**Two doses of parainfluenza are required for prophylaxis.
Precautions: The use of any biological may produce anaphylactoid reactions.
Antidote: Epinephrine.
The vaccine contains gentamicin and a fungistat as preservatives. Leptobac diluent contains thimerosal as a preservative. Store at 2-7° C. Burn this container and all unused contents.
How Supplied: Box of 50 single doses.
*Patent No. 4303645

GALAXY® 6 MP-L
Canine Distemper-Adenovirus Type 2-Parainfluenza-Parvovirus Vaccine, Modified Live Virus, Chicken Tissue Culture and Cell Line Origin, Leptospira Bacterin

Indications: Galaxy 6 MP-L is a modified live virus vaccine for immunization against canine distemper, adenovirus type 2, adenovirus type 1 (hepatitis), parainfluenza and parvovirus, combined with inactivated Leptospira canicola and Leptospira icterohaemorrhagiae bacterin (Leptobac) as a diluent. The canine distemper fraction is propagated in chicken embryo cell cultures; canine adenovirus type 2 and parainfluenza fractions in cell line cultures. The parvovirus is of feline origin and is propagated in cell line cultures. Data indicates that the development of corneal opacity is not associated with the use of this product. The vaccine strain of adenovirus type 2 has been demonstrated to be non-oncogenic.
Galaxy 6 MP-L provides excellent protection against canine infectious diseases including Canine Parvovirus Infection.
Corneal opacity ("Blue Eye") does not occur with the use of Galaxy 6 MP-L.
Galaxy 6 MP-L protects against canine adenovirus type 1 (Hepatitis) infection.
Galaxy 6 MP-L provides excellent protection against canine respiratory disease associated wih adenoviruses and/or parainfluenza virus.
Studies have shown no post-vaccinal sequelae, reversion to virulence or shed to contact dogs.
This product can be used in any age dog (not pregnant dogs).
Dosage and Administration: Rehydrate each vaccine vial with 1 ml. of LEPTOBAC diluent. Inject intramuscularly or subcutaneously. Repeat the dose in 3–4 weeks.** Puppies should receive an initial vaccination at 8–9 weeks of age; a second dose at 12–13 weeks of age; and a final booster at 16–18 weeks of age. If pups are presented at a younger age, they should receive a first dose at 7–9 weeks of age, a second dose at 10–12 weeks of age, a third dose at 13–15 weeks of age, and a final booster at 16–18 weeks of age. **Annual revaccination with one dose is recommended.** Vaccinate only healthy nonparasitized dogs. Transfer the contents of the LEPTOBAC to the vaccine vial aseptically. Do not chemically sterilize the needles and syringes.
**Two doses of parainfluenza are required for prophylaxis.
Precautions: The use of any biological may prodce anaphylactoid reactions.
Antidote: Epinephrine.
The vaccine contains gentamicin and a fungistat as preservatives. Leptobac diluent contains thimerosal as preservatives. **Store at 2–7° C.** Burn this container and all unused contents.
How Supplied: Box of 50 single doses

PANODRY®
Ear Drying Solution for Dogs

Product Description: Panodry is a clear blue solution containing 2.7% boric acid in a fragrant vehicle consisting of not more than 90% (V/V) isopropyl alcohol and silicone-fluid base.
Indications: Panodry is designed to be part of the Solvay ear care program for maintaining healthy ears in dogs. Certain canine breeds have ears which retain high amounts of moisture. This provides a warm moist environment in which certain pathogenic bacteria and yeast can grow and cause infection and/or inflammation. Following proper cleansing, a drying solution can be applied into the ear canal on a regular basis.
Directions for Use: Fill each ear canal with Panodry and wipe away the excess with a piece of cotton or other suitable material, such as facial tissue. Apply twice weekly.
Additional Information: Other available ear care products from Solvay Veterinary, Inc., are Panoprep® (ear cleaning solution), which is designed to clean wax, dirt and debris from the external ear canal, Panolog® Ointment (nystatin-neomycin sulfate-thiostrepton-triamcinolone acetonide ointment), and Xenodine® (polyhydroxydine® solution), for the treatment of ear infections in dogs and cats. See these product listings for complete information.
Cautions: Keep out of reach of children. In case of accidental contact with eyes, flush with water immediately. Accidental ingestion: seek professional assistance or contact a poison control center immediately.
Flammable—keep away from open flame and heat.
Storage: Store at room temperature; avoid excessive heat.
How Supplied: Panodry is supplied in 2 fl. oz. bottles.

Xenodine and Polyhydroxydine are trademarks of Xenovet Division, eMDee Corporation.

PANOLOG® CREAM VETERINARY

Nystatin—Neomycin Sulfate—Thiostrepton—Triamcinolone Acetonide Cream

For Topical Use on Dogs and Cats

Description: Panolog Cream combines nystatin, neomycin sulfate, thiostrepton, and triamcinolone acetonide.

Each gram contains 100,000 units nystatin, neomycin sulfate equivalent to 2.5 mg. of neomycin base, 2,500 units thiostrepton, and 1.0 mg. triamcinolone acetonide in an aqueous, nonirritating vanishing cream base with cetearyl alcohol (and) ceteareth-20, ethylenediamine hydrochloride, methylparaben, propylparaben, propylene glycol, sorbitol solution, titanium dioxide, sodium citrate, citric acid, white petrolatum, glyceryl monostearate, polyethylene glycol monostearate, sorbic acid and simethicone.

Actions: By virtue of its four active ingredients, Panolog Cream (Nystatin—Neomycin Sulfate—Thiostrepton—Triamcinolone Acetonide Cream) provides four basic therapeutic effects: anti-inflammatory, antipruritic, antifungal and antibacterial. Triamcinolone acetonide is a potent synthetic corticosteroid providing rapid and prolonged symptomatic relief on topical administration. Inflammation, edema, and pruritus promptly subside, and lesions are permitted to heal. Nystatin is the first well-tolerated antifungal antibiotic of dependable efficacy for the treatment of cutaneous infections caused by *Candida albicans* (Monilia). Nystatin is fungistatic *in vitro* against a variety of yeast and yeast-like fungi including many fungi pathogenic to animals. No appreciable activity is exhibited against bacteria. Thiostrepton has a high order of activity against gram-positive organisms, including many which are resistant to other antibiotics; neomycin exerts antimicrobial action against a wide range of gram-positive and gram- negative bacteria. Together they provide comprehensive therapy against those organisms responsible for most superficial bacterial infections.

Indications: Panolog Cream (Nystatin—Neomycin Sulfate—Thiostrepton—Triamcinolone Acetonide Cream) is indicated in the management of dermatologic disorders in dogs and cats, characterized by inflammation and dry or exudative dermatitis, particularly those caused, complicated, or threatened by bacterial or candidal *(Candida albicans)* infections. It is also of value in eczematous dermatitis, contact dermatitis, and seborrheic dermatitis; and as an adjunct in the treatment of dermatitis due to parasitic infestation.

Contraindications: Panolog Cream (Nystatin—Neomycin Sulfate—Thiostrepton—Triamcinolone Acetonide Cream) should not be used ophthalmically.

Warnings: Panolog Cream (Nystatin—Neomycin Sulfate—Thiostrepton—Triamcinolone Acetonide Cream) is indicated for use in dogs and cats only. Not for use in animals which are raised for food.

Absorption of triamcinolone acetonide through topical application and by licking may occur. Therefore, animals should be observed closely for signs of polydipsia, polyuria and increased weight gain particularly when the preparation is used over large areas or for extended periods of time.

Precautions: Panolog Cream (Nystatin—Neomycin Sulfate—Thiostrepton—Triamcinolone Acetonide Cream) is not intended for the treatment of deep abscesses or deep-seated infections such as inflammation of the lymphatic vessels. Parenteral antibiotic therapy is indicated in these infections.

Panolog Cream (Nystatin—Neomycin Sulfate—Thiostrepton—Triamcinolone Acetonide Cream) has been extremely well tolerated. The occurrence of systemic reactions is rarely a problem with topical administration.

Sensitivity to neomycin may occur. If redness, irritation, or swelling persists or increases, discontinue use. Do not use if pus is present since the drug may allow the infection to spread.

Dosage and Administration: Frequency of administration is dependent on the severity of the condition. For mild inflammations, application may range from once daily to once a week; for severe conditions Panolog Cream (Nystatin—Neomycin Sulfate—Thiostrepton—Triamcinolone Acetonide Cream) may be applied as often as 2 to 3 times daily, if necessary. Frequency of treatment may be decreased as improvement occurs.

Clean affected areas, removing any encrusted discharge or exudate. Apply Panolog Cream sparingly in a thin film.

Caution: Federal law restricts this drug to use by or on the order of a licensed veterinarian.

How Supplied: Panolog Cream (Nystatin—Neomycin Sulfate—Thiostrepton—Triamcinolone Acetonide Cream) is supplied in 7.5 gram and 15 gram tubes.

Storage: Store at room temperature; avoid excessive heat (104°F).

PANOLOG® OINTMENT VETERINARY

Nystatin—Neomycin Sulfate—Thiostrepton—Triamcinolone Acetonide Ointment

For Use in Dogs and Cats Only

Description: Panolog Ointment combines nystatin, nemoycin sulfate, thiostrepton, and triamcinolone acetonide in a non-irritating protective vehicle, Plastibase® (Plasticized Hydrocarbon Gel), a polyethylene and mineral oil gel base.

Each ml. contains 100,000 units nystatin, neomycin sulfate equivalent to 2.5 mg. neomycin base, 2,500 units thiostrepton, and 1.0 mg. triamcinolone acetonide.

The preparation is intended for local therapy in a variety of cutaneous disorders of cats and dogs; it is especially useful in disorders caused, complicated or threatened by bacterial and/or candidal (monilial) infection.

Actions: By virtue of its four active ingredients, Panolog Ointment (Nystatin—Neomycin Sulfate—Thiostrepton—Triamcinolone Acetonide Ointment) provides four basic therapeutic effects: anti-inflammatory, antipruritic, antifungal and antibacterial. Triamcinolone acetonide is a potent synthetic corticosteroid providing rapid and prolonged symptomatic relief on topical administration. Inflammation, edema, and pruritus promptly subside, and lesions are permitted to heal. Nystatin is the first well-tolerated antifungal antibiotic of dependable efficacy for the treatment of cutaneous infections caused by *Candida albicans* (Monilia). Nystatin is fungistatic *in vitro* against a variety of yeast and yeast-like fungi, including many fungi pathogenic to animals. No appreciable activity is exhibited against bacteria.Thiostrepton has a high order of activity against gram-positive organisms, including many which are resistant to other antibiotics; neomycin exerts antimicrobial action against a wide range of gram-positive and gram-negative bacteria. Together they provide comprehensive therapy against those organisms responsible for most superificial bacterial infections.

Indications: Panolog Ointment (Nystatin—Neomycin Sulfate—Thiostrepton—Triamcinolone Acetonide Ointment) is particularly useful in the treatment of acute and chronic otitis of varied etiologies, in interdigital cysts in cats and dogs, and in anal gland infections in dogs.

The preparation is also indicated in the management of dermatologic disorders characterized by inflammation and dry or exudative dermatitis, particularly those caused, complicated, or threatened by bacterial or candidal *(Candida albicans)* infections. It is also of value in eczematous dermatitis, contact dermatitis, and seborrheic dermatitis; and as an adjunct in the treatment of dermatitis due to parasitic infestation.

Precautions: Panolog Ointment is not intended for the treatment of deep abscesses or deep-seated infections such as inflammation of the lymphatic vessels. Parenteral antibiotic therapy is indicated in these infections.

Panolog Ointment (Nystatin—Neomycin Sulfate—Thiostrepton—Triamcinolone Acetonide Ointment) has been extremely well tolerated. Cutaneous reactions attributable to its use have been extremely rare. The occurence of systemic reactions is rarely a problem with topical administration. There is some evidence that corticosteroids can be absorbed after topical application and cause systemic effects. Therefore, an animal receiving Panolog Ointment therapy should be observed closely for signs such as polydipsia, polyuria, and increased weight gain.

Panolog Ointment (Nystatin—Neomycin Sulfate—Thiostrepton—Triamcinolone Acetonide Ointment) is not generally recommended for the treatment of deep or puncture wounds or serious burns.

Continued on next page

S

Solvay—Cont.

Sensitivity to neomycin may occur. If redness, irritation, or swelling persists or increases, discontinue use. Do not use if pus is present since the drug may allow the infection to spread. Keep this and all medications out of the reach of children.

Dosage and Administration: Frequency of administration is dependent on the severity of the condition. For mild inflammations, application may range from once daily to once a week; for severe conditions Panolog Ointment may be applied as often as two to three times daily, if necessary. Frequency of treatment may be decreased as improvement occurs.

Otitis: Clean ear canal of impacted cerumen. Inspect canal and remove any foreign bodies such as grass awns, ticks, etc. Instill three to five drops of Panolog Ointment (Nystatin—Neomycin Sulfate—Thiostrepton—Triamcinolone Acetonide Ointment).

Preliminary use of a local anesthetic such as Ophthaine® Solution Veterinary (Proparacaine Hydrochloride Ophthalmic Solution) may be advisable. The suggested dosage for Ophthaine is two drops instilled into the ear every five minutes for three doses just prior to cleaning—see package insert accompanying that product for complete information.

Infected Anal Glands, Cystic Areas, etc.: Drain gland or cyst and then fill with Panolog Ointment.

Other Dermatologic Disorders: Clean affected areas, removing any encrusted discharge or exudate. Apply Panolog Ointment sparingly in a thin film.

How Supplied: Panolog Ointment (Nystatin—Neomycin Sulfate—Thiostrepton—Triamcinolone Acetonide Ointment) is supplied in tubes of ¼fl. oz. (7.5 ml.), ½fl. oz. (15 ml.) and 1 fl. oz. (30 ml.), each with an elongated tip for easy application, and in dispensing packages of 8 fl. oz. (240 ml.).

Caution: Federal law restricts this drug to use by or on the order of a licensed veterinarian.

PARVOID™ 2
Modified Live Canine Origin Parvovirus Vaccine, Cell Line Origin

Indications: Parvoid 2 is a modified live virus vaccine for the immunization of dogs against canine parvovirus. The parvovirus is a large plaque variant (LP). Cornell Strain* of canine origin.

Parvoid 2 contains a CORNELL STRAIN* of modified live canine origin parvovirus (HOMOTYPIC) which has been extensively tested for safety, efficacy, and durable immunity against canine parvovirus disease.

The parvovirus fraction has been further selectively attenuated by Solvay's exclusive high technology cell line system.

No reversion to virulence.

No post-vaccinal sequelae.

Annual revaccination recommended.

Only one dose needed in adult dogs.

Dosage and Administration: The recommended vaccine dosage is 1.0 ml. ***Adult dogs*** should received a single 1 ml dose administered intramuscularly or subcutaneously. ***Puppies*** should receive an initial vaccination at 8-9 weeks of age; a second dose at 12-13 weeks of age, and a final booster at 16-18 weeks of age. If pups are presented at a younger age, they should receive a first dose at 7-9 weeks of age, a second dose at 10-12 weeks of age, a third dose at 13-15 weeks of age, and a final booster at 16-18 weeks of age. Annual revaccination with one dose is recommended. Vaccinate only healthy non-parasitized dogs. Transfer the contents of the vaccine vial to the syringe aseptically. Do not chemically sterilize needles and syringes.

Precautions: The use of any biological may produce anaphylactoid reactions.

Antidote: Epinephrine.

The vaccine should be stored at 2-7°C. Parvoid 2 contains gentamicin and a fungistat as preservatives. Burn this container and all unused contents.

How Supplied: Box of 20 single 1 ml doses. Box of 100 single 1 ml doses. Bottle of 10 x 1 ml doses. (Multidose Vial)

*Patent No. 4303645

PRINCILLIN® BOLUSES
Ampicillin Boluses Veterinary For Oral Use in Non-Ruminating Calves Only

Description: Princillin Boluses (Ampicillin Boluses Veterinary) contain the crystalline trihydrate of [D(-)-α- aminobenzyl] penicillin, a semisynthetic penicillin possessing an antibacterial spectrum which extends beyond the spectrum of activity of penicillin G.

Each Princillin Bolus provides ampicillin trihydrate equivalent to 400 mg. of ampicillin activity.

Actions: Ampicillin is clinically effective against the gram-positive organisms usually susceptible to penicillin G plus a variety of gram-negative organisms. *In vitro,* ampicillin is bactericidal even at low concentrations.

The following organisms show *in vitro* sensitivity to ampicillin:

Gram-Positive —strains of hemolytic and non-hemolytic *Streptococcus sp.,* those strains of *Staphylococcus sp.* which do not produce penicillinase, *Clostridium sp., Bacillus anthracis,* and most strains of enterococci.

Gram-Negative —*Brucella sp., Proteus mirabilis, Pasteurella sp.* and many strains of *Salmonella sp.* and *Escherichia sp.*

Note: Some bacteria produce an enzyme known as penicillinase which destroys or inactivates ampicillin. This phenomenon is responsible for ampicillin not being effective against penicillinase- producing organisms including certain strains of *Staphylococcus sp., Pseudomonas aeruginosa, P. vulgaris, Aerobacter aerogenes* and some strains of *E. coli.* Ampicillin is not active against Rickettsia, Mycoplasma and viruses.

Ampicillin is well absorbed from the gastrointestinal tract and rapidly produces adequate blood concentrations.

Indications: In non-ruminating calves, Princillin Boluses (Ampicillin Boluses Veterinary) are indicated for the treatment of the following diseases susceptible to ampicillin: colibacillosis caused by *E. coli,* bacterial enteritis caused by *Salmonella sp.,* and bacterial pneumonia caused by *Pasteurella sp.*

Ampicillin is a bactericidal antibiotic *in vitro* with a broad spectrum of activity, thus it may be used prior to completion of appropriate laboratory tests. *In vitro* culturing and susceptibility tests should be conducted on samples collected before treatment. Based on these tests depending on the nature and severity of the condition, usage should be reevaluated.

Contraindications: Ampicillin is contraindicated in infections caused by penicillinase-producing organisms. It is also contraindicated in non-ruminating calves known to be allergic to any of the penicillins.

Warnings: For use in non-ruminating calves only. Not for use in animals which are raised for food production.

Treated calves must not be slaughtered for food during treatment and for 15 days after the last treatment.

Precautions: With the use of any antibiotic preparation, constant alertness for signs of overgrowth of nonsusceptible organisms, including fungi, is essential. Should superinfection occur, the antibiotic should be discontinued and/or other appropriate measures taken.

If no response to treatment is obtained within three to five days, reestablish the diagnosis. Failure to respond may be related to ampicillin resistance.

Adverse Reactions: As with other penicillins, sensitivity reactions to ampicillin, such as hives or difficult respiration, may occur in some animals.

Dosage and Administration: The oral dosage is 5 mg per pound of body weight twice daily (one bolus for each 80 pounds of calf body weight twice daily) for not more than 5 days.

Storage: Store at room temperature; avoid excessive heat.

How Supplied: Princillin Boluses (Ampicillin Boluses Veterinary), providing ampicillin trihydrate equivalent to 400 mg. of ampicillin activity in each bolus, are supplied in 48-bolus packages.

Caution: Federal law restricts this drug to use by or on the order of a licensed veterinarian.

PRINCILLIN® '125' CAPSULES
PRINCILLIN® '250' CAPSULES
PRINCILLIN® '500' CAPSULES
Ampicillin Capsules U.S.P. Veterinary
PRINCILLIN® '125' FOR ORAL SUSPENSION
Ampicillin for Oral Suspension U.S.P. Veterinary For Oral Use in Dogs and Cats Only

Description: Princillin Capsules (Ampicillin Capsules U.S.P. Veterinary) contain the crystalline trihydrate of [D(-)-α-

aminobenzyl] penicillin, a semisynthetic penicillin possessing an antibacterial spectrum which extends beyond the spectrum of activity of penicillin G. It is available for oral administration as Princillin '125' Capsules, Princillin '250' Capsules, and Princillin '500' Capsules providing ampicillin trihydrate equivalent to 125 mg., 250 mg., and 500 mg. of ampicillin activity, respectively. (NOTE: Princillin '500' Capsules are for use in dogs only because of the size of the capsules.)
Princillin '125' for Oral Suspension (Ampicillin for Oral Suspension U.S.P. Veterinary) contains the crystalline trihydrate of [D(-)-α-aminobenzyl] penicillin, a semisynthetic penicillin possessing an antibacterial spectrum which extends beyond the spectrum of activity of penicillin G. After mixing, the suspension contains the equivalent of 125 mg. ampicillin per 5 ml. teaspoonful.
Actions: Ampicillin is clinically effective against the gram-positive organisms usually susceptible to penicillin G plus a variety of gram-negative organisms. In contrast to chloramphenicol and tetracyclines, which are bacteriostatic, ampicillin is bactericidal *in vitro* even at low concentrations.
The following organisms show *in vitro* sensitivity to ampicillin:
GRAM-POSITIVE—strains of hemolytic and non-hemolytic *Streptococcus sp.*, those strains of *Staphylococcus sp.* which do not produce penicillinase, *Clostridium sp.*, *Bacillus anthracis*, and most strains of enterococci.
GRAM-NEGATIVE—*Brucella sp.*, *Proteus mirabilis* and many strains of *Salmonella sp.* and *Escherichia sp.*
NOTE: Some bacteria produce an enzyme known as penicillinase which destroys or inactivates ampicillin. This phenomenon is responsible for ampicillin not being effective against penicillinase-producing organisms including certain strains of *Staphylococcus sp.*, *Pseudomonas aeruginosa*, *P. vulgaris*, *Aerobacter aerogenes* and some strains of *E. coli.* Ampicillin is not active against Rickettsia, Mycoplasma and viruses.
Ampicillin is well absorbed from the gastrointestinal tract and rapidly reaches adequate blood concentrations.
Indications: Princillin Capsules (Ampicillin Capsules U.S.P. Veterinary) and Princillin '125' for Oral Suspension (Ampicillin for Oral Suspension U.S.P. Veterinary) are indicated in the treatment of the following disease conditions:
Dogs:
1. Respiratory tract infections [tracheobronchitis (kennel cough) and tonsillitis] due to *E. coli*, *Pseudomonas sp.*, *Proteus sp.*, *Staphylococcus sp.*, and *Streptococcus sp.*
2. Urinary tract infections (cystitis) due to *E. coli*, *Staphylococcus sp.*, *Streptococcus sp.*, and *Proteus sp.*
3. Bacterial gastroenteritis due to *E. coli*
4. Generalized infections (septicemia) associated with abscesses, lacerations and wounds due to *Staphylococcus sp.* and *Streptococcus sp.*
5. Bacterial dermatis due to *Staphylococcus sp.*, *Streptococcus sp.*, *Proteus sp.* and *Pseudomonas sp.* (Appropriate adjunctive therapy to be used where indicated.)

Cats:
1. Respiratory tract infections (bacterial pneumonia) due to *Staphylococcus sp.*, *Streptococcus sp.*, *E. coli* and *Proteus sp.*
2. Urinary tract infections (cystitis) due to *E. coli*, *Staphylococcus sp.*, *Streptococcus sp.*, *Proteus sp.*, and *Corynebacterium sp.*
3. Generalized infections (septicemia) associated with abscesses, lacerations and wounds due to *Staphylococcus sp.*, *Streptococcus sp.*, *Bacillus sp.* and *Pasteurella sp.*

Since ampicillin is a bactericidal antibiotic *in vitro* with a wide spectrum of activity, it may be used as an emergency measure. However, appropriate laboratory tests should be conducted including *in vitro* culturing and susceptibility tests on samples collected prior to treatment. Based on these tests and depending on the nature and severity of the condition being treated, usage and dosage should be re-evaluated.
Contraindications: Ampicillin is contraindicated in infections caused by penicillinase-producing organisms. It is also contraindicated in dogs and cats known to be allergic to any of the penicillins.
Warnings: For use in dogs and cats only. Not for use in animals which are raised for food production.
Precautions: With the use of any antibiotic preparation, constant alertness for signs of overgrowth of nonsusceptible organisms, including fungi, is essential. Should superinfection occur, the antibiotic should be discontinued and/or other appropriate measures taken.
If no response to treatment is obtained within 3 to 5 days, reestablish the diagnosis. Failure to respond may be related to ampicillin resistance.
Adverse Reactions: As with other penicillins, sensitivity reactions to ampicillin, such as hives or difficult respiration, may occur in some animals. In a few instances, vomiting or diarrhea may occur while dogs or cats are on ampicillin medication.
Dosage and Administration: The usual dosage for dogs is 5 to 10 mg. (0.2 to 0.4 ml. of the oral suspension) per pound of body weight given two or three times daily. In severe or acute conditions, 10 mg. per pound of body weight should be given three times daily. (The mixed suspension contains 125 mg. ampicillin activity per 5 ml.)
The usual dosage for cats is 10 to 30 mg. (0.4 to 1.2 ml. of the oral suspension) per pound of body weight given two to three times daily. NOTE: Some cats may object to administration of the oral suspension because of the fruit flavoring. In these instances, administration may be accomplished by use of a plastic dropper or the medication should be changed to Princillin Capsules (Ampicillin Capsules U.S.P. Veterinary).
Administer required dosage one to two hours prior to feeding.
The duration of treatment required depends on the severity and nature of the condition being treated. In clinical cases, the usual duration of treatment is three to five days. Daily treatment should be continued for at least 48 hours after the animal's temperature has returned to normal and all other signs of infection have subsided.
How Supplied: Princillin Capsules (Ampicillin Capsules U.S.P Veterinary) are available as follows: 125 mg. capsules in bottles of 1000; 250 mg. capsules in bottles of 500; and 500 mg. capsules in bottles of 500.
Princillin '125' for Oral Suspension (Ampicillin for Oral Suspension U.S.P. Veterinary) is available in bottles of 80 ml.
Caution: Federal law restricts this drug to use by or on the order of a licensed veterinarian.

PRINCILLIN® SOLUBLE POWDER
Ampicillin Soluble Powder Veterinary
For Oral Use in Swine Only

Description: Princillin Soluble Powder (Ampicillin Soluble Powder Veterinary) provides the crystalline trihydrate of [D(-)-α-aminobenzyl] penicillin, a semisynthetic penicillin possessing an antibacterial spectrum which extends beyond the spectrum of activity of penicillin G.
Each bottle of Princillin Soluble Powder (Ampicillin Soluble Powder Veterinary) contains 4 oz. (113.4 grams) soluble powder providing ampicillin trihydrate, dispersed in an inert carrier, equivalent to 10 grams of ampicillin activity. One gram of Princillin Soluble Powder is equivalent to 88.2 mg. ampicillin activity.
Actions: Ampicillin is clinically effective against the gram-positive organisms usually susceptible to penicillin G plus a variety of gram-negative organisms. Ampicillin is bactericidal *in vitro* even at low concentrations.
The following organisms show *in vitro* sensitivity to ampicillin:
GRAM-POSITIVE—strains of hemolytic and nonhemolytic *Streptococcus sp.*, those strains of *Staphylococcus sp.* which do not produce penicillinase, *Clostridium sp.*, *Bacillus anthracis*, and most strains of enterococci.
GRAM-NEGATIVE—*Brucella sp.*, *Proteus mirabilis* and many strains of *Salmonella sp.* and *Escherichia sp.*
Note: Some bacteria produce an enzyme known as penicillinase which destroys or inactivates ampicillin. This phenomenon is responsible for ampicillin not being effective against penicillinase-producing organisms including certain strains of *Staphylococcus sp.*, *Pseudomonas aeruginosa*, *P. vulgaris*, *Aerobacter aerogenes* and some strains of *E. coli.* Ampicillin is not active against Rickettsia, Mycoplasma and viruses.
Ampicillin is well absorbed from the gastrointestinal tract and rapidly produces adequate blood concentrations.
Indications: Princillin Soluble Powder (Ampicillin Soluble Powder Veterinary) is indicated in the treatment of porcine colibacillosis *(E. coli)* and salmonel-

Continued on next page

S

Solvay—Cont.

losis *(Salmonella sp.)* infections in swine up to 75 pounds in body weight. It is also indicated in the treatment of bacterial pneumonia in swine, caused by *Pasteurella multocida, Staphylococcus sp., Streptococcus sp.* and *Salmonella sp.*
Ampicillin is a bactericidal antibiotic *in vitro* with a wide spectrum of activity, thus it may be used prior to completion of appropriate laboratory tests. *In vitro* culturing and susceptibility tests should be conducted on samples collected before treatment. Based on these tests and depending on the nature and severity of the condition, usage should be reevaluated.
Contraindications: Ampicillin is contraindicated in infections caused by penicillinase-producing organisms. It is also contraindicated in swine known to be allergic to any of the penicillins.
Warnings: For use in swine only. Not for use in other animals which are raised for food production. Treated swine must not be slaughtered for food during treatment and for 24 hours following the last treatment.
Precautions: With the use of any antibiotic preparation, constant alertness for signs of overgrowth of nonsusceptible organisms, including fungi, is essential. Should superinfection occur, the antibiotic should be discontinued and/or other appropriate measures taken.
If no response to treatment is observed within three to five days, reestablished the diagnosis. Failure to respond may be related to ampicillin resistance.
Adverse Reactions: As with other penicillins, sensitivity reactions to ampicillin, such as hives or difficult respiration, may occur in some animals.
Dosage and Administration: The dosage is 5 mg., per pound of body weight twice daily administered orally by gavage or in the drinking water for up to five days.
Individual or Gavage Treatment: Add one level measuring spoonful of Princillin Soluble Powder (Ampicillin Soluble Powder Veterinary) to 60 ml. (2 oz.) of water. Shake gently until all of the powder is in solution. Solutions prepared in this manner contain approximately 5 mg. of ampicillin per ml. Administer 1 ml. of solution per pound of body weight twice daily.
Drinking Water Treatment (Herd): Daily Treatment. *First 6-hour period:* prepare fresh medicated water to supply dosage of 5 mg./lb. B.W.
Second 6-hour period: prepare fresh medicated water to supply dosage of 5 mg./lb. B.W.
Balance of day: unmedicated water.
Repeat the above treatment regimen every 24 hours for up to five days. Start medication at the same time each day. For complete directions on preparing medicated water to supply the above dosage recommendations see the Directions and Dosage Table below.
Directions and Dosage:
FOR EACH 6-HOUR TREATMENT PERIOD

Small Group of Pigs

Pig body Weight	Add to 2 gal. Water	Approx. No. of Pigs Treated
25 lbs.	3 spoonfuls	7
50 lbs.	5 spoonfuls	6
75 lbs.	6 spoonfuls	5

[See table below].
Note: One measuring spoonful of Princillin Soluble Powder (Ampicillin Soluble Powder Veterinary) treats approximately 60 lbs. of pig body weight for six hours.
One 4 oz. bottle of Princillin Soluble Powder (Ampiciilin Soluble Powder Veterinary) treats approximately 2000 lbs of pig body weight for six hours.
Add the Princillin Soluble Powder (Ampicillin Soluble Powder Veterinary) to the designated quantity of water and stir gently until all the powder is in solution.
If medicating via the drinking water, no other source of water should be available. Swine should consume sufficient medicated drinking water to provide 10 mg. of ampicillin activity per pound of body weight daily. Since sick animals may not consume normal quantities of drinking water, it may be necessary to adjust the above recommended concentrations of ampicillin in the drinking water to assure the correct daily intake of ampicillin medication.
How Supplied: Each bottle of Princillin Soluble Powder (Ampicillin Soluble Powder Veterinary) contains 4 oz. (113.4 grams) soluble powder providing ampicillin trihydrate equivalent to 10 grams of ampicillin activity.
A measuring spoon is packaged with each bottle; one level spoonful will provide approximately 300 mg ampicillin activity.
Caution: Federal law restricts this drug to use by or on the order of a licensed veterinarian.

Large Group of Pigs

Pig Body Weight	Mix one 4 oz. Bottle Water	Approx No. of Pigs Treated	Usual Water Consumption Per Pig/6 hrs.
25 lbs.	20 gallons	80	0.25 gal.
50 lbs.	12 gallons	40	0.3 gal.
75 lbs.	11 gallons	27	0.4 gal.

PSITTACOID
Feline Chlamydia Vaccine-Modified Live Chlamydia-Cell Line Origin

Indications: Psittacoid is a modified live feline chlamydia vaccine for immunizing cats against feline chlamydiosis (pneumonitis). Feline Chlamydia is propagated in an approved cell line.
Dosage and administration: Rehydrate each vaccine vial with 1 ml of diluent. Inject intramuscularly or subcutaneously. Revaccinate those cats vaccinated before 12 weeks of age when 16 weeks old. Annual revaccination with one dose is recommended. Transfer diluent vial contents to vaccine vial aseptically. Do not chemically sterilize needles and syringes.
Precautions: Use of any biological may produce anaphylactoid reactions.
Antidote: Epinephrine.
The vaccine contains gentamicin and fungistat as preservatives. Store at 2-7° C. Burn the container and all unused contents. *CHLAMYDIA PSITTACI (MIYAGAWANELLA FELIS; BEDSONIA FELIA)* is only one of several respiratory infections. This vaccine can be expected to be effective only against the *CHLAMYDIA PSITTACI* infection.
How Supplied: Box of 10 single 1 ml dose vials

RABVAC™ 1
Rabies Vaccine-Killed Virus-Feline Cell Line Origin.

Indications: Rabvac 1 contains rabies virus propagated in feline cell line cultures. The virus is chemically inactivated and is recommended for immunizing dogs and cats against rabies. Rabvac 1 can be used in combination with these Solvay vaccines: Eclipse 3 KP and Eclipse 4 KP.
Dosage & Administration: Inject one dose (1ml) intramuscularly at one site in the thigh. Vaccinate dogs and cats at three months of age or older. Revaccinate annually thereafter to maintain a high level of immunity.
Restricted to use by or under the supervision of a veterinarian.
Precautions: Use entire contents when first opened. The use of any biological may produce anaphylactoid reactions.
Antidote: Epinephrine.
The vaccine contains gentamicin, a fungistat, and thimerosal as preservatives; and β-propiolactone for inactivation.
Store at 2–7° C. Do not freeze.
How Supplied: Box of 20 single 1 ml dose vials, multiple dose vials containing 10—1 ml doses.

RABVAC™ 3
Rabies Vaccine-Killed Virus-Feline Cell Line Origin.

Indications: Rabvac 3 is a rabies vaccine that meets the three-year duration-of-immunity requirements and is recommended for immunizing dogs and cats against rabies. The virus is propagated in feline cell line cultures and has been chemically inactivated.
Dosage & Administration: Inject one dose (1 ml) intramuscularly at one site in the thigh. Vaccinate dogs and cats at three months of age or older. Revaccination thereafter is recommended every three years for dogs and cats.
Restricted to use by or under the supervision of a veterinarian.
Precautions: Use entire contents when first opened. The use of any biological may produce anaphylactoid reactions.

Antidote: Epinephrine.
The vaccine contains gentamicin, a fungistat, and thimerosal as preservatives; and β-propiolactone for inactivation.
Store at 2–7° C. Do not freeze.
How Supplied: Box of 20 single 1 ml dose vials, multiple dose vials containing 10—1 ml doses.

RE-COVR® INJECTION
Tripelennamine Hydrochloride Injection

Description: Tripelennamine hydrochloride is a white, crystalline material which is stable, nonhygroscopic, and readily soluble in water. It is supplied in multiple dose vials containing 20 mg of Tripelennamine Hydrochloride USP per mL.
Action: Tripelennamine hydrochloride is characterized by its capacity to antagonize many of the pharmacologic effects of histamine.
Indications: For use in cattle, horses, dogs, and cats in conditions in which antihistaminic therapy may be expected to lead to alleviation of some signs of disease.
Warning: Do not use in horses intended for food purposes.
Milk that has been taken during treatment and for 24 hours (two milkings) after the last treatment must not be used for food.
Treated cattle must not be slaughtered for food during treatment and for four days following the last treatment.
Caution: Central nervous system stimulation in the form of hyperexcitability, nervousness, and muscle tremors lasting up to 20 minutes have been noted in horses, particularly following intravenous administration; therefore, only the intramuscular route of administration should be used in horses.
Overdosage of tripelennamine hydrochloride may give rise to excitement, ataxia, and convulsions.
Depression of the central nervous system and incoordination may occur when the drug is used at therapeutic dose levels.
Disturbances in gastrointestinal function may occur in some instances.
While poisonous snake bites have been treated with antihistaminic drugs, other conjunctive therapy is required because of toxic reactions associated with the protein complex of venom.
Dosage and Administration: Warm the solution to near body temperature. Using aseptic precautions, administer intravenously or intramuscularly as specified below. Intramuscular injections should be made into the heavy musculature of the hind leg or cervical area. The doses specified below may be repeated in 6 to 12 hours if necessary.
Cattle—Administer intravenously or intramuscularly at a dose of 0.5 mg per lb of body weight (2.5 mL for each 100 lbs of body weight). For a more rapid onset of action, the intravenous route of administration is recommended.
Horses—Administer *intramuscularly only* at a dose of 0.5 mg per lb of body weight (2.5 mL for each 100 lbs of body weight).
Dogs and Cats—Administer *intramuscularly only* at a dose of 0.5 mg per lb of body weight (0.25 mL for each 10 lbs of body weight).
Caution: Federal law restricts this drug to use by or on the order of a licensed veterinarian.
How Supplied: Re-Covr Injection (Tripelennamine Hydrochloride Injection) is supplied in 20 mL, 100 mL, 250 mL, and 500 mL multiple dose vials containing 20 mg Tripelennamine Hydrochloride USP per mL.
Storage: Protect from light. Store at room temperature; avoid excessive heat (104°F).

TASK®
(dichlorvos)
Dog Anthelmintic

Description: The Task (dichlorvos) Dog Anthelmintic formulation is a nondigestible, beadshaped resin pellet, approximating 0.05 inch in length and 0.05 inch in diameter, the active ingredient of which is dichlorvos (2, 2-dichlorovinyl dimethyl phosphate). Dichlorvos is released slowly from the resin pellets as they pass through the dog's gastrointestinal tract. The rate of drug release is designed to provide maximum anthelmintic activity and toxicologic safety in the dog.
Spectrum: Task is effective in removing *Toxocara canis, toxascaris leonina* (roundworms), *Ancylostoma caninum, Uncinaria stenocephala* (hookworms), and *Trichuris vulpis* (whipworm) residing in the lumen of the gastrointestinal tract. The drug is vermicidal. There is little or no activity against the migrating larval forms of these parasites.
Contraindications: Do not administer Task (dichlorvos) Dog Anthelmintic in conjunction with other anthelmintics, taeniacides, antifilarial agents (diethylcarbamazine excepted), muscle relaxants, or tranquilizers. Do not administer to dogs showing signs of severe constipation, mechanical blockage of the intestinal tract, impaired liver function, circulatory failure, or to dogs recently exposed to or showing signs of infectious disease.
Dogs over one year of age in endemic heartworm areas or dogs originating from such areas should be examined for the presence of *D. immitis* prior to the administration of Task. Do not use in dogs infected with *Dirofilaria immitis*.
Do not use in animals other than the dog.
Rapidity of Action: Expulsion of drug-sensitive nematodes is generally initiated within three to twelve hours following dosage and for all practical purposes is complete within 24 hours. Dead, unattached hookworms have been found in the small intestine of puppies within one hour following Task dosage.
Stability: The active ingredient dichlorvos is a volatile substance which is easily destroyed by oxidizing agents and/or moisture (hydrolysis). All Task product labels bear an expiration date. The Task packets are stable for the period of time preceding that date, if stored at temperatures below 80°F. The gelatine capsule form of the drug must be stored under refrigeration to assure proper shelf-life. OUTDATED MATERIALS OR PRODUCT WHICH IS WET OR STICKY SHOULD NOT BE USED.
Toxicology: The acute oral LD_{50} for drug-grade, unformulated dichlorvos if dogs falls in the range of 28-45 milligrams per kilogram of body weight. The acute oral LD_{50} for Task (dichlorvos) Dog Anthelmintic (formulated dichlorvos) in the young adult dog ranges from 387 to 1,262 total milligrams active ingredient per kilogram body weight. The minimum lethal dose (i.e., the LD^1) is calculated to be between 182 and 384 total milligrams active ingredient per kilogram of body weight. The single recommended therapeutic dosage of Task is 27-33 total milligrams active ingredient per kilogram of body weight, of which an average 10-12 milligrams per kilogram (35% of the total) is available to the dog over the normal 24-hour digestive tract residency time.
The cardinal signs of acute toxicity in dogs resulting from dichlorvos overdosage are excessive salivation, pupillary contraction, retching, emesis, frequent defecation of watery stools, muscular fasciculations, neurological disturbances such as ataxia, general muscular weakness progressing toward paralysis, depressed blood pressure and a drop in the respiratory rate with dyspnea. The latter sign, if sufficiently severe, appears to be the ultimate cause of death.
Single sublethal doses of Task® capable of producing many of the cardinal signs of organophosphate toxicity, short of general paralysis, usually have no effects lasting beyond 24 hours.
Repeated oral administration of the drug at recommended levels does not result in gross, histopathological or functional damage to any of the major organs. Single or repeated dosages of dichlorvos given at varying stages of gestation to bitches, queens, mares, sows, rabbits, rats, or mice have shown no interference with reproductive performance, or the numbers and health of their offspring.
Pharmacology/Physiological: Dosage limitations with Task (dichlorvos) Dog Anthelmintic, insofar as it is known, are due solely to the drug's action on the nervous system where it depresses the activity of the enzyme cholinesterase. This action allows for an accumulation of acetylcholine at the neuronal junctions, with a resultant overstimulation of skeletal muscle, smooth muscle, and the parasympathetic end-organs. The severity of this effect is directly related to dosage. A transient increase in the peristaltic rate of the intestine is sometimes evident at the single therapeutic dose, and this may produce one or two loose stools within 2-6 hours following treatment.
When administered the recommended dosage of Task, dogs have generally shown a slight drop in plasma and/or red-cell cholinesterase activities. Normal values were regained or exceeded within seven to fourteen days. The exact significance of plasma and/or red blood cell

Continued on next page

Solvay—Cont.

Packet Color	Label Number	Active Ingredient (mg)	Lbs. Body Weight Treatment/Packet
Yellow	10	136 mg	10 lb
Green	15	204 mg	15 lb
Black	40	544 mg	40 lb

cholinesterase depression is not known since animals have been observed to survive long periods of time on chronic toxicological studies with little or no detectable circulating cholinesterase activity. Such measurements serve only to indicate that small, but significant, amounts of the intact drug are absorbed from the digestive tract.

Repeated large dosages, of Task have shown some anthelmintic activity against adult *Dirofilaria immitis* and their microfilariae. The administration of the single recommended dose of Task, however, has no practical effectiveness against these parasites. The irreversible pathologic changes associated with *D. immitis* may reduce the subject's metabolic and excretory capacity for the drug. Such alterations sometimes result in dichlorvos blood levels high enough to cause signs of drug toxicity or a migration of worms from the heart ventricle into the pulmonary artery and the lungs. Additional studies have shown that Task (dichlorvos) Dog Anthelmintic, in conjunction with or following the use of standard antifilarial agents, will on occasion produce mortality, especially in older dogs. This is believed to be the result of (a) accelerated parasite migration or kill, and (b) a reduced tolerance to the combination of drugs. Recent studies have shown that Task is compatible with diethylcarbamazine when this drug is used continuously for heartworm prophylaxis.

Some investigators have reported toxicologic interaction between cholinesterase-inhibiting compounds and the various muscle relaxants and central nervous system depressants (e.g., phenothiazine-derived tranquilizers). The use of Task concurrently with these drugs is not necessary or recommended.

Pathology: Gross lesions in animals succumbing to high oral doses of unformulated dichlorvos or Task (formulated dichlorvos) are limited to severe hyperemia and occasional hemorrhage into the G.I. tract, petechiation of the lungs, and congestion of the liver and kidneys. Intestinal intussusception has occurred in a small number of the test animals.

Studies in the pig and chicken have shown that repeated doses of dichlorvos do not cause demyelination of nerve fibers.

Dosage Forms: Two dosage forms of Task (dichlorvos) Dog Anthelmintic are available. The gelatin capsule form is recommended for direct veterinary administration, while the packet form is designed for use in canned dog food or ground meat and may conveniently be dispensed for use at home by the client.

Use Directions: The capsule form of Task is recommended for use at the following dosage rates:

[See table below].

The packet form of Task is designed for hospital, kennel, or home use. The Task pellets should be administered in about one-third of the regular canned dog food ration or in ground meat as follows:

[See table above].

Dogs may be treated with one or any combination of capsules or packets so that the active ingredient dosage falls within the range 12 to 15 milligrams per pound of body weight. The drug should not be used in dogs weighing less than two pounds.

Critical anthelmintic studies have shown that the administration of one-half the above single recommended dosage of Task (dichlorvos) Dog Anthelmintic, and repeated 8-24 hours later, provides the efficacy and spectrum equivalent to the single full dose.

This split dosage schedule should be used in "risk" animals which are very old, heavily parasitized, anemic, or otherwise debilitated. It is also useful in dogs which have the tendency to vomit all forms of oral medication.

The occasional dog that shows emesis one to two hours following administration of Task should not be retreated immediately; high anthelmintic efficacy against roundworms and hookworms is generally obtained. Those dogs that do not develop a negative stool for drug-sensitive nematode ova are best retreated 10-14 days later with the recommended split-dose schedule.

In some dogs, the efficacy of Task against *Trichuris vulpis* (whipworms) may be erratic. The possible edematous and inflamed condition of the cecum may limit the access of Task to the parasites. Stool samples of all dogs infected with *Trichuris vulpis* (whipworms) should be examined 10-14 days following initial treatment. Dogs that do not develop a negative stool for *Trichuris vulpis* (whipworm) ova should then be retreated and a stool sample checked 10-14 days following the repeat treatment. If at that time a negative stool is not obtained, consideration should be given to alternate means of therapy. Task in the control of gastrointestinal nematodes of the dog is not a substitute for good sanitary practices, but rather should be used to complement such practices. Dogs or puppies that are returned to parasite-contaminated areas after administration of Task will become reinfected. The rate and degree of reinfection will be related to the life cycle of the parasite(s) and the exposure level. Retreatment schedules with Task are at the discretion of the veterinarian.

Capsule Color	Label Number	Active Ingredient (mg)	Lbs. Body Weight Treatment/Capsule
Blue	5	68 mg	5 lb
Yellow	10	136 mg	10 lb
Green	15	204 mg	15 lb

Observe the expiration date on each container. Outdated drug should not be used.

Warning: Between capsule withdrawal, store bottles under refrigeration and keep tightly capped. Use packet contents shortly after opening; do not store unused drug. Keep out of reach of children. Avoid pellet contact with the skin. Task is a cholinesterase inhibitor. Do not use this product in animals simultaneously or within a few days before or after treatment with or exposure to cholinesterase-inhibiting drugs, pesticides, or chemicals. Atropine is antidotal.

Caution: U.S. Federal law restricts this drug to use by or on the order of a licensed veterinarian.

How Supplied: Package Sizes:

Capsules	Packets
68 mg dichlorvos	136 mg dichlorvos
136 mg dichlorvos	204 mg dichlorvos
204 mg dichlorvos	544 mg dichlorvos
25 capsules per bottle	25 packets per box

Task® is a trademark of SDS Biotech Corp.

STORE PACKETS AT LESS THAN 80°F
STORE CAPSULES UNDER REFRIGERATION

TASK® TABS
(dichlorvos)
Anthelmintic
For Cats And Puppies

Indications: Task Tabs (dichlorvos) is an anthelmintic product recommended for the removal and control of roundworms (*Toxocara canis, Toxocara cati, Toxascaris leonina*) and hookworms (*Ancylostoma caninum, Ancylostoma tubaeforme, Uncinaria stenocephala*) occurring in the intestinal tracts of cats and puppies. The drug is vermicidal.

Contraindications: Do not administer other anthelmintics concurrently with Task Tabs. Do not administer to puppies or cats showing signs of constipation, mechanical blockage of the intestinal tract, impaired liver function, or to animals recently exposed to or showing signs of infectious disease. Do not use the product in animals simultaneously or within a few days before or after treatment with or exposure to cholinesterase-inhibiting drugs, pesticides, or chemicals. Do not use in dogs infected with *D. immitis*. Task Tabs are not recommended for use in animals other than cats or dogs.

Rapidity of Action: Task Tabs have demonstrated extremely rapid vermicidal properties. In two-month-old puppies dead, unattached hookworms have been found in the small intestine within one hour following dosage. Parasite expulsion from cats and puppies generally begins within six hours and for all practical purposes is complete within 24 hours following treatment.

Stability: The active ingredient dichlorvos (2, 2-dichlorovinyl dimethyl phosphate) is a volatile substance which is easily destroyed by oxidizing agents and by hydrolysis. Task Tabs should be stored under refrigeration (40°F) to insure proper shelf life. Between tablet withdrawals, the bottle must be tightly capped.

Toxicology: The acute oral LD_{50} for Task Tabs (formulated dichlorvos) approximates 38 mg dichlorvos per pound of body weight in kittens and young adult cats and 111 mg dichlorvos per pound of body weight in 3-week-old puppies. The minimum lethal dosages for cats and puppies have been determined to be 25 mg/lb and 45 mg/lb respectively. The recommended therapeutic dosage for cats and puppies is 5 mg/lb. Profuse vomiting tends to limit the amount of formulated drug which can be administered in acute toxicity studies.

The cardinal signs of toxicity from dichlorvos overdose in puppies are excessive salivation, pupillary contraction, dyspnea, retching, emesis, watery diarrhea, muscular fasciculations, evidence of abdominal pain, ataxia, and general weakness progressing toward paralysis. In kittens and cats high dosages of the drug will cause apprehension and convulsive muscular activity in addition to the other cholinergic signs. This formulation provides a very rapid release of the active ingredient; when the tablets are given at elevated non-lethal dosages, all signs of toxicity generally regress without antidotal therapy in 2–4 hours.

Task Tabs were administered to puppies at three times the therapeutic dose, twice weekly from three weeks of age through nine weeks of age, weaning being accomplished at six weeks. Emesis was common (23%) but when compared to control and placebo-treated groups there were no detrimental effects noted on survival growth, or on the hematology and serum chemistry measured. After the six weeks of continuous therapy, average RBC acetylcholinesterase activity was depressed 30% below the controls, whereas plasma cholinesterase activity in some puppies had rebounded to twice that of the controls. In another treatment group, one of seven pups succumbed after six continuous weeks of six times the therapeutic dosage, given twice weekly.

Task Tabs were administered to young adult cats at the recommended therapeutic dose twice weekly for ten weeks. Clinical side reactions were minimal (less than 5% emesis) and when compared to control cats, there were no detrimental effects noted on general clinical condition, or on the hematology and serum chemistry measured. At the conclusion of the test average whole blood cholinesterase activity was depressed 15–20% below the control values. Some of these test cats became pregnant, and the Task Tabs treatments were continued throughout their gestation; no reproductive problems were encountered.

Pharmacology and Physiology: Dosage limitations with Task Tabs insofar as it is known, are due to the drug's action on the nervous system, where it depresses the enzyme acetylcholinesterase. This allows for an accumulation of the substrate acetylcholine at the neuronal junctions, with a resultant overstimulation of the motor and parasympathetic fibers. The severity of this effect is directly related to dosage.

Cats and puppies when administered the recommended dosage of Task Tabs have shown a small but detectable drop in circulating (blood) cholinesterase activities. Normal values are regained within five to ten days. Fifty ppm of unformulated dichlorvos in the ration of dogs for 40 consecutive days were required to effect a significant drop in red blood cell and plasma cholinesterase activities. Sixty days of 15 and 25 ppm continuous feeding of unformulated dichlorvos were required to cause comparable cholinesterase depressions. These drug levels did not produce visible signs of toxicity, and weight gains were not reduced.

The exact significance of plasma, red blood cell, and/or platelet cholinesterase depression is not known since animals have been observed to survive long periods of time in chronic toxicological studies with near zero levels of detectable circulating cholinesterase activity. Such measurements serve only to indicate that very small amounts of the intact drug are absorbed from the digestive tract.

Single or repeated (weekly) recommended dosages of Task Tabs to puppies and/or cats have not produced abnormal changes in the erythrocyte count, leukocyte count, leukocyte differential, hemoglobin, hematocrit, blood glucose, blood urea nitrogen, alkaline phosphatase, lactic dehydrogenase, serum glutamic-oxalacetic transaminase, serum cholesterol, serum uric acid, serum calcium, serum inorganic phosphorus, or total serum protein.

Reproduction: Single or repeated recommended dosages of dichlorvos have been administered to sows, bitches, queens, and rats in various stages of pregnancy, indicating no interference with gestation, parturition, or the subsequent performance of their offspring. Rat, dog, and swine studies have included chronic feeding of the drug for two years or more, through two or more generations, with no adverse effects on the overall reproductive scheme.

Task Tabs have been administered twice weekly to queens from the onset of estrus continuing throughout their gestation. Again, there was no apparent interference with gestation, parturition, or the health of the kittens.

Pathology: The administration of varying dosages of dichlorvos for varying periods of time to rats, rabbits, dogs, cats, and swine has produced no distinctive gross or histopathological changes in any of the organs or tissues. Occasionally large single dosages of the active ingredient have caused hyperemia and congestion of the intestinal mucosa.

Post-mortem examinations of puppies, kittens, and cats succumbing acutely to lethal doses of Task Tabs have shown minimal gross pathology. Typical of the lesions seen are: engorgement of intestinal vessels, inflammation and congestion of the intestinal mucosa with occasional hemorrhage, and congestion of the liver and/or lungs. Studies in the pig and chicken have shown that single or repeated doses of dichlorvos do not cause demyelination of nerve fibers.

Usage: Task Tabs are available in two tablet sizes, containing 10 mg and 25 mg dichlorvos respectively. The product is designed for use in cats and in puppies according to the following table:

Dosage Table

Number Imprinted on Tablet	Active Ingredient (Dichlorvos)	Body Weight Dosage/Tablet
"2"	10 mg	2 lb.
"5"	25 mg	5 lb.

WEIGH EACH ANIMAL PRIOR TO DOSING

The small tablet is scored. Accordingly, one-half of this tablet will treat 1 lb of body weight. Cats or puppies may be treated with one-half, one, or a combination of tablets which will provide the therapeutic dosage of 5 mg dichlorvos per lb body weight. Task Tabs should not be used in animals under 10 days of age or under 1 lb body weight.

Pretreatment fasting is not necessary, although feeding simultaneously with tablet dosage may tend to hold the drug in the stomach and reduce its effectiveness down the tract. Since the drug is not active against migrating tissue-phase larvae, a second treatment 2-3 weeks after the first is advisable.

Occasionally a cat or a puppy may show signs of emesis within 30 to 90 minutes after dosing. This animal should not be retreated immediately; the product's effectiveness against roundworms and hookworms is usually not altered. Those subjects that do not show a negative fecal egg count within a few days, because of emesis or any other reason, may then be retreated with the drug. In clinical trials mild emesis was reported in 3% of the cats and in 8% of the preweaned puppies.

Laboratory and field trials have indicated that puppies known to be maintained in a high hook worm exposure en-

Continued on next page

Solvay—Cont.

vironment are best treated with Task Tabs in advance of severe clinical signs. Once hookworm disease has progressed to the clinical stage, then supportive therapy (blood) should precede worming if the pup is to have a chance for survival. In case of accidental overdose, atropine and 2-PAM are antidotal.

Attention: Task Tabs used in the control of gastrointestinal nematodes of cats or puppies are not a substitute for good sanitary practices, but rather should be used in conjunction with such practices. Retreatment schedules with Task Tabs are at the discretion of the veterinarian. Cats or puppies which are returned to parasite-contaminated areas will become reinfected. The rate and degree of reinfection will be related to the life cycle of the parasite(s) and the exposure level.

Warning: Keep out of reach of children. Between tablet withdrawal, keep bottle tightly capped. Store under refrigeration. This drug is a cholinesterase inhibitor; atropine and 2-PAM are antidotal.

Caution: Veterinary Use Only. U.S. Federal law restricts this drug to use by or on the order of a licensed veterinarian.

How Supplied: Package Sizes: 10 mg dichlorvos/tablet or 25 mg. dichlorvos/tablet, 100 tablets/bottle, 12 bottles per case.

Task® is a trademark of SDS Biotech Corp.

STORE UNDER REFRIGERATION (40°F)

S

VETALOG® CREAM
Triamcinolone Acetonide Cream U.S.P.
For Topical Use on Dogs Only

Description: Vetalog Cream (Triamcinolone Acetonide Cream U.S.P.) provides 1 mg. triamcinolone acetonide per gram (0.1%) in a vanishing cream base containing propylene glycol, cetearyl alcohol (and) ceteareth-20, white petrolatum, sorbitol solution, glyceryl monostearate, polyethylene glycol monostearate, simethicone, sorbic acid and purified water.

Actions: Vetalog (Triamcinolone Acetonide) is a corticosteroid that provides prompt relief of itching, burning, inflamed skin lesions by virtue of its anti-inflammatory, antipruritic, and antiallergic effects.

Indications: Vetalog Cream (Triamcinolone Acetonide Cream U.S.P.) is indicated for topical treatment of allergic dermatitis and summer eczema in dogs.

Contraindications: Vetalog Cream (Triamcionolone Acetonide Cream U.S.P.) should not be used ophthalmically.

Warnings: Vetalog Cream (Triamcinolone Acetonide Cream U.S.P.) is indicated for use on dogs only. Do not use this preparation on animals which are raised for food production.

Absorption of triamcinolone acetonide through topical application on the skin and by licking does occur. Therefore, dogs receiving Vetalog Cream (Triamcinolone Acetonide Cream U.S.P.) therapy should be observed closely for signs of polydipsia, polyuria and increased weight gain, particularly when used over large areas or for extended periods of time.

Precautions: If local infection exists, suitable concomitant antimicrobial therapy should be administered. If a favorable response does not occur promptly, application of the cream should be discontinued until the infection is adequately controlled by appropriate measures.

Dosage and Administration: Apply Vetalog Cream (Triamcinolone Acetonide Cream U.S.P.) by rubbing into the affected areas 2 to 4 times daily for 4 to 10 days.

How Supplied: In tubes of 15 grams.

Caution: Federal law restricts this drug to use by or on the order of a licensed veterinarian.

VETALOG® ORAL POWDER
Triamcinolone Acetonide Powder Veterinary
For Oral Use in Horses Only

Description: Vetalog Oral Powder is available for oral administration in 15 g foil packets providing 10 mg triamcinolone acetonide in lactose.

Actions: Triamcinolone acetonide is a highly potent synthetic glucocorticoid which is primarily effective because of its anti-inflammatory activity. The apparent analgesic effect is a result of the anti-inflammatory properties of the drug.

Inflammation and Related Disorders: Vetalog Oral Powder (Triamcinolone Acetonide Powder Veterinary) provides rapid relief from pain and reduces inflammation and swelling. The usual pattern of response is improvement of motion and decrease of pain within 24 hours, followed by diminution of swelling.

The extent of return to normal is limited by the degree of irreversible pathologic change present. Triamcinolone acetonide will not reverse permanent pathologic changes.

Indications: Vetalog Oral Powder (Triamcinolone Acetonide Powder Veterinary) is indicated for use in horses for the treatment of inflammation and related disorders.

Contraindications: Do not use in viral infections. Except for emergency therapy, do not use in animals with tuberculosis or chronic nephritis. Existence of congestive heart failure and osteoporosis are relative contraindications.

Warnings: Not for use in horses intended for food.

Usage in Pregnancy: The safety of most corticosteroid drugs for use during all stages of pregnancy has not been adequately established. However, clinical and experimental data have demonstrated that corticosteroids administered orally or parenterally to animals may induce the first stage of parturition when administered during the last trimester of pregnancy and may precipitate premature parturition followed by dystocia, fetal death, retained placenta, and metritis. Additionally, corticosteroids administered to dogs, rabbits, and rodents during pregnancy have resulted in cleft palate in offspring. Corticosteroids administered to dogs during pregnacy have also resulted in other congenital anomalies including deformed forelegs, phocomelia, and anasarca. Therefore, before use of corticosteroids in pregnant animals, the possible benefits to the pregnant animal should be weighed against potential hazards to its developing embryo or fetus.

Precautions: Vetalog Oral Powder (Triamcinolone Acetonide Powder Veterinary) should not be used to alleviate pain or reduce inflammation arising from infectious states unless concomitant antimicrobial therapy is given.

Because of the anti-inflammatory action of corticosteroids, signs of infection may be hidden and it may be necessary to stop treatment until diagnosis is made.

Overdosage of some glucocorticoids may result in sodium retention, fluid retention, potassium loss, and weight gains.

Corticosteroids have been used in the treatment of laminitis; Vetalog Oral Powder (Triamcinolone Acetonide Powder Veterinary) is not recommended for that use. Care is necessary when using any corticosteroid in the equine species.

Adverse Reactions: As with any corticosteroid, polydipsia or polyuria may occur with high dosage or frequent administration of triamcinolone acetonide. The likelihood of their occurrence may be minimized by giving as brief a course of corticosteroid therapy as possible, and by waiting for the reappearance of symptoms before repeating therapy. If polydipsia or polyuria should occur, therapy should be discontinued until these unwanted effects have disappeared; therapy should then be resumed at a lower dosage level.

Other adverse reactions that have occurred with the use of corticosteroids are weight loss, anorexia, and diarrhea.

Dosage and Administration: Each 15 g packet provides 10 mg of triamcinolone acetonide in lactose.

Vetalog Oral Powder (Triamcinolone Acetonide Powder Veterinary) is administered at a dosage of 0.005 mg to 0.01 mg triamcinolone acetonide per pound of body weight twice daily (½ to 1 packet twice daily for a 1,000 lb horse). The recommended dose should be sprinkled on a small portion of the feed given twice daily.

Depending on the nature or severity of the condition, it may be desirable to initiate treatment with Vetalog Parenteral Veterinary (Sterile Triamcinolone Acetonide Suspension USP); see package insert accompanying that product for complete information. If additional steroid therapy is needed after three or four days, Vetalog Oral Powder (Triamcinolone Acetonide Powder Veterinary) may be administered.

Caution: Federal law restricts this drug to use by or on the order of a licensed veterinarian.

How Supplied: Vetalog Oral Powder (Triamcinolone Acetonide Powder Veter-

inary) is supplied for oral administration in 15 g foil packets providing 10 mg triamcinolone acetonide in lactose.
Storage: Store at room temperature; avoid excessive heat.

VETALOG® PARENTERAL VETERINARY
SterileTriamcinolone Acetonide Suspension USP

Description: Vetalog Parenteral (Sterile Triamcinolone Acetonide Suspension USP) is available for veterinary use as a sterile suspension in vials providing 2 mg or 6 mg triamcinolone acetonide per ml with 0.9% (w/v) benzyl alcohol as a preservative, sodium chloride for isotonicity, 0.75% sodium carboxymethylcellulose, and 0.04% polysorbate 80. Sodium hydroxide or hydrochloric acid may be present to adjust the pH. At the time of manufacture, the air in the container is replaced by nitrogen.
Actions: Triamcinolone acetonide is a highly potent synthetic glucocorticoid which is primarily effective because of its anti-inflammatory activity. The apparent analgesic effect is a result of the anti-inflammatory properties of the drug.
Rationale For Use:
Inflammation and Related Disorders: ***Dogs, Cats and Horses***—Injection of Vetalog Parenteral (Sterile Triamcinolone Acetonide Suspension USP) provides rapid relief from pain and reduces inflammation and swelling.
Depending on the nature of the condition, Vetalog Parenteral may be injected intramuscularly, intraarticularly or intrasynovially. The usual pattern of response is improvement of motion and decrease of pain within 24 hours, followed by diminution of swelling.
The extent of return to normal is limited by the degree of irreversible pathologic change present. Triamcinolone acetonide will not reverse permanent pathologic changes.
Allergic and Dermatologic Disorders: ***Dogs and Cats***—Intramuscular or subcutaneous administration of Vetalog Parenteral (Sterile Triamcinolone Acetonide Suspension USP) has been found to provide prompt and prolonged relief in the management of allergic symptoms such as conjunctivitis or reactions to insect bites, and in various dermatoses. Inflammation, edema, and pruritus are suppressed and discomfort is eased, usually within 24 hours. Since scratching is reduced or eliminated, lesions are permitted to heal more rapidly. In many cases a single injection is sufficient to terminate symptomatology. If necessary, repeat treatments can be administered.
Intralesional administration of Vetalog Parenteral (Sterile Triamcinolone Acetonide Suspension USP) is effective for treatment of dermatological disorders such as moist eczema, frictional acanthosis, and other dermatitides in dogs and cats. Inflammation and pruritus are often abated within one to three days. A single intralesional injection is often sufficient to effect remission or elimination of the lesion within a period of one to two weeks.
Indications: Vetalog Parenteral (Sterile Triamcinolone Acetonide Suspension USP) is indicated for the treatment of inflammation and related disorders in *dogs, cats* and *horses*. It is also indicated for use in *dogs* and *cats* for the management and treatment of acute arthritis, allergic, and dermatologic disorders.
Contraindications: Do not use in viral infections. Except for emergency therapy, do not use in animals with tuberculosis, chronic nephritis, or cushingoid syndrome. Existence of congestive heart failure, diabetes, and osteoporosis are relative contraindications.
Warnings: Not for use in horses intended for food.
Usage in Pregnancy: The safety of most corticosteroid drugs for use during all stages of pregnancy has not been adequately established. However, clinical and experimental data have demonstrated that corticosteroids administered orally or parenterally to animals may induce the first stage of parturition when administered during the last trimester of pregnancy and may precipitate premature parturition followed by dystocia, fetal death, retained placenta, and metritis. Additionally, corticosteroids administered to dogs, rabbits, and rodents during pregnancy have resulted in cleft palate in offspring. Corticosteroids administered to dogs during pregnancy have also resulted in other congenital anomalies including deformed forelegs, phocomelia, and anasarca. Therefore, before use of corticosteroids in pregnant animals, the possible benefits to the pregnant animal should be weighed against potential hazards to its developing embryo or fetus.
Precautions: Vetalog Parenteral (Sterile Triamcinolone Acetonide Suspension USP) should not be used to alleviate pain or reduce inflammation arising from infectious states unless concomitant antimicrobial therapy is given. Because of the anti-inflammatory action of corticosteroids, signs of infection may be hidden and it may be necessary to stop treatment until diagnosis is made.
Overdosage of some glucocorticoids may result in sodium retention, fluid retention, potassium loss, and weight gains.
Corticosteroids have been used in the treatment of laminitis; Vetalog Parenteral (Sterile Triamcinolone Acetonide Suspension USP) is not recommended for that use. Cases of laminitis have been reported following the administration of Vetalog Parenteral (Sterile Triamcinolone Acetonide Suspension USP); the mechanism of that response has not been fully elucidated. Care is necessary when using any corticosteroid in the equine species.
Adverse Reactions: As with any corticosteroid, polydipsia or polyuria may occur with high dosage or frequent administration of triamcinolone acetonide. The likelihood of their occurrence may be minimized by giving as brief a course of corticosteroid therapy as possible, and by waiting for the reappearance of symptoms before repeating therapy. If polydipsia or polyuria should occur, therapy should be discontinued until these unwanted effects have disappeared; therapy should then be resumed at a lower dosage level.
Other adverse reactions that have occurred with the use of corticosteroids are weight loss, anorexia, and diarrhea. Anaphylactoid reactions have occasionally been seen following administration.
Intra-articular injection in leg injuries of the horse may produce osseous metaplasia.
Dosage and Administration: Intramuscular or Subcutaneous: ***Dogs and Cats***—The dose is a single injection of 0.05 mg. to 0.1 mg. triamcinolone acetonide per pound of body weight in inflammatory or allergic disorders and 0.1 mg. per pound of body weight in dermatologic disorders. Remission of symptoms, if not permanent, usually lasts 7 to 15 days. After this time, if symptoms recur, the dose may be repeated or oral corticosteroid therapy may be instituted.
Horses—The dose is 0.01 mg. to 0.02 mg. triamcinolone acetonide per pound of body weight as a single injection; the usual range is 12 mg. to 20 mg.
Dogs and Cats—Intralesional: The usual intralesional dosage is 1.2 mg. to 1.8 mg. triamcinolone acetonide. Injections should be circumscribed around the lesion in various sites to insure adequate distribution of the dose. Injections should be spaced 0.5 cm. to 2.5 cm. apart depending on the size of the lesion. The spacing of the dose also reduces pain and/or pressure necrosis.
The dose injected at any one site should not exceed 0.6 mg. to minimize local tissue intolerance and atrophy, and should be made well into the cutis to prevent subsequent rupture of the epidermis. When treating dogs and cats with multiple lesions, do not exceed a total dose of 6 mg. Repeat courses of treatment may be administered if necessary.
It is preferable to employ a tuberculin syringe with a small bore needle (23-25 gauge) for accuracy of dose measurement and ease of administration.
Dogs, Cats, and Horses—Intra-Articular and Intrasynovial: The dose for intra-articular or intrasynovial administration is dependent on the size of the joint to be treated and on the severity of symptoms. A single injection of 1 mg. to 3 mg. triamcinolone acetonide for cats and dogs and 6 mg. to 18 mg. for horses is recommended. After three or four days injections may be repeated depending on the severity of symptoms and the clinical response. If initial results are inadequate or too transient, dosage may be increased, but the recommended dose should not be exceeded.
Routine aseptic preparation of the area should be made prior to all intra-articular injections. A thorough understanding of the pertinent anatomic relationships is essential. The inadvertent administration of the corticosteroid into the soft tissues surrounding a joint is not harmful, but is the most common cause of failure to achieve the desired local results.

Continued on next page

Solvay—Cont.

Following intra-articular administration, pain and other local symptoms may continue for a short time before effective relief is obtained, but an increase in joint discomfort is rare. A marked increase in pain accompanied by local swelling, further restriction of joint motion, fever, and malaise are suggestive of a septic arthritis. If these complications should occur, and the diagnosis of sepsis is confirmed, antimicrobial therapy should be instituted immediately and continued until all evidence of infection has disappeared.

How Supplied: Vetalog Parenteral (Sterile Triamcinolone Acetonide Suspension USP) is supplied for veterinary use in vials providing 2 mg. or 6 mg. triamcinolone acetonide per ml. The 2 mg. per ml. is available in vials of 25 ml. and 100 ml.; the 6 mg. per ml. is available in vials of 5 and 25 ml.

Storage: Store at room temperature; avoid freezing.

Caution: Federal law restricts this drug to use by or on the order of a licensed veterinarian.

S

VETALOG® TABLETS
Triamcinolone Acetonide Tablets

Description: Triamcinolone acetonide is a highly potent synthetic glucocorticoid and anti-inflammatory agent for the treatment of various arthritides and dermatoses in dogs and cats.

Indications: Because of its anti-inflammatory properties Vetalog Tablets (Triamcinolone Acetonide Tablets) are recommended for use in dogs and cats in the symptomatic treatment of arthritic and related conditions; in the management of such dermatologic disorders as summer eczema, non-specific pruritus, and allergic dermatoses; and as supportive therapy in allergic reactions.

Rationale For Use: *Arthritis and Related Disorders*—Vetalog Tablets (Triamcinolone Acetonide Tablets) provide rapid relief from pain and reduce inflammation and swelling. The usual pattern of response is improvement of motion and decrease of pain generally seen within 24 hours, followed by diminution of swelling.

The extent of return to normal is limited by the degree of irreversible pathologic change present. Triamcinolone acetonide will not reverse permanent pathologic changes of rheumatoid arthritis.

Allergic and Dermatologic Conditions: Administration of Vetalog Tablets (Triamcinolone Acetonide Tablets) has been found to provide anti-inflammatory action and as supportive therapy provides prompt relief in the management of allergic reactions and in various dermatoses. Inflammation, edema, and pruritus are suppressed and discomfort is eased, usually within 24 hours. Since scratching is reduced or eliminated, lesions usually heal more rapidly. A single treatment with Vetalog Tablets (Triamcinolone Acetonide Tablets) as supportive therapy may suffice to terminate symptomatology. Subsequent therapy, if necessary, is as effective as the initial administration.

Contraindications: Do not use in viral infections. Except for emergency therapy, do not use in animals with tuberculosis, chronic nephritis, cushingoid syndrome, and peptic ulcers. Existence of congestive heart failure, diabetes, and osteoporosis are relative contraindications.

Warning: Usage in Pregnancy—The safety of most corticosteroid drugs for use during all stages of pregnancy has not been adequately established; therefore, before use in pregnant animals the possible benefits to the pregnant animals should be weighed against potential hazards to its developing embryo or fetus. Clinical and experimental data have demonstrated that corticosteroids administered orally or parenterally to animals may induce the first stage of parturition when administered during the last trimester of pregnancy and may precipitate premature parturition followed by dystocia, fetal death, retained placenta, and metritis. Additionally, corticosteroids administered to dogs, rabbits, and rodents during pregnancy have resulted in cleft palate in offspring. Corticosteroids administered to dogs during pregnancy have also resulted in other congenital anomalies including deformed forelegs, phocomelia, and anasarca.

Precautions: Vetalog Tablets (Triamcinolone Acetonide Tablets) should not be used to alleviate pain or reduce inflammation arising from infectious states unless concomitant antimicrobial therapy is given.

Because of the anti-inflammatory action of corticosteroids, signs of infection may be hidden and it may be necessary to stop treatment until diagnosis is made. Overdosage of some glucocorticoids may result in sodium retention, fluid retention, potassium loss, and weight gains.

Adverse Reactions: As with any corticosteroid, polydipsia or polyuria may occur with high dosage or frequent administration of triamcinolone acetonide. The likelihood of their occurrence may be minimized by giving as brief a course of corticosteroid therapy as possible, and by waiting for the reappearance of symptoms before repeating therapy. If polydipsia or polyuria should occur, therapy should be discontinued until these unwanted effects have disappeared; therapy should then be resumed at a lower dosage level. Other side reactions that have been seen with the use of corticosteroids are weight loss, anorexia, and diarrhea.

Dosage and Administration: Initial daily dosage of 0.05 mg per pound of body weight is usually sufficient to control symptoms, although up to 0.1 mg. per pound may be given daily if response to the smaller dose is inadequate. As soon as feasible, and in any case within 2 weeks, dosage should be reduced gradually to maintenance levels of 0.0125 to 0.025 mg. per pound of body weight per day. In general, therapy should be discontinued by a gradual reduction in dosage after the condition has been controlled for several days.

If desired, therapy may be initiated with a single dose of Vetalog Parenteral (Sterile Triamcinolone Acetonide Suspension U.S.P.) for veterinary use (see package insert accompanying that product for complete information). In this case, the following dosage regimen for Vetalog Tablets (Triamcinolone Acetonide Tablets) should be followed, beginning 5 to 7 days after the injection of Vetalog Parenteral (Sterile Triamcinolone Acetonide Suspension U.S.P), or when symptoms reappear.

[See table below].

REPRESENTATIVE ORAL DOSAGES

Body Weight	Initial Dosage (daily)	Maintenance Dosage
5 lb.	½ to 1 0.5 mg tablets	¼ 0.5 mg. tablet every 1 or 2 days
10 lb.	1 to 2 0.5 mg. tablets	¼ to ½ 0.5 mg. tablet
20 lb.	2 to 4 0.5 mg. tablets	½ to 1 0.5 mg. tablet
30 lb.	1 to 2 1.5 mg. tablets	¼ to 1½ 0.5 mg. tablet or ¼ to ½ 1.5 mg. tablet
60 lb.	2 to 4 1.5 mg. tablets	½ to 1 1.5 mg. tablet

How Supplied: Vetalog Tablets (Triamcinolone Acetonide Tablets) are intended for veterinary use. They are supplied for oral administration in potencies of 0.5 mg triamcinolone acetonide and 1.5 mg triamcinolone acetonide per tablet. The 0.5 mg tablets are available in bottles of 100 and 1000. The 1.5 mg tablets are available in bottles of 100 and 500.

Storage: Store at room temperature; avoid excessive heat.

Caution: Federal law restricts this drug to use by or on the order of a licensed veterinarian.

VETISULID® INJECTION
Sodium Sulfachlorpyridazine Injection
VETISULID® POWDER
Sodium Sulfachlorpyridazine Powder
VETISULID® BOLUSES
Sulfachlorpyridazine Boluses
VETISULID® ORAL SUSPENSION
Sulfachlorpyridazine Oral Suspension
For Veterinary Use Only

Description: Vetisulid Injection (Sodium Sulfachlorpyridazine Injection) is a sterile, aqueous solution for intravenous

use. Each ml. provides 215 mg. (21.5%) sodium sulfachlorpyridazine (equivalent to 200 mg. sulfachlorpyridazine), 16 mg. benzyl alcohol, and sodium hydroxide to adjust the pH.
Bottles of Vetisulid Powder for oral use contain 54 g. sodium sulfachlorpyridazine powder (equivalent to 50 g. sulfachlorpyridazine).
Vetisulid Boluses for oral administration contain 2 g. sulfachlorpyridazine per bolus.
Vetisulid Oral Suspension provides 50 mg. (5%) sulfachlorpyridazine per ml. A pump that is calibrated to deliver approximately 1.2 ml. (60 mg.) of sulfachlorpyridazine with each complete compression is supplied for convenient oral administration.

Actions: Sulfachlorpyridazine is a broad spectrum antibacterial compound which is effective in the treatment of infections caused by gram-positive and gram-negative organisms that are commonly susceptible to sulfonamide therapy and which has been proven by laboratory and field experiments to be highly effective against diseases caused by *Escherichia coli.*
Sulfachlorpyridazine has a rapid onset of action in several species of animals following both oral and parenteral administration. In comparison with other sulfonamides, the administration of equi-effective oral doses of sulfachlorpyridazine to dogs produces blood concentrations that reach maximum levels in 1 to 3 hours. The blood level declines to 1 to 2 mg.-percent after 12 hours and the drug is completely excreted in the urine within 48 hours. In experimental studies in which cattle are given the recommended dosage of sulfachlorpyridazine intravenously, the blood level rises to above 12 mg.-percent within 1 hour and 6 hours later it falls to 3 to 4 mg.-percent; after 18 hours no sulfonamide can be detected. In swine given the recommended dosage of sulfachlorpyridazine either intramuscularly or orally, the blood level reaches 5.5 mg percent after 1.5 hours. The blood level declines to 1 to 2 mg.- percent within 6 hours; after 12 hours practically no sulfonamide can be detected. Laboratory studies with other species of animals have demonstrated similar responses in blood and urine following oral or parenteral administration of sulfachlorpyridazine.
Sulfachlorpyridazine is readily soluble at normal urinary pH making it unlikely that crystallization of the free and acetylated forms will occur.
Studies with laboratory animals indicate that sulfachlorpyridazine attains a high concentration in the bile; the concentrations in the liver and kidneys approximately parallel that of the blood thus demonstrating excellent penetration of tissues.
Veterinary laboratories have confirmed the exceptional activity of sulfachlorpyridazine against *E. coli* by both *in vitro* and *in vivo* tests. In one study, 64 out of 70 *E. coli* strains that were isolated from clinical cases of colibacillosis in calves were sensitive to sulfachlorpyridazine. Another sensitivity study involving calves revealed 225 isolates of *E. coli* that were sensitive to sulfachlorpyridazine out of a total of 226 isolates examined. Pretreatment and posttreatment identifications of various serotypes of *E. coli* were made in this study. In all serotypes, except one, the number of isolates cultured from the feces of treated calves was reduced following treatment with sulfachlorpyridazine. Results from a study in swine revealed that 110 out of 118 strains of *E. coli* isolated from swine enteritis were sensitive to sulfachlorpyridazine. Clinical studies confirm its efficacy in treating *E. coli* infections.

Indications: Vetisulid Injection (Sodium Sulfachlorpyridazine Injection), Vetisulid Powder (Sodium Sulfachlorpyridazine Powder), and Vetisulid Boluses (Sulfachlorpyridazine Boluses) are especially indicated for the treatment of diarrhea caused or complicated by *E. coli* (colibacillosis) in calves under 1 month of age; Vetisulid Powder (Sodium Sulfachlorpyridazine Powder) is also indicated for the treatment of colibacillosis in swine.
Vetisulid Oral Suspension (Sulfachlorpyridazine Oral Suspension) is indicated for the treatment of diarrhea caused or complicated by *E. coli* (colibacillosis) in baby pigs.

Warning: Treated calves must not be slaughtered for food during treatment and for 5 days after the last intravenous or 7 days after the last oral treatment. Treated swine must not be slaughtered for food during treatment and for 4 days after the last treatment.

Caution: The diagnosis should be reconfirmed if symptoms persist for 2 to 3 days.
To insure adequate urine flow and to prevent crystalluria, water should be readily available to animals receiving sulfachlorpyridazine therapy.

Dosage and Administration: ***Calves:*** The recommended daily dose is 30 to 45 mg. of sulfachlorpyridazine per lb. of body weight administered in 2 divided doses for 1 to 5 days, as follows:
Vetisulid Injection —Administer intravenously 1 ml. per 10 lb. body weight morning and night.
Vetisulid Boluses —Administer 1 bolus orally for each 100 lb. of body weight twice daily.
Vetisulid Powder —Mix the contents of a 54 g. bottle of Vetisulid Powder (equivalent to 50 g. sulfachlorpyridazine) with sufficient milk or milk substitute to treat a number of calves totaling 1100 to 1650 lb. of body weight (e.g. 10 calves from 110 to 165 lb. each) and divide into 2 doses for oral administration morning and night.
It is suggested that therapy be initiated by administering Vetisulid Injection intravenously and continuing therapy with the oral administration of either Vetisulid Boluses or Vetisulid Powder.
Swine: Vetisulid Powder —the recommended daily oral dose is 20 to 35 mg. of sulfachlorpyridazine per lb. of body weight for 1 to 5 days. The dose may be administered either individually or by herd treatment.
Individual Pig Treatment: To prepare a solution for treatment, add the contents of a 54 g. bottle of Vetisulid Powder to 5 cups (40 ounces) of water. Draw the prepared solution into a syringe graduated in mls and administer it to each pig orally using the following dosage schedule:

Pig Weight in Pounds	Dose per Pig
5.0	2 ml twice daily
10.0	4 ml twice daily

Important: When treating the pigs individually, make certain the entire recommended dose is swallowed by each pig.
Herd Treatment: To prepare a solution for treatment, add the contents of a 54 g. bottle of Vetisulid Powder to 15 gallons of water. Since the daily water consumption of pigs varies tremendously, that quantity of Vetisulid Powder (Sodium Sulfachlorpyridazine Powder) medicated drinking water will treat the following number of pigs daily according to their body weight.

Pig Weight in Pounds	Number of Pigs Treated
12.5	110 to 200
25.0	55 to 100
50.0	30 to 50
100.0	15 to 25

If the recommended quantity of medicated drinking water is consumed, replace it with normal or unmedicated water for the rest of the day.
Vetisulid Oral Suspension: The recommended daily dose is 20 to 35 mg of sulfachlorpyridazine per lb. of body weight, in 2 divided doses, for 1 to 5 days. A single complete compression of the pump will provide approximately 1.2 ml. (60 mg.) of sulfachlorpyridazine; therefore, a representative dosage is one compression for each 4 pounds of body weight twice daily.

Note: When treating pigs over 20 lbs. in weight, water treatment with Vetisulid Powder is recommended instead of Vetisulid Oral Suspension.

How Supplied: Vetisulid Injection (Sodium Sulfachlorpyridazine Injection) is supplied in 100 ml. and 250 ml. multiple dose vials. Vetisulid Powder (Sodium Sulfachlorpyridazine Powder) is available in 54 g. bottles. Vetisulid Boluses (Sulfachlorpyridazine Boluses) are supplied in packages of 100 boluses. Vetisulid Oral Suspension (Sulfachlorpyridazine Oral Suspension) is available in 180 ml. multiple dose bottles with a calibrated dispensing pump.

Storage: Vetisulid Injection: Protect from light. Store at room temperature; avoid freezing.
Vetisulid Oral Suspension: Store at room temperature; avoid freezing.
Vetisulid Boluses and Vetisulid Powder: Store at room temperature; avoid excessive heat (104°F).

Continued on next page

Solvay—Cont.

XENODINE®
Polyhydroxydine™ Solution

Product Description: Xenodine (Polyhydroxydine Solution), is a unique topical microbicide, providing a form of iodine 1% in a greaseless solution.
Actions: Clinical and/or *in vitro* studies confirm first-line antimicrobial activity against Gram-positive and Gram-negative bacteria, fungi and viruses.
Xenodine, in an *in vitro* study has shown to be at least three times as active as Povidone Iodine solution (Betadine®) and tincture of iodine against both Gram-positive and Gram-negative strains.[1]
Indications: As an aid in wound healing, prevention of topical infections, and reduction of fungal growth.
1. Topical Infections: Otitis externa infections including *Pseudomonas aeruginosa;* Acute and chronic bacterial infections, including pyoderma, and/or mixed infections of the skin caused by bacteria and fungi; Interdigital infections.
2. Wounds: Abscess lavage; Wound dressing.
3. Surgical Site Preparation.

S

Directions for Use: Cleanse affected area thoroughly and apply two or three times daily, or as directed by veterinarian. May be covered or bandaged after application.
Specific: 1. *Topical Infections: Otitis externa* —3-5 drops in affected ear, two or three times daily. Massage ear following appliction to assure even distribution throughout the ear canal; *Acute and chronic bacterial skin infections* —Apply directly to affected area, two or three times daily until healed. May be covered with gauze or bandge if necessary; *Interdigital infections in dogs and cats*— Flush the lesion with Xenodine two or three times daily. Also apply a small amount over the surface of the lesion. Rub in well. May be bandaged if necessary.
2. *Wounds: Abscess lavage* —Instill amount of Xenodine into abscess that is necessry to flush the lesion adequately. This should be done at least once daily, or more frequently depending on severity and size of abscess; *Wound dressing* —Apply Xenodine full strength on the wound, two or three times daily. If wound is bandaged, less frequency will be required. Each change of bandage will require a new application of Xenodine.
3. *Surgical Site Preparation:* Prepare the surgical site in the normal manner. Xenodine should be applied last in the normal preoperative site preparation. This can be accomplished by saturating a sterile gauze sponge and applying Xenodine to the entire surgical site. Do not wipe off. Xenodine can also be applied directly from the dispenser bottle onto the surgical site. Spread with a sterile gauze sponge.

Warnings: For external use only on non-food animals. Keep out of the reach of children.
Caution: Use caution in cases of deep or puncture wounds or serious burns.
How Supplied: Xenodine (polyhydroxydine solution) is supplied in 1 oz., 4 oz., and 8 oz. bottles.

1. Tindall, E.E.: Evaluation of a new iodophor antiseptic. *Modern Veterinary Practice:* 675-677, August 1983.

Xenodine, Polyhydroxydine and Polyhydroxydine Complex are trademarks of the Xenovet Division, eMDee Corporation.

XENODINE® SPRAY
Polyhydroxydine™ Solution
Topical Microbicide for Cats, Dogs and Horses

Product Description:
Xenodine (Polyhydroxydine Solution), is a unique topical microbicide, providing a form of iodine 1% in a greaseless solution.
Actions:
Clinical and/or in vitro studies confirm first-line antimicrobial activity against Gram-positive and Gram-negative bacteria, fungi and viruses.
Xenodine in an in vitro study has shown to be at least three times as active as Povidone Iodine solution and tincture of iodine against both Gram-positive and Gram-negative strains.[1]
Uses: As an aid in wound healing, prevention of topical infections, and reduction of fungal growth.
Directions: Cleanse affected area thoroughly and apply Xenodine two or three times daily, or as directed by veterinarian. Hold container 10 to 12 inches from skin; press spray pump sufficient number of compressions to cover the desired area. May be covered or bandaged after application.
Caution: In case of deep or puncture wounds or serious burns, consult veterinarian. If redness, irritation or swelling persists or increases, discontinue use and consult veterinarian.
Warnings: AVOID SPRAYING IN EYES. FOR EXTERNAL USE ONLY ON NONFOOD ANIMALS. KEEP OUT OF REACH OF CHILDREN.
Contains: A greaseless solution of Polyhydroxydine Complex® providing a form of Iodine-1%.
How Supplied: Xenodine Spray (polyhydroxydine solution) is supplied in 12 oz. bottles.

1. Tindall, E.E.: Evaluation of a new iodophor antiseptic. Modern Veterinary Practice: 675–677, August 1983.

Xenodine, Polyhydroxydine and Polyhydroxydine Complex are trademarks of the Xenovet Division, eMDee Corporation.
US Patent: 4,297,232

Products are cross-indexed by generic and chemical names in the
Active Ingredients Section

E.R. Squibb & Sons, Inc.
See SOLVAY VETERINARY, INC.

Syntex Animal Health, Inc.
4800 WESTOWN PARKWAY, SUITE 200
WEST DES MOINES, IA 50265
Subsidiary of Syntex Agribusiness, Inc.
PALO ALTO, CA

ANAPRIME®
(flumethasone with neomycin sulfate and polymyxin B sulfate)
Opthakote®
(hydroxypropyl methylcellulose vehicle)
Ophthalmic Solution

Description: The active ingredients of Anaprime® Ophthalmic Solution Veterinary are flumethasone, neomycin sulfate and polymyxin B sulfate. Flumethasone occurs as a white to creamy white, odorless, crystalline powder. The appearance of Anaprime® Solution with the Opthakote® vehicle, is a clear odorless to slightly yellowish mobile liquid.
Composition: Each ml of the ophthalmic preparation contains 0.10 mg flumethasone; 5.0 mg neomycin sulfate (3.5 mg neomycin base); 10,000 units polymyxin B sulfate; in an aqueous vehicle containing polyethylene glycol 3350, propylene glycol, hydroxypropyl methylcellulose, methylparaben, propylparaben and citric acid with sodium hydroxide and/or sulfuric acid added to adjust the pH if necessary.
Physiological Effects: Flumethasone has been reported[2] to possess 700 times the glucocorticoid activity of cortisol (hydrocortisone) as measured in the liver glycogen deposition assay in the rat, 120 times that of cortisol in the cotton pellet assay in the rat, and in the same animal, shows a net excretion of sodium.
In similar tests in rats, another report[3] showed flumethasone to be 730 times more potent than cortisol in the granuloma inhibition assay and 165 times the activity of cortisol in the glycogen deposition assay. The same report showed that in man the compound possessed 7.8 times the potency of prednisolone.
An additional report[4] indicated that flumethasone possessed 677 times the potency of cortisol in the liver glycogen deposition test in the rat, and 30, 25, and 31 times respectively, the eosinopenic, hyperglycemic and antirheumatic potency of cortisol, as measured in man.
In comparison tests involving prednisone and dexamethasone, experimental studies utilizing the eosinophil depression test in normal dogs and blood glucose elevation and eosinophil depression in normal cattle as parameters of drug activity indicate that flumethasone possesses greater anti-inflammatory and gluconeogenic activity than either of these compounds, on an equivalent basis.

General Effects of Adrenocorticoids: The adrenocorticoids are divided into two main classes; e.g., mineralocorticoids and glucocorticoids, based on their major physiologic and pharmacologic actions. Mineralocorticoids such as the naturally occurring desoxycorticosterone and aldosterone, are mainly concerned with hydration, sodium and potassium regulation, and the normal renal glomerular filtration of these two electrolytes. The mineralocorticoids have little if any effect as anti-inflammatory agents, and are not widely used in medicine.

Glucocorticoids include the naturally occurring compounds, cortisone and hydrocortisone. Their major effects are as follows:

1. Increase protein catabolism and gluconeogenesis.
2. Depression of lymphoid tissue, fibroblasts and eosinophils.
3. Increase the sense of well being and tolerance to pain.
4. Depress thyroid function and anterior pituitary function through reciprocal influences.
5. Influence vasoconstrictive response of the circulatory system to norepinephrine, helping to maintain blood pressure.
6. Increase renal flow.
7. Influence gastric HCl and pepsin production.
8. Reduces the secretion of mucus from respiratory and enteric mucosa.
9. Affect to some degree sodium retention and potassium excretion.
10. Stimulate erythropoiesis and myelopoiesis.

Synthetic analogues of cortisone and hydrocortisone containing a double bond between carbon 1 and 2 of the corticosteroid nucleus, resulted in compounds with a greatly decreased effect on electrolyte metabolism. Additional molecular changes present in other synthetic corticoids presently used in medicine, such as methylation at carbons 6 or 16 and hydroxylation at carbon 16, have led to a further decrease in the electrolyte imbalance frequently noted with the use of the naturally occurring glucocorticoids. Fluorination at carbon 6 and/or 9 have led to a marked increase in anti-inflammatory activity.

The synthetic glucocorticoids exhibit a marked increase in potency in that a smaller amount of drug is required to elicit the same effects seen only with larger amounts of the natural glucocorticoids. It is also noted that the synthetic analogues persist for a longer period of time in the body. This is believed to be due to their slower metabolism and excretion.

In general, the ocular effects of corticosteroid therapy are to:

1. suppress hypersensitivity reactions
2. suppress ocular reactions to irritants
3. suppress inflammatory processes created as a result of infection
4. suppress neovascularization of the cornea
5. reduce fibroblastic activity in the cornea

Organism	Neomycin Sensitivity	Polymyxin Sensitivity
	mcg./ml.	mcg./ml.
Aerobacter aerogenes	10.0	3.0
Alcaligenes spp.	10.0	0.5
Bacillus subtilis	3.0	10.0
Brucella abortus	8.0	10.0
Corynebacterium diphtheriae	1.0	—
Diplococcus pneumoniae	10.0	—
Escherichia coli	—	1.0
Hemophilus influenzae	—	5.0
Hemophilus pertussis	8.0	2.5
Klebsiella Pneumoniae	5.0	1.5
Micrococcus flavus	10.0	—
Micrococcus pyogenes		
var. albus	3.0	—
var. aureus	10.0	—
Mycobacterium phlei	0.3	—
Mycobacterium smegmatis	0.5	—
Neisseria meningitidis	—	5.0
Pasteurella multocida	—	5.0
Proteus vulgaris	8.0	—
Pseudomonas aeruginosa	5.0	12.0
Pseudomonas spp.	5.0	31.2
Salmonella spp.	5.0	5.0
Shigella dysenteriae	2.0	5.0
Shigella paradysenteriae	5.0	5.0
Shigella sonnei	2.0	5.0
Streptococcus pyogenes, Group A	10.0	—
Vibrio comma	—	5.0

The primary effect of corticosteroids in the treatment of ocular conditions is aimed, not at treatment of the causative agents, but rather at the tissue response to those agents.[5]

Antibiotic Sensitivity: Studies designed to evaluate the sensitivity of neomycin sulfate and polymyxin B sulfate indicate that the following organisms are sensitive to these antibiotics at the following concentrations.[6]

[See table above].

Indications: For Ophthalmic Use Only—Anaprime® Ophthalmic Solution Veterinary with the Opthakote® vehicle, is recommended for the treatment of the inflammation, edema and secondary bacterial infections associated with topical ophthalmological conditions of the eye such as corneal injuries, incipient pannus, superficial keratitis, conjunctivitis, acute nongranulomatous anterior uveitis, keratoconjunctivitis, and blepharitis in the dog.

The drug is intended for use in those disease states where neomycin sulfate and /or polymixin B sulfate provide specific and effective antimicrobial coverage, except in those situations where the drug is used as adjunctive therapy combined with standard primary therapy.

Dosage and Administration: Prior to the administration of Anaprime® with the Opthakote® vehicle, the hair in the adjacent areas should be clipped closely. The ocular area should be properly cleansed prior to treatment.

The recommended dosage for Anaprime® Ophthalmic Solution Veterinary with the Opthakote® vehicle, is one to two drops per eye every six hours.

Precautions and Contraindications: Anaprime® Ophthalmic Solution Veterinary with the Opthakote® vehicle, is contraindicated in infectious tuberculosis lesions of the eye, early acute stages of viral diseases of the cornea and conjunctiva, Herpes simplex lesions of the eye, and fungal infections of the conjunctiva and eyelids.

In treating ophthalmological conditions associated with bacterial infections, this preparation is contraindicated in those cases in which the micro-organisms are non-susceptible to the antibiotics incorporated into this formulation.

The usual precautions and contraindications for adrenocorticoids are applicable with this compound. Corticosteroids may inhibit essential inflammatory responses intrinsic to the fundamental healing mechanism. Adrenocorticoid compounds have been reported to cause an increase in intraocular pressure. Intraocular pressure should be checked frequently. Ocular re-examinations should be made at frequent intervals during long-term therapy.

Storage: Not to be stored at temperatures exceeding 25°C (77°F).

How Supplied: Anaprime® Ophthalmic Solution Veterinary with Opthakote® vehicle: vials containing 5 ml, in cartons of 12.

Caution: Federal (U.S.A.) Law restricts this drug to use by or on the order of a licensed veterinarian.

For Veterinary Use Only.

BENZELMIN®
(oxfendazole)
Equine Anthelmintic Paste

Description: Benzelmin Equine Anthelmintic Paste is a broad spectrum anthelmintic which has been specially de-

Continued on next page

S

Syntex—Cont.

veloped to provide maximum efficacy, ease of administration, and safety.
Indications: Benzelmin Equine Anthelmintic Paste is effective in horses for the removal of most gastrointestinal worms:

Ascarids (large roundworms)	*Parascaris equorum*
Pinworms (mature and 4th stage larvae)	*Oxyuris equi*
Large Strongyles (blood worms, red worms, or palisade worms)	*Strongylus edentatus* *Strongylus vulgaris* *Strongylus equinus*
Small Strongyles	

Safety: When used as directed, Benzelmin® (oxfendazole) Equine Anthelmintic Paste has an ample safety margin for all practical conditions of use in horses.
Dosage and Administration: The recommended dose of oxfendazole is 10 mg per kg of body weight. Benzelmin Equine Anthelmintic paste is formulated to deliver 4.5 g of oxfendazole or 12 g of paste per 1000 lb of body weight.
Horses maintained on premises where reinfection is likely to occur should be retreated in 6–8 weeks.
Method of Administration: The paste is readily administered directly into the horse's mouth. Withholding feed or water prior to administration is not necessary. The recommendations for administration are as follows:

1. Remove cap from the end of the syringe.
2. "Zero" the syringe by turning the dial ring (the side of the ring facing the barrel) to zero, and advancing the plunger.
3. Following determination of the weight of the horse, select the proper dosage to administer (one mark on the plunger for each 250 pounds of body weight—12 g syringe . . . and one mark on the plunger for each 500 pounds of body weight—72 g syringe).
4. Confirm that the horse's mouth is free of grass, hay or grain.
5. Insert the syringe tip into the side of the horse's mouth, direct tip through the interdental space (space between incisor and premolar teeth) and quickly deposit the drug as far back on the base of the tongue as possible.

Partially Used Syringes—Multi-dose syringes that are partially used, if recapped, may be stored for up to one year provided the expiration date on the labeling is not exceeded.
Precautions: It is recommended that this drug be administered with caution to sick or severely debilitated horses. Consult your veterinarian for assistance in the diagnosis, treatment and control of parasitism.
How Supplied: 12 g and 72 g syringes.
Warning: USE STRICTLY AS DIRECTED. KEEP OUT OF REACH OF CHILDREN. NOT FOR HUMAN USE. NOT FOR USE IN HORSES INTENDED FOR FOOD.

BENZELMIN®
(oxfendazole)
Equine Anthelmintic Suspension

Description: Benzelmin® Equine Anthelmintic Suspension is a broad spectrum anthelmintic which has been specially developed to provide maximum efficacy, safety, and ease of administration either by a stomach tube or by dose syringe.
Indications: Benzelmin® Equine Anthelmintic Suspension is effective in horses for the removal of most gastrointestinal worms:

Ascarids (large roundworms)	*Parascaris equorum*
Pinworms (mature and 4th stage larvae)	*Oxyuris equi*
Large Strongyles (blood worms, red worms or palisade worms)	*Strongylus edentatus* *Strongylus vulgaris* *Strongylus equinus*
Small Strongyles	

Safety: When used as directed, Benzelmin® Equine Anthelmintic Suspension has an ample safety margin for all practical conditions of use in horses.
Dosage and Administration: Benzelmin® Equine Anthelmintic Suspension is supplied in one liter bottles containing 90.6 grams oxfendazole per liter. The recommended dose of oxfendazole is 10 mg per kg of body weight. Benzelmin Equine Anthelmintic Suspension may be administered either by stomach tube or by dose syringe at the rate of 25 ml per 500 lbs (227 kg) of body weight. This product should be shaken well prior to use.
Horses maintained on premises where reinfection is likely to occur should be retreated in 6–8 weeks.
Precautions: It is recommended that this drug be administered with caution to sick or severely debilitated horses.
How Supplied: One liter bottles. (Treats 20–1000 lb. horses)
Warning: USE STRICTLY AS DIRECTED, KEEP OUT OF REACH OF CHILDREN. NOT FOR HUMAN USE. NOT FOR USE IN HORSES INTENDED FOR FOOD.
Caution: Federal (U.S.A.) law restricts this drug to use by, or on the order of a licensed veterinarian.
U.S. Patent No. 3,929,821

BENZELMIN® PLUS
(oxfendazole and trichlorfon)
Equine Anthelmintic and Boticide Paste

Description: Benzelmin Plus Equine Anthelmintic and Boticide Paste is a broad spectrum anthelmintic in combination with a potent boticide which has been specially developed to provide maximum efficacy, ease of administration and safety.
Indications: Benzelmin Plus Equine Anthelmintic and Boticide Paste is effective for the removal of most gastrointestinal worms and bots:

Ascarids (large round worms)	*Parascaris equorum*
Pinworms (adult and 4th stage larvae)	*Oxyuris equi*
Large Strongyles (blood worms, red worms, or palisade worms)	*Strongylus edentatus* *Strongylus vulgaris* *Strongylus equinus*
Small Strongyles	
Bots	*Gasterophilus intestinalis* *Gasterophilus nasalis* (1st, 2nd and 3rd instars)

Safety: When used as directed, Benzelmin® Plus Equine Anthelmintic and Boticide Paste has an ample safety margin for all practical conditions of use in horses.
Dosage and Administration: Benzelmin Plus Equine Anthelmintic and Boticide Paste is supplied in 40 g tubes. Each gram of paste contains 28.5 mg oxfendazole and 454.5 mg trichlorfon, enough to treat 1000 lb. (454 kg) of horse body weight.
The recommended dose of oxfendazole in this combination is 2.5 mg/kg; the recommended dose of trichlorfon is 40 mg/kg. Benzelmin Plus Equine Anthelmintic and Boticide Paste is formulated to deliver 1.14 g of oxfendazole and 18.18 g of trichlorfon in 40 g of paste per 1000 lb. of body weight. The syringe is designed to provide sufficient medication to treat 250 pounds of body weight for each mark on the plunger.
Horses maintained on premises where reinfection is likely to occur should be retreated in 6–8 weeks.
Method of Administration: The paste is readily administered directly into the horse's mouth. Feed or water should NOT be withheld prior to administration. The recommendations for administration are as follows:

1. Remove cap from the end of the syringe.
2. "Zero" the syringe by turning the dial ring (the side of the ring facing the barrel) to zero and advancing the plunger.

3. Following determination of the weight of the horse, select the proper dosage to administer (one mark of the plunger for each 250 pounds of body weight).
4. Confirm that the horse's mouth is free of grass, hay or grain.
5. Insert the syringe tip into the side of the horse's mouth, direct tip through the interdental space (space between incisor and premolar teeth) and quickly deposit the drug as far back on the base of the tongue as possible.
6. Immediately following administration, raise the horse's head for a few seconds to facilitate swallowing.

Precautions: Use strictly as directed. It is recommended that this drug be administered with caution to sick or severely debilitated horses. Administration to mares during the last month of pregnancy is not recommended. Symptoms of overdose are ataxia, colic, and diarrhea. Atropine is antidotal.
Consult your veterinarian for assistance in the diagnosis, treatment, and control of parasitism.
Warning: Not for use in humans. Keep out of reach of children. If swallowed by a human, IMMEDIATELY call physician or hospital emergency room.
Not for use in horses intended for food.
Trichlorfon is a cholinesterase inhibitor. Do not use this product simultaneously with, or within a few days before or after treatment with or exposure to, cholinesterase inhibiting drugs, pesticides, or chemicals. Do not administer in conjunction with, or within one week of administration of succinylcholine chloride, phenothiazine-derived tranquilizers or anesthetics. Avoid prolonged or repeated contact with skin. Wash hands after use.
Notice to Physicians and Veterinarians: Trichlorfon is a cholinesterase inhibitor. Administer atropine as an antidote; give after cyanosis has been overcome, and administer to effect. 2-PAM is a supplemental treatment.
How Supplied: 40 g syringes.

BENZELMIN®
(oxfendazole)
Equine Anthelmintic
Top Dress Pellets

Description: Benzelmin® (oxfendazole) Equine Anthelmintic Top Dress is a palatable broad spectrum anthelmintic, which has been specially developed to provide maximum efficacy, ease of administration, and safety.
Indications: Benzelmin® (oxfendazole) Equine Anthelmintic Top Dress is effective in horses for the removal of most gastrointestinal worms:

Ascarids (large roundworms)	*Parascaris equorum*
Pinworms (mature and 4th stage larvae)	*Oxyuris equi*
Large Strongyles (blood worms, red worms, or palisade worms)	*Strongylus edentatus* *Strongylus vulgaris*
Small Strongyles	

Safety: When used as directed, Benzelmin® Equine Anthelmintic Top Dress has an ample safety margin for practical conditions of use in horses.
Dosage and Administration: The recommended dose of oxfendazole is 10 mg per kg of body weight. Benzelmin® Equine Anthelmintic Top Dress is supplied in 35 g packets of pellets. Each 35 g packet contains 2.27 g of oxfendazole or sufficient oxfendazole to treat a 500 lb (227 kg) horse. For the average mature horse (1,000 lb or 454 kg) two packets are recommended.
Use directions: Sprinkle required amount of pellets on feed. Withholding feed or water is not necessary.
Caution: Use strictly as directed. Keep out of reach of children. Store at room temperature, not to exceed 40°C (104°F).
Warning: Not for use in horses intended for food.
Precaution: Consult your veterinarian for assistance in the diagnosis, treatment and control of parasitism. It is recommended that this drug be administered with caution to sick or severely debilitated horses.
How Supplied: Net Contents: 35 g
For Veterinary Use Only

BENZELMIN®
(oxfendazole)
Equine Anthelmintic
Powder for Suspension

Description: Benzelmin® (oxfendazole) Equine Anthelmintic Powder for Suspension is a broad spectrum anthelmintic, which has been specially developed for safety, efficacy, and ease of reconstitution for administration by stomach tube.
Indications: Benzelmin (oxfendazole) Equine Anthelmintic Powder for Suspension is effective in horses for the removal of most gastrointestinal worms:

Ascarids (large roundworms)	*Parascaris equorum*
Pinworms (mature and 4th stage larvae)	*Oxyuris equi*
Large Strongyles (blood worms, red worms, or palisade worms)	*Strongylus edentatus* *Strongylus vulgaris* *Strongylus equinus*
Small Strongyles	

Dosage and Administration: The recommended dose of oxfendazole is 10 mg per kg of body weight. A 30 g measuring scoop is provided. Use the following dosing schedule with the clear plastic scoop to treat the animal:

Estimated Weight	Measured Amount Drug Product
250 lb	½ scoop or 15 g
500 lb	1 scoop or 30 g
750 lb	1½ scoops or 45 g
1000 lb	2 scoops or 60 g

For Gravity Administration via stomach tube—To prepare the suspension for stomach tube administration place the contents of the measured amount of product into a clean container. Add one half to one pint of warm (tepid) water per packet and mix by swirling for 30 to 60 seconds.
For Positive Administration via stomach tube and dose syringe—Add 5 fl. oz. warm (tepid) water per level scoop and mix. Administer to the animal.
Precautions: Unused portions of the suspension should not be stored beyond 24 hours. It is recommended that this drug be administered with caution to sick or debilitated horses.
Caution: Use strictly as directed. Keep out of reach of children. Store at room temperature, not to exceed 40°C (104°F).
Warning: Not for use in horses intended for food.
NOTE: Contents of each opened packet should be used within 24 hours.
For Veterinary Use Only

BOVILENE®
(fenprostalene)
Sterile Solution

Description: Fenprostalene is a synthetic compound, (1) 4,5-Heptadienoic acid, 7[3,5-dihydroxy-2-(3-hydroxy-4-phenoxy-1-butenyl) cyclopentyl]-methyl ester. (2) Methyl (±)-7-[1R*, 2R* 3R*, 5S*)-3,5-dihydroxy-2-[(E)-(3R*)-3-hydroxy-4-phenoxy-1-butenyl]-cyclopentyl]-4, 5-heptadienoate.

Fenprostalene, developed by Syntex Research, is an analogue of the naturally occurring prostaglandin $PGF_{2}\alpha$ While related chemically to $PGF_{2}\alpha$, it is the methyl ester of a synthetic prostaglandin.
Each ml of Bovilene® contains 0.5 mg fenprostalene, 0.5 mg dl-alpha tocopherol and polyethylene glycol 400 qs.
General Biological Activity: Prostaglandins are widely distributed in mammalian tissues but vary considerably among species in amount and quality. In general, individual prostaglandins within a group have the same biological action on any one system but may differ in quantitative response. However, prostaglandins of the same group may elicit different responses depending on the tissue, and prostaglandins from different groups may cause markedly different responses. For example, PGE_1 relaxes umbilical blood vessels whereas PGE_2

Continued on next page

Syntex—Cont.

has a stimulatory effect. Both prostaglandins, E_1 and E_2 are bronchodilators whereas $PGF_1\alpha$ and $PGF_2\alpha$ are bronchoconstrictors, cause an increase in blood pressure, and stimulate smooth muscle. Prostaglandin $F_2\alpha$ causes regression of the corpus luteum in non-primate animals where luteal maintenance depends on the presence of the uterus. However, luteolysis in the normal primate cycle is not controlled by the uterus and thus the corpus luteum is not affected by prostaglandins.

Fenprostalene is a synthetic analogue of the naturally occurring $PGF_2\alpha$ and is approximately 750 times more active than $PGF_2\alpha$ based on the hamster antifertility assay. In the bovine, fenprostalene is approximately twenty five times more potent than $PGF_2\alpha$ in causing lysis of the corpus luteum.

Safety and Toxicity: The LD_{50} of fenprostalene in rats has been found to be 1.26 mg/kg subcutaneously and 1.82 mg/kg orally. In dogs the lethal dose was found to be 0.125 mg/kg subcutaneously. Dogs administered 10 mg/kg orally died within 6 hours of treatment. The clinical changes observed in dogs included: pallor, decreased activity, ataxia, salivation, emesis, defecation, urination, dyspnea, cold extremities, collapse and death.

S

Fenprostalene was examined for mutagenic activity in a series of *in vitro* microbial assays employing *Salmonella* and *Saccharomyces* indicator organisms. The drug was also studied in the Syrian hamster embryo cell assay. No genetic activity was demonstrated in any of these assays.

The no-effect levels of fenprostalene in three-month oral dosing studies were found to be 20 mcg/kg/day for rats and 30 mcg/kg/day for monkeys.

Fenprostalene was nonteratogenic in rats when administered orally at doses of 1, 10 and 100 mcg/kg/day from day 6 through day 15 of pregnancy. In rabbits, no teratogenic effects attributable to fenprostalene were seen when the drug was administered orally at 0.1, 0.5 and 2.0 mcg/kg/day from day 6 through day 18 of pregnancy. In pregnant rabbits, given orally 2, 10 or 50 mcg/kg/day from day 6 to day 18 of pregnancy, a slight to marked embryolethal effect and/or abortions were noted. This is an expected pharmacological effect since fenprostalene is a potent luteolytic compound.

Male rats were administered fenprostalene orally at doses of 4, 20, 100 or 500 mcg/kg/day for more than 60 days. The males were then mated to untreated female rats. Daily oral administration of fenprostalene in dosages up to 500 mcg/kg/day for more than 60 days did not affect the fertility and the reproductive capacity of male rats.

In peri- and post-natal study in rats, fenprostalene in dosages up to and including 10 mcg/kg/day was well tolerated when given orally to pregnant rats daily from day 14 of pregnancy until the pups were weaned at 21 days post-partum. In pregnant rats given 100 mcg/kg/day, decreased lengths of gestation and high pup mortality were noted; these changes are consistent with the abortifacient action of the compound.

A two-generation fertility and reproduction study in female rats administered 1, 10 or 100 mcg/kg of fenprostalene daily from 14 days before mating until 21 days post-partum revealed no abnormal effects in either the first or second generation offspring. A study was conducted in normally cycling rhesus monkeys to evaluate the effect of fenprostalene upon the menstrual cycle. Comparison of pretreatment and treatment cycle data from the high dose group (8 mcg/kg) with control group cycles revealed no statistically significant differences in menstrual cycle length or changes in steroid hormone and gonadotropin levels.

In cattle, a single subcutaneous administration of 1, 3 or 5 mg of fenprostalene failed to cause any adverse effects as determined by hematology, or blood chemistry. Animals beyond 120 days of gestation treated with 3 or 5 mg of fenprostalene exhibited retained placenta with vaginal discharge. There was no indication of this at the recommended use level of 1 mg either in this study or in the clinical trials. The incidence of retained placenta approximated 1%, at or below the normally expected rate. Single doses of 10 mg or 23.5 mg caused a transient 2–4°F rise in body temperature which returned to normal within 48 hours. Heifers treated with subcutaneous doses of 1, 5, or 25 mg of fenprostalene twice with 11-day intervals between treatments showed no meaningful changes in hematology, blood chemistry, urinalysis or gross and histopathology. A transient rise in body temperature was noted in the clinical observations.

Luteolytic doses of fenprostalene administered to pregnant cattle have no effect on the offspring provided the pregnant cattle do not abort. However, it must be remembered that a 1 mg dose of fenprostalene results in abortion over 90% of the time in cattle less than 150 days pregnant.

No abnormal increases in plasma progesterone or estradiol 17β levels have been noted in fenprostalene-treated cattle. The only effect is to reset the estrous cycle.

Metabolic studies conducted in the bovine indicate the plasma half-life of a subcutaneously administered dose of fenprostalene to be 18 to 23 hours. Fenprostalene is a methyl ester which is rapidly converted to the acid form by the body. The upper side chain contains an allene group between carbons 4 and 6 preventing further oxidation at the β position. The lower side chain contains a phenoxy group which prevents reduction of the 13, 14 double bond and oxidation of the hydroxyl at carbon 15. The only metabolite of fenprostalene is its acid form with 57% of the dose found in the urine, 42.6% in the feces and 0.4% in the milk.

Indications and Instruction for Use for Subcutaneous Use for:

1. Abortion in feedlot heifers pregnant 150 days or less.
   Fenprostalene was tested as an abortifacient in pregnant feedlot heifers using a single, subcutaneous dose of 1 mg.
   In animals pregnant 150 days or less, the resulting abortion rate averaged 91.6%. The abortion is usually uncomplicated with the fetus and its associated membranes expelled at an average of 5 days following treatment.
2. Estrus Synchronization in Beef Cattle and Non-Lactating Dairy Heifers.
   The luteolytic action of Bovilene® Sterile Solution causes the induction of estrus and ovulation in an individual cycling animal or a group of animals. This allows control of the breeding time in cycling cows or heifers. It should be remembered that Bovilene is effective only on those normally cycling females having a corpus luteum (ovulation having occurred at least 5 days prior to treatment). Treatment of such animals with Bovilene usually results in estrus 1 to 5 days following administration with a majority of animals showing heat in 3 to 4 days. Bovilene has been successfully used in the commonly recommended controlled breeding programs. Some of these programs are:

1. Single Bovilene® Sterile Solution Injection: In order to obtain the maximum response from a single injection, only non-pregnant, normal, cycling females with a mature corpus luteum should be selected and injected with fenprostalene subcutaneously. Animals should then be bred at the usual time relative to detected estrus.
   When using the single injection program, it may be advantageous to estimate the percentage of cycling animals in the herd before treatment with Bovilene. This can be done by observing for estrus and breeding at the usual time for a 5-day period prior to injection. If on the sixth day normal estrus events are detected in approximately 25% of the animals (5% per day), those animals that are non-pregnant, normal, and cycling with active corpora lutea should be selected and injected subcutaneously with Bovilene. Breeding should occur at the usual time following estrus detection on days 6 through 11.
2. Double Bovilene Sterile Solution Injections: Normal, non-pregnant, cycling females should be selected and injected subcutaneously with Bovilene. It is not necessary that animals have a mature corpus luteum at the time of the first injection when employing a double injection regimen. The animals should be retreated with Bovilene 11 to 13 days after the first injection. All animals should be bred at the usual time relative to detected estrus. If estrus detection is not feasible, treated animals should be bred once at about 80 hours or preferably twice at approximately 72 and 96 hours after the second injection.

A high percentage of animals will be detected in estrus following the first Bovilene® Sterile Solution treatment. These animals can be bred at the usual time relative to detected estrus. Those animals not bred after 11 days should be retreated with Bovilene Sterile Solution and inseminated at the usual time relative to detected estrus or may be inseminated once at about 80 hours or twice at approximately 72 and 96 hours after the second injection.

For maximum success, any of the preceding breeding programs should be completed by either (1) continued estrus detection (particularly during the third week after treatment) and breeding any animals returning to estrus or (2) expose the cattle to clean-up bulls.

Bovilene can be successfully employed as part of an effective breeding program. However, if corrective measures are not instituted in any deficient area, an artificial insemination program, which has produced poor results in the past, will continue to produce poor results when used in conjunction with Bovilene. Bovilene should not be viewed as a fertility-enhancing drug. It is a luteolytic drug designed to be used as a management tool by allowing for reduction in the time required for heat detection, breeding, and calving, which may result in increased conception rates in a shorter period of time.

Precautions:

1. While this drug has been shown to be highly efficacious in cattle at up to 150 days of pregnancy, care should be taken to confirm through palpation that the duration of pregnancy does not exceed this figure. In cattle pregnant more than 150 days, the production of progesterone necessary for maintenance of pregnancy shifts from the corpus luteum to the placenta. Therefore fenprostalene is not recommended for use in pregnant feedlot Heifers beyond 150 days of gestation.
2. Non-steroidal anti-inflammatory drugs inhibit the synthesis and release of prostaglandins.
3. Do not administer to pregnant animals unless abortion is desired.
4. *Aggressive antibiotic therapy should be employed at the first sign of infection at the injection site whether localalized or diffuse. As with all parenteral products careful aseptic techniques should be employed to decrease the possibility of post-injection bacterial infections.*
5. Bovilene® Sterile Solution should be administered only by the subcutaneous route with a 16 gauge ½ to ¾ inch needle. Injection should be made only in the areas of the body with freer movement between the skin and the underlying tissues, such as the neck, the area behind the shoulder, or the escutcheon. Do not administer by the intramuscular route.

Adverse Reactions:

Localized post-injection bacterial infections that may become generalized have been reported. In rare instances such infections have terminated fatally.

Warning:

For veterinary use only. Women of child-bearing age, asthmatics, and persons with bronchial and other respiratory problems should exercise extreme caution when handling this product. In the early stages women may be unaware of their pregnancies.

Fenprostalene is readily absorbed through the skin and can cause abortion and/or bronchiospasms. Direct contact with the skin should therefore be avoided. Accidental spillage on the skin should be washed off immediately with soap and water.

Dosage and Administration

Bovilene® (fenprostalene) Sterile Solution is to be administered by subcutaneous injection ONLY using aseptic techniques at a dose rate of 2 ml (1 mg) per injection to:

1. Induce abortion in feedlot cattle pregnant 150 days or less.
2. To regulate the timing of estrus and ovulation in cycling beef cattle and non-lactating dairy heifers that have a corpus luteum.

Bovilene® is supplied in multidose vials at a concentration of 0.5 mg of fenprostalene per ml. Adequate safeguards should be taken to preserve the sterility of the multidose vial by disinfecting the vial seal and using a sterile needle each time. This product may tend to congeal at colder temperatures (below 40°F, 4–5°C). Stability and potency, however, are unaffected.

How Supplied:

Bovilene® is supplied as a sterile solution in 20 ml (10 dose) vials, each in an individual carton.

Caution:

Federal (U.S.A.) law restricts this drug to use by or on the order of a licensed veterinarian.

DI-TRIM® TABLETS
For Veterinary Use Only.

Description: Di-Trim is a synthetic antibacterial combination product which provides effective antibacterial activity for a wide range of bacterial infections in animals.

Trimethoprim is 2,4 diamino-5(3,4,5-trimethoxybenzyl)-pyrimidine.

It was developed to interfer with bacterial purine metabolism, selectively inhibiting the enzyme dihydrofolate reductase, thereby blocking the conversion of folic to folinic acid.

Sulfadiazine, in common with other sulfonamides, interrupts bacterial metabolism by inhibiting the use of *para* -aminobenzoic acid in the synthesis of folic acid. Di-Trim thus imposes a sequential double blockade on bacterial metabolism. This deprives bacteria of nucleic acids and proteins essential for multiplication and life, and produces a high level of antibacterial activity which is usually bactericidal.

Although both sulfadiazine and trimethoprim are antifolate, neither affects the folate metabolism of animals. The reasons are: animals do not synthesize folic acid and cannot, therefore, be directly affected by sulfadiazine; and although animals must reduce their dietary folic acid to folinic acid, trimethoprim does not affect this reduction because its affinity for dihydrofolate reductase of mammals is some 5,000 times less than for the corresponding bacterial enzyme.

Bacteriology: Di-Trim is active against a wide spectrum of common bacterial pathogens, both gram-negative and gram-positive. In general, species of the following genera are sensitive to Di-Trim.

Very Sensitive
Escherichia
Streptococcus
Proteus
Salmonella
Pasteurella
Shigella

Sensitive
Staphylococcus
Neisseria
Klebsiella
Fusiformis
Corynebacterium
Clostridium
Bordetella

Moderately Sensitive
Moraxella
Nocardia
Brucella

Not Sensitive
Mycobacterium
Leptospria
Pseudomonas
Erysipelothrix

As a result of the sequential double blockade by trimethoprim and sulfadiazine of the metabolism of susceptible organisms, the minimum inhibitory concentration (MIC) of Di-Trim® is markedly less than that of either of the components used sepoarately. Many straims of bacteria that are not susceptible to one of the components are susceptible to Di-Trim.

In vitro sulfadiazine is usually only bacteriostatic. Di-Trim is bactericidal against susceptible strains. It is often effective against sulfonamide-resistant organisms.

The precise *in vitro* MIC of the combination varies with the ratio of the drugs present but action of Di-Trim occurs over a wide range of ratios with an increase in the concentration of one of its components compensating for a decrease in the other. It is usual, however, to determine MIC's using a constant ratio of one part trimethoprim in twenty parts of the combination.

The following table shows MIC's, using the above ratio, of bacteria which were susceptible to both trimethoprim (TMP) and sulfadiazine (SDZ). The organisms are those most commonly involved in conditions for which Di-Trim is indicated.

[See table on next page].

The following table demonstrates the marked effect of the trimethoprim and sulfadiazine combination against sulfadi-

Continued on next page

Syntex—Cont.

azine resistant strains of normally susceptible organisms.
[See table above].

Absorption, distribution and excretion: Following oral administration, Di-Trim is rapidly absorbed and widely distributed throughout body tissues. Concentrations of trimethoprim are usually higher in tissues than in serum. The levels of trimethoprim are high in lung, kidney and liver, as would be expected from its physical properties.

Studies with labeled trimethoprim in dogs have shown that about two-thirds of the dose is excreted mainly in the urine, as unchanged drug, in 24 hours.

Therapeutic serum levels are detected one to three hours after dosing. In dogs, peak blood levels occur three to four hours after oral administration.

Usually, the concentration of an antibacterial in the blood and the *in vitro* MIC of the infecting organism indicate an appropriate period between doses of a drug. This does not hold entirely for Di-Trim because trimethoprim, in contrast to sulfadiazine, localizes in tissues and, therefore, its concentration and ratio to sulfadiazine are higher there than in blood. Serum levels following dosing give an indication, however, of the probable duration of effectiveness of a single dose. The following table shows the average serum concentrations of trimethoprim and sulfadiazine in six adult dogs following administration of single oral dose of 30mg/kg on two separate occasions.
[See table on next page].

Excretion of Di-Trim® is chiefly by the kidneys, by both glomerular filtration, and tubular secretion. Urine concentrations of Di-Trim are severalfold higher than blood concentrations. Neither trimethoprim or sulfadiazine interferes with the excretion pattern of the other.

Susceptibility Testing: In testing susceptibility to Di-Trim, it is essential that the medium used does not contain significant amounts of interfering substances which can bypass the metabolic blocking action, e.g., thymidine or thymine. Further details are available on request.

Indications: Di-Trim is indicated in dogs where potent systemic anti-bacterial action against sensitive organisms is required, either alone or as an adjunct to surgery or debridement with associated infection.

Di-Trim tablets are indicated where control of bacterial infections is required during treatment of:

AVERAGE MINIMUM INHIBITORY CONCENTRATION OF SULFADIAZINE RESISTANT STRAINS (MIC-mcg./ml)

Bacteria	TMP Alone	SDZ Alone	TMP/SDZ TMP	SDZ
Escherichia coli	0.32	>245	0.27	5.0
Proteus species	0.66	>245	0.32	6.2

- Acute urinary tract infections
- Acute bacterial complications of distemper
- Acute respiratory tract infections
- Acute alimentary tract infections
- Wound infections and abscesses

Contraindications: Di-Trim should not be used in dogs showing marked liver parenchymal damage or blood dyscrasias nor in those with a history of sulfonamide sensitivity.

Precautions: Water should be readily available to dogs receiving sulfonamide therapy.

Adverse Reactions: Keratitis sicca, possibly due to prolonged use of Di-Trim has been reported. This condition has also been associated with the prolonged use of other sulfonamide-containing products.

Hepatitis possibly due to sulfonamide hypersensitivity has been diagnosed following Di-Trim therapy.

Dogs can tolerate up to ten times the recommended therapeutic dose without exhibiting ill effects. Dogs dosed at 300 mg/kg per day for a period of 20 days revealed only slight changes in hematologic values.

Slight to moderate reductions in hemopoietic activity following high, prolonged dosage in several species have been recorded. This is usually reversible by folinic acid administration or by stopping the drug. During long-term treatment of dogs, periodic platelet counts and white and red blood cell counts are advisable.

Teratology: Dogs given therapeutic doses (30 mg/kg per day) of Di-Trim™ continuously and at interrupted intervals throughout pregnancy gave birth to normal progeny. From these studies, it appears that Di-Trim can safely be given to gestating dogs.

Dosage and Administration: The schedule below provides for a dose of approximately 30 mg/kg per day (14 mg/lb per day) or as follows:

WEIGHT OF DOG (lb.)	Di-Trim® Tablets
2.2 lb	1 tablet
4.4 lb	2 tablets
6.6 lb	3 tablets
8.8 lb	4 tablets

The recommended dose may be given once daily. Alternatively, especially in severe infections, the initial dose may be followed by one-half the recommended daily dose every 12 hours.

Administer for two to three days after symptoms have subsided. Do not extend therapy for more than 14 consecutive days.

If no improvement is seen in three (3) days discontinue Di-Trim therapy and reevaluate diagnosis.

How Supplied:

30 mg Tablets	Bottles of 500
120 mg Tablets	Bottles of 100 and 1000
480 mg Tablets	Bottles of 100 and 250
960 mg Tablets	Bottles of 100

120 mg tablets (Each sugar-coated tablet contains 20 mg trimethoprim and 100 mg sulfadiazine). 480 mg Tablets (Each scored tablet contains 80 mg trimethoprim and 400 mg sulfadiazine).

Caution: Federal (U.S.A.) law restricts this drug to use by or on the order of a licensed veterinarian.

DI-TRIM® 24% INJECTION STERILE
(trimethoprim and sulfadiazine)
For Use In Dogs

Description: Di-Trim 24% Injection is a sterile aqueous suspension of trimethoprim* in a solution of the sodium salt of sulfadiazine for subcutaneous administration. Each ml contains: trimethoprim 40 mg and sulfadiazine 200 mg. Vehicle contains the inactive ingredients diethanolamine 6 mg. polyvinylpyrrolidone 25 mg. sodium hydroxide 32.8 mg (additional may be added to adjust pH), polysorbate 80 0.1 mg, sodium metabisulfite 1 mg (at time of manufacture) and water for injection, q.s. Di-Trim is a combination of trimethoprim and sulfadiazine in the ratio of 1 part to 5 parts by weight, which provides effective antibacterial activity against a wide range of bacterial infections in animals.

Trimethoprim is 2,4 diamino-5-(3,4,5-trimethoxybenzyl)-pyrimidine.

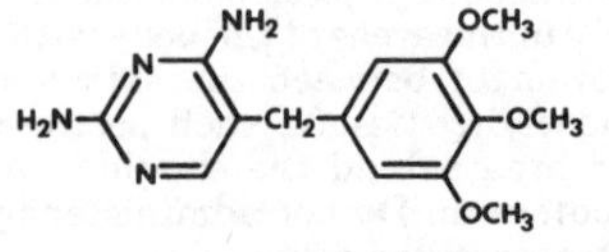

Actions: *Microbiology:* Trimethoprim blocks bacterial production of tetrahydrofolic acid from dihydrofolic acid by binding to and reversibly inhibiting the enzyme dihydrofolate reductase.

AVERAGE MINIMUM INHIBITORY CONCENTRATION (MIC-mcg./ml)

Bacteria	TMP Alone	SDZ Alone	TMP/SDZ TMP	SDZ
Escherichia coli	0.31	26.5	0.07	1.31
Proteus species	1.3	24.5	0.15	2.85
Staphylococcus aureus	0.6	17.6	0.13	2.47
Pasteurella species	0.06	20.1	0.03	0.56
Salmonella species	0.15	61.0	0.05	0.95
β Streptocaccus	0.5	24.5	0.15	2.85

Sulfadiazine, in common with other sulfonamides, inhibits bacterial synthesis of dihydrofolic acid by competing with *para-* aminobenzoic acid.
Di-Trim thus imposes a sequential double blockade on bacterial metabolism. This deprives bacteria of nucleic acids and proteins essential for survival and multiplication and produces a high level of antibacterial activity which is usually bactericidal.
Although both sulfadiazine and trimethoprim are antifolate, neither affects the folate metabolism of animals. The reasons are: animals do not synthesize folic acid and cannot, therefore, be directly affected by sulfadiazine; and although animals must reduce their dietary folic acid to tetrahydrofolic acid, trimethoprim does not affect this reduction because its affinity for dihydrofolate reductase of mammals is significantly less than for the corresponding bacterial enzyme.
Di-Trim is active against a wide spectrum of bacterial pathogens, both gram-negative and gram-positive. In general, species of the following genera are sensitive to Di-Trim:
[See table below].
As a result of the sequential double blockade of the metabolism of susceptible organisms by trimethoprim and sulfadiazine, the minimum inhibitory concentration (MIC) of Di-Trim® is markedly less than that of either of the components used separately. Many strains of bacteria that are not susceptible to one of the components are susceptible to Di-Trim. A synergistic effect between trimethoprim and sulfadiazine in combination has been shown experimentally both *in vitro* and *in vivo* (in dogs).
Di-Trim is bactericidal against susceptible strains and is often effective against sulfonamide-resistant organisms. *In vitro,* sulfadiazine is usually only bacteriostatic.
The precise *in vitro* MIC of the combination varies with the ratio of the drugs present but action of Di-Trim occurs over a wide range of ratios with an increase in the concentration of one of its components compensating for a decrease in the other. It is usual, however, to determine MIC's using a constant ratio of one part trimethoprim in twenty parts of the combination.
The following table shows MIC's, using the above ratio, of bacteria which were susceptible to both trimethoprim (TMP) and sulfadiazine (SDZ). The organisms are those most commonly involved in conditions for which Di-Trim is indicated.
[See table on next page].
The following table demonstrates the marked effect of the trimethoprim and sulfadiazine combination against sulfadiazine-resistant strains of normally susceptible organisms:
[See table on next page].
Susceptibility Testing: In testing susceptibility to Di-Trim®, it is essential that the medium used does not contain significant amounts of interfering substances which can bypass the metabolic blocking action, e.g., thymidine or thymine.
The standard SDT disc is appropriate for testing by the disc diffusion method.
Pharmacology: Following parenteral administration, Di-Trim is rapidly absorbed and widely distributed throughout body tissues. Concentrations of trimethoprim are usually higher in tissues than in blood. The levels of trimethoprim are high in lung, kidney and liver, as would be expected from its physical properties.
Studies with labeled trimethoprim in dogs have shown that about two-thirds of the dose is excreted in the urine in 24 hours.
In dogs, therapeutic levels in serum are detected 30 to 60 minutes after dosing with peak levels occurring two to four hours after parenteral administration.
Usually, the concentration of an antibacterial in the blood and the *in vitro* MIC of the infecting organism indicate an appropriate period between doses of a drug. This does not hold entirely for Di-Trim® because trimethoprim, in contrast to sulfadiazine, localizes in tissues and, therefore, its concentration and ratio to sulfadiazine are higher there than in blood. Serum levels following dosing give an indication, however, of the probable duration of effectiveness of a single dose.
The following table shows the average serum concentration of trimethoprim and sulfadiazine in five adult dogs following a once daily 30 mg/kg subcutaneous injection of Di-Trim for three consecutive days:
[See table on next page].

AVERAGE SERUM CONCENTRATION (mcg./ml)

Trimethoprim (5mg/kg)				Sulfadiazine (25 mg/kg)			
1 hr	3 hr	6 hr	24 hr	1 hr	3 hr	6 hr	24 hr
1.36	1.52	0.51	>0.047	21.6	30.1	27.3	9.8

Excretion of Di-Trim is chiefly by the kidneys, by both glomerular filtration, and tubular secretion. Urine concentrations of Di-Trim are severalfold higher than blood concentrations. Neither trimethoprim or sulfadiazine interferes with the excretion pattern of the other.
Indications and Usage: Di-Trim 24% Injection is indicated in dogs where potent systemic antibacterial action against sensitive organisms is required.
Di-Trim 24% Injection is indicated where control of bacterial infections is required during treatment of:

Acute Urinary Tract Infections	Acute Alimentary Tract Infections
Acute Bacterial Complications of Canine Distemper	Wound Infections and Abscesses
Acute Respiratory Tract Infections	Acute Septicemia due to *Streptococcus zooepidemicus*

Contraindications: Di-Trim should not be used in dogs showing marked liver parenchymal damage, blood dyscrasias, or in those with a history of sulfonamide sensitivity.
Adverse Reactions: Conditions reported following use of trimethoprim/sulfadiazine include polyarthritis, urticaria, facial swelling, fever, hemolytic anemia, polydypsia/polyuria, vomiting, anorexia, diarrhea, and seizures. Keratitis sicca, possibly due to prolonged use of trimethoprim/sulfadiazine, has been reported. This condition has also been associated with the prolonged use of other sulfonamide-containing products.
Hepatitis, possibly due to sulfonamide hypersensitivity, has been diagnosed following trimethoprim/sulfadiazine therapy.
Individual animal hypersensitivity may result in local or generalized reactions, sometimes fatal.
Anaphylactoid reactions, although rare, may also occur—Antidote: epinephrine.
Precautions: Water should be readily available to dogs receiving sulfonamide therapy.
Toxicity and Side Effects: Toxicity is low. The acute toxicity (LD_{50}) of Di-Trim is more than 5 g/kg orally in rats and mice. No significant changes were recorded in rats given doses of 600 mg/kg per day for 90 days.
Dogs can tolerate up to 10 times the recommended therapeutic dose without exhibiting ill effects. Dogs dosed at 300 mg/kg per day for a period of 20 days revealed only slight changes in hematologic values.
Slight to moderate reductions in hemopoietic activity following high, prolonged dosage in several species have been recorded. This is usually reversible by folinic acid (leucovorin) administration or by stopping the drug. During long-term treatment of dogs, periodic platelet counts and white and red blood cell counts are advisable.
Teratology: Dogs given therapeutic doses (30 mg/kg per day) of Di-Trim® continuously and at interrupted intervals throughout pregnancy gave birth to normal progeny. From these studies, it

Very Sensitive	Sensitive	Moderately Sensitive	Not Sensitive
Escherichia	*Staphylococcus*	*Moraxella*	*Mycobacterium*
Streptococcus	*Neisseria*	*Nocardia*	*Leptospira*
Proteus	*Klebsiella*	*Brucella*	*Pseudomonas*
Salmonella	*Fusiformis*		*Erysipelothrix*
Pasteurella	*Corynebacterium*		
Shigella	*Clostridium*		
	Bordetella		

Continued on next page

Syntex—Cont.

appears that Di-Trim can safely be given to dogs during gestation.

Dosage and Administration: The recommended dose is 1 ml Di-Trim 24% Injection per 20 lb (9 kg) body weight per day.

Shake well before using.

Administer by subcutaneous injection.

The dose should be given once every 24 hours. Alternatively, for severe infections, the initial dose may be followed by one-half the normal daily dose every 12 hours.

Continue acute infection therapy for two or three days after clinical signs have subsided.

If no improvement of acute infections is seen in three to five days, re-evaluate diagnosis.

Di-Trim 24% Injection may be used alone or in conjunction with oral dosing. Following an initial injection, therapy can be maintained using Di-Trim Tablets.

Therapy with Di-Trim Injection is not recommended for more than 14 days. A complete blood count should be done periodically in patients receiving Di-Trim for prolonged periods. If significant reduction in the count of any formed blood element is noted, treatment with Di-Trim should be discontinued.

How Supplied: Di-Trim 24% Injection is available in 30 ml multiple dose vials, twelve vials to a carton.

Also available: Di-Trim 30 mg Tablets in bottles of 500, 120 mg Tablets in bottles of 100 and 1000, Di-Trim 480 mg. Tablets in bottles of 100 and 250 and Di-Trim 960 mg in bottles of 100.

Caution: Federal law restricts this drug to use by or on the order of a licensed veterinarian.

® Mfg under Pat. 3,956,327

DI-TRIM® 48% Injection STERILE (trimethoprim and sulfadiazine) For Use in Horses

Description: Di-Trim® 48% Injection is a sterile aqueous suspension of trimethoprim* in a solution of the sodium salt of sulfadiazine for intravenous administration. Each ml contains: trimethoprim 80 mg and sulfadiazine 400 mg. Vehicle contains the inactive ingredients diethanolamine 6 mg, sodium hydroxide 55 mg (additional may be added to adjust pH), polysorbate 80 0.2 mg, sodium metabisulfite 1 mg (at time of manufacture) and water for injection, q.s.

AVERAGE MINIMUM INHIBITORY CONCENTRATION OF SULFADIAZINE-RESISTANT STRAINS (MIC—mcg/ml)

Bacteria	TMP Alone	SDZ Alone	TMP/SDZ	
			TMP	SDZ
Escherichia coli	0.32	>245	0.27	5.0
Proteus species	0.66	>245	0.32	6.2

Di-Trim® is a combination of trimethoprim and sulfadiazine in the ratio of 1 part to 5 parts of weight, which provides effective antibacterial activity against a wide range of bacterial infections in animals.

Trimethoprim is 2,4 diamino-5-(3,4,5-trimethoxybenzyl) pyrimidine.

[structural formula: pyrimidine ring with NH_2 groups, CH_2 bridge to benzene ring bearing CH_3O, OCH_3, OCH_3]

Actions: *Microbiology:* Trimethoprim blocks bacterial production of tetrahydrofolic acid from dihydrofolic acid by binding to and reversibly inhibiting the enzyme dihydrofolate reductase.

Sulfadiazine, in common with other sulfonamides, inhibits bacterial synthesis of dihydrofolic acid by competing with *para* -aminobenzoic acid.

Di-Trim® thus imposes a sequential double blockade on bacterial metabolism. This deprives bacteria of nucleic acids and proteins essential for survival and multiplication and produces a high level of antibacterial activity which is usually bactericidal.

Although both sulfadiazine and trimethoprim are antifolate, neither affects the folate metabolism of animals. The reasons are: animals do not synthesize folic acid and cannot, therefore, be directly affected by sulfadiazine; and although animals must reduce their dietary folic acid to tetrahydrofolic acid, trimethoprim does not affect this reduction because its affinity for dihydrofolate reductase of mammals is significantly less than for the corresponding bacterial enzyme.

Di-Trim® is active against a wide spectrum of bacterial pathogens, both gram-negative and gram-positive. In general, species of the following genera are sensitive to Di-Trim®.

[See table on next page].

As a result of the sequential double blockade of the metabolism of susceptible organisms by trimethoprim and sulfadiazine, the minimum inhibitory concentration (MIC) of Di-Trim® is markedly less than that of either of the components used separately. Many strains of bacteria that are not susceptible to one of the components are susceptible to Di-Trim®. A synergistic effect between trimethoprim and sulfadiazine in combination has been shown experimentally both *in vitro* and *in vivo* (in dogs).

Di-Trim® is bactericidal against susceptible strains and is often effective against sulfonamide-resistant organisms. *In vitro* sulfadiazine is usually only bacteriostatic.

The precise *in vitro* MIC of the combination varies with the ratio of the drugs present, but action of Di-Trim® occurs over a wide range of ratios with an increase in the concentration of one of its components compensating for a decrease in the other. It is usual, however, to determine MIC's using a constant ratio of one part trimethoprim in twenty parts of the combination.

The following table shows MIC's, using the above ratio, of bacteria which were susceptible to both trimethoprim (TMP) and sulfadiazine (SDZ). The organisms are those most commonly involved in conditions for which Di-Trim® is indicated.

[See table on next page].

The following table demonstrates the marked effect of the trimethoprim and sulfadiazine combination against sulfadiazine-resistant strains of normally susceptible organisms:

[See table on next page].

Susceptibility Testing: In testing susceptibility to Di-Trim®, it is essential that the medium used does not contain significant amounts of interfering substances which can bypass the metabolic blocking action, e.g., thymidine or thymine.

The Di-Trim® sensitivity disc is appropriate for testing by the disc diffusion method.

Pharmacology: Following parenteral administration, Di-Trim® is rapidly absorbed and widely distributed throughout body tissues. Concentrations of trimethoprim are usually higher in tissues than in blood. The levels of trimethoprim are high in lung, kidney and liver, as would be expected from its physical properties.

Serum concentrations in horses following intravenous administration indicate rapid dissolution of trimethoprim particles and a steady rate of elimination of

AVERAGE MINIMUM INHIBITORY CONCENTRATION (MIC—mcg/ml)

Bacteria	TMP Alone	SDZ Alone	TMP/SDZ	
			TMP	SDZ
Escherichia coli	0.31	26.5	0.07	1.31
Proteus species	1.3	24.5	0.15	2.85
Staphylococcus aureus	0.6	17.6	0.13	2.47
Pasturella species	0.06	20.1	0.03	0.56
Salmonella species	0.15	61.0	0.05	0.95
β Streptococcus	0.5	24.5	0.15	2.85

both components, with half lives of about three hours and clearance within 24 hours.
Usually, the concentration of an antibacterial in the blood and the MIC of the infecting organism indicate an appropriate period between doses of a drug. This does not hold entirely for Di-Trim® because trimethoprim, in contrast to sulfadiazine, localizes in tissues and, therefore, its concentration and ratio to sulfadiazine are higher there than in blood. Serum levels following dosing give an indication, however, of the probable duration of effectiveness of a single dose.
The following table shows the average serum concentration of trimethoprim and sulfadiazine in eleven adult horses following administration of a single IV dose of 22 mg/kg.
[See table on next page].
Excretion of Di-Trim® is chiefly by the kidneys, by both glomerular filtration and tubular secretion. Urine concentrations of both trimethoprim and sulfadiazine are severalfold higher than blood concentrations. Neither trimethoprim nor sulfadiazine interferes with the excretion pattern of the other.
Indications and Usage: Di-Trim ® 48% Injection is indicated in horses where potent systemic antibacterial action against sensitive organisms is required. Di-Trim® 48% Injection is indicated where control of bacterial infections is required during treatment of:
Acute Strangles
Respiratory Tract Infections
Acute Urogenital Infections
Wound Infections and Abscesses
Di-Trim® is well tolerated by foals.
Contraindications: Di-Trim® should not be used in horses showing marked liver parenchymal damage, blood dyscrasias or in those with a history of sulfonamide sensitivity.
Warning: Not for use in horses intended for food.
Adverse Reactions: Transient pruritus has been reported following the first dose in a small number of horses. This resolved spontaneously within 24 hours and did not recur after subsequent doses.
Following administration intramuscularly, subcutaneously or by accidental perivascular infiltration, swelling, pain and minor tissue damage have occasionally been observed.
Individual animal hypersensitivity may result in local or generalized reactions, sometimes fatal. Anaphylactoid reactions although rare, may also occur—Antidote: Epinephrine.
Precaution: Water should be readily available to horses receiving sulfonamide therapy.
Toxicity and Side Effects: Toxicity is low. The acute toxicity (LD_{50}) of Di-Trim® is more than 5 g/kg orally in rats and mice. No significant changes were recorded in rats given doses of 600 mg/kg per day for 90 days.
Horses have tolerated up to five times the recommended daily dose for seven days or the recommended daily dose for 21 consecutive days without clinical effects or histopathological changes.
Lengthening of clotting time was seen in some of the horses on high or prolonged dosing in one of two trials. The effect, which may have been related to a resolving infection, was not seen in a second similar trial.
Slight to moderate reductions in hematopoietic activity following high, prolonged dosage in several species have been recorded. This is usually reversible by folinic acid (leucovorin) administration or by stopping the drug. During long-term treatment of horses, periodic platelet counts and white and red blood cell counts are advisable.
Teratology: The effect of Di-Trim® 48% Injection on pregnancy has not been determined. Studies to date show there is no detrimental effect on stallion spermatogenesis with or following the recommended dose of Di-Trim® 48% Injection.
Dosage and Administration: The recommended dose is 2 ml Di-Trim® 48% Injection per 100 lb (45 kg) body weight per day.
Shake well before using.
Administer by intravenous injection.
The usual course of treatment is a single, daily dose for 5 to 7 days.
The daily dose may be halved and given morning and evening.
Continue acute infection therapy for two to three days after clinical signs have subsided.
A convenient dosage guide is:
250 lb body weight—5 ml daily
500 lb body weight—10 ml daily
750 lb body weight—15 ml daily
1000 lb body weight—20 ml daily
1250 lb body weight—25 ml daily
If no improvement of acute infections is seen in three to five days, reevaluate diagnosis.
A complete blood count should be done periodically in patients receiving Di-Trim® for prolonged periods. If significant reduction in the count of any formed blood element is noted, treatment with Di-Trim® should be discontinued.

AVERAGE SERUM CONCENTRATION (mcg/ml)

TMP/SDZ (30 mg/kg)	Trimethoprim (5 mg/kg)			Sulfadiazine (25 mg/kg)		
	3 h	6 h	24 h	3 h	6 h	24 h
	0.28	0.24	0.18	38.7	23.7	4.3

Very Sensitive	Sensitive	Moderately Sensitive	Not Sensitive
Escherichia	*Staphylococcus*	*Moraxella*	*Mycobacterium*
Streptococcus	*Neisseria*	*Nocardia*	*Leptospira*
Proteus	*Klebsiella*	*Brucella*	*Pseudomonas*
Salmonella	*Fusiformis*		*Erysipelothrix*
Pasteurella	*Corynebacterium*		
Shigella	*Clostridium*		
	Bordetella		

How Supplied: Di-Trim® 48% Injection is available in 100 ml multiple dose vials.
Caution: Federal law restricts this drug to use by or on the order of a licensed veterinarian.
*Mfd. under Pat. 3,956,327

DI-TRIM® 400
(trimethoprim* and sulfadiazine)
Oral Paste
For Use in Horses

Description: Di-Trim® 400 Oral Paste contains 67 mg trimethoprim and 333 mg sulfadiazine per gram.
Di-Trim is a combination of trimethoprim and sulfadiazine in the ratio of 1 part to 5 parts by weight, which provides effective antibacterial activity against a wide range of bacterial infections in animals.
Trimethoprim is 2,4 diamino-5-(3,4,5-trimethoxybenzyl) pyrimidine.

NH_2 N N CH_2 NH_2 CH_3O OCH_3 OCH_3

Actions:
Microbiology: Trimethoprim blocks bacterial production of tetrahydrofolic acid from dihydrofolic acid by binding to and reversibly inhibiting the enzyme dihydrofolate reductase.
Sulfadiazine, in common with other sulfonamides, inhibits bacterial synthesis of dihydrofolic acid by competing with *para*-aminobenzoic acid.
Di-Trim® thus imposes a sequential double blockade on bacterial metabolism. This deprives bacteria of nucleic acids and proteins essential for survival and multiplication and produces a high level of antibacterial activity which is usually bactericidal.
Although both sulfadiazine and trimethoprim are antifolate, neither affects the folate metabolism of animals. The reasons are: animals do not synthesize folic acid and cannot, therefore, be directly affected by sulfadiazine; and although animals must reduce their dietary folic acid to tetrahydrofolic acid, trimethoprim does not affect this reduction because its affinity for dihydrofolate reductase of mammals is significantly less than for the corresponding bacterial enzyme.
Di-Trim® is active against a wide spectrum of bacterial pathogens, both gram-negative and gram-positive. The follow-

Continued on next page

Syntex—Cont.

ing *in vitro* are available, but their clinical significance is unknown. In general, species of the following genera are sensitive to Di-Trim:

Very Sensitive	**Sensitive**
Escherichia	*Staphylococcus*
Streptococcus	*Neisseria*
Proteus	*Klebsiella*
Salmonella	*Fusiformis*
Pasteurella	*Corynebacterium*
Shigella	*Clostridium*
Haemophilus	*Bordetella*
Moderately Sensitive	**Not Sensitive**
Moraxella	*Mycobacterium*
Nocardia	*Leptospira*
Brucella	*Pseudomonas*
	Erysipelothrix

As a result of the sequential double blockade of the metabolism of susceptible organisms by trimethoprim and sulfadiazine, the minimum inhibitory concentration (MIC) of Di-Trim is markedly less than that of either of the components used separately. Many strains of bacteria that are not susceptible to one of the components are susceptible to Di-Trim. A synergistic effect between trimethoprim and sulfadiazine in combination has been shown experimentally both *in vitro* and *in vivo* (in dogs).

Di-Trim is bactericidal against susceptible strains and is often effective against sulfonamide-resistant organisms. *In vitro* sulfadiazine is usually only bacteriostatic.

The precise *in vitro* MIC of the combination varies with the ratio of the drugs present, but action of Di-Trim occurs over a wide range of ratios with an increase in the concentration of one of its components compensating for a decrease in the other. It is usual, however, to determine MIC's using a constant ratio of one part of trimethoprim in twenty parts of the combination.

The following table shows MIC's, using the above ratio, of bacteria which were susceptible to both trimethoprim (TMP) and sulfadiazine (SDZ). The organisms are those most commonly involved in conditions for which Di-Trim® is indicated.

[See table on next page].

The following table demonstrates the marked effect of the trimethoprim and sulfadiazine combination against sulfadiazine-resistant strains of normally susceptible organisms:

[See table on next page].

Susceptibility Testing: In testing susceptibility to Di-Trim, it is essential that the medium used does not contain significant amounts of interfering substances which can bypass the metabolic blocking action, e.g. thymidine or thymine.

The standard SDT disc is appropriate for testing by the disc diffusion method.

Pharmacology: Following oral administration, Di-Trim is rapidly absorbed and widely distributed throughout the body tissues. Concentrations of trimethoprim are usually higher in tissues than in blood. The levels of trimethoprim are high in lung, kidney and liver, as would be expected from its physical properties.

Serum trimethoprim concentrations in horses following oral administration indicate rapid absorption of the drug; peak concentrations occur in 2–3 hours. The mean serum elimination half-life is 2 to 3 hours. Sulfadiazine absorption is slower, requiring 3 to 6 hours to reach peak concentrations. The mean serum elimination half-life for sulfadiazine is about 7 hours.

Usually, the concentration of an antibacterial in the blood and the *in vitro* MIC of the infecting organism indicate an appropriate period between doses of a drug. This does not hold entirely for Di-Trim® because trimethoprim, in contrast to sulfadiazine, localizes in tissues and therefore its concentration and ratio to sulfadiazine are higher there than in blood. The following table shows the average serum concentration of trimethoprim and sulfadiazine in eleven adult horses observed on Day Three of three consecutive daily doses of Di-Trim 400 Oral Paste.

[See table on next page].

Excretion of Di-Trim is chiefly by the kidneys, by both glomerular filtration and tubular secretion. Urine concentrations of both trimethoprim and sulfadiazine are severalfold higher than blood concentrations. Neither trimethoprim nor sulfadiazine interferes with the excretion pattern of the other.

Indications and Usage: Di-Trim therapy is indicated in horses where potent systemic antibacterial action against sensitive organisms is required. Di-Trim 400 Oral Paste is indicated where control of bacterial infections is required during treatment of:

Acute Strangles
Respiratory Tract Infections
Acute Urogenital Infections
Wound Infections and Abscesses

Di-Trim is well tolerated by foals.

Contraindications: Di-Trim should not be used in horses showing marked liver parenchymal damage, blood dyscrasias or in those with a history of sulfonamide sensitivity.

Warning: Not for use in horses intended for food.

Adverse Reactions: No adverse reactions of consequence have been noted following the use of Di-Trim 400 Oral Paste. During clinical trials, one case of anorexia and one case of loose feces following treatment with the drug were reported. Individual animal hypersensitivity may result in local or generalized reactions, sometimes fatal. Anaphylactoid reactions, although rare, may also occur —Antidote: Epinephrine.

Precaution: Water should be readily available to horses receiving sulfonamide therapy.

Toxicity and Side Effects: Toxicity is low. The acute toxicity (LD_{50}) of Di-Trim® is more than 5 g/kg orally in rats and mice. No significant changes were recorded in rats given doses of 600 mg/kg per day for 90 days.

Horses treated intravenously with Di-Trim 48% Injection have tolerated up to five times the recommended daily dose for seven days or the recommended daily dose for 21 consecutive days without clinical effects or histopathological changes. Lengthening of clotting time was seen in some of the horses on high or prolonged dosing in one of two trials. The effect, which may have been related to a resolving infection, was not seen in a second similar trial.

Slight to moderate reductions in hematopoietic activity following high, prolonged dosage in several species have been recorded. This is usually reversible by folinic acid (leucovorin) administration or by stopping the drug. During long-term treatment of horses, periodic platelet counts and white and red blood cell counts are advisable.

Teratology: The effect of Di-Trim 400 Oral Paste on pregnancy has not been determined. Studies to date show there is no detrimental effect on stallion spermatogenesis with or following the recommended dose of Di-Trim 400 Oral Paste.

AVERAGE MINIMUM INHIBITORY CONCENTRATION OF SULFADIAZINE-RESISTANT STRAINS (MIC—mcg/ml)

			TMP/SDZ	
Bacteria	TMP Alone	SDZ Alone	TMP	SDZ
Escherichia coli	0.32	> 245	0.27	5.0
Proteus species	0.66	> 245	0.32	6.2

AVERAGE MINIMUM INHIBITORY CONCENTRATION (MIC—mcg/ml)

			TMP/SDZ	
Bacteria	TMP Alone	SDZ Alone	TMP	SDZ
Escherichia coli	0.31	26.5	0.07	1.31
Proteus species	1.3	24.5	0.15	2.85
Staphylococcus aureus	0.6	17.6	0.13	2.47
Pastuerella species	0.06	20.1	0.03	0.56
Salmonella species	0.15	61.0	0.05	0.95
β Streptococcus	0.5	24.5	0.15	2.85

AVERAGE SERUM CONCENTRATION (mcg/ml)

Trimethoprim (3.6 mg/kg)					Sulfadiazine (18 mg/kg)				
1 h	3 h	6 h	8 h	24 h	1 h	3 h	6 h	8 h	24 h
1.15	0.64	0.17	0.07	<0.02	27.2	16.4	7.5	4.5	0.09

Dosage and Administration: The recommended dose is 5 g Di-Trim 400 Oral Paste per 150 lb (68 kg) body weight per day.
Administer orally once a day by means of the Dial-A-Dose®** syringe. Each marking on the syringe doses 150 lbs body weight. When administering Di-Trim 400 Oral Paste, the oral cavity should be empty. Deposit paste on back of tongue by depressing plunger that has been previously set to deliver the correct dose.
The usual course of treatment is a single, daily dose for five to seven days.
Continue acute infection therapy for two to three days after clinical signs have subsided.
If no improvement of acute infections is seen in three to five days, reevaluate diagnosis.
Di-Trim 400 Oral Paste may be used alone or in conjunction with intravenous dosing. Following treatment with Di-Trim 48% Injection, therapy can be maintained using the oral paste.
A complete blood count should be done periodically in patients receiving Di-Trim for prolonged periods. If significant reduction in the count of any formed blood element is noted, treatment with Di-Trim should be discontinued.
How Supplied: Di-Trim 400 Oral Paste is available in 30 g Dial-A-Dose®** syringes.
Caution: Federal (U.S.A.) law restricts this drug to use by or on the order of a licensed veterinarian.
KEEP OUT OF REACH OF CHILDREN
*Mfd. under Pat. 3,956,327
**Trademark—Silver Industries, Inc.

AVERAGE MINIMUM INHIBITORY CONCENTRATION (MIC—mcg/ml)

Bacteria	TMP Alone	SDZ Alone	TMP/SDZ TMP	TMP/SDZ SDZ
Escherichia coli	0.31	26.5	0.07	1.31
Proteus species	1.3	24.5	0.15	2.85
Staphylococcus aureus	0.6	17.6	0.13	2.47
Pasteurella species	0.06	20.1	0.03	0.56
Salmonella species	0.15	61.0	0.05	0.95
β Streptococcus	0.5	24.5	0.15	2.85

DOMOSO®
(dimethyl sulfoxide, medical grade) Gel
(90% dimethyl sulfoxide)

Composition: Dimethyl sulfoxide (DMSO), an oxidation product of dimethyl sulfide, is an exceptional solvent possessing a number of commercial uses.
DMSO is the lowest member of the group of alkyl sulfoxides with a general formula of RSOR.
It freely mixes with water with the evolution of heat and lowers the freezing point of aqueous solutions. It is soluble in many other compounds including ethanol, acetone, diethyl ether, glycerin, toluene, benzene and chloroform. DMSO is a solvent for many aromatic and unsaturated hydrocarbons as well as inorganic salts and nitrogen-containing compounds. DMSO has a high dielectric constant due to the polarity of the sulfur-oxygen bond. Its basicity is slightly greater than water due to enhanced electron density at the oxygen atom. It forms crystalline salts with strong protic acids and coordinates with Lewis acids. It modifies hydrogen bonding.
DMSO is a hygroscopic stable organic liquid essentially odorless and water white in color. Other physical characteristics include:
Molecular Weight 78.13
Melting Point ....18.45°C
Boiling Point ....189°C
Domoso® Gel Veterinary contains 90.0% dimethyl sulfoxide. Carbopol 934, disodium edetate, NaOH and/or HCl for pH adjustment, and purified water q.s.
Indications: *Canine and Equine: Domoso® (dimethyl sulfoxide) Gel Veterinary, is recommended as a topical application to reduce acute swelling due to trauma.*
Pharmacology: The original biological applications of DMSO were primarily confined to its use in preserving various tissues and cellular elements including blood[1], blood cells and bone marrow[2], leukocytes[3], lymphocytes[4], platelets[5], spermatozoa[6,7,8], corneal grafts[9,10], skin[11], tissue culture cells[12,13,14,15] and trypanosomes[16], by freezing techniques. DMSO has also been investigated as a radio-protective agent[17,18].
DMSO has been stated to increase the penetration of low molecular weight allergens such as penicillin G but not large molecular weight allergens such as house dust[19].
The rate of passage of tritiated water in the presence of DMSO on the epidermis of the hairless mouse was measured in vitro. DMSO did not appear to promote the passage of water by its presence, but when concentrated solutions (60% to 100%) were used, permanent changes were produced in the rate of passage of water. It was concluded that the concentration of DMSO used seemed more significant than the time of exposure in establishing the effect on the water barrier[20].
When the tails of the mice were immersed in a 5% solution of various psychoactive drugs in DMSO, the drugs appeared to exert their usual pharmacological effects indicating drug penetration as judged by the behavioral effects observed in the experimental subjects. Other solvents, including water, also appeared to permit some drug penetration in this study[21].
Using ten quaternary ammonium salts as test compounds and either water or DMSO as solvents, the oral LD50 values were determined in rats and mice. Toxicity changes were obtained in some instances by 50% DMSO and more changes were observed in rats than mice although the results in the two species were not always parallel. When toxicity was altered by DMSO it increased in all instances except one.[22].
When administered systemically in another study, however, various drugs dissolved in DMSO did not differ significantly in their lethality or cellular penetration as compared to the same drugs administered in saline[23].
When evaluated as a solvent for biologic screening tests, low doses of hormones in DMSO stimulated a response similar to that of the hormone in the control vehicle. Higher doses of hormone, however, failed to give the expected response suggesting a partition coefficient in favor of the solvent[24]. DMSO was also shown to carry physostigmine and phenylbutazone through the skin of the rat[25].
The absorption of phenylbutazone dissolved in an aqueous solution of DMSO was impaired when administered orally to the rabbit. Absorption of the same drug was not improved using the subcutaneous route simultaneously with DMSO. However, phenylbutazone could be detected in rabbit's blood for several hours when an ointment containing DMSO and 5% phenylbutazone was applied to the skin. When the DMSO content of the ointment was increased, the phenylbutazone levels increased. An increase of phenylbutazone in the muscle tissues underlying the site of application over a control ointment containing phenylbutazone without DMSO could be demonstrated in rats[26].
In a number of other studies in experimental animals[21,25,27] where DMSO has been chiefly administered orally or by injection, no anti-inflammatory or analgesic activity could be established.
Following experimental hypersensitization to human gamma globulin, in the horse, antigen challenge resulted in massive erythema, necrosis and slough. This reaction could be markedly reduced by the hourly application of undiluted DMSO to the reaction site, after challenge[19].
DMSO, by itself, at concentrations of 100%, 66% and 33% has been shown to produce neurolysis following perineural injection in the rat's sciatic nerve[28].

Continued on next page

Syntex—Cont.

AVERAGE SERUM CONCENTRATION (mcg/ml)

Trimethoprim (5 mg/kg)					Sulfadiazine (25 mg/kg)				
1 h	3 h	6 h	10 h	24 h	1 h	3 h	6 h	10 h	24 h
0.71	0.95	0.37	0.04	<0.04	8.0	15.8	9.9	5.6	0.6

The conflicting reports cited above for the anti-inflammatory and analgesic properties of DMSO are partially dependent upon the experimental models and methods used to measure these parameters. DMSO fails to show analgesic or anti-inflammatory activity in certain of these situations, particularly when used by the systemic route or when administered topically preceded by an irritant substance. In clinical studies in the horse, it was noted that when iodine, liniments or other strong irritants were present on the skin from previous therapy and DMSO applied, a temporary but marked local reaction would occur. This was due to the ability of DMSO to carry these substances into the underlying skin tissues where their irritant actions could be displayed.

Using the isolated guinea pig heart it was found that DMSO (dimethyl sulfoxide) did not influence the amplitude of cardiac contractions, heart rate or coronary flow although high intravenous doses in the rat and cat resulted in a transient lowering of blood pressure[25].

Isolated, innervated guinea pig preparations were also used to study the effects of DMSO on skeletal, smooth and cardiac muscles. The compound depressed diaphragm response to both muscle and nerve stimulation and also caused spontaneous skeletal muscle fasciculation. Actual contraction amplitude was augmented although contraction rate appeared unaffected. Vagal threshold was lowered almost 50% by a bath concentration of 6% DMSO. The fasciculations and increased tone of skeletal muscle and lowering of the vagal threshold by DMSO could be due to cholinesterase inhibition[29].

The in vitro oxygen consumption of liver, brain and hemidiaphragm tissues of rats is not affected by the intravenous administration of 75 mg. DMSO/100 gm. body weight during the 7 subsequent days.

Urease, trypsin and chymotrypsin are inhibited by DMSO dependent upon its concentration. The in vitro metabolism of corticosterone by rat liver slices is not affected by the intravenous administration of 100 mg. DMSO/100 gm. body weight during 3 subsequent days[30].

DMSO treatment administered intraperitoneally to rats for 35 days decreased experimentally induced intestinal adhesions by 80% over controls as compared to saline, cortisone acetate or a combination of cortisone and DMSO administered separately[31].

In rabbits the application of 70% DMSO, adjacent to but not on the wound incision site, appeared to increase the development of wound tensile strength over controls[32].

Increasing the concentration of DMSO resulted in an increasing inhibition of fibroblast proliferation, in vitro, which was reversible[19].

Toxicology: In a study designed to evaluate the effect of Domoso® (dimethyl sulfoxide) Solution Veterinary at a total daily dose of 100–300 ml. administered for a total period of 90 days, no essential or clinically meaningful ophthalmological effects were seen in the horse. There were no significant variations in glucose, sodium, potassium SGOT, or SGPT measurements. There were a few fluctuations in hematologic values but no changes appear drug-related or of significance.

Another study was conducted in the dog to determine the effects of Domoso® Solution Veterinary at a total daily dose of 20–60 ml administered topically for 21 consecutive days. No clinically meaningful ophthalmological effects were noted. No significant variations were observed in blood measurements, including glucose, BUN, SGOT and plasma electrophoresis. Hematologic values were similar to control animals used in the study.

Long term topical applications of the drug to guinea pigs resulted in histopathologic changes similar to those observed in allergic contact dermatitis. The observed clinical changes were compatible with either an allergic contact dermatitis or a primary irritant effect[33]. DMSO was shown to cause erythema and blistering of human and rat skin resulting in increased permeability of venules and capillaries[34].

In most cases the local irritation of the skin characterized by erythema, vesicle or blister formation and scurfing abates even with continued treatment. This phenomenon has been described as "accommodation" or "hardening" of the skin, and has been noted with other solvents.

The undiluted compound has low systemic toxicity but a marked local necrotizing and inflammatory effect when it is injected subcutaneously. In rats the subcutaneous injection of 10 gm/kg or the intravenous injection of 2.5 gm/kg of undiluted DMSO for 2 weeks showed no definite indication of systemic toxicity. The local necrotizing effects produced at these dose levels, however, prevented a longer period of treatment. No significant hematologic or biochemical changes were noted in 3 dogs receiving 0.4 gm/kg for 33 days[24].

Four dogs were administered topical DMSO at 1 gm/kg body weight, 5 days weekly for 18 months. Serum glutamic oxaloacetic transaminase (SCOT), serum glutamic pyruvic transaminase (SGPT), prothrombin time, alkaline phosphatase, bilirubin, total protein and albumin, globulin (AG) ration, and blood urea nitrogen (BUN) were determined at the beginning of treatment and at monthly intervals. Significant abnormalities did not occur[41].

Upon injection of DMSO in the rat pleura, there is an accumulation of fluid, initially appearing as a transudate, but later as a protein-rich exudate. Exudate formation is thought to be due to increased vascular permeability, predominantly in venules, brought about by a delayed release of histamine together with activation of a vasoactive slow contracting substance[34].

Hemolysis resulting in hemoglobinuria and methemoglobinuria was noted in anesthetized cats following single intravenous doses of 200 mg/kg DMSO. The intraperitoneal administration of DMSO or the dilution of DMSO with isotonic saline prior to intravenous administration reduced its hemolytic activity[39].

Tests in vitro showed that washed rabbit erythrocytes are hemolyzed in a short time with 40% to 60% DMSO solutions. Higher concentrations caused, without hemolysis, an agglutination of the erythrocytes[40].

A compliation of the results for a number of acute toxicity (LD^{50}) determinations derived from several published reports (24, 42, 43, 44, 40) in several experimental animal species are as follows:

[See table on next page].

Teratology: The intraperitoneal administration of 5.5 gm/kg of DMSO as a single dose to pregnant hamsters induced developmental malformations of their embryos[35].

Bot dimethyl sulfoxide and diethyl sulfoxide are teratogenic whn injected into the chick embryo, the classification of malformations being dependent upon the stage of embryonic development at the time of treatment. The same drugs when administered by various techniques to mice, rats and rabbits in which fertility had been established, did not cause any embryonic malformations[36].

Ocular Effects: In a variety of experimental animals including rats, dogs, swine, rabbits and primates, following oral or topical administration of DMSO certain eye changes have been noted. These consist mainly of a change in the refractive index of the lens described as a "lens within a lens". The lens changes are characterized by a decrease in the

AVERAGE MINIMUM INHIBITORY CONCENTRATION OF SULFADIAZINE-RESISTANT STRAINS (MIC—mcg/ml)

Bacteria	TMP Alone	SDZ Alone	TMP/SDZ TMP	TMP/SDZ SDZ
Escherichia coli	0.32	> 245	0.27	5.0
Proteus species	0.66	> 245	0.32	6.2

normal relucency of the lens cortex, causing the normal central zone of the lens to act as a biconvex lens. When viewing the fundus of affected animals, it is necessary to interpose biconcave lenses in order to see the retinal vessels clearly. The functional effect would be a tendency toward myopia[37].

The lens changes were first observed in dogs receiving 5 gm DMSO/kg after 9 weeks of administration. At lower dose levels the change was observed later, in rabbits these changes were seen after 90 days of dermal application, (8 mg. 50% DMSO/kg day and 4 mg 100% DMSO /kg day and higher). In swine, dermal application of 4.5 gm 90% DMSO/kg twice daily caused similar lens changes by 90 days of treatment[38].

The lens changes appear earlier with oral administration, and also bear a relation to the dosage employed; the higher the dose the more rapid their appearance.

The eye changes are slowly reversible but with a definite species difference, the dog being the slowest to exhibit improvement.

No effects were seen following direct application of aqueous solutions varying from 10% to full strength into the eyes of albino rabbits for a total dosage of DMSO between 0.1 and 0.2 gm/kg body weight per day for six months. Rabbits which received daily doses as high as 10 gm/kg orally or topically showed lines of discontinuity in their lenses. No cataract was seen after ten weeks of such daily treatment, although discontinuous lens lines could be detected in about two weeks by slit lamp examination. Chemical studies on these lenses revealed reduction in the usual concentrations of urea, glutathione, uric and amino acids[19].

Dosage and Administration: Domoso® Gel Veterinary is to be administered topically to the skin over the affected area.

Dogs—Liberal application should be administered three to four times daily. Total daily dosage should not exceed 20 g. Total duration of therapy should not exceed 14 days.

Horses—Liberal application should be administered two to three times daily. Total daily dosage should not exceed 100 g. Total duration of therapy should not exceed 30 days.

Side Effects: In general, adverse reactions are local, and while they may prove annoying to some patients, they are usually not of a serious nature. Upon topical application, an occasional animal may develop transient erythema, associated with local "burning" or "smarting". Even when erythema or vesiculation occur, they are self-limiting reversible states, and not necessarily an indication to discontinue medication. Dryness of the skin and an oyster-like breath odor has been reported. These effects are temporary and are not considered to be of serious consequence. Changes in the refractive index of the lens of the eye and nuclear cataracts have been observed in animals, with the use of this drug. This appears to be related to dosage and duration of therapy.

Species	Rt. of Administr	LD^{50} gm/kg
Mouse	SQ	13.9–20.5
Mouse	IV	3.82–10.73
Mouse	Oral	15.0–22
Mouse	IP	20.06
Rat	IV	6.25–5.36
Rat	Oral	16.0–28.3
Rat	IP	6.5 –13.621
Dog	IV	2.5
Guinea Pig	IP	6.5
Chicken	Oral	12.5

Precautions and Contraindications: Contact between Domoso® Gel, and the skin should be avoided. Rubber gloves should be worn while applying this drug. Forceps and swabs may be used to facilitate application. If absorbed through the skin, Domoso® Gel will cause odorous breath and unpleasant mouth taste. Mild sedation or drowsiness, sensations of warmth, burning, irritation, itching and mild erythematous localized or generalized dermatitis have been reported in some persons following exposure to Domoso® Gel. Treatment of such side effects is symptomatic. Consult a physician immediately if adverse effects appear.

Domoso® Gel Veterinary may mask certain disease signs such as seen in fractures etc.; this does not obviate the need for specific therapy in such conditions.

Since Domoso® Gel Veterinary effectively alters the biologic membrane, it will in some cases facilitate the systemic absorption of other topically applied drugs and may have a potentiating effect on drugs administered systemically.

Domoso® Gel Veterinary should be judiciously used when administered in conjunction with other pharmaceutical preparations especially those affecting the cardiovascular and central nervous system.

Domoso® Gel Veterinary may enhance the absorption of other materials into the skin. The veterinarian should make certain that other medications are not present prior to its application.

Keep Domoso® Gel out of the reach of children.

Domoso® Gel Veterinary is recommended for topical application only. *DO NOT ADMINISTER BY ANY OTHER ROUTE.*

Domoso® Gel Veterinary should not be used under occlusive dressings.

Domoso® Gel Veterinary is contraindicated in horses and dogs intended for breeding purposes.

Domoso® Gel Veterinary is a potent solvent and may have a deleterious effect on fabrics, plastics and other materials. Care should be taken to prevent physical contact with Domoso® Gel Veterinary.

Domoso® Gel Veterinary should not be administered to horses that are to be slaughtered for food.

Precaution: Hygroscopic. Close cap tightly after use. Avoid freezing. Due to the rapid penetrating ability of Domoso® Gel Veterinary, rubber gloves should be worn when applying this drug.

Caution: Federal (USA) law restricts this drug to use by or on the order of a licensed veterinarian.

How Supplied: Domoso® Gel Veterinary. Containers of 60 g and 120 g collapsible tubes and 425 gm containers.

For Veterinary Use Only.

DOMOSO®
(dimethyl sulfoxide)
Solution
90% dimethyl sulfoxide
Medical Grade
For veterinary use only

Composition: Each ml. of Domoso® Solution Veterinary contains 90.0% dimethyl sulfoxide and 10.0% water.

Metabolism: Dimethyl sulfoxide when administered topically or orally is rapidly absorbed and distributed in living material.

Using S^{35}-labeled DMSO[1] the maximal blood concentration after cutaneous application was achieved in approximately 10 minutes in rats and less than 1 hour in dogs. In rats and dogs the substance did not accumulate in the organs but the concentration in the treated skin and underlying muscle was increased. The main route of excretion is via the urine partially dependent on the species and route of application. In rats there was no significant difference in the elimination half time of 6 to 8 hours after intravenous or cutaneous administration; in the dog, the elimination half time was 1.5 to 2 days after intravenous or oral administration. In the dog, however, after cutaneous application about 55% of the administered material was eliminated within 14 days. The radioactivity eliminated via the lungs, and identified as dimethyl sulfide, was about 3% of the administered dose.

In another S^{35}-labeled study[2] with DMSO, following intravenous or cutaneous administration, the only metabolite detectable in the urine of humans and rats, was dimethyl sulfone ($DMSO_2$).

In another S^{35}-labeled rat study[3], DMSO was administered by the oral, intraperitoneal and dermal routes at a level of 500 mg/kg body weight. Plasma radioactivity after an intraperitoneal dose was highest at 0.5 hours, the half-time being 5 to 6 hours. When applied dermally, levels remained constant for 6 hours. Radioactivity in the urine collected for 22 hours represented 60% to 85% of the intraperitoneal and oral doses and 36% to 50% of the dermal dose. The skin contained 3% to 7% of the labeled dosage in all cases.

Continued on next page

Syntex—Cont.

A peculiar sweetish odor was noted in the exhaled breath of cats treated with dimethyl sulfoxide[4]. The compound responsible for this was identified as dimethyl sulfide. The same odor has been noted in all species treated with the compound.
In rabbits, dimethyl sulfone was detected in the urine following treatment of DMSO[5].
It has been shown that dimethyl sulfone is a constituent of normal cow's milk[6].
Pharmacology: The original biological applications of DMSO were primarily confined to its use in preserving various tissues and cellular elements including blood[7], blood cells and bone marrow[8], leukocytes[9], lymphocytes[10], platelets[11], spermatozoa[12,13,14], corneal grafts[15,16], skin[17], tissue culture cells[18,19,20,21] and trypanosomes[22], by freezing techniques. DMSO has also been investigated as a radioprotective agent[23,24].
In early studies with plants it was claimed that DMSO exerted a profound effect on the biologic membrane, altering their natural selectivity and enhancing the penetration of antibiotics and fungicides[25].
In one of the first studies reported in animals, various drugs were added to 15% solution of DMSO instilled into the urinary bladder of intact, anesthetized dogs through which an enhancement of absorption was demonstrated[25]. Utilizing a similar technique the transport of physiologically active insulin across the intact bladder mucosa was demonstrated. Results were judged on a decrease in blood sugar levels over that of controls[26].
In vivo and in vitro methods demonstrated that DMSO enhanced human percutaneous absorption of various compounds including steroids, vasoconstrictors, antiperspirants and dyes, as well as an anthelmintic (thiabendazole) and a skin antiseptic (hexachlorophene)[27,28,29,60,61,62]. Enhancement was not due to irreversible damage to the stratum corneum[28].
DMSO has been stated to increase the penetration of low molecular weight allergens such as penicillin G but not large molecular weight allergens such as house dust[30].
The rate of passage of tritiated water in the presence of DMSO on the epidermis of the hairless mouse was measured in vitro. DMSO did not appear to promote the passage of water by its presence, but when concentrated solutions (60% to 100%) were used, permanent changes were produced in the rate of passage of water. It was concluded that the concentration of DMSO used seemed more significant than the time of exposure in establishing the effect on the water barrier[31].
When the tails of mice were immersed in a 5% solution of various psychoactive drugs in DMSO, the drugs appeared to exert their usual pharmacological effects, indicating drug penetration as judged by the behavioral effects observed in the experimental subjects. Other solvents, including water, also appeared to permit some drug penetration in this study[32].
Using ten quaternary ammonium salts as test compounds and either water or DMSO as solvents, the oral LD50 values were determined in rats and mice. Toxicity changes were obtained in some instances by 50% DMSO and more changes were observed in rats than mice although the results in the two species were not always parallel. When toxicity was altered by DMSO it increased in all instances except one[33].
When administered systemically in another study, however, various drugs dissolved in DMSO did not differ significantly in their lethality or cellular penetration as compared to the same drug administered in saline[34].
When evaluated as a solvent for biologic screening tests, low doses of hormones in DMSO stimulated a response similar to that of the hormone in the control vehicle. Higher doses of hormone, however, failed to give the expected response, suggesting a partition coefficient in favor of the solvent[35]. DMSO was also shown to carry physostigmine and phenylbutazone through the skin of the rat[36].
The absorption of phenylbutazone dissolved in an aqueous solution of DMSO was impaired when administered orally to the rabbit. Absorption of the same drug was not improved using the subcutaneous route simultaneously with DMSO.
However, phenylbutazone could be detected in rabbit's blood for several hours when an ointment containing DMSO and 5% phenylbutazone was applied to the skin. When the DMSO content of the ointment was increased, the phenylbutazone levels increased. An increase of phenylbutazone in the muscle tissues underlying the site of application over a control ointment containing phenylbutazone without DMSO could be demonstrated in rats[37].
When 1% fluorescein was injected intradermally at several different concentrations of DMSO in man, the dermal clearance of this substance was considerably decreased as compared to saline control solutions. This was believed due to reduced diffusion through the dermis[29].
The addition of 50% DMSO to solutions containing 1% old tuberculin (OT) abolished positive patch test reactions in tuberculin sensitive human subjects, and 50% DMSO also prevented the dermatitis produced by 1% trypsin. A possible explanation of these phenomena is the formation of complexes with proteins causing their denaturation[28]. DMSO has also been reported to alter the Schwartzman reaction[30]. It is believed that, similar to chelating agents, DMSO can form complexes with certain metallic salts[25,38].
Based on the above evidence as well as gas chromatographic and radio-isotope studies it is established that DMSO can effectively penetrate the stratum corneum of the epidermis and enter the systemic circulation. DMSO also has the ability to allow some substances ordinarily unable to penetrate the skin barrier to be carried through it. The mechanism of penetrant action is not yet understood although some theories have been advanced as explanations[25,38].
DMSO has been claimed to show anti-inflammatory activity against the baker's yeast granuloma in guinea pigs, and when administered orally, against the carrageenin granuloma in rats. The dose needed to achieve these effects is quite high, requiring 1 to 5 gm./kg. body weight[39].
In a number of other studies in experimental animals[32,36,40] where DMSO has been chiefly administered orally or by injection, no anti-inflammatory or analgesic activity could be established.
Following experimental hypersensitization to human gamma globulin in the horse, antigen challenge resulted in massive erythema, necrosis and slough. This reaction could be markedly reduced by the hourly application of undiluted DMSO to the reaction site, after challenge[30].
In the human, DMSO did not exert any beneficial effects on experimentally induced thermal burns, contact dermatitis or ultraviolet burns. It was noted in this study that the burns were of a non-infected nature[28,29].
In experimentally induced thermal edema of the legs of rabbits, the leg volume was the same for DMSO treated and untreated groups at 3 and 24 hours, but less at 6 hours for the treated group. The DMSO in this experiment was applied at a site distant to the injury[30].
Sedative effects have been noted in dogs when 90% DMSO was administered at 10 mg/kg dosage levels and mild reserpine-like actions of the drug have also been described in mice[30].
DMSO, by itself, at concentrations of 100%, 66%, and 33%, has been shown to produce neurolysis following perineural injection in the rat's sciatic nerve[41].
The conflicting reports cited above for the anti-inflammatory and analgesic properties of DMSO are partially dependent upon the experimental models and methods used to measure these parameters. DMSO fails to show analgesic or anti-inflammatory activity in certain of these situations, particularly when used by the systemic route or when administered topically preceded by an irritant substance. In clinical studies in the horse, it was noted that when iodine, liniments or other strong irritants were present on the skin from previous therapy and DMSO applied, a temporary but marked local reaction would occur. This was due to the ability of DMSO to carry these substances into the underlying skin tissues where their irritant actions could be displayed. When DMSO was used clinically, it was applied topically to the involved area, while in the experimental situation this procedure was seldom used. In clinical situations, a marked reduction of pain and edema has often been noted following topical application. The mechanism of action, although not understood, may be partially

related to the heat of dissolution of DMSO. It has been demonstrated that following cutaneous application of DMSO in dogs, the skin, dermis and underlying muscle tissues show a local rise in temperature[30].

The analgesic and anti-inflammatory activity of DMSO, as observed clinically and the differences noted by classical pharmacological methods, may be partially due to the ability of the compound to alter the underlying pathology of the disease state under treatment[42].

Using the isolated guinea pig heart it was found that DMSO did not influence the amplitude of cardiac contractions, heart rate, or coronary flow, although high intravenous doses in the rat and cat resulted in a transient lowering of blood pressure[36].

Isolated, innervated guinea pig preparations were also used to study the effects of DMSO on skeletal, smooth and cardiac muscles. The compound depressed diaphragm response to both muscle and nerve stimulation and also caused spontaneous skeletal muscle fasciculation. Acutal contraction amplitude was augmented although contraction rate appeared unaffected. Vagal threshold was lowered almost 50% by a bath concentration of 6% DMSO. The fasciculations and increased tone of skeletal muscle, and lowering of the vagal threshold by DMSO could be due to cholinesterase inhibition[43]. Intravenous doses of 50% DMSO in doses as high as 1 gm/kg failed to alter the EKG of anesthetized dogs and monkeys[26].

With single intravenous doses of 200 mg/kg of DMSO to anesthetized cats, apnea and a transient fall in blood pressure were produced. Subsequent doses caused only a transient hypotension and apnea was no longer observed. Vagotomy failed to influence the course of DMSO-induced hypotension and bradycardia but atropine (1 mg/kg) significantly attenuated these effects. Repeated intravenous administration of DMSO where each succeeding dose was doubled, led to a gradually lowered blood pressure until death ensued at about 4 gm/kg. Myoneural transmission, ganglionic transmission and force of cardiac contraction also deteriorated gradually with repeated doses until death. The transient fall in blood pressure occurred only rarely after intraperitoneal administration. One cat exhibited hypotension following a 1 gm/kg dose of DMSO but the remainder received dosages of 4 gm/kg without showing this effect[44].

The in vitro oxygen consumption of liver, brain and hemidiaphragm tissues of rats is not affected by the intravenous administration of 75 mg DMSO/100 gm. body weight during the 7 subsequent days. Urease, trypsin and chymotrypsin are inhibited by DMSO, dependent upon its concentration. The in vitro metabolism of corticosterone by rat liver slices is not affected by the intravenous administration of 100 mg DMSO/100 gm body weight during 3 subsequent days[2].

DMSO treatment administered intraperitoneally to rats for 35 days decreased experimentally induced intestinal adhesions by 80% over controls as compared to saline, cortisone actetate or a combination of cortisone and DMSO administered separately[45].

In rabbits, the application of 70% DMSO, adjacent to but not on the wound incision site, appeared to increase the development of wound tensile strength over controls[46].

Increasing the concentration of DMSO resulted in an increasing inhibition of fibroblast proliferation in vitro, which was reversible[30].

There is an increase in urinary production following the dermal or systemic administration of DMSO, and a transient doubling of urine volume after the intravenous administration of the drug[48].

Some studies have indicated that DMSO may potentiate the action of certain compounds including insulin[39], endogenous steroids and others. It was suggested that in the case of steroids it might be due to improved penetration at their sites of action on lysosomal membranes[30].

The minimal inhibitory concentration (MIC) of DMSO to the nearest 10% was determined for two isolates each of *Staphylococcus aureus, Staphylococcus aureus* var. *albus, b*-hemolytic Streptococci, Corynebacterium acnes, *Corynebacterium* species, *Alcaligenes faecalis, Escherichia coli* and proteus species. Twenty percent DMSO was found to be bacteriostatic. For *Staphylococcus aureus,* the bactericidal concentration of 50% was 2.5 times that of the MIC: for the remainder, it ranged from 30% to 40% with the gram negative bacteria being somewhat more susceptible[29].

No growth of Staphylococci, Pseudomonas or *Escherichia coli* occurred in the presence of 36%, 25%, 33% or greater concentrations, respectively, of DMSO[49].

The minimal inhibitory concentration of DMSO in Sabouraud's broth to the nearest 10% was determined for three dermatophytes: *Trichophyton mentagrophytes, Microsporum gypseum,* and *Microsporum canis.* Ten percent DMSO was inhibitory to all three species. The fungicidal concentrations were 30% for the *Microsporum* species, while *T. mentagrophytes* survived the highest test concentrations of 50%[29].

Toxicology: Absorption of topically applied DMSO results in degranulation of the mast cells at the site of application and a release of histamine followed by characteristic histamine whealing of the overlying skin. Following repeated applications of the compound to the same skin area, the mast cells are eventually depleted and the wheal no longer occurs[28].

The erythema of the skin following topical application of DMSO is considered to be partially due to the release of histamine. In addition, DMSO has the typical action of most solvents in causing drying and defatting of the skin.

In a study designed to evaluate the effects of Domoso® (dimethyl sulfoxide) Solution Veterinary at a total daily dose of 100–300 ml administered for a total period of 90 days, no essential or clinically meaningful ophthalmological effects were seen in the horse. There were no significant variations in glucose, sodium, potassium SGOT, or SGPT measurements. There were a few fluctuations in hematologic values but no changes appear to be drug-related or of significance.

Another study was conducted in the dog to determine the effects of Domoso® Solution Veterinary at a total daily dose of 20–60 ml. administered topically for 21 consecutive days. No clinically meaningful ophthalmological effects were noted. No significant variations were observed in blood measurements, including glucose, BUN, SGOT and plasma electrophoresis. Hematologic values were similar to control animals used in the study.

Long-term topical applications of the drug to guinea pigs resulted in histopathologic changes similar to those observed in allergic contact dermatitis. The observed clinical changes were compatible with either an allergic contact dermatitis or a primary irritant effect[50]. DMSO was shown to cause erythema and blistering of human and rat skin resulting in increased permeability of venules and capillaries[51].

In most cases the local irritation of the skin characterized by erythema, vesicle or blister formation and scurfing abates even with continued treatment. This phenomenon has been described as "accommodation" or "hardening" of the skin, and has been noted with other solvents.

The undiluted compound has low systemic toxicity but a marked local necrotizing and inflammatory effect when it is injected subcutaneously. In rats the subcutaneous injection of 10 gm/kg or the intravenous injection of 2.5 gm/kg of undiluted DMSO for 2 weeks showed no definite indication of systemic toxicity. The local necrotizing effects produced at these dose levels, however, prevented a longer period of treatment. No significant hematologic or biochemical changes were noted in 3 dogs receiving 0.4 gm/kg for 33 days[35].

Four dogs were administered topical DMSO at 1 gm/kg body weight, 5 days weekly for 18 months. Serum glutamic oxaloacetic transmaniase (SGOT), serum glutamic pyruvic transmaniase (SGPT), prothrombin time, alkaline phosphatase, bilirubin, total protein and albumin: globulin (AG) ratio, and blood urea nitrogen (BUN) were determined at the beginning of treatment and at monthly intervals. Significant abnormalities did not occur[39].

Upon injection of DMSO into the rat pleura, there is an accumulation of fluid, initially appearing as a transudate, but later as a protein-rich exudate. Exudate formation is thought to be due to increased vascular permeability, predominantly in venules, brought about by a delayed release of histamine together with activation of a vasoactive slow contracting substance[51].

Rats were orally dosed 5 days a week for 2 weeks at levels of 1, 3, 5, 5 and 10

Continued on next page

Syntex—Cont.

mg/kg of DMSO. The only deaths in this group were due to dosing injuries. No signs of dermal sensitization were noted following a course of intradermal injection of a 10% V/V aqueous solution of DMSO in guinea pigs, nor did the same species show signs of injury following 28 daily applications of the undiluted drug to the clipped skin of the back[52].
A compilation of the results for a number of acute toxicity (LD50) determinations derived from several published reports[35,52,53,54,55] in several experimental animal species are as follows:
[See table below].
Hemolysis resulting in hemoglobinuria and methemoglobinuria was noted in anesthetized cats following single intravenous doses of 200 mg/kg DMSO. The intraperitoneal administration of DMSO or the dilution of DMSO with isotonic saline prior to intravenous administration reduced its hemolytic activity[44].
Tests in vitro showed that washed rabbit erythrocytes are hemolyzed in a short time with 40% to 60% DMSO solution. Higher concentrations caused, without hemolysis, an agglutination of the erythrocytes[55].
Teratology: The intraperitoneal administration of 5.5 gm/kg of DMSO as a single dose to pregnant hamsters induced developmental malformation of their embryos[56]. Both dimethyl sulfoxide and diethyl sulfoxide are teratogenic when injected into the chick embryo, the classification of malformations being dependent upon the stage of embryonic development at the time of treatment. The same drugs when administered by various techniques to mice, rats and rabbits in which fertility had been established did not cause any embryonic malformations[57].
Ocular Effects: In a variety of experimental animals including rats, dogs, swine, rabbits and primates, following oral or topical administration of DMSO, certain eye changes have been noted. These consist mainly of a change in the refractive index of the lens described as a "lens within a lens." The lens changes are characterized by a decrease in the normal relucency of the lens cortex, causing the normal central zone of the lens to act as a biconvex lens. When viewing the fundus of affected animals, it is necessary to interpose biconcave lenses in order to see the retinal vessels clearly. The functional effect would be a tendency toward myopia[58].
The lens changes were first observed in dogs receiving 5 gm/kg after 9 weeks of administration. At lower dose levels the change was observed later. In rabbits these changes were seen after 90 days of dermal application, (8 mg 50% DMSO/kg/day and 4 mg 100% DMSO/kg/day and higher). In swine, dermal application of 4.5 gm 90% DMSO/kg twice daily caused similar lens changes by 90 days of treatment[59].
The lens changes appear earlier with oral administration, and also bear a relation to the dosage employed; the higher the dose the more rapid their appearance.
The eye changes are slowly reversible but with a definite species difference, the dog being the slowest to exhibit improvement.
No effects were seen following direct application of aqueous solutions varying from 10% to full strength into the eyes of albino rabbits for a total dosage of DMSO between 0.1 to 0.2 gm/kg body weight per day for six months. Rabbits which received daily doses as high as 10 gm/kg orally or topically showed lines of discontinuity in their lenses. No cataract was seen after ten weeks of such daily treatment, although discontinuous lens lines could be detected in about two weeks by slit lamp examination.
Chemical studies on these lenses revealed reduction in the usual concentrations of urea, glutathione, uric and amino acids[30].
Indications—Canine and Equine: Domoso® (dimethyl sulfoxide) Solution Veterinary, is recommended as a topical application to reduce acute swelling due to trauma.
Dosage and Administration: Domoso® (dimethyl sulfoxide) Solution Veterinary, is to be administered topically to the skin over the affected area.
Dogs—Liberal application should be administered three to four times daily. Total daily dosage should not exceed 20 ml. Total duration of therapy should not exceed 14 days.
Horses—Liberal application should be administered two to three times daily. Total daily dosage should not exceed 100 ml. Total duration of therapy should not exceed 30 days.
Side Effects: In general, adverse reactions are local, and while they may prove to be annoying to some patients, they are usually not of a serious nature. Upon topical application, an occasional animal may develop transient erythema, associated with local "burning" or "smarting." Even when erythema or vesiculation occur, they are self-limiting reversible states, and not necessarily an indication to discontinue medication. Dryness of the skin and an oyster-like breath odor have been reported. These effects are temporary and are not considered to be of serious consequence. Changes in the refractive index of the lens of the eye and nuclear cataracts have been observed in animals, with the use of this drug. This appears to be related to dosage and duration of therapy.
Precautions and Contraindications: Contact between Domoso® Solution and the skin should be avoided. Rubber gloves should be worn while applying this drug. Forceps and swabs may be used to facilitate application. If absorbed through the skin, Domoso® Solution will cause odorous breath and unpleasant mouth taste. Mild sedation or drowsiness, sensations of warmth, burning, irritation, itching and mild erythematous localized or generalized dermatitis have been reported in some persons following exposure to Domoso® Solution. Treatment of such side effects is symptomatic. Consult a physician immediately if adverse effects appear.
Domoso® Solution Veterinary may mask certain disease signs such as are seen in fractures etc.; this does not obviate the need for specific therapy in such conditions, Domoso® should not be used directly prior to racing or other physical stress wherein the drug might mask existing pathology, such as a fracture.
Since Domoso® Solution Veterinary effectively alters the biologic membrane, it will in some cases facilitate the systemic absorption of other topically applied drugs and may have a potentiating effect on drugs administered systemically. Therefore, great care should be exercised in use of other drugs at the Domoso® application site because of the demonstrated—if variable—ability of DMSO to carry other chemicals through the dermis into the general circulation. If other topical medications are indicated they should not be applied until Domoso® (dimethyl sulfoxide) Solution Veterinary is thoroughly dry. Frequently, due to the heat of resolution, a "smoking" effect following application is noted due to vaporization of the drug.
Domoso® Solution Veterinary should also be judiciously used when administered in conjunction with other pharmaceutical preparations, especially those affecting the cardiovascular and central nervous system. DMSO may potentiate the activity of atropine, insulin, endogenous steroids, and certain other drugs.
Lowering of the vagal threshold, spontaneous skeletal muscle fasciculation, and increased smooth muscle tone in the stomach following DMSO exposure may be due to cholinesterase inhibition. Therefore, Domoso® should not be used on dogs, or horses, simultaneously or within a few days before or after treatment with, or exposure to, cholinesterase-inhibiting pesticides or drugs.
Domoso® Solution Veterinary is recommended for topical application only. The application of Domoso® should take

Species	Rt. of Administr.	LD^{50} gm./kg.
Mouse	— SQ	—13.9–20.5
Mouse	— IV	—3.82–10.73
Mouse	— Oral	—15.0–22
Mouse	— IP	—20.06
Rat	— IV	—5.25–5.36
Rat	— Oral	—16.0–28.3
Rat	— IP	—5.5–13.621
Dog	— IV	—2.5
Guinea Pig	— IP	—5.5
Chicken	— Oral	—12.5

place only in well ventilated quarters. Inhalation of the drug should be avoided. Avoid contact of the medication with the eyes.
Keep Domoso® Solution out of the reach of children.
Do not administer by any other route.
Domoso® Solution Veterinary should not be used under occlusive dressings.
Domoso® Solution Veterinary is contraindicated in horses and dogs intended for breeding purposes.
Domoso® Solution Veterinary is a potent solvent and may have a deleterious effect on fabrics, plastics and other materials. Care should be taken to prevent physical contact with Domoso® Solution Veterinary and these materals, either alone or until drying of the treated skin surface has occurred when applied to an animal.
Precaution: Extremely hygroscopic! Close bottle cap tightly after use. Avoid freezing. Due to the rapid penetrating ability of Domoso®, rubber gloves should be worn when applying this drug.
Caution: Federal (U.S.A.) law restricts this drug to use by or on the order of a licensed veterinarian.
How Supplied: Domoso® Solution Veterinary available in 4 oz bottles with sprayer, 16 oz bottles and gallon jugs.

EQUIPROXEN®
(naproxen)
10% Solution and Granules
For veterinary use only

Description: Equiproxen® (naproxen) is a new and unique non-steroidal anti-inflammatory agent developed by Syntex Research. It is unrelated to salicylates or the corticosteroid hormones, but is related chemically to the arylacetic acid class of drugs. Naproxen is an odorless white to creamy white powder which is practically insoluble in water. Chemically, it is (+)-6-methoxy-α-methyl-2-naphthaleneacetic acid with the following structural formula:

CH₃
C–COOH
C
CH₃O

When reconstituted with 19.0 ml of sterile water for injection each ml will contain 100.0 mg naproxen; 24.13 mg potassium hydroxide U.S.P.; 1.0 mg sodium benzoate U.S.P. with sodium phosphate, dibasic as buffer; potassium hydroxide and/or hydrochloric acid for pH adjustment, if necessary, and sterile water for injection q.s.
Each 8 g. granule packet contains 4 g. naproxen.
Actions: Naproxen has been shown to have striking anti-inflammatory properties when tested in classical animal test systems. In addition, it has marked analgesic and antipyretic actions.
Since naproxen raises the pain threshold only in those states involving inflammation, the apparent analgesic effect in horses is the result of the drug's anti-inflammatory properties. It exhibits its anti-inflammatory effect even in adrenalectomized animals, indicating that its action is not mediated through the pituitary-adrenal axis. It inhibits prostaglandin synthesis, as do other non-steroidal anti-inflammatory agents; however, the exact mechanism of its anti-inflammatory action is not known.
Safety Data and Metabolism: Naproxen exhibits a low order of toxicity in single-dose studies in hamsters, rats, dogs and mice. The oral LD_{50} in these species is 4110 mg/kg, 543 mg/kg, > 1000 mg/kg and 1234 mg/kg respectively.
In subacute and chronic oral studies with naproxen in a variety of species, the principal pathologic effects observed were gastrointestinal irritation and ulceration. The lesions were predominately in the small intestine and ranged from hyperemia to perforation and peritonitis. Similar results have been reported with other nonsteroidal and anti-inflammatory agents such as phenylbutazone[1], aspirin[2], indomethacin[3], and mefenamic acid[4].
Neuropathy was seen occasionally in rats, mice and rabbits as high dose levels of naproxen, but not in monkeys or miniature pigs. A variety of neuropathies has been reported in laboratory animals with other non-steroidal anti-inflammatory agents[5,6,7,8]. Other pathologic changes seen with naproxen were considered to be clealy secondary to its effects on the gastrointestinal tract.
In two laboratory animals studies (mice) at 30 and 60 times the single therapeutic intravenous horse dose, naproxen significantly augmented chloral hydrate induced sleep.
In the horse no lesions were observed that could be attributed to Equiproxen® when administered intravenously or orally even at three times the recommended dose for forty-two consecutive days.
Studies in mares administered Equiproxen® in late pregnancy showed no effect upon either the mare or the newborn foal following parturition. Mares were re-bred and conceived without undue difficulty.
Stallions treated with Equiproxen® showed no subsequent interference with libido nor their ability to impregnate mares.
Naproxen has a half-life of approximately four hours in the horse. Isotope studies indicate complete elimination in about 48 hours after the last treatment (I.V. or oral), with 90% being excreted in the urine.
Indications: Equiproxen® (naproxen) is recommended for the relief of inflammation and associated pain and lameness exhibited with myositis and other soft tissue diseases of the musculoskeletal system of the horse.
Myositis, sometimes referred to as "tying up", is commonly seen in horses put into rigorous training or following the stress of being moved via a van or trailer. Horses so affected will show lameness and rigidity of the croup or loin muscles accompanied by pain and reluctance to move. This usually appears at the end of or following strenuous exercise. In a milder form, the horse may be "sore" and not performing up to its capability.
The oral regimen will usually provide therapeutic results in from 5-7 days, although the drug may be fed orally for 14 consecutive days.
Dosage and Administration: Either of two therapeutic regimens may be followed when using Equiproxen®:

1. **Intravenous and oral combination:**
   The recommended intravenous dosage is 5 mg./kg. For the average 400 kg. (880 lb.) horse, administer an initial dose of 2 gm. Equiproxen Injectable (rehydrated to 20 ml 10% sterile solution) by slow intravenous injection.
   When reconstituted use entire contents immediately. Avoid saving fractional contents for later use.
   For maintenance therapy **via** the oral route, administer 10 mg. naproxen/kg. twice daily for up to 14 consecutive days. Therefore, for the average 400 kg. (880 lb.) horse, the contents of one 8 gram packet of Equiproxen® Granules (4 grams of naproxen) top dressed on the feed twice daily will provide the desired dosage and are readily accepted by the horse.
2. **Oral Only:**
   Administer 10 mg. naproxen/kg. as a top dressing twice daily for up to 14 consecutive days. Therefore, for the average 400 kg. (880 lb.) horse, the contents of one 8 gram packet of Equiproxen® Granules (4 grams naproxen) should be top dressed on the feed twice daily. Equiproxen® Granules are readily accepted by the horse.

Precaution: In the treatment of inflammatory conditions associated with infections, specific anti-infective therapy is required.
Warning: NOT FOR USE IN HORSES INTENDED FOR FOOD.
Store at Room Temperature. Avoid Excessive Heat (104°F).
How Supplied:
Granules
Cartons of 14 × 8 gram packets, each packet containing 4 grams of naproxen.
Injectable
2 gm vial with 19 ml vial Sterile Water for Injection.
Caution: Federal (U.S.A.) law restricts this drug to use by or on the order of a licensed veterinarian.

FLUCORT® SOLUTION
(flumethasone)
0.5 mg. per ml.

Composition: The active ingredient of Flucort® Solution Veterinary is flumethasone which occurs as a white to creamy white, odorless, crystalline powder. The appearance of Flucort® Solution Veterinary is a clear colorless to slightly yellowish mobile liquid.
Each ml. of the injectable preparation contains 0.5 mg. flumethasone, 420 mg. polyethylene glycol 400, 9 mg. benzyl alcohol as a preservative, 8 mg. sodium

Continued on next page

Syntex—Cont.

chloride, 0.1 mg. citric acid, Sodium Hydroxide and/or Hydrochloric Acid for pH adjustment when necessary, and purified water U.S.P., q.s.

Physiological Effects: Flumethasone has been reported[1] to possess 700 times the glucocorticoid activity of cortisol (hydrocortisone) as measured in the liver glycogen deposition assay in the rat; 120 times that of cortisol in the cotton pellet assay in the rat; and also in the same animal, shows a net excretion of sodium.

In similar tests in rats, another report[2] showed flumethasone 730 times more potent than cortisol in the granuloma inhibition assay and 165 times the activity of cortisol in the glycogen deposition assay. The same report showed that in man, the compound possessed 7.8 times the potency of prednisolone.

An additional report[3] indicated that flumethasone possessed 677 times the potency of cortisol in the liver glycogen deposition test in the rat, and 30, 25, and 31 times respectively, the eosinopenic, hyperglycemic and antirheumatic potency of cortisol, as measured in man.

Veterinary experimental studies utilizing the eosinophil depression test in normal dogs and blood glucose elevation and eosinophil depression in normal cattle as parameters of drug activity, in comparison tests involving prednisone and dexamethasone, indicate that flumethasone possesses greater anti-inflammatory and gluconeogenic activity than these compounds, on an equivalent basis.

Clinical evidence of drug potency obtained during evaluation of the compound and based upon effective drug dosage levels further substantiates the above experimental findings.

General Effects of Adrenocorticoids

The adrenocorticoids are divided into two main classes: mineralocorticoids and glucocorticoids, based on their major physiologic and pharmacologic actions.

Mineralocorticoids such as the naturally occurring desoxycorticosterone and aldosterone are mainly concerned with hydration, sodium and potassium regulation and the normal renal glomerular filtration of these two electrolytes. The mineralocorticoids have little if any effect as anti-inflammatory agents, and are not widely used in medicine.

Glucocorticoids include the naturally occurring compounds, cortisone and hydrocortisone. Their major effects are as follows:

1. Increase protein catabolism and gluconeogenesis.
2. Depression of lymphoid tissues, fibroblasts and eosinophils.
3. Increase the sense of well being and tolerance to pain.
4. Depress thyroid function and anterior pituitary function through reciprocal influences.
5. Influence vasoconstrictive response of the circulatory system to norepinephrine, helping to maintain blood pressure.
6. Increase renal flow.
7. Influence gastric HCI and pepsin production.
8. Reduces the secretion of mucus from respiratory and enteric mucosa.
9. Affect to some degree sodium retention and potassium excretion.
10. Stimulate erythropoiesis and myelopoiesis.

Synthetic analogues of cortisone and hydrocortisone containing a double bond between carbon 1 and 2 of the corticosteroid nucleus, resulted in compounds with a greatly decreased effect on electrolyte metabolism. Additional molecular changes present in other synthetic corticoids presently used in medicine such as methylation at carbons 6 or 16 and hydroxylation at carbon 16, have led to a further decrease in electrolyte imbalance noted with the naturally occurring glucocorticoids. Fluorination at carbon 6 and/or 9 have led to a marked increase in anti-inflammatory activity.

The synthetic glucocorticoids exhibit a marked increase in potency in that a smaller amount of drug is required to elicit the same effects seen only with large amounts of the natural glucocorticoids. It is also noted that the synthetic analogues persist for a longer period of time in the body which is believed due to their slower metabolism and excretion.

Indications: Flucort® (Flumethasone) Solution Veterinary is recommended for the various rheumatic, allergic, dermatologic and other disease states which are known to be responsive to the anti-inflammatory corticoids.

Equine Indications:

1. Musculoskeletal conditions due to inflammation, where permanent structural changes do not exist, such as bursitis, carpitis, osselets, and myositis. Following therapy an appropriate period of rest should be instituted to allow a more normal return to function of the affected part.
2. In allergic states such as hives, urticaria and insect bites.

Canine Indications.

1. Musculoskeletal conditions due to inflammation of muscles or joints and accessory structures, where permanent structural changes do not exist, such as arthritis, osteoarthritis, the disc syndrome and myositis. In septic arthritis appropriate antibacterial therapy should be concurrently administered.
2. In certain acute and chronic dermatoses of varying etiology to help control the pruritis, irritation and inflammation associated with these conditions. The drug has proven useful in otitis externa in conjunction with topical medication for similar reasons.
3. In allergic states such as hives, urticaria and insect bites.
4. Shock and shock-like states,[4] by intravenous administration.

Feline Indications:

1. In certain acute and chronic dermatoses of varying etiology to help control the pruritus, irritation and inflammation associated with these conditions.

Dosage and Administration: Flucort® (Flumethasone) Solution Veterinary is recommended for administration by injection using various routes depending on the animal species and conditions under treatment. Injection should be accomplished slowly, with the drug at or near body temperature.

The following recommended dosages should be used as therapeutic guides. Each animal should be treated on an individual basis and dosage adjusted according to the response noted.

Dosage of Flucort® Solution Veterinary:

Equine: 1.25 to 2.5 mg. daily by intravenous, intramuscular or intra-articular injection. If necessary, the dose may be repeated.

Canine: 0.0625 to 0.25 mg. daily by intravenous, intramuscular or subcutaneous injection. If necessary, the dose may be repeated. With chronic conditions, the preceding doses may be used and oral maintenance therapy with Flucort® (Flumethasone) Tablets Veterinary instituted at a daily dose of 0.0625 to 0.25 mg. Intralesional dosages in the dog have ranged from 0.125 to 1.0 mg depending on the size and location of the lesion under treatment. Intra-articular dosages in the dog have ranged from 0.166 to 1.0 mg depending on the severity of the condition under treatment and the size of the involved joint.

Feline: 0.03125 to 0.125 mg by intravenous, intramuscular or subcutaneous injection. If necessary, the dose may be repeated. With chronic conditions, the preceding injectable doses may be used and oral maintenance therapy with Flucort® (Flumethasone) Tablet Veterinary instituted at a daily dosage of 0.03125 to 0.125 mg.

Directions: The use of a microsyringe or standard tuberculin syringe may facilitate the accurate administration of small amounts of the drug.

If desired, therapy with Flucort® (Flumethasone) Solution Veterinary may be substituted for other corticoids by the appropriate adjustment of dose levels.

Precautions: The usual precautions and contraindications for adrenocorticoid hormones are applicable with this compound. The close observation of animals under treatment with this drug is necessary, since the usual signs of adrenocorticoid overdosage which include sodium retention, potassium loss, fluid retention, weight gain, etc., may not be readily observed.

The most commonly observed side effects with corticosteroid therapy in animals are polydipsia, polyuria, and on occasion, a gain in weight. Under clinical and experimental trials with Flucort® Solution Veterinary, only a few such side effects have been noted. If they occur, the veterinarian should be prepared to take the necessary steps to correct them, which consist of temporarily discontinuing therapy with the drug until the effects disappear, when therapy may be resumed at a lower dose level.

Warning: Clinical and experimental data have demonstrated that corticosteroids administered orally or parenterally to animals may induce the first stage of parturition when administered during the last trimester of pregnancy and may precipitate premature parturition followed by dystocia, fetal death, retained placenta, and metritis.

When long-term therapy with corticosteroids is used, as is necessary on occasion in the dog and cat, the dose should be individually adjusted so that the minimum maintenance dose (which will keep the condition being treated under control) is desirable. In dogs and cats on long-term therapy with these drugs, a protein-rich diet is useful to counteract nitrogen loss if it should occur.

Similarily, a small amount of potassium chloride daily in the diet will counteract excessive potassium loss if this is present. Some natural dietary sources of potassium include dry non-fat milk solids, citrus juice, bran flakes, meat, fish and light cane molasses.

Experimentally, it has been demonstrated that corticosteroids especially at high dose levels may result in delayed wound healing. An increase in the incidence of osteoporosis may be noted, mainly in the elderly, with the prolonged use of these compounds. Their use in older dogs and cats, during the healing stages of a bone fracture is not indicated for the reason listed above.

In man, corticosteroid therapy especially of a prolonged nature has been reported to induce a number of side effects. These include hypertension or elevation of blood pressure, obesity of the Cushingoid type, plethora, weakness, striae, hirsutism in females, virilism, psychotic states, osteoporosis, ankle edema, purpura, exophthalmos, posterior subcapsular cataracts, peptic ulcers, etc. Side effects of a similar nature during or following corticoid therapy in animals have rarely, if ever, been reported. The veterinarian, however, should be aware of the possible occurrence of such drug induced changes, in animals on long-term corticosteroid therapy.

Continuous therapy with Flucort® (Flumethasone) Solution Veterinary, especially at high dose levels, may result in suppression of adrenal cortical function. In such cases, temporary suspension of therapy and stimulation of the adrenal cortex by the use of ACTH may be advisable. Following prolonged therapy with the drug, it is recommended that the drug be withdrawn gradually. If such animals are later subjected to stressful situations (trauma, surgery, etc.), it is advisable to institute a temporary course of therapy with Flucort® Solution Veterinary.

Flucort® Solution Veterinary may be administered to animals with bacterial diseases provided that specific and appropriate antibacterial therapy with antibiotic is administered simultaneously. In the absence of specific concomitant anitimicrobial therapy, the prolonged use of corticosteroids is likely to lead to the spread of pathogenic microorganisms. The use of corticosteroids in such situations is not indicated. It should be borne in mind that flumethasone, like cortisone, through its anti-inflammatory action, may mask the usual signs of an infection such as pyrexia, inappetence, lassitude, etc. In the course of therapy with Flucort® Solution Veterinary, should the question of determining the presence of an infectious disease arise, the drug should be withheld temporarily until a diagnosis or rediagnosis establishes the facts.

Contraindications: Do not use in viral infections. Except for emergency therapy, do not use in animals with tuberculosis, chronic nephritis, cushingoid syndrome, and peptic ulcers. Existence of congestive heart failure, diabetes and osteoporosis are relative contraindications.

How Supplied: Flucort® Solution Veterinary: Vials of 100 ml.

Caution: Federal (U.S.A.) law restricts this drug to use by or on the order of a licensed veterinarian.

For Veterinary Use Only.

FLUCORT®
(Flumethasone)
Tablets
(0.0625 mg./tablet)
For veterinary use only

General: Flucort® is a chemical modification of prednisolone which possesses greater anti-inflammatory and gluconeogenic properties than the parent compound when compared on an equivalent basis. Due to the potency of Flucort® Tablets Veterinary, dosage recommendations should be consulted prior to drug administration. Chemically, it is 6α,9α-difluoro-16α methylprednisolone. The structural formula is as follows:

Description: The active ingredient of Flucort® Tablets is flumethasone which occurs as a white to creamy white, odorless, crystalline powder. Each tablet contains 0.0625 mg. flumethasone, 143.34 mg. spray-dried lactose, 6 mg. starch, and 0.25 to 0.75 mg. magnesium stearate.

Physiological Effects: Flumethasone has been reported (1) to possess 700 times the glucocorticoid activity of cortisol (hydrocortisone) as measured in the liver glycogen deposition assay in the rat; 120 times that of cortisol in the cotton pellet assay in the rat; and also in the same animal, shows a net excretion of sodium.

In similar tests in rats, another report (2) showed flumethasone 730 times more potent than cortisol in the granuloma inhibition assay and 165 times the activity of cortisol in the glycogen deposition assay. The same report showed that in man the compound possesses 7.8 times the potency of prednisolone.

An additional report (3) indicated that flumethasone possesses 677 times the potency of cortisol in the liver glycogen deposition test in the rat, and 30, 25, and 31 times respectively, the eosinopenic, hyperglycemic and anti-rheumatic potency of cortisol, as measured in man.

Veterinary experimental studies utilizing the eosinophil depression test in normal dogs and blood glucose elevation and eosinophil depression in normal cattle as parameters of drug activity, in comparison tests involving prednisone and dexamethasone, indicate that flumethasone possesses greater anti-inflammatory and gluconeogenic activity than these compounds, on an equivalent basis.

Clinical evidence of drug potency obtained during evaluation of the compound and based upon effective drug dosage levels further substantiates the above experimental findings.

General Effects of Adrenocorticoids

The adrenocorticoids are divided into two main classes: mineralocorticoids and glucocorticoids, based on their major physiologic and pharmacologic actions.

Mineralocorticoids such as the naturally occuring desoxycorticosterone and aldosterone are mainly concerned with hydration, sodium and potassium regulation and the normal renal glomerular filtration of these two electrolytes. The mineralocorticoids have little if any effect as anti-inflammatory agents, and are not widely used in medicine.

Glucocorticoids include the naturally occurring compounds, cortisone and hydrocortisone. Their major effects are as follows:

1. Increase protein catabolism and gluconeogenesis.
2. Depression of lymphoid tissue, fibroblasts and eosinophils.
3. Increase the sense of well being and tolerance to pain.
4. Depress thyroid function and anterior pituitary function through reciprocal influences.
5. Influence vasoconstrictive response of the circulatory system to norepinephrine, helping to maintain blood pressure.
6. Increase renal flow.
7. Influence gastric HCl and pepsin production.
8. Reduces the secretion of mucus from respiratory and enteric mucosa.
9. Affect to some degree sodium retention and potassium excretion.
10. Stimulate erythropoiesis and myelopoiesis.

Synthetic analogues of cortisone and hydrocortisone containing a double bond between carbon 1 and 2 of the corticosteroid nucleus, result in compounds with a greatly decreased effect on electrolyte metabolism. Additional molecular changes present in other synthetic corticoids presently used in medicine, such as methylation at carbons 6 or 16 and hydroxylation at carbon 16, have led to a further decrease in electrolyte imbalance noted with the naturally occurring glucocorticoids. Fluorination at carbon 6

Continued on next page

Syntex—Cont.

and/or 9 have led to a marked increase in anti-inflammatory activity.
The synthetic glucocorticoids exhibit a marked increase in potency in that a smaller amount of drug is required to elicit the same effects seen only with large amounts of the natural glucocorticoids. It is also noted that the synthetic analogues persist for a longer period of time in the body which is believed due to their slower metabolism and excretion.
Indications: Flucort® (Flumethasone) Tablets Veterinary is recommended for the various rheumatic, allergic, dermatologic and other disease states which are known to be responsive to the anti-inflammatory corticoids.
Canine Indications:
1. Musculoskeletal conditions due to inflammation of muscles or joints and accessory structures, where permanent structural changes do not exist, such as arthritis, the disc syndrome and myositis. In septic arthritis appropriate antibacterial therapy should be concurrently administered.
2. In certain acute and chronic dermatoses of varying etiology to help control the pruritis, irritation and inflammation associated with these conditions. The drug has proven useful in otitis externa in conjunction with topical medication for similar reasons.

Feline Indications:
1. In certain acute and chronic dermatoses of varying etiology to help control the pruritus, irritation and inflammation associated with these conditions.

Dosage and Administration: Flucort® Tablets are recommended for oral administration to small animals.
The following recommended doses should be used as therapeutic guides. Each animal should be treated on an individual basis and dosage adjusted according to the response noted.
Oral dosage of Flucort® Tablets:
Canine: 0.0625 to 0.25 mg. daily in divided doses. The dose used is dependent on the size of the animal, the stage (acute or chronic) and severity of the disease under consideration.
Injection of 0.625 to 0.25 mg. of Flucort® (Flumethasone) Solution Veterinary may be preferred as initial therapy and desired drug levels maintained with subsequent oral administration of the tablets.
Feline: 0.03125 to 0.25 mg. daily in divided doses. The dose used is dependent on the size of the animal, the stage (acute or chronic) and severity of the disease under consideration.
Injection of 0.03125 to 0.125 mg. of Flucort® (Flumethasone) Solution Veterinary may be preferred as initial therapy and desired drug levels maintained with subsequent oral administration of the tablet.
If desired, therapy with Flucort® Tablets may be substituted for other corticoids by the appropriate adjustment of dose levels.
Precautions: The usual precautions and contraindications for adrenocorticoid hormones are applicable with this compound. Close observation of animals under treatment with this drug is necessary, since the usual signs of adrenocorticoid overdosage which include sodium retention, potassium loss, fluid retention, weight gain, etc., may not be readily observed.
The most commonly observed side effects with corticosteroid therapy in animals are polydipsia, polyuria, and on occasion, a gain in weight. Under clinical and experimental trials with Flucort® (Flumethasone) Tablets Veterinary, only a few such side effects have been noted. If they occur, the veterinarian should be prepared to take the necessary steps to correct them, which consist of temporarily discontinuing therapy with the drug until the effects disappear, when therapy may be resumed at a lower dose level.
When long-term therapy with corticosteroids is used, as is necessary on occasion in the dog and cat, the dose of the drug should be individually adjusted so that the minimum maintenance dose which will keep the condition being treated under control, is desirable. In dogs and cats on long-term therapy with these drugs, a protein-rich diet is useful to counteract nitrogen loss, if it should occur.
Similarly, a small amount of potassium chloride daily in the diet, will counteract excessive potassium loss, if this is present.
Experimentally it has been demonstrated that corticosteroids especially at high dose levels may result in delayed wound healing. An increase in the incidence of osteoporosis may be noted, mainly in the elderly, with the prolonggd use of these compounds. Their use in older dogs and cats, during the healing stages of a bone fracture is not indicated for the reason listed above.
In man, corticosteroid therapy especially of a prolonged nature has been reported to induce a number of side effects. These include: hypertension or elevation of blood pressure, obesity of the Cushingoid type, plethora, weakness striae, hirsutism in females, virilism, psychotic states, osteoporosis, ankle edema, purpura, exophthalmos, posterior subcapsular cataracts, peptic ulcers etc. Side effects of a similar nature during or following corticoid therapy in animals have rarely, if ever, been reported. The veterinarian, however, should be aware of the possible occurrence of such drug induced changes, in animals on long-term corticosteroid therapy.
Continuous therapy with Flucort® Tablets especially at high dose levels, may result in suppression of adrenal cortical function. In such cases temporary suspension of therapy and stimulation of the adrenal cortex by the use of ACTH may be advisable. Following prolonged therapy with the drug, it is recommended that the drug be withdrawn gradually. If such animals are later subjected to stressful situations (trauma, surgery, etc.) it is advisable to institute a temporary course of therapy with Flucort® (Flumethasone) Solution.
Flucort® Tablets may be administered to animals with bacterial diseases provided that specific and appropriate antibacterial therapy with antibiotic is administered simultaneously. In the absence of specific concomitant antimicrobial therapy, the prolonged use of corticosteroids is likely to lead to the spread of pathogenic microorganisms. The use of corticosteroids in such situations is not indicated. It should be borne in mind that flumethasone, like cortisone, through its anti-inflammatory action, may mask the usual signs of an infection such as pyrexia, inappetence, lassitude, etc. In the course of therapy with Flucort® Tablets, should the question of determining the presence of an infectious disease arise, the drug should be withheld temporarily until a diagnosis or rediagnosis establishes the facts.
Warning: Clinical and experimental data have demonstrated that corticosteroids administered orally or parentally to animals may induce the first stage of parturition when administered during the last trimester of pregnancy and may precipitate premature parturition followed by dystocia, fetal death, retained placenta, and metritis.
Caution: Federal (U.S.A.) law restricts this drug to use by or on the order of a licensed veterinarian.
How Supplied: Bottles of 1000.

NEO-SYNALAR® CREAM (neomycin sulfate 0.5%) (0.35% neomycin base) Fluocinolone Acetonide 0.025%

Composition: Neo-Synalar® Cream Veterinary contains 0.5% neomycin sulfate (equivalent to 0.35% base) and 0.025% fluocinolone acetonide (6α, 9α-difluoro-16α-hydroxyprednisolone-16, 17-acetonide) in a bland, non-sensitizing, hydrophilic base.
Indications: Neo-Synalar® Cream is indicated in the relief of pruritis and inflammation associated with superficial acute and chronic dermatoses in the dog. It has been proven beneficial in the dog, in the treatment of such conditions as allergic and acute moist dermatitis, and to a lesser degree in nonspecific dermatitis, probably due to the multiplicity of causes. It has been shown to be beneficial in the treatment of wound infections in dogs and cats.
Administration: For best results, particularly in areas of heavy hair covering and in the long-haired breeds, the area around the lesion should be clipped, and the lesion cleaned before treatment. Apply a small amount of cream to the area under treatment and gently rub it on. This should be repeated two to three times daily.
Precautions: Topical steroid therapy generally will cause remission of allergic dermatoses. However, until the specific causative agent is identified and removed from the animal's environment, the condition may be expected to recur when therapy is terminated.

Neo-Synalar® Cream Veterinary is virtually nonsensitizing and nonirritating. The neomycin, incorporated in Neo-Synalar® Cream Veterinary, rarely produces allergic reactions.
In chronic conditions treatment should be withdrawn by gradually decreasing the frequency of application. Although side effects are not ordinarily encountered with topically applied steroids, as with all drugs, a few animals may react unfavorably under certain conditions. If such reactions or idiosyncrasies are seen, Neo-Synalar® Cream Veterinary should be discontinued and appropriate steps taken.
Antibiotic susceptibility of the pathogenic organism(s) should be determined prior to use of this preparation. Use of topical antibiotics may permit overgrowth of non-susceptible bacteria, fungi, or yeasts. If this occurs, treatment should be instituted with other appropriate agents as indicated. Where there is severe local infection, the use of systemic antibiotics should be considered in conjunction with NEO-SYNALAR cream veterinary.
Warning: Clinical and experimental data have demonstrated that corticosteroids administered orally or parenterally to animals may induce the first stage of parturition when administered during the last trimester of pregnancy and may precipitate premature parturition followed by dystocia, fetal death, retained placenta and metritis.
Additionally, corticosteroids administered to dogs, rabbits, and rodents during pregnancy have resulted in cleft palate in offspring. Corticosteroids administered to dogs during pregnancy have also resulted in other congenital anomalies, including deformed forelegs, phocomelia, and anasarca.
Caution: Federal (U.S.A.) law restricts this drug to use by or on the order of a licensed veterinarian.
How Supplied: Neo-Synalar® Cream Veterinary, 5 g. Collapsible Tubes and 15 g. Collapsible Tubes.
For Veterinary Use Only

OPTIPRIME®
(neomycin sulfate and polymyxin B sulfate)
OPTHAKOTE®
(hydroxypropyl methylcellulose vehicle)
(Ophthalmic Solution)

Composition: The active ingredients of Optiprime® Ophthalmic Solution Veterinary are neomycin sulfate and polymyxin B sulfate. The appearance of Optiprime® Solution with the Opthakote® vehicle is a clear colorless to slightly yellowish mobile liquid.
Each ml. of the ophthalmic preparation contains 5.0 mg. neomycin sulfate (3.5 mg. neomycin base); 10,000 units polymyxin B sulfate; in an aqueous vehicle containing polyethylene glycol 3,350. propylene glycol, hydroxypropyl methylcellulose, methylparaben propylparaben and citric acid with sodium hydroxide and/or sulfuric acid added to adjust the pH if necessary.

Organism	Neomycin Sensitivity mcg./ml	Polymyxin Sensitivity mcg./ml.
Aerobacter aerogenes	10.0	3.0
Alcaligenes spp.	10.0	0.5
Bacillus subtilis	3.0	10.0
Brucella abortus	3.0	10.0
Corynebacterium diphtheriae	1.0	—
Diplococcus pneumoniae	10.0	—
Escherichia coli	—	1.0
Hemophilus influenzae	—	5.0
Hemophilus pertussis	8.0	2.5
Klebsiella Pneumoniae	5.0	1.5
Micrococcus flavus	10.0	—
Micrococcus pyogenes		
var. albus	3.0	—
var. aureus	10.0	—
Mycobacterium phlei	0.3	—
Mycobacterium smegmatis	0.5	—
Neisseria meningitidis	—	5.0
Pasteurella multocida	—	5.0
Proteus vulgaris	8.0	—
Pseudomonas aeruginosa	5.0	12.0
Pseudomonas spp.	5.0	31.2
Salmonella spp.	5.0	5.0
Shigella dysenteriae	2.0	5.0
Shigella paradysenteriae	5.0	5.0
Shigella sonnei	2.0	5.0
Streptococcus pyogenes, Group A	10.0	—
Vibrio comma	—	5.0

Pharmacological Effects: Combinations of neomycin and polymyxin B are of value in the topical treatment of diseases of the eyelid, conjunctiva, cornea, and anterior segment.[2]
For ophthalmic therapy it is frequently recommended to employ antibiotics that are seldom used systemically, (such as neomycin and polymyxin B) to minimize the possiblity of development of bacterial resistance.[3,4]
Antibiotic Sensitivity: Studies designed to evaluate the sensitivity of neomycin sulfate and polymyxin B sulfate indicate that the following organisms are sensitive to these antibiotics at the following concentrations.[5]
[See table above].
Indications: *For Ophthalmic Use Only*—Optiprime® Ophthalmic Solution Veterinary is recommended for the treatment of bacterial infections associated with topical ophthalmological conditions such as corneal injuries, superficial keratitis conjunctivitis, keratoconjunctivitis, and blepharitis in the dog.
The drug is intended for use in those disease sttes where neomycin sulfate and /or polymyxin B sulfate provide specific and effective antimicrobial coverage, except in those situations where the drug is used as adjunctive therapy combined with standard primary therapy.
Dosage and Administration: Prior to the administration of Optiprime® Solution, the ocular area should be properly cleansed.
The recommended dosage for Optiprime® Solution is one to two drops per eye, every six hours.
Precautions and Contraindications: In treating ophthalmological conditions associated with bacterial infections, Optiprime® is contraindicated in those cases in which the microorganisms are non-susceptible to the antibiotics incorporated into this formulation.
Storage: Not to be stored at temperatures exceeding 25°C. (77°F.).
Caution: Federal (U.S.A.) law restricts this drug to use by or on the order of a licensed veterinarian.
How Supplied: Optiprime® Ophthalmic Solution Veterinary with Opthakote® vehicle: Vials containing 5 ml. in cartons of 12.
For Veterinary Use Only

REPOSE® Ⓒ
Euthanasia Solution
For Dogs Only

Description: Repose is a non-sterile solution containing secobarbital sodium and dibucaine hydrochloride as the active ingredients, and is intended for humane euthanasia in the dog.
Each ml contains: **Active ingredients**—sodium secobarbital 400 mg and dibucaine hydrochloride 25 mg.; **Inactive ingredients**—Propylene glycol 0.15 ml, Boric Acid 3.09 mg*, Sodium Hydroxide 1.36 mg*, Potassium Chloride 3.75 mg, Phenolphthalein 0.01 mg, Isopropyl Alcohol 0.002 ml, and Purified Water q.s.
*Additional amounts may be added to adjust pH.
Actions: Repose provides a unique combination of the anesthetic effect of secobarbital sodium with the cardiotoxic effect of dibucaine hydrochloride. The result is humane, painless, and rapid euthanasia.
Euthanasia is effected in the following sequence:

Continued on next page

Syntex—Cont.

1. Anesthesia by the secobarbital component concurrent with marked respiratory depression.
2. Cardiac arrest due to the combined effect of secobarbital and dibucaine. Secobarbital desensitizes the cardiac musculature sufficiently to prevent fibrillation while the cardiotoxic effect of dibucaine causes rapid cardiac arrest.

Indications: Repose® is intended for intravenous use in dogs to induce rapid, painless euthanasia.

POISON

Warning: For euthanasia in dogs only. This drug must not be used for therapeutic purposes nor in animals intended for human consumption.
Caution: Caution should be exercised against accidental self-administration or contact of the drug with open wounds. Keep out of the reach of children.

Precautions: As with all agents intended for euthanasia, precautions should be taken to adequately restrain the animal during administration.
Dosage and Administration: Administer intravenously to dogs at the rate of 1 ml per 10 pounds of body weight.
After establishing that the needle of appropriate size is properly located within the lumen of the vessel, administer Repose smoothly and continuously to anesthetic effect, then inject the balance of the dose.
If other than disposable needles and syringes are used, they should be cleaned thoroughly with 70% isopropyl alcohol.
How Supplied: 100 ml multiple dose vials.
Caution: Federal (U.S.A.) law restricts this drug to use by or on the order of a licensed veterinarian.

SPECTINOMYCIN ORAL LIQUID

Composition: Spectinomycin Oral Liquid is a new antibiotic that is active against a variety of gram-negative and gram-positive organisms. This oral liquid is a convenient dosage form of Spectinomycin for baby pigs.
Indications: Spectinomycin Oral Liquid is indicated for oral administration to control infectious bacterial enteritis (white scours) associated with *Escherichia coli* in pigs under four weeks of age.
Dosage and Administration: The plastic doser supplied with Spectinomycin Oral Liquid makes it easy to give to baby pigs. After inserting the doser in the bottle, making sure the cap is secure, press plunger a few times to fill the pump and the clear plastic tube with the medication. To adminster Spectinomycin Oral Liquid, insert the plastic tube in the pig's mouth and press the plunger to obtain the desired dose. The recommended dosage is:
Pigs under 10 lb.—1 pump (1 ml.), twice daily.
Pigs over 10 lb.—2 pumps (2 ml.), twice daily.
Each pump of the plunger delivers one ml. of solution containing 50 mg. of Spectinomycin Oral Liquid. Treatment may be continued twice daily for 3 to 5 days. If pigs do not improve within 48 hours, rediagnosis is suggested.
When not in use, remove the plunger from the bottle. Put the clear plastic tube in the neck of the bottle and press the plunger a few times to remove the medication from the pump. Replace the original cap on the bottle and then rinse out the doser with water to prevent sticking.
Caution: This product is intended for use only in pigs under four weeks of age or weighing less than 15 lb. Do not administer within 21 days of slaughter.
How Supplied: Spectinomycin Oral Liquid is supplied in 240 ml, 480 ml and 960 ml. multiple-dose plastic bottles, packaged 12 per case. The 240 ml. is packed with handy, individual plastic dosers.

For Veterinary Use Only.

SYNALAR® CREAM (fluocinolone acetonide) 0.025% For Topical Use Only

General: Synalar® cream veterinary contains 0.025% fluocinolone acetonide (6α, 9α-difluoro-16α-hydroxyprednisolone-16, 17-acetonide) in a water-washable aqueous base of stearyl alcohol, propylene glycol, cetyl alcohol, polyoxyl 20 cetostearyl ether, mineral oil, white wax, simethicone, butylated hydroxytoluene, edetate disodium, citric acid, and purified water, with methylparaben and propylparaben as preservatives. Synalar® possesses over 100 times the anti-inflammatory activity of hydrocortisone and provides important advantages in topical therapy. It decreases edema, inflammation, erythema, infiltration and pruritus, lessens scratching and excoriation, and thus the possibility of infection associated with pruritus. Lesions under treatment with Synalar® fade and become flattened. Synalar® is effective in sparing amounts and is easily applied. The specially formulated hydrophilic base used in Synalar® is odorless, nonstaining, and cosmetically appealing to the most particular client.
Description: Synalar® contains 0.025% Fluocinolone Acetonide, an odorless crystalline powder essentially white in color, and having a melting point between 265° and 277° Centigrade and a molecular weight of 452.50.
Indications: Synalar® (fluocinolone acetonide) Cream Veterinary is indicated for the relief of pruritus and inflammation associated with certain superficial acute and chronic dermatoses in the dog.
It has been proven specifically beneficial in the dog in such conditions as allergic and acute moist dermatitis, and to a lesser degree in nonspecific dermatitis, probably due to the multiplicity of causes.
It has been proven beneficial, also, in the relief of superficial inflammation caused by chemical and physical abrasions and burns in the dog.
Administration: For best results, particularly in areas of heavy hair covering and in the longhaired breeds, the area around the lesion should be clipped, and the lesion cleaned before treatment. Apply a small amount of cream to the area under treatment and gently rub it on. This should be repeated two to three times daily.
Precautions: Topical steroid therapy generally will cause remission of allergic dermatoses. However, until the specific causative agent is identified and removed from the animal's environment, the condition may be expected to recur when therapy is terminated. In chronic conditions, treatment should be withdrawn by gradually decreasing the frequency of application. Although side effects are not ordinarily encountered with topically applied steroids, as with all drugs, a few animals may react unfavorably under certain conditions. If such reactions or idiosyncrasies are seen, Synalar® (fluocinolone acetonide) Cream Veterinary should be discontinued and appropriate steps taken.
Antibiotic susceptibility of the pathogenic organism(s) should be determined prior to the use of this preparation. Use of topical antibiotics may permit overgrowth of non-susceptible bacteria, fungi or yeasts. If this occurs, treatment should be instituted with other appropriate agents as indicated. Where there is severe local infection the use of systemic antibiotics should be considered in conjunction with Synalar cream veterinary.
Warning: Clinical and experimental data have demonstrated that corticosteroids administered orally or parenterally to animals may induce the first stage of parturition when administered during the last trimester of pregnancy and may precipitate premature parturition followed by dystocia, fetal death, retained placenta and metritis.
Additionally, corticosteroids administered to dogs, rabbits, and rodents during pregnancy have resulted in cleft palate in offspring. Corticosteroids administered to dogs during pregnancy have also resulted in other congenital anomalies, including deformed forelegs, phocomelia, and anasarca.
Caution: Federal (U.S.A.) law restricts this drug to use by or on the order of a licensed veterinarian.
How Supplied: 5 g. collapsible tubes and 15 g. collapsible tubes.
For Veterinary Use Only.

SYNOTIC® (fluocinolone acetonide 0.01% and dimethyl sulfoxide 60%) Otic Solution

Composition: Each ml. of the solution contains 0.01% fluocinolone acetonide (6α, 9α-difluoro-11β, 16α, 17, 21-tetrahydroxypregna-1, 4-diene-3, 20-dione, cyclic 16, 17-acetal with acetone) and 60% dimethyl sulfoxide in propylene glycol and citric acid.

Indications: Synotic® Otic Solution Veterinary is indicated for the relief of pruritus and inflammation associated with acute and chronic otitis in the dog.

Pharmacology: Fluocinolone acetonide is chemically related to prednisolone and possesses marked anti-inflammatory properties when applied topically. It has been shown to have over 100 times the anti-inflammatory activity of hydrocortisone. Fluocinolone acetonide decreases edema, inflammation, erythema, infiltration and pruritus with its associated scratching and excoriation. Following topical application of fluocinolone acetonide, especially at elevated dosage levels, systemic effects such as some adrenal suppression and weight loss have been observed. These effects, however, have been demonstrated to be reversible.

It has been demonstrated in the human, by both *in vivo* and *in vitro* methods, the DMSO enhances the percutaneous absorption of various compounds including steroids, vasoconstrictors, anti-perspirants and dyes, as well as an anthelmintic (thiabendazole) and a skin antiseptic (hexachlorophene) (1, 2, 3, 4, 5). It was also shown in immature female rats that both estrogens and corticoids applied topically in DMSO exerted some of their usual biological effects. (6, 7).

Toxicology: *Dimethyl sulfoxide:* Changes in the refractive index of the lens of the eye and nuclear cataracts have been observed in animals with the oral use of DMSO and appeared to be related to high daily doses or a long duration of daily therapy. The lens changes were first observed in dogs receiving 5 g/kg of DMSO orally daily after 9 weeks of administration. Later studies revealed ocular effects at 4.5 ml/kg in 5-9 weeks and at 0.5-1.0/ml/kg for 19 weeks. These eye changes were slowly reversible but with a definite species difference, the dog being the slowest to exhibit improvement.

In a subsequent study conducted in dogs to determine the effects of a 90% dimethyl sulfoxide solution applied topically at a total daily dose of 20-60 ml for 21 consecutive days, no clinically meaningful ophthalmological effects were noted. No significant variations were observed in hematologic values or in other blood measurements including glucose, BUN, SGOT and plasma electrophoresis. DMSO may facilitate the systemic absorption of other topically-applied drugs and may have a potentiating effect on drugs administered systemically. Medications containing DMSO as a vehicle should be used judiciously when administered in conjunction with other pharmaceutical preparations especially those affecting the cardiovascular and central nervous systems. Other medication should not be present at the site of its topical application. If other topical medications are indicated they should not be applied until after the medication containing DMSO is thoroughly dry.

DMSO is a potent solvent and may have a deleterious effect upon fabrics, plastics and other materials. Care should be taken to prevent physical contact with Synotic® (fluocinolone acetonide and dimethyl sulfoxide) Otic Solution Veterinary when the drug is applied. Contact with the treated area should be avoided until drying of the treated ear canal has occurred.

Fluocinolone Acetonide: It is estimated that the maximum dosage dogs will tolerate, when fed fluocinolone acetonide daily for a period of 2 weeks, is less than 0.125 mg/kg. At this dose level animals lost weight and displayed diarrhea and intestinal inflammation. When dogs were fed fluocinolone acetonide daily for a period of three months the maximum daily dose tolerated is estimated to be between 0.05 and 0.125 mg/kg. At the lower dose the adrenal glands of treated dogs appeared somewhat smaller than the controls.

The intravenous lethal dose of fluocinolone acetonide in 50% aqueous-propylene glycol is in excess of 50 mg/kg in mice and rabbits, in excess of 40 mg/kg in dogs, and in excess of 30 mg/kg in rats. The compound induced no pyrogenic response in rabbits nor sensitizing effects in guinea pigs. Gross or histologic effects were not encountered.

The lethal dose orally in dogs and cats exceeds 1.0 g/kg. There was lymphocytopenia in all animals and erythrocytosis in cats employed in this study.

Two g/kg of 0.05 to 0.2% fluocinolone acetonide applied daily 5 days per week for 3 weeks to the abraded skin of rabbits, resulted in neither local nor systemic toxicity.

Similar applications to intact skin for 13 weeks, including an additional group at 0.025%, resulted only in decreased body weight and adrenal size.

A small decrease in body weight was seen in dogs treated for 7 days with 0.5 ml (15 drops)/ear/day of Synotic® (fluocinolone acetonide and dimethyl sulfoxide) Otic Solution Veterinary. In dogs which were treated for 21 days with 1.5 ml (45 drops)/ear/day of this formulation there was a slight loss of weight with changes in the adrenal glands consistent with corticosteroid treatment. This indicates absorption from the dogs' ears. This absorption, and concomitant effects, are probably enhanced by the action of DMSO.

In a subsequent study, dogs were treated with the recommended therapeutic dose of Synotic® Otic Solution Veterinary, at the rate of 12 drops (0.4 ml) per ear daily for 21 consecutive days. No significant changes were detected in clinical chemistry, urinalysis, or hematology. A reversible adrenal cortical atrophy with cortical cytoplasmic vacuolization was noted. An equivocal response was noted following ACTH administration on the day after Synotic® Otic Solution Veterinary treatment was suspended, but after a one week recovery period, there was a definite eosinophile depression and recovery following ACTH administration, indicating normal adrenal function.

Dosage and Administration: The recommended dose of Synotic® Otic Solution Veterinary is 4 to 6 drops (0.2 ml) per ear administered twice daily into the ear canal for a maximum period of 14 days. The total dosage used should not exceed 17 ml. It is recommended that the affected ear canal be cleansed by some appropriate method prior to the instillation of the solution. Following instillation, gentle external massage of the ear canal may aid in promoting an even distribution of the medication. Care should be taken to avoid contact of the medication with the dog's eyes. Contact of the bare hand with the medication should also be avoided.

Side Effects: A transient, but mild, stinging sensation may be experienced by some animals when the solution is applied to denuded areas. The effect will disappear as healing progresses. A temporary increase in temperature of the area may also be noted.

Corticosteroid therapy will generally cause a remission of signs of allergic origin. However, until the causative agent is identified and removed from the animal's environment, the condition may recur when therapy is terminated.

Ordinarily, side effects are not encountered with topically applied corticosteroids; but as with all drugs, some animals may exhibit unfavorable local and/or systemic reactions. A local reaction may be due to sensitization to the corticosteroid or one of the other components of the solution.

It is known that DMSO enhances the percutaneous absorption of topically applied corticosteroids and the veterinarian should be aware of possible systemic reactions in this situation. Accordingly, this product is contraindicated wherever systemic corticosteroids would be dangerous. Adrenal suppression, weight loss and increased susceptibility to infections may be evidenced with the use of this drug, especially in overdosage. Therefore, care should be taken to assure that the recommended dosage is not exceeded. In the presence of local and/or systemic side effects, the drug should be withdrawn. When a local reaction occurs other therapeutic measures should be instituted. Therapy can usually be resumed at a lower dose once systemic signs abate, without further recurrence of the problem.

Absorption of DMSO following topical application may result in an odorous breath described as oyster or garlic-like with an unpleasant taste. Some animals and clients may find this objectionable but these effects are transient and not considered to be of serious consequence.

Precautions: There should be careful initial evaluation and follow-up of infected ears. Incomplete response or exacerbation of corticosteroid responsive lesions may be due to the presence of an infection which requires identification or antibiotic sensitivity testing, and the use of the appropriate antimicrobial agent. As with any corticosteroid, animals with a generalized infection should not be treated with this product without proper supportive antimicrobial therapy. Preparations with DMSO should not be used in

Continued on next page

Syntex—Cont.

pregnant animals since studies in chick embryos and guinea pigs have indicated it is teratogenic and embryo-toxic.
Synotic® (fluocinolone acetonide and dimethyl sulfoxide) Otic Solution Veterinary is recommended for topical application to the ear canal of the dog only.
Do not administer by any other route.
Caution: Very hygroscopic. Close vial tightly after use. Avoid freezing and excessive heat.
How Supplied: Synotic® (fluocinolone acetonide and dimethyl sulfoxide) Otic Solution Veterinary:
Dropper vials of 8 ml. and 60 ml.
Caution: Federal law restricts this drug to use by or on the order of a licensed veterinarian.
For Veterinary Use Only.

SYNOVEX® C
Calf Implants
For Improved
Growth Promotion
For Animal Use Only

Composition: Each dosage consists of 4 pellets containing 100 mg Progesterone and 10 mg Estradiol Benzoate per implantation.
How To Implant With Synovex® Pellets: Study the following instructions carefully, then proceed step by step, until the technique becomes routine. Many head can be implanted per hour by an experienced team, one member of which should be assigned to do nothing but the implantation. He should keep his hands clean and use sanitary instruments only.
SYNOVEX®C is recommended for use in suckling beef calves weighing up to approximately 400 lbs. SYNOVEX® C may be used in both steer and heifer calves including heifers intended for breeding later.

DO NOT USE IN VEAL CALVES OR IN CALVES LESS THAN 45 DAYS OLD.

Warning: Implant pellets in the ear only. Any other location may result in violation of Federal law. Do not attempt salvage of implanted site for human or animal food.
Caution: Bulling, rectal prolapse, ventral edema and elevated tailheads have been occasionally reported in calves administered with SYNOVEX® C implants.
Keep this and all drugs out of the reach of children.
Restricted drug — use only as directed.
See diagram for implantation.
STEP 1 Loading The Implanter Load the implanter following the directions outlined in the instruction manual accompanying each implanter.
STEP 2 Restraint Calves must be adequately restrained prior to implantation to minimize movement of the head. Heavier calves may be confined in a restraint mechanism (squeeze chute or head gate). The implant site on the back of the ear should be prepared by scrubbing with a generous-sized piece of cotton that has been soaked in a germicidal solution.
STEP 3 Implant Site Divide the ear into three imaginary sections as illustrated. The implanted pellets should be deposited in the center one-third of the ear as shown. To accomplish this, the implanter needle should be inserted in the outer one-third of the ear as indicated by the "X" in the iullustration. Implanting too close to the head may cause side effects. Care should be taken to avoid severing the major arteries of the ear.
STEP 4 Insert Needle Grasp the ear with one hand. Holding the implanter firmly with the other hand, penetrate the skin at the point shown by the "X". Thrust the needle under the skin taking care not to penetrate the cartilage. Ease the implanter forward (toward the base of the ear) until the full needle length is beneath the skin.
STEP 5 Pellet Implantation When the needle is completely inserted, withdraw the needle approximately one-half inch. Then with continuous gentle pressure on the trigger, expel the pellets while continuing to slowly withdraw the needle. This technique allows the implant pellets to be deposited in a straight line in the path of the needle.
STEP 6 Inspection Check the implant site. If properly administered, the implants should lie in a straight line under the skin.
Disinfect the implanter needle in a germicidal solution. You are now ready to implant the next animal.
[See table below].

SYNOVEX® H
Heifer Implants
For Improved
Growth Promotion
and Feed Efficiency
For Animal Use Only

Composition: Each dosage consists of 8 pellets containing 200 mg. Testosterone

SYNOVEX® C
SYNOVEX® H
SYNOVEX® S

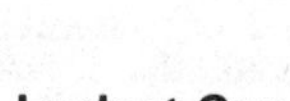
Implant Gun

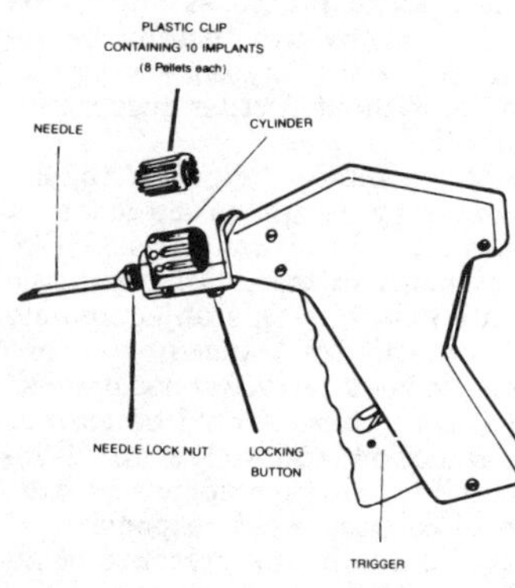

Step 1
Loading The Implanter

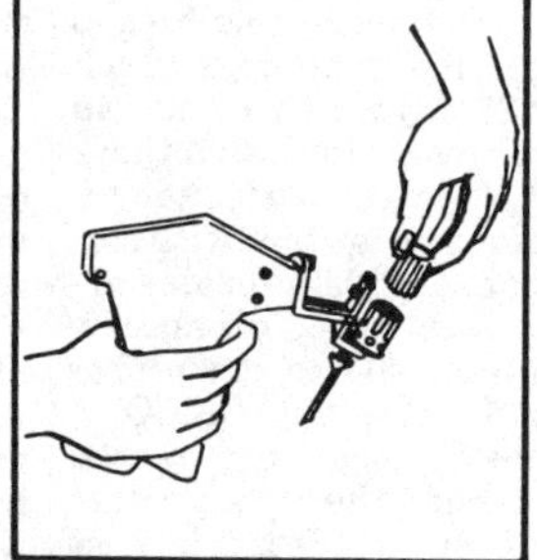

Step 2
Restraint

Step 3
Implant Site

Step 4
Insert Needle

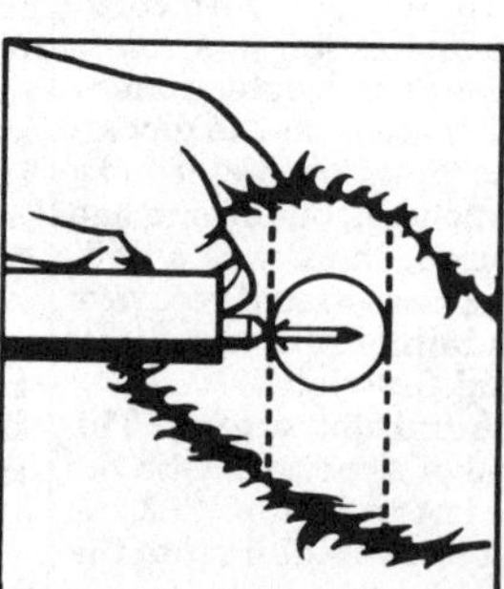

Step 5
Pellet Implantation

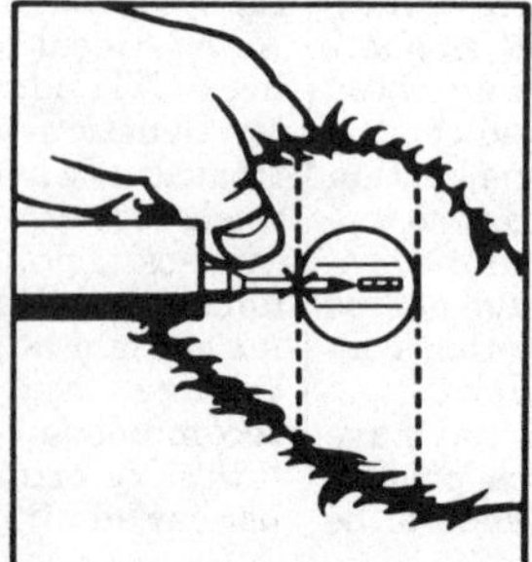

Step 6
Inspection

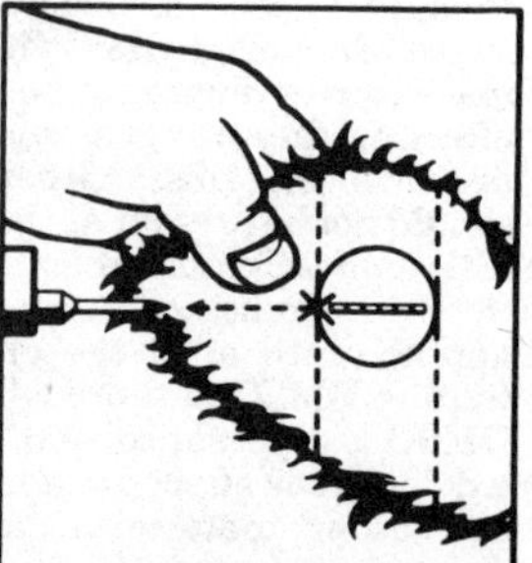

Propionate and 20 mg. Estradiol Benzoate per implantation.

How To Implant With Synovex® Pellets: Study the following instructions carefully, then proceed step by step, until the technique becomes routine. Many head can be implanted per hour by an experienced team, one member of which should be assigned to do nothing but the implantation. He should keep his hands clean and use sanitary instruments only.

SYNOVEX® H is recommended for use in heifers weighing 400 lbs or more.

When properly administered, SYNOVEX® H implants can help increase rate of weight gain, and improve feed efficiency.

Warning: Not for dairy or beef replacement heifers. Implant pellets in the ear only. Any other location may result in violation of Federal law. Do not attempt salvage of implanted site for human or animal food.

Caution: Bulling, vaginal and rectal prolapse, udder development, ventral edema and elevated tailheads have been occasionally reported in heifers administered with SYNOVEX® H implants.

Keep this and all drugs out of the reach of children.

Restricted drug—use only as directed.

See diagram for implantation.

STEP 1 Loading The Implanter Load the implanter following the directions outlined in the instruction manual accompanying each implanter.

STEP 2 Restraint The animal must be confined in a restraint mechanism (squeeze chute or head gate). The implant site on the back of the ear should be prepared by scrubbing with a generous-sized piece of cotton that has been soaked in a germicidal solution.

Note: If implanting horned cattle, greater safety is provided when the head is controlled by the use of a bull lead (nose tongs).

STEP 3 Implant Site Divide the ear into three imaginary sections as illustrated. The implanted pellets should be deposited in the center one-third of the ear as shown. To accomplish this, the implanter needle should be inserted in the **outer** one-third of the ear as indicated by the "X" in the illustration. Implanting too close to the head may cause abnormal sexual behavior Care should be taken to avoid severing the major arteries of the ear.

STEP 4 Insert Needle Grasp the ear with one hand. Holding the implanter firmly with the other hand, penetrate the skin at the point shown by the "X". Thrust the needle under the skin taking care not to penetrate the cartilage. Ease the implanter forward (toward the base of the ear) until the full needle length is beneath the skin.

STEP 5 Pellet Implanation When the needle is completely inserted, withdraw the needle approximately one-half inch. Then with continuous gentle pressure on the trigger, expel the pellets while continuing to slowly withdraw the needle. This technique allows the implant pellets to be deposited in a straight line in the path of the needle.

STEP 6 Inspection Check the implant site. If properly administered, the implants should lie in a straight line under the skin.

Disinfect the implanter needle in a germicidal solution. You are now ready to implant the next animal.

SYNOVEX® S
Steer Implants For Improved Growth Promotion and Feed Efficiency

Each dosage consists of 8 pellets containing 200 mg. Progesterone and 20 mg. Estradiol Benzoate per implantation.

For Animal Use Only

How To Implant With Synovex® Pellets: Study the following instructions carefully, then proceed step by step, until the technique becomes routine. Many head can be implanted per hour by an experienced team, one member of which should be assigned to do nothing but the implantation. He should keep his hands clean and use sanitary instruments only.

SYNOVEX® S is recommended for use in steers weighing 400 lbs or more.

When properly administered, SYNOVEX® S implants can help increase rate of weight gain, and improve feed efficiency.

Warning: Implant pellets in the ear only. Any other location may result in violation of Federal law. Do not attempt salvage of implanted site for human or animal food.

Caution: Bulling, rectal prolapse, ventral edema and elevated tailheads have been occasionally reported in steers administered with SYNOVEX® S implants.

Keep this and all drugs out of the reach of children.

Restricted drug—use only as directed.

See diagram for implantation.

STEP 1 Loading The Implanter Load the implanter following the directions outlined in the instruction manual accompanying each implanter.

STEP 2 Restraint The animal must be confined in a restraint mechanism (squeeze chute or head gate). The implant site on the back of the ear should be prepared by scrubbing with a generous-sized piece of cotton that has been soaked in a germicidal solution.

Note: If implanting horned cattle, greater safety is provided when the head is controlled by the use of a bull lead (nose tongs).

STEP 3 Implant Site Divide the ear into three imaginary sections as illustrated. The implanted pellets should be deposited in the center one-third of the ear as shown. To accomplish this, the implanter needle should be inserted in the **outer** one-third of the ear as indicated by the "X" in the illustration. Implanting too close to the head may cause abnormal sexual behavior. Care should be taken to avoid severing the major arteries of the ear.

STEP 4 Insert Needle Grasp the ear with one hand. Holding the implanter firmly with the other hand, penetrate te skin at the point shown by the "X". Thrust the needle under the skin taking care not to penetrate the cartilage. Ease the implanter forward (toward the base of the ear) until the full needle length is beneath the skin.

STEP 5 Pellet Implantation When the needle is completely inserted, withdraw the needle approximately one-half inch. Then with continuous gentle pressure on the trigger, expel the pellets while continuing to slowly withdraw the needle. This technique allows the implant pellets to be deposited in a straight line in the path of the needle.

STEP 6 Inspection Check the implant site. If properly administered, the implants should lie in a straight line under the skin.

Disinfect the implanter needle in a germicidal solution. You are now ready to implant the next animal.

TRANVET® CHEWABLE TABLETS
(propiopromazine hydrochloride)

Composition: Tranvet® is a phenothiazine derivative and has a generic name, propiopromazine hydrochloride and chemical name, 1-Propanone, 1-1-[10-[3-(dimethylamino) propyl] phenothiazin-2yl]-, monohydrochloride. It is a yellow, odorless powder and exists in two crystalline forms: the one form melts between 144° and 149°C. and the other melts between 155° and 160° C. It is readily soluble in water (greater than 350 mg per ml.)

Tranvet® is an effective tranquilizer designed for veterinary use in dogs. The phenothiazine derivatives have assumed an important position as animal tranquilizers, and their use is well recognized as a valuable addition to the armamentarium of the veterinarian. Tranvet® (propiopromazine hydrochloride) is recommended as a method of "chemical restraint." It reduces, and in some instances completely eliminates, the need for manual or physical restraint ordinarily required to subdue vicious, nervous or unruly animals. It facilitates physical examination, reduces struggling, and eases handling and transporting of animals. Tranvet® allays apprehension, and, with anxiety and excitement reduced, the animal is relaxed, quiet, and more easily handled.

When Tranvet® is administered at recommended levels, the desired effects on behavioral mechanisms is usually accomplished without undesirable side effects. Drugs of the phenothiazine type are believed to exert their effect by action on certain metabolic functions of cells, particularly those of nervous tissue. Reduction in anxiety and apprehension is accomplished while the animal remains alert. Tranvet® enables animals to adapt more easily to a new and strange environment. Tranquilization may be apparent for a period of from several hours following administration to as long as two to three days. It facilitates handling and transporting without loss of normal responses and in addition, anorexia, vomiting and hyperexcitability,

Continued on next page

Syntex—Cont.

often the result of exposure to new surroundings, are curtailed. Tranvet® is not an analgesic but the apparent mental detachment produced in the animal seemingly makes pain more bearable. In chewable tablet form, Tranvet® is paticularly useful for controlling fractious dogs.

Indications: Tranvet® is indicated in clinical circumstances which require the aid of a tranquilizer. Tranvet® (propiopromazine hydrochloride) is an effective aid in the handling of difficult, excited and unruly animals, controlling excessive kennel barking, car sickness and severe dermatitis cases. It is indicated prior to routine examinations; laboratory and diagnostic procedures; and in minor surgery. With adjunctive Tranvet® pretreatment, it is less difficult to: groom, clean teeth, clip hair and nails, treat and dress wounds, lesions and skin abrasions, apply splints, bandages and remove sutures, remove skin warts, cysts and tumors, examine and medicate eyes, and administer oral anthelmintics. Cauterization and other minor surgical or laboratory procedures, including urological procedures, radiography, catheterization, rectal palpation and examination of genitalia, are facilitated.

Pharmacology: Pharmacological studies of Tranvet® in mice, rats, dogs, cats, rabbits and monkeys reveal a picture of a typical phenothiazine tranquilizer. However, it appears to be somewhat more sedative, produces greater potentiation of barbiturates, and the degree of motor deficit is slightly greater than chlorpromazine. Tranvet® has an adrenergic blocking action, causing epinephrine reversal in a manner similar to chlorpromazine. In addition, this drug has marked, but not unlimited, antimetic effect against apomorphine and produces a lowering of blood pressure in cats and rats under pentobarbital anesthesia.

Mice. The LD_{50} of Tranvet® (propiopromazine hydrochloride) was determined in white mice. The oral LD_{50} is 650 mg/kg ($\pm$ 53 mg/kg) and the LD_{50} intraperitoneally is 170 mg/kg. ($\pm$ 8 mg/kg.) The fatal dose in mice is at least 40 times greater than the minimal effective dose necessary to elicit decreased activity. Manifestations resulting from Tranvet® in mice are typical of phenothiazine tranquilizers. A long-lasting decrease in motor activity is the most striking effect and is observed in doses as low as 10 mg/kg intraperitoeally. As the dose is increased, jerking movements, slowing of respiration, and terminal clonic convulsions appear. Surviving animals exhibit marked depression and decrease in activity, which may persist for 24 to 48 hours.

Rats: The LD_{50} intraperitoneally was found to be 160 mg/kg. Orally, the LD_{50} is 1100 mg/kg and none of the oral doses produced any excitement. Intraperitoneally, a dose of 100 mg/kg produced decreased activity. At doses of 150 mg/kg and 200 mg/kg, jumping from a resting position and gasping were observed.

Monkey: Administered intramuscularly at 2 mg/kg, decreased activity and decreased aggressiveness were noted.

Subacute Toxicity Studies: Subacute parenteral toxicity studies were conducted with rats. Comparisons were made during a five-week period, between three groups of rats, one group receiving Tranvet® at 20 mg/kg, one group at 10 mg/kg, and one group maintained as controls. All injections were made by the intraperitoneal route. Both levels of the drug resulted in ataxia, depression, and decrease in activity. However, all rats gained weight and terminal hematological and urinary findings were all within normal limits. At sacrifice, histological studies were conducted of brain, heart, lung, liver, spleen, kidney, adrenals, gastrointestinal tract, pancreas, genital organs and bone marrow. There were no morphological changes attributable to the drug.

In another study, 24 dogs were divided into four groups. Seven dogs received oral Tranvet® (propiopromazine hydrochloride) once daily, five days each week for eight to 14 weeks at a level of 1 mg/lg. A similar group of seven dogs received 3 mg/lb and a third group of five dogs received 5 mg/lg five days each week for just eight weeks. A fourth group of five dogs remained untreated. None of the dogs showed adverse reactions to the drug and weight gains of treated dogs were comparable to weight gains of untreated dogs. Continued tranquilization was evident throughout the test.

Doses in these studies reached two and one-half to ten times the recommended level.

Dosage and Administration: Tranvet® Chewable Tablets are specially flavored so that most dogs will readily accept them. They are available in two strengths; 10 mg of Tranvet® per tablet and 20 mg of Tranvet® per tablet.

Tranquilization Dosage: The recommended dosage for dogs is 0.5 to 2 mg of Tranvet® per pound body weight given once or twice daily, depending upon degree of tranquilization desired. The dose of Tranvet® must be adjusted for each animal according to body weight, the degree of tranquilization desired and the anticipated response of the individual animal. Obese and older animals may require less Tranvet® per pound of body weight to achieve the desired response than young, underweight or nervous individuals.

Responses to Tranvet® Chewable Tablet may vary from patient to patient. In clinical trials the desired calming effect generally occurred within 60 minutes after oral administration of 0.5-2 mg per pound and lasted from 12 to 24 hours.

Precautions: When Tranvet® (propiopromazine hydrochloride) Chewable Tablets are administered at recommended levels, they enjoy a comfortable margin of safety and no undesirable effects are to be anticipated. Since Phenothiazine has been reported to cause blood dyscrasias when administered over extended periods, it is advisable to follow the blood picture where Tranvet® is required for a prolonged period. Overdosage in hypersentisitive animals may produce prolonged depression accompanied by psychomotor hyperactivity. The dose of Tranvet® must be adjusted for each animal according to body weight, the degree of tranquilization desired and the anticipated response of the individual patient. Obese and older dogs may require less Tranvet® per pound of body weight to achieve the desired result than do young, underweight or nervous animals. Tranvet® produces a relatively long lasting effect (12 to 24 hours) in most animals and this quality is deemed to be an advantage.

Warning: Do not use this product with organophosphates and/or procaine hydrochloride. A phenothiazine may potentiate the toxicity of organophosphates and the activity of procaine hydrochloride.

Epinephrine is contraindicated when phenothiazine derivatives are used. If an adrenergic drug is desired, norepinephrine should be used.

This drug is contraindicated in the presence of pre-existing severe central nervous system depression such as following large doses of barbiturates or opiates.

Caution: Federal (U.S.A.) law restricts this drug to use by or on the order of a licensed veterinarian.

How Supplied: Tranvet® Chewable Tablets are availabe as follows:
10 mg. Bottles of 120 Tablets
20 mg. Bottles of 60 Tablets.
For Veterinary Use Only.

TechAmerica Group, Inc.

15TH & OAK
P.O. BOX 338
ELWOOD, KS 66024

ACEPROMAZINE MALEATE INJECTION

Description: Acepromazine Maleate, a potent neuroleptic agent with a low order of toxicity, is of particular value in the tranquilization of dogs. Its rapid action and lack of hypnotic effect are added advantages.

Indications: As an aid in tranquilization and as a preanesthetic agent in dogs. Acepromazine Maleate Injection can be used as an aid in controlling intractable animals during examination, treatment, grooming, x-ray and minor surgical procedures.

Acepromazine Maleate Injection is particularly useful as a preanesthetic agent; (1) to enhance and prolong the effects of barbiturates, thus reducing the requirements for general anesthesia; (2) as an adjunct to surgery under local anesthesia.

Contraindications: Phenothiazines may potentiate the toxicity of organophosphates. Therefore, do not use Acepromazine Maleate to control tremors associated with organic phosphate poisoning.

Do not use in conjunction with organophosphorus vermifuges or ectoparasiticides, including flea collars.
Do not use with procaine hydrochloride.
Cautions: Tranquilizers are potent central nervous system depressants, and they can cause marked sedation with suppression of the sympathetic nervous system.
Tranquilizers can produce prolonged depression or motor restlessness when given in excessive amounts or when given to sensitive animals.
Tranquilizers are additive in action to the actions of other depressants and will potentiate general anesthesia. Tranquilizers should be administered in smaller doses and with greater care during general anesthesia and also to animals exhibiting symptoms of stress, debilitation, cardiac disease, sympathetic blockade, hypovolemia or shock. Acepromazine, like other phenothiazine derivatives, is detoxified in the liver; therefore, it should be used with caution on animals with a previous history of liver dysfunction or leukopenia.
Hypotension can occur after rapid intravenous injection causing cardiovascular collapse.
Epinephrine is contraindicated for treatment of acute hypotension produced by phenothiazine derivative tranquilizers since further depression of blood pressure can occur.
Phenothiazines should be used with caution when followed by epidural anesthetic procedures because they may potentiate the arterial hypotensive effects of local anesthetics.
Dosage and Administration: Acepromazine Maleate Injection is a sterile solution which may be given intravenously, intramuscularly or subcutaneously. The dosage should be individualized, depending upon the degree of tranquilization required. As a general rule, the dosage requirement in mg/lb of body weight decreases as the weight of the animal increases. The following schedule may be used as a guide to intravenous, intramuscular or subcutaneous injections:
Dogs: 0.25–0.5 mg per lb of body weight. Intravenous doses should be administered slowly, and a period of at least 15 minutes should be allowed for the drug to take full effect.
Warning: Federal law restricts this drug to use by or on the order of a licensed veterinarian.
How Supplied: 50 ml vials: Each ml contains 10 mg Acepromazine Maleate, sodium citrate 0.36%, citric acid 0.075%, benzyl alcohol 1.0% and water for injection q.s.

ACEPROMAZINE MALEATE TABLETS

Description: Acepromazine Maleate, a potent neuroleptic agent with a low order of toxicity, is of particular value in the tranquilization of dogs. Its rapid action and lack of hypnotic effect are added advantages.
Indications: As an aid in tranquilization and as a preanesthetic agent in dogs. Acepromazine Maleate Tablets can be used as an aid in controlling intractable animals during examination, treatment, grooming, x-ray and minor surgical procedures.
Contraindications: Phenothiazines may potentiate the toxicity of organophosphates. Therefore, do not use Acepromazine Maleate to control tremors associated with organic phosphate poisoning.
Do not use in conjunction with organophosphorus vermifuges or ectoparasiticides, including flea collars.
Do not use with procaine hydrochloride.
Cautions: Tranquilizers are potent central nervous system depressants, and they can cause marked sedation with suppression of the sympathetic nervous system.
Tranquilizers can produce prolonged depression or motor restlessness when given in excessive amounts or when given to sensitive animals.
Tranquilizers are additive in action to the actions of other depressants and will potentiate general anesthesia. Tranquilizers should be administered in smaller doses and with greater care during general anesthesia and also to animals exhibiting symptoms of stress, debilitation, cardiac disease, sympathetic blockade, hypovolemia or shock. Acepromazine, like other phenothiazine derivatives, is detoxified in the liver; therefore, it should be used with caution on animals with a previous history of liver dysfunction or leukopenia.
Hypotension can occur after rapid intravenous injection causing cardiovascular collapse.
Epinephrine is contraindicated for treatment of acute hypotension produced by phenothiazine derivative tranquilizers since further depression of blood pressure can occur.
Phenothiazines should be used with caution when followed by epidural anesthetic procedures because they may potentiate the arterial hypotensive effects of local anesthetics.
Dosage and Administration: Acepromazine Maleate Tablets:
Dogs: 0.25–1.0 mg/lb of body weight. Dosage may be repeated as required.
Warning: Federal law restricts this drug to use by or on the order of a licensed veterinarian.
How Supplied: Acepromazine Maleate tablets are available in 10 & 25mg. concentrations, and are quarter scored for convenience of administration and imprinted to indicate tablet strength. Both concentrations are available in bottles of 100 and 500 tablets.

ADENOMUNE™-7
Canine Distemper-Hepatitis-Parainfluenza-Adenovirus Type 2-Parvovirus Vaccine
Modified Live and Killed Virus Canine and Feline Cell Line Origin
Leptospira Bacterin

Composition: Adenomune™-7 is a multiple immunogen product containing desiccated modified canine distemper, canine hepatitis and canine parainfluenza viruses of Canine Perma-Cell Line™ Origin, to be rehydrated with inactivated Parvovirus of Feline Perma-Cell Line Origin, Canine Adenovirus Type 2 of Canine Perma-Cell Line Origin *Leptospira Canicola Icterohaemorrhagiae* Bacterin.
Data indicates that the development of corneal opacity is not associated with the use of this product.
The bacterin is prepared from inactivated whole cultures of *L. canicola* and *L. icterohaemorrhagiae* grown in a specially developed medium designed to assure high immunogenicity and to reduce the possibility of allergic reactions. Each 1 ml. dose contains a full immunizing dose of each of the component fractions. Each serial meets or exceeds all standards prescribed for this product by the U.S. Department of Agriculture.
Indications: For the immunization of normal, healthy puppies and dogs against canine distemper, canine hepatitis, canine parainfluenza, canine parvovirus, canine adenovirus type 2 and canine leptospirosis caused by either *Leptospira canicola* or *Leptospira icterohaemorrhagiae.*
Dosage and Administration: Using aseptic technique, rehydrate the canine distemper, hepatitis, parainfluenza desiccated portion with the accompanying parvovirus, canine adenovirus type 2, Leptospira Bacterin and inject the entire contents of the vial subcutaneously or intramuscularly.
Research has shown that the persistence of maternal antibodies to canine parvovirus may be as long as twenty weeks in some puppies. The presence of maternal antibodies is known to interfere with the development of active immunity and should receive the veterinarians consideration as immunization programs are planned. Puppies of any age may be safely vaccinated. A recommended vaccination of puppies should start at or about nine weeks of age in order to provide as much protection as possible as the chances of exposure are increased. Puppies should ideally be re-vaccinated every two to four weeks until they are at least 16 weeks of age. Puppies from nonimmune bitches and orphan puppies should be immunized at an earlier age.
All dogs over 16–20 weeks of age should initially receive one dose of Adenomune-7 and a booster two to four weeks later in order to develop an adequate level of immunity.
Annual revaccination of all dogs with Adenomune-7 is recommended.
For Veterinary Use Only.
How Supplied: 25 × 1 dose (Bio Paks) with each pack containing 25 doses desiccated vaccine and 1 tray respectively of 25 1 ml. killed CAV2, Parvovirus and Lepto C & I as diluent.

Continued on next page

T

TechAmerica—Cont.

ADENOMUNE™7-L
Canine Distemper-Adenovirus Type 2-Hepatitis-Parainfluenza-Parvovirus Vaccine
Modified Live and Killed Virus Canine and Feline Cell Line Origin
Leptospira Bacterin

Composition: Adenomune™7-L is a multivalent, highly antigenic immunogen for protection of puppies and adult dogs against the diseases caused by the viral and bacterial fractions represented. The live viruses contained have been so attenuated as to assure safety upon administration without destroying their antigenicity. All virus fractions represented are modified live antigens with the exception of the Adenovirus Type 2 which is inactivated to assure complete safety while retaining a high level of immunogenicity. The parvovirus is the highly antigenic Gorham Strain propogated in a Feline Perma-Cell Line.™ The attenuated virus provides complete safety and a lack of virus shedding following vaccination.
Indications: For the immunization of normal, healthy puppies and dogs against canine distemper, canine hepatitis, canine parainfluenza, canine parvovirus, canine adenovirus type 2 and leptospirosis caused by either *Leptospira canicola* or *Leptospira icterohaemorrhagiae.*
Dosage and Administration: Aseptically rehydrate the desiccated vaccine using the accompanying fluid Adenovirus Type 2-Parvovirus Vaccine-Lepto C & I bacterin as the diluent. Inject 1 ml. subcutaneously or intramuscularly. Puppies of any age may be safely vaccinated. Puppies 9–14 weeks old are the ideal age at which to begin the vaccination schedule. Repeat every 2 to 4 weeks until 16 weeks of age. Annual revaccination is recommended. Persistence of maternal origin antibody in puppies should receive consideration in determining vaccination programs.
For Veterinary Use Only.
How Supplied: 25 × 1 (Bio-Pak) with each pack containing 25 doses desiccated vaccine and 1 tray respectively of 25 1 ml. killed CAV_2, MLV parvovirus and Lepto C & I as diluent.

AMINOPLEX-C
(34X Concentrate)

Composition: A combination of pure and essential crystalline amino acids, crystalline B-Vitamins, electrolytes and dextrose in concentrated solution.
Each 100 ml. contains:

Dextrose-H_2O	5 g
Sodium Acetate	0.25 g
Calcium Chloride-$2H_2O$	150 mg
Potassium Chloride	200 mg
Magnesium Sulfate-$7H_2O$	200 mg
Vitamin B_2	4 mg
d-Panthenol	5 mg
Niacinamide	150 mg
Vitamin B_6	10 mg
Vitamin B_{12}	5 mcg
Valine	136 mg
Leucine	187 mg
Isoleucine	85 mg
Arginine, HCl	85 mg
Histidine HCl-H_2O	59.5 mg
Methionine	51 mg
Phenylalanine	119 mg
Threonine	78.2 mg
Tryptophan	34 mg
Lysine-HCl	170 mg
Methyl Paraben	0.18%
Ethly Paraben	0.01%
Propyl Paraben	0.02%
Cysteine-HCl	0.05%
Sodium metabisulfite	0.02%
Water	q.s.

Indications: As an aid in the supportive treatment of debilitated (weakened) cattle, horses, sheep and swine.
Dosage and Administration: 1 to 3 ml. per 10 pounds of body weight depending on size and condition of the animal, 1 to 3 times daily. Warm to body temperature and administer slowly. Product may be administered intravenously, intraperitoneally, intramuscularly or subcutaneously. Intravenous route is recommended where severity of condition requires availability of formula.
Warning: Do not administer intraperitoneally in horses.
Store at controlled room temperature (59–86°F).
How Supplied: 500 ml.

AMINOPLEX SOLUTION
(Amino Acid Solution with Electrolytes, Vitamin B Complex and Dextrose 5%)

Composition: Each 100 ml. contains:
PURE CRYSTALLINE AMINO ACIDS
Valine 8 mg; Leucine 11 mg; Isoleucine 5 mg; Arginine-HCl 5 mg; Histidine-HCl-H_2O 3.5 mg; Methionine 3 mg; Phenylalanine 7 mg; Threonine 4.6 mg; Tryptophan 2 mg; Lysine-HCl 10 mg.
B-VITAMINS, ELECTROLYTES AND DEXTROSE Riboflavin 4 mg; d-Panthenol 5 mg; Niacinamide 150 mg; Pyridoxine HCl 10 mg; Cyanocobalamin 5 mcg; Sodium Acetate 0.25 g; Calcium Chloride-$2H_2O$ 150 mg; Potassium Chloride 200 mg; Magnesium Sulfate-$7H_2O$ 200 mg; Dextrose-H_2O 5 g.
PRESERVATIVES
Methyl Paraben 0.18%; Ethyl Paraben 0.01%; Propyl Paraben 0.02%; Cysteine-HCl 0.005%; Sodium meta-Bisulfite 0.002%; water q.s.
Indications: An aid in the supportive treatment of debilitated cattle, horses, sheep and swine.
Dosage and Administration: Administer parenterally (intravenously, intraperitoneally or subcutaneously) 1 to 5 ml. per pound of body weight depending on size and condition of the animal. Warm to body temperature and administer slowly. Product may be administered intravenously, intraperitoneally, intramuscularly or subcutaneously. Intravenous route is recommended where severity of condition requires availability of formula.
Warning: Do not administer intraperitoneally in horses.
Store at controlled room temperature (59–86°F).
How Supplied: 500 ml and 950 ml.

ANESTATAL™
Sodium Thiamylal for Injection

Indications: Sodium Thiamylal for Injection is an ultra-short action thiobarbiturate anesthetic for use in dogs, cats, swine, horses and cattle to accomplish interferences and examinations of short duration (10–15 minutes), for induction of anesthesia prior to intubation for administration of a volatile anesthetic and for anesthesia in major surgery by administration of additional amounts as necessary.
[See table below].
Sodium Thiamylal solutions should be prepared under aseptic conditions. Solution cannot be heated for sterilization. The solutions should be stored in a refrigerator, and used within six days. If kept at room temperature, the solution should be used within twenty-four hours. Only clear solutions should be used; discard if cloudiness or a precipitate forms. Refrigeration of the reconstituted sodium thiamylal contributes to maintenance of a clear solution.
Dosage and Administration: For intravenous administration only. The first one-third to one-half of the calculated dose should be administered rather rapidly to carry the patient through the excitement stage. Should apnea or severe respiratory depression occur, suspend injection until rhythmic respiration resumes. Then continue to slowly inject the Sodium Thiamylal for Injection solution until the desired stage of surgical anesthesia is reached, as determined by lack of appropriate reflexes. For best results, Sodium Thiamylal for Injection should be administered to fasted animals, since emesis may occasionally occur.
Caution: Federal law restricts this drug to use by or on the order of a licensed veterinarian.
How Supplied: Sodium Thiamylal for Injection is available in 50 ml. vial con-

Quantities of Solvent Required to Prepare Solutions of Desired Strength

Percent Solution	Calculated mg/cc	Sodium Thiamylal for Inj. 1 GRAM	Sodium Thiamylal for Inj. 5 GRAM
2.0%	20	50 ml	250 ml
2.5%	25	40 ml	200 ml
4.0%	40	25 ml	125 ml

taining 1 gram or 250 ml. vial containing 5 grams.

BORDITECH™-P
Bordetella Bronchiseptica, Pasteurella Multocida Bacterin Aluminum Hydroxide Adsorbed

Composition: This product is prepared from chemically inactivated cultures of *B. bronchiseptica* and *P. multocida.* The strains used in the product have been selected especially for their immunogenic characteristics.
Protection: Turbinate damage often results in a higher incidence of pneumonia due to the decreased ability of the nasal turbinates to filter foreign materials, thus preventing their access to the lungs. Studies have shown that *B. bronchiseptica* itself can be a cause of pneumonia in pigs. *P. multocida* is considered to be an opportunistic secondary invader, causing pneumonia only when other predisposing stress factors (such as turbinate atrophy) are present. Pulmonary pasteurellosis is, nevertheless, a disease of high incidence which results in great economic loss to the swine industry.
Indications: For use in healthy swine as an aid in the control or prevention of atrophic rhinitis (AR) due to *Bordetella bronchiseptica* and pasteurellosis due to *Pasteurella multocida.*
Dosage and Administration:
1. Shake well before using. The product may be given subcutaneously or intramuscularly. Use aseptic precautions throughout the inoculation procedures.
2. For subcutaneous inoculation, the usual site in sows/gilts is behind one of the ears, in the neck region. In piglets, the product is injected into the fold of the flank, or inner side of the front leg.
3. For intramuscular inoculation, inject pigs in the ham region.
4. Vaccinate according to the following schedule:
   a. *Sows/Gilts:* 2 ml. dosage. For initial vaccination give two doses, at least two weeks apart. The last dose should be given 1–3 weeks prior to farrowing. Revaccinate 1–3 weeks prior to each subsequent farrowing.
   b. *Piglets:* 1 ml. dosage. Vaccinate at 3–7 days of age. Repeat dosage at 14–21 days of age.
   c. *Boars:* 2 ml. dosage. To reduce the possibility of boars being a source of infection they should be given two doses at least 2 weeks apart. Revaccinate every 6 months.

For Veterinary Use Only
How Supplied: 100 ml. plastic vials.

BORDITECH™P–E
Bordetella Bronchiseptica, Pasteurella Multocida, Erysipelothrix Rhusiopathiae Bacterin Aluminum Hydroxide Adsorbed

Composition: BordiTech-P-E™ is prepared from chemically inactivated cultures of *B. bronchiseptica, P. multocida* and *E. rhusiopathiae.* The strains used in the product have been selected especially for their immunogenic characteristics.
BordiTech-P-E, as a trivalent bacterin, is designed as an aid in the protection of sows against infection by the organisms represented, during periods of stress encountered through gestation, parturition and immediately following when their resistance may be lowered.
It has been demonstrated that transfer of maternal antibody through the colostrum confers a degree of passive immunity against infection of the very young by *Bordetella bronchiseptica.* There is insufficient data available to know if such passive protection against *E. rhusiopathiae* is transferred.
The *B. bronchiseptica* bacterium is recognized as the primary cause of infectious atrophic rhinitis. Although *B. bronchiseptica* strains vary greatly in their virulence and immunogenic abilities, the actual immunogen (factor on the bacterial cell responsible for eliciting immunity) is felt to be common among strains *P. multocida* is considered to be an opportunistic secondary invader, causing pneumonia only when other predisposing factors (such as turbinate atrophy) are present. Pulmonary pasteurellosis is, nevertheless, a disease of high incidence which results in great economic loss to the swine industry.
The erysipelas bacterin in BordiTech-P-E is an excellent prophylactic agent which will adequately protect vaccinates against the disease. The bacterin contains a highly antigenic strain of *Erysipelothrix rhusiopathiae.*
Indications: BordiTech-P-E is indicated as an aid in the protection of sows against infection by *B. bronchiseptica, P. multocida* and *E. rhusiopathiae.* If, in the opinion of the user, use of this product in young pigs will be deemed beneficial in preventing disease, it may be used in that manner.
Dosage and Administration:
1. Shake well before using. The product may be given subcutaneously or intramuscularly. Use aseptic precautions throughout the inoculation procedures.
2. For subcutaneous inoculation, the usual site in sows/gilts is behind one of the ears, in the neck region. In piglets, the product is injected into the fold of the flank, or inner side of the front leg.
3. For intramuscular inoculation, inject pigs in the ham region.
4. Vaccinate according to the following schedule:
   a. Sows/Gilts: 2 ml dosage. For initial vaccination give two doses, at least two weeks apart. The last dose should be given 1–3 weeks prior to farrowing. Revaccinate 1–3 weeks prior to each subsequent farrowing.
   b. Piglets: 1 ml. dosage. Vaccinate 3–7 days of age. Repeat dosage at 14–21 days of age.
   c. Boars: 2 ml. dosage. To reduce the possibility of boars being a source of infection they should be given two doses at least 2 weeks apart. Revaccinate every 6 months.

For Veterinary Use Only
How Supplied: 100 ml. plastic vials.

BOVA CREME

Composition: Vitamins A, D_3, E, B_2 (Riboflavin), B_5 (Panthenol), B_6 (Pyridoxine), H (d-Biotin), and B_3 (Niacinamide) in a specially compounded base stabilized at pH of normal animal skin.
Indications: Bova Creme with Multi Vitamins for use as an aid in reducing dry, cracked and chapped udders in cattle. Contains humectants which assist in maintaining skin and tissue in natural moisture balance.
Milking machines, inclement weather and other factors strip natural moisture from the udders, leaving them dry and chapped. Bova Creme is a unique blend of 8 vitamins which are naturally present in healthy skin. Helps promote natural moisture balance of chapped udders in cattle.
The non-sticky, disappearing cream base discourages dirt and manure from sticking to udders.
Directions: Apply daily or as needed after milking to aid in reducing dryness, cracking and chapping associated with chapped udders in cattle.
Precautions: Bova Creme is not a substitute for balanced nutrition. Animals with signs of nutritional deficiency in the skin may require injections of therapeutic levels of vitamins. Consult your veterinarian for assistance in the diagnosis and treatment of nutritional deficiency.
Caution: If animal shows signs of uncontrolled generalized infections, consult your veterinarian. Wash the teats and udders thoroughly before milking. Keep out of reach of children. For animal use only.
How Supplied: 1 lb. and 5 lb.

BRONCHICINE™
Bordetella Bronchiseptica Bacterin Extracted Cellular Antigens

Composition: Bronchicine™ is prepared from antigenic material extracted from the cells of the *Bordetella bronchiseptica* organism.
Starting with a highly immunogenic strain of *B. bronchiseptica* the organism is grown to a high yield, then subjected to a unique process which extracts the antigens from the bordetella cells. The residual cell debris is then removed, resulting in a product which retains the desirable immunogenic qualities of the whole cell, while reducing the toxic and other undesirable side affects associated with whole cell bacterins.
The product is not adjuvanted, as studies have shown that such is not necessary for efficacy of this product. Thimersol (merthiolate) has been added as a preservative.
As a federally licensed product, Bronchicine meets or exceeds all U.S. Department of Agriculture requirements for sterility, safety, potency, and efficacy.
The Disease: Canine Infectious Tracheobronchitis (CITB; Canine Cough) is a

Continued on next page

TechAmerica—Cont.

highly contagious respiratory tract disease which may last from several days to several weeks. It is generally a mild, self-limiting disease characterized by a harsh, dry, hacking cough. Retching or vomiting may follow the periods of paroxysmal coughing spasms. Occasionally the disease may present a more severe clinical picture, progressing to bronchial pneumonia.
Canine cough has been considered a disease of complex etiology involving bacterial, viral or mycoplasma agents, acting either alone or synergistically to produce the clinical picture. Studies by several investigators have indicated, however, that *B. bronchiseptica* is one of the etiological agents in the kennel cough syndrome. The disease can be experimentally reproduced by challenge with this agent alone.
Close confinement of dogs, such as in breeding or boarding kennels, or in dog shows, facilitates the transmission of the disease. Conventional antibiotic therapy has been shown to be generally unsuccessful in reducing or eliminating bordetella infection in dogs.
Protection: In Bronchicine, the development of an extracted immunogen has resulted in a product with unsurpassed safety and efficacy. Controlled challenge studies indicate that dogs given two vaccinations are significantly protected from a challenge which produced a typical clinical picture in the nonvaccinated control dogs. Vaccinated dogs were protected from both experimental aerosol challenge, and continuous reexposure by comingling with infected control dogs. Accelerated clearance of the challenge organisms from the respiratory tract was also evidenced in the vaccinated dogs.
Significant humoral antibody titers were evident in vaccinated dogs as early as 7 days following one vaccination with Bronchicine. The product needs no adjuvant for efficacy and this fact may, in part, explain the rapid antibody response. While agglutinating antibody titers do not rise significantly after revaccination, studies indicate the IgG titers to rise significantly after a second vaccination, thus, the recommendation for two vaccinations for primary immunization.
Challenge studies clearly indicate a rise in humoral IgG antibody titers following aerosol challenge of both vaccinates and controls, demonstrating the importance of the humoral immune system as both a response to challenge exposure and a protective mechanism against the clinical disease picture.
Indications: A nonadjuvanted, antigenic product extracted from the cells of *B. bronchiseptica*. For use in the immunization of normal, healthy puppies and dogs against canine bordetella infection, as an aid in the control of canine infectious tracheobronchitis (canine cough).
Dosage and Administration: Shake well. Using aseptic technique, inject the 1 ml. dose subcutaneously. For primary immunization, inject two doses 2 to 4 weeks apart. Annual revaccination is recommended, in order to maintain a high level of immunity.
Initial vaccination of puppies is recommended at or about 6–8 weeks of age, in order to provide as much protection as possible as the chances of exposure are increased. The effect of the presence of maternal antibodies to *B. bronchiseptica* upon the ability of the puppy to develop an active immune response has not been ascertained, however, puppies from immune bitches usually have low titers to *B. bronchiseptica* and this antibody usually disappears by the time the puppy is 4 to 6 weeks old.
For Veterinary Use Only
Precautions:
1. Store at 35°F to 45°F (2°C–7°C).
2. Use entire contents when first opened. Care should be taken to avoid microbial contamination of the product.
3. If allergic response occurs, symptomatic treatment should be provided immediately.
4. Transient local irritation at the site of injection, though rare, may occur subsequent to use of this product.

How Supplied: 10 ml/10 dose and 25 × 1 dose carton.

CALCIUM GLUCONATE
23% Solution

Composition:
*Calcium Gluconate .... 23% w/v
Water .... q.s.
*Present as salts of boryl esters of gluconic acid.
Indications: For use as an aid in the treatment of calcium deficiencies in horses, cattle, swine and sheep including parturient paresis (milk fever) in cattle.
Dosage and Administration: *Horses, and cattle,* 250 ml. to 500 ml. *Swine and sheep,* 25 ml. to 50 ml.
Administer intravenously, intramuscularly, or subcutaneously. If given subcutaneously or intramuscularly, divide the dosage among several locations. Massage the point of injections, to aid in absorption.
Cautions: Solution should be warmed to room temperature and administered slowly. This product contains no preservative. Entire contents should be used upon entering. Discard any unused portion.
Keep out of reach of children.
How Supplied:
500 ml.

CAL-PHOS #2
Reinforced

Composition: Each 500 ml. Contains:
Calcium .... 10.00 grams
(Stabilized with boryl esters of gluconic acid)
Magnesium .... 2.76 grams
(Obtained from 23.07 grams of magnesium chloride hexahydrate)
Phosphorus .... 6.03 grams
(Obtained from 20.65 grams of sodium hypophosphite $\cdot H_2O$)
Dextrose $\cdot H_2O$ .... 75.00 grams
Water .... q.s.
Indications: For use in cattle exhibiting deficiencies of Calcium (milk fever or parturient paresis, hypocalcemia), Magnesium (grass tetany) or hyperpotassemia (wheat pasture poisoning). Administer intravenously, intramusculary, intraperitoneally or subcutaneously. If given subcutaneously or intramuscularly, divide the dosage among several locations. Massage the point of injections to aid in absorption.
Dosage and Administration: *Cattle:* 250 to 500 ml. If there is no noticeable improvement in the condition within 24 hours following treatment, consult your veterinarian. Aseptic precautions should be observed such as using sterile needle and syringe. Disinfect the site of injection.
Caution: Solution should be warmed to room temperature and administered slowly. This product contains no preservative. Entire contents should be used upon entering. Discard any unused portion.
Keep Out of Reach of Children
How Supplied: 500 ml.
For Veterinary Use Only.

C.C.S.N.S.
Clostridium
Chauvoei-Septicum-Novyi-Sordellii
Bacterin-Toxoid
Aluminum Hydroxide Adsorbed

Composition: A formaldehyde-inactivated, aluminum hydroxide adsorbed bacterin-toxoid prepared from cultures of *C. chauvoei, C. septicum, C. novyi* and *C. sordellii* specifically chosen for their immunogenicity.
Indications: For use in the immunization of healthy cattle and sheep against infections causes by *C. chauvoei* (Blackleg), *C. septicum* (Malignant Edema), *C. novyi* (Black Disease) and *C. sordellii.*
Dosage and Administration: Shake well, administer 5 ml subcutaneously using aseptic technique. For Black Disease, repeat the dose every 5 to 6 months in animals subject to reexposure. Revaccination for C. sordellii is recommended at 2 to 4 weeks. Calves vaccinated under 3 months of age should be revaccinated at weaning or 4 to 6 months of age.
Protection: The use of this product is indicated whenever it is desired to immunize concurrently against *C. chauvoei, C. septicum, C. novyi* and *C. sordellii* infections.
The isolation of *C. septicum* and *C. sordellii* from cases of sudden death in feedlot or pasture calves has become increasingly frequent. Where this problem is encountered the combined C.C.S.N.S. bacterin should be administered.
C. novyi infection (Black Disease) once believed a disease of sheep has been increasingly diagnosed in cattle. Whether the incidence of the disease is increasing or the improved diagnostic procedures are responsible for increased incidence is not clear. There exists the probability that Black Disease has always been a major problem and has in the past been the

actual cause of some suspected outbreaks of Blackleg and Malignant Edema.

Black Disease seemingly is especially prevalent in areas where water sufficient to support a snail population is present. Liver damage resulting from fluke infestation creates a situation favorable for growth of *C. noyvi*. In such areas early preventative vaccination should be employed.

Studies have shown that vaccination with C.C.S.N.S. Bacterin-Toxoid, according to the above recommendations, produces protection in the host ruminant against subsequent challenge with the virulent organisms. However, lethal toxins play a major role in the pathology of the clostridial infections, and because of the immunological principle that a two-dose vaccination regime is usually superior to a one-dose regime for bacterin-toxoids, a second vaccination, given 3 to 4 weeks after the first, is recommended in order to establish a higher, long-lasting level of immunity.

Precautions: Do not vaccinate within 21 days before slaughter.

For Veterinary Use Only

How Supplied: 10 dose (50 ml) and 50 dose (250 ml) plastic vials.

CLOSTRIDIAL 7-WAY
Clostridium Chauvoei-Septicum-Novyi-Sordellii-Perfringens Types C & D Bacterin-Toxoid Aluminum Hydroxide Adsorbed

Composition: Clostridial 7-Way is a formaldehyde-inactivated and aluminum hydroxide gel adjuvanted bacterin-toxoid prepared from cultures of *Cl. chauvoei* (blackleg), *Cl. Septicum* (malignant edema), *Cl. novyi* (black disease), *Cl sordellii* and *Cl. perfringens* Type C & D (enterotoxemia). The product meets all potency standards for clostridial vaccines established by the U.S.D.A.

Fermentor production assures a highly immunogenic, uniformly consistent vaccine serial to serial. Precise control of temperature, pH, nutrient medium, anaerobic conditions, agitation and inactivation for each serial is assured.

The alhydrogel brand of aluminum hydroxide gel adjuvant provides uniformly high absorption capacity, more uniform distribution of antigen, more standardized antigen content per dose and better vaccine stability. Alhydrogel also reduces reaction potential when compared to other adjuvants.

Indications: Clostridial 7-Way is indicated for immunization of healthy cattle and sheep against diseases caused by *Cl. chauvoei, Cl septicum, Cl. novyi, Cl. sordellii* and *Cl. perfringens* Types C & D. Although *Cl. Perfringens* Type D is not a significant problem in the U.S.A., immunity may be provided against the beta and epsilon toxins elaborated by *Cl. perfringens* Type B. This immunity is derived from the combination of Type C (beta) and Type D (epsilon) fractions.

Dosage and Administration: Shake well. Using aseptic technique, inject subcutaneously or intramuscularly. Dosage: 5 ml for cattle and 2 ml for sheep. Revaccinate in 2 to 6 weeks for *Cl. sordellii* and *Cl. perfringens* Types C & D. For *Cl. novyi*, repeat the dose every 5 to 6 months in animals subjected to reexposure. For animals vaccinated before 3 months, revaccinate at weaning or 4 to 6 months of age. Annual revaccination is recommended for breeding animals.

Precautions: Do not vaccinate within 21 days of slaughter.

For Veterinary Use Only.

How Supplied: 10 ds/50 ml.; 50 ds/250 ml.; 200 ds/1000 ml.

CMPK
(Cal-Phos #2 w/Potassium)

Description:

Each 500 ml. Contains:

Calcium ....10.00 grams
(Stabilized with boryl esters of gluconic acid)

Magnesium ....2.76 grams
(Obtained from 23.07 grams of magnesium chloride hexahydrate)

Phosphorus ....6.03 grams
(Obtained from 20.65 grams of sodium hypophosphite $\cdot H_2O$)

Potassium ....0.525 gram
(Obtained from 1.00 gram of potassium chloride)

Dextrose $\cdot H_2O$ ....75.00 grams

Water ....q.s.

Indications: For treatment of hypocalcemia (milk fever, etc.) complicated with deficient amounts of potassium. Also contains magnesium for treatment of grass tetany and wheat pasture poisoning and necessary for use in geographical area of magnesium deficiency. The addition of potassium is a further aid to parenteral therapy for the purpose of increasing recovery rates and preventing relapses.

Suggested Dosage: Standard procedure in treating an average case of milk fever is to administer 1 gram of Calcium per 100 lbs. body weight (1000 lb. cow).

How Supplied: 500 ml.

COMBIPLEX-B
Injectable

Composition: Each ml. contains:

Thiamine HCl U.S.P. ....12.5 mg
Riboflavin (as 5' Phosphate Sodium) ...2 mg
Niacinamide U.S.P. ....100 mg
d-Panthenol ....10 mg
Pyridoxine HCl U.S.P. ....5 mg
Cyanocobalamin (Cryst.) U.S.P. ...5 mcg
Benzyl Alcohol (Preservative) 1.5%
Water ....q.s.

Indications: For use in Multiple B Complex deficiencies in both large and small animals.

Dosage and Administration: Administer intramuscularly or intravenously. Dogs and Cats: ½ to 2 ml; Sheep and Swine: 5 to 10 ml; Horses and Cattle: 10 to 20 ml. Repeat daily as indicated.

Caution: Anaphylactogenesis to parenteral Thiamine HCl has been reported. Administer slowly and with caution in doses over 50 mg. Federal law restricts this drug to use by or on the order of a licensed veterinarian.

How Supplied: 100 ml., 250 ml. and 500 ml.

CONTROLLER® FLEA-KILL MIST
(For dogs, cats and horses)

Composition:

Pyrethrins	0.15%
*Piperonyl butoxide, technical	1.50%
n-Octyl bicycloheptene dicarboximide	0.50%
2,3,4,5-bis (2-butylene) tetrahydro-2-furaldehyde	0.50%
Petroleum distillate	1.35%
**Inert Ingredients	96.00%
Total	100.00%

*Equivalent to 1.2% (butylcarbityl) (6-propyl piperonyl) ether and 0.3% related compounds.

**Inert ingredients include a grooming agent to ease combing and brushing of coat to remove dead fleas and lice.

Indications: For the control of Fleas, Ticks and Lice on Dogs, Cats and Horses, and for temporarily repelling Gnats, Mosquitoes and Biting Flies.

Directions: It is a violation of Federal law to use this product in a manner inconsistent with its labeling.

Cats and Dogs: Remove cap and insert sprayer. Cover animal's eyes with hand and with firm fast stroke, to get a proper spray mist, spray head, ears, and chest until damp. With finger tips rub into face around mouth, nose and eyes. Then spray neck, middle and hind quarters, finishing legs last. For best penetration of spray to the skin, direct spray against the natural lay of the hair. On long haired dogs rub your hand against the natural lay of the hair, spraying the ruffled hair directly behind the hand. Make sure spray thoroughly wets ticks. Repeat treatment as needed.

Puppies and Kittens: Treat same as cats and dogs except nursing puppies and kittens, spray only along back or on your finger tips and rub in with your finger tips. Do not use on puppies or kittens under 4 weeks of age.

Pet Sleeping Quarters: Spray around baseboards, windows, door frames, wall cracks and local area of floors. If mosquitoes, gnats or flies are present, spray lightly into the air. Repeat as needed. The bedding should be sprayed and then replaced with fresh bedding for best results.

Horses: To control stable flies, horse flies, deer flies and face flies apply to face, legs, flanks, topline and other body areas commonly attacked by these flies. Repeat treatment as needed.

Warning: *Humans:* Harmful if swallowed or inhaled. Avoid breathing spray mist. Avoid contact with skin or eyes. Avoid contamination of feed or foodstuffs.

Animals: Avoid contact with animal's eyes. Do not use on nursing animals.

Environmental Hazards: This product is toxic to aquatic organisms. Do not apply directly to water. Do not contaminate water by cleaning of equipment or disposal of wastes.

Continued on next page

T

TechAmerica—Cont.

How Supplied: 16 oz w/trigger sprayer, 32 oz, gallon refills.

CONTROLLER™ FLEA & TICK COLLAR

Kills fleas and ticks for up to 5 months on medium and large dogs, and up to 6 months on small dogs and cats

Available Only Through Veterinarian

Active Ingredient:
2-(1-Methylethoxy) phenol methylcarbonate 10.0%
Inert Ingredients: 90.0%
Total 100.0%

CONTROLLER™ FLEA & TICK COLLAR uses a patented controlled release system to dispense an insecticide which kills fleas and ticks continuously for up to 5 months. This multilayered CONTROLLER FLEA & TICK COLLAR is a reinforced laminate so it may be used as a restraining collar.

Precautionary Statements
HAZARDS TO HUMANS & DOMESTIC ANIMALS.
Caution: May be harmful if swallowed or chewed. Avoid breathing dust. Avoid direct contact with eyes, skin or clothing. Do not allow children to handle this collar. Do not open protective pouch until ready to use. Wash thoroughly after handling. Some animals may be sensitive to this product. When collar is first worn, observe neck area and remove collar at first sign of adverse reactions such as skin irritation or any other symptoms. Collar is intended for use as an insecticide dispenser and is not to be taken internally by man or animals. Do not use on sick or convalescing animals. Do not use other pesticides on animals while collar is worn. Do not use on animals under 6 weeks of age.

Statement of Practical Treatment
If swallowed: Call a physician or Poison Control Center. Drink 1 or 2 glasses of water and induce vomiting by touching finger to back of throat.
If on skin: Wash with soap and water.
If in eyes: Flush eyes with plenty of water.
Note to Physicians: This product contains a cholinesterase inhibitor. Atropine is antidotal if symptoms of cholinesterase inhibition are present.

Storage and Disposal
Storage: Store in a cool dry place.
Product Disposal: Securely wrap used collar in several layers of newspaper and discard in trash.
Container Disposal: Do not reuse empty pouch. Wrap pouch in newspaper and discard in trash.

U.S. Pat. Nos. 3,864,468; 4,102,991; 4,160,335; 4,284,444; 3,852,416
EPA Reg. No. 8730-43-48808
EPA Est. No. 6175-LA-01

Directions for Use
It is a violation of Federal Law to use this product in a manner inconsistent with its labeling. Remove collar, buckle and "D" ring from package. Attach one end of the collar into one end. Slip D-ring on loose end of collar. Measure collar on pet's neck. (When attached, allow room to insert two fingers easily between collar and pet's neck.) Cut off excess length so that ends of collar will meet at mid-point of buckle. (Warning: Do not overlap. Overlapping will cause collar to fall off.) Place collar on pet and clamp securely. The collar starts starts killing fleas as soon as it is placed around the animal's neck. Fleas on the animal will be killed and new ones which may temporarily appear will also be killed while collar is worn. Replace collar after 5 months or when effectiveness diminishes.
Remove collar when bathing animals or when animals are likely to become wet. When collar is first placed on the animal, adult ticks will be killed in a few days and will fall off or may then be easily removed. Immature ticks which are small and difficult to see are also killed by the CONTROLLER FLEA & TICK COLLAR. The insecticide released continuously by the collar will also kill ticks that may carry and transmit Rocky Mountain Spotted Fever and tularemia.
How Supplied: Cat, 14″; small dog, 14″; medium dog, 22″; large dog, 30″.

CONTROLLER® HOUSE AND CARPET SPRAY

Composition:

Chlorpyrifos (0,0-diethyl 0-(3,5,6-trichloro-2-pyridyl) phosphorothioate)	0.50%
Xylene range aromatic solvent	0.33%
Inert Ingredients:	99.17%
Total	100.00%

Indications: Controls fleas, brown dog ticks and numerous pests in and around households.
Caution: Harmful if swallowed. Avoid contact with eyes, skin and clothing. Avoid breathing vapors or spray mist. Keep away from food, feedstuffs and domestic water supplies. Wash thoroughly with soap and water after handling.
Directions for Use: It is a violation of Federal law to use this product in a manner inconsistent with its labeling.
General Information: Use this insecticide at full strength to control the pests indicated in the areas listed. Repeat the treatment as needed. When spraying indoors, cover aquaria and fish bowls and remove birds such as canaries from area prior to treating. DO NOT PERMIT HUMANS OR PETS TO CONTACT TREATED SURFACES UNTIL SPRAY HAS DRIED.
For Control of Fleas and Brown Dog Ticks: Thoroughly apply as a spray for spot treatment to infested areas such as pet beds and resting quarters; nearby cracks and crevices; along and behind baseboards, window and door frames and localized areas of floor and floor covering where these pests may be present. THE PERIOD OF ACTIVITY OF THIS PRODUCT TO KILL FLEA LARVA IS UP TO 42 DAYS. Old bedding of pets should be removed and replaced with clean, fresh bedding after treatment of pet area. Do Not Treat Pets With This Product. To control the source of flea infestation, pets inhabiting the treated premises should be treated with a product registered for application to animals.
For Spot Treatment Only: Apply as a course spray or with a paint brush to localized areas where cockroaches (including strains resistant to other insecticides) ants, clover mites, crickets, firebrats, silverfish, and spiders are found or normally occur including dark corners of rooms and closets; around plumbing and other utility installations; cracks and crevices in walls; along and behind baseboards; beneath and behind sinks, stoves, refrigerators and cabinets. For ants apply to ant trails, also around doors and windows and wherever else these pests may find entrance. Note: A period of 4 to 7 days is normally required for maximum effect on cockroaches. Apply spray until area is moist or damp, avoid excessive wetting.
How Supplied: 32 oz w/trigger.

DELTOX™ C & D

Clostridium Perfringens
Types C & D
Bacterin-Toxoid
Aluminum Hydroxide Adsorbed

Composition: Clostridium Perfringens Type C & D Bacterin-Toxoid is a combination product containing toxoids and cellular antigens of *Cl. perfringens* Type C and *Cl. perfringens* Type D. The cultures are formalin inactivated, aluminum hydroxide adsorbed and blended in proper proportions to assure maximum efficacy in each production serial.
Each culture is grown separately in Fermentation Design Equipment, tested in process for purity, and toxigenicity before combining the two fractions in proper proportions to make the combination product.
Clostridium Perfringens Type C and D combines in a single dose antigens protecting against both beta and epsilon toxins (produced by *Cl. perfringens* Type B, C and D).
Indications: For the immunization of healthy cattle and sheep against Types C & D enterotoxemia.
Dosage and Administration: Shake well. Administer subcutaneously, 5 ml. to cattle, 2 ml. to sheep. Repeat in 21 days. For feedlot animals, give the last injection 10 days prior to intensive feeding. For breeding females, yearly boosters are recommended during the last third of pregnancy. Vaccinate sheep and lambs before placing them on concentrated rations, or before turning on lush pastures in the spring.
Precautions: Do not vaccinate within 21 days of slaughter.
For Veterinary Use Only.
How Supplied: 10 dose (50 ml.) and 50 dose (250 ml.) plastic bottles.

DERMAQUEL™ PET SHAMPOO

(With Complex Iodine 1%)

Contains: Complex Iodine 1% in an anionic shampoo base, providing 0.2% titratable iodine.
Indications: A deep cleaning, nonstaining, medicated shampoo for sham-

pooing dogs and cats. Very helpful for cleaning soiled or contaminated wounds.
Use: External application.
Directions: Wet the animal with warm water, then apply shampoo to the entire body. Massage well and rinse. Repeat application; then rinse again. For maximum effect the second application may be allowed to remain in contact with the skin and hair 5 to 10 minutes before rinsing. Repeat application as indicated.
How Supplied: 6 fl. oz., Gallon.

DERMAQUEL™ PET SHAMPOO
(A concentrated neutral shampoo)

Description: Dermaquel concentrated neutral shampoo has been designed for use by the veterinarian to leave a luster or sheen to the hair-coat. It is an excellent shampoo, general cleaner for equipment, field and obstetrical use. This product is not heavily perfumed and leaves a clean smell. This is a low sudsing, highly effective shampoo that rinses easily and quickly. Not necessary to rewash to remove suds from coat.
Indications: It may be used just as it is for maximum cleaning or untangling of matted hair-coat. However, for routine shampooing, it may be diluted up to 6 times.
For routine equipment or hospital cleaning, add tablespoonful of Dermaquel Shampoo per gallon of water.
For obstetrical use, use undiluted as needed and wash off with warm water when completed. This shampoo and cleaner contains no insecticides or antiseptics of any kind.
Directions For Use: For shampooing, wet coat with warm water, apply shampoo and work into a lather with hands or brush. When dealing with matted hair or difficult odors, allow patient to stand with suds in coat for a few minutes. Then rinse.
How Supplied: 6 fl. oz., Gallon, 5 Gallon.

DERMAQUEL™ PET SHAMPOO
(With Sulfa-Tar)

Contains:

Coal Tar Solution	2.5%
Colloidal Sulfur	5%
Salicylic Acid	1%
Parachlorometaxylenol	0.1%

Combined with the cleansing action of surface active agents.
Indications: As a therapeutic shampoo to be used to remove dry, scaling skin, and to relieve itching and related symptoms associated with eczema and psoriasis. Combines effective cleansing agents with active ingredients useful in the treatment of skin disorders caused by surface parasites.
Medicated skin shampoo provides supportive therapy in the treatment of sarcoptic mange and ringworm.
Use: For external use only.
Directions: Thoroughly wet the entire hair-coat with warm water and apply enough shampoo to make a lather, and work thoroughly into the hair-coat. For best results, repeat application and allow lather to remain on pet for 10 to 15 minutes before rinsing, or as directed by your veterinarian.
How Supplied: 6 fl. oz., Gallon.

DEXAMYCIN

Composition: This product is a sterile aqueous suspension for intramuscular injection in which each milliliter contains: 200,000 units penicillin G procaine, 10 mg. chlorpheniramine maleate, 0.5 mg. dexamethasone, 10 mg. sodium citrate, 20 mg. procaine hydrochloride, 1 mg. lecithin in 250 mg. dihydrostreptomycin solution (as the sulfate), 1.0 mg. propylparaben sodium and 0.25% phenol (as preservative), water for injection q.s.
Indications: For use only in horses, dogs, and cats for treating infections in which the invading organisms are known to be sensitive to penicillin or dihydrostreptomycin and when stress due to infection necessitates the administration of a corticosteroid as adjuvant therapy. This product is useful in the following conditions in cats, dogs and horses. It should not be used in horses which are to be slaughtered for human consumption.
Dogs and Cats
1. Respiratory tract infections, pneumonia, bronchitis, tracheobronchitis and tonsillitis.
2. Supportive therapy and prevention of complications of the distemper complex and infectious hepatitis.
3. All bacterial infections susceptible to penicillin and/or dihydrostreptomycin.
4. Infections of the reproductive tract.
5. Pre- or post-operative prophylaxis for stress or infection.
6. Lesions of allergy, eczema or dermatitis showing secondary infection.
7. Phlegmon, cellulitis, pyemia.
8. Infected wounds.

Horses
1. Respiratory tract infections, pneumonia.
2. Bacterial septicemias, pyogenic infections, cellulitis, phlegmon, etc. due to organisms susceptible to penicillin and /or dihydrostreptomycin.
3. Wound infection.
4. Pre- or post-operative prophylaxis for stress or infection.

Dosage and Administration: Administer Dexamycin by intramuscular injection only.
Dogs and Cats: under 10 lb., 0.5 ml.; 10-20 lb., 1 ml.; 20-30 lb., 1.5 ml.; over 30 lb., 2 ml.
Horses: 1 to 1.5 ml. per 100 lb. body weight.
Warning: Clinical and experimental data have demonstrated that corticosteroids administered orally or parenterally to animals may induce the first stage of parturition when administered during the last trimester of pregnancy and may precipitate premature parturition followed by dystocia, fetal death, retained placenta, and metritis.
Dexamycin is for intramuscular use only. *Do not Use Intravenously* or *Subcutaneously.* Keep under refrigeration until used. Store below 15°C. (59°F). Shake well before using. Keep out of reach of children.
Caution: Federal law restricts this drug to use by or on the order of a licensed veterinarian.
How Supplied 100 ml.

DEXASONE
(Dexamethasone Solution 2 mg./ml.)

Important Notice: Dexamethasone is a synthetic analogue of prednisolone having similar but more potent anti-inflammatory therapeutic action, and diversified hormonal and metabolic effects.
Composition: Each ml. contains 2 mg. 9-alpha-fluoro-16-alpha-methylprednisolone, 500 mg. polyethylene glycol 400, 9 mg. benzyl alcohol, ethyl alcohol 0.05 ml., 1.8 mg. methylparaben and 0.2 mg. propylparaben, as preservatives, water q.s.
All of the precautions and contraindications for adrenocortical hormones apply at this time to the drug.
The dosage of Dexamethasone required is markedly lower than that of prednisone or prednisolone. The sections on indications, dosage, and precautions should be read before this drug is used.
Indications: Small animal indications include inflammatory conditions involving the joints and accessory structures where structural changes such as ankylosing joints, ruptured ligaments, sheaths, etc. do not exist; nonspecific dermatitis.
Dexamethasone Solution is indicated as an anti-inflammatory agent in canine, feline and equine.
Equine indications include acute musculoskeletal conditions such as bursitis, carpitis, osslets, tendonitis, myositis, sprains, rattlesnake bite, and as supportive therapy in fatigue, heat exhaustion and influenza.
If bony changes exist in any of these conditions, responses to dexamethasone cannot be expected.
Dosage and Administration: Therapy with dexamethasone should be individualized according to the severity of the condition being treated, anticipated duration of steroid therapy and the patient's threshold or tolerance for steroid excess. The lowest dose that will offer adequate relief in chronic conditions should be the dose employed. The use of large doses in chronic conditions may produce polyuria and polydipsia. Large doses, however, may be necessary and in such instances, the patient must be closely observed for the occurrence of side effects. Acute conditions sometimes demand the use of larger doses for a short period of time in order to obtain the necessary degree of relief. When side effects occur, it may be necessary to reduce the dose of the drug or to discontinue therapy.
Treatment may be changed over to dexamethasone from any other glucocorticoid with proper reduction and adjustment of dosage.
Dosage: *Canine* — 0.25 to 1 mg. intravenously or intramuscularly. The dose may be repeated if necessary.

Continued on next page

T

TechAmerica—Cont.

Feline — 0.125 to 0.5 mg. intravenously or intramuscularly. The dose may be repeated if necessary.
Equine — 2.5 to 5 mg. intravenously or intramuscularly.
Warning: Clinical and experimental data have demonstrated that corticosteroids administered orally or parenterally to animals may induce the first stage of parturition when administered during the last trimester of pregnancy and may precipitate premature parturition followed by dystocia, fetal death, retained placenta, and metritis.
Not To Be Used in Horses Intended For Food.
Caution: Federal law restricts this drug to use by or on the order of a licensed veterinarian.
How Supplied: 100 ml.

DEXTROSE SOLUTION, 50%
Sterile

Composition:
Dextrose $\cdot H_2O$ ....50% w/v
Water...q.s
Indications: As a fluid and nutrient replenisher in cattle. For use in supportive therapy when intake is restricted or inadequate to maintain nutritional requirements.
Suggested Dosage: The usual dose is 50 ml. per 100 lbs. of body weight. It may be injected intravenously, intramuscularly, intraperitoneally or subcutaneously. May be repeated in 8 to 10 hours or on successive days. If there is no noticeable improvement in the condition being treated after 3 to 4 days of treatment, consult your veterinarian.
Directions: If administered intramuscularly or subcutaneously, the dosage should be divided among several locations and the point of injections massaged to aid in absorption.
Aseptic precautions should be observed such as withdrawing from the bottle through a sterile 14 or 16-gauge needle into a sterile syringe. Disinfect the site of injection.
Caution: Solution should be warmed to room temperature and administered slowly. This product contains no preservative. Entire contents should be used upon entering. Discard any unused portion.
Keep out of Reach of Children.
How Supplied: 500 ml.
For Veterinary Use Only.

T

DISAL® (FUROSEMIDE) INJECTION 5%
A diuretic saluretic for prompt relief of edema.

Contents: Each ml. contains: 50 mg. furosemide as a monoethanolamine salt preserved and stabilized with myristyl-gamma-picolinium chloride 0.02%, EDTA sodium 0.1%, sodium sulfite 0.1% with sodium chloride 0.2% q.s. with water for injection. pH adjusted with sodium hydroxide and/or hydrochloride acid.
Indications: Disal® (Furosemide) is an effective diuretic-saluretic for use in the treatment of acute inflammatory tissue edema in dogs and horses, and for use in the treatment of edema (pulmonary congestion, ascites) associated with cardiac insufficiency in the dog.
Contraindications: Because animal reproductive studies have shown that furosemide may cause fetal abnormality, the drug is contraindicated in pregnant bitches, mares and stallions at stud.
Dosage and Administration: Administer either intramuscularly or intravenously. Dogs: 0.25 to 0.50 ml per 10 pounds body weight once or twice daily at 6 to 8 hour intervals. Horses: Approximately 0.50 mg/lb body weight (1.0 mg/kg) once or twice daily at 6 to 8 hour intervals.
Caution: Federal law restricts this drug to use by or on the order of a licensed veterinarian.
How Supplied: 50 and 100 ml. Multidose vial.

DISAL® TABLETS
A diuretic saluretic for prompt relief of edema.

Ingredients: Furosemide (4-chloro-N-furfuryl-5-sulfamoylanthranilic acid).
Indications: *Dogs* —Disal® is an effective diuretic saluretic for oral use in the treatment of edema (pulmonary congestion, ascites) associated with cardiac insufficiency and acute non-inflammatory tissue edema.
Contraindications: Because animal reproductive studies have shown that furosemide may cause fetal abnormality, the drug is contraindicated in pregnant animals.
Dosage and Administration: *Dogs:* One 50 mg. scored tablet per 25 to 50 pounds body weight. Administer once or twice daily at 6–8 hour intervals. The dosage may be doubled or increased by increments of 1 mg. per pound body weight in refractory or severe edema cases.
How Supplied: 12.5 mg. in 100 and 500 Tablet Containers; 50 mg. in 100 and 500 Tablet Containers.

DIZAN® TABLETS
(Dithiazanine Iodide)

Actions: Dizan, dithiazanine iodide, is an effective broad spectrum anthelmintic, that has shown therapeutic activity for the removal of many intestinal helminths in dogs. The anthelmintic potential of the cyanine dyes, including Dizan, is thought to be due to the amidinium ion system which interferes with enzyme maintenance of oxygen uptakes and carbohydrate metabolism of a number of parasites.
Indications: Dizan, dithiazanine iodide, is indicated for the removal of large roundworms *(Toxocara canis, Toxascaris leonina)*, hookworms *(Ancylostoma caninum, Uncinaria stenocephala)*, heartworm microfilariae *(Dirofilaria immitis)*, strongyloides *(Strongyloides canis, Strongyloids stercoralis)* and whipworms *(Trichuris vulpis)* from dogs.
Dosage and Administration: Administer orally according to the following dosage table.
Tablets: Administer immediately after feeding.
Large roundworms 10 mg./lb. 3–5 days.
Hookworms and whipworms 10 mg./lb. 7 days.
Strongyloides 10 mg./lb. 10–12 days.
Heartworm microfilariae 3–5 mg./lb. 7–10 days.
Treatment with Dizan for heartworm microfilariae should follow six weeks after therapy for adult heartworms.
How Supplied: 50 mg. coated, bottles of 100 and 500; 100 mg. coated, bottles of 100 and 500; 200 mg. coated, bottles of 100 and 500.

DUAL-PEN
(Sterile Benzathine Penicillin G and Procaine Penicillin G in aqueous suspension)

Description: Each ml. of suspension contains: 150,000 units penicillin G benzathine; 150,000 units penicillin G procaine; 3.0 mg. sodium formaldehyde sulfoxylate; 14.0 mg. lecithin; 1.20 mg. methylparaben (as preservative); 0.14 mg. propylparaben (as preservative); 0.25% Phenol (as preservative); 7.0 mg. tween 40; 10.0 mg. span 40; 10.0 mg. sodium citrate; 20.0 mg. procaine hydrochloride; 1.5 mg. sodium carboxymethylcellulose; 3.5 mg. povidone; 0.15 ml. sorbitol solution; and water for injection q.s.
Action: Penicillin G is an antibiotic which shows a marked bactericidal effect against certain organisms during their growth phase. It is relatively specific in its action against Gram-positive bacteria but is usually ineffective against Gram-negative organisms.
When treating an animal for a bacterial infection, it is advisible to isolate and identify the causitive organism and conduct appropriate in vitro susceptibility tests. In cases where organisms other than those susceptible to penicillin are present, re-evaluation of treatment should be made. Organisms normally considered susceptible to penicillin include *Clostridium septicum, Corynebacterium pyogenes, Staphylococcus aureus, Streptococcus canis, Streptococcus equi* and *Streptococcus pyogenes.*
Indications
This product is indicated for treatment of the following bacterial infections in dogs, horses and beef cattle due to pencillin G susceptible micro-orgasnisms that are susceptible to the serum levels common to this particular dosage form, such as:
1. Bacterial Pneumonia *(Streptococcus spp., Corynebacterium pyogenes, Staphylococcus aureus)*
2. Upper Respiratory Infections such as Rhinitis or Pharyngitis *(Corynebacterium pyogenes)*
3. Equine Strangles *(Streptococcus equi)*
4. Blackleg *(Clostridium chauvoei)*
5. Anthrax *(Bacillus anthracis)*
6. Prophylaxis of Bovine Shipping Fever in 300–500 pound beef calves.

Contraindications: This product is contraindicated in patients which have shown hypersensitivity to penicillin.

Warning: Beef cattle should be withheld from slaughter for food use for 30 days following last treatment. Treatment in beef cattle must be limited to two (2) doses. Not to be used in horses intended for food purposes.
Caution: Federal law restricts this drug to use by or on the order of a licensed veterinarian.
Adverse Reaction: Anaphylactic reactions have been reported in cattle given penicillin. Treated animals should be closely observed and if allergic or anaphylactic reactions occur, administer epinephrine or antihistamines immediately.
Administration: This product should be given by intramuscular injection to horses. In beef cattle the recommended dosage should be administered by subcutaneous injection only. Dogs may be injected by either the intramuscular or subcutaneous route.
Dosage: *Horses:* 2 ml. per 150 lb. body weight given intramuscularly (2,000 units penicillin G procaine and 2,000 units penicillin G benzathine per lb. body weight). Treatment should be repeated in 48 hours.
Beef Cattle: 2 ml. per 150 lb. body weight given subcutaneously only (2,000 units penicillin G procaine and 2,000 units penicillin G benzathine per lb. body weight). Treatment should be repeated in 48 hours.
Important: Treatment in beef cattle should be limited to two (2) doses of this product, given by subcutaneous injection only.
Dogs: 1 ml. per 10 to 25 lb. body weight given intramuscularly or subcutaneously (6,000 to 15,000 units penicillin G procaine and 6,000 to 15,000 units penicillin G benzathine per lb. body weight). Treatment should be repeated in 48 hours.
Keep in a cool place—store below 15°C(59 °F).
How Supplied: 100 ml.; 250 ml.

ELECTRO SOLUTION
w/Dextrose

Composition: Dextrose 5.0% w/v, Sorbitol 2.5% w/v, and Electrolytes; Sodium Lactate, Sodium Chloride, Potassium Chloride, Calcium Chloride, Magnesium Chloride in proper proportions.
Indications: As a fluid and nutrient replenisher in the treatment of dehydration and electrolyte depletion accompanying diarrhea or severe hemorrhage in cattle, sheep, swine and horses.
Dosage and Administrations: 100 to 250 ml. per 100 lbs. body weight. Administer intravenously. May be repeated in 18 to 24 hours.
Caution: Solution should be warmed to room temperature and administered slowly.
How Supplied: 950 ml.

EROCON®
Erysipelothrix Rhusiopathiae Bacterin

Composition: Erysipelas Bacterin is a concentrated formalin inactivated, aluminum hydroxide absorbed culture of a highly antigenic strain of *Erysipelothrix rhusiopathiae (insidiosa).*
Uniform suspension is accomplished and maintained with a minimum of agitation, assuring total uniformity from dose to dose, and excellent syringeability.
Swelling at the site of injection is virtually nonexistant.
Indications: For the protection of swine against Swine Erysipelas.
Dosage and Administration: Shake well. The dosage for swine of all ages is 2 ml. injected subcutaneously. To insure continuous high levels of protection animals held for breeding stock should be revaccinated before breeding.
In very young animals (8 weeks or less) the level of immunity resulting from one vaccination may be variable due to presence of interfering maternal antibody levels or the inherent inability of the very young to develop immunity. Swine vaccinated prior to that age should be revaccinated after weaning to assure maximum protection.
Erysipelas Bacterin is an excellent prophylactic agent which will provide adequate protection from weaning time to market age in swine.
Precautions: Do not vaccinate within 21 days of slaughter. Refer to label for recommended precautions.
For Veterinary Use Only.
How Supplied: 50 dose (100 ml.), 125 dose (250 ml.), and 250 dose (500 ml.) plastic vials.

GENTAMICIN SULFATE INJECTION
Sterile

Composition: Gentamicin Sulfate Injection is a clear, colorless to pale yellow, sterile solution for intramuscular or subcutaneous injection.
Each ml contains gentamicin sulfate equivalent to 50 mg gentamicin base, 3.2 mg sodium bisulfite, 0.1 mg disodium edetate, 1.8 mg methylparaben and 0.2 mg propylparaben as preservatives and water for injection, qs. Glacial acetic acid and/or sodium hydroxide may be used for pH adjustment.
Actions: Gentamicin sulfate is a member of a group of broad-spectrum antibiotics referred to as the aminoglycosides. It is a mixture of gentamicin C_1, C_{1A} and C_2 sulfate salts and is derived from the growth of **micromonospora purpurea.**[1]
The aminoglycosides exert their inhibitory action on bacteria by binding to ribosomes and interfering with protein synthesis.[1,2,3] Gentamicin is effective against a wide range of gram-negative and gram-positive bacteria.
In Vitro Susceptibility Testing: The following gentamicin **in vitro** data are available but their clinical significance are unknown.
In vitro antibacterial activity has shown that gentamicin is active against non-resistant **Staphylococcus aureus,** most indole positive and some indole negative Proteus species, alpha hemolytic Streptococcus spp. (beta hemolytic Streptococcus are not susceptible including **Strep. pneumoniae), Pseudomonas aeruginosa, Escherichia coli.**[1,2]
In one clinical study, the **in vitro** activity of gentamicin against 1,160 organisms isolated from dogs was determined. Using a 10 mcg antibiotic disc, 98% of the total gram-positive and gram-negative bacteria tested were susceptible to gentamicin.[2] The presence of serum inhibits the activity of gentamicin; the destruction of microorganisms may be up to 12 times slower. Sodium bicarbonate enhances the activity of gentamicin 8 to 32 fold, since gentamicin is most active at pH 7.5[4]
Pharmacokinetics: In dogs, intramuscular administration of gentamicin at a dosage of 0.73 mg/lb resulted in peak serum and urine concentrations averaging approximately 11 and 14 mcg/ml within 60 minutes. Serum and urine concentration time profiles in dogs following intramuscular administration are illustrated graphically in the following figure.[5,6]

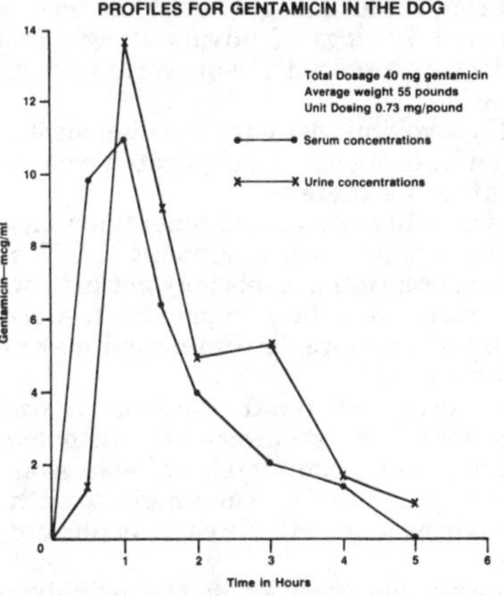

Toxicology: A safety study was conducted in 22 dogs where gentamicin was administered intramuscularly at 0, 1x, 3x and 5x (0, 2, 6 and 10 mg/lb body weight) the recommended dosage. All groups were dosed for 3x the normal duration of therapy (21 days). At 1x, a mild interstitial nephritis resulted, at 3x, more pronounced signs of toxicity were noted and at 5x, 50% of the dogs were moribund by day nineteen. There was also a dose related trend of albuminuria and a decrease in urine specific gravity in all treated groups.
One hundred two dogs were treated in the clinical trials. Sixty-six percent (67/102) of the dogs exhibited pretreatment albuminuria and 24% (24/102) exhibited low urine specific gravity, indicating impaired renal function prior to treatment. Posttreatment (day 7) urinalyses, performed on 66 of the dogs, revealed that an additional 3% (2/66) of the dogs, which were normal prior to treatment, demonstrated albuminuria and that 26% (11/42) of those with pretreatment albuminuria continued to exhibit it posttreatment. Day 7 urinalyses also indicated that an additional 17%

Continued on next page

TechAmerica—Cont.

(11/66) of the dogs, which were normal prior to treatment, had low urine specific gravity and that 73% (11/15) of those with low urine specific gravity prior to treatment remained low posttreatment.

Indications: Gentamicin Sulfate Injection is indicated for use in the treatment of cystitis in dogs caused by **Proteus mirabilis.** As with all antibiotics, pretreatment cultures and sensitivity testing should be done on samples collected prior to treatment to determine the susceptibility of the microorganisms to gentamicin.

Contraindications: Gentamicin is contraindicated in dogs with renal azotemia.

Precautions: The safety of gentamicin in dogs with impaired renal function has not been demonstrated.

The following conditions have been found to contribute to the toxicity of gentamicin in dogs:

- —Prior renal damage (most commonly found in dogs of advanced age) and dogs infected with heartworm microfilaria.[7]
- —Hypovolemic dehydration (dehydrated patients should be rehydrated prior to initiating therapy).[8]

In dogs where decreased renal function is suspected prior to treatment, BUN or serum creatinine levels may not indicate the degree of kidney impairment. A creatinine clearance determination may be more useful.

Monitoring of renal function during treatment is recommended. Although there is not a completely reliable monitoring program for gentamicin toxicity, urinalysis may indicate early nephrotoxicity.

Unfavorable changes in the urinalysis which may indicate toxicity include:

- —Decreased specific gravity in the absence of fluid therapy.[9,10]
- —Appearance in the urine of casts, albumin, glucose or blood.[9,10]

Continued use of gentamicin where any functional renal impairment has occurred may lead to enhanced renal damage as well as increased likelihood of ototoxicity and/or neuromuscular blockade.[10]

Dogs receiving a full course of gentamicin therapy may develop signs of nephrotoxicity at 1–3 weeks after therapy has terminated. Tests to determine renal function should be considered at 3 weeks posttreatment.[11]

Gentamicin sulfate should not be administered in conjunction with other nephrotoxic, ototoxic or neruromuscular blocking drugs.[1,10,12]

Concurrent administration of furosemide and/or cephalosporins with gentamicin may enhance nephrotoxicity.[8,11,12,13]

Not for use in breeding dogs as reproductive studies have not been conducted.

Neurotoxic and nephrotoxic antibiotics may be absorbed in significant quantities from body surfaces after local irrigation or application. The potential toxic effect of antibiotics administered in this fashion should be considered.[12]

If hypersensitivity develops, treatment with Gentamicin Sulfate Injection should be discontinued and appropriate therapy instituted.

Caution: Federal law restricts this drug to use by or on the order of a licensed veterinarian.

Warning: Aminoglycosides, including gentamicin, are not indicated in uncomplicated episodes of cystitis unless causative agents are susceptible to them and are not susceptible to antibiotics having less potential for toxicity.[14]

Gentamicin should be used with extreme caution in dogs in which hearing acuity is required for functioning, such as seeing eye, hearing ear or military patrol, as the auditory and vestibular impairment tends not to be reversible.[10]

Toxicity manifested by the loss of righting ability and kidney dysfunction, including death, were observed when the label recommended dose of gentamicin (2 mg/lb body weight) and the label recommended duration of treatment (7 days) were concurrently exceeded.

To maintain the integrity of the septum and insure the sterility of the product, no more than 50 entries should be made into a single vial.

Adverse Reactions: Gentamicin auditory damage is dose related. Initial effects are associated with high frequency hearing loss. Total hearing loss can follow.[1]

Early signs of ototoxicity can include ataxia, nausea and vomiting. Auditory and vestibular impairment may be reversible in the very early stages, but if treatment is continued the conditions will become irreversible.[1,10]

Accumulation of gentamicin in the kidney proximal tubule cells can lead to acute renal failure.[15,16]

Based on adverse drug reactions received by FDA, in many of the dogs in which non-fatal nephrotoxicity was associated with gentamicin therapy, drug withdrawal was followed by a decrease in the level of the BUN.

Injection site irritation has been observed in dogs.

Dosage and Administration: Gentamicin Sulfate Injection, 50 mg/ml may be administered by intramuscular or subcutaneous injection.

The recommended dosage for cystitis in dogs is 2 mg per pound of body weight twice the first day then once per day thereafter. Treatment should not exceed 7 days.

If no improvement is seen after 3 days, treatment should be discontinued and the diagnosis reevaluated.

How Supplied: Gentamicin Sulfate Injection, 50 mg/ml is available in 50cc multiple dose vials.

For Veterinary Use Only.

Keep out of reach of children

HERD-VAC™ 10
Bovine Rhinotracheitis-Virus Diarrhea-
Parainfluenza 3 Vaccine-
Haemophilus
Somnus-Campylobacter Fetus-
Leptospira Canicola-Grippotyphosa-
Hardjo-Icterohaemorrhagiae-
Pomona Bacterin
Aluminum Hydroxide Adsorbed

Description: For use in the immunization of healthy cattle against bovine rhinotracheitis virus diarrhea and parainfluenza 3 infections *haemophilus somnus, campylobacter fetus,* caused by *Leptospira canicola, Leptospira grippotyphosa, Leptospira hardjo, Leptospira icterohaemorrhagiae* and *Leptospira pomona.*

Dosage and Adminsitration: Rehydrate vial of vaccine with the accompanying vial of bacterin. Shake well and administer 5 ml IM or SC. Annual revaccination is recommended. In areas where vibriosis is endemic, a second vaccination with campylobacter fetus bacterin in 21 days is recommended for primary immunization. Calves vaccinated under 3 months of age should be revaccinated at 4 to 6 months of age or at weaning because of the possible interfering influence of passive immunity.

Precautions: Do not vaccinate pregnant cows or calves nursing pregnant cows. Do not vaccinate within 21 days before slaughter.

Storage: Store at 35°F–45°F (2°C–7°C). Protect the vaccine from the direct rays of the sun. Use entire contents without delay after rehydration. Rehydrate to 50 ml. Care should be taken to avoid chemical or microbial contamination of the product. Burn each vaccine container and unused contents. If allergic response occurs symptomatic treatment should be provided. The viral vaccine contains gentamicin and amphotericin B as preservatives.

Scientific evidence demonstrates the inability of some animals of an occasional herd to develop antibodies to bovine virus diarrhea after vaccination. The affected animal may exhibit symptoms similar to mucosal disease. Research data is on file at Biologics Corporation indicating Bacterin used as diluent has no virucidal or other deleterious effects upon the viral vaccine fraction. This data likewise demonstrates no immunogenic interference upon administration of the multiple antigen vaccine.

How Supplied: 10 Doses (50 ml) and 20 dose (100 ml) plastic vials.

IBR-BVD-PI 3
Bovine Rhinotracheitis-Virus
Diarrhea Parainfluenza 3 Vaccine
Modified Live Virus
Bovine Cell Line Origin

Composition: This product is a multiple immunogen product containing desiccated bovine rhinotracheitis (IBR), virus diarrhea (BVD) and parainfluenza 3 (PI 3) modified live viruses.

Multiple passages in tissue culture have modified the viruses to a level where they are safe and yet have retained their

immunogenicity. The Perma-Cell™ Line is of Bovine Origin. It is tested by U.S.D.A. approved methods and has been shown to be free of adventitious agents. The use of a Perma-Cell Line makes possible the production of a consistently safe, high titered, immunogenic virus vaccine.
Each serial meets or exceeds all standards prescribed for this product by the U.S. Department of Agriculture.
Indications: For the immunization of healthy cattle against bovine rhinotracheitis, bovine virus diarrhea and parainfluenza 3 infections.
Dosage and Administration: Rehydrate vial of vaccine with accompanying vial of diluent. Shake well and administer 2 ml. intramuscularly or subcutaneously to each animal.
Protection: Bovine rhinotracheitis virus, virus diarrhea virus and parainfluenza 3 virus are important caustic factors in the bovine respiratory disease complex. Susceptible animals will usually develop a satisfactory immune response from one vaccination with the modified live virus vaccine.
Calves vaccinated under 3 months of age should be revaccinated at 4 to 6 months of age or at weaning because of the possible interfering influence of passive maternal immunity. Calves suffering from stresses such as disease, malnutrition or weaning may not develop or maintain a satisfactory immune response and when any of these conditions are present, a second vaccination is recommended. The vaccine is most effective when administered to healthy, susceptible calves, which are not in the incubation stage of the diseases. Vaccination of exposed calves may be of value as long as it is realized that those already incubating the infections may evidence clinical illness even after vaccination.
Precautions:
1. Do not vaccinate pregnant cows or calves nursing pregnant cows.
2. Do not vaccinate within 21 days before slaughter.

For Veterinary Use Only.
How Supplied: 5 dose, 10 dose, and 50 dose packages with corresponding 20 ml. and 100 ml. vials of diluent.

IBR-BVD-PI 3-Lepto 5
Bovine Rhinotracheitis-Virus Diarrhea-Parainfluenza 3 Vaccine-Modified Live Virus
Bovine Cell Line Origin
Leptospira Canicola-Grippotyphosa-Hardjo-Icterohaemorrhagiae-Pomona Bacterin
Aluminum Hydroxide Adsorbed

Composition: This product is a multiple immunogen product containing bovine rhinotracheitis (IBR), virus diarrhea (BVD) and parainfluenza 3 (PI 3) modified live viruses to be rehydrated with Leptospira Canicola-Grippotyphosa-Hardjo-Icterohaemorrhagiae-Pomona Bacterin.
Protection: Bovine rhinotracheitis virus, virus diarrhea virus, parainfluenza 3 virus and *L. canicola, L. grippotyphosa, L. hardjo, L. icterohaemorrhagiae* and *L. pomona* are important causative factors in the bovine disease complex. Susceptible animals will usually develop a satisfactory immune response from one vaccination with the modified live virus vaccine. Annual revaccination with the Leptospira Canicola-Grippotyphosa-Hardjo-Icterohaemorrhagiae-Pomona Bacterin is recommended in order to assure the development of a lasting high level of immunity.
Calves vaccinated under 3 months of age should be revaccinated at 4 to 6 months of age or at weaning because of the interfering influence of passive maternal immunity.
Calves suffering from stresses such as disease, malnutrition or weaning may not develop or maintain a satisfactory immune response and when any of these conditions are present, a second vaccination is recommended. The vaccine is most effective when administered to healthy, susceptible calves which are not in the incubation stage of the diseases. Vaccination of exposed calves may be of value as long as it is realized that those already incubating the infections may evidence clinical illness even after vaccination.
Indications: For the immunization of healthy cattle against bovine rhinotracheitis, virus diarrhea and parainfluenza 3 infections and leptospirosis caused by *L. canicola, L. grippotyphosa, L. hardjo, L. icterohaemorrhagiae* and *L. pomona.*
Dosage and Administration: Rehydrate vial of vaccine with accompanying vial of bacterin. Shake well and administer 2 ml. intramuscularly or subcutaneously to each animal.
Precautions:
1. Do not vaccinate pregnant cows or calves nursing pregnant cows.
2. Do not vaccinate within 21 days before slaughter.

For Veterinary Use Only.
How Supplied: 5 dose, 10 dose and 50 dose vials with corresponding 10 ml., 20 ml., and 100 ml. vials of Leptospira grippotyphosa, hardjo, pomona, canicola and icterohaemorrhagiae bacterin as diluent.

IBR-BVD-PI 3-PASTEURELLA
Bovine Rhinotracheitis-Virus Diarrhea-Parainfluenza 3 Vaccine
Modified Live Virus
Bovine Cell Line Origin
Pasteurella Haemolytica-Multocida Bacterin
Aluminum Hydroxide Adsorbed

Composition: This product is a multiple immunogen product containing desiccated bovine rhinotracheitis (IBR), virus diarrhea (BVD) and parainfluenza 3 (PI 3) modified live viruses to be rehydrated with Pasteurella Haemolytica-Multocida Bacterin.
Indications: For the immunization of healthy cattle against bovine rhinotracheitis, bovine virus diarrhea and parainfluenza 3 infections and *P. haemolytica* and *P. multocida.*
Dosage and Administration: Rehydrate vial of vaccine with accompanying vial of bacterin. Shake well and administer 2 ml. intramuscularly or subcutaneously to each animal.
Protection: Bovine rhinotracheitis virus, virus diarrhea virus, parainfluenza 3 virus, *P. haemolytica* and *P. multocida* are important causative factors in the bovine respiratory disease complex. Susceptible animals will usually develop a satisfactory immune response from one vaccination with the modified live virus vaccine. Revaccination with the Pasteurella Haemolytica-Multocida Bacterin is recommended at 2 to 4 weeks.
Calves vaccinated under 3 months of age should be revaccinated at 4 to 6 months of age or at weaning because of the possible interfering influence of passive maternal immunity. Calves suffering from stresses such as disease, malnutrition or weaning may not develop or maintain a satisfactory immune response and when any of these conditions are present, a second vaccination is recommended. The vaccine is most effective when administered to healthy, susceptible calves, which are not in the incubation stage of the disease. Vaccination of exposed calves may be of value as long as it is realized that those already incubating the infections may evidence clinical illness even after vaccination.
Precautions:
1. Do not vaccinate pregnant cows or calves nursing pregnant cows.
2. Do not vaccinate within 21 days before slaughter.

For Veterinary Use Only.
How Supplied: 10 dose and 50 dose vials with corresponding 20 ml. and 100 ml. vials of Pasteurella Haemolytica-Multocida Bacterin to be used as a diluent.

IBR-BVD-PI3-SOMNUTECH®
Bovine Rhinotracheitis-Virus Diarrhea-Parainfluenza 3 Vaccine
Modified Live Virus
Bovine Cell Line Origin
Haemophilus Somnus Bacterin

Composition: This product is a multiple immunogen product containing Bovine Rhinotracheitis (IBR), Virus Diarrhea (BVD), and Parainfluenza 3 (PI3) modified live viruses to be rehydrated with SomnuTech (Haemophilus Somnus) Bacterin.
Indications: For the immunization of healthy cattle of all ages against Bovine Rhinotracheitis, Bovine Virus Diarrhea, and Parainfluenza infections and *Haemophilus somnus.*
Dosage and Administration: Rehydrate vial of vaccine with accompanying vial of bacterin. Shake well and administer 2 ml. intramuscularly or subcutaneously to each animal.
Protection: Bovine Rhinotracheitis Virus, Parainfluenza 3 Virus, Virus Diarrhea Virus, and *Haemophilus somnus* are important causative factors in the bovine disease complex. Susceptible animals will usually develop a satisfactory immune response from one vaccination with the modified live virus vaccine. Revaccination with the *Haemophilus somnus* bacterin is recommended in 14–28

Continued on next page

TechAmerica—Cont.

days to insure adequate immunity against this organism. Annual revaccination is recommended thereafter.
Calves vaccinated under 3 months of age should be revaccinated at 4–6 months of age or at weaning, because of the possible interfering influence of passive maternal immunity. Calves suffering from stresses such as disease, malnutrition, or weaning may not develop or maintain a satisfactory immune response and when any of these conditions are present, a second vaccination is recommended. The vaccine is most effective when administered to healthy, susceptible calves which are not in the incubation stage of the diseases. Vaccination of exposed calves may be of value as long as it is realized that those already incubating the infections may evidence clinical illness after vaccination.
Precautions:
1. Do not vaccinate pregnant cows or calves nursing pregnant cows.
2. Do not vaccinate within 21 days before slaughter.

For Veterinary Use Only
How Supplied: 5 dose, 10 dose, and 50 dose vials, corresponding 10 ml., 20 ml., and 100 ml. vials of *Haemophilus somnus* bacterin to be used as diluent.

T

IBR-BVD-PI3-VIBRIO-LEPTO 5 (HERD-VAC™9)
Bovine Rhinotracheitis-Virus Diarrhea-Parainfluenza 3 Vaccine Modified Live Virus Bovine Cell Line Origin Campylobacter Fetus-Leptospira Canicola-Grippotyphosa-Hardjo-Icterohaemorrhagiae-Pomona Bacterin Aluminum Hydroxide Adsorbed

Composition: For use in the immunization of healthy cattle against bovine rhinotracheitis, virus diarrhea and parainfluenza 3 infections, campylobacter fetus and leptospirosis caused by *Leptospira canicola, Leptospira grippotyposa, Leptospira hardjo, Leptospira icterohaemorrhagiae* and *Leptospira pomona.*
Dosage and Administration: Rehydrate vial of vaccine with the accompanying vial of bacterin. Shake well and administer 5 ml. IM or SC. Annual revaccination is recommended. In areas where vibriosis is endemic a second vaccination with Vibrio Fetus Bacterin in 21 days is recommended for primary immunization. Calves vaccinated under 3 months of age should be revaccinated at 4 to 6 months of age or at weaning because of the possible interfering influence of passive immunity.
Precautions:
1. Do not vaccinate pregnant cows or calves nursing pregnant cows.
2. Do not vaccinate within 21 days before slaughter.

Scientific evidence demonstrates the inability of some animals of an occasional herd to develop antibodies to bovine virus diarrhea after vaccination. The affected animal may exhibit symptoms similar to mucosal disease. Research data is on file at Biologics Corporation indicating the Bacterin used as diluent has no virucidal or other deleterious effects upon the viral vaccine fraction. This data likewise demonstrates no immunogenic interference upon administration of the multiple antigen vaccine.
For Veterinary Use Only.
How Supplied: 5ds(25ml); 10ds(50ml); 20ds(100ml).

IBR-PI 3
Bovine Rhinotracheitis Parainfluenza 3 Vaccine Modified Live Virus Bovine Cell Line Origin

Composition: This product is a double immunogen product containing desiccated bovine rhinotracheitis (IBR) and parainfluenza 3 (PI 3) modified live viruses.
Indications: For the immunization of healthy cattle against bovine rhinotracheitis and parainfluenza 3 infections.
Dosage and Administration: Rehydrate vial of vaccine with accompanying vial of diluent. Shake well and administer 2 ml. intramuscularly or subcutaneously to each animal.
Protection: Bovine rhinotracheitis virus and parainfluenza 3 virus are important causative factors in the bovine respiratory disease complex. Susceptible animals will usually develop a satisfactory immune response from one vaccination. Calves vaccinated under 3 months of age should be revaccinated at 4 to 6 months of age or at weaning because of the possible interfering influence of passive maternal immunity. Calves suffering from stresses such as disease, malnutrition or weaning may not develop or maintain a satisfactory immune response and when any of these conditions are present, a second vaccination is recommended. The vaccine is most effective when administered to healthy, susceptible calves which are not in the incubation stage of the diseases. Vaccination of exposed calves may be of value as long as it is realized that those already incubating the infections may evidence clinical illness even after vaccination.
Precautions:
1. Do not vaccinate pregnant cows or calves nursing pregnant cows.
2. Do not vaccinate within 21 days before slaughter.

For Veterinary Use Only.
How Supplied: 10 dose and 50 dose packages with corresponding 20 ml. and 100 ml. vials as diluent.

IODO-CAM
(Injection)

Composition: Each ml. contains:

Camphor	60 mg. w/v
Menthol	60 mg. w/v
Iodoform	40 mg. w/v
Eucalyptus Oil	0.01 ml. v/v
Benzyl Alcohol	4.0% v/v
Sesame Oil	q.s.

Indications: A sterile solution for use as supportive treatment in respiratory conditions where an expectorant and anti-inflammatory action is desired.
Directions: Administer intramuscularly only.
Suggested Daily Dosage:

Dogs and Cats	1 to 5 ml.
Sheep	5 to 10 ml.
Swine	5 to 10 ml.
Horses	10 to 20 ml.
Cattle	10 to 20 ml.

If symptoms persist 3 to 5 days after administration, consult your veterinarian.
Warning: Milk taken from treated dairy animals within 96 hours (8 milkings) after latest injection must not be used for human consumption.
How Supplied: 250 ml.

IRON DEXTRAN COMPLEX INJECTION
(Iron Hydrogenated Dextran)

Composition: Iron Dextran Complex is a sterile solution containing Ferric hydroxide in complex with a low molecular weight dextran fraction equivalent to 200 mg. or 100 mg. elemental iron per ml. with 0.5% phenol as a preservative.
Injectable Iron Dextran Complex is easy and economical to use. Injection into the ham is rapid, safe, effective, quickly absorbed by the blood and goes to work immediately. With injectable Iron Dextran Complex the right dosage can be given to every animal with assurance that it will be utilized.
Treatment of baby pigs with Iron Dextran Complex prevents anemia and reduces losses due to iron deficiency. Adequate iron is necessary for normal, healthy, vigorous growth.
Indications: Iron Dextran Complex is intended for the prevention or treatment of iron deficiency anemia in baby pigs. Iron deficiency anemia occurs commonly in the suckling pig, often within the first few days following birth. As body size and blood volume increase rapidly from the first few days following birth, hemoglobin levels in the blood fall due to diminishing iron reserves which cannot be replaced adequately from iron in the sow's milk. This natural deficiency lowers the resistance of the pig and scours, pneumonia or other infections may develop and lead to death of the animal. Pigs not hampered by iron deficiency anemia are more likely to experience normal growth and to maintain their normal level of resistance to disease.
Dosage: For Intramuscular Use Only. Intramuscular Injection. Prevention: 1 ml. (200 mg.) at 1–3 days of age or 1 ml. (100 mg). at 2–4 days of age. Treatment: 1 ml. (100 mg. or 200 mg.) at first sign of iron deficiency.
Directions For Use: Disinfect rubber stopper of vial as well as site of injection. Use small needle (20 gauge ⅝) inch that has been sterilized (boiled in water for 20 minutes). Injection should be intramuscular into the back of the ham.
Iron Dextran Complex cannot be considered a substitute for sound animal husbandry. If disease is present in the litter, consult a veterinarian.
Side Effects: Occasionally pigs may show a reaction to injectable iron, clini-

cally characterized by prostration with muscular weakness. In extreme cases, death may result.
Notice: Organic iron preparation injected intramuscularly into pigs beyond 4 weeks of age may cause staining of muscle tissue.
How Supplied:
100 mg/cc in 100 ml vials
200 mg/cc in 100 ml vials

LEPTO 5, 2 ml
Leptospira Canicola - Grippotyphosa - Hardjo - Icterohaemorrhagiae - Pomona Bacterin Aluminum Hydroxide Adsorbed

Composition: Lepto 5 is a chemically inactivated bacterin prepared from whole cultures of *L. canicola, L. gripp., L. hardjo, L. icterohaemorrhagiae,* and *L. pomona.*
This bacterin is grown in a specially developed medium designed to assure high immunogenicity and to reduce the possibility of allergic reactions to an absolute minimum.
The inactivated cultures are adsorbed onto aluminum hydroxide gel and blended under constant agitation in order to assure that each 2 ml dose contains a fully immunizing dose to each of the component fractions. Each serial is tested for potency, safety and sterility in accordance with the U.S.D.A. requirements.
Indications: For use in the immunization of healthy cattle and swine against leptospirosis caused by *L. canicola, L. grippotyphosa, L. hardjo, L. icterohaemorrhagiae* and *L. pomona.*
Dosage and Administration: *Cattle and swine:* Shake well. Inject 2 ml intramuscularly or subcutaneously.
Precautions: If allergic response occurs symptomatic treatment should be provided immediately.
For Veterinary Use Only
How Supplied: 10 dose (20 ml), 50 dose (100 ml) plastic vials.

MEDAMYCIN®
(Oxytetracycline Hydrochloride Injection 50 mg./ml.)

Composition:
EACH ml CONTAINS:
Oxytetracycline HCl........................50 mg
Water for Injection 17.7%
Magnesium chloride
hexahydrate............................3.1% w/v
Propylene glycol..................................q.s.
With Sodium Formaldehyde Sulfoxylate, 0.656% w/v as a preservative and Monoethanolamine for pH adjustment.
For animal use only in beef cattle, beef calves, non-lactating dairy cattle and dairy calves.
Indications: No refrigeration required. Concentrated and ready to use for high blood levels and fast effective action against a wide variety of disease causing organisms in cattle which are sensitive to oxytetracycline.
This product may tend to darken on standing. This will not affect the potency of oxytetracycline.

Each ml contains:

	20mg/ml	40mg/ml
Methylprednisolone Acetate	20.0mg	40.0mg
Polyethylene Glycol 3350	30.0mg	30.0mg
Sodium Chloride	9.0mg	9.0mg
Myristyl-gamma-picolinium Chloride as a preservative	0.200mg	0.200mg
Water for Injection	qs	qs

If necessary, pH is adjusted with either hydrochloric acid or sodium hydroxide.

Occasional local tissue reaction or anaphylactic reactions may be observed. Consult your veterinarian if severe.
See accompanying literature for complete directions.
Dosage and Administration: The injection of 3 to 5 mg. of oxytetracycline intramuscularly per pound of body weight per day (6 to 10 ml. per 100 lbs. body weight) is the recommended dosage.
Caution: Do not inject more than 10 ml of MEDAMYCIN per site in adult cattle. When administered intramuscularly to animals within 30 days of slaughter, muscle discoloration may necessitate trimming of the injection site(s) and surrounding tissues during the dressing procedure.
Warning: Discontinue treatment at least 22 days prior to slaughter. Not for use in lactating dairy cattle.
How Supplied: 500 ml.

MEDAMYCIN®-100
(Oxytetracycline Hydrochloride Injection 100 mg./ml.)

Description: Oxytetracycline Hydrochloride Injection is for the treatment of diseases in beef cattle, beef calves, non-lactating dairy cattle and dairy calves caused by pathogens sensitive to Oxytetracycline HCl.
Contents: Each ml. contains:
Oxytetracycline HCl ....100 mg
Magnesium Chloride-6H_2O ..5.75% w/v
Water for Injection ....17.0% v/v
Propylene Glycol ....q.s.
With Sodium Formaldehyde Sulfoxylate, 1.3% w/v, as a preservative and Monoethanolamine for pH adjustment.
Note: Solution may darken on storage but potency remains unaffected.
Storage Temperature: 59°–86°F.
Dosage: 3–5 mg./lb. body weight per day for a maximum of 4 consecutive days. For intravenous administration only.
Warning: Discontinue treatment at least 22 days prior to slaughter. Not for use in lactating dairy cattle.
Caution: If no improvement occurs within 24 to 48 hours, consult a veterinarian.
Do not use the drug for more than 4 consecutive days. Use beyond 4 days or dosage higher than the maximum recommended dose may result in antibiotic residue in the tissues beyond the withdrawal time.
How Supplied: 500 ml.

METHYLPREDNISOLONE ACETATE INJECTABLE
Sterile Aqueous Suspension

Description: Methylprednisolone Acetate Injectable is available in two concentrations containing 20mg and 40mg/ml methylprednisolone acetate. The product is recommended for intramuscular or intrasynovial injection in dogs and horses and intramuscular injection in cats.
[See table above].
Actions: Methylprednisolone, a potent glucocorticoid and anti-inflammatory agent, is a synthetic 6-methyl derivative of prednisolone. Exceeding prednisolone in anti-inflammatory potency and having even less tendency than prednisolone to induce sodium and water retention, methylprednisolone offers the advantage over older corticosteroids of affording equally satisfactory anti-inflammatory effect with the use of lower doses and with an enhanced split between anti-inflammatory and mineralocorticoid activities.[1,2,3] In anti-inflammatory activity, as measured by the granuloma pouch assay, methylprednisolone is twice as active as prednisolone.[4] In mineralocorticoid activty (i.e., the capacity to induce retention of sodium and water in the adrenalectomized rat) methylprednisolone is slightly less active than prednisolone.[4]
The duration of plasma steroid levels following rapid intravenous injection in intact dogs is appreciably longer for methylprednisolone than for prednisolone, the respective "half-life" value for the two steroids being 80.9 ± 7.5 minutes for methylprednisolone and 71.3 ± 1.7 minutes for prednisolone.[4]
Glucocorticoids exert a regulatory influence on lymphocytes, erythrocytes and eosinophils of the blood and on the structure and function of lymphoid tissues.[1,5,6] A primary feature of the glucocorticoids is their anti-inflammatory activity with minimum sodium and water retention which is often associated with the mineralocorticoids.[1,2,3,5,6,7] Glucocorticoids not only inhibit the early phases of the inflammatory process (edema, fibrin deposition, capillary dilatation, migration of leukocytes into the inflamed area and phagocytic activity) but also the later manifestations (capillary proliferation, fibroblast proliferation and deposition of collagen). [3,5,7] The exact mechanism is not known, but the glucocorticoids obviously suppress normal tissue response to injury and alleviate symptoms from many conditions.[2]
Indications: Musculoskeletal Conditions. As with other adrenal steroids, methylprednisolone acetate has been found useful in alleviating the pain and lameness associated with acute localized arthritic conditions and generalized arthritic conditions. It has been used successfully to treat rheumatoid arthritis,

Continued on next page

TechAmerica—Cont.

traumatic arthritis, osteoarthritis, periostitis, tendinitis, synovitis, tenosynovitis, bursitis and myositis in horses and traumatic arthritis, osteoarthritis and generalized arthritic conditions in dogs. Remission of musculoskeletal conditions may be permanent, or symptoms may recur, depending on the cause and extent of structural degeneration.[1,2,3,5,6]

Dermal Conditions and Allergic Manifestations. Methylprednisolone acetate relieves pruritus and inflammation of allergic dermatitis, acute moist dermatitis, dry eczema, urticaria, bronchial asthma, pollen sensitivities and otitis externa in dogs and allergic dermatitis and moist and dry eczema in cats. Onset of relief may begin within a few hours to a few days following injection and may persist for a few days to six weeks. Symptoms may be expected to recur if the cause of the allergic reaction is still present, in which case retreatment may be indicated. In treating acute hypersensitivity reactions, such as anaphylactic shock, appropriate treatment such as prednisolone sodium succinate should be used.[1,2,3,5,6]

Overwhelming Infections with Severe Toxicity. In dogs and cats moribund from overwhelmingly severe infections for which antibacterial therapy is available (e.g., critical pneumonia, pyometritis), methylprednisolone acetate may be lifesaving, acting to inhibit the inflammatory reaction, which itself may be lethal; preventing vascular collapse and preserving the integrity of the blood vessels; modifying the animal's reaction to drugs; and preventing or reducing the exudative reaction which often complicates certain infections. As supportive therapy, it improves the general attitude of the animal being treated. All necessary procedures for the establishment of a bacterial diagnosis should be carried out whenever possible before institution of therapy. Corticosteroid therapy in the presence of infection should be administered for the shortest possible time compatible with maintenance of an adequate response, and antibacterial therapy should be continued for at least three days after the hormone has been withdrawn. Combined hormone and antibacterial therapy does not obviate the need for indicated surgical treatment.[1,2,3,4,5,6,7]

Other Conditions. In certain conditions where it is desired to reduce inflammation, vascularization, fibroblastic infiltration and scar tissue, the use of Methylprednisolone Acetate Injectable should be considered. Snakebite of dogs also is an indication for the use of this suspension because of its antitoxemic, antishock and anti-inflammatory activity. It is particularly effective in reducing swelling and preventing sloughing. Its employment in the treatment of such conditions is recommended as a supportive measure to standard procedures and time-honored treatments and will give comfort to the animal and hasten complete recovery.[1,2,3,4,5,6,7]

Contraindications: Do not use in viral infections. Systemic therapy with methylprednisolone acetate, as with other corticoids, is contraindicated in animals with arrested tuberculosis, peptic ulcer, acute psychoses, corneal ulcer and Cushingoid syndrome. The presence of active tuberculosis, diabetes mellitus, osteoporosis, renal insufficiency, predisposition to thrombophlebitis, hypertension or congestive heart failure necessitates carefully controlled use of corticosteroids. Intrasynovial, intratendinous or other injections of corticosteroids for local effect are contraindicated in the presence of acute infectious conditions. Exacerbation of pain, further loss of joint motion, with fever and malaise following injection may indicate that the condition has become septic. Appropriate antibacterial therapy should be instituted immediately.

Caution: Federal law restricts this drug to use by or on the order of a licensed veterinarian.

Warning: Clinical and experimental data have demonstrated that corticosteroids administered orally or parenterally to animals may induce the first stage of parturition when administered during the last trimester of pregnancy and may precipitate premature parturition followed by dystocia, fetal death, retained placenta and metritis. Not for human use.

Additionally, corticosteroids administered to dogs, rabbits and rodents during pregnancy have produced cleft palate. Other congenital anomalies including deformed forelegs, phocomelia and anasarca have been reported in the offspring of dogs which received corticosteroids during pregnancy.

To maintain the integrity of the septum and insure the sterility of the product, no more than 50 entries should be made into a single vial.

DO NOT USE IN HORSES INTENDED FOR FOOD.

Precautions: Methylprednisolone acetate exerts an inhibitory influence on the mechanisms and the tissue changes associated with inflammation. Vascular permeability is decreased, exudation diminished and migration of the inflammatory cells markedly inhibited. In addition, systemic manifestations such as fever and signs of toxemia may also be suppressed. While certain aspects of this alteration of the inflammatory reaction may be beneficial, the suppression of inflammation may mask the signs of infection and tend to facilitate spread of microorganisms. Hence, all animals receiving this drug should be watched for evidence of intercurrent infection. Should infection occur, it must be brought under control by the use of appropriate antibacterial measures or administration of this preparation should be discontinued. However, in infections characterized by overwhelming toxicity, methylprednisolone acetate therapy in conjunction with appropriate antibacterial therapy is effective in reducing mortality and morbidity. Without concomitant use of an antibiotic to which the invader-organism is sensitive, imprudent use of the adrenal hormones in animals with infections can be hazardous. As with other corticoids, continued or prolonged use is discouraged.

While no sodium retention or potassium depletion has been observed at the doses recommended, animals receiving methylprednisolone acetate, as with all corticoids, should be under close observation for possible untoward effects. If symptoms of hypopotassemia (hypokalemia) should occur, corticoid therapy should be discontinued and potassium chloride administered by continuous intravenous drip.

Since this drug lacks significant mineralocorticoid activity in usual therapeutic doses, it is not likely to afford adequate support in states of acute adrenocortical insufficiency. For treatment of the latter, the parent adrenocortical steroids, hydrocortisone or cortisone, should be used.

Use of corticosteroids may result in the inhibition of endogenous steroid production which sometimes persists for weeks following drug withdrawal. In patients presently receiving or recently withdrawn from corticosteroid treatment, administration of a rapidly acting corticosteroid before, during and after an unusually stressful situation is recommended.

Side Effects: Side effects such as SAP and SGPT enzyme elevations, weight loss, anorexia, polydipsia and polyuria have occurred following the use of synthetic corticosteroids in dogs. Vomiting and diarrhea (occasionally bloody) have been observed in dogs and cats.

Cushing's syndrome in dogs has been reported in association with prolonged or repeated therapy.

Intramuscular Dosage and Administration: Following intramuscular injection of methylprednisolone acetate, a prolonged systemic effect results. The dose varies with the size of the animal, the severity of the condition under treatment and the animal's response to therapy.

Dogs and Cats. The average intramuscular dose for dogs is 20mg. In accordance with the size of the dog and severity of the condition under treatment, the dose may range from 2mg in miniature breeds to 40mg in medium breeds and even as high as 120mg in extremely large breeds or dogs with severe involvement. The average intramuscular dose for cats is 10mg with a range up to 20mg.

Injections may be made at weekly intervals or in accordance with the severity of the condition and clinical response.

Horses. The usual intramuscular dose for horses is 200mg repeated as necessary.

For maintenance therapy in chronic conditions, initial doses should be reduced gradually until the smallest effective (i.e., individualized) dose is established. Methylprednisolone Tablets may also be used for maintenance in dogs and cats, administered according to the recommended dose.

T

When treatment is to be withdrawn after prolonged and intensive therapy, the dose should be reduced gradually.

If signs of stress are associated with the condition being treated, the dose should be increased. If a rapid hormonal effect of maximum intensity is required, as in anaphylactic shock, the intravenous administration of prednisolone sodium succinate is indicated.

Intrasynovial Dosage and Administration: Methylprednisolone acetate, a slightly soluble ester of methylprednisolone, is capable of producing a more prolonged local anti-inflammatory effect than equimolar doses of hydrocortisone acetate. Following intrasynovial injection, relief from pain may be experienced within 12 to 24 hours. The duration of relief varies, but averages three to four weeks, with a range of one to five or more weeks. Injections of methylprednisolone acetate have been well tolerated. **Intrasynovial (intra-articular) injections may occasionally result in an increased localized inflammatory response.**

Intrasynovial injection is recommended as an adjuvant to general therapeutic measures to effect suppression of inflammation in one or a few peripheral structures when (1) the disease is limited to one or a few peripheral structures; (2) the disease is widespread with one or a few peripheral structures actively inflamed; (3) systemic therapy with other corticoids or corticotropin controls all but a few of the more actively involved structures; (4) systemic therapy with cortisone, hydrocortisone or corticotropin is contraindicated; (5) joints show early but actively progressing deformity (to enhance the effect of physiotherapy and corrective procedures) and (6) surgical or other orthopedic corrective measures are to be or have been done.

The action of Methylprednisolone Acetate Suspension injected intrasynovially appears to be well localized since significant metabolic effects characteristic of systemic administration of adrenal steroids have not been observed. In a few instances mild and transient improvement of structures other than those injected have been reported. No other systemic effects have been noted. However, it is possible that mild systemic effects may occur following intrasynovial administration, and this possibility is greater the larger the number of structures injected and the higher the total dose employed.

Procedure for Intrasynovial Injection. The anatomy of the area to be injected should be reviewed in order to assure that the suspension is properly placed and to determine that large blood vessels or nerves are avoided. The injection site is located where the synovial cavity is most superficial. The area is prepared for aseptic injection of the medicament by the removal of hair and cleansing of the skin with alcohol or other suitable antiseptics. A sterile 18 to 21 gauge needle for horses, 20 to 22 gauge needle for dogs, on a dry syringe is quickly inserted into the synovial space and a small amount of synovial fluid withdrawn. If there is an excess of synovia and more than 1 ml of suspension is to be injected, it is well to aspirate a volume of fluid comparable to that which is to be injected. With the needle in place, the aspirating syringe is removed and replaced by a second syringe containing the proper amount of suspension which is then injected. In some animals a transient pain is elicited immediately upon injection into the affected cavity. This pain varies from mild to severe and may last for a few minutes up to 12 hours. After injection, the structure may be moved gently a few times to aid mixing of the synovial fluid and the suspension. The site may be covered with a small sterile dressing.

Areas not suitable for injection are those that are anatomically inaccessible such as spinal joints and those like the sacroiliac joints, which are devoid of synovial space. Treatment failures are most frequently the result of failure to enter the synovial space. If failures occur when injections into the synovial spaces are certain, as determined by aspiration of fluid, repeated injections are usually futile. Local therapy does not alter the underlying disease process, and whenever possible, comprehensive therapy including physiotherapy and orthopedic correction should be employed.

The single intrasynovial dose depends on the size of the part, which corresponds to the size of the animal. The interval between repeated injections depends on the duration of relief obtained.

Dogs. The average initial dose for a large synovial space in dogs is 20mg. Smaller spaces will require a correspondingly lesser dose.

Horses. The average initial dose for a large synovial space in horses is 120mg with a range from 40 to 240mg. Smaller spaces will require a correspondingly lesser dose.

How Supplied: Methylprednisolone Acetate Injectable, 20mg/ml is available in 10ml and 30ml vials.

Methylprednisolone Acetate Injectable, 40mg/ml is available in 5ml and 30ml vials.

For Veterinary Use Only.

Keep out of reach of children.

METHYLPREDNISOLONE TABLETS
For Oral Use in Dogs and Cats Only.

Description: Methylprednisolone, a potent glucocorticoid and anti-inflammatory agent, is a synthetic 6-methyl derivative of prednisolone. It has a greater anti-inflammatory potency than prednisolone and is less likely to induce sodium and water retention. Its advantage over the older corticoids lies in its ability to achieve equal anti-inflammatory effect with a lower dose, while at the same time enhancing the split between anti-inflammatory and mineralocorticoid activities.[1,2,3] Each tablet contains 1mg or 2 mg of methylprednisolone.

Actions: Glucocorticoids exert a regulatory influence on lymphocytes, erythrocytes and eosinophils of the blood and on the structure and function of lymphoid tissues.[1,4,5] A primary feature of the glucocorticoids is their anti-inflammatory activity with minimum sodium and water retention which is often associated with the mineralocorticoids.[2,3,4,5,6] Glucocorticoids not only inhibit the early phases of the inflammatory process (edema, fibrin deposition, capillary dilatation, migration of leukocytes into the inflamed area and phagocytic activity) but also the later manifestations (capillary proliferation, fibroblast proliferation and deposition of collagen).[3,4,6] The exact mechanism is not known, but the glucocorticoids obviously suppress normal tissue response to injury and alleviate symptoms from many conditions.[2]

Indications: The indications are the same as those for other anti-inflammatory steroids and comprise the various collagen, dermal, allergic, ocular, otic and musculoskeletal conditions known to be responsive to the anti-inflammatory corticosteroids. Representative of the conditions in which the use of steroid therapy and the benefits to be derived therefrom have had repeated confirmation in the veterinary literature are:

Dermal Conditions, such as non-specific eczema and summer dermatitis.[1,2,4]

Allergic Manifestations, such as acute urticaria, allergic dermatitis, drug and serum reactions, non-specific pruritus, bronchial asthma and pollen sensitivities.[1,2,3,4,5]

Ocular Conditions, such as iritis, iridocyclitis, secondary glaucoma, uveitis and chorioretinitis.[1,3,4,5]

Otic Conditions, such as otitis externa.[4]

Musculoskeletal Conditions, such as myositis, rheumatoid arthritis, osteoarthritis and bursitis.[1,2,3,4,5]

Various chronic or recurrent diseases of unknown etiology such as ulcerative colitis and nephrosis.[1,2,3,5]

In acute adrenal insufficiency, methylprednisolone may be effective because of its ability to correct the defect in carbohydrate metabolism and relieve the impaired diuretic response to water, characteristic of primary or secondary adrenal insufficiency. However, because this agent lacks significant mineralocorticoid activity, hydrocortisone sodium succinate or cortisone should be used when salt retention is indicated.[6]

Contraindications: Do not use in viral infections. Methylprednisolone, like prednisolone, is contraindicated in animals with arrested tuberculosis, peptic ulcer, acute psychoses, corneal ulcer and Cushingoid syndrome. The presence of diabetes, osteoporosis, chronic psychotic reactions, predisposition to thrombophlebitis, hypertension, congestive heart failure, renal insufficiency and active tuberculosis necessitates carefully controlled use. Some of the above conditions occur only rarely in dogs and cats but should be kept in mind.

Caution: Federal law restricts this drug to use by or on the order of a licensed veterinarian.

Continued on next page

TechAmerica—Cont.

Warning: Because of its inhibitory effect on fibroplasia, methylprednisolone may mask the signs of infection and enhance dissemination of the infecting organism. Hence, all animals receiving methylprednisolone should be watched for evidence of intercurrent infection. Should infection occur, it must be brought under control by use of appropriate antibacterial measures or administration of methylprednisolone should be discontinued.

Not for human use. Clinical and experimental data have demonstrated that corticosteroids administered orally or parenterally to animals may induce the first stage of parturition when administered during the last trimester of pregnancy and may precipitate premature parturition followed by dystocia, fetal death, retained placenta and metritis.

Additionally, corticosteroids administered to dogs, rabbits and rodents during pregnancy have produced cleft palate. Other congenital anomalies including deformed forelegs, phocomelia and anasarca have been reported in offspring of dogs which received corticosteroids during pregnancy.

Precautions: Methylprednisolone, like prednisolone and other adrenocortical steroids, is a potent therapeutic agent influencing the biochemical behavior of most, if not all, tissues of the body. Because this anti-inflammatory steroid manifests little sodium-retaining activity, the usual early sign of cortisone or hydrocortisone overdosage (i.e., increase in body weight due to fluid retention) is not a reliable index of overdosage. Hence, recommended dosage levels should not be exceeded, and all animals receiving methylprednisolone should be under close medical supervision. All precautions pertinent to the use of prednisolone apply to methylprednisolone. Moreover, the veterinarian should endeavor to keep informed of current studies with methylprednisolone as they are reported in the veterinary literature.

Use of corticosteroids, depending on dose, duration and specific steroid, may result in inhibition of endogenous steroid production following drug withdrawal. In patients presently receiving or recently withdrawn from systemic corticosteroid treatments, therapy with a rapid acting corticosteroid should be considered in unusually stressful situations.

Adverse Reactions: Methylprednisolone is similar to prednisolone in regard to kinds of side effects and metabolic alterations to be anticipated when treatment is intensive or prolonged. In animals with diabetes mellitus, use of methylprednisolone may be associated with an increase in the insulin requirement. Negative nitrogen balance may occur, particularly in animals that require protracted maintenance therapy; measures to counteract persistent nitrogen loss include a high protein intake and the administration, when indicated, of a suitable anabolic agent. Excessive loss of potassium, like excessive retention of sodium, is not likely to be induced by effective maintenance doses of methylprednisolone. However, these effects should be kept in mind and the usual regulatory measures employed as indicated. Ecchymotic manifestations, **while not noted during the clinical evaluation in dogs and cats,** may occur. If such reactions do occur and are serious, reduction in dosage or discontinuance of methylprednisolone therapy may be indicated. Concurrent use of daily oral supplements of ascorbic acid may be of value in helping to control ecchymotic tendencies.

Side effects, such as SAP and SGPT enzyme elevations, weight loss, anorexia, polydipsia and polyuria have occurred following the use of synthetic corticosteroids in dogs. Vomiting and diarrhea (occasionally bloody) have been observed in dogs and cats. Cushing's syndrome in dogs has been reported in association with prolonged or repeated steroid therapy.

Dosage and Administration: The keystone of satisfactory therapeutic management with methylprednisolone, as with its steroid predecessors, is individualization of dosage in reference to the severity of the disease, the anticipated duration of steroid therapy and the animal's threshold or tolerance for steroid excess. The prime objective of steroid therapy should be to achieve a satisfactory degree of control with a minimum effective daily dose.

The dosage recommendations are suggested **average total daily doses and are intended as guides.** As with other orally administered corticosteroids, the total daily dose of methylprednisolone tablets should be given in equally divided doses. The initial suppressive dose level is continued until a satisfactory clinical response is obtained, a period usually of 2 to 7 days in the case of musculoskeletal diseases, allergic conditions affecting the skin or respiratory tract and ocular inflammatory diseases. If a satisfactory response is not obtained in 7 days, reevaluation of the case to confirm the original diagnosis should be made. As soon as a satisfactory clinical response is obtained, the daily dose should be reduced gradually, either to termination of treatment in the case of acute conditions (e.g., seasonal asthma, dermatitis, acute ocular inflammations) or to the minimal effective maintenance dose level in the case of chronic conditions (e.g., rheumatoid arthritis). In chronic conditions, and in rheumatoid arthritis especially, it is important that the reduction in dosage from initial to maintenance dose levels be accomplished slowly. The maintenance dose level should be adjusted from time to time as required by fluctuation in the activity of the disease and the animal's general status. Accumulated experience has shown that the long-term benefits to be gained from continued steroid maintenance are probably greater the lower the maintenance dose level. In rheumatoid arthritis in particular, maintenance steroid therapy should be at the lowest possible level.

IMPORTANT: In the therapeutic management of animals with chronic diseases, such as rheumatoid arthritis, methylprednisolone should be regarded as a highly valuable adjunct, to be used in conjunction with but not as a replacement for standard therapeutic measures.

RECOMMENDED DOSAGE SCHEDULE

Average, total daily doses for dogs and cats are as follows:

5 to 15 lb body wt. ..... 2 mg
15 to 40 lb body wt ...... 2 to 4 mg
40 to 80 lb body wt ...... 4 to 8 mg

The total daily dose should be given in divided doses, 6 to 10 hours apart.

How Supplied:
Methylprednisolone Tablets, 2 mg Bottles of 1000 Tablets
Keep out of reach of children
For Veterinary Use Only.

MULTI-B SUPER
(Injectable)

Composition: Each ml. contains:
Thiamine HCl U.S.P. ....100 mg
Riboflavin
(as 5′ Phosphate Sodium)..........5 mg
Niacinamide U.S.P. ....100 mg
d-Panthenol ....10 mg
Pyridoxine HCl U.S.P. ....10 mg
Cyanocobalamin (Cryst)
U.S.P. ....100 mcg
Benzyl Alcohol...............................1.5%
(Preservative)
Water ....q.s

Indications: A sterile solution for use in Vitamin B deficiencies in dogs, cats, swine, sheep, cattle and horses.

Dosage and Administration: Administer intramuscularly or intravenously. Dogs and Cats, ½ to 2 ml.; Swine and Sheep, 5 to 10 ml; Cattle and Horses, 10 to 20 ml. Repeat daily as indicated.

Caution: Anaphylactogenesis to parenteral Thiamine HCl has been reported. Administer slowly and with caution in doses over 50 mg. Federal law restricts this drug to use by or on the order of a licensed veterinarian.

How Supplied: 100 ml; 250 ml.

NEMACIDE® -C
(Film-Coated Diethylcarbamazine Citrate Tablets)

Indications: For the prevention of heartworm disease (*Dirofilaria immitis*) in dogs, as an aid in the treatment of ascarid infections in dogs (*Toxocara canis*) and cats (*Toxocara canis* and *Toxascaris leonina*) and as an aid in the control of ascarid infections (*Toxocara canis*) in dogs.

Dosage and Administration: Nemacide® -C is preferably given orally immediately after feeding. This reduces the possibility of vomiting which occasionally occurs if the animal's stomach is empty.

For prevention of heartworm disease in dogs: Administer orally at a dosage rate of 3 mg. diethylcarbamazine citrate per pound of body weight daily.

For treatment of Ascarid infection in dogs and cats: Administer orally at a dosage rate of 25 mg. to 50 mg. of diethylcarbamazine citrate per pound of body weight. A repeat dose should be given in 10 to 20 days to remove immature worms that enter the intestines from the lungs after the first dose.

For control of Ascarid infections in dogs: Daily dosage at a rate of 3 mg./lb. of body weight prevents the establishment of canine ascarid infections.

Caution: Federal law restricts this drug to use by or on the order of a licensed veterinarian. Do not use in dogs that may be harboring adult heartworms.

Not for human use.

How Supplied:
50 mg. Bottles of 200's, and 500's
100 mg. Bottles of 200's, and 500's
200 mg. Bottles of 200's, and 1000's
300 mg. Bottles of 100's, and 200's
400 mg. Bottles of 100's, and 200's

NEMACIDE® CHEWABLE TABLETS (MICROENCAPSULATED)
(Diethylcarbamazine Citrate)

Indications: For the prevention of heartworm disease (*Dirofilaria immitis*) in dogs, as an aid in the treatment of ascarid infections in dogs (*Toxocara canis*) and cats (*Toxocara canis* and *Toxascaris leonina*) and as an aid in the control of ascarid infections (*Toxocara canis*) in dogs.

Dosage and Administration: NEMACIDE Chewable Diethylcarbamazine Citrate Tablets are palatable to most dogs. Tablets may be fed free choice immediately after feeding or crumbled and placed on food. This reduces the possibility of vomiting which occasionally occurs if the stomach is empty.

TechAmerica's new microencapsulation process makes Nemacide Chewable Tablets extremely palatable. Independent studies show 98% of the dogs studied readily accepted the palatable Nemacide Chewable Tablets on a regular basis.

For prevention of heartworm disease in dogs:
Administer at a dosage rate of 3 mg. diethylcarbamazine citrate per pound of body weight daily.

Recommended Dosage Schedule Nemacide Chewable Tablets:

Tablets (daily)	Body Weight (lbs.)
1- 30 mg.	10
1- 60 mg.	20
1-120 mg.	40
1-180 mg.	60

For treatment of Ascarid infections in dogs and cats: Oral dose rate of 25 mg. to 50 mg./lb. of body weight in dogs and cats in a single dose.

Tablet Size	Tablet Dosage
60 mg	1 tablet for each 1.2-2.4 pounds body weight
120 mg	1 tablet for each 2.4-4.8 pounds body weight
180 mg	1 tablet for each 3.6-7.2 pounds body weight

Roundworms may be expelled dead or living. They should be promptly removed to prevent reinfestation.

A repeat dose should be given in 10 to 20 days to remove immature worms which may enter the intestine from the lungs after the first dose.

How Supplied:
60 mg. Bottles of 100's and 200's
120 mg. Bottles of 100's
180 mg. Bottles of 50's, 100's and 200's

NEMACIDE® ORAL SYRUP
(Diethylcarbamazine Citrate Syrup)

Description: Each ml. provides 60 mg. Diethylcarbamazine Citrate U.S.P. in a palatable syrup base.

Indications: For the removal of roundworms (ASCARIDS-*TOXOCARA CANIS*) in dogs and for the prevention of heartworm disease (*DIROFILARIA IMMITIS*) in dogs.

Use: Oral administration only.

Dosage for Ascarids: 50 mg. per pound of body weight divided into two equal doses and given 8–12 hours apart. May be dosed directly or by mixing with the regular ration.

Recommended Dosage Schedule
1 lb. ....0.5 ml. morning and eve.
2–3 lbs. ....1 ml. morning and eve.
4–5 lbs. ....2 ml. morning and eve.
6 lbs. ....2 ½ ml. morn. and eve.
9–10 lbs. ....4 ml. morning and eve.
12 lbs. ....5 ml. (1 teaspoonful) morning and evening
24 lbs. ....10 ml. (2 teaspoonsful) morning and evening.

Dosage for Heartworms: The optimum dosage is 3 mg. diethylcarbamazine citrate per pound of body weight daily. One ml. per 20 pounds of body weight.

Warning: Do not use in dogs that may be harboring adult heartworms.

How Supplied: 4 oz., 8 oz., and Gallon.

NEMACIDE® TABLETS
(Diethylcarbamazine Citrate)

Indications: For the prevention of heartworm disease (*Dirofiliaria immitis*) in dogs, as an aid in the treatment of ascarid infection in dogs (*Toxocara canis*) and cats (*Toxocara canis* and *Toxascaris leonina*) and as an aid in the control of ascarid infections (*Toxocara canis*) in dogs.

Dosage and Administration: NEMACIDE Diethylcarbamazine Citrate is administered orally, preferably given immediately after feeding. This reduces the possibility of vomiting which occasionally occurs if the stomach is empty. If administration of tablets is difficult, NEMACIDE may be pulverized and given in the feed.

For prevention of heartworm disease in dogs:
Daily administration of 3 mg./lb. of body weight provides the optimum dosage of diethylcarbamazine citrate for effectively preventing the maturation of recently inoculated heartworm larvae into adults (*Dirofilaria immitis*).

Administration of NEMACIDE Tablets should start one month before the beginning of mosquito activity and be continued for approximately two months thereafter. Young dogs may be started on the preventive program at two months of age.

Recommended Dosage Schedule for Prevention of Heartworms

Tablets (daily)	Body Weight (lbs.)
1- 50 mg.	16
1-100 mg.	32
1-200 mg.	65
1-300 mg.	100
1-400 mg.	130

For Treatment of Ascarid Infections in dogs and cats: Oral dose at rate of 25 mg. to 50 mg./lb. of body weight in dogs and cats in a single dose.

Tablet Size	Tablet Dosage
50 mg	½ to 1 tablet per pound body weight
100 mg	½ to 1 tablet for each 2 pounds body weight
200 mg	½ to 1 tablet for each 4 pounds body weight
300 mg	½ to 1 tablet for each 6 pounds body weight
400 mg	½ to 1 tablet for each 8 pounds body weight

How Supplied:
50 mg. Bottles of 200's, and 500's
100 mg. Bottles of 100's, 200's, and 500's
200 mg. Bottles of 200's and 1000's
300 mg. Bottles of 100's, 200's, and 1000's
400 mg. Bottles of 100's, and 1000's.

NEO–SUL™ JR.
(Calf Scour Bolus)

Composition: Each bolus contains:
Neomycin Sulfate ....500 mg.
(equivalent to 350 mg. Neomycin Base)
Sulfamethazine........................37.5 grains
Sulfathiazole ....37.5 grains

Indications: For the treatment of *colibacillosis* (bacterial scours) caused by *Escherichia coli* and bacterial pneumonia caused by *Pasteurella spp.* in calves and sheep.

Dosage Schedule and Administration: Lubricate bolus with mineral oil and administer orally. Give 1 bolus per 50 lbs. body weight as initial dose followed by 1 bolus per 50 lbs. body weight every 24 hours preferably in divided doses of ½ bolus every 12 hours. Treatment should be instituted early and should continue 24 to 48 hours beyond the remission of the disease symptoms but not to exceed 4 consecutive days.

Caution: This preparation, like all sulfonamides, is a dangerous drug and may cause toxic reactions. It should be administered under adequate supervision. Provide ample drinking water at all times. If any signs of toxicity appear, discontinue the drug. If symptoms persist after 2 or 3 days, consult your veterinarian for further instruction.

Warning: Discontinue treatment with this drug at least 30 days before slaughtering animals for food. Do not treat lactating dairy animals.

How Supplied: 25's, 50's , and 100's.

NEO–SUL,™ SR.
(Cattle Scour Bolus)

Description: For the treatment of *colibacillosis* (bacterial scours) caused by *Escherichia coli* and bacterial pneumonia caused by *Pasteurella spp.* in calves and cattle.

Continued on next page

TechAmerica—Cont.

Contents:
Each bolus contains:
Neomycin Sulfate ....2000 mg.
(Equivalent to 1400 mg Neomycin Base)
Sulfamethazine.........................150 grains
Sulfathiazole ....150 grains
Dosage: Lubricate bolus with mineral oil and administer orally. Give 1 bolus per 200 lbs. body weight as initial dose followed by 1 bolus per 200 lbs. body weight every 24 hours preferably in divided doses of ½ bolus every 12 hours. Treatment should be instituted early and should continue 24 to 48 hours beyond the remission of the disease symptoms but not to exceed 4 consecutive days.
Caution: This preparation, like all sulfonamides, is a dangerous drug and may cause toxic reactions. It should be administered under adequate supervision. Provide ample drinking water at all times. If any signs of toxicity appear, discontinue the drug. If symptoms persist after 2 or 3 days, consult your veterinarian for further instruction.
Warning: Discontinue treatment with this drug at least 30 days before slaughtering animals for food. Do not treat lactating animals.
How Supplied: 50's.

NEUROSYN™
(Primidone)

Description: Primidone, 5-Ethyldihydro-5-phenyl-4, 6 (1H, -5H)-pyrimidinedione, is a white crystalline substance, and a pyrimidine derivative. Studies of chronic administration of primidone indicate it can metabolize into two active metabolites, phenobarbital and phenylethylmalonamide (PEMA).
Primidone acts upon the central nervous system to raise the seizure threshold, hence its value as an anticonvulsant, whether the seizure is induced electrically or is a symptom of a primary disease process.
Warning: For use only in dogs.
Indications: For the control of convulsions associated with idiopathic epilepsy, epileptiform convulsions, virus encephalitis, distemper, and hardpad disease that occurs as a clinically recognizable lesion in certain disease entities in dogs.
Precautions: Do not use in feline species, as Primidone appears to have a specific neurotoxicity in cats.
Dosage and Administration: Usual daily dosage—25 mg./lb. of body weight (55 mg./kg.). Tablets may be administered whole or crushed and mixed with food. When convulsions are frequent, the daily dosage should be divided and administered at intervals. Reduction in dosage should be made gradually and never be discontinued abruptly.
How Supplied: Each Neurosyn tablet contains 250 mg. of primidone (scored), in bottles of 100's and 1000's.
Caution: Federal Law restricts this drug to use by or on the order of a licensed veterinarian.

NITROFURAZONE DRESSING 0.2%
Antibacterial Preparation for Topical Application

Composition: 0.2% Nitrofurazone in a Water Soluble base of Polyethylene Glycols.
Indications: For prevention or treatment of surface bacterial infections of wounds, burns and cutaneous ulcers in dogs, cats and horses (not for food use.)
Administration: Apply directly on the lesion with a spatula, or first place on a piece of gauze. Use of a bandage is optional. The preparation should remain on the lesion for at least 24 hours. The dressing may be changed several times daily or left on the lesion for a longer period.
Cautions: Not for use in horses intended for food. In case of deep or puncture wounds or serious burns, consult veterinarian. If redness, irritation or swelling persists or increases, discontinue use; consult veterinarian. Avoid exposure to alkaline material and fluorescent lighting.
How Supplied: 4 oz and 16 oz.

NITROFURAZONE SOLUBLE POWDER
Antibacterial Preparation for Topical Application

Contents: 0.2% Nitrofurazone in a water soluble base.
Indications: For prevention or treatment of surface bacterial infections of wounds, burns, skin ulcers and abscesses after incision in dogs, cats, and horses (not for food use).
Administration: Apply several times daily to the lesion or affected area.
Caution: Not for use in horses intended for food. In case of deep or puncture wounds or serious burns, consult veterinarian. If redness, irritation or swelling persists or increases, discontinue use; consult veterinarian. Avoid exposure to alkaline material and fluorescent lighting.
KEEP AWAY FROM EXCESSIVE HEAT OR DIRECT SUNLIGHT.
How Supplied: 15 gm., 50 gm., 75 gm. Containers.

NITROFURAZONE SOLUTION 0.2%
Antibacterial Preparation

Composition: 0.2% Nitrofurazone in a water miscible vehicle.
Indications: For prevention or treatment of surface bacterial infections of wounds, burns and cutaneous ulcers in dogs, cats and horses (not for food use). Also for the treatment of genital tract infections and impaired fertility of female horses caused by strains of *Staphylococcus, Streptococcus, Escherichia coli, Salmonella, Pseudomonas* and *Vibrio fetus*, sensitive to nitrofurazone.
Dosage and Administration: For treatment of surface bacterial infections, apply directly to the lesion. In the case of wet dressings, it may be diluted with two or three parts of sterile water or saline solution. This may be applied several times daily or left beneath occlusive dressing for several days.
To treat obvious female genital tract infections in horses, aseptically instill 30 to 90 ml into the affected portions of the genital tract once daily. Continue treatment 48 hours after clinical signs subside or until negative bacteriological findings indicate recovery. In cases of impaired fertility, aseptically instill 30 ml into the uterus 4 to 48 hours after breeding.
Caution: Not for use in horses intended for food. Avoid exposure to alkaline material and fluorescent lighting.
How Supplied: Gallons.

OMNIVAC™–PRV
Pseudorabies Virus Vaccine Modified Live Virus

Composition: OMNIVAC™-PRV contains a modified live pseudorabies virus, further attenuated by a genetically engineered gene deletion to increase safety. OMNIVAC™-PRV is recommended for immunizing healthy swine against disease caused by Pseudorabies Virus.
Dosage and Administration: Rehydrate with accompanying fluid, mix well, and aseptically inject 2 ml. intramuscularly. Piglets farrowed by suspectible sows may be vaccinated when 3 days old; those nursing immune sows should be vaccinated at 3–8 weeks of age when maternal antibody levels have declined. For breeding animals, semi-annual revaccination is recommended.
Storage: Store at 35°F–45°F (2°C–7°C). Use entire contents when first rehydrated.
Precautions: Do not vaccinate within 21 days before slaughter. Vaccination may induce antibody responses that may restrict subsequent movement of vaccinated swine. Contains gentamicin and amphotericin B as preservatives. Burn this container and all unused contents.
How Supplied: 10 dose (20 ml) and 50 dose (100 ml)
For Veterinary Use Only

OXYTOCIN
(Injection 20 U.S.P. Units/ml Double U.S.P. Potency)

Composition: Each ml. contains:
Oxytoxin (Synthetic)
20 U.S.P. units per ml.
Sodium Chloride .... 0.9% w/v
Chlorobutanol .... 0.5% w/v
Water for Injection U.S.P. .... q.s.
ph adjusted with Acetic Acid
Dosage and Administration: For obstetrical use: See insert prior to use. Keep refrigerated: 36–46°F. Do not freeze. Intravenous, intramuscular or subcutaneous.
How Supplied: 30 ml., 100 ml.

PARAMUNE™–5
Canine-Distemper-Hepatitis-Parainfluenza Vaccine, Modified Live Virus, Canine Perma-Cell Line™ Origin Leptospira Canicola-Icterohaemorrhagiae Bacterin

Composition: Paramune™-5 is a combination of three stable, modified live viruses of Perma-Cell Line™ Origin with inactivated *Leptospira Canicola Ic-*

terohaemorrhagiae Bacterin as diluent. Multiple passes in tissue culture have modified the viruses to a level where they are both immunogenic and safe.
Protection: Convenience in Combinations.
Flexibility of Use.
Ultimate Uniformity—Resulting from Perma-Cell Process.
Maximum Immunogenicity.
Painless Injection
Fast Rehydration.
Indications: Paramune-5 is indicated for the immunization of healthy, unexposed puppies and dogs against Canine Distemper, Infectious Canine Hepatitis, Canine Parainfluenza (CPI), and leptospirosis caused by *L. canicola* and *L. icterohaemorrhagiae.*
Dosage and Administration: Using aseptic technique, rehydrate the vaccine with accompanying L.C.I. diluent and inject the entire contents of the vial subcutaneously or intramuscularly.
The first vaccination is recommended at or before nine weeks of age in order to provide as much protection as possible as the chances of exposure to disease are increased. A second inoculation should be given 2–4 weeks later. Such a two-dose vaccination schedule should protect practically all puppies; however, in rare cases, interfering levels of passive immunity may persist for as long as 16 weeks. Two doses of Paramune-5 are recommended in the initial immunization to best provide the maximum level of immunity against canine parainfluenza. Thus, ideally all dogs over 16 weeks of age should initially receive 1 dose of Paramune-5 vaccine plus a booster with any of Biologics Corporation's canine parainfluenza vaccines four weeks later. Annual revaccination of all dogs with Paramune-5 is recommended. Revaccination with Biologics Corporation canine parainfluenza vaccine prior to placing dogs in shows, kennels, or veterinary hospitals, where chances of exposure are increased, is recommended.
For Veterinary Use Only
How Supplied: 25 × 1 dose (Bio-Pak) with each pack containing 25 doses desiccated vaccine and 1 tray respectively of 25 × 1 ml. L.C.I. Bacterin as diluent.

PARVOCINE™
Parvovirus Vaccine
Killed Virus
Feline Cell Line Origin

Composition: Parvocine™ is a stable parvovirus vaccine produced in a Perma-Cell Line™ which is tested by U.S.D.A. approved methods and has been shown to be free of adventitious agents. The use of a Perma-Cell Line makes possible the production of a consistently safe, immunogenic virus vaccine.
Each serial meets or exceeds all standards prescribed for this product by the U.S. Department of Agriculture.
Indications: For the immunization of normal, healthy puppies and dogs against diarrhea caused by canine parvovirus.
Dosage and Administration: Using aseptic technique, inject the entire contents of the vial (1 ml) intramuscularly or subcutaneously.
Research has shown that the persistence of maternal antibodies to canine parvovirus may be as long as sixteen weeks in some puppies. The presence of maternal antibodies is known to interfere with development of active immunity and should receive the veterinarian's consideration as immunization programs are planned. Puppies of any age may be safely vaccinated. A recommended vaccination of puppies should start at or about nine weeks of age in order to provide as much protection as possible as the chances of exposure are increased. Puppies should ideally be revaccinated every two to four weeks until they are at least 16 weeks of age. Puppies from nonimmune bitches and orphan puppies should be immunized at an earlier age.
Dogs over 16 weeks of age should receive two doses of Parvocine two to four weeks apart to develop a maximum level of immunity. Annual revaccination is recommended. Since Parvocine is an inactivated virus it may be administered safely to pregnant bitches.
For Veterinary Use Only
How Supplied: 10 dose vials and 25×1 dose carton.

PARVOTECH™-LEPTO 5
Porcine Parvo - Vaccine
Porcine Cell Line
Killed Virus
Leptospira Canicola
Grippotyphosa-Hardjo-
Icterohaemorrhagiae Pomona
Bacterin

Composition: This product contains inactivated Porcine Parvo virus and inactivated Leptospira canicola-grippotyphosa-hardjo-icterohaemorrhagiae pomona bacterin.
Indications: Porcine Parvo-Lepto 5 is a killed virus, adjuvanted product recommended for the immunization of swine against infection by swine parvovirus and the leptospira serovar represented.
Dosage and Administration: Inject 2 ml intramuscularly to sows and gilts 4 to 6 weeks prior to breeding followed by a second vaccination 2 to 4 weeks later. A single revaccination 2 to 6 weeks prior to subsequent breedings is recommended.
Precautions: Store at 35°F–45°F (2°C–7°C). Use entire contents when first opened. Do not vaccinate within 21 days of slaughter. Anaphyloctoid reactions, though rare, can occur. In such instances, symptomatic treatment should be quickly provided.
For Veterinary Use Only.
How Supplied: 10 dose (20 ml) and 50 dose (100 ml) plastic vials.

PARVOCINE™-MLV
Modified Live Virus
Feline Cell Line Origin

Composition: Parvocine™-MLV is a stable parvovirus vaccine produced in a Perma-Cell Line™ which is tested by U.S.D.A. approved methods and has been shown to be free of adventitious agents. The use of a Perma-Cell Line™ makes possible the production of a consistently safe, immunogenic virus vaccine.
Indications: For the immunization of healthy puppies and dogs against diarrhea caused by canine parvovirus.
Dosage and Administration: Using aseptic technique, inject one dose (1 ml.) intramuscularly or subcutaneously.
Parvocine-MLV has been thoroughly tested in susceptible puppies to assure total safety. Puppies given multiple doses developed no leukopenia when observed for 21 days post vaccination. Virus could not be isolated from fecal material when checked for a similar period. Likewise, histopathological examination of lymphatics, thymus, heart muscle and other organs revealed no residual virus upon micropsy 27 days post vaccination.
For Veterinary Use Only
How Supplied: 10 dose vials.

PEN-AQUEOUS

Composition: Procaine Penicillin G U.S.P. in Aqueous Suspension.
Each ml. contains: 300,000 I.U. Procaine Penicillin G with 0.12% Methylparaben and 0.014% Propylparaben, and 0.25% phenol as preservatives, 0.8% sodium citrate, 0.15% sodium carboxymethylcellulose, 15.0% sorbitol solution, 0.06% polyvinylpyrrolidone and 0.6% lecithin.
Dosage and Administration: Refer to package insert.
How Supplied: 100 ml. and 250 ml. glass vials.

PEN-STREP

Composition: Procaine Penicillin G in Dihydrostreptomycin Sulfate Solution.
Each ml. contains: Procaine Penicillin G 200,000 I.U.; Dihydrostreptomycin Sulfate equivalent to 0.25 gm. Dihydrostreptomycin Base with 0.015% Butylparaben and 0.37% Sodium Formaldehyde sulfoxylate and 0.25% phenol as preservatives, 2% procaine hydrochloride, 1.25% sodiun citrate, 2% dibasic sodium phosphite, 0.5% povidone, 0.25% lecithin, 0.21% urea, and sodium hydroxide.
Dosage and Administration: Refer to package insert.
How Supplied: 100 ml. glass vials, 250 ml. glass vials.

PREMIER®
(Killed BVD)
Bovine Virus Diarrhea Vaccine
Killed Virus

Composition: Bovine Virus Diarrhea Vaccine is an adjuvanted, killed virus vaccine containing the New York plus Singer Strain of BVD virus. The viruses are grown on a bovine cell line. The vaccine is indicated for the immunization of healthy cattle against the Bovine Viral Diarrhea-Mucosal Disease complex.
Dosage and Administration: Shake well and inject 5 ml SC or IM to cattle of any age. For complete immunization, inject a second dose in 2 to 4 weeks. Animals vaccinated at 6 months of age or

Continued on next page

TechAmerica—Cont.

older should be revaccinated annually with a single dose. If calves are vaccinated earlier than 6 months of age, a repeat vaccination should be administered after they reach that age with annual revaccination with a single dose. Being a killed virus vaccine, this product may be safely administered to pregnant cattle at any stage of gestation and their calves.
Precaution: Store at 35°F–45°F (2°C–7°C). Use entire contents when first opened. Avoid freezing. Do not vaccinate within 21 days of slaughter. Anaphylactoid reactions can occur following use of products of this nature. Should such occur, symptomatic treatment should be quickly applied. Contains gentamicin, a fungistat and merthiolate as preservatives.

For Veterinary Use Only

How Supplied: 10 dose (50 ml) and 50 dose (250 ml) plastic vials.

PREMIER®–IB
Bovine Rhinotracheitis - Virus Diarrhea Vaccine Killed Virus

Composition: Premier™-IB vaccine is an inactivated virus vaccine containing the highly antigenic Cooper Strain of Bovine Rhinotracheitis virus and New York plus Singer Strains of BVD virus. The viruses are produced in a cell line substrate of bovine origin approved for vaccine production by APHIS-USDA. Viral fluids are adjuvanted assuring increased immune response.
Indications: For the immunization of healthy cattle against bovine rhinotracheitis and bovine virus diarrhea infections.
Dosage and Administration: Shake well. For primary immunization give 2 doses 2 to 4 weeks apart. Inject SC or IM. To maintain a high level of immunity, revaccinate with a single 5 ml dose annually.
Being a killed virus vaccine, Premier-IB may be safely used in pregnant cows at any stage of gestation or very young animals nursing pregnant cows. Two doses are recommended for calves 6 months or older. Calves vaccinated before 6 months of age should be revaccinated at 6 months of age with 2 doses. Annual revaccination with a single dose is recommended.
Precaution: Store at 35°F–45°F (2°C–7°C). Avoid freezing. Use entire contents when first opened. Do not vaccinate within 21 days of slaughter. In case of anaphylactoid reactions, symptomatic treatment should be quickly applied. Contains gentamicin, a fungistat and thimerosal as preservatives.

For Veterinary Use Only.

How Supplied: 10 dose (50 ml) and 50 dose (250 ml) plastic vials.

PREMIER® IBL-5
Bovine Rhinotracheitis-Virus Diarrhea Vaccine Killed Virus Leptospira Canicola-Grippotyphosa-Hardjo-Icterohaemorrhagiae-Pomona Bacterin

Composition: Premier™ IBL-5 is a multivalent immunogen containing inactivated, adjuvanted, highly antigenic Cooper Strain of IBR virus, and New York plus Singer Strains of BVD virus in combination with the 5 Serovars of Leptospira, canicola, grippotyphosa, hardjo, icterohaemorrhagiae and pomona. The viruses represented are grown in a Bovine Cell Line approved for vaccine production by APHIS-USDA. The Leptospira are produced in a medium designed to assure maximum growth and antigenicity. The product is adjuvanted to procure increased immune response by all fractions.
Dosage and Administration: Administer 5 ml SC or IM to calves or cattle of any age. For initial immunization, a second dose of the viral fractions is required 2 to 4 weeks later. Annual vaccination with a single 5 ml dose is recommended for maintenance of a satisfactory immune level.
Being a killed virus vaccine, Premier IBL-5 may be safely used in pregnant cows at any stage of gestation or very young animals nursing pregnant cows. Two doses are recommended for calves 6 months or older. Calves vaccinated before 6 months of age should be revaccinated at 6 months of age with 2 doses. Annual revaccination with a single dose is recommended.
Precaution: Store at 35°F–45°F (2°C–7°C). Avoid freezing. Use entire contents when first opened. Do not vaccinate within 21 days of slaughter. Anaphylactoid reactions, though rare, can occur. Should such occur, symptomatic treatment should be quickly administered. Contains gentamicin, a fungistat and thimerosal as preservatives.

For Veterinary Use Only

How Supplied: 10 dose (50 ml) and 50 dose (250 ml) plastic vials.

PREMIER® IBL-SOMNUTECH®
Bovine Rhinotracheitis-Virus Diarrhea Vaccine Killed Virus Haemophilus Somnus-Leptospira Pomona Bacterin

Composition: Premier IBL-SomnuTech is a multivalent immunogen containing inactivated, highly antigenic Cooper strain of IBR virus and New York plus Singer Strains of BVD virus in combination with Haemophilus Somnus-Leptospira Pomona Bacterin. Premier IBL SomnuTech is intended for use in cattle of all ages for protection against disease caused by the organisms represented.
Dosage and Administration: Administer 5 ml. subcutaneously or intramuscularly to calves or cattle of any age. For initial immunization a second dose is required 2 to 4 weeks later. Annual vaccination with a single 5 ml. dose is recommended for maintenance of a satisfactory immune level. Two doses are recommended for calves 6 months or older. Calves vaccinated before 6 months of age should be revaccinated at 6 months of age with 2 doses. Annual revaccination is recommended.
Storage: Store at 35°F–45°F (2°C–7°C). Avoid freezing. Use entire contents when first opened.
Precautions: Do not vaccinate within 21 days of slaughter. Anaphylactoid reactions, though rare, can occur. Should such occur, symptomatic treatment should be quickly administered. Contains gentamicin and amphotericin B as preservatives.
How Supplied: 50 dose (250 ml.).
For Veterinary Use Only

PREMIER® IBP
Bovine Rhinotracheitis-Virus Diarrhea-Parainfluenza 3 Vaccine Killed Virus

Composition: Premier IBP is an inactivated virus vaccine containing the highly antigenic Cooper Strain of Bovine Rhinotracheitis virus and New York plus Singer Strains of BVD and PI3 virus. The viruses are produced in a cell line substrate of bovine origin approved for vaccine production by APHIS-USDA. Viral fluids are adjuvanted assuring increased immune response.
Dosage and Administration: Shake well. For primary immunization give 2 doses 2 to 4 weeks apart. Inject SC or IM. To maintain a high level of immunity, revaccinate with a single 5 ml dose annually.
Being a killed virus vaccine, Premier IBP may be safely used in pregnant cows at any stage of gestation or very young animals nursing pregnant cows. Two doses are recommended for calves 6 months or older. Calves vaccinated before 6 months of age should be revaccinated at 6 months of age with 2 doses. Annual revaccination with a single dose is recommended.
Storage: Store at 35°F–45°F (2°C–7°C). Avoid freezing. Use entire contents when first opened. Do not vaccinate within 21 days of slaughter. In case of anaphylactoid reactions, symptomatic treatment should be quickly applied. Contains gentamicin and amphotericin B as preservatives.
How Supplied: 10 doses (50 ml) and 50 doses (250 ml)

PREMIER IBPL$_5$®
Bovine Rhinotracheitis-Virus Diarrhea-Parainfluenza 3 Vaccine-Leptospira Canicola-Grippotyphosa-Hardjo-Icterohaemorrhagiae-Pomona Bacterin Killed Virus

Composition: Premier IBPL$_5$ is a multivalent immunogen containing inactivated, adjuvanted, highly antigenic strains of IBR virus, BVD and PI3 virus in combination with the 5 Serovars of Leptospira canicola, grippotyphosa, hardjo, icterohaemorrhagiae and pomona. The viruses represented are grown in a Bovine Cell Line approved for vaccine production by APHIS-USDA. The Leptospira are produced in a medium designed to assure maximum growth and antigenicity. The product is adjuvanted to procure increased immune response by all fractions.

Dosage and Administration: Administer 5 ml SC or IM to calves or cattle of any age. For initial immunization a second dose of the viral fractions is required 2 to 4 weeks later. Annual vaccination with a single 5 ml dose is recommended for maintenance of a satisfactory immune level.

Being a killed virus vaccine, Premier $IBPL_5$ may be safely used in pregnant cows at any stage of gestation or very young animals nursing pregnant cows. Two doses are recommended for calves 6 months or older. Calves vaccinated before 6 months of age should be revaccinated at 6 months of age with 2 doses. Annual revaccination with a single dose is recommended.

Storage: Store at 35°F–45°F (2°C–7°C). Avoid freezing. Use entire contents when first opened. Do not vaccinate within 21 days of slaughter. Anaphylactoid reactions, though rare, can occur. Should such occur, symptomatic treatment should be quickly administered. Contains gentamicin and amphotericin B as preservatives. Burn this container and all unused contents.

How Supplied: 10 doses (50 ml) and 50 doses (250 ml)

RESPOMUNE®–CP

Feline Rhinotracheitis-Calici-Panleukopenia Vaccine Modified Live and Killed Virus Feline Perma-Cell Line™ Origin

Composition: Respomune®-CP is a combination of Feline Rhinotracheitis (FVR)-Calicivirus (FCV), modified live viruses, with inactivated Feline Panleukopenia Virus as a diluent. All have been propagated on feline Perma-Cell Line.™ Multiple passes in tissue culture have modified the FVR and FCV to levels at which they are safe yet have retained their immunogenicity. The inactivated panleukopenia portion is also selected for safety and immunogenicity.

Protection: Maximum Protection—Protects 100% of cats and kittens tested.

No Post-Vaccinal Reactions—Clients remain satisfied.

Can be safely administered subcutaneously or intramuscularly with equal effectiveness.

Painless Injection—1 ml. dose.

Uniformity of Product—From common host Perma-Cell Line.

Safe—Free of any adverse reactions and shedding. Proven free of leukemia virus.

Indications: For the immunization of healthy, unexposed kittens and cats against Feline Viral Rhinotracheitis, Feline Calicivirus, and Feline Panleukopenia infections.

Dosage and Administration: Using aseptic technique, rehydrate the desiccated fraction with the accompanying inactivated Feline Panleukopenia Vaccine and inject the entire contents of the vial (1 ml.) subcutaneously or intramuscularly.

Kittens may be safely vaccinated at any age. Routinely, the first vaccination is recommended at or before nine weeks of age to provide as much protection as possible as chances of exposure are increased.

A second inoculation should be given three to four weeks later in case persistent maternal antibody has interfered with development of active immunity from the first vaccination. Present indications are that maternal antibodies to FVR and FCV endure approximately eight weeks and maternal antibody to Panleukopenia Virus somewhat longer. These probabilities should receive the veterinarian's consideration in planning any immunization program. Kittens born of susceptible queens may be immunized at an earlier age.

Adult cats should receive two doses, three to four weeks apart in order to develop a maximum level of immunity. Annual revaccination of all cats with Respomune®-CP is recommended.

For Veterinary Use Only.

How Supplied: 25 × 1 dose (Bio-Pak) with each pack containing 25 doses desiccated vaccine and 1 tray respectively of 25 × 1 ml. Inactivated Feline Panleukopenia vaccine as diluent.

REVIVE™

(Oral Electrolyte Replacement for Diarrhea)

Contents: Dextrose, Citric Acid, Glycine, Potassium Chloride, Sodium Acetate, Sodium Chloride.

Indications: Revive™ is a water soluble preparation of highly superior absorption characteristics for use as an aid in the replacement of normal body fluids and electrolytes and for energy rich nutritional support in young diarrheic calves, lambs and foals.

Dosage and Administration: Revive™ should be fed or drenched according to the following schedule; add the entire contents of the packet to two quarts of warm water and mix until dissolved. This solution should be prepared just prior to use and may be routinely administered with nursing bottles and pails. Administer two quarts of this solution to each calf or foal two times each day for the first two days. Discontinue milk or milk replacer feedings for these first two days. On the third and fourth days administer one quart of Revive™ mixed with either one quart of milk or one quart of milk replacer to each calf or foal two times a day. Lambs will require approximately one fourth of the above dosage. Most treated animals are returned to normal feeding on the fifth day, however, treatment with the mixture may be continued on the fifth, sixth and seventh days if desired.

NOTE: In cases of severe dehydration or large neonatal animals, two quarts of Revive™ solution should be administered to each calf or foal three or four times each day for the first two days of treatment. Again, lambs will require approximately one fourth of this higher dosage regimen. Use the same treatment regimen for the third and fourth days as previously recommended.

Store in a cool, dry place.

For Veterinary Use Only.

How Supplied: 50, 162.5 gm packets per bucket, and 12, 162.5 gm. packet per box.

RHINOPAN®-MLV

Feline Rhinotracheitis-Calici-Panleukopenia Vaccine Modified Live Virus Feline Cell Line Origin

Composition: Rhinopan®-MLV is a combination of three stable, modified live feline viruses of feline Perma-Cell Line™ Origin. Multiple passes in tissue culture have modified the viruses to a level at which they are safe yet have retained their immunogenicity.

Indications: For the immunization of healthy, unexposed kittens and cats against feline viral rhinotracheitis, feline calicivirus infection, and feline panleukopenia.

Dosage and Administration: Using aseptic technique, rehydrate the desiccated fraction with the accompanying Feline Panleukopenia Vaccine and inject the entire contents of the vial (1 ml.) subcutaneously or intramuscularly.

Kittens of any age may be safely vaccinated. Routinely, the first vaccination is recommended at or before nine weeks of age to provide as much protection as possible as chances of exposure are increased. Kittens vaccinated before nine weeks of age should ideally receive a dose of vaccine every three to four weeks until they are at least twelve weeks of age. Present indications are that maternal antibodies to feline rhinotracheitis virus and calicivirus may persist approximately eight weeks in kittens from immune queens and maternal antibodies against feline panleukopenia virus persist somewhat longer. These conditions should receive the veterinarian's consideration as immunization programs are planned. The presence of maternal antibody is known to interfere with development of active immunity. Kittens from nonimmune queens and orphan kittens should be immunized at an earlier age.

For Veterinary Use Only

How Supplied: 25 × 1 dose (Bio-Pak) with each pack containing 25 doses desiccated vaccine and 1 tray respectively of 25 × 1 ml. Modified Live Feline Panleukopenia vaccine as diluent.

SOMNUTECH®

Haemophilus Somnus Bacterin

Composition: Haemophilus Somnus Bacterin is prepared from highly immunogenic strains of *Haemophilus somnus* grown in a specially designed medium under carefully controlled conditions in a closed fermentation system. They are harvested in a manner designed to maintain their immunogenic character. The

Continued on next page

T

TechAmerica—Cont.

product is evaluated for purity, safety and potency before release to market.
For the protection of healthy calves against infection by *Haemophilus somnus* organisms.
Dosage and Administration: Shake well and administer 2 ml. IM or SC to healthy calves. Repeat in 14–28 days. Annual revaccination is recommended. Ideally calves should be 4 months of age or older when immunization procedures are instituted.
Precautions: Do not vaccinate within 21 days before slaughter.
For Veterinary Use Only
How Supplied: 10ds(20ml); 50ds(100ml).

TANISOL
(Astringent and Drying Agent)

Composition: Each ml. contains:
Salicylic Acid.................................10.0 mg.
Tannic Acid....................................57.4 mg.
Boric Acid......................................26.4 mg.
In a modified base of Propylene Glycol and Isopropanol.
Indications: As an aid in the management of moist dermatitis in dogs and cats and as an astringent and drying agent for weeping wounds in large animals.
This preparation will sting for a short time when applied to a sensitive lesion. This reaction should be expected, but is not usually apparent on subsequent applications as drying and healing advances.
Directions for Use: Topical application. Apply to skin lesion with cotton pledget or dauber. Repeat at 6 to 8 hour intervals until lesion is dry. Continue one application daily until healing is complete. Apply to foot pads or between toes with dauber, or by dipping pad in an undiluted solution of TANISOL.
Caution
Do not apply in or near eye or on mucous membrane. Store out of direct light.
How Supplied: 4 oz.; Gallon.

TYLOSIN INJECTION
Antibiotic
Sterile

Description: Tylosin Injection is available in two concentrations containing 50 mg and 200 mg/ml tylosin base. The product is recommended for intramuscular injection only in beef cattle, nonlactating dairy cattle and swine.
Each ml Contains:

	50 mg/ml	200 mg/ml
Tylosin base	50.0 mg	200.0 mg
Propylene Glycol	50.0% v/v	50.0% v/v
Benzyl Alcohol	4% v/v	4% v/v
Water for Injection	qs	qs

Indications: Tylosin Injection is indicated for use in the treatment of bovine respiratory complex (shipping fever, pneumonia) usually associated with **Pasteurella multocida** and **Corynebacterium pyogenes;** foot rot (necrotic pododermatitis) and calf diphtheria caused by **Fusobacterium necrophorum** and metritis caused by **Corynebacterium pyogenes** in beef cattle and nonlactating dairy cattle.
In swine, Tylosin Injection is indicated for the treatment of swine arthritis caused by **Mycoplasma hyosynoviae;** swine pneumonia caused by **Pasteurella** spp.; swine erysipelas caused by **Erysipelothrix rhusiopathiae;** acute swine dysentery associated with **Treponema hyodysenteriae** when followed by appropriate medication in the drinking water and/or feed.
Dosage and Administration: For intramuscular injection only.
Beef Cattle and Nonlactating Dairy Cattle—Inject intramuscularly 8 mg per pound of body weight once daily (1 ml of the 50 mg product per 6.25 pounds or 1 ml of the 200 mg product per 25 pounds.) Treatment should be continued 24 hours after symptoms of the disease have stopped, not to exceed 5 days. Do not inject more than 10 ml per site. The 50 mg formulation is recommended for use in calves weighing less than 200 pounds.
Swine—Inject intramuscularly 4 mg per pound of body weight (1 ml of the 50 mg per 12.5 pounds or 1 ml of the 200 mg product per 50 pounds) twice daily. Treatment should be continued 24 hours after symptoms of the disease have stopped, not to exceed 3 days. Do not inject more than 5 ml per site.
Side Effects: Side effects consisting of edema of the rectal mucosa, anal protrusion, diarrhea, erythema and pruritus have been observed in some hogs following the use of tylosin. Discontinuation of treatment effected an uneventful recovery.
Caution: Do not mix Tylosin Injection with other injectable solutions as this may cause precipitation of the active ingredients,. Do not administer to horses or other equines. Injection of tylosin in equines has been fatal.
Precautions: Adverse reactions including shock and death may result from overdosage in baby pigs.
Do not attempt injection of the 50 mg product into pigs weighing less than 6.25 pounds (0.5 ml) unless the syringe is capable of accurately delivering 0.1 ml. Do not attempt injection of the 200 mg product into pigs weighing less than 25 pounds (0.5 ml). It is recommended that the 50 mg formulation be used in pigs weighing less than 25 pounds.
If tylosin medicated drinking water is used as follow-up treatment for swine dysentery, the animal should thereafter receive feed containing 40 to 100 grams of tylosin per ton for 2 weeks to assure depletion of tissue residues.
Warning: Discontinue use in cattle 21 days before slaughter. Discontinue use in swine 14 days before slaughter. Do not use in lactating dairy cattle.
Store at 72°F (22°C) or below.
How Supplied: Tylosin Injection, 50 mg/ml is available in 100 ml vials. Tylosin Injection, 200mg/ml is available in 100 ml, 250 ml and 500 ml vials.
For Veterinary Use Only
Keep out of reach of children

VIBRIO–LEPTO 5
Campylobacter Fetus-Leptospira Canicola-Grippotyphosa-Hardjo-Icterohaemorrhagiae-Pomona Bacterin
Aluminum Hydroxide Adsorbed

Composition: The product is chemically inactivated, aluminum hydroxide adjuvanted bacterin prepared from antigenic cultures of *Campylobacter fetus* (previously called Vibrio fetus), *L. canicola, L. grippotyphosa, L. hardjo, L. icterohaemorrhagiae* and *L. pomona.*
The *C. fetus* strain used in production of the bacterin was chosen especially for its immunogenicity. It contains a broad spectrum of the heat-labile factors (K antigens) responsible for eliciting immunity. The cultures are fermenter-grown in a medium designed to produce maximum growth (a high antigen mass) and optimal immunogenicity.
The leptospira cultures are grown in a medium designed to support immunogenicity and the reduce the possibility of allergic reaction. The medium does not contain whole serum but rather an albumin fraction as a growth nutrient.
In-process testing and quality control checks for all cultures used in the bacterin assure lot-to-lot uniformity. The cultures are adsorbed onto aluminum hydroxide gel and blended in a manner which assures that the final product contains the optimal dose for each fraction. The product contains formaldehyde and merthiolate as preservatives.
As a federally licensed product, each serial meets or exceeds all standards set by the U.S. Department of Agriculture for purity, safety, potency and efficacy.
Indications: For the immunization of healthy cattle against vibriosis due to *Campylobacter (vibrio) fetus* and leptospirosis due to *Leptospira canicola, Leptospira grippotyphosa, Leptospira hardjo, Leptospira icterohaemorrhagiae* and *Leptospira pomona.*
Description of the Disease: Bovine genital vibriosis is considered to be a primary cause of infertility. It is caused by the bacterium *Campylobacter fetus,* previously called Vibrio fetus. The organism is transmitted by sexual contact. A cyclic pattern is established, where infected bulls will transmit the organism to clean heifers/cows, which in turn infect clean bulls. A superficial infection is established in the genital tract of the heifer/cow, which can cause early death of the embryo and a subsequent return to estrus. The primary clinical sign of vibriosis in a range herd is repeat breeding, resulting in extended calving and a reduced calf crop.
Leptospirosis is a widespread disease of cattle and other domestic and wild animals. It is caused by bacteria belonging to several serotypes (serovars) of the genus Leptospira. *L. canicola, L. grippotyphosa, L. hardjo, L. icterohaemorrhagiae* and *L. pomona* have been associated with the disease in cattle. Exposure is by direct contact with urine or water contaminated with the bacterium. If infection occurs during the last trimester of gesta-

T

tion, fetal death may result in abortion or stillbirth, surviving fetuses may be born as weak calves. Leptospira infections are also associated with long-term sterility problems in mature females, reduced milk production in dairy cattle, and occasionally acute disease in young animals. However, the primary clinical sign of leptospirosis in cattle is abortion and stillbirth.

Protection: The heat-labile surface antigens (K antigens) of *C. fetus* have been shown to be responsible for eliciting immunity after vaccination. Several of these heat-labile antigens have been characterized. The ability of the organism to alter its antigenic makeup during infection has also been reported. The strain used in production of the bacterin was chosen specifically because it contains a broad spectrum of these antigenic factors. In an experimental challenge of heifers the bacterin was shown to elicit significant protection against a virulent NADC challenge culture, different from the strain used in the bacterin. Thus, a high degree of immunity can be expected against field strains which may contain various antigenic makeups. Circulating antibody has been shown to be protective against bovine vibriosis due to the "spill-over" into the genital tract, and this is likely the mechanism of protection after vaccination. Because vibrio infection is limited to the superficial layers of the genital tract, exposure is not likely to stimulate a humoral anamnestic antibody response. Thus, it is important to have a high level of circulating protective antibody at the time of possible exposure and the optimal time to vaccinate is just prior to the breeding season.

Dosage and Administration: Shake well. Inject 5 ml intramuscularly or subcutaneously 2 to 6 weeks prior to breeding or being added to the breeding herd. Revaccinate once annually to maintain a high level of immunity.

In vibrio infected herds or endemic areas, two doses at least 3 weeks apart, are recommended for primary immunization.

Precautions:

1. Store at 35°F to 45°F (2°C to 7°C). Do not freeze.
2. Use entire contents when first opened. Care should be taken to avoid microbial contamination of this product.
3. Do not vaccinate within 21 days before slaughter.
4. If allergic response occurs, symptomatic treatment should be provided immediately.

How Supplied: 10 dose (50 ml) and 50 dose (250 ml) plastic vials.

VITAMIN A-D_3 INJECTABLE

Composition: Each ml. contains:

Vitamin A	500,000 IU
Vitamin D_3	75,000 IU
Benzyl alcohol	2% v/v
Ethyl alcohol	10%
Vitamin E	
BHA (as preservative)	0.75%
BHT (as preservative)	0.75%

Indications: A sterile solution of vitamins in oil for use as a source of vitamins A and D_3 in cattle, sheep, and swine.

Administration: For intramuscular, subcutaneous and intrarumenal administration.

Suggested Dosage: May be repeated in two to three months, as needed:

Calves	½ to 1 ml.
Yearlings	1 to 2 ml.
Adult cattle	2 to 4 ml.
Lambs	¼ to ½ ml.
Growing lambs	½ to 1 ml.
Adult sheep	1 to 2 ml.
Weaning pigs	¼ to ½ ml.
Growing pigs	½ to 1 ml.
Adult swine	1 to 2 ml.

Cautions: If symptoms of deficiencies persist after 7 days, the diagnosis should be reevaluated.

Store in cool dry place—Keep partially used vial under refrigeration.

Keep from freezing.

For veterinary use only.

Keep out of reach of children.

How Supplied: 100 ml., 250 ml., and 500 ml.

VITAMINO® 4X
(Concentrated Pediatric Drops for Small Animals)

Composition: Each ounce contains:

Cyanocobalamin	400 mcg.
Niacinamide	80 mg.
Riboflavin	8 mg.
Thiamine HCl	32 mg.
Pyridoxine HCl	16 mg.
d-Calcium Pantothenate	48 mg.
Liver	3 g.
Amino Acids (as protein hydrolysate)	4.5 g.
Iron (as ferrous sulfate U.S.P.)	48 mg.
Aromatic Syrup base	q.s.
Sodium Benzoate as preservative	

Indications: As an oral iron, B vitamin, liver, and balanced amino acid supplement for young and orphaned small animals.

Directions for Use: oral administration.

Dosage: Up to 3 pounds body weight: ½ ml. two to three times daily. Over 3 pounds body weight: 1 ml. (dropperful) two or three times daily. One teaspoonful per 20 pounds two times daily.

How Supplied: 1 fluid ounce and gallon.

IDENTIFICATION PROBLEM?
Consult the
Product Identification Section
where you'll find
products pictured
in full color.

3M/Animal Care Products
225-1N 3M CENTER
ST. PAUL, MN 55144

SECTROL®
Concentrate No. 1490 Microencapsulated Pyrethrins Insecticide

Description: SECTROL Concentrate No. 1490 is an undiluted form of SECTROL Pet and Household Flea Spray No. 1495, listed elsewhere in this directory. See that listing for description, indications, directions for use and precautionary statements.

Composition: Active Ingredients:

Pyrethrins	1.1%
*Piperonyl Butoxide, Technical	2.2%
N-Octyl Bicycloheptene Dicarboximide	3.7%
Petroleum Distillate	4.5%
Inert Ingredients	88.5%
Total	100.0%

*Equivalent to 1.76% Butylcarbityl (6-propylpiperonyl) ether and to 0.44% related compounds.

Directions For Use: Dilution Instructions: Shake SECTROL Concentrate well before diluting. Mix well after diluting, remove screen from sprayer.

For General Use Including Preventative Maintenance: Dilute one part SECTROL Concentrate with 9 parts water. (12.8 fl. oz./gallon).

For Severe Infestations: Dilute one part SECTROL Concentrate with 4 parts water. (12.8 fl. oz./one-half gallon).

*A 1:12 dilution may also be used for some preventative maintenance treatments.

See application directions for SECTROL Pet and Household Flea Spray No. 1495.

How Supplied: One gallon (3.785 l) plastic bottle. Makes 10 gallons ready-to-use.

12.8 fl. oz. (378.5 ml) plastic bottle. Makes 1 gallon ready-to-use.

U.S. Patent 4,056,610

SECTROL®
Pet and Household Flea Spray No. 1495
Ready-to-use microencapsulated natural pyrethrins insecticide for extended residual control of fleas and ticks indoors and on dogs and cats.

(Formerly No. 1494 Premise Flea Spray and No. 1496 Pet Spray—now combined into one product)

Description: Clinically proven to provide timed-release residual activity against fleas for 30 days in the home and for 8 days on dogs and cats. Microencapsulated natural pyrethrins insecticide provides timed-release activity with extremely low mammalian toxicity (oral LD_{50} >34,600 mg/kg). SECTROL Pet and Household Flea Spray is not a cholinesterase inhibitor. If label directions are followed, it can be used on puppies and kittens. Safety for animals younger than 6 weeks has not been determined.

Continued on next page

T

3M—Cont.

Features important for home use include its water-based, non-staining virtually odorless formula. Safe for household furnishings, houseplants, and carpets.

Composition: Active Ingredients:

Pyrethrins	0.11%
*Piperonyl Butoxide, Technical	0.22%
N-Octyl Bicycloheptene Dicarboximide	0.37%
Petroleum Distillate	0.45%
Inert Ingredients	98.85%
Total	100.00%

*Equivalent to 0.18% butylcarbityl (6-propylpiperonyl) ether and to 0.04% related compounds.

Indications: For long-lasting effective flea and tick control on dogs and cats. Also for general control on premises of:

fleas	weevils
cockroaches	spiders
ants	beetles
crickets	waterbugs
flies	gnats
silverfish	centipedes
firebrats	ticks
moths	

Directions for Use: Before use, shake thoroughly and adjust sprayer to deliver a coarse spray.

On Cats and Dogs—For best results, shampoo pet with product recommended by veterinarian. Towel dry. Hold sprayer a few inches from pet. Start by spraying pet's head (avoiding contact with the eyes) and work your way back to the hind quarters. Spray under the haircoat by backcombing against the direction of hair growth with your other hand. It is important to wet the entire haircoat and any exposed skin thoroughly to assure adequate coverage. Allow pet to dry or use blow dryer. Do not towel dry as this will remove many of the microcapsules. Reapply weekly or as needed.

On Household Surfaces—Thoroughly vacuum all carpeting, upholstered furniture, along baseboards, under furniture and in closets. Seal vacuum bag and dispose. Mop hard floors. Replace pet bedding. Using a smooth back-and-forth motion, spray all floors and other aforementioned areas thoroughly, especially pet resting areas and other areas your pet frequents. Repeat application after 30 days or as needed.

Refrain from vacuuming treated areas until flea cycle is broken (normally 10–14 days). If you vacuum, retreat vacuumed areas. Apply at the rate of one gallon per 1000 square feet of surface area. If product begins to run off or leave pools, you are spraying too heavily. SECTROL Pet and Household Flea Spray will not damage surfaces that are unaffected by water.

Caution: Keep out of reach of children.

Precautionary Statements:

Hazards to Humans and Domestic Animals: Avoid contact with eyes. Avoid breathing spray mist. Keep container closed when not in use.

Environmental Hazards: This product is toxic to fish. Cover or remove fish bowls and aquaria. May be used in food areas, but food, food contact surfaces, and cooking utensils should be removed or covered during treatment or thoroughly cleaned before using.

Statement of Practical Treatment: If on skin: Remove contaminated clothing and immediately wash skin with soap and water. **If in eyes:** Immediately flush eyes with plenty of water. Get medical attention if irritation persists.

How Supplied: 15 fl. oz. (444 ml) and 1 gal. (3.785 liter) trigger spray plastic bottles.

U.S. Patent 4,056,610

DURATROL™
Household Flea Spray No. 1488
Contains microencapsulated Dursban® insecticide for residual control of fleas and ticks indoors.

Description: Duratrol Household Flea Spray is a unique microencapsulated formulation for the residual control of fleas and ticks. The microcapsules provide a "timed release" mechanism for the active ingredient, chlorpyrifos, to provide long-lasting control of pests. This product provides clinically-proven 60–90 day flea control in the home, even after vacuuming. It helps break the flea life cycle by killing both adult fleas and flea larvae. And the unique microencapsulation of the active ingredient reduces mammalian toxicity (oral LD_{50} > 25,850 mg/kg).

Composition: Active Ingredient:

Chlorpyrifos [0,0-Diethyl 0-(3,5,6-Trichloro-2-Pyridyl)-Phosphorothioate]	0.50%
Inert Ingredients:	99.50%
Total	100.00%

Indications: For long-lasting flea and tick control in homes, apartments and clinics.

Directions For Use:

1. **SHAKE WELL BEFORE USING** to obtain a uniform dispersion of microcapsules. Adjust sprayer to deliver coarse wet spray.
2. Thoroughly apply the spray to infested areas, such as pet beds and resting quarters, along baseboards, and localized areas of floor and floor coverings where fleas and ticks may be present. Old bedding should be removed and replaced with clean, fresh bedding after treatment. **Do not treat pets with this product.**
3. Spray with a smooth back-and-forth motion to deposit product uniformly. It is not necessary to soak the treated surface, but an even treatment is desirable.
4. As fleas pick up or are bombarded by microcapsules of insecticide, the capsules begin to release their active ingredient. Noticeable flea reductions will be observed within 24 hours.

Caution: Keep out of reach of children.

Precautionary Statements

Hazards To Humans and Domestic Animals: Avoid breathing spray mist. Avoid contact with skin and eyes. Harmful if absorbed through skin. Wash hands thoroughly with soap and water after handling and before eating. Do not spray directly on pets or humans. Do not allow spray to contact food or food-contacting surfaces, feedstuffs, or water supplies. Do not use in food preparation areas of commercial establishments. Do not use in serving areas while food is exposed.

Statement of Practical Treatment—If Swallowed: Call a physician or Poison Control Center. Drink 1 or 2 glasses of water and induce vomiting by touching finger to back of throat. Never give anything by mouth to an unconscious person.

If on skin: remove contaminated clothing and wash skin with soap and water. **If in eyes:** flush eyes with plenty of water. If irritation persists, call physician.

Note to Physician: Chlorpyrifos is a cholinesterase inhibitor, treat symptomatically. Atropine only by injection is an antidote.

Environmental Hazards: This product is toxic to fish, wildlife, and birds. Keep out of any body of water. Do not contaminate lakes or streams by cleaning of equipment or disposal of wastes.

How Supplied: No. 1488T—30 fl. oz. plastic trigger-spray bottle; No. 1488K—kit which contains one 30 oz. bottle of spray and one 1-liter pump-up sprayer; and No. 1488R 30 oz. refill.

Patent pending.

"Duratrol" is a trademark of 3M.

"Dursban" is a trademark of the Dow Chemical Co.

DURATROL™
Yard and Kennel Concentrate Flea Spray No. 1489
Contains microencapsulated Dursban® insecticide for residual control of fleas and ticks on lawns, concrete and kennels.

Description: Timed-release formula provides 30-day flea control, even after it rains. Unique microencapsulation of active ingredient reduces mammalian toxicity (oral LD_{50} > 25,850 mg/kg). Helps break the flea life cycle by killing both adult fleas and flea larvae. Easy to apply with most garden hose sprayers or pump-up type tank sprayers.

Composition: Active Ingredient:

Chlorpyrifos [0, 0-Diethyl 0-(3,5,6-Trichloro-2-Pyridyl)-Phosphorothioate]	1.70%
Inert Ingredients	98.30%
Total	100.00%

Indications: For long-lasting flea and tick control on lawns, concrete and kennels.

Directions For Use: Shake well before using!

In Yards—Use 2 fl. oz. (4 tbsp.) of concentrate in 1 gallon of water for 160 sq. ft. of area to be treated. This bottle (30 fl. oz.) treats up to 2400 sq. ft., diluted in 15 gals. water. A garden hose spray attachment (such as the Ortho 1 qt. Lawn Sprayer) makes application easy because no premixing is necessary—the sprayer automatically siphons and dilutes the concentrate with the water from the garden hose. Use a coarse, low-pressure spray in a smooth back-and-forth motion to uniformly apply product. Repeat treatment as necessary to maintain effectiveness.

For Kennels and Dog Houses—Mix 20 fl. oz. of concentrate and water to make 1 gal. of spray. Apply to buildings, resting areas, and floors. Do not apply directly to pets.

Caution: Keep out of reach of children.

Precautionary Statements

Hazards To Humans and Domestic Animals:

CAUTION: May be harmful if swallowed. Avoid breathing spray mist. Avoid contact with eyes, skin or clothing. Wash thoroughly after handling. Avoid contaminaion of feed and food utensils. Do not spray directly on humans or pets.

Statement of Practical Treatment—

If Swallowed: Call a physician or Poison Control Center. Drink 1 or 2 glasses of water and induce vomiting by touching finger to back of throat. Never give anything by mouth to an unconscious person. **If on skin:** remove contaminated clothing and wash skin with soap and water. **If in eyes:** flush eyes with plenty of water. If irritation persists, call physician.

Note To Physician: Chlorpyrifos is a cholinesterase inhibitor, treat symptomatically. Atropine only by injection is an antidote.

Environmental Hazards: This product is toxic to fish, wildlife, and birds. Do not apply directly to water. Do not contaminate lakes or streams by cleaning of equipment or disposal of wastes.

How Supplied: 30 fl. oz. plastic concentrate bottle.

Patent pending.

"Duratrol" is a trademark of 3M.

"Dursban" is a trademark of the Dow Chemical Co.

SECTROL®
Two-Way™ Pet Spray No. 1497
Residual Flea and Tick Spray with Quick Kill for Use on Dogs and Cats

Description: SECTROL Two-Way Pet Spray combines microencapsulated natural pyrethrins for timed-release residual activity and unencapsulated natural pyrethrins for quick kill. Clinical studies show that Two-Way Pet Spray provides 98% control of new flea infestations for at least a week after initial application and starts killing fleas within 60 seconds of application.

The water-based SECTROL Two-Way Pet Spray contains no alcohol and is extremely low in mammalian toxicity (oral LD_{50} > 30,000 mg/kg). It is virtually odorless, non-oily and won't stain an animal's coat or irritate its skin. SECTROL Two-Way Pet Spray is not a cholinesterase inhibitor. It may be used on puppies and kittens 6 weeks or older if label directions are followed. Safety for animals younger than 6 weeks has not been determined.

Composition: Active Ingredients:

Pyrethrins	0.21%
*Piperonyl Butoxide Technical	0.42%
N-Octyl Bicycloheptene Dicarboximide	0.70%
Inert Ingredients	98.67%
Total	100.00%

*Equivalent to 0.336% Butylcarbityl (6-propylpiperonyl) ether and to 0.084% related compounds.

Indications: For fast acting, long lasting flea and tick control.

Directions For Use: Before use, shake thoroughly and adjust spayer to deliver a coarse spray. For best results, shampoo pet with product recommended by veterinarian. Towel dry. Hold sprayer a few inches from pet. Apply Sectrol Two-Way Pet Spray so that pet is moist—not soaked. When applying to cats, do not exceed 10 grams (10 squeezes of the trigger sprayer) for each pound your cat weighs.

Start by spraying pet's head (avoiding eyes) and work your way back to the hind quarters. Spray under the haircoat by backcombing against the direction of hair growth with your other hand. Rough up the hair as needed to expose skin to insecticide. Allow pet to dry or use blow dryer. Do not towel dry as this will remove many of the microcapsules. Reapply weekly or as needed.

Applying this product at the level described above will provide rapid flea kill and at least 8 days residual activity. Because some animals, particularly cats and kittens, may be sensitive to insecticides, do not exceed the recommended application rate on cats and kittens unless so advised by your veterinarian.

Caution: Keep out of reach of children.

Precautionary Statements:

Hazards to Humans and Domestic Animals: Avoid contact with eyes. Avoid breathing spray mist. Keep container closed when not in use.

Some animals, particularly cats and kittens, may be sensitive to insecticides. See "Directions for Use" for specific application information. If adverse reactions are observed (e.g., heavy salivation, lethargy, breathing difficulties, or other unusual reactions), bathe pet immediately in warm, soapy water. If symptoms persist, seek medical attention.

Environmental Hazard: This product is toxic to fish. Cover or remove fish bowls and aquaria. Food and food utensils should be removed or covered during treatment or thoroughly cleaned before using.

Statement of Practical Treatment: If on skin: Remove contaminated clothing and immediately wash skin with soap and water. **If in eyes:** Immediately flush eyes with plenty of water. Get medical attention if irritation persists.

How Supplied: 15 fl. oz (444 ml) plastic bottle with trigger action spray pump.

U.S. Patent: 4,056,610

SECTROL®
Two-Way™ Flea Foam No. 1498
Residual Flea and Tick Treatment with Quick Knockdown. For use on cats. Also for dogs that are sensitive to conventional sprays.

Description: SECTROL Two-Way Flea Foam combines microencapsulated natural pyrethrins for timed-release residual activity and unencapsulated natural pyrethrins for quick kill. Clinical studies show that Two-Way Flea Foam provides 98% control of new flea infestations for at least a week after initial application and starts killing within 60 seconds of application.

The water-based SECTROL Two-Way Flea Foam contains no alcohol and is extremely low in mammalian toxicity (oral LD_{50} > 30,000 mg/kg). It is virtually odorless, non-oily, and won't stain an animal's coat or irritate its skin. SECTROL Two-Way Flea Foam is not a cholinesterase inhibitor. If label directions are followed it may be used on puppies and kittens 6 weeks or older. Safety for use on animals younger than 6 weeks has not been determined.

Excellent for use on pets sensitive to sprays because it can be applied first into your palm while you face away from the animal.

Composition: Active Ingredients:

Pyrethrins	.15%
*Piperonyl Butoxide, Technical	0.70%
N-Octyl Bicycloheptene Dicarboximide	0.34%
Petroleum Distillate	0.61%
Inert Ingredients	98.20%
Total	100.00%

*Equivalent to 0.56% butylcarbityl (6-propylpiperonyl) ether and to 0.14% related compounds.

Indications: For fast acting, long lasting flea and tick control on cats and on dogs that are sensitive to ordinary sprays.

Directions For Use: Shake well before using.

Start by applying a one-second burst of foam to haircoat near the pet's head (avoiding eyes). Massage foam into haircoat until it disappears.

Repeat this procedure making sure to thoroughly moisten, but not soak, the entire haircoat. When applying to cats, use a one-second burst for each pound your cat weighs. Usually 4–5 one-second bursts will cover a 5–7 pound cat. Allow pet to dry or use blow dryer. Do not towel dry as this will remove many of the microcapsules. Reapply weekly or as needed.

Applying this product at the level described above will provide rapid flea kill and at least 8 days residual activity. Because some animals, particularly cats and kittens, may be sensitive to insecticides, do not exceed the recommended application rate on cats and kittens unless so advised by your veterinarian.

Caution: Keep out of reach of children.

Precautionary Statements

Hazards to Humans and Domestic Animals: Avoid contact with eyes. Some animals, particularly cats and kittens, may be sensitive to insecticides. See "Directions for Use" for specific application information. If adverse reactions are observed (e.g., heavy salivation, lethargy, breathing difficulties, or other unusual reactions), bathe pet immediately in warm, soapy water. If symptoms persist, seek medical attention.

Physical or Chemical Hazards: Contents under pressure. Do not puncture or incinerate container. Do not use or store near heat or open flame. Do not store be-

Continued on next page

T

3M—Cont.

low 32° F. Exposure to temperatures above 130° F may cause bursting.
Environmental Hazard: This product is toxic to fish. Do not contaminate water, food, or feed by storage or disposal.
Statement of Practical Treatment: If in eyes: Immediately flush eyes with plenty of water, get medical attention if irritation persists.
How Supplied: Net Weight: 10 oz. (283 g), in spray can.
U.S. Patent: 4,056,610

The Upjohn Company
7000 PORTAGE ROAD
KALAMAZOO, MICHIGAN 49001

ALBAPLEX® TABLETS
(tetracycline hydrochloride and novobiocin)

Composition: Albaplex Tablets, designed for use in dogs, contains a combination of two antibiotics—Panmycin® Hydrochloride (tetracycline hydrochloride) and Albamycin® (novobiocin sodium)—which supply additive antibacterial effects against certain bacterial pathogens. Each tablet contains: Panmycin Hydrochloride (tetracycline hydrochloride) . . . 60 mg; Albamycin (novobiocin sodium) . . . 60 mg

T

Actions: Panmycin Hydrochloride (tetracycline hydrochloride)
Panmycin Hydrochloride is an odorless, yellow, fine crystalline powder which is freely soluble in water and gastric juice. Panmycin Hydrochloride is absorbed readily from the gastrointestinal tract. Following oral administration to dogs, peak blood concentrations are obtained within two to four hours, effective concentrations are found at 12 hours and detectable amounts remain in the serum for at least 24 hours. The antibiotic is excreted principally through the kidney.
The range of antimicrobial activity of Panmycin Hydrochloride includes a broad range of gram-positive and gram-negative bacteria such as alpha and beta streptococci; some strains of staphylococci, Klebsiella pneumoniae, certain clostridia, Shigella, *Aerobacter aerogenes* and some strains of Salmonella. The clinical significance of this has not been determined.
In an *in vivo* study, it was shown that tetracycline was significantly less effective than novobiocin in eliminating pathogenic staphylococci organisms from the throats of dogs suffering from upper respiratory infections. However, it was also shown that tetracycline was significantly more effective than novobiocin in eliminating pathogenic streptococci.
Studies show that Panmycin Hydrochloride has a low order of toxicity comparable to that of other tetracycline.
Albamycin (novobiocin sodium)
Albamycin is an antibiotic produced by *Streptomyces niveus* and developed in the Research Laboratories of The Upjohn Company. The crystalline antibiotic has a light yellow to white color depending upon the state of subdivision. In contrast to most antibiotics produced by actinomycetes, Albamycin, like penicillin, is acidic in nature and is stable to the degree of acidity or alkalinity present in the gastrointestinal tract. Following oral administration to dogs, peak blood concentrations are obtained within one to two hours and significant levels are found at twelve hours. When appreciable amounts of Albamycin are present in the serum, the drug diffuses into the pleural and ascitic fluids. Albamycin does not diffuse into the cerebrospinal fluid. The antibiotic is concentrated in the liver and bile and is excreted in the feces and urine. As determined by tests in animals, Albamycin has a relatively low order of toxicity.
In vitro studies show that Albamycin is active against both gram-positive and gram-negative bacteria including *Staphylococcus aureus, Streptococcus hemolyticus, Diplococcus pneumoniae,* and some strains of *Proteus vulgaris*. The drug is particularly active against *Staphylococcus aureus*. Albamycin shows no cross resistance with penicillin against resistant strains of *M. pyogenes*, var. *aureus*. However, *in vitro* studies indicate that *M. pyogenes* var. *aureus* may develop resistance to Albamycin as with other antibiotics. The clinical significance of these *in vitro* results has not been determined.
Combined Antibiotic Therapy: Albaplex (tetracycline hydrochloride and novobiocin) therapy offers a wider range of antimicrobial activity than does therapy with either single antibiotic.
As *in vivo* clinical study in dogs with upper respiratory infections showed Albaplex was significantly more effective in eliminating *Staphylococcus spp.* and *E. coli* organisms from throat tissues than was tetracycline or novobiocin administered singly. Treatment failure was significantly reduced by use of Albaplex when compared to treatment with either single antibiotic. This *in vivo* clinical study demonstrated that the two antibiotics had complementary spectra of activities with significantly fewer organisms resistant to the combination of tetracycline and novobiocin than to either single antibiotic.
Note: The prednisolone component of Delta Albaplex (tetracycline, novobiocin and prednisolone) has been shown to contribute to clinical response if administered for the first *48 hours* of treatment. Subsequent antibacterial treatment is to be continued with Albaplex® (tetracycline and novobiocin). See **Indications** and **Dosage** Sections following.
Indications: Albaplex (tetracycline hydrochloride and novobiocin) Tablets are indicated for use in the treatment of acute or chronic canine respiratory infections such as tonsillitis, bronchitis, and tracheobronchitis when caused by pathogens susceptible to tetracycline and/or novobiocin such as *Staphylococcus spp.* and *E. coli.* As with all antibiotics, appropriate in vitro culturing and susceptibility tests of samples taken before treatment should be conducted.
Dosage and Administration: The recommended dose of Albaplex (tetracycline hydrochloride and novobiocin) Tablets for dogs is: 10 mg of each antibiotic per lb of body weight (one tablet for each 6 lbs) repeated at 12 hour intervals. This dose can be given as follows:

Body Weight	Tablets Every 12 Hours
5 to 8 lb	1
9 to 15 lb	2
16 to 24 lb	3
25 to 40 lb	5
41 to 65 lb	8

Treatment should be continued for at least 48 hours after the temperature has returned to normal and all evidence of infection has disappeared.
Warning: Not for Human Use.
Caution: Federal (U.S.A.) law restricts this drug to use by or on the order of a licensed veterinarian.
Side Effects: Since the use of any broad spectrum antibiotic may result in overgrowth of nonsusceptible organisms, constant observation of the animal patient is essential. If new infections appear during therapy, appropriate measures should be taken.
Because of the wide antibacterial effect of this antibiotic combination on intestinal flora, a change in the character of the stools may be anticipated in certain animals; however, administration of novobiocin and tetracycline, combined, to dogs at exaggerated dosages daily for six months caused no significant toxic effects. If allergic reactions develop during treatment with Albaplex Tablets, use should be discontinued.
How Supplied: Albaplex (tetracycline hydrochloride and novobiocin) Tablets are supplied in bottles of 500.

BIO-DELTA®
brand of penicillin G procaine, dihydrostreptomycin sulfate, and prednisolone sterile aqueous suspension
For Veterinary Use Only

Description:
Bio-Delta Sterile Aqueous Suspension, designed for use in horses and foals, contains a combination of two antibiotics—penicillin G procaine and dihydrostreptomycin sulfate, which supply complementary antibacterial effect against certain bacterial pathogens—and prednisolone, which supplies anti-stress and anti-inflammatory effects. It is a free-flowing sterile aqueous suspension ready for immediate use.
Each ml contains:
penicillin G procaine..200,000 Int. units
dihydrostreptomycin sulfate
equiv. to dihydro-
streptomycin ....250 mg
prednisolone anhydrous
(as prednisolone hydrous)..........10 mg
also
lecithin..2.8 mg
sodium citrate hydrous..................10 mg
povidone.......................................3.17 mg
methylparaben ....1.05 mg

propylparaben ....0.105 mg
added as preservatives

Combined Penicillin-Dihydrostreptomycin Therapy

Since the antibacterial spectra of penicillin and dihydrostreptomycin are, in general, complementary, the combined range of antibacterial activity of this effective antibiotic combination includes both gram-positive and gram-negative organisms. Moreover, bacteriologic studies have demonstrated enhancement of bactericidal effect against certain organisms as well as marked delay in the development of bacterial resistance.

Prednisolone

Prednisolone, a derivative of hydrocortisone, has greater glucocorticoid activity, greater anti-inflammatory activity, less sodium-retaining effect, and less potassium-losing effect than the parent compound. The glucocorticoid activity of prednisolone is approximately three times that of hydrocortisone.

Combined Antibiotic-Adrenocortical Therapy

Bio-Delta Sterile Aqueous Suspension has been purposefully formulated to facilitate the combined use of penicillin, dihydrostreptomycin, and prednisolone. It provides the complementary antibacterial effects of the antibiotics plus the metabolic supportive and anti-inflammatory actions of prednisolone in a convenient injectable form. By virtue of the antibiotic-adrenocortical ratio employed, Bio-Delta retains the advantage of adaptable therapeutic control, i.e., when the infection is more severe, the accompanying stress and manifestation of systemic toxicity are generally greater, thus increasing the need for more intensive antibiotic therapy and adrenocortical support. The development of Bio-Delta was prompted by the growing emphasis that the role of corticosteroids in the management of bacterial infections accompanied by stress, toxemia, and inflammation is an adjuvant one, and that they should be used to supplement standard antibacterial therapy. With this combined formulation, it is possible to circumvent some of the very real stress and inflammatory problems encountered in animals ill with acute or chronic bacterial infections.

Indications

This preparation is indicated in the treatment of acute and chronic bacterial infections due to organisms susceptible to penicillin G and dihydrostreptomycin, or to organisms more susceptible to the combination than to either antibiotic alone, and in which stress and inflammation are important contributing factors. It is indicated in the following infections when caused by penicillin G-sensitive or dihydrostreptomycin-sensitive organisms and when accompanied by undue stress, toxemia, or inflammation: ***Horses***—pneumonia and postoperative prophylaxis. Not to be used in horses to be slaughtered for purposes of human consumption.

While mortality and morbidity have been decreased in such viral diseases as equine distemper, this must be attributed to control of secondary bacterial invaders rather than to any specific antiviral effect, and to established antistress and anti-inflammatory effects.

All necessary procedures for establishment of bacterial diagnosis should be carried out whenever possible before institution of therapy. Combined antibiotic-corticosteroid therapy does not obviate the need for indicated surgical procedures.

Contraindications

As with cortisone, hydrocortisone, and their adrenocortical derivatives, use of this product is contraindicated in the presence of tuberculosis, Cushingoid syndrome, and peptic ulcer. Congestive heart failure, and osteoporosis are relative contraindications.

Bio-Delta Sterile Aqueous Suspension should not be administered to animals known to be sensitive to penicillin G procaine, or dihydrostreptomycin.

Warnings

For veterinary use in horses only; not for use in horses to be slaughtered for human consumption.

While rare in animals, if allergic reactions that are not readily controlled by antihistaminic drugs develop during treatment, use of this product should be discontinued. In animals with impaired renal function, care must be taken in adjusting dosage since retention of the dihydrostreptomycin with subsequent toxic manifestations may develop.

Dihydrostreptomycin, particularly when used in high doses for prolonged periods, is associated with eighth nerve toxicity (i.e., impairment of hearing and to a lesser extent vertigo). The smaller doses of dihydrostreptomycin required in combined penicillin-dihydrostreptomycin therapy reduce the risk of toxic reactions associated with larger doses of the antibiotic. Animals receiving Bio-Delta Sterile Aqueous Suspension should be watched for signs of eighth nerve toxicity. If loss of hearing or vestibular disturbances occur, use of this product should be discontinued, unless the animal's condition justifies the risk of continuing therapy. In order to obviate these effects, strict adherence to the dosage schedule is recommended.

Clinical and experimental data have demonstrated that corticosteroids administered orally or parenterally to animals may induce the first stage of parturition when administered during the last trimester of pregnancy and may precipitate premature parturition followed by dystocia, fetal death, retained placenta, and metritis.

Additionally, corticosteroids administered to dogs, rabbits, and rodents during pregnancy have resulted in cleft palate in offspring. Corticosteroids administered to dogs during pregnancy have also resulted in other congenital anomalies including deformed forelegs, phocomelia, and anasarca.

Precautions

Since the use of penicillin procaine G and dihydrostreptomycin may result in overgrowth of nonsusceptible organisms, particularly monilia, constant observation of the animal patient is essential. If new infections appear during therapy, appropriate measures should be taken.

Adverse Reactions

The over-all incidence of troublesome side effects is less with prednisolone than with therapeutically equivalent doses of hydrocortisone. While the use of Bio-Delta Sterile Aqueous Suspension in the doses recommended is not likely to induce the side effects commonly associated with prolonged or intensive adrenocorticoid therapy, overdosage may give rise to the following: glycosuria and hyperglycemia; nitrogen loss; epigastric distress; psychic effects, such as depression; and suppression of endogenous adrenocortical activity.

Prednisolone inhibits the processes involved in the production of inflammation and also suppresses or corrects the associated tissue changes. Vascular permeability is decreased, exudation diminished, migration of inflammatory cells markedly suppressed, and antibiotics thus permitted to exert their full effects. While in certain aspects this alteration of the inflammatory reaction by corticosteroid therapy may be beneficial, the suppression of inflammation, particularly locally, may mask signs of infection and facilitate spread of micro-organisms. However, in infections characterized by undue stress and overwhelming toxicity, prednisolone therapy, in conjunction with appropriate antibacterial therapy, is effective in combating stress, reducing mortality and morbidity, and improving the general attitude and appetite of the animal being treated. In addition, systemic manifestations, such as fever and signs of toxemia, may be suppressed. However, without conjoint use of an antibiotic to which the invading organism is sensitive, the injudicious use of adrenal hormones in animals with infections can be hazardous. A retardant effect on wound healing has not been encountered with prednisolone, but such a possibility should be considered when it is used following surgery.

Although penicillin is virtually nontoxic, it possesses a significant index of sensitization and may produce urticaria, anaphylaxis and skin rash in some subjects. Resuscitative drugs, such as epinephrine, antihistamines and intravenous corticosteroids should be readily available for emergency administration.

Administration and Dosage

The size of the animal, the severity of the infection, stress, and inflammation, and the effect desired should be considered in determining the dose. In order to provide high blood levels, th following recommended doses should be administered once or twice daily.

Horses.......................................6 to 10 ml
Foals...2 to 6 ml

Administer by deep ***intramuscular injection only;*** continue therapy for the shortest possible time compatible with maintenance of adequate clinical response. When antibacterial effect is not prompt, the dosage should be increased temporarily, with subsequent reduction

Continued on next page

Upjohn—Cont.

to the above recommended average dose as soon as the desired clinical effect is obtained. Antibacterial treatment should be continued for at least 48 hours after the temperature has returned to normal and all evidence has disappeared, and for at least three days after Bio-Delta Sterile Aqueous Suspension and other corticosteroid therapy have been withdrawn.

If prolonged therapy is anticipated, a high protein intake should be provided to keep the animal in positive nitrogen balance. In such cases, when discontinuing therapy, withdrawal should be accomplished by a gradual stepwise reduction in the daily dose.

How Supplied

Bio-Delta Sterile Aqueous Suspension is available in vials of 100 ml.

BIOLYTE™

Calf Electrolyte Formula

Description: Each 800 gram bottle of BIOLYTE Calf Electrolyte Formula contains: dextrose anhydrous, sodium bicarbonate, sodium chloride, potassium chloride, magnesium sulfate anhydrous. Each 80 grams of BIOLYTE provides: sodium, 134.0 mEq; potassium, 22.8 mEq; magnesium, 6.6 mEq; bicarbonate, 81.0 mEq; chloride, 75.8 mEq; dextrose, 68 grams.

Indications: BIOLYTE Calf Electrolyte Formula is recommended for oral use for nutritional support and re-establishment and maintenance of electrolyte balance in neonatal calves.

Directions for Use:

Warnings: Not for human use.

Preparation of Solution: Dissolve 80 grams (1/3 cup) of BIOLYTE Calf Electrolyte Formula in water and dilute to a total volume of 1 quart or dissolve 240 grams (1 cup) of BIOLYTE in water and dilute to a total volume of 3 quarts.

Dosage and Administration: Administer the solution by feeding or drench at the rate of 1 quart per 60 pounds bodyweight 3–4 times daily for 2 days as the only source of oral fluids. For the following 2 days the solution should be diluted 1:1 with the milk replacer and given at feeding time.

Caution: Avoid exposure to excessive heat. Store in dry place. Keep container tightly closed.

How Supplied: BIOLYTE Calf Electrolyte Formula is available in 800 gram, (28 oz) plastic bottles. U.S. Patent No. 3,928,574.

BIOSOL®

(neomycin sulfate) Liquid

Composition: Each ml contains: Neomycin Sulfate (commercial grade), 200 mg (equivalent to 140 mg neomycin).

Indications: For treatment of bacterial diarrheas and bacterial enteritis in cattle, swine, sheep, horses, poultry, and dogs.

Administration: Biosol Liquid may be given undiluted or diluted with water for individual treatment. For herd or flock treatment, it may be added to the drinking water that will be consumed by the affected animals or birds in 12 hours. It may also be given in the milk. When administered in the drinking water, no other water should be allowed during or just prior to the treatment period. Usually 1 day or 24 hours treatment is sufficient. Not for use in liquid feed supplements.

Caution: If symptoms persist after using this preparation for 2 or 3 days, the diagnosis should be redetermined.

Warning: Not for human use. Discontinue treatment prior to slaughter by at least the number of days listed below for the appropriate species:

Cattle	30 days
Swine and Sheep	20 days
Turkeys and Laying Hens	14 days
Broilers	5 days

Dosage: Dosage schedule for treatment of bacterial diarrheas—Oral use

Total Body Weight	*Daily Dose*
40 lb	16 drops
75 lb	1½ teaspoonful
150 lb	1 teaspoonful
500 lb	1 tablespoonful
1000 lb	1 fluid ounce

How Supplied: 16 oz (480 ml) bottle.

BIOSOL®

brand of neomycin sulfate tablets For Oral Veterinary Use Only

BIOSOL Tablets contain neomycin sulfate and are designed especially for use in dogs and cats. Each tablet contains neomycin sulfate 100 mg (equivalent to 70 mg neomycin).

Actions: Neomycin: a wide-spectrum antibiotic derived from the soil isolate *Streptomyces fradiae,* is not inactivated by gastrointestinal secretions, bacteria, or enzymes and is only sparingly absorbed into the systemic circulation. The antibacterial effect of orally administered neomycin is not diverted from the gut by absorption, or inactivatied by gastrointestinal secretions, bacteria, or enzymes.

Neomycin

Neomycin is bactericidal in low concentration against many Gram-positive and Gram-negative intestinal pathogens. Microorganisms do not readily develop resistance to neomycin. Recently, however, resistance to neomycin has been reported more frequently than in the past. It is relatively nonirritating. Neomycin possesses no known antiprotozoal, antifungal, or antiviral action. The results of *in vitro* studies of the effectiveness of neomycin in inhibiting representative specimens of both Gram-positive and Gram-negative organisms are listed in the following chart.

Minimum Inhibitory Concentration, Expressed in Micrograms per Ml, Required to Inhibit Test Organisms

A. aerogenes	0.14
E. coli	0.06
Paracolobactrum spp.	0.4
Past. multocida	0.3
Pr. vulgaris	0.13
Ps. aeruginosa	0.33
Sal. enteritidis	12.5
Sal. Typhimurium	2.1
Staph. albus	0.01
Staph. aureus	0.01
Strep. pyogenes	0.5
alpha-streptococci	0.01
beta-streptococci	0.03

Neomycin is stable to wide fluctuations in temperature. Important therapeutically is the fact that neomycin is essentially unabsorbed from the gastrointestinal tract, allowing full utilization against the offending bacteria within the gut. Also, neomycin is stable in the gastrointestinal tract in the presence of food, digestive ferments and enzymes, bacteria, products of bacterial growth, pus and pus-forming organisms, necrotic tissue, and changes in pH. Further, neomycin is nontoxic and nonirritating to sensitive tissue.

Indications: BIOSOL Tablets are indicated for the treatment of bacterial diarrheas of dogs and cats. BIOSOL Tablets are useful and effective in treating epizootic outbreaks of infectious diarrhea caused by bacteria sensitive to neomycin. BIOSOL Tablets are also of value as an aid in preventing enteric infections in animals known to be exposed or susceptible to organisms sensitive to neomycin.

Precautions: BIOSOL Tablets are intended for *oral use only.* Inasmuch as neomycin is only sparingly absorbed from the gastrointestinal tract, the antibacterial action of orally administered neomycin is concentrated within the gut. **BIOSOL Tablets do not provide systemic antibacterial effect when given orally.**

Dosage and Administration: The usual dose of BIOSOL Tablets for dogs and cats is one tablet per 20 lb. body weight, or according to the following average dosage schedule:

Total Body Weight	*Daily Dose*
5 lb	¼ tablet
10 lb	½ tablet
20 lb	1 tablet
40 lb	2 tablets
60 lb. and over	3 tablets

In **severe cases,** it may be necessary or desirable to repeat the dose at 8- to 12-hour intervals. If improvement is not noted in 2 to 3 days, the diagnosis should be redetermined, and appropriate therapeutic measures initiated.

Other accepted therapeutic procedures for the treatment of diarrheas and enteritis, such as the administration of parenteral infusion fluids to correct dehydration, the administration of parenteral vitamins to compensate for loss of B vitamins, and the parenteral use of antibiotics to combat generalized infections should be employed when indicated.

BIOSOL Tablets have the Following Advantages in Treating Gastrointestinal Infections:

1. Wide-spectrum effect against many enteric bacterial infections.
2. Bactericidal in low concentrations against many common intestinal path-

U

ogens, does not favor development of resistant strains.
3. Antibacterial action restricted to and concentrated in the gut.
4. Fully active in presence of gastrointestinal contents.
5. Nontoxic and nonirritating to sensitive tissues.
6. Allows intake of food and fluids.

How Supplied: BIOSOL Tablets are available in bottles of 1000.

BIOSOL AQUADROPS®
brand of neomycin sulfate liquid
For Oral Veterinary Use Only

Description: BIOSOL AQUADROPS Liquid contains neomycin sulfate and is designed for oral administration to dogs and cats for the treatment of bacterial enteric infection and bacterial diarrhea. Each ml contains neomycin sulfate, 50 mg (equivalent to 35 mg neomycin).

Actions: Neomycin: a wide-spectrum antibiotic derived from the soil isolate, *Streptomyces fradiae,* is not inactivated by gastrointestinal secretions, bacteria, or enzymes and is only sparingly absorbed into the systemic circulation. The antibacterial effect of orally administered neomycin is not diverted from the gut by absorption or inactivated by gastrointestinal secretion, bacteria, or enzymes.

Neomycin sulfate has a very wide antibacterial spectrum and is effective *in vitro* against *Staph. aureus,* hemolytic streptococci, *Pasteurella multocida, E. coli, Klebsiella spp., A. Aerogenes,* and other Gram-positive and Gram-negative bacteria. It is often bactericidal *in vitro* even in low concentrations. Microorganisms do not readily develop resistance to neomycin. Recently, however, resistance to neomycin has been reported more frequently than in the past. It is relatively nonirritating. Neomycin possesses no known antiprotozoal, antifungal or antiviral action.

Neomycin sulfate is unusually stable under many physical and chemical conditions. It is stable under wide fluctuations in temperature, in alkaline solution, in the presence of bacteria, bacterial byproducts, pus, exudates, or enzymes.

Indications: BIOSOL AQUADROPS Liquid is indicated for treatment of bacterial diarrheas of dogs and cats. It is useful and effective in treating epizootic outbreaks of infectious diarrhea caused by bacteria sensitive to neomycin. BIOSOL AQUADROPS is also of value as an aid in preventing enteric infections in animals known to be exposed or susceptible to organisms sensitive to neomycin.

Precautions: BIOSOL AQUADROPS Liquid is intended for *oral use only.* Inasmuch as neomycin is only sparingly absorbed from the gastrointestinal tract, the antibacterial action of orally administered BIOSOL AQUADROPS is concentrated within the gut and does not provide systemic antibacterial effect when given orally.

Warning: Not for Human Use.

Dosage and Administration: The recommended dosage for treatment of bacterial enteritis in dogs and cats is 5 mg (0.1 ml) neomycin sulfate per pound per day in divided doses every twelve hours. This dosage level is attained by the use of 1 ml per 20 lb of body weight given twice daily. The daily dosage may be measured as follows, using the enclosed calibrated dropper.

Total Body Weight	Dosage
5 lb	¼ ml B.I.D.
10 lb	½ ml B.I.D.
20 lb	1 ml B.I.D.

BIOSOL AQUADROPS Liquid may be given directly to the individual animal or may be added to the milk or feed.

If improvement is not noted in 2 to 3 days, the diagnosis should be redetermined, followed by appropriate therapeutic measures. Other accepted therapeutic procedures for the treatment of diarrheas and enteritis, such as the administration of parenteral infusion fluids to correct dehydration, the administration of parenteral vitamins to compensate for loss of B vitamins, and the parenteral use of antibiotics to combat generalized infections, should be employed when indicated.

BIOSOL AQUADROPS has the Following Advantages in Treating Gastrointestinal Infections:
1. May be given individually to animals or may be added to the milk or feed. BIOSOL AQUADROPS is palatable.
2. Wide-spectrum effect against many enteric bacterial infections.
3. Bactericidal in low concentrations against many intestinal pathogens; does not favor development of resistant strains.
4. Antibacterial action restricted to and concentrated in the gut.
5. Fully active in presence of gastrointestinal contents.
6. Nontoxic and nonirritating to sensitive tissues.
7. Allows intake of food and fluids.

How Supplied: BIOSOL AQUADROPS Liquid—50 mg neomycin sulfate per ml. Available in 10 ml bottles with direction labels and calibrated droppers.

BIOSOL® Bolus 500 mg
(neomycin sulfate)

Composition: Each bolus contains: Neomycin Sulfate 500 mg (equivalent to 350 mg neomycin).

A wide-spectrum antibiotic bolus for intrauterine or oral use in livestock.

Indications: Intra-uterine use—Biosol Bolus 500 mg is indicated in the treatment and control of bacterial infections of the uterus, vagina, and vulvovaginal area. It is particularly effective in preventing postparturient bacterial infections of the uterus.

Oral use: Biosol Bolus 500 mg is also indicated in the treatment and control of bacterial diarrheas and infectious enteritis—white scours in calves, foal dysentery, swine enteritis, and bacillary diarrheas of sheep and vibrio enteritis in cattle. It is particularly effective in treating enteric infections prevalent in the young of each species.

Warning: Not for human use. Discontinue treatment prior to slaughter by at least 30 days for cattle and calves and by at least 20 days for swine and sheep.

Milk that has been taken from animals during treatment and within 48 hours (4 milkings) after the latest treatment must not be used for food.

Caution: If symptoms persist after using this preparation for two or three days, the diagnosis should be redetermined. If the diarrhea condition is complicated with upper respiratory infections, systemic antibacterial treatment should be given. Biosol is intended for intra-uterine or oral use only and does not provide systemic antibacterial effect when given by these methods. Neomycin is only sparingly absorbed from the gastrointestinal tract, the antibacterial action of orally administered Biosol being concentrated within the gut.

Dosage and Administration: *Intrauterine use:* Cattle—2 to 4 boluses in the uterus or vagina. Repeat in 24 to 48 hours, if necessary. Swine and Sheep—for postparturient uterine use, insert ½ to 1 bolus into the uterus.

Oral use: Up to 50 pounds, ½ bolus daily; 50 to 100 pounds, 1 bolus daily; for each additional 100 pounds, 1 bolus daily. Where possible, best results are obtained when the daily dose is given in two to four divided doses. Three days of therapy are recommended for the average case, but treatment may be continued for five days, if necessary.

How Supplied: Bottles 100 boluses.

BIOSOL® 325
(neomycin sulfate)
Soluble Powder

Composition: Each pound contains: Neomycin Sulfate (commercial grade equiv. to 227.5 Gm. Neomycin), 325 Gm.

Dosage and Administration: Dosage Schedule and Administration for the treatment of bacterial enteritis in livestock and poultry.

The recommended daily oral dose of neomycin sulfate is 5 mg. per pound of body weight.

One level tablespoonful (U.S. Std. Measure) will deliver 10 Gm. Biosol 325 Powder, equal to 7 Gm. neomycin sulfate—the daily dose for 1,400 pounds of body weight.

The appropriate dose should be added to the drinking water which will be consumed by the animals in 12 hours. Water freshly medicated with the powder should be prepared daily. Allow no other source of water during the treatment period.

For swine under average conditions, the recommended dose will be consumed if one level tablespoonful is added to each 14 gallons of drinking water. For use in automatic proportiners delivering 1 ounce of stock solution per gallon of drinking water, dissolve 9 level tablespoonful in a gallon of water to make the stock solution. This water dosage may need to be varied under extreme temperature conditions. The dosage per pound of body weight as given above should be the basic guide for dosage.

Continued on next page

Upjohn—Cont.

The powder may also be mixed with milk or dry feed. Not for use in liquid feed supplements. In dry feed, Biosol 325 should be used as follows:
Treatment of bacterial enteritis—5 or 10 oz. (14 or 28 level tablespoonsful) Biosol 325 per ton of feed (100 or 200 Gm. neomycin sulfate).
To aid in thorough mixing, Biosol 325 should be blended with about 50 lb. of feed prior to mixing into larger quantities. One lb. of Biosol 325 may be mixed with 31.5 lb. of feed and this mixture added at the rate of 5, 10, or 20 lb. per ton of complete ration to provide 50, 100, or 200 grams neomycin sulfate.
For the treatment of bacterial enteritis, use medicated feed or water for 3 to 5 days.
Caution: If no improvement is seen within 3 days, redetermine the diagnosis.
Warning: Not for human use. Discontinue treatment prior to slaughter by at least the number of days listed below for appropriate species:

Cattle	30 days
Swine and Sheep	20 days
Turkeys and Laying Hens	14 days
Broilers	5 days

How Supplied: 1 lb. jar.

CHEQUE® DROPS
(mibolerone)
For canine estrus prevention
For oral use in adult female dogs

Composition: Cheque (mibolerone) Drops are 17-β-hydroxy-7α, 17-dimethylestr-4-en-3-one, generic name mibolerone, a non-progestational steroid. In its pure form, mibolerone is a white crystalline solid. The compound is stable under ordinary conditions and temperatures.
Actions: More than 90 percent of normal, mature cycling bitches did not exhibit estrus when administered Cheque (mibolerone) Drops in adequate doses.
Mibolerone has been shown to be an anabolic and androgenic steroid in rats. When compared to methyltestosterone, it is 41 times more potent as an anabolic agent and 16 times more potent as an androgen. Mibolerone has no estrogenic activity in mice when used at levels up to 1.0 mg per animal per day. It is antiestrogenic in mice in intravaginal tests at 0.9 mcg and in subcutaneous tests at 10 mcg or less when tested against estradiol.
In the bitch, mibolerone has androgenic, anabolic and antigonadotrophic activity. Mibolerone selectively blocks the luteinizing hormone (LH) peak thereby preventing estrual activity. No significant progestational nor estrogenic activity has been demonstrated in the canine.
Metabolism: Based on tritium labeled studies in the bitch, approximately equal quantities of mibolerone were excreted via the urine and feces. Mibolerone was extensively metabolized, being excreted as over 10 metabolites. Mibolerone was present in most tissues with highest concentrations being in the liver, anal glands and reproductive organs. Significant levels of radioactivity occurred along the digestive tract.
Canine Efficacy: Mibolerone dosage for estrous prevention was evaluated in 13 breeds of purebred dogs in kennels. It was also field tested in a substantial number of bitches. Based on kennel trials and in home evaluations for various periods of time, more than 90 percent of normal, mature cycling bitches did not exhibit estrus when administered Cheque (mibolerone) Drops in adequate dosage.
Animal Toxicology: Beagles treated orally for 28 days with mibolerone at a level of 300 mcg/kg had no drug related alterations in hematology or blood chemistry and no toxic symptoms were observed.
In a subsequent test, mibolerone was administered orally to Beagles at the rate of 3,000 to 30,000 mcg/kg daily for 28 days. Clinical chemistry, hematology, urinalysis, including urine concentration test, gross pathology and histopathology showed no drug related toxic effects. The only drug related effects included a reduction of the stainable lipid in the adrenal cortices, enlargement of the clitoris, thickening of the myometrium and endometrium, and inhibition of spermatogenesis (3,000 mcg/kg level). All treated dogs had periodic episodes of epiphora. There was an apparent drug related increase in renal, uterine, and prostatic weights and a decrease in the ovarian, testicular and thymic weights.
Beagles, male and female, have been treated with levels of mibolerone of up to 500 mcg per day for 240 days and 200 mcg per day for up to 730 days. The incidence of vaginal irritation and clitoral enlargement was more pronounced in the immature than mature bitch. Other effects included: (1) blockage of tertiary but not primary or secondary follicular development, (2) maintenance of prepubertal ovarian and uterinecervical weights in the immature treated bitches, (3) a slight decrease in adrenal weights without evidence of altered morphology or function, (4) an increase in kidney weight without evidence of altered morphology or function, (5) a decrease in prostate weight in high dose immature dogs. Treated males and females had slight increases in mean SGOT (serum glutamic oxalacetic transaminase, or aspartate transaminase) and SGPT (serum glutamic pyruvic transaminase or alanine transaminase) without evidence of hepatocellular damage (based on light microscopy) or alteration of hepatic function (based on BSP retention and clinical chemistry).
After terminating mibolerone treatment, Beagle bitches returned to cyclic estrous activity as soon as 7 days after last treatment with the longest interval being somewhat over 200 days. In a study involving 96 bitches bred starting their first estrus after the end of mibolerone treatment, bitches had a normal pregnancy and delivery and had normal pups. Mibolerone bitches had a lower conception rate for all breedings compared to untreated bitches (76% vs 100%). However, percent mibolerone treated bitches whelping of those conceiving (97%) was similar to untreated bitches (90%).
Weaned Beagle puppies (7–15 weeks of age, averaging 6.36 kg in weight) were treated daily with levels of mibolerone up to 200,000 mcg per day for 30 days. During the fourth week of treatment, the animals receiving 200,000 mcg per day showed excessive lacrimation, depression, anorexia, weight loss and myalgia. No gross lesions occured at necropsy. An expected dose related uterotropic resonse occurred as well as marked increase in prostate weight. A dose related decrease occurred in adrenal weight at 4,000 and 200,000 mcg/animal/day. Histologically there was a slight fatty change in the livers of 3 of 4 females receiving 200,000 mcg per day.
Mibolerone was administered six times a week for up to 9.6 years (average 6.1 years) to bitches of seven breeds of dogs. The average of all dogs at time of their termination was 9.7 years. Sixty-three bitches served as nontreated controls, 103 bitches received 30 to 180 mcg mibolerone per day to approximate the efficacious dose, and 61 bitches were given 90 to 900 mcg mibolerone per day as an exaggerated dose. Study bitches were evaluated with physical examinations, hematology, and clinical chemistry. Tissues of dogs which died during the study and those of dogs killed at study termination were evaluated histopathologically. Dogs were tested also for changes in peripheral circulation concentrations of both cortisol in response to ACTH and triiodothyronine and thyroxin to TSH.
Chronic oral administration of mibolerone was associated with an increased incidence of chronic liver disease with controls, 1X, and the exaggerated dose groups showing 57, 91, and 93 percent of the dogs with diseased livers, respectively. Drug administration was also associated with cirrhosis with controls, 1X, and exaggerated dose groups having 4, 10, and 28 percent of the dogs with cirrhosis, respectively. An increased prevalence of hepatocellular intranuclear crystalline inclusion bodies was found in many treated bitches.
Treatment related reproductive tract lesions included ovarian arterial mineralization, endometrial atrophy, endometrial cysts, endocervical cysts, vaginal mucosal atrophy, invaginations and cysts of the vaginal mucosa, vaginitis , clitoral ossification and clitoritis at the efficacious and exaggerated doses. A 10% incidence of ovarian fibroma was found in bitches given the approximate efficacious dose, only; an increased incidence of ovarian folllicular cysts was found in bitches given the exaggerated dose.
Chronic mibolerone exposure was also associated with decreased numbers of corpora lutea and vaginal fibromas at the efficacious and exaggerated doses.
Treatment related findings from other organs included increased incidences of mineral deposition in the kidneys, adre-

nal cortical lipidosis and a reduction in the incidence of mammary neoplasms and total neoplasms, all at the efficacious and exaggerated doses.

The Beagle, but not the other six breeds, appeared to have a reduced response to ACTH challenge. Epiphora appeared to be mibolerone related in Toy Poodles and Beagles.

The therapeutic dose of mibolerone kept females out of heat and did not elicit side effects or clinical health problems that would prevent the animal from being a functional pet. The dogs fed mibolerone at exaggerated doses were not compromised as judged by their fitness to be a functional pet, based on clinical evaluations.

Adult bitches of mixed breeding receiving 60 mcg of mibolerone daily for up to 1,574 days showed no signs of toxicity. A drug related increase in clitoral size occurred but it was not deemed to be objectionable.

Adult Beagle bitches were started on mibolerone treatment orally at 20 or 60 mcg per animal per day starting 1, 3 or 6 days after the first two breedings and were continued on treatment until weaning. Conception and implantation were not prevented in bitches started on treatment after breeding. Gestation, parturition, and lactation were normal in all bitches. Female pups from the animals receiving mibolerone were masculinized. No other lesions were observed.

One study indicated liver tissue changes such as cellular swelling, obliterations of sinusoids, vascular degeneration, leukocyte infiltration and fibrosis.

The acute oral LD_{50} in the rat is greater than 1,600,000 mcg/kg while the intraperitoneal LD_{50} in the mouse is 555,600 mcg/kg.

Mibolerone has been well tolerated in rats at levels of 3,000 or 10,000 or 30,000 mcg/kg orally for up to 28 days. Changes observed included hypertrophy of the myometrium, reduction of the amount of stainable lipid in all three zones of the adrenal cortices, arrest of spermatogenesis and atrophy of the accesory sex gland of male rats at 3,000 and 10,000 mcg/kg. Treated animals ate less than the controls and required more food per unit of body weight gain.

The dose of mibolerone was increased at equal increments weekly from 600 mcg/kg the first week to 4,800 mcg/kg the fourth week in rats. A reduction in food consumption and a reduction in weight gain were noted. Treated males had a leukocytosis. No other toxic effects or changes in hemotology or in gross or microscopic pathology were observed in either males or females. Rats exposed under dynamic conditions for one hour to a dust aerosol of mibolerone at a concentration of 5.03 mg/liter of air did not have any signs of toxicity during exposure or during a 14 day post treatment observation period.

Ointment containing mibolerone at a concentration of 0.25% was applied to abraded and unabraded rabbit skin daily for five days. The ointment was slightly irritating to the unbraded skin of the abdomen while it was not irritating to abraded skin.

Indications: Cheque (mibolerone) Drops are administered orally for estrous (heat) prevention in adult female dogs not intended primarily for breeding purposes. Cheque Drops dosage should be discontinued after 24 months of use.

Cheque Drops are effective in preventing estrus only when drug administration is initiated 30 days prior to the start of the proestrus. It should not be used in an attempt to abbreviate an estrous period. It should not be used in bitches prior to the first estrous period.

Contraindications: (Also See Warnings) Cheque (mibolerone) Drops should not be used in a pregnant bitch or female dogs with perianal adenoma, perianal adenocarcinoma, or other androgen dependent neoplastic conditions. Cheque should not be administered to any animal with a prior history of liver or kidney disease.

Warning: Not for human use. One study in humans indicated a potential altered liver function that resulted in termination of the study.

Do Not Administer For More Than 24 Months.

Precautions: Cheque (mibolerone) Drops should be administered only to normal, mature, nonpregnant, nonlactating bitches, as directed and should not be administered to immature bitches, male dogs, puppies or cats. Cheque Drops should not be administered to bitches intended primarily for breeding purposes.

Cheque Drops should not be administered to any animal with prior history of liver or kidney disease. Liver serum enzyme elevations may be encountered. Some androgens may result in jaundice in particularly sensitive animals. This effect has been observed in a few animals administered Cheque Drops at the therapeutic level. If jaundice does occur, Cheque Drops treatment should be discontinued. Periodic liver function tests are recommended under prolonged administration. SGPT values were evaluated and appear to be an appropriate criterion for monitoring liver changes.

Cheque Drops should be used with caution in the younger mature bitch (approximately 7 months old or less) in that steroids with androgenic activity can result in early epiphyseal closure. This effect on skeletal development has, however, not been observed with mibolerone treatment. Some immature bitches are especially responsive to the androgenicity of Cheque Drops with marked clitoral enlargement and low grade vaginitis resulting from prolonged therapy. Topical antibiotic-corticosteroid ointments for genital application may be used if the irritation results in problem discharges. Failure to respond to topical treatment indicates the animal is no longer a candidate for Cheque Drops.

Cheque Drops should be used with caution in animals with chronic epiphora or other conditions involving the lacrimal apparatus. Testing in miniature and Toy Poodles has, however, not resulted in detectable aggravation of existing epiphora.

If Cheque Drops dosage is started and then the bitch comes into estrus, Cheque Drops may be continued but caution should be taken to prevent breeding. If breeding occurs, Cheque Drops dosage should be stopped until such time as the bitch is determined not to be pregnant.

Cheque Drops should not be used concurrently with or following use of any progestational or estrogenic compound until potential clinical abnormalities associated with use of those compounds are eliminated.

Drug Interactions: The following classes of drugs have been administered concurrently during mibolerone therapy without apparent problems being observed: general and local anesthetics, analgesic/antipyretics, anthelmintics—parasitacides, antibacterials—fungicides, corticosteroids and biologicals. However, dogs administered pharmaceuticals or biologicals concurrrent with Cheque (mibolerone) Drops should be carefully monitored for possible interactions.

Data from a well controlled study support the concurrent uses of mibolerone and styrylpyridinium chloride-diethylcarbamazine citrate when the latter is used for prevention of heart worm infections. Concurrent therapy of the pharmaceuticals altered neither the efficacy nor safety of mibolerone or of styrylpyridinium chloride-diethylcarbamazine citrate.

Seizure activity has been reported in a previously controlled epileptic patient while simultaneously receiving mibolerone and diphenylhydantoin.

Adverse Reactions: Some animals, particularly immature females, have shown increased sensitivity to mibolerone. This sensitivity has been expressed by clitoral enlargement and white viscid discharge consisting of leukocytes originating from the clitoral fossa. If irritation of the vaginal vestibule persists some bitches may develop mounting behavior. Occasional bitches have had a musky body odor.

In clinical evaluation of Cheque (mibolerone) Drops the following side effects have been attributed to Cheque at estrus inhibiting doses (listed as a % of total clinical cases reporting): Clitoral enlargement (20%); vaginal discharge (10%); riding behavior (1.6%); epiphora (5.6%), objectionable body odor (4.3%). Percent of all reported side effects was 45.4. A common finding after prolonged dosage was the presence of small (<1 mm diameter) vesicles on the vaginal mucosa posterior to the urethral orifice. The clinical significance of these vesicles has not been determined.

Since the market introduction of Cheque Drops, certain clinical signs have been reported as being associated with dogs receiving the drug. The actual role of mibolerone in the ellicitation of those signs has not in all cases been determined. In decreasing order of frequency, they are:

Continued on next page

U

Upjohn—Cont.

1. Expression of estrus—generally due to failure to receive proper dose.
2. Vaginal/uterine discharge—may lead to diagnostic problems: e.g. mimic heat, confuse diagnosis of uterine disease.
3. Mating—may occur during estrus break or false estrus due to genital discharge.
4. Hepatic dysfunction as evidenced by jaundice, hepatomegaly, cirrhosis, and occasional deaths have been reported.
5. Increased aggressiveness—a recognizable side effect of androgenic substances.

Dosage and Administration: Cheque (mibolerone) Drops dosage is as follows (administer orally once each day by adding to a small amount of food or directly to the mouth):

Weight of Bitch (Lbs)	Cheque Drops Daily Dosage ml	mcg
1 to 25	0.3	30
26 to 50	0.6	60
51 to 100	1.2	120
101 and over	1.8	180
German Shepherd Dog or German Shepherd Mix (All Weights)	1.8	180

Cheque Drops Volume Dispensed (Bottle Size)	Approximate Days of Treatment For Different Dose Levels Daily Dose (ml) .3	.6	1.2	1.8
55.0 ml	180	90	45	30

How Supplied: Cheque (mibolerone) Drops are available in bottles of 55 ml fill with graduated dropper. Each ml contains 100 mcg mibolerone and propylene glycol, qs.

Caution: Federal (U.S.A.) law restricts this drug to use by or on the order of a licensed veterinarian.

U

CORTABA®
(methylprednisolone and acetylsalicylic acid) Compressed Tablets

Composition: Each tablet contains Medrol® (methylprednisolone), 0.5 mg.; aspirin, 300 mg. (5 gr); preserved with ascorbic acid.

This oral formulation, especially suitable for use in dogs, combines the unique anti-inflammatory action of Medrol and the effective analgesic action of aspirin.

Actions: Methylprednisolone. Methylprednisolone, an anti-inflammatory steroid synthesized and developed in the Research Laboratories of The Upjohn Company, is the 6-methyl derivative of prednisolone. Exceeding prednisolone in anti-inflammatory potency and having even less tendency than prednisolone to induce sodium and water retention, methylprednisolone offers the advantage over older corticosteroids of affording equally satisfactory anti-inflammatory effect with the use of lower doses and with an enhanced split between anti-inflammatory and mineralocorticoid activities.

The glucocorticoid activity of methylprednisolone in the liver-glycogen deposition test in adrenalectomized rats is three times that of prednisolone. In anti-inflammatory activity, as measured by the granuloma pouch assay, methylprednisolone is twice as active as prednisolone. In mineralocorticoid activity, methylprednisolone is slightly less active than prednisolone. The duration of plasma steroid levels following rapid intravenous injection in intact dogs is appreciably longer for methylprednisolone than for prednisolone, the respective "half-life" value for the two steroids being 80.9± 7.5 minutes for methylprednisolone and 71.3± 1.7 for prednisolone.

Aspirin. Aspirin continues to be one of the most useful drugs available for controlling pain in canine practice. Its efficiency in suppressing pain is well recognized, but the mechanism of this action remains unexplained. Certain experimental studies suggest a direct anti-inflammatory effect at the cellular level. Aspirin is absorbed rapidly from the upper gastrointestinal tract and is excreted principally in the urine; in the presence of impaired renal function, salicylism or salicylate intoxication may occur on doses smaller than those generally conceded tolerable for long-term use. Compared with sodium salicylate, aspirin is a more potent analgesic (on a weight basis) and has less local irritant effect on the gastrointestinal tract. Serious reactions to aspirin occur infrequently in dogs. **Vomiting will occur on overdosing.**

Indications for Dogs: These tablets are indicated whenever the anti-inflammatory effect of methylprednisolone and the analgesic effect of aspirin are desired. The following conditions when of mild to moderate severity are indications: (1) musculoskeletal conditions, such as myositis, fibrositis, neuritis, rheumatoid arthritis, osteoarthritis, spondylitis, bursitis and tenosynovitis; (2) ocular conditions, such as iritis, iridocyclitis, secondary glaucoma, uveitis, chorioretinitis; (3) otic conditions, such as otitis externa; (4) dermal conditions, such as non-specific dermatitis, and burns; (5) allergic manifestations, such as acute uticaria, allergic dermatitis, summer eczema, drug and serum reactions, bronchial asthma, and pollen sensitivities.

Contraindications: As with other adrenocorticosteroid hormones, methylprednisolone is contraindicated in the presence of tuberculosis, chronic nephritis, Cushingoid syndrome, and peptic ulcer. Presence of diabetes mellitus, osteoporosis, predisposition to thrombophlebitis, hypertension, and congestive heart failure necessitates carefully controlled use of this product.

CORTABA SHOULD NOT BE ADMINISTERED TO CATS. Because of the intolerance of cats and other felines to salicylates, this preparation should not be used on these species.

Warning: Clinical and experimental data have demonstrated that corticosteroids administered orally or parenterally to animals may induce the first stage of parturition when administered during the last trimester of pregnancy and may precipitate premature parturition followed by dystocia, fetal death, retained placenta, and metritis. Additionally, corticosteroids administered to dogs, rabbits and rodents during pregnancy have resulted in cleft palate in offspring. Corticosteroid administered to dogs during pregnancy have also resulted in other congenital anomalies including deformed forelegs, phocomelia, and anasarca.

Precautions: Because methylprednisolone manifests little sodium-retaining activity, the usual early sign of adrenocorticoid overdosage (i.e., increase in body weight due to fluid retention) is not a reliable index of methylprednisolone overdosage. Hence, recommended dose levels should not be exceeded.

Canine patients receiving Cortaba should have close medical supervision, and the same precautions that apply to other adrenocorticoids should be observed, namely: (1) symptoms of infection may be masked; (2) co-existent or intercurrent acute infectious diseases should be treated promptly and adequately with appropriate antibacterial measures; and (3) in the event of any unusual stress, adequate adrenocortical reserve should be insured by the supplemental use of cortisone or hydrocortisone.

Adverse Reactions: Use in the dosages herein recommended is not likely to induce undesirable effects associated with adrenocorticoid therapy or administration of salicylates. Undesirable effects of adrenocorticoid administration are sodium and water retention, potassium loss, glycosuria, hyperglycemia, polyuria, and polydipsia. Those of salicylism are vomiting and weakness.

Doses for Dogs: The dosage will vary according to the size of the animal, the nature and severity of the condition being treated, and the effect desired. Suggested dosage is as follows: for dogs under 15 lb, from ¼ to 1 tablet daily; for dogs 15 to 60 lb, 1 to 2 tablets daily; or dogs 60 lb. and over, 2 tablets daily.

The total daily dose should be administered in divided doses, if possible, along with a light feeding. The starting dosage may be continued until a satisfactory clinical response has been obtained, at which time gradual reduction in dosage should be attempted in order to determine the minimal effective dose level. When long-term treatment is discontinued, it should be accomplished by a gradual stepwise reduction of the daily dose.

How Supplied: Bottles 1000 tablets.

DELTA ALBAPLEX®
(tetracycline hydrochloride, novobiocin, and prednisolone) Tablets

Important Note: The prednisolone component of Delta Albaplex (tetracycline, novobiocin and prednisolone) has been shown to contribute to clinical response if administered only for the first *48 hours* of treatment. Subsequent antibacterial treatment is to be continued with Albaplex® (tetracycline and novobiocin). See *Indications* and *Dosage* Sections following.

Description: This oral antibiotic corticosteroid formulation contains prednisolone, which provides a faster clinical response in the indicated conditions, and a combination of two antibiotics—tetracycline and novobiocin—which supplies additive antibacterial effect against certain bacterial pathogens. Each tablet contains: tetracycline hydrochloride 60 mg; Novobiocin sodium equiv. to novobiocin 60 mg; prednisolone anhydrous 1.5 mg.

Actions

Tetracycline hydrochloride is an odorless, yellow, fine crystalline powder which is freely soluble in water and gastric juice. It is absorbed readily from the gastrointestinal tract. Following oral administration to dogs, peak blood concentrations are obtained within two to four hours, high levels are found at twelve hours, and detectable amounts remain in the serum for at least 24 hours. The antibiotic is excreted principally through the kidney.

The *in vitro* spectrum of antimicrobial activity of tetracycline hydrochloride includes a broad range of gram-positive and gram-negative bacterial such as alpha and beta streptococci, some strains of staphylococci, *Klebsiella pneumoneia*, certain clostridia, Shiegella, *Aerobacter aerogenes*, and some strains of Salmonella. The clinical significance of this has not been determined.

In an *in vivo* study, it was shown that tetracycline hydrochloride is significantly more effective than novobiocin in eliminating pathogenic streptococci.

Studies conducted in laboratory animals show that tetracycline hydrochloride has a low order of toxicity comparable to that of the other tetracyclines.

Novobiocin is an antibiotic produced by *Streptomyces niveus* and developed in the Research Laboratories of The Upjohn Company. The crystalline antibiotic has a light yellow to white color, depending upon the state of subdivision. In contrast to most antibiotics produced by actinomycetes, novobiocin, like penicillin, is acidic in nature and is stable to the degree of acidity or alkalinity present in the gastrointestinal tract. Following oral administration of 10 mg per kg to dogs, peak blood concentrations are obtained within one or two hours, significant levels are found at twelve hours. When an appreciable amount of Albamycin (novobiocin) is present in the serum, the drug diffuses into the pleural and ascitic fluids. Novobiocin does not diffuse into the cerebrospinal fluid. The antibiotic is concentrated in the liver and bile and is excreted in the feces and urine. As determined by tests in animals, Albamycin has a relatively low order of toxicity.

In vitro studies show that novobiocin is active against both gram-positive and gram-negative bacteria, including some strains of *Staphylococcus aureus*, *Streptococcus hemolyticus*, *Diplococcus pneumoniae*, and some strains of *Proteus vulgaris*. The clinical significance of this has not been determined, novobiocin shows no cross-resistance with penicillin against resistant strains of *Staphylococcus aureus*. However, *in vitro* studies indicate that *Staphylococcus aureus* may develop resistance to novobiocin as with other antibiotics.

Prednisolone

Prednisolone, a derivative of hydrocortisone, has greater glucocorticoid activity, greater antiinflammatory activity, less sodium-retaining effect, and less potassium-losing effect than the parent compound. The glucocorticoid activity of prendisolone is approximately three times that of hydrocortisone, and the dose required to produce a given anti-inflammatory effect in dogs is of the order of one-fourth to one-third the required dose of hydrocortisone (or about one-fifth the required dose of cortisone).

Prednisolone exerts an inhibitory influence on the cellular, fibrous, and amorphous components of connective tissue and thereby suppresses the basic processes of inflammation. Vascular permeability is decreased, exudation diminished, migration of inflammatory cells markedly impaired. In infections characterized by stress and/or toxicity, prednisolone therapy, in conjunction with properly indicated antibacterial therapy, is helpful in combating stress, reducing clincial signs and in speeding the recovery of the animal being treated.

Combined Antibiotic-Adrenocortical Therapy

Delta Albaplex Tablets have been formulated to provide for the use of tetracycline hydrochloride, novobiocin, and prednisolone. It provides a broad antibacterial effect from the combined antibiotics plus the anti-inflammatory effects of prednisolone.

Combined antibiotic therapy offers a wider range of antibacterial activity than therapy with single antibiotics. *In vitro* studies with tetracycline hydrochloride and novobiocin have indicated that this antibiotic combination is effective against such organisms as *Staphylococcus aureus*, *Streptococcus fecalis*, and *Proteus rettgeri*. Moreover, *in vitro* studies have shown that the development of resistance by *Staphylococcus aureus* to a combination of tetracycline hydrochloride and novobiocin occurs at a markedly slower rate than to either antibiotic alone. Studies in mice infected with *Staphylococcus aureus* have indicated that tetracycline hydrochloride and novobiocin are compatible *in vivo* against the strains tested.

An *in vivo* clinical study in dogs has shown that the combination of novobiocin and tetracycline hydrochloride is significantly more effective than either single antibiotic in eliminating pathogenic *Staphylococcus spp.* and *E. coli* from the throats of dogs suffering from upper respiratory disease. This study also showed that the incidence of treatment failure is significantly reduced when novobiocin and tetracyclilne hydrochloride are administered concurrently.

In dogs with upper respiratory infections, the prednisolone component of Delta Albaplex results in a significantly faster reduction in the clinical signs of illness in the first 48 hours of treatment than is achievable by therapy with novobiocin and tetracycline, either singly or in combination. After 48 hours, treatment is to be continued for 3 days with Albaplex (tetracycline-novobiocin).

Indications: Delta Albaplex tablets are indicated in the treatment of acute or chronic upper respiratory conditions, i.e. tonsilitis, bronchitis, and tracheobronchitis, when it is necessary to initially reduce the severity of associated clinical signs and when caused by pathogens susceptible to novobiocin and tetracycline such as *Staphyloccus spp.* and *E. Coli.*

The product has been shown to be of maximum benefit when used during the first 48 hours of treatment. Subsequently therapy should be continued with Albaplex (novobiocin-tetracycline) for an additional 3 days or longer as needed.

As with all antibiotics, appropriate *in vitro* culturing and susceptibility tests should be conducted on samples taken before treatment is started.

Contraindications: As with other adrenocorticordal steroids, this product is contraindicated in animals with tuberculosis, hyperadrenocorticism and peptic ulcer.

Warning: Clinical and experimental data have demonstrated that corticosteroids administered orally or parenterally to animals may induce the first stage of parturition when administered during the last trimester of pregnancy and may precipitate premature parturition followed by dystocia, fetal death, retained placenta, and metritis. Additionally, corticosteroids administered to dogs, rabbits, and rodents during pregnancy have resulted in cleft palate in offspring. Corticosteroids administered to dogs during pregnancy have also resulted in other congenital anomalies, including deformed forelegs, phocomelia, and anasarca.

Caution: Federal (USA) law restricts this drug to use by or on the order of a licensed veterinarian.

Precautions: In the following conditions this product should be used with caution; diabetes mellitus, osteoporosis, predisposition to thromobophlebitis, hypertension, congestive heart failure, and renal insufficiency.

All necessary procedures for establishment of a bacterial diagnosis should be carried out whenever possible before institution of therapy. Combined antibiotic corticosteroid therapy does not obviate the need for indicated surgical procedures.

Side Effects: Because of the wide antibacterial effect of this antibiotic combination on intestinal flora, a change in the character of the stools may be anticipated in certain animals; however, administration of novobiocin and tetracycline, combined, to dogs at exaggerated doses for six months caused no significant toxicity. If allergic reactions develop during treatment with this product, use of it should be discontinued.

Continued on next page

Upjohn—Cont.

Since the use of any broad spectrum antibiotic may result in overgrowth of nonsusceptible organisms, constant observation of the animal patient is essential. If new infections appear during therapy, appropriate measures should be taken.
Injudicious use of adrenal hormones in animals with infections can be hazardous. It is therefore essential that the effective antibacterial agents be administered concurrently. Alteration of the inflammatory reaction by corticosteroid therapy may be beneficial; however, it may also mask signs of infection and facilitate spread of microorganisms. In addition, systemic manifestations, such as fever and signs of toxemia, may be suppressed. A retardant effect on wound healing has not been encountered with prednisolone, but such a possiblitiy should be considered when it is used in conjunction with surgery.
While the use of Delta Albaplex Tablets in recommended doses is not likely to induce the side effects commonly associated with prolonged or intensive adrenocorticoid therapy, overdosage may give rise to the following: hyperglycemia and glycosuria; nitrogen loss; and suppression of endogenous adrenocortical activity. The most commonly observed symptoms of overdosage in the dog are polydipsia and polyuria.
Dosage: The dosage for dogs is 10 mg of each antibiotic per lb of body weight (one tablet for each 6 lbs of body weight) repeated at 12 hour intervals for 48 hours. This dose can be given as follows:

Body Weight	*Tablets per Dose*
2.5 to 4 lb	½
5 to 8 lb	1
9 to 15 lb	2
16 to 24 lb	3
25 to 40 lb	5
41 to 65 lb	8

U

Antibacterial treatment is to be continued with Albaplex Tablets containing novobiocin and tetracycline at the same dose schedule for an additional 3 days.
How Supplied: Bottles of 500 tablets.
For Veterinary Use Only

DEPO-MEDROL® brand of methylprednisolone acetate sterile aqueous suspension 20 mg per ml and 40 mg per ml

Description: These preparations are recommended for intramuscular and intrasynovial injection in horses and dogs, and intramuscular injection in cats. Depo-Medrol Sterile Aqueous Suspension is available in two concentrations, 20 mg per ml and 40 mg per ml. Each ml of these preparations contains:

	20 mg	*40 mg*
Methyl-prednisolone Acetate	20 mg	40 mg
Polyethylene Glycol 3350	29.6 mg	29 mg
Sodium Chloride	8.9 mg	8.7 mg
Myristyl-gamma-picolinium chloride added as preservative	0.198 mg	0.195 mg

When necessary, pH was adjusted with sodium hydroxide and/or hydrochloric acid.
Metabolic and Hormonal Effects: Methylprednisolone, an anti-inflammatory steroid synthesized and developed in the Research Laboratories of The Upjohn Company, is the 6-methyl derivative of prednisolone. Exceeding prednisolone in anti-inflammatory potency and having even less tendency than prednisolone to induce sodium and water retention, methylprednisolone offers the advantage over older corticosteroids of affording equally satisfactory anti-inflammatory effect with the use of lower doses and with an enhanced split between anti-inflammatory and mineralocorticoid activities. Estimates of the relative potencies of methylprednisolone and prednisolone range from 1.13 to 2.1, with an average of 1.5. In anti-inflammatory activity, as measured by the granuloma pouch assay, methylprednisolone is twice as active as prednisolone. In mineralocorticoid activity (i.e., the capacity to induce retention of sodium and water in the adrenalectomized rat) methylprednisolone is slightly less active than prednisolone. The duration of plasma steroid levels following rapid intravenous injection in intact dogs is appreciably longer for methylprednisolone than for injection in intact dogs is appreciably longer for methylprednisolone than for prednisolone, the respective "half-life" value for the two steroids being 80.9 ± 7.5 minutes for methylprednisolone and 71.3 ± 1.7 minutes for prednisolone.
While the effect of parenterally administered Depo-Medrol (methylprednisolone acetate) is prolonged, it has the same metabolic and antiinflammatory actions as orally administered methylprednisolone acetate.
Indications: *Musculoskeletal Conditions.* As with other adrenal steroids, Depo-Medrol (methylprednisolone acetate) has been found useful in alleviating the pain and lameness associated with acute localized arthritic conditions and generalized arthritic conditions. It has been used successfully to treat rheumatoid arthritis, traumatic arthritis, osteoarthritis, periostitis, tendinitis, synovitis, tenosynovitis, bursitis, and myositis of horses; traumatic arthritis, osteoarthritis, and generalized arthritic conditions of dogs. Remission of musculoskeletal conditions may be permanent, or symptoms may recur, depending on the cause and extent of structural degeneration.
Allergic Conditions. This preparation is especially beneficial in relieving pruritus and inflammation of allergic dermatitis, acute moist dermatitis, dry eczema, urticaria, bronchial asthma, pollen sensitivities and otitis externa in dogs; allergic dermatitis and moist and dry eczema in cats. Onset of relief may begin within a few hours to a few days following injection and may persist for a few days to six weeks. Symptoms may be expected to recur if the cause of the allergic reaction is still present, in which case retreatment may be indicated. In treating acute hypersensitivity reactions, such as anaphylactic shock, intravenous Solu-Delta-Cortef® (prednisolone sodium succinate), as well as other appropriate treatments, should be used.
Overwhelming Infections with Severe Toxicity. In dogs and cats moribound from overwhelmingly severe infections for which antibacterial therapy is available (e.g. critical pneumonia, pyometritis), Depo-Medrol may be lifesaving, acting to inhibit the inflammatory reaction, which itself may be lethal; preventing vascular collapse and preserving the integrity of the blood vessels; modifying the patients reaction to drugs; and preventing or reducing the exudative reaction which often complicates certain infections. As supportive therapy, it improves the general atitude of the animal being treated.
All necessary procedures for the establishment of a bacterial diagnosis should be carried out whenever possible before institution of therapy. Corticosteroid therapy in the presence of infection should be administered for the shortest possible time compatible with maintenance of an adequate response, and antibacterial therapy should be continued for at least three days after the hormone has been withdrawn. Combined hormone and antibacterial therapy does not obviate the need for indicated surgical treatment.
Other conditions. In certain conditions where it is desired to reduce inflammation, vascularization, fibroblastic infiltration, and scar tissue, the use of Depo-Medrol should be considered. Snakebite of dogs is also an indication for the use of this suspension because of its antitoxemic, antishock, and anti-inflammatory activity. It is particularly effective in reducing swelling and preventing sloughing. Its employmentment in the treatment of such conditions is recommended as a supportive measure to standard procedure and time honored treatments and will give comfort to the animal and hasten complete recovery.
Contraindications: Systemic therapy with methylprednisolone acetate, as with other corticosteroids, is contraindicated in animals with arrested tuberculosis, peptic ulcer, and Cushing's syndrome. The presence of active tuberculosis, diabetes mellitus, osteoporosis, renal insufficiency, predisposition to thrombophlebitis, hypertension, or congestive heart failure necessitates carefully controlled use of corticosteroids. Intrasynovial, intratendinous, or other injections of corticosteroids for local effect are contraindicated in the presence of acute infectious conditions. Exacerbation of pain, further loss of joint motion, with fever and malaise following injection may indicate that the condition has become septic. Appropriate antibacterial therapy should be instituted immediately.
Warning: Clinical and experimental data have demonstrated that corticosteroids administered orally or parenterally to animals, may induce the first stage of

parturition when administered during the last trimester of pregnancy and may precipitate premature parturition followed by dystocia, fetal death, retained placenta and metritis. Additionally, corticosteroids administered to dogs, rabbits, and rodents during pregnancy have resulted in cleft palate in offspring. Corticosteroids administered to dogs during pregnancy have also resulted in other congenital anomalies, including deformed forelegs, phocomelia, and anasarca.
Not for human use.

Precautions: Depo-Medrol Sterile Aqueous Solution exerts an inhibitory influence on the mechanisms and the tissue changes associated with inflammation. Vascular permeability is decreased, exudation diminished, and migration of the inflammatory cells markedly inhibited. In addition, systemic manifestations such as fever and signs of toxemia may also be suppressed. While certain aspects of this alteration of the inflammatory reaction may be beneficial, the ression of inflammation may mask the signs of infection and tend to facilitate spread of microorganisms. Hence, all patients receiving this drug should be watched for evidence of intercurrent infection. Should infection occur, it must be brought under control by the use of appropriate antibacterial measures, or administration of this preparation should be discontinued. However, in infections characterized by overwhelming toxicity, methylprednisolone acetate therapy in conjunction with appropriate antibacterial therapy is effective in reducing mortality and morbidity. Without conjoint use of an antibiotic to which the invader-organism is sensitive, injudicious use of the adrenal hormones in animals with infections can be hazardous. As with other corticoids, continued or prolonged use is discouraged.

While no sodium retention or potassium depletion has been observed at the doses recommended, animals receiving methylprednisolone acetate, as with all corticoids, should be under close observation for possible untoward effects. If symptoms of hypopotassemia (hypokalemia) should occur, corticoid therapy should be discontinued and potassium chloride administered by continuous intravenous drip.

Since this drug lacks significant mineralocorticoid activity in usual therapeutic doses, it is not likely to afford adequate support in states of acute adrenocortical insufficiency. For treatment of the latter, the parent adrenocortical steroids, hydrocortisone or cortisone, should be used.

Intramuscular Administration and Dosage: Following intramuscular injection of methylprednisolone acetate, a prolonged systemic effect results. The dose varies with the size of the animal patient, the severity of the condition under treatment, and the animals response to therapy.

Dogs and Cats. The average intramuscular dose for dogs is 20 mg. In accordance with the size of the dog and severity of the condition under treatment, the dose may range from 2 mg in miniature breeds to 40 mg in medium breeds, and even as high as 120 mg in extremely large breeds or dogs with severe involvement.

The average intramuscular dose for cats is 10 mg with a range up to 20 mg.

Injections may be made at weekly intervals or in accordance with the severity of the conditions and clinical response.

Horses. The usual intramuscular dose for horses in 200 mg repeated as necessary.

For maintenance therapy in chronic conditions, initial doses should be reduced gradually until the smallest effective (i.e., individualized) dose is established. Medrol (methylprednisol one) Tablets may also be used for maintenance in dogs and cats, administered according to the recommended dose.

When treatment is to be withdrawn after prolonged and intensive therapy, the dose should be reduced gradually.

If signs of stress are associated with the condition being treated, the dose should be increased. If a rapid hormonal effect of maximum intensity is required, as in anaphylactic shock, the intravenous administration of highly soluble Solu-Delta-Cortef (prednisolone sodium succinate) is indicated.

Intrasynovial Administration and Dosage: Methylprednisolone acetate, a slightly soluble ester of methylprednisolone, is capable of producing a more prolonged local anti-inflammatory effect than equimolar doses of hydrocortisone acetate. Following intrasynovial injection, relief from pain may be experienced within 12 to 24 hours. The duration of relief varies, but averages three to four weeks, with a range of one to five or more weeks. Injections of methylprednisolone acetate have been well tolerated. Intrasynovial (intraarticular) injections may occasionally result in an increased localized inflammatory response.

Intrasynovial injection is recommended as an adjuvant to general therapeutic measures to effect suppression of inflammation in one or a few peripheral structures when (1) the disease is limited to one or a few peripheral structures; (2) the disease is widespread with one or a few peripheral structures actively inflamed; (3) systemic therapy with other corticoids or corticotropin controls all but a few or the more actively involved structures; (4) systemic therapy with cortisone, hydrocortisone, or corticotropin is contraindicated; (5) joints show early but actively progressing deformity (to enhance the effect of physiotherapy and corrective procedures); and (6) surgical or other orthopedic corrective measures are to be or have been done.

The action of Depo-Medrol Sterile Aqueous Solution injected intrasynovially appears to be well localized since significant metabolic effects characteristic of systemic administration of adrenal steroids have not been observed. In a few instances mild and transient improvement of structures other than those injected have been reported. No other systemic effects have been noted. However, it is possible that mild systemic effects may occur following intrasynovial administration, and this possibility is greater the larger the number of structures injected and the higher the total dose employed.

Procedure for Intrasynovial Injection. The anatomy of the area to be injected should be reviewed in order to assure that the suspension is properly placed and to determine that large blood vessels or nerves are avoided. The injection site is located where the synovial cavity is most superficial. The area is prepared for aseptic injection of the medicament by the removal of hair and cleansing of the skin with alcohol or Mercresin® tincture. A sterile 18 to 21-gauge needle for horses, 20 to 22-gauge needle for dogs, on a dry syringe is quickly inserted into the synovial space and a small amount of synovial fluid withdrawn. If there is an excess of synovia and more than 1 ml of suspension is to be injected, it is well to aspirate a volume of fluid comparable to that which is to be injected. With the needle in place, the aspirating syringe is removed and replaced by second syringe containing the proper amount of suspension which is then injected. In some animals a transient pain is elicited immediately upon injection into the affected cavity. This pain varies from mild to severe and may last for a few minutes up to 12 hours. After injection, the structure may be moved gently a few times to aid mixing of the synovial fluid and the suspension. The site may be covered with a small sterile dressing.

Areas not suitable for injection are those that are anatomically inaccessible such as spinal joints and those like the sacroiliac joints, which are devoid of synovial space. Treatment failures are most frequently the result of failure to enter the synovial space. If failures occur when injections into the synovial spaces are certain, as determined by aspiration of fluid, repeated injections are usually futile. Local therapy does not alter the underlying disease process, and whenever possible comprehensive therapy including physiotherapy and orthopedic correction should be employed.

The single intrasynovial dose depends on the size of the part, which corresponds to the size of the animal. The interval between repeated injections depends on the duration of relief obtained.

Horses: The average initial dose for a large synovial space in horses is 120 mg with a range from 40 to 240 mg. Smaller spaces will require a correspondingly lesser dose.

Dogs: The average initial dose for a large synovial space in dogs is 20 mg. Smaller spaces will require a correspondingly lesser dose.

How Supplied: 20 mg/ml, 10 ml sterile vial and 20 ml sterile vial; 40 mg/ml, 5 ml sterile vial.

Continued on next page

Upjohn—Cont.

DEPO®-PENICILLIN
brand of penicillin G benzathine and penicillin G procaine sterile suspension (For Veterinary Use in Beef Cattle, Horses and Dogs)

Description
Each ml of DEPO-Penicillin Sterile Suspension contains: 150,000 units penicillin G benzathine; 150,000 units penicillin G procaine; 11.7 mg lecithin; 1.75 mg sodium formaldehyde sulfoxylate; 1.20 mg methylparaben (as preservative); 0.14 mg propylparaben (as preservative); 8.19 mg tween 40; 11.3 span 40; 3.98 mg sodium citrate anhydrous; 20.0 mg procaine hydrochloride; 1.04 mg sodium carboxymethylcellulose; and water for injection, qs.

Action
Penicillin G is an antibiotic which shows a marked bactericidal effect against certain organisms during their growth phase. It is relatively specific in its action against gram-positive bacteria but is usually ineffective against gram-negative organisms.

When treating an animal for a bacterial infection, it is advisable to isolate and identify the causative organism and conduct appropriate *in vitro* susceptibility tests. In cases where organisms other than those susceptible to penicillin are present, re-evaluation of treatment should be made. Organisms normally considered susceptible to penicillin include *Clostridium septicum, Corynebacterium pyogenes, Staphylococcus aureus, Streptococcus canis, Streptococcus equi* and *Streptococcus pyogenes.*

It is normally recommended that any bacterial infection be treated as early as possible and with a dosage which will give effective blood levels. Although the recommended dosage of DEPO-Penicillin Sterile Suspension will give longer detectable penicillin blood levels than penicillin G procaine alone, it is recommended that a second dose be administered at 48 hours when treating a penicillin-susceptible bacterial infection.

If no definite improvement is noted following the second dose of DEPO-Penicillin, the diagnosis should be re-evaluated and use of another chemotherapeutic agent considered.

Indications
DEPO-Penicillin Sterile Suspension is indicated for treatment of the following bacterial infections in dogs, horses and beef cattle due to penicillin G susceptible microorganisms that are susceptible to the serum levels common to this particular dosage form, such as:

1. Bacterial Pneumonia *(Streptococcus spp., Corynebacterium pyogenes, Staphylococcus aureus)*
2. Uppler Respiratory Infections such as rhinitis or pharyngitis *(Corynebacterium pyogenes)*
3. Equine Strangles *Streptococcus equi)*
4. Blackleg *(Clostridium chauvoei)*

Contraindications
DEPO-Penicillin Sterile Suspension is contraindicated in patients which have shown hypersensitivity to penicillin.

Warning
Beef cattle should be withheld from slaughter for food use for thirty (30) days following last treatment. Treatment in beef cattle must be limited to two (2) doses. Not to be used in horses intended for food purposes.

Adverse Reactions
Anaphylactic reactions have been reported in cattle given penicillin. Treated animals should be closely observed and if allergic or anaphylactic reactions occur, administer epinephrine or antihistamines immediately.

Administration
DEPO-Penicillin Sterile Suspension should be given by intramuscular injection to horses. In beef cattle the recommended dosage should be administered by subcutaneous injection only. Dogs may be injected by either the intramuscular or subcutaneous route.

Dosage:
Horses: 2 ml per 150 lb body weight given intramuscularly (2,000 units penicillin G procaine and 2,000 units penicillin G benzathine per lb body weight). Treatment should be repeated in 48 hours.

Beef Cattle: 2 ml per 150 lb body weight given subcutaneously only (2,000 units penicillin G procaine and 2,000 units penicillin G benzathine per lb body weight). Treatment should be repeated in 48 hours.

Important: Treatment in beef cattle should be limited to two (2) doses of DEPO-Penicillin, given by subcutaneous injection only.

Dogs: 1 ml per 10 to 25 lb body weight given intramuscularly or subcutaneously (6,000 to 15,000 units penicillin G procaine and 6,000 to 15,000 units penicillin G benzathine per lb body weight). Treatment should be repeated in 48 hours.

Store in a refrigerator 2°–8° C (36°–46°F)
Shake Well Before Each Use

Caution
Federal law restricts this drug to use by or on the order of a licensed veterinarian.

How Supplied
DEPO-Penicillin Sterile Suspension is supplied in multiple dose vials of aqueous suspension. Each ml of suspension contains 150,000 units of penicillin G benzathine and 150,000 units of penicillin G procaine.

DRYGARD®
(novobiocin oil suspension)
For Udder Instillation in Dry Cows Only.
For the Treatment of Mastitis in Dry Cows.

Composition: Each 10 ml Plastet® contains: Sodium Novobiocin equiv. to Albamycin® (novobiocin) . . . 400 mg; Chlorobutanol Anhydrous (chloral derivative—used as preservative) . . . 50 mg; In a special bland vehicle. Store at controlled room temperature 15°–30°C (59°–86°F). Shake Well Before Using.

Indications: Drygard (novobiocin oil suspension) is indicated for the treatment, in dry cows only, of mastitis caused by susceptible strains of Staphylococcus aureus and Streptococcus agalactiae.

Warning: 1. Do not use less than 30 days prior to calving. 2. Treated animals must not be slaughtered for human consumption for 30 days following udder infusion. 3. Not for human use.

Caution: For use in dry cows only. Discard empty container; do not reuse.

Dosage: Infuse the contents of one (1) plastet of Drygard (novobiocin oil suspension) into each quarter of the cow udder at the initiation of the dry period.

Directions for Use: At the time of drying off, but not less than 30 days prior to calving, milk the udder dry. Wash the teats and udder thoroughly with warm water containing a suitable dairy antiseptic. Dry the teats and udder thoroughly. Treat all four quarters using the following procedure. Using the alcohol pads provided, wipe each teat end clean using a separate pad for each teat. Warm Drygard (novobiocin oil suspension) to body temperature and shake thoroughly. Remove cap from tip of plastet and insert tip into the teat canal. Instill entire contents of plastet into the quarter. Massage the udder after treatment to distribute the Drygard throughout the quarters. Using a suitable teat dip, dip all teats following treatment.

How Supplied: Drygard (novobiocin oil suspension) is available in unbroken packages of 12—10 ml plastets® with 12 individually wrapped 70% isopropyl alcohol pads.

ECP®
(estradiol cypionate)
Sterile Solution

Composition: This is the oil-soluble 17β-cyclopentylpropionate ester of "alpha" estradiol. It provides estradiol-17β, believed to be most potent of the naturally occurring estrogens, in the form of the cyclopentylpropionate ester, a highly fat-soluble derivative with profound estrogenic effect.

The sterile solution contains per ml: 2 mg estradiol cypionate, also 5.4 mg chlorobutanol anhydrous (chloral deriv.), in 916 mg cottonseed oil.

Actions: Comparative studies have demonstrated that estradiol cypionate produces estrogenic effects which are qualitatively the same as those produced by other estradiol esters.

Indications: ECP (estradiol cypionate) offers all of the functional activity of natural estrogenic substances with the advantage of a prolonged action.

The indications in bovine medicine are:

To correct anestrus (absence of heat period) in the absence of follicular cysts in some cases.

To treat cattle having a persistent corpus luteum due to certain causes.

To expel purulent material from the uterus in pyometra of cows.

To stimulate uterine expulsion of retained placentas and mummified fetuses.

U

Contraindications: As with all products of this nature, a complete examination to determine the status of the reproductive tract should be undertaken prior to administration of this drug. Pregnancy may be the prime reason for either anestrus or the persistence of the corpus luteum. Since pregnancy may be terminated by estrogens, ECP (estradiol cypionate) is contraindicated where a desired pregnancy exists.

Warning: Estrogens used in the canine may produce a gradual anemia and a profound leukocytosis which is followed by leukopenia. Thrombocytopenia may result with a concomitant alteration in the clotting mechanisms. First gross signs of alteration of the clotting mechanisms would include petechial and/or ecchymotic hemorrhage of mucus membranes and may result in frank hemorrhage in some animals. The possibility of endometritis and pyometritis following the use of estrogens is always present in the bitch. It has been demonstrated that endometrial hyperplasia is produced more consistently when estrogen and progesterone are given to the bitch. Theoretically then, estrogen given during late estrus or in metestrus in the presence of endogenous progesterone, which is being produced at near maximal rate by the recently developed corpora lutea, could result in endometrial proliferation and pyometra.

Not for human use.

ECP is intended for use only in cattle used for breeding purposes.

Precautions: Administration of an estrogenic substance to an animal may result in development of follicular cysts.

In the case of prolonged persistence of the corpus luteum in cows, thorough examinations should also be made of the uterus to determine the presence of an endometritis or a fetus. Use of appropriate antimicrobial agents, in addition to ECP (estradiol cypionate) should be considered if endometritis exists.

In the absence of normally developing follicles on the ovaries, estrus may be produced, but ovulation may not accompany estrus.

Because it is impossible to determine exactly if and when ovulation may occur in treated females during an induced heat period, it may help to breed the female frequently throughout the induced heat periods in order to improve the possibility of conception.

Repeat breeding will improve the chance of conception only if ovulation occurs.

Adverse Reactions: Prolonged estrus, precocious development, genital irritation, follicular cysts, and a reduction of milk flow may occur following estrogen therapy, frequently as a result of overdosage. If any of these phenomena are observed, the dosage should be reduced accordingly.

Newer Concepts of Anestrus In Cattle: Recent research findings indicate the necessity for a reappraisal of the causes and effects of anestrus in cattle. Two recent reports have suggested that frequently cows with a follicular cyst may be more inclined to be anestrual than nymphomaniac. Many cows will recover spontaneously from anestrus (if due to follicular cysts) if less than 60 days postparturient. In cases of anestrus due to follicular cysts, estrogens are not usually indicated.

Frequently, anestrus or follicular cysts have developed in association with a marked loss in body condition due to disease or high milk production.

Anestrus in conjunction with a persistent corpus luteum probably reflects some interference with normal function of the uterine endometrium. As indicated earlier, pregnancy must be considered as a cause of the persistence of the corpus luteum. Prolonged maintenance of the corpus luteum has also occurred following hysterectomy or experimental induction of endometritis. It is doubtful that corpora lutea are retained indefinitely in cattle with normal uterine function. It has been demonstrated that some estrogen esters will cause regression of the corpus luteum in cycline, pregnant or hysterectomized cattle. The response of the corpus luteum of pregnancy may differ with different estrogen esters. In the absence of a pregnancy or a detectable uterine malfunction, repeated rectal palpations will be required to establish a diagnosis of persistent corpus luteum. Although some estrogen esters may produce luteal regression, consideration of proper uterine treatment should also be given.

The proper diagnosis of anestrus without frequent rectal palpation is difficult since normal ovarian cycles can occur without accompanying estrus. It has been reported that such "silent heat" is more frequent at the first postpartum estrus.

The induced estrus in cows or heifers may not be fertile. Regular cyclic activity may not follow an ECP (estradiol cypionate) induced estrus.

Dosage and Administration: Sterile Solution ECP (estradiol cypionate) is *for intramuscular injection only.* Average doses for cows may be repeated, if necessary, in one week.

Do not overdose. If this product is exposed to temperature of less than 7°C (45°F), some constituents of the vehicle will solidify. If this should occur, warm the vial to room temperature before using:

Cows: Anestrus 3 to 5 mg; Pyometra 10 mg; Retained placenta 10 mg; Persistent corpus luteum 4 mg; Mummified fetus 10 mg; *Heifers:* Anestrus 3mg.

How Supplied: 2mg/ml 50 ml. Sterile Vials.

Caution: Federal (U.S.A.) law restricts this drug to use by or on the order of a licensed veterinarian.

FORTE-TOPICAL®
(procaine penicillin G, neomycin sulfate, polymyxin B sulfate, hydrocortisone acetate, and hydrocortisone sodium succinate) Suspension

Composition: Forte-Topical contains per ml: 2 mg hydrocortisone acetate; 1.25 mg hydrocortisone sodium succinate; 25 mg neomycin sulfate (equivalent to 17.5 mg of neomycin); 10,000 International units penicillin G procaine; 5,000 units polymyxin B sulfate; and 5 mg chlorobutanol anhydrous (chloral derivative); in a special bland vehicle. This combination of two forms of hydrocortisone and three antibiotics is ideal for the treatment of dermatitis, otitis externa, infected wounds, and genital infections because of the prompt, potent, and definitive action of the individual components.

Antibacterial Activity

Neomycin Sulfate. It has been established by both laboratory and clinical studies that neomycin sulfate is effective in the treatment of topical infections and that the antibiotic exerts high antibacterial activity against streptococci, staphylococci, coliform, and Pseudomonas organisms. These studies also prove that neomycin in therapeutic concentrations is nonirritating to dermal and genital tissues. Expressed in micrograms per milliliter required to inhibit test organisms, neomycin exerts the following antibacterial activity:

Organism	
Str. hemolyticus	1.6
Staph. aureus	0.01
Staph. albus	0.01
Esch. coli	0.06
Corynebacterium	0.3
Ps. aeruginosa	0.33
A. aerogenes	0.14

This chart demonstrates clearly that those bacteria commonly associated with dermal, otic, genital infections are highly susceptible to the antibacterial action of neomycin.

Neomycin sulfate is an antibacterial substance that Waksman and Lechevalier (*Science,* **109**:305, 1949) derived from culturing a strain of the soil organism *Streptomyces fradiae.* These investigators became interested in the antibiotic originally because it was active against pathogens that had become streptomycin-resistant. Also, neomycin, being effective against both gram-positive and gram-negative organisms, was found to possess a wider range of antibacterial activity than bacitracin, streptomycin, or penicillin.

Penicillin G Procaine. Penicillin is incorporated in Forte-Topical as the relatively insoluble penicillin G procaine. This is a stable chemical combination of penicillin and procaine which disintegrates slowly, achieving therapeutic levels of the antibiotic over prolonged periods.

Penicillin G procaine possesses the potent antibacterial action of penicillin. This antibiotic reinforces the action of neomycin.

Polymyxin B Sulfate. Polymyxin is highly active against *Pseudomonas aeruginosa.* It is also effective against many other gram-negative and gram-positive organisms, including *Aerobacter aerogenes* and *Escherichia coli.* Polymyxin possesses antifungal properties comparable, *in vitro,* to those agents commonly used for treatment of superficial mycotic infections. Thus, the possibility of fungal

Continued on next page

U

Upjohn—Cont.

overgrowth following the pronounced antibacterial effects of Forte-Topical is markedly reduced.

In addition to the complementary and additive effects of polymyxin when combined with penicillin and neomycin, it has been demonstrated that polymyxin and neomycin act synergistically.

Also, *in vitro* studies indicate that certain strains of susceptible micrococci have been found to be made more sensitive to neomycin or polymyxin by the addition of hydrocortisone sodium succinate.

Anti-Inflammatory Activity: Hydrocortisone, recognized as the principal steroid hormone of the adrenal gland, exerts a direct and potent anti-inflammatory effect when used locally. Topically applied hydrocortisone markedly inhibits inflammatory reaction through its controlling influence on the vascular and connective tissue components. It has been demonstrated that the anti-inflammatory effects of hydrocortisone are prompt and that it does not interfere with the established antibactetial effects of penicillin, neomycin, or polymyxin.

Forte-Topical contains the rapid anti-inflammatory activity of the water-soluble hydrocortisone sodium succinate, plus the time-proven sustained anti-inflammatory activity of hydrocortisone acetate.

Rapid diminution of the cardinal signs of inflammation (redness, swelling, heat, and pain) has been observed upon post-treatment physical examination following application of Forte-Topical.

U

Indications: Dermal Use. Forte-Topical may be used in large and small animal medicine for a wide variety of dermal conditions. The antibiotic combination in this product will prevent and treat infections caused by bacteria susceptible to neomycin, penicillin, and polymyxin B. In, dogs and cats, the indications for Forte-Topical include summer eczema, atopic dermatitis, and interdigital eczema; in large animals, such conditions as allergic dermatitis, harness galls, infected wounds, and pustular dermatitis.

Otic Use. Forte-Topical is recommended for the treatment of otitis externa in dogs and cats when caused or complicated by bacteria susceptible to neomycin, penicillin, and polymyxin B.

Genital Use. Forte-Topical has been found effective for the treatment of cervicitis, vaginitis, metritis , and pyometra.

Not for intramammary use in dairy animals.

Directions for Topical Use: This product should be shaken thoroughly before using. After cleansing the lesions, a small amount of the suspension should be rubbed gently into the involved area one to three times a day. When definite improvement is observed, application may be reduced to once a day or every other day.

In severely infected dermatitides, systemic therapy with appropriate antibiotics, such as Biosol® Sterile, should be used in addition to topical therapy with Forte-Topical. In severe or widespread dermatitides in small animals, orally administered corticoid tablets such as Medrol® or Delta Albaplex® may be used for systemic effect. In ear conditions, "the ear canal should be cleansed and dried. Forte-Topical may be used for the cleaning procedure. Forte-Topical should be expressed into the external ear canal, the ears folded down and gently massaged to distribute the preparation to all parts of the ear canal. If considerable inflammatory debris is present, the ears may be swabbed again and the procedure repeated until the ear canals are satisfactorily cleaned. Treatment may be applied one or two times a day and continued in accordance with clinical judgement.

Warning—If redness, irritation, or swelling persists or increase, discontinue use and redetermine diagnosis.

Directions for Genital Use: In large animals, 20 to 100 ml of this product is administered into the vagina and around the cervix, or into the uterus, depending on the condition to be treated. This product is administered at the time the animal is examined, and the animal is bred at the following heat period. If the animal is treated at estrus, she is bred at the following estrus.

Warning: This medication contains penicillin. Allergic reactions in humans are known to occur from topical exposure to penicillin. Not for human use.

How Supplied: 10 ml Applicator Tubes.

Caution: Federal (U.S.A.) law restricts this drug to use by or on the order of a licensed veterinarian.

LINCOCIN®
(lincomycin hydrochloride)
For intramuscular, intravenous, and oral use in dogs and cats

Composition: Lincomycin, an antibiotic produced by *Streptomyces lincolnensis var. lincolnensis,* is chemically distinct from all other clinically available antibiotics and is isolated as a white crystalline solid. It is stable in the dry state and in aqueous solution for at least 24 months. Lincomycin is readily soluble in water at room temperature in concentrations up to 500 mg/ml. Physical stability of aqueous solutions can be maintained at drug concentrations up to 345 mg/ml at temperatures as low as 4°C. The solubility in 95 percent ethanol is 80 mg/ml.

Lincocin (lincomycin hydrochloride) has been shown to be effective against most of the common gram-positive pathogens. Depending on the sensitivity of the organism and concentration of the antibiotic, it may be either bactericidal or bacteriostatic. It has not shown cross resistance with other available antibiotics. Microorganisms have not developed resistance to Lincocin rapidly when tested by *in vitro* or *in vivo* methods.

Actions: *Animal Toxicology*—The acute LD_{50} intraperitoneally in mice is 1000 mg/kg and orally in rats is 15,645 mg/kg. Lincocin (lincomycin hydrochloride) was well tolerated orally in rats and dogs at doses up to 300 mg/kg/day for periods up to one year. Parenteral dosages of up to 60 mg/kg/day for 30 days subcutaneously in the rat and intramuscularly in the dog produced no significant systemic effects of pathological findings at necropsy.

Swine receiving Lincocin intramuscularly at 10, 25, and 50 mg/lb (two, five, and ten times overdose) for 14 days tolerated all injections well, gained weight normally, and showed normal hematology, urinalysis, and blood chemistry values. Diarrhea was noted in the 50 mg/lb group with a lessening gradation of soft stools seen in the 25 mg/lb and 10 mg/lb groups. These changes in stool consistency did not adversely affect performance or blood electrolyte values. By the tenth day of the trial period, all stools were again normal.

Lincocin at a daily dose level of 75 mg/kg subcutaneously was injected into mature male and female rats during a prebreeding period of 60 days and throughout two mating cycles (84 days). No evidence was obtained that Lincocin exerted any effect on breeding performance and no drug-induced anomalies were discovered in the young. Similarly no evidence was obtained that Lincocin, when given in sustained parenteral dosage of 50 mg/kg daily to pregnant bitches, produced a teratogenic effect on the canine embryo.

The subcutaneous LD_{50} value in the newborn rat was determined to be 783 mg/kg. Newborn rats and canine pups have tolerated multiple doses of 30-90 mg/kg/day of the drug without evidence of ill effects.

Biological Studies—*In vitro* studies indicate that the spectrum of activity includes *Staphylococcus aureus, Staphylococcus albus, β-hemolytic Streptococcus, Streptococcus viridans, Clostridium tetani, Erysipelothrix insidiosa, Mycoplasma spp., and Clostridium perfringens.* The drug is not active against gram-negative organisms or yeasts.

In vivo experimental animal studies demonstrated Lincocin's effectiveness in protecting animals infected with *Streptococcus viridans, β-hemolytic Streptococcus, Staphylococcus aureus, Erysipelothrix insidiosa, Mycopiasma spp., and Leptospira pomona.* It was ineffective in *Klebsiella, Pasteurella, Pseudomonas,* and *Salmonella* infections.

Cross resistance has not been demonstrated with penicillin, erythromycin, triacetyloleandomycin, chloramphenicol, novobiocin, streptomycin, or the tetracyclines. Staphylococci develop resistance to Lincocin in a slow, stepwise manner based on *in vitro,* serial subculture experiments. This pattern of resistance development is unlike that shown for streptomycin.

Clinical Absorption and Excretion—Administered intramuscularly, Lincocin Sterile Solution is very rapidly absorbed. In studies with dogs, peak serum levels were reached in from ten minutes to two hours with detectable levels for 16 to 24 hours. The concentration of Lincocin in the blood serum varies with the dose administered and with the individual animal. Levels are maintained above the *in vitro* minimum inhibitory concentration for most gram-positive organisms for six to eight hours following a therapeutic dose. Intravenous administration also provides very rapid absorption, but should be administered with normal saline or 5% glucose as an intravenous drip infusion.

In swine, when Lincocin was administered intramuscularly at various dose levels, high levels were found in peritoneal fluid, pericardial fluid, and bile at five to six hours. At 24 hours, detectable levels were still present in these fluids. At 48 hours, all tissues were free of drug.

Administered orally to dogs, Lincocin was also rapidly absorbed with serum levels present within one-half hour; peak values were reached at two to four hours; and detectable levels persisted for 16 to 24 hours.

Tissue level studies indicate that bile is an important route of excretion. Significant levels of Lincocin have been demonstrated in the majority of body tissues. After a single oral administration of Lincocin to a dog, fecal excretion amounted to 77 percent of the dose; urinary excretion to 14 percent. After a single intramuscular injection, fecal excretion equaled 38 percent of the dose; and urinary excretion, 49 percent. Urinary excretion was essentially complete in less than 24 hours and fecal excretion by 48 hours after either route of administration. Lincocin has also been shown to be excreted in the milk of lactating cows, goats, rats, and women.

Indications: *Dogs and Cats* —Lincocin (lincomycin hydrochloride) is indicated in infections caused by gram-positive organisms which are sensitive to its action, particularly streptococci and staphylococci. The drug has proven effective in eradicating causative organisms in most of the common upper respiratory tract infections, in septicemia, and in infections of the skin and adjoining tissues. Systemic therapy with Lincocin has been shown to be of benefit in many animals with pustular dermatitis. As with all antibiotics, *in vitro* sensitivity studies should be performed before Lincocin is utilized as sole antibiotic therapy.

Lincocin has been demonstrated to be effective in the treatment of staphylococcal infections resistant to other antibiotics and sensitive to lincomycin. The drug may be administered in combination therapy with other antimicrobial agents when indicated.

No serious hypersensitivity reactions have been reported and many animals have received Lincocin repeatedly without developing evidence of hypersensitivity.

In dogs, Lincocin has demonstrated excellent efficacy in the treatment of upper respiratory infections and of skin diseases, particularly those caused by staphylococcus and streptococcus organisms. Lincocin has demonstrated efficacy even in some chronic conditions of long standing and in infections which have resisted treatment with other antibacterial agents.

Infections successfully treated with Lincocin include pustular dermatitis, abscesses, infected wounds (including bite and fight wounds), tonsillitis, laryngitis, metritis, and secondary bacterial infections associated with the canine distemper-hepatitis complex.

In cats, Lincocin has demonstrated efficacy in the treatment of localized infections, such as abscesses following fight wounds, pneumonitis, and feline rhinotracheitis.

Contraindications: As with all drugs, the use of Lincocin (lincomycin hydrochloride) is contraindicated in animals previously found to be hypersensitive to the drug.

Lincocin should not be given to animals with known preexisting monilial infections.

The following species are sensitive to the gastrointestinal effects of lincomycin: rabbits, hamsters, guinea pigs and horses. Therefore, the administration of Lincocin should be avoided in these species.

Warning: Not for human use. Swine intended for human consumption should not be slaughtered within 48 hours of latest treatment.

Precautions: The use of antibiotics occasionally results in overgrowth of nonsusceptible organisms—particularly yeasts. Should superinfections occur, appropriate measures should be taken.

Adverse Reactions: Loose stools occasionally have been observed in dogs and cats on oral doses. Vomiting in cats has occasionally been reported following oral administration.

Intramuscularly and intravenously, Lincocin (lincomycin hydrochloride) has demonstrated excellent local tolerance with no reports of pain or inflammation following injection.

The intramuscular administration to swine may cause a transient diarrhea or loose stools. Although this effect has rarely been reported, one must be alert to the possibility that it may occur. Should this occur, it is important that the necessary steps be taken to prevent the effects of dehydration.

Dosage and Administration: *Dogs and Cats* —Oral: 10 mg per pound of body weight every 12 hours or 7 mg per pound every 8 hours.

*Intramuscular** 10 mg per pound of body weight once a day or 5 mg per pound every 12 hours.

Intravenous: 5 to 10 mg per pound of body weight one or two times per day diluted with 5 percent glucose in water or normal saline and given as a drip infusion.

Treatment with Lincocin (lincomycin hydrochloride) may be continued for periods as long as 12 days if clinical judgment indicates.

As with any multi-dose vial, practice aseptic techniques in withdrawing each dose. Adequately clean and disinfect the vial closure prior to entry with a sterile needle and syringe.

How Supplied: 100 mg/ml 20 ml sterile vial; 500 mg tablets, bottle of 100; 100 mg tablets, bottle of 500; 200 mg tablets, bottles of 250; 50 mg/ml, 20 ml dropper bottle.

Store at controlled room temperature 15°–30° (59°–86°F).

LINCOCIN® Soluble Powder
(lincomycin hydrochloride)

Composition: Each packet contains: 1.41 oz (40 gm) lincomycin hydrochloride equivalent to 16 gm linocomycin.

Dosage: Lincocin® Soluble Powder should be administered at a dose rate of 250 mg of lincomycin HCl per gallon of drinking water. In clinical studies, this dose rate provided an average of 3.8 mg of lincomycin HCl per pound of body weight per day.

Treatment Period: The drug should be administered for a minimum of 5 consecutive days beyond the disappearance of symptoms (bloody stools) up to a maximum of 10 consecutive days.

Administration: Each packet will medicate 64 gallons of drinking water providing 250 mg gallon.

A dose of 3.8 mg lincomycin HCl per pound of body weight may be maintained by medicating the drinking water at a concentration of 250 mg per gallon of drinking water when pigs are consuming 1.5 gallons per 100 lbs of body weight per day. Under these circumstances, the concentration of lincomycin required in medicated water may be adjusted to compensate for variations in age and weight of animals, the nature and severity of disease symptoms, environmental temperature and humidity, each of which affects water consumption.

Note: After water treatment is discontinued, a control program for swine dysentery may be followed by feeding 40 grams of lincomycin feed additive per ton of complete feed as the sole ration.

Cautions:

1. Discard medicated drinking water if not used within 2 days. Fresh stock solution should be prepared daily.
2. If clinical signs of bloody scours (watery, mucoid or bloody stools) have not improved during the first 6 days of medication, discontinue treatment and redetermine the diagnosis.
3. Occasionally, swine fed lincomycin may within the first two days after the onset of treatment develop diarrhea and/or swelling of the anus. On rare occassions, some pigs may show reddening of the skin and irritable behavior. These conditions have been self-correcting within five to eight days without discontinuing the lincomycin treatment.
4. Not for use in swine weighing more than 250 pounds.

Warning: Do not slaughter swine for human consumption for 6 days following last treatment.

Not for human use.

Store at Controlled Room Temperature 15°–30°C (59°–86°F)

Restricted Drug-Use Only as Directed.

Continued on next page

Upjohn—Cont.

LINCOCIN®
(lincomycin hydrochloride injection) Sterile Solution
For Intramuscular use in swine.

Composition: Lincomycin, an antibiotic produced by *Streptomyces lincolnensis var. lincolnensis,* is chemically distinct from all other clinically available antibiotics and is isolated as a white crystalline solid. It is stable in the dry state and in aqueous solution for at least 24 months. Lincomycin is readily soluble in water at room temperature in concentrations up to 500 mg/ml. Physical stability of aqueous solutions can be maintained at drug concentrations up to 345 mg/ml at temperatures as low as 4°C. The solubility in 95 percent ethanol is 80 mg/ml.

Lincocin has been shown to be effective against most of the common gram-positive pathogens. Depending on the sensitivity of the organism and concentration of the antibiotic, it may be either bactericidal or bacteriostatic. It has not shown cross resistance with other available antibiotics. Microorganisms have not developed resistance to Lincocin rapidly when tested by *in vitro* or *in vivo* methods.

Indications for swine: Lincocin (lincomycin hydrochloride injection) is indicated for the treatment of infectious forms of arthritis caused by organisms sensitive to its activity. This includes most of the organisms responsible for the various infectious arthritides in swine, such as staphylococci, streptococci, *Erysipelothrix* and *Mycoplasma spp.*

It is also indicated for the treatment of *Mycoplasma pneumonia.*

Dosage and Administration: For arthritis or mycoplasma pneumonia—5 mg. per pound of body weight intramuscularly once daily for three to seven days as needed. When using *Lincocin* containing 25 mg/ml, 1 ml/5 lb body weight will provide 5 mg/lb; when using *Lincocin* containing 50 mg/ml, 1 ml/10 lb body weight will provide 5 mg/lb; when using *Lincocin* containing 100 mg/ml, 1 ml/20 lb body weight will provide 5 mg/lb.

For optimal results in infectious forms of arthritis, initiate treatment as soon as possible.

As with any multi-dose vial, practice aseptic techniques in withdrawing each dose. Adequately clean and disinfect the vial closure prior to entry with a sterile needle and syringe.

Warning: Not for Human Use.

Swine intended for human consumption should not be slaughtered within 48 hours of latest treatment.

Contraindications: As with all drugs, the use of Lincocin (lincomycin hydrochloride injection) is contraindicated in animals previously found to be hypersensitive to the drug.

Lincocin should not be given to animals with known preexisting monilial infections.

The following species are sensitive to the gastrointestinal effects of lincomycin: rabbits, hamsters, guinea pigs and horses. Therefore, the administration of Lincocin should be avoided in these species.

Caution: If no improvement is noted within 48 hours, consult a veterinarian.

Adverse Reactions: The intramuscular administration to swine may cause a transient diarrhea or loose stools. Although this effect has rarely been reported, one must be alert to the possibility that it may occur.

Should this occur, it is important that the necessary steps be taken to prevent the effects of dehydration.

Actions: *Animal Toxicology*—The acute LD_{50} intraperitoneally in mice is 1000 mg/kg and orally in rats is 15,645 mg/kg. Lincocin (lincomycin hydrochloride injection) was well tolerated orally in rats and dogs at doses up to 300 mg/kg/day for periods up to one year. Parenteral dosages of up to 60 mg/kg/day for 30 days subcutaneously in the rat and intramuscularly in the dog produced no significant systemic effects or pathological findings at necropsy.

Swine receiving Lincocin intramuscularly at 10, 25, and 50 mg/lb (two, five; and ten times overdose) for 14 days tolerated all injections well, gained weight normally, and showed normal hematology, urinalysis, and blood chemistry values. Diarrhea was noted in the 50 mg/lb group with a lessening gradation of soft stools seen in the 25 mg/lb and 10 mg/lb groups. These changes in stool consistency did not adversely affect performance or blood electrolyte values. By the tenth day of the trial period, all stools were again normal.

Lincocin at a daily dose level of 75 mg/kg subcutaneously was injected into mature male and female rats during a prebreeding period of 60 days and throughout two mating cycles (84 days). No evidence was obtained that Lincocin exerted any effect on breeding performance and no drug-induced anomalies were discovered in the young. Similarly no evidence was obtained that Lincocin, when given in sustained parenteral dosage of 50 mg/kg daily to pregnant bitches, produced a teratogenic effect on the canine embryo. The subcutaneous LD_{50} value in the newborn rat was determined to be 783 mg/kg. Newborn. rats and canine pups have tolerated multiple doses of 30–90 mg/kg/day of the drug without evidence of ill effects.

Biological Studies—*In vitro* studies indicate that the spectrum of activity includes *Staphylococcus aureus, Staphylococcus albus,* β-hemolytic Streptococcus, Streptococcus viridans, Clostridium tetani, Erysipelothrix insidiosa, Mycoplasma spp. and *Clostridium perfringens.* The drug is not active against gram-negative organisms or yeasts.

In vivo experimental animal studies demonstrated Lincocin is effective in protecting animals infected with *Streptococcus viridans,* β-hemolytic Streptococcus, Staphylococcus aureus, Erysipelothrix insidiosa, Mycoplasma spp. and *Leptospira pomona.* It was ineffective in *Klebsiella, Pasteurella, Pseudomonas* and *Salmonella* infections.

Cross resistance has not been demonstrated with penicillin, erythromycin, triadetyloleandomycin, chloramphenicol, novobiocin, streptomycin, or the tetracyclines. Staphylococci develop resistance to Lincocin in a slow, stepwise manner based on *in vitro,* serial subculture experiments. This pattern of resistance development is unlike that shown for streptomycin.

When Lincocin was administered intramuscularly in swine at various dose levels, high levels were found in peritoneal fluid, pericardial fluid, and bile at five to six hours. At 24 hours, detectable levels were still present in these fluids. At 48 hours, all tissues were free of drug.

Tissue level studies indicate that bile is an important route of excretion. Significant levels of Lincocin have been demonstrated in the majority of body tissues. After a single oral administration of Lincocin to a dog, fecal excretion amounted to 77 percent of the dose; urinary excretion to 14 percent. After a single intramuscular injection, fecal excretion equaled 38 percent of the dose; and urinary excretion, 49 percent. Urinary excretion was essentially complete in less than 24 hours and fecal excretion by 48 hours after either route of administration. Lincocin has also been shown to be excreted in the milk of lactating cows, goats, rats and women.

How Supplied: 20 ml Sterile Vial (100 mg); 100 ml Sterile Vial (100 mg).

Veterinary
LUTALYSE® Sterile Solution
(dinoprost tromethamine)

Veterinary: For intramuscular use for estrus synchronization, treatment of unobserved (silent) estrus and pyometra (chronic endometritis) in cattle; for abortion of feedlot and other non-lactating cattle and for parturition induction in swine.

Description: This product contains the naturally occurring prostaglandin F2 alpha (dinoprost) as the tromethamine salt. Each ml contains dino prost tromethamine equivalent to 5 mg dinoprost; also, benzyl alcohol, 9.45 mg added as preservative. When necessary, pH was adjusted with sodium hydroxide and/or hydrochloric acid. Dinoprost tromethamine is a white or slightly offwhite crystalline powder that is readily soluble in water at room temperature in concentrations to at least 200 mg/ml.

General Biologic Activity: Prostaglandins occurs in nearly all mammalian tissues. Prostaglandins, especially PGE's and PGF's, have been shown, in certain species, to 1) increase at time of parturition in amniotic fluid, maternal placenta, myometrium, and blood, 2) stimulate myometrial activity, and 3) to induce either abortion or parturition. Prostaglandins, especially $PGF_{2}\alpha$, have been shown to 1) increase in the uterus and blood to levels similar to levels achieved by exogenous administration which elicited luteolysis, 2) be capable of crossing from the iterine vein to the ovarian artery (sheep), 3) be related to IUD induced luteal regression (sheep), and 4) be capable of regressing the corpus luteum of most mammalian species studied to date. Prostaglandins, especially PGE's, may be involved in the process of ovulation and gamate transport. Also, $PGF_{2}\alpha$ has been reported to cause increase in blood pressure, bronchoconstriction, and smooth muscle stimulation in certain species.

Safety and Toxicity: Dinoprost was nonteratogenic in rats when administered orally at 1.25, 3.2, 10.0 and 20.0 mg/kg/day from day 6th –15th of gestation or when administered subcutaneously at 0.5 and1.0 mg/kg/day on gestation days 6, 7 and 8 or 9, 10 and 11 or 12, 13 and 14. Dinoprost was non-teratogenic in the rabbit when administered either subcutaneously at doses of 0.5 and 1.0 mg/kg/day on gestation days 6, 7 and 8 or 9, 10 and 11 or 12, 13 and 14 or 15, 16 and 17 orally at doses of 0.01 0.1 and 1.0 mg/kg/day on days 6–18 or 5.0 mg/kg/day on days 8–18 of gestation. A slight and marked embryo lethal effect was observed in dams given 1.0 and 0.5 mg/kg/day respectively. This was due to the expected luteolytic properties of the drug.

A 14-day continuous intravenous infusion study in rats at 20 mg $PGF_{2}\alpha$ per kg body weight indicated prostaglandins of the F series could induce bone deposition. However, such bone changes were not observed in monkeys similarly administered *Lutalyse (dinoprost tromethamine)* at 15 mg $PGF_{2}\alpha$ per kg body weight for 14 days.

In cattle, evaluation was made of clinical observations, clinical chemistry, hematology, urinalysis, organ weights, and gross plus microscopic measurements following treatment with various doses up to 250 mg dinoprost administered twice intramuscularly at a 10 day interval or doses of 25 mg administered daily for 10 days. There was no unequivocal effect of dinoprost on the hematology or clinical chemistry parameters measured. Clinically, a slight transitory increase in heart rate was detected. Rectal temperature was elevated about 1.5°F through the 6th hour after injection with 250 mg dinoprost but had returned to baseline at 24 hours after injection. No dinoprost associated lesions were detected. There was no evidence of toxicological effects. Thus, dinoprost had a safety factor of **at least 10x** on injection (25 mg luteolytic dose vs. 250 mg safe dose), based on studies conducted with cattle. At luteolytic doses, dinoprost had no effect on progeny. If given to a pregnant cow, it may cause abortion; the dose required for abortion varies considerably with the stage of gestation.

Induction of abortion in feedlot cattle at stages of gestation up to 100 days of gestation did not result in dystocia, retained placenta or death of heifers in the field studies. The smallness of the fetus at this early stage of gestation should not lead to complications at abortion. However, induction of parturition or abortion with any exogenous compound may precipate dystocia, fetal death, retained placenta and/or metritis, especially at latter stages of gestation.

In pigs, evaluation was made of clinical observations, food consumption, clinical pathologic determinations, body weight changes, urinalysis, organ weights, and gross and microscopic observations following treatment with single doses of 10, 30, 50 and 100 mg dinoprost administered intramuscularly. The results indicated no treatment related effects from dinoprost treatment that were deleterious to the health of the animals or to their offspring.

A number of metabolism studies have been done in laboratory animals. The metabolism of tritum labeled dionprost ($^{3}H\ PGF_{2}\alpha$) in the rat and in the monkey was similar. Although quantitative differences were observed, qualitatively similar metabolites were produced. A study demonstrated that equimolar doses of ^{3}H PGF2 alpha Tham and ^{3}H PGF2 alpha free acid administered intravenously to rats demonstrated no significant differences in blood concentration of dinoprost. An interesting observation in the above study was that the radioactive dose of $^{3}H\ PGF_{2}\alpha$ rapidly distributed in tissues and dissipated in tissues with almost the same curve as it did in the serum. The half-life of dinoprost in bovine blood has been reported to be on the order of minutes. A complete study on the distribution of decline of ^{3}H PGF2 alpha Tham in the tissue of rats was well correlated with the work done in the cow. Cattle serum collected during 24 hours after doses of 0 to 250 mg dinoprost have been been assayed by RIA for dinoprost and the 15-keto metabolite. These data support previous reports that dinoprost has a half-life of minutes.

Dinoprost is a natural prostaglandin. All systems associated with dinoprost metabolism exist in the body; therefore, no new metabolic, transport, excretory, binding or other systems need be established by the body to metabolize injected dinoprost.

Indications and Instruction for Use: *Cattle*—Lutalyse (dinoprost tromethamine) sterile solution is indicated as a luteolytic agent.

Lutalyse is effective only in those cattle having a corpus luteum, i.e., those which ovulated at least five days prior to treatment. Future reproductive performance of animals that are not cycling will be unaffected by Lutalyse injection.

1. **For Intramuscular Use for Estrus Synchronization in Beef Cattle and Non-Lactating Dairy Heifers.** Lutalyse is used to control the timing of estrus and ovulation in estrous cycling cattle that have a corpus luteum.
   Inject a dose of 5 ml lutalyse (25 mg $PGF\alpha$) intramuscularly either once or twice at a 10- to 12-day interval.
   With the single injection, cattle should be bred at the usual time relative to estrus.
   With the two injections cattles can be bred after the second injection either at the usual time relative to detected estrus or about 80 hours after the second Lutalyse injection.
   Estrus is expected to occur 1 to 5 days after injection if a corpus luteum was present. Cattle that do not become pregnant to breeding at estrus on days 1 to 5 after injection wil be expected to return to estrus in about 18 to 24 days.
2. **For Intramuscular Use for Unobserved (Silent) Estrus in Lactating Dairy Cows with a Corpus Luteum.** Inject a dose of 5 ml Lutalyse (25 mg $PGF_{2}\alpha$) intramuscularly. Breed cows as they are detected in estrus. If estrus has not been observed by 80 hours after injection, breed at 80 hours. If the cow returns to estrus breed at the usual time relative to estrus.

Management Considerations: Many factors contribute to success and failure of reproduction management, and these factors are important also when time of breeding is to be regulated with Lutalyse. Some of these factors are:

a. Cattle must be ready to breed—they must have a corpus luteum and must be healthy;
b. Nutritional status must be adequate as this has a direct effect on conception and the initiation of estrus in heifers or return of estrous cycles in cows following calving;
c. Physical facilities must be adequate to allow cattle handling without being detrimental to the animal;
d. Estrus must be detected accurately if timed A1 is not employed;
e. Semen of high fertility must be used;
f. Semen must be inseminated properly.

A sucessful breeding program can employ Lutalyse effectively, but a poorly managed breeding program will continue to be poor when Lutalyse is employed unless other management deficiencies are remedied first.

Cattle expressing estrus following Lutalyse are receptive to breeding by a bull. Using bulls to breed large numbers of cattle in heat following Lutalyse will require proper management of bulls and cattle.

3. **For Intramuscular Use for Treatment of Pyometra (chronic endometritis) in Cattle.** Inject a dose of 5 ml *Lutalyse* (25 mg $PGF_{2}\alpha$) intramuscularly. In studies conducted with *Lutalyse,* pyometra was defined as presence of a corpus luteum in the ovary and uterine horns containing fluid but not a conceptus based on palpation *per rectum.* Return to normal was defined as evacuation of fluid and return to uterine horn size to 40mm or less based on palpation *per rectum* at 14 and 28 days. Most cattle that recovered in response to *Lutalyse* recovered within 14 days after injection. After 14 days, recovery rate of treated cattle was no different than that in nontreated cattle.
4. **For Intramuscular Use for Abortion of Feedlot and Other Non-Lactating Cattle.** Lutalyse is indicated for its abortifacient effect in feedlot and other non-lactating cattle during the first 100 days of gestation. Inject a dose of 25 mg intramuscularly. Cattle that

Continued on next page

Upjohn—Cont.

abort will abort within 35 days of injection.
Commercial cattle were palpated per rectum for pregnancy in six feedlots. The percent of pregnant cattle in each feedlot less than 100 days of gestation ranged between 26 and 84; 80% or more of the pregnant cattle were less than 150 days of gestation. The abortion rates following injection of Lutalyse increased with increasing doses up to about 25 mg. As examples, the abortion rates, over 7 feedlots on the dose titration study, were 22%, 50%, 71%, 90% and 78% for cattle up to 100 days of gestation when injected IM with Lutalyse doses of 0, 1 (5 mg), 2 (20 mg), 4 (20 mg), and 8 (40 mg) ml, respectively. The statistical predicted relative abortion rate based on the dose titration data, was about 93% for the 5 ml (25 mg) Lutalyse dose for the cattle injected up to 100 days of gestation.

Swine—For Intramuscular Use for Parturition Induction in Swine. *Lutalyse* Sterile Solution (dinoprost tromethamine) is indicated for parturition induction in swine when injected within 3 days of normal predicted farrowing.
The response to treatment varies by individual animals with a mean interval from administration of 2 ml *Lutalyse* (10 mg dinoprost) to parturition of approximately 30 hours. This can be employed to control the time of farrowing in sows and gilts in late gestation.

Management Considerations—Several factors must be considered for the successful use of *Lutalyse* for parturition induction in swine. The product must be administrered at a relatively specific time (treatment earlier than 3 days prior to normal predicted farrowing may result in increased piglet mortality). It is important that adequate records be maintained on (1) the average length of gestation period for the animals on a specific location, and (2) the breeding and projected farrowing dates for each animal. This information is essential to determine the appropriate time for *Lutalyse* administration.

Warning: Not for human use.
Women of child-bearing age, asthmatics, and persons with bronchial and other respiratory problems should exercise **extreme caution** when handling this product. In the early stages, women may be unaware of their pregnancies. Dinoprost tromethamine is readily absorbed through the skin and can cause abortion and/or bronchiospasms. Direct contact with the skin should, therefore, be avoided. Accidental spillage on the skin should be washed off **immediately** with soap and water.
Use of this product in excess of the approved dose may result in drug residues.

Precautions: Do not administer to pregnant cattle unless abortion is desired.
Do not administer intravenously (I.V.) as this route might potentiate adverse reactions.
Cattle administered a progestogen would be expected to have a reduced response to Lutalyse.
Aggressive antiobiotic therapy should be employed at the first sign of infection at the injection site whether localized or diffuse. As with all parenteral products careful aseptic techniques should be employed to decrease the possibility of post injection bacterial infections.
Swine—Do not administer to sows and/or gilts prior to 3 days of normal predicted farrowing, as increased number of stillborn and postnatal mortality may result.

Adverse Reactions:
Cattle
1. The most frequently observed side effect is in creased rectal temperature at a 5x or 10x overdose. However, rectal temperature change has been transient in all cases observed and has not been detrimental to the animal
2. Limited salivation has been reported in some instances.
3. Intravenous administration might increase heart rate.
4. Localized post injection bacterial infections that may become generalized have been reported. In rare instances such infections have terminated fatally. See PRECAUTIONS.

Swine—The most frequently observed side effects were erythema and pruritus, slight incoordination, nesting behavior, itching, urination, defecation, abdominal muscle spasms, tail movements, hyperpnea or dyspnea, increased vocalization, salivation, and at the 100 mg (10X) dose only, vomition. These side effects are transitory, lasting from 10 minutes to 3 hours, and were not detrimental to the health of the animal.

IMPORTANT: Cattle—No milk discard or preslaughter drug withdrawal period is required for labeled uses.
Swine—No preslaughter drug withdrawal period is required for labeled uses.

Dosage and Administration: *Cattle*—Lutalyse (dinoprost tromethamine) is supplied at a concentration of 5 mg dinoprost per ml. Lutalyse is luteolytic in cattle at 25 mg (5 ml) administered intramuscularly. As with any multidose vial, practice aseptic techniques in withdrawing each dose. Adequately clean and disinfect the vial closure prior to entry with a sterile needle.
Swine—*Lutalyse* will induce parturition in swine at 10 mg (2 ml) when injected intramuscularly. As with any multidose vial, practice aseptic techniques in withdrawing each dose. Adequately clean and disinfect the vial closure prior to entry with a sterile needle.

Caution: Federal (U.S.A.) law restricts this drug to use by or on the order of a licensed veterinarian.

How Supplied: Lutalyse (dinoprost tromethamine) Sterile Solution is available in 10 and 30 ml vials.

MEDROL® brand of methylprednisolone 1 mg. Tablets
For use in dogs and cats only.

Composition: Methylprednisolone, a potent antiinflammatory steroid synthesized and developed in the Research Laboratories of The Upjohn Company is the 6-methyl derivative of prednisolone. It has a greater anti-inflammatory potency than prednisolone and even less tendency than prednisolone to induce sodium and water retention. Its advantage over the older corticoids lies in its ability to achieve equal antiinflammatory effect with lower dose, while at the same time enhancing the split between antiinflammatory and mineralocorticoid activities.

Indications: The indications are the same as those for other anti-inflammatory steroids and comprise the various collagen, dermal, allergic, ocular, otic, and musculoskeletal conditions known to be responsive to the anti-inflammatory corticosteroids. Representative of the conditions in which the use of steroid therapy and the benefits to be derived therefrom have had repeated confirmation in the veterinary literature: (1) dermal conditions, such as nonspecific eczema, summer dermatitis, and burns; (2) allergic manifestations, such as acute urticaria, allergic dermatitis, drug and serum reactions, bronchial asthma, and pollen sensitivities; (3) ocular conditions, such as iritis, iridocyclitis, secondary glaucoma, uveitis, and chorioretinitis; (4) otic conditions, such as otitis externa; (5) musculoskeletal conditions, such as myositis, rheumatoid arthritis, osteoarthritis, and bursitis; (6) various chronic or recurrent diseases of unknown etiology such as ulcerative colitis and nephrosis.
In acute adrenal insufficiency, Medrol (methylprednisolone) may be effective because of its ability to correct the defect in carbohydrate metabolism and relieve the impaired diuretic response to water characteristic of primary or secondary adrenal insufficiency. However, because this agent lacks significant mineralocorticoid activity, the parent hormones, Solu-Cortef® (hydrocortisone sodium succinate), Cortef® (hydrocortisone), or cortisone should be used when salt retention is indicated.

Contraindications: Medrol Tablets, like prednisolone, are contraindicated in animals with arrested tuberculosis, peptic ulcer, acute psychoses, and Cushingoid syndrome. The presence of diabetes, osteoporosis, chronic psychotic reactions, predisposition to thrombophlebitis, hypertension, congestive heart failure, renal insufficiency, and active tuberculosis necessitates carefully controlled use. Some of the above conditions occur only rarely in dogs and cats but should be kept in mind.

Caution: Because of its inhibitory effect on fibroplasia, methylprednisolone may mask the signs of infection and enhance dissemination of the infecting organism. Hence, all animal patients receiving methylprednisolone should be watched for evidence of intercurrent infection. Should infection occur, it must be brought under control by use of appropriate antibacterial measures, or administration of methylprednisolone should be discontinued.

Warning: Not for human use. Clinical and experimental data have demonstrated that corticosteroids administered orally or parenterally to animals may induce the first stage of parturition when administered during the last trimester of pregnancy and may precipitate premature parturition followed by dystocia, fetal death, retained placenta, and metritis. Additionally, corticosteroids administered to dogs, rabbits and rodents during pregnancy have resulted in cleft palate in offspring. Corticosteroids administered to dogs during pregnancy have also resulted in other congenital anomalies including deformed forelegs, phocomelia, and anasarca.

Precautions: Medrol Tablets, like prednisolone and other adrenocortical steroids, is a potent therapeutic agent influencing the biochemical behavior of most, if not all, tissues of the body. Because this anti-inflammatory steroid manifests little sodium-retaining activity, the usual early sign of cortisone or hydrocortisone overdosage (i.e. increase in body weight due to fluid retention) is not a reliable index of overdosage. Hence, recommended dose levels should not be exceeded, and all animal patients receiving Medrol should be under close medical supervision. All precautions pertinent to the use of prednisolone apply to methylprednisolone. Moreover, the veterinarian should endeavor to keep informed of current studies with Medrol as they are reported in the veterinary literature.

Adverse Reactions: With therapeutically equivalent doses, the likelihood of occurrence of troublesome side effects is less with methylprednisolone than with prednisolone; moreover, side effects actually have been conspicuously absent during clinical trials with Medrol (methylprednisolone) in dogs and cats. However, methylprednisolone is similar to prednisolone in regard to kinds of side effects and metabolic alterations to be anticipated when treatment is intensive or prolonged. In animal patients with diabetes mellitus, use of methylprednisolone may be associated with an increase in the insulin requirement. Negative nitrogen balance may occur, particularly in animals that require protracted maintenance therapy; measures to counteract persistent nitrogen loss include a high protein intake and the administration, when indicated, of a suitable anabolic agent. Excessive loss of potassium, like excessive retention of sodium is not likely to be induced by effective maintenance doses of Medrol. However, these effects should be kept in mind and the usual regulatory measures employed as indicated. Ecchymotic manifestations, *while not noted during the clinical evaluation* in dogs and cats, may occur. If such reactions do occur and are serious, reduction in dosage or discontinuance of methylprednisolone therapy may be indicated. Concurrent use of daily oral supplements of ascorbic acid may be of value in helping to control ecchymotic tendencies.

Since methylprednisolone, like prednisolone, suppresses endogenous adrenocortical activity, *it is highly important that the animal patient receiving Medrol be under careful observation, not only during the course of treatment but for some time after treatment is terminated. Adequate adrenocortical supportive therapy with cortisone or hydrocortisone, and including ACTH, must be employed promptly if the animal is subjected to any unusual stress such as surgery, trauma, or severe infection.*

Administration: The keystone of satisfactory therapeutic management with Medrol Tablets, as with its steroid predecessors, is individualization of dosage in reference to the severity of the disease, the anticipated duration of steroid therapy, and the animal patient's threshold or tolerance for steroid excess. The prime objective of steroid therapy should be to achieve a satisfactory degree of control with a minimum effective daily dose.

The dosage recommendations are suggested *average total daily doses and are intended as guides.* As with other orally administered corticosteroids, the total daily dose of Medrol should be given in equally divided doses. The initial suppressive dose level is continued until a satisfactory clinical response is obtained, a period usually of 2 to 7 days in the case of musculoskeletal diseases, allergic conditions affecting the skin or respiratory tract, and ocular inflammatory diseases. If a satisfactory response is not obtained in 7 days, reevaluation of the case to confirm the original diagnosis should be made. As soon as a satisfactory clinical response is obtained, the daily dose should be reduced gradually, either to termination of treatment in the case of acute conditions (e.g., seasonal asthma, dermatitis, acute ocular inflammations) or to the minimal effective maintenance dose level in the case of chronic conditions (e.g. rheumatoid arthritis). In chronic conditions, and in rheumatoid arthritis especially, it is important that the reduction in dosage from initial to maintenance dose levels be accomplished slowly. The maintenance dose level should be adjusted from time to time as required by fluctuation in the activity of the disease and the animal's general status. Accumulated experience has shown that the long-term benefits to be gained from continued steroid maintenance are probably greater the lower the maintenance dose level. In rheumatoid arthritis in particular, maintenance steroid therapy should be at the lowest possible level.

Important: In the therapeutic management of animal patients with chronic diseases such as rheumatoid arthritis, methylprednisolone should be regarded as a highly valuable adjunct, to be used in conjuction with but *not as replacement* for standard therapeutic measures.

Dosage: Average total daily doses for dogs and cats are as follows: 5 to 15 lbs body weight 2 mg; 15 to 40 lbs body weight 2 to 4 mg; 40 to 80 lbs body weight 4 to 8 mg.

The total daily dose should be given in divided doses, 6 to 10 hours apart.

How Supplied: Bottles of 1000 tablets.

Caution: Federal (U.S.A.) law restricts this drug to use by or on the order of a licensed veterinarian.

MITABAN® LIQUID CONCENTRATE
(amitraz)
For Topical Use on Dogs

Warning: Toxicology studies conducted in the dog and other species suggest amitraz may alter the animal's ability to maintain homeostasis. Animals treated with Mitaban (amitraz) should not be subjected to stress for a period of at least 24 hours posttreatment. Adverse reactions including three fatalities were reported during the clinical studies. In excess of 1100 patients with generalized demodicosis were topically treated with Mitaban.

Description: Mitaban Liquid Concentration (amitraz) contains 19.9% N^1-(2, 4-dimethylphenyl)-N-[[(2, 4-dimethylphenyl) imino] methyl]-N-methylmethanimidamide (w/w), and also xylol, propylene oxide, and a blend of alkyl benezene sulfonates and exthoxylated polyethers. Amitraz, a diamide, is pale yellow, has a melting point of 86° to 87°C, is not hygroscopic, is stable to heating, soluble in most organic solvents, and sparingly soluble in water.

Pharmacology: Amitraz is hydrolyzed to 2,4-dimethyl-formanilide and N-(2, 4-dimethylphenyl)-N^1-methylformamidine; these metabolites are further metabolized to 2,4-dimethylaniline and ultimately to 4-amino-3-methlbenzoic acid, which was the principle metabolite in the urine and liver.

Radiolabeled amitraz was administered to beagles as a single oral treatment at a level of 4 mg/kg. Peak blood levels were reached between 1.5 and 6 hours posttreatment; the half-life was approximately 12 hours during the initial 48 hours. Radioactivity was extremely low in whole blood and plamsa at 72 (0.05–0.06 ppm) and 96 (0.03–0.06 ppm) hours. The organs having residues at levels greater than plasma concentrations at 96 hours included: liver, skin, eyes, bile, kidney, medulla, cerebrum, lungs, gonads, fat, thyroid, spleen, and large intestine. The main metabolite isolated from these tissues was identified as 4-amino-3-methylbenzoic acid, which is nontoxic for the dog.

Studies have not been conducted to quantitatively determine absorption by the dog following topical or dermal treatment with amitraz. The technical drug (amitraz) and formulated material (Mitaban Liquid Concentrate) have been extensively evaluated in laboratory and domesticated animals in a series of acute, subchronic and chronic studies.

The mechanism of action for amitraz is unknown, however, data currently available suggest the drug may act on the cen-

Continued on next page

Upjohn—Cont.

tral nervous system. *In vitro* housefly tests indicated amitraz does not have significant cholinesterase inhibitory activity.

Indications: Mitaban (amitraz) is indicated for treatment of generalized demodicosis *(Demodex canis)* in dogs. Current data do not support use for treatment of localized demodicosis or scabies.

Contraindications: Fertility impairment studies have not been conducted in the canine with Mitaban (amitraz). It is not known whether Mitaban) may cause impairment of ferility in dogs.

Reproduction studies during pregnancy have not been conducted with Mitaban. It is not known whether Mitaban may harm the embryo or fetus.

The safety of Mitaban has not been established for dogs less than four months of age.

Warnings: Please refer to warning at the beginning of the package insert.

Not for human use. Keep out of reach of children.

Mitaban (amitraz) may be harmful if swallowed by humans. If swallowed, do not induce vomiting (contains xylol) and immediately call a physician. Avoid inhalation of vapors (xylol) and contamination of feed and food stuffs.

Mitaban is flammable; when diluted with water, the mixture is not flammable.

Mitaban (concentrate or diluted) may cause eye or skin irritation in sensitive persons. Do not get in eyes, on skin or on clothing. If in eyes, wash with water for 15 minutes and call a physician immediately.

Protect exposed skin (e.g. with rubber gloves, etc) when mixing Mitaban with water and treating animals. Wash hands and arms with soap and water after treatment of the pet(s). Dispose of unused Mitaban-water solution by flushing down the drain. Rinse the Mitaban container with water and do not reuse. Avoid handling the pet(s) immediately after treatment.

Precautions: Though eye or dermal irritation was not reported during controlled experiments, such effects have been infrequently reported from clinical use. Consistent with good veterinary practice, it is recommended that a protectant be used in the eyes of patients prior to facial treatment with any topical therapy.

Well-controlled experiments with Mitaban (amitraz) have not been conducted to determine the compatibility range with other products.

Adverse Reactions and Side Effects

Ingestion of *Mitaban* may increase the risk of adverse effects. Therefore, appropriate care should be exercised both during and immediately after *Mitaban* application to minimize the opportunity for exposure by the oral route. The most frequently observed adverse reaction in the clinical studies was transient sedation, which occurred in approximately 8% of the generalized demodicosis patients. This effect was observed within 2 to 6 hours posttreatment, and usually dissipated within 24 to 72 hours. In approximately 40% of the affected generalized demodicosis patients, the effect dissipated in less than 24 hours. Sedation often was less apparent when additional *Mitaban* (amitraz) treatments were applied, however in approximately 35% of the generalized demodicosis patients sleepiness was observed after each treatment. Transient pruritus, which clinical investigators considered to be an indirect effect due to an inflammatory reaction associated with dead mites, occurred in less than 3% of the generalized demodicosis patients. This effect usually occurred and dissipated within 24–48 hours posttreatment. Other observations noted by the clinical investigators and /or clients were a low incidence (less than 1%) of convulsions, ataxia, hyperexcitability, personality change, hypothermia, appetite stimulation, bloat, polyuria, vomition, diarrhea, anorexia, edema and erythema and other varying degrees of skin irritation. Three fatalities were recorded.

Toxicology:

Dermal Studies—Dog: Acute and subchronic dermal toxicity studies were conducted with nondiseased beagles using the recommended concentration (250 ppm active drug) and exaggerated concentrations of Mitaban (amitraz). A single treatment with 250 ppm, 1250 ppm or 2500 ppm was topically applied to healthy dogs. Transient sedation was observed within 8 hours posttreatment in 1 of 6 dogs at 250 ppm, and all of the animals at 1250 ppm and 2500 ppm; all of the animals were normal at 24 hours posttreatment. There was a significant depression of rectal temperatures at 4 hours posttreatment in the 1250 ppm and 2500 ppm groups. Blood glucose values were elevated at 4 hours posttreatment in the 250 ppm female group, and in both sexes at the 1250 ppm and 2500 ppm concentrations. Rectal tem peratures and glucose values returned to normal within 24 hours posttreatment.

In another study, groups of healthy beagles were topically treated with either 250 ppm, 750 ppm or 1250 ppm of active drug at 14 day intervals and for 12 weeks. Blood glucose values were elevated at the 750 ppm concentration at 4 hours posttreatment after 3 to 6 treatments, and after 5 of 6 treatments at the 1250 ppm level. In the 750 ppm group, serum glucose values returned to normal at 24 hours posttreatment, however for the 1250 ppm group, at 24 hour and after 3 of 6 treatments the levels remained significantly elevated.

Dermal or ocular responses were not observed when *Mitaban* was applied at recommended or exaggerated concentrations to the skin and incidentally to the eyes of dogs controlled experiments stimulating recommended use. However, such responses have been infrequently reported from clinical use (see **PRECAUTIONS**).

Oral Studies—Dog: An acute oral toxicity study was conducted with amitraz utilizing nondiseased beagles. Death occurrred in one of two dogs given a single oral dose of 100 mg/kg. Clinical signs included CNS depression, ataxia, hypothermia, bradycardia, muscular weakness, vomition, uncontrolled vocal spasm and micturition. Clinical laboratory data indicated a hemoconcentration, and transient elevations in blood glucose, blood urea nitrogen, serum potassium and alkaline phosphate values. Dogs given 20 mg/kg (single oral dose) showed similar, though less pronounced, clinical signs and were clinically normal at three days posttreatment. Hemoconcentration and increased blood urea nitrogen were noted in both dogs; increased and transient blood glucose and serum alkaline phosphatase values were observed in one dog. Dogs given 4 mg/kg (single oral dose) had decreased rectal temperatures within three hours and were normal at 24 hours posttreatment.

Amitraz was orally administered to nondiseased beagles at levels of 0, 0.25, 1 and 4 mg/kg once daily for 90 days. There were no deaths in any of the groups. At 3 hours posttreatment and for only the initial three days of the 90 day experiment, dogs treated with 4 mg/kg exhibited CNS depression and ataxia; the effects remained for 3 to 6 hours and the dogs were normal within 24 hours posttreatment. Vomition occurred in two dogs on only the initial two days of the study. Thereafter (days 4 through 90) the dogs appeared to be subdued for approximately 6 hours after dosing, and ataxia was nearly impossible to detect. In the initial 48 to 72 hours, dogs treated with 1 mg/kg/day exhibited signs of depression (without ataxia) for 4–6 hours; subsequently the depression became less marked and of shorter duration. At 3 hours after dosing, dogs treated with 1 or 4 mg/kg consistently had subnormal rectal temperatures and pulse rates; both parameters returned to normal within 24 hours posttreatment. At 0.25 mg/kg/day, the dogs appeared normal throughout the experiment. Hyperglycemia consistently occurred in dogs treated with 1 and 4 mg/kg/day and rarely occurred in dogs at the 0.25 mg/kg level; this response was maximal within 6 hours posttreatment and serum glucose values returned to normal within 24 hours after treatment. Grossly there was a significant increase in liver weights for dogs treated at the 4 mg/kg level, however mircroscopically the findings were miminal and consisted of a slight enlargement of the central and midzonal hepatocytes; the degree of enlargement was not dose related. However, at the two higher doses the area affected appeared more prominen t as reflected by an increase of the periportal hepatocytes. In the adrenal gland, several dogs treated with the two higher levels had thinning of the zonae fasiculata and reticularis, which may be associated with slight hyperplasia of the zone glomerulosa. (see **PRECAUTIONS**)

Information for Clients: Clients should be informed that animals treated with Mitaban (amitraz) should not be subjected to additional stress for a period of at least 24 hours posttreatment. Refer to information in italics under **WARNINGS.**

Dosage and Administration: Long and medium-haired dogs should be clipped closely before treating. Prior to the initial treatment, all dogs should be bathed with mild soap and water and towel dried. The entire animal should then be topically treated with Mitaban (amitraz) at a rate of 10.6 milliliters (contents of one bottle) per 2 gallons of warm water (250 pmm active drug). Two bottles (21.2 milliliters) per four gallons of water may be necessary to treat large dogs. The entire dog should be thoroughly and completely wetted with the mixture, and then allowed to air dry. Do not rinse or towel dry the dog after treatment with Mitaban. A fresh Mitaban-water mixture should be prepared for each patient: using the same mixture for more than one patient can spread other dermal infections and also the concentration of Mitaban could be reduced to a level which would be less effective than recommended concentration.

Three to six topical treatments (14 days apart) are recommended for the treatment of generalized demodicosis. It is important to continue treatment until no viable (alive) mites are found in the skin scrapings at two successive treatments, or until six treatments have been applied. Severe (chronic) cases and dogs which are reinfested may require a second and third series of treatments, and again the treatment should be applied at 14 days intervals. Discontinue treatment of dogs which do not respond clinically.

When employing Mitaban for treatment of demodicosis, other dogs in the home also should be examined for lesions to ascertain whether treatment of these animals is warranted.

Canine Efficacy

Controlled Studies: The efficacy of Mitaban(amitraz) was extensively evaluated on dogs experimentally or naturally parasitized with *Demodex canis.* Three to six Mitaban treatments (250 ppm active drug), at 14 day intervals, were highly efficacious for treatment of naturally acquired demodicosis. Mitaban treatment was continued until all Demodex in the skin scrapings were dead or the dogs no longer harbored mites at two successive treatments, or the animal received six treatments. Ninety-six percent of the dogs were cleared of mites.

Clinical Studies: Investigators at university veterinary clinics, small animal practitioners, and dermatology specialists clinically evaluated Mitaban. A total of 1107 generalized demodicosis patients were included in these investigations. A variety of breeds, ages, hair conditions and lengths, and weights of dogs were included in these field investigations. The pre- and posttreatment demodicosis indices were used to quantify the degree and extent of involvement. Of the generalized cases, greater than 95% clinically improved (posttreatment clinical condition better than pretreatment condition), and the average clinical response [(mean pretreatment index − mean posttreatment index) × 100 ÷ mean pretreatment index] was greater than 90%; these patients received an average of 5 treatments. Seventy-five percent of the generalized demodicosis patients were negative for viable mites prior to administration of the final Mitaban treatment. Eighty percent of the generalized demodicosis patients were returned to clinical normalcy and did not require additional therapy after receiving one treatment series. Twenty percent of all patients with generalized demodicosis required a second treatment series. When retreated, the 14 day treatment interval was again followed, and these patients received an average of 5 treatments. Greater than 90% of the dogs clinically improved, and the average clinical response of these patients was approximately 80%. Greater than 96% of all generalized demodicosis patients returned to normalcy after receiving one or two treatment series and did not require further therapy. Between 3 and 4% of all generalized demodicosis patients were returned to the investigators and required therapy beyond the second treatment series; these patients received a third and fourth series of Mitaban treatments. Greater than 99% of all generalized demodicosis patients returned to normalcy after receiving one, two, or three treatment series and did not require further therapy; less than 1% of the patients required additional therapy.

Caution: Federal (U.S.A.) law restricts this drug to use by or on the order of a licensed veterinarian.

How Supplied: Mitaban Liquid Concentrate (amitraz) is available in cartons of 12—10.6 ml bottles.

For Veterinary Use Only

MYCITRACIN® Sterile Ointment (bacitracin-polymyxin B sulfate-neomycin sulfate) Sterile Ophthalmic Ointment

Composition: Each gram contains: Bacitracin, 500 units, neomycin sulfate, 5 mg (equivalent to 3.5 mg neomycin base); polymyxin B sulfate, 5,000 units; also anhydrous lanolin, mineral oil, and white petrolatum; chlorobutanol (chloral derivative) 0.65% added as preservative.

Action: The three antibiotics present in Mycitracin Sterile Ointment (bacitracin, polymyxin B sulfate and neomycin sulfate) provide a broad spectrum of activity against the gram-positive and gram-negative bacteria commonly involved in superficial infections of the eyelid, conjunctiva. Polymyxin B sulfate is bactericidal to gram-negative bacteria especially Pseudomonas. No resistant strains have been found to develop in vivo. Bacitracin is effective against gram-positive bacteria including hemolytic and non-hemolytic streptococci and staphylococci. Resistant strains rarely develop. Neomycin is effective against both gram-positive and gram-negative bacteria including staphylococci, Escherichia coli, and influenza and many strains of Proteus and Pseudomonas.

Indications: In the treatment of superficial bacterial infections of the eyelid and conjunctiva in dogs and cats when due to organisms susceptible to the antibiotics contained in the ointment. Laboratory tests should be conducted including in vitro culturing and susceptibility tests on samples collected prior to treatment.

Precautions: Sensitivity To Mycitracin Sterile Ointment (bacitracin, polymyxin B sulfate and neomycin sulfate) is rare; however, if a reaction occurs, discontinue use of the preparation, prolonged use may result in the overgrowth of nonsusceptible organisms including fungi. Appropriate measures should be taken if this occurs. If infection does not respond to treatment in two or three days, the diagnosis and therapy should be reevaluated. Mycitracin should not be relied upon as the sole therapy for deep ocular infections. Appropriate systemic therapy should also be employed in such conditions.

Care should be taken not to contaminate the applicator tip of the tube during application of the preparation. Do not allow the applicator tip to come in contact with any tissue.

Caution: Federal (U.S.A.) law restricts this drug to use by or on the order of a licensed veterinarian.

Caution: This product is not for use in food producing animals.

Adverse Reactions: Itching, burning or inflammation may occur in animals sensitive to the product. Discontinue use in such case.

Dosage and Administration: Apply a thin film over the cornea three or four times daily in dogs and cats. The area should be properly cleansed prior to the use of Mycitracin Sterile Ointment (bacitracin, polymyxin B sulfate and neomycin sulfate). Foreign bodies, crusted exudates and debris should be carefully removed.

How Supplied: 3.5 gm tubes.

U

NEO–DELTA–CORTEF® brand of neomycin sulfate-prednisolone acetate sterile suspension For Veterinary Use Only

Description: Eye-Ear Sterile Suspension Neo-Delta-Cortef contains in each ml prednisolone acetate, 2.5 mg; and neomycin sulfate, 5 mg (equivalent to 3.5 mg neomycin). Also, sodium citrate, polyethylene glycol 3350 added as preservative, povidone, myristyl-gamma-picolinium chloride 0.2 mg added as a preservative. When necessary, pH was adjusted with sodium hydroxide and/or hydrochloric acid. This combination of prednisolone and neomycin is well suited for the treatment of certain eye and ear conditions in dogs and cats.

Actions: Prednisolone exerts a marked anti-inflammatory effect in the same manner as does hydrocortisone, that is, through a controlling influence on vascular permeability and on the cellular, fibrous, amorphous components of conective tissue. In anti-inflammatory activ-

Continued on next page

Upjohn—Cont.

ity, prednisolone is more potent than hydrocortisone, and a concentration of 0.25% of prednisolone acetate is highly effective when applied topically in inflammatory conditions of the conjunctiva and the external ear.
Local application to the eye often gives rapid relief of pain, particularly in lesions of the cornea. This effect is believed due to the controlling action of the hormone on the inflammatory process rather than to a specific analgesic effect. By inhibiting fibroblastic proliferation, symblepharon formation in chemical and thermal burns may be prevented: through decreased scar formation and reduced formation of new blood vessels, clearer corneas may result.
Topically applied prednisolone acetate is usually rapidly effective, particularly in acute inflammatory conditions of the conjunctiva, sclera and cornea, and in otitis externa. Chronic conditions respond more slowly and relapses are more frequent.
Neomycin is an antibacterial substance derived from cultures of the soil organism *Streptomyces fradiae.* Its antimicrobial range includes both gram-positive and gram-negative organisms commonly responsible for ocular and otic infections, such as staphylococci, *Escherichia coli,* and many strains of Proteus and Pseudomonas organisms. It is not active against fungi. Neomycin is unusually nontoxic for epithelial cells in tissue culture and is nonirritating in therapeutic concentrations. The presence of neomycin in Neo-Delta-Cortef (neomycin sulfate-prednisolone acetate) affords control of infections caused by neomycin-susceptible organisms.

U

Indications: Neo-Delta-Cortef (neomycin sulfateprednisolone acetate) is indicated for treating infectious, allergic and traumatic keratitis and conjunctivitis, acute otitis externa, and, to a lesser degree, chronic otitis externa in dogs and cats.
Contraindications: All topical ophthalmic preparations containing corticosteroids, with or without an antimicrobial agent, are contraindicated in the initial treatment of corneal ulcers. They should not be used until infection is under control and corneal regeneration is well under way.
Caution: Topical ophthalmic preparations containing corticosteroids without an antimicrobial agent are generally contraindicated for the treatment of infectious diseases of the eye. Purulent and chronic catarrhal conjunctivitis are usually associated with bacterial infections. In these the steroid may mask the signs or enhance the activity of the infectious agent. Note: Neomycin susceptibility tests should be conducted prior to the use of Neo-Delta-Cortef (neomycin sulfate-prednisolone acetate).
Precautions: Incomplete response or exacerbation of corticosteroid responsive lesions may be due to the presence of non-susceptible organisms or to prolonged use of antibiotic-containing preparations resulting in overgrowth of non-susceptible organisms, particularly Monilia. Thus, if improvement is not noted within two or three days, or if redness, irritation, or swelling persists or increases, the diagnosis should be redetermined and appropriate therapeutic measures initiated.
Warning
Not for human use. Clinical and experimental data have demonstrated that corticosteroids administered orally or by injection to animals may induce the first stage of parturition if used during the last trimester of pregnancy and may precipitate premature parturition followed by dystocia, fetal death, retained placenta, and metritis.
Additionally, corticosteroids administered to dogs, rabbits, and rodents during pregnancy have resulted in cleft palate in offspring. Corticosteroids administered to dogs during pregnancy have also resulted in other congenital anomalies, including deformed forelegs, phocomelia, and anasarca.
Dosage and Administration: For beginning treatment in acute ocular inflammations, 1 or 2 drops may be placed in the conjunctival sac three to six times during a 24-hour period. When improvement occurs, the dosage may be reduced to 1 drop two to four times daily. In otitis externa, 2 to 6 drops may be placed in the external ear canal two or three times daily.
Advantages of Neo-Delta-Cortef:
(neomycin sulfate-prednisolone acetate)
1. Potent anti-inflammatory effect of prednisolone.
2. Wide spectrum antibacterial effect of neomycin.
3. Usually prompt relief of symptoms.
4. Ease of applications.

How Supplied: 5.0 ml plastic dropper bottle.

NEO–PREDEF® brand of neomycin sulfate and isoflupredone acetate sterile ointment For Veterinary Use Only

NEO-PREDEF Sterile Ointment is for ophthalmic, otic and topical use in horses, cattle, dogs and cats. Each gram contains the potent anti-inflammatory agent isoflupredone acetate 1 mg (0.1%); and the antibiotic neomycin sulfate, 5 mg (0.5%) (equivalent to 3.5 mg neomycin); also anhydrous lanolin, white petrolatum, and mineral oil. Chlorobutanol (chloral derivative) 0.65% added as preservative. This combination is well suited for the treatment or adjunctive therapy of many eye, ear, and skin conditions, as well as a dressing for superficial wounds occurring in horses, cattle, dogs and cats. Its action is prompt, potent, and specific as to antiinflammatory and bactericidal properties.
Isoflupredone
It has been reported by research workers that isoflupredone (Predef) is 14 times as potent as hydrocortisone as an anti-inflammatory steroid as measured by the cotton pellet implantation assay. Isoflupredone markedly inhibits inflammatory reaction through its controlling influence on connective tissue and vascular components. Topically applied isoflupredone is rapidly effective. In otitis externa, wounds of the concha, ulcerations of the ear flaps, and irritated lesions of the skin, the inflammatory response may also be effectively inhibited by isoflupredone. Chronic conditions respond more slowly and relapses are more frequent.
Neomycin
Neomycin is an antibiotic substance derived from cultures of the soil organism *Streptomyces fradiae.* Its antimicrobial range includes both gram-positive and gram-negative organisms commonly responsible for or associated with ocular and otic infections, such as staphylococci, streptococci, *Escherichia coli, Aerobacter aerogenes,* and many strains of Proteus and Pseudomonas organisms. It is not active against fungi. Neomycin rarely induces sensitization or causes resistant strains of microorganisms to develop. It is unusually nontoxic for epithelial cells in tissue culture and is nonirritating in therapeutic concentrations. The presence of neomycin in Neo-Predef (neomycin sulfate and isoflupredone acetate ointment) affords prophylactic as well as therapeutic control of secondary infection caused by neomycin-sensitive organisms.
Advantages of Neo-Predef:
1. Potent anti-inflammatory effect of isoflupredone.
2. Wide-spectrum bactericidal effect of neomycin.
3. Prompt relief of symptoms.
4. Ease of application.
5. No pupillary dilation or influence on accommodation.

Indications: Neo-Predef Sterile Ointment is indicated as treatment or adjunctive therapy of certain eye, ear, and skin conditions in horses, cattle, dogs and cats caused by or associated with neomycin susceptible organisms and/or allergy. In addition it is indicated as superficial dressing applied to minor cuts, wounds, lacerations, abrasions, and for postsurgical application where reduction of inflammatory response is deemed desirable.
Neo-Predef is useful in treating such conditions as keratitis and conjunctivitis in dogs, keratoconjunctivitis (pink-eye) in cattle, and acute otitis externa in dogs and to a lesser degree, chronic olitis externa in dogs. It also is effective in treating anal gland infections and moist dermatitis in the dog and is a useful dressing for minor cuts, lacerations, abrasions, and post-surgical therapy in the horse, cat, and dog.
Neo-Predef may also be used following amputation of dewclaws, tails and claws, following ear trimming, castrating, and dehorning operations.
General Contraindications For Ophthalmic Preparations Containing Corticosteroids
1. Corneal Ulcers
All topical ophthalmic preparations containing corticosteroids, with or

without an antimicrobial agent, are contraindicated in the initial treatment of corneal ulcers. They should not be used until infection is under control and corneal regeneration is well under way.
2. Infectious Diseases of the Eyeball and Accessory Structures.
Topical ophthalmic preparations containing corticosteroids without an antimicrobial agent* are generally contraindicated for the treatment of infectious diseases of the eye. Purulent and chronic catarrhal conjunctivitis are usually associated with bacterial infections. In these the steroid may mask the signs or enhance the activity of the infectious agent.

Note: Susceptibility tests for the selection of a proper antimicrobial agent should be conducted prior to the use of topical ophthalmic preparations containing both a corticosteroid and an antimicrobial agent. Inactivity of the antimicrobial agent would mask the signs and enhance the infectious agent as stated above.

The preceding caution does not pertain to those bacterial infections of the eyeball and accessory structure where the etiological agent is known and a specific effective antimicrobial agent is employed.

*This preparation does contain the broad-spectrum antimicrobial agent neomycin sulfate; thus, this contraindication does not apply to this preparation.

Warning

Clinical and experimental data have demonstrated that corticosteroids administered orally or by injection to animals may induce the first stage of parturition if used during the last trimester of pregnancy and may precipitate premature parturition followed by dystocia, fetal death, retained placenta, and metritis.

Additionally, corticosteroids administered to dogs, rabbits, and rodents during pregnancy have resulted in cleft palate in offspring. Corticosteroids administered to dogs during pregnancy have also resulted in other congenital anomalies, including deformed forelegs, phocomelia, and anasarca.

Not for human use.

Caution: Incomplete response or exacerbation of corticosteroid responsive lesions may be due to the presence of nonsusceptible organisms or to prolonged use of antibiotic-containing preparations resulting in overgrowth of non-susceptible organisms, particularly Monilia. Thus, if improvement is not noted within two or three days, or if redness, irritation, or swelling persist or increases, the diagnosis should be redetermined and appropriate therapeutic measure initiated.

When used for cuts and abrasions on the teats of dairy animals, the udder and teats should be thoroughly cleaned prior to milking.

Dosage and Administration: Neo-Predef Sterile Ointment may be placed in the conjunctival sac three or four times daily. When improvement occurs, the frequency of application may be reduced to two or three times daily. In treatment of otitis externa and other inflammatory conditions of the external ear canal, a quantity of ointment sufficient to fill the external ear canal may be applied one to three times daily. When used on the skin or mucous membranes, cleanse the affected area, apply a small amount of the ointment and spread or rub in gently. The involved area may be treated one to three times a day and continue these daily applications in accordance with the clinical response.

How Supplied: 3.5 and 5 gm tubes each with special applicator tip.

Caution: Federal (U.S.A.) law restricts this drug to use by or on the order of a licensed veterinarian.

NEO–PREDEF® with TETRACAINE (neomycin sulfate, isoflupredone acetate, and tetracaine hydrochloride) Topical Powder

For topical ear and skin use in dogs, cats and horses.

Composition: Neo-Predef with Tetracaine contains in each gram neomycin sulfate, 5 mg (equivalent to 3.5 mg neomycin); isoflupredone acetate, 1 mg; tetracaine hydrochloride, 5 mg; myristyl-gamma-picolinium chloride, 0.2 mg; also lactose hydrous. Because of the prompt, potent, and specific actions of the individual components, this combination is well suited for the treatment of certain ear and skin conditions occurring in dogs, cats and horses.

Advantages of Neo-Predef with Tetracaine:
1. Highly potent anti-inflammatory effect of isoflupredone acetate.
2. Wide-spectrum bactericidal effect of neomycin.
3. Rapid anesthetic effect of tetracaine.
4. Prompt relief of symptoms.
5. Reduces further self-inflicted trauma.
6. Ease of application.
7. Adherent to moist surfaces.

Isoflupredone Acetate

Isoflupredone acetate markedly inhibits inflammatory reaction through its controlling influence on connective tissue and vascular components. Topically applied isoflupredone acetate is usually rapidly effective. In otitis externa, wounds of the concha, ulcerations of the ear flaps, and irritated lesions of the skin, the inflammatory response may also be effectively inhibited by isoflupredone acetate. Chronic conditions respond more slowly and relapses are more frequent.

Neomycin

Neomycin is an antibiotic substance derived from cultures of the soil organism *Streptomyces fradiae.* Its antimicrobial range includes both gram-positive and gram-negative organisms commonly responsible for or associated with otic infections, such as staphylococci, streptococci, *Escherichia coli, Aerobacter aerogenes,* and many strains of Proteus and Pseudomonas organisms. It is not active against fungi. Neomycin is unusually nontoxic for epithelial cells in tissue culture and is nonirritating in therapeutic concentrations. The presence of neomycin in Neo-Predef with Tetracaine affords control of neomycin-sensitive organisms.

Tetracaine

Tetracaine hydrochloride is a topical anesthetic agent that is more potent than either procaine or cocaine in comparable concentration. The duration of anesthetic action of tetracaine exceeds that produced by either butacaine or phenacaine.

Many investigators have demonstrated that local anesthesia plays a significant part in the promotion of healing, especially where pain is a prominent factor. It is believed that trauma stimulates local pain receptors, which results in reflex vasodilation, edema, tenderness, and muscular spasm.

If the reflex is abolished through use of a local anesthetic such as tetracaine, amelioration of these tissue changes that interfere with healing is favored. The local anesthetic action of tetracaine has proved to be of great value in alleviating the pain reflex in painful skin and ear conditions.

Myristyl-Gamma-Picolinium Chloride

Myristyl-gamma-picolinium Chloride is highly germicidal, nonirritating and relatively nontoxic. In solution it reduces surface tension (a surfactant), possesses detergent and emulsifying actions, and exhibits properties which favor the penetration and wetting of tissue surfaces. The drug is effective against a wide range of organisms, its active ingredient killing in ten minutes *Staphylococcus aureus* in dilutions up to 1:85,000 at 37 degrees Centigrade; *E. typhosa* in dilutions up to 1:140,000; *Esch. Coli.* in dilutions up to 1:40,000, and *S. dysenteriae* in dilutions up to 1:80,000.

Myristyl-gamma-picolinium Chloride has been used, per se, for preoperative disinfection of the skin, for application to superficial injuries, for irrigating deep wounds, and for application to infections and wounds of mucous membranes.

Indications: Neo-Predef with Tetracaine Topical Powder is indicated in the treatment for adjunctive therapy of certain ear and skin conditions in dogs, cats and horses caused by or associated with neomycin-susceptible organisms and/or allergy. In addition, it is indicated as superficial dressing applied to minor cuts, wounds, lacerations, abrasions, and for post-surgical application where reduction of pain and inflammatory response is deemed desirable. Neo-Predef with Tetracaine may be used as a dusting powder following amputation of tails, claws, and dewclaws; following ear trimming and castrating; and following such surgical procedure as ovariohysterectomies.

Applied superficially, it has been used successfully in the treatment of acute otitis externa in dogs, acute moist dermatitis and interdigital dermatitis in the dog, and as a dusting powder to various

Continued on next page

U

Upjohn—Cont.

minor cuts, lacerations, and abrasions in the horse, cat and dog.
Precautions: Incomplete response or exacerbation of corticosteroid-response lesions may be due to the presence of non-susceptible organisms or to prolonged use of antibiotic-containing preparations resulting in overgrowth of non-susceptible organisms, particularly Monilia. Thus, if improvement is not noted within two or three days, or if redness, irritation, or swelling persists or increases, the diagnosis should be redetermined and appropriate therapeutic measures initiated.
Applications: After cleansing the affected area, Neo-Predef with Tetracaine is applied by compressing the sides of the container with short, sharp squeezes. In most instances a single daily application will be sufficient; however, it may be applied one to three times daily, as required.
How Supplied: 15 gm plastic insufflator bottles.
Caution: Federal (U.S.A.) law restricts this drug to use by or on the order of a licensed veterinarian.

PANMYCIN Aquadrops®
(tetracycline oral suspension U.S.P.)
For oral veterinary use in dogs and cats only.

Composition: Tetracycline is a broad spectrum antibiotic that can be conveniently administered to dogs and cats in a palatable liquid preparation, Panmycin Aquadrops. Panmycin Aquadrops contains in each ml. tetracycline base equivalent to 100 mg of tetracycline hydrochloride, suspended in a chocolate-mint flavored aqueous vehicle. Methylparaben, 0.075%; propylparaben, 0.025%; and sodium metabisulfite, 0.5%; are present as preservatives. Panmycin Aquadrops is stable at room temperature.
Panmycin (tetracycline) is a bright yellow, crystalline, broad spectrum antibiotic produced by a species of *Streptomyces.* Although its chemical and physical properties as well as its antibacterial spectrum resemble those of oxytetracycline and chlortetracycline, tetracycline hydrochloride offers the advantage of greater stability in plasma and, on oral administration, fewer gastrointestinal side effects.
Action: Panmycin (tetracycline) has a wide range of antibacterial activity against gram-positive and gram-negative bacteria. These include *Streptococcus spp., Staphylococcus spp., Aerobacter aerogenes, E. coli, Klebsiella spp., Salmonella spp., (Haemophilus)* and *Pasteurella spp.* The antimicrobial activity of Panmycin also includes rickettsia and agents belonging to the psittacosis-lymphogranuloma group.
Administered by mouth, Panmycin is absorbed from the gastrointestinal tract and readily diffuses into various body fluids including blood serum, spinal fluid, pleural fluid, and peritoneal fluid, cord serum, and saliva. Maximum blood levels of the antibiotic are reached at about two hours after administration and are maintained at high levels for 6 to 8 hours. The blood levels were observed to be somewhat higher than those obtained with similar doses of oxytetracycline or chlortetracycline. Spinal fluid concentrations were found to be notably higher than those produced by the other tetracyclines indicating the greater ease of tetracycline to pass the blood-brain barrier. The urinary excretion of tetracycline is rapid, the rate being approximately equal to that of the other tetracyclines. A significent portion of the dose is not absorbed and appears in the feces.
Indications: Panmycin (tetracycline) Aquadrops is indicated for oral administration to dogs and cats in the treatment of infections caused by organisms sensitive to tetracycline hydrochloride such as:

1. Bacterial gastroenteritis due to *E. coli.*
2. Urinary tract infections due to *Staphylococcus spp.* and *E. coli.*

Appropriate laboratory tests should be conducted including in vitro culturing and susceptibility tests on samples collected prior to treatment.
Warning: For oral use in dogs and cats only. *Not for use in animals raised for food production.*
Not for human use.
Caution: Use of tetracycline hydrochloride during tooth development (late prenatal, neonatal and early postnatal periods) may cause discoloration of the teeth (yellow-grey-brownish). This effect occurs mostly during long-term use of the drug. But it has also been observed following short treatment courses.
With the use of any broad spectrum antibiotic, prolonged use may result in overgrowth of nonsusceptible organisms, including *Candida (monilia) albicans.* Constant observation is essential. Should superinfection occur, the antibiotic should be discontinued and/or other appropriate measures taken.
Adverse Reactions: Tetracycline hydrochloride is generally well tolerated; however, in some instances a change in consistency of the stool may occur due to the wide antibacterial effects of tetracycline on the intestinal flora.
If allergic reactions occur or if individual idiosyncrasy appears, discontinue medication.
Dosage and Administration: The dosage of Panmycin (tetracycline), as with other tetracycline drugs, will vary in different animal patients according to the severity of the infection, response to treatment, and susceptibility of the causative bacteria. The following average dosage is suggested:
Dogs and Cats—25 mg (5 drops) per pound of body weight, per day, in divided doses every 6 hours.
Treatment should be continued until the temperature has been normal for 48 hours or characteristic symptoms of the disease have subsided. In dogs and cats Panmycin is usually well tolerated, but, if necessary, the drug may be given with cold milk or a light diet.
To assure even distribution of the Panmycin the bottle should be shaken thoroughly before each dose.
How Supplied: 15 ml bottles with calibrated dropper; 30 ml bottles with calibrated dropper.
Each ml of product contains tetracycline base equivalent to 100 mg tetracycline hydrochloride.
Caution: Federal (U.S.A.) law restricts this drug to use by or on the order of a licensed veterinarian.

PANMYCIN® HYDROCHLORIDE
(tetracycline hydrochloride) 500 mg. Bolus

Composition: Each bolus contains: Tetracycline hydrochloride, 500 mg.
For oral use in calves.
Indications: For treatment of bacterial pneumonia caused by organisms susceptible to tetracycline and bacterial enteritis caused by E. coli and Salmonella organisms susceptible to tetracycline.
Dosage: Administer orally 10 mg. per pound of body weight per day divided into two daily doses (1 bolus per 100 lb. twice daily).
Precautions: The use of broad-spectrum antibiotics may result in gastrointestinal disturbances. They may be minimized by reducing the individual dose and administering the drug at more frequent intervals. Allergic manifestations are rare. If adverse reactions occur, discontinue medication. Intestinal protectants containing aluminum hydroxide or salts of calcium or magnesium given with tetracyclines have been shown to decrease absorption and hence are contraindicated.
Caution: If symptoms persist after using this product for two or three days the diagnosis should be redetermined.
Warning: Do not use for more than 5 days. Use as the sole source of tetracycline. Do not slaughter animals for food within 12 days of treatment. Not for human use.
How Supplied: bottle of 100.

PREDEF® 2X brand of
isoflupredone acetate
sterile aqueous suspension
For intramuscular or intrasynovial use only.
For Veterinary Use Only

Composition: Each ml contains 2 mg of isoflupredone acetate; also 4.5 mg sodium citrate hydrous; 120 mg polyethylene glycol 3350; 0.2 mg myristyl-gamma-picolinium chloride added as preservative; 1 mg povidone. When necessary, pH was adjusted with hydrochloric acid and/or sodium hydroxide. It is for intramuscular or intrasynovial injection in animals and is indicated in situations requiring glucocorticoid, anti-inflammatory, and/or supportive effect.
Metabolic and Hormonal Effects: Predef 2X (isoflupredone acetate), a potent corticosteroid developed in the Research Laboratories of The Upjohn Company, has greater glucocorticoid activity than an equal quantity of prednisolone.

The glucocorticoid activity of Predef 2X is approximately 10 times that of prednisolone, 50 times that of hydrocortisone, and 67 times that of cortisone as measured by liver glycogen deposition in rats. The gluconeogenic activity is borne out by its hyperglycemic effect in both normal and ketotic cattle.

Indications: Bovine Ketosis. Predef 2X, by its gluconeogenic and glycogen deposition activity, is an effective and valuable treatment for the endocrine and metabolic imbalance of primary bovine ketosis. The stresses of parturition and high milk production predispose the dairy cow to this condition. This adrenal steroid causes a prompt physiological effect, with blood glucose levels returning to normal or above within 8 to 24 hours following injection. There is a decrease in circulating eosinophils, followed by a reduction in blood and urine ketones. Usually the general attitude of the cow is much improved, appetite returns, and milk production rises to previous levels within 3 to 5 days. In secondary bovine ketosis, where the condition is complicated by pneumonia, mastitis, endometritis, traumatic gastritis, etc., Predef 2X should be used concurrently with proper local and parenteral antibacterial therapy, infusion solutions, and other accepted treatments for the primary conditions.

Musculoskeletal Conditions: As with other adrenal steroids, this preparation has been found useful in alleviating the pain and lameness associated with generalized and acute localized arthritic conditions in large animals. Predef 2X (isoflupredone acetate) has been used successfully to treat laminitis, rheumatoid and traumatic arthritis, osteoarthritis, periostitis, tendinitis, tenosynovitis, bursitis, and myositis. Generalized muscular soreness, stiffness, depression, and anorexia resulting from overwork, shipping, unusual physical exertion, etc., respond promptly. Remission of symptoms may be permanent, or symptoms may recur, depending on the cause and extent of structural degeneration.

Allergic Reactions. Predef 2X (isoflupredone acetate) is especially beneficial in treating acute hypersensitivity reactions resulting from treatment with a sensitizing drug or exposure to other allergenic agents. Usual manifestations are anaphylactoid reactions and urticaria. Less severe allergic manifestations, such as atopic and contact dermatitis, summer eczema, and conjunctivitis, may also be treated. Response is usually rapid and complete, although in severe cases with extensive lesions, more prolonged adrenocorticoid therapy and other appropriate treatment may be indicated.

Overwheiming Infections with Severe Toxicity. In animals moribund from overwhelmingly severe infections for which specific antibacterial therapy is available (e.g., critical pneumonia, peritonitis, endometritis, septic mastitis), intensive Predef 2X (isoflupredone acetate) therapy may aid in correcting the circulatory defect by counteracting the responsible inflammatory changes, thereby permitting the antibacterial agent to exert its full effect. As supportive therapy, this steroid combats the stress and improves the general attitude of the animal being treated. All necessary procedures for the establishment of a bacterial diagnosis should be carried out whenever possible before institution of therapy. Predef 2X therapy in the presence of infection should be administered for the shortest possible time compatible with maintenance of an adequate response, and antibacterial therapy should be continued for at least three days after the hormone has been withdrawn. Combined hormone and antibacterial therapy does not obviate the need for indicated surgical treatment.

Shock: Predef 2X is indicated in adrenal failure and shocklike states occurring in association with severe injury or other trauma, emergency surgery, anaphylactoid reactions, and elective surgery in poor surgical risks. It is recommended as an adjuvant to standard methods of combating shock, including use of plasma expanders. Because of interrelated physiologic activities, beneficial effects may not be exhibited until all such procedures have been employed.

Other Indications. Exhaustion following surgery or dystocia, retained placenta, inflammatory ocular conditions, snakebite, and other stress conditions are also indications for use. Its employment in the treatment of these conditions is recommended as a supportive measure to standard procedures and time-honored treatments and will give comfort to the animal and hasten complete recovery.

Predef 2X (isoflupredone acetate) has been found useful as supportive therapy in the treatment of the stress associated with parturient paresis i.e., milk fever. It should be given intramuscularly, before or after the administration of the calcium infusion solutions commonly employed in treating the disease. Predef 2X is not to be added to the infusion solutions.

Warning: Not for human use. Animals intended for human consumption should not be slaughtered within 7 days of last treatment.

Clinical and experimental data have demonstrated that corticosteroids administered orally or parenterally to animals may induce the first stage of parturition when administered during the last trimester of pregnancy and may precipitate premature parturition followed by dystocia, fetal death, retained placenta, and metritis. Additionally, corticosteroids administered to dogs, rabbits, and rodents during pregnancy have resulted in cleft palate in offspring. Corticosteroids administered to dogs during pregnancy have also resulted in other congenital anomalies, including deformed forelegs, phocomelia, and anasarca.

Precautions: Predef 2X (isoflupredone acetate) exerts an inhibitory influence on the mechanisms and the tissue changes associated with inflammation. Vascular permeability is decreased, exudation diminished, and migration of the inflammatory cells markedly inhibited. In addition, systemic manifestations such as fever and signs of toxemia may also be suppressed. While certain aspects of this alteration of the inflammatory reaction may be beneficial, the suppression of inflammation may mask the signs of infection and tend to facilitate spread of microorganisms. However, in infections characterized by overwhelming toxicity, Predef 2X therapy in conjunction with appropriate antibacterial therapy is effective in reducing mortality and morbidity. Without concurrent use of an antibiotic to which the invaderorganism is sensitive, injudicious use of the adrenal hormones in animals with infections can be hazardous. As with other corticoids, continued or prolonged use is discouraged.

While no sodium retention nor potassium depletion has been observed at the doses recommended in animals rceeiving 9-fluoro-prednisolone acetate, as with all corticoids, animals should be under close observation for possible untoward effects. If symptoms of hypopotassemia should occur, corticoid therapy should be discontinued and 5% solution of potassium chloride administered by continuous intravenous drip.

Dosage and Administration: Sterile Aqueous Suspension Predef 2X is administered by deep intramuscular injection for systemic effect, or into joint cavity, tendon sheath, or bursa for local effect.

Cattle: The usual intramuscular dose for cattle is 10 to 20 mg, according to the size of the animal and severity of the condition. This dose may be repeated in 12 to 24 hours if indicated.

Ketosis studies have demonstrated that relatively high initial doses of corticoids produce a more prompt recovery with a lower incidence of relapse than when relatively low doses are used, even when these are repeated. Response of ketosis to Predef 2X therapy parallels that derived with prednisolone. Predef 2X is 10 times more glucogenic than prednisolone. Thus, 10 mg of isoflupredone acetate therapeutically equals 100 mg of prednisolone.

In the event of poor response or relapse, diagnosis should be reconfirmed by reexamining the animal for complications (i.e., pneumonia, metritis, traumatic gastritis, mastitis).

Horses. The usual intramuscular dose for horses is 5 to 20 mg repeated as necessary. The usual intrasynovial dose in joint inflammation, tendinitis, or bursitis is 5 to 20 mg or more, depending on the size of the cavity to be injected.

Swine. The usual intramuscular dose for swine is 5 mg for a 300 pound animal. The dose for larger or smaller pigs is proportional to the weight of the animal.

How Supplied: 2 mg per ml, 10 ml sterile vial, 100 ml sterile vial.

Continued on next page

Upjohn—Cont.

PROSTIN F2 ALPHA®
(dinoprost tromethamine)
Sterile Solution
For intramuscular use
For use in mares

Composition: This product contains Prostin F2 alpha (dinoprost tromethamine) as the tromethamine salt of the naturally occurring prostaglandin F2 alpha (PGF2α).
Chemical Name: 7-[3α, 5α-dihydroxy-2β-[(3S)-3 hydroxytrans-1-octenyl]-1α-cyclopentyl]-*cis* -5-heptenoic acid compound with 2-amino-2(hydroxymethyl)-1,3- propanediol.
Molecular Formula equals $C_{20}H_{34}O_5 \cdot C_4H_{11}NO_3$.
Prostin F2 alpha is a white or slightly off-white crystalline powder that is readily soluble in water at room temperature in concentrations to at least 200 mg/ml.
General Biologic Activity: Prostaglandins occur in nearly all mammalian tissues. Prostaglandins, especially PGE's and PGF's, have been shown, in certain species, to 1) increase at time of parturition in amniotic fluid, maternal placenta, myometrium, and blood, 2) stimulate myometrial activity, and 3) to induce either abortion or parturition. Prostaglandins, especially PGF_2, have been shown to 1) increase in the uterus and blood to levels similar to levels achieved by exogenous administration which elicited luteolysis, 2) be capable of crossing from the uterine vein to the ovarian artery (sheep), 3) be related to IUD induced luteal regression (sheep), and 4) be capable of regressing the corpus luteum of most mammalian species studied to date. Prostaglandins have been reported to result in release of pituitary tropic hormones. Data suggest prostaglandins, especially PGE's and PGF's, may be involved in the process of ovulation and gamete transport. Also, $PGF_{2}\alpha$ has been reported to cause increase in blood pressure, bronchoconstriction, and smooth muscle stimulation in certain species.
Safety and Toxicity: Prostin F2 alpha (dinoprost tromethamine) was administered to adult mares (weighing 320 to 485 kg; 2 to 20 years old), at the rates of 0, 100, 200, 400, and 800 mg per mare per day for 8 days. Route of administration for each dose group was both intramuscularly (2 mares) and subcutaneously (2 mares). Changes were detected in all treated groups for clinical (reduced sensitivity to pain; locomotor incoordination; hypergastromotility; sweating; hyperthermia; labored respiration), blood chemistry (elevated cholesterol, total bilirubin, LDH, and glucose), and hematology (decreased eosinophils; increased hemoglobin, hematocrit, and erythrocytes) measurements. The effects in the 100 mg dose, and to a lesser extent, the 200 mg dose groups were transient in nature, lasting for a few minutes to several hours. Mares did not appear to sustain adverse effects following termination of the side effects. Mares treated with either 400 mg or 800 mg exhibited more profound symptoms. The excessive hyperstimulation of the gastrointestinal tract caused a protracted diarrhea, slight electrolyte imbalance (decreased sodium and potassium), dehydration, gastrointestinal irritation, and slight liver malfunction (elevated SGOT, SGPT at 800 mg only). Heart rate was increased but pH of the urine was decreased. Other measurements evaluated in the study remained within normal limits. No mortality occurred in any of the groups. No apparent differences were observed between the intramuscular and subcutaneous routes of administration. Luteolytic doses of Prostin F2 alpha are on the order of 5 to 10 mg administered on one day, therefore, Prostin F2 alpha was demonstrated to have a wide margin of safety. Thus, the 100 mg dose gave a safety margin of 10 to 20X for a single injection or 80 to 160X for the 8 daily injections.
Additional studies investigated the effects of single intramuscular doses of 0, 0.25, 1.0, 2.5, 3.0, 5.0, and 10.0 mg Prostin F2 alpha. Heart rate, respiration rate, rectal temperature, and sweating were measured at 0, 0.25, 0.50, 0.75, 1.0, 1.5, 2.0, 3.0, 4.0, 5.0, and 6.0 hr after injection. Neither heart rate nor respiration rates were significantly altered ($P > 0.05$) when compared to contemporary control values. Sweating was observed for 0 of 9, 2 of 9, 7 of 9, 7 of 9, 9 of 9, and 8 of 9 mares injected with 0.25, 1.0, 2.5, 3.0, 5.0, or 10.0 mg Prostin F2 alpha, respectively. Sweating was temporary in all cases and was mild for doses of 3.0 mg or less but was extensive (beads of sweat over the entire body and dripping) for the 10 mg dose. Sweating after the 5.0 mg dose was intermediate between that seen for mares treated with 3.0 and 10.0 mg. Sweating began within 15 minutes after injection and ceased by 45 to 60 minutes after injection. Rectal temperature was decreased during the interval 0.5 until 1.0, 3 to 4, or 5 hr. after injection for 0.25 and 1.0 mg, 2.5 and 3.0, or 5 and 10.0 mg dose groups, respectively. Average rectal temperature during the periods of decreased temperature was on the order of 97.5 to 99.6, with the greatest decreases observed in the 10 mg dose group.
Indications: Prostin F2 alpha (dinoprost tromethamine) is indicated for its luteolytic effect in mares. This luteolytic effect can be utilized to control the timing of estrus in estrous cycling and clinically anestrous mares that have a corpus luteum in the following circumstances:

1. *Controlling time of estrus of estrous cycling mares:* Mares treated with Prostin F2 alpha during diestrus (4 or more days after ovulation) will return to estrus within 2 to 4 days in most cases and ovulate 8 to 12 days after treatment. This procedure may be utilized as an aid to scheduling the use of stallions.
2. *Difficult-to-Breed Mares:* In extended diestrus there is failure to exhibit regular estrous cycles which is different from true anestrus. Many mares described as anestrus during the breeding season have serum progesterone levels consistent with the presence of a functional corpus luteum.

A proportion of "barren," maiden, and lactating mares do not exhibit regular estrous cycles and may be in extended diestrus. Following abortion, early fetal death and resorption, or as result of "pseudopregnancy," there may be serum progesterone levels consistent with a functional corpus luteum.
Treatment of such mares with Prostin F2 alpha usually results in regression of the corpus luteum followed by estrus and/or ovulation. In one study with 122 Standardbred and Thoroughbred mares in clinical anestrus for an average of 58 days and treated during the breeding season, behavioral estrus was detected in 81 percent at an average time of 3.7 days after injection with 5 mg. Prostin F2 alpha; ovulation occurred an average of 7.0 days after treatment. Of those mares bred, 59 percent were pregnant following an average of 1.4 services during that estrus.
Treatment of "anestrous" mares which abort subsequent to 36 days of pregnancy may not result in return to estrus due to presence of functional endometrial cups.
Contraindications and Precautions:

1. Prostin F2 alpha (dinoprost tromethamine) is ineffective when administered prior to day-5 after ovulation.
2. Pregnancy status should be determined prior to treatment, since Prostin F2 alpha has been reported to induce abortion and parturition when sufficient doses were administered.
3. Mares should not be treated if they suffer from either acute or subacute disorders of the vascular system, gastrointestinal tract, respiratory system, or reproductive tract.
4. Do not administer by intravenous route.
5. Non steroidal anti-inflammatory drugs (i.e. indomethacin) may inhibit prostaglandin synthesis, therefore these drugs should not be administered concurrently.

Warning:

1. Not for human use.
2. Not for use in horses intended for food.
3. Women of child-bearing age, asthmatics, and persons with bronchial and other respiratory problems should exercise **extreme caution** when handling this product. In the early stages, women may be unaware of their pregnancies. Prostin F2 alpha is readily absorbed through the skin and can cause abortion and/or bronchiospasms. Direct contact with the skin should therefore be avoided. Accidental spillage on the skin should be washed off **immediately** with soap and water.

Note: Spills of Prostin F2 alpha on the skin should immediately be washed off with soap and water.
Side Effects: The most frequently observed side effects are sweating and decreased rectal temperature. However, these have been transient in all cases observed and have not been detrimental to

the animal. Other reactions seen have been increase in heart rate, increase in respiration rate, some abdominal discomfort, locomotor incoordination, and lying down. These effects are usually seen within 15 minutes of injection and disappear within one hour. Mares usually continue to eat during the period of expressison of side effects. One anaphylactic reaction of several hundred mares treated with Prostin F2 alpha (dinoprost tromethamine) was reported but was not confirmed.

Instructions for Use:

1. Evaluate the reproductive status of the mare.
2. Administer a single intramuscular injection of 1 mg per 100 lbs (45.5 kg) body weight which is usually 1 ml to 2 ml. Prostin F2 alpha.
3. Observe for signs of estrus by means of daily teasing with a stallion, and evaluate follicular changes on the ovary by palpation of the ovary per rectum.
4. Some clinically anestrous mares will not express estrus but will develop a follicle which will ovulate. These mares may become pregnant if inseminated at the appropriate time relative to rupture of the follicle.
5. Breed mares in estrus in a manner consistent with normal management.

Dosage: Prostin F2 alpha (dinoprost tromethamine) is administered once as a single intramuscular injection of 1 mg per 100 lbs (45.5 kg) body weight which is usually 1 ml to 2 ml of Prostin F2 alpha containing 5 mg dinoprost as the tromethamine salt per milliliter.

How Supplied: 10 ml vials.

Caution: Federal (U.S.A.) law restricts this drug to use by or on the order of a licensed veterinarian.

QUARTERMASTER* SUSPENSION (penicillin-dihydrostreptomycin in oil)

Composition: Each 10 ml disposable syringe contains 1,000,000 units of Procaine Penicillin G, micronized, and 1 gram Dihydrostreptomycin base, as Dihydrostreptomycin Sulfate, micronized, in an extended action base consisting of 1% w/v Hydrogenated Peanut Oil, 3% w/v Aluminum Monostearate, and Peanut Oil, USP, q.s.

Actions: Infusion of antibiotics at the start of the drying off period has the following advantages: (1) it is active against existing infections; (2) it is prophylactic against new infections, during the time when cattle are likely to become infected[1]; (3) the antibiotic remains in the udder for a sufficiently long period to accomplish the intended objective and is not diluted with milk, as is the case in lactation therapy; (4) the danger of drug residues in the milk is reduced.

Antibiotic control is to be considered an adjunct to good herd hygiene management and milking management. Detailed field studies in England and the United States have demonstrated that a program consisting of treatment, at the time of drying off, with a highly effective antibiotic preparation in a slow-release base, and routine dipping of teats after each milking with an effec tive disinfectant, markedly reduces the incidence of all udder infections at calving.[2,3,4]

It has recently been recommended that a disinfectant teat dip be used on unmilked cows, or at least be used for 10 days before parturition[5] to reduce the bacterial challenge to the depleted levels of antibiotic in the teat as freshening is approached.[6]

When the herd infection level has been reduced, or when herds are not heavily infected initially, it may be desirable to be selective in treating dry quarters.[7]

Indications: For use at drying off to reduce the frequency of existing infection, and to prevent new infection with *Staphylococcus aurea.*

Directions for Use: At the last milking prior to drying off completely milk out cow. Warm the Quartermaster syringe to the body temperature; slowly infuse entire contents. Instill the contents of one syringe into each quarter. Discard the syringe after use. Treated teats should then be dipped into an effective teat dip. The teat or quarter should not be manipulated again until the cow freshens. To achieve and maintain a lower frequency of infection, proper dipping of teats during lactation is recommended.

Warnings: For udder instillation upon drying off only. Not to be used within 6 weeks of freshening. Not for use in lactating cows. Milk taken from animals within 96 hours (8 milkings) after calving must not be used for food. Animals infused with this product must not be slaughtered for food within 60 days from time of infusion nor within 96 hours after calving.

Caution: Federal law restricts this drug to use by or on the order of a licensed veterinarian.

How Supplied: Disposable 10 ml syringes.

Attention Doctor: It is your responsibility to inform your client of the warnings stated above so to avoid adulteration of meat or milk and possible prosecution under Federal law.

References:

1. Smith, A.; Westgarth, D.R.; Jones, M.R.; Neave, F.K.; Dodd, F.H. & Brander, G.C., Methods of Reducing the Incidence of Udder Infection in Dry Cows. *Veterinary Record* 81:504–510, 1967.
2. Dodd, F.H. & Neave, F.K., Mastitis Control, N.I.R.D. *Biennial Reviews* 1970, pp. 21–60.
3. Roberts, S.J.; Meek, A.M.; Natzke, R. & Guthrie, R. A Mastitis Control Program Combining Teat Dipping & Dry Cow Therapy. *XIX World Veterinary Congress* (Mexico City, 8/15–21/71). *Proceedings* 3:935–939, 1971.
4. Newbould, F.H.S.; Carey, P.G. & Barnum, D.A., The Numbers of Intramammary Infections & Teat Duct Colonizations in a Herd of Twins During a Hygiene Experiment. *Canadian Journal of Comparative Medicine 34:203–208, 1970.*
5. Neave, F.K. & Jackson, E.R., The Prevention of Intramammary Infection, pp. 15–24 in *The Control of Bovine Mastitis* Proceedings, Joint Meeting, British Cattle Veterinary Association & the Agricultural Development Association, Reading University, 1/5–6/71.) N.I.R.D., 1971.
6. Feagan, J.T.; Hehir, A.F. & White, B.R., The Effectiveness in Control of Mastitis of Iodine as a Post Milking Teat Dip. *Australian Journal of Dairy Technology* 25:87–90, 1970.
7. *Supplement to Current Concepts of Bovine Mastitis.* The National Mastitis Council Inc, Washington, D.C. 22003, 1972, page 7.

Quartermaster is manufactured for the Upjohn Company, Kalamazoo, MI

NDC 3267-1

*Quartermaster is a registered trademark of Alfa Laval, AB.

SOLU–DELTA–CORTEF® brand of prednisolone sodium succinate sterile powder

100 mg and 500 mg per 10 ml*

For intravenous or intramuscular use

Composition: Solu-Delta-Cortef sterile powder contains prednisolone sodium succinate which is a salt of prednisolone that is particularly suitable for intravenous or intramuscular injection because it is highly water soluble, permitting administration of relatively large doses in a small volume of diluent. It is especially designed for intravenous use in situations requiring rapid and intense glucocorticoid and/or anti-inflammatory effect; however, it may be used by the intramuscular route in less acute conditions.

*Each ml (when mixed) of these preparations contains:

	100 mg	500 mg
Prednisolone Sodium Succinate equivalent to prednisolone	10 mg	50 mg
Monobasic Sodium Phosphate Anhydrous	0.075 mg	0.075 mg
Diabasic Sodium Phosphate Dried	0.81 mg	0.81 mg
Lactose Hydrous	19.6 mg	19.6 mg
Tyloxapol	4.9 mg	4.9 mg
Chlorobutanol Anhydrous	3.08 mg	3.08 mg

(chloral deriv.) added as preservative

When necessary, pH was adjusted with sodium hydroxide and/or hydrochloric acid.

Metabolic and Hormonal Effects: Prednisolone a derivative of hydrocortisone, has greater glucocorticoid activity, greater anti-inflammatory activity, less sodium-retaining effect, and less potassium-losing effect than the parent compound.

The glucocorticoid activity of prednisolone is approximately 4 times that of hydrocortisone and 5 times that of cortisone as measured in experimental animals in terms of liver glycogen deposition,

Continued on next page

Upjohn—Cont.

eosinopenic response, and thymic involution.
The anti-inflammatory activity of prednisolone is at least 4 times that of hydrocortisone. Solu-Delta-Cortef exerts an inhibitory influence on the cellular, fibrous and amorphous components of connective tissue and thereby suppresses the basic processes of inflammation. Vascular permeability is decreased, exudation deminished, and the migration of inflammatory cells markedly impaired.
Indications: Solu-Delta-Cortef (prednisolone sodium succinate) is indicated for use in situations in which a rapid and intense adrenal glucocorticoid and/or anti-inflammatory effect is necessary. If the intravenous route is impracticable or the need is not so urgent, the intramuscular route may be used.
Inflammatory Conditions: As with the other adrenal steroids, Solu-Delta-Cortef has been found useful in alleviating lameness associated with acute localized and generalized arthritic conditions in horses, dogs, and cats. Treatment is usually required daily or on alternate days, depending on the severity or duration of the condition. Prednisolone sodium succinate has been used successfully to treat bursitis, carpitis, tendinitis, and myositis. Remission of the symptoms may be permanent, or symptoms may recur, depending on the cause and the extent of structural degeneration.
Generalized muscular soreness, stiffness; depression, and anorexia as a result of overtraining, shipping, unusual physical exertion, etc., respond promptly to prednisolone sodium succinate.
The intravenous administration is of particular value in treating acute laminitis (founder) in horses. It is important that the condition be detected early so that therapy may be instituted before there is irreparable damage to the laminae. It may be given at intervals of 12 to 24 hours, depending upon the response. Correction and/or treatment of the etiological factors is imperative and routine local antiphlogistic measures should be employed.
Allergic Reactions. Solu-Delta-Cortef is especially beneficial in treating acute hypersensitivity reactions resulting from treatment with a sensitizing drug or exposure to other allergic agents. Usual manifestations are anaphylactoid reactions and urticaria. Less severe allergic manifestations, such as atopic and contact dermatitis, summer eczema, and conjunctivitis also may be treated. Response is usually rapid and complete, although in severe cases with extensive lesions, more prolonged adrenocorticoid therapy and other appropriate treatment may be indicated.
Overwhelming Infections with Severe Toxicity. In animals moribund from overwhelmingly severe infections for which specific antibacterial therapy is available (e.g., critical pneumonia, peritonitis, endometritis, mastitis), intensive prednisolone sodium succinate therapy may aid in correcting the circulatory defect by counteracting the responsible inflammatory changes, thereby permitting the antibacterial agent to exert its full effect. As supportive therapy, this product combats the stress and improves the general attitude of the animal being treated. All necessary procedures for the establishment of a bacterial diagnosis should be carried out whenever possible before institution of therapy. In the presence of infection, prednisolone sodium succinate should be administered for the shortest possible time compatible with maintenance of an adequate clinical response, and antibacterical therapy should be continued for at least three days after the hormone has been withdrawn. Combined hormone and antibacterial therapy does not obviate the need for indicated surgical treatment.
Shock. For dogs, intravenous Solu-Delta-Cortef is indicated in the prevention and treatment of adrenal failure and shocklike states occurring in association with severe injury or other trauma, emergency surgery, anaphylactoid reactions and elective surgery in poor surgical risks. This hormone is recommended as an adjuvant to standard methods of combating shock, including use of plasma expanders. Because of interrelated pysiologic activities, beneficial effects may not be exhibited until all such procedures have been employed. Solu-Delta-Cortef is an invaluable emergency kit drug.
Other Indications. Solu-Delta-Cortef has been found useful as supportive therapy in the treatment of stress-induced exhaustion, rattlesnake bite, toxemia, inflammatory ocular conditions and other stress conditions. Its employment in the treatment of these conditions is recommended as a measure supportive to standard procedures and time-honored treatments and will aid in recovery of the animal.
Contraindications: Except when used for emergency therapy, prednisolone sodium succinate is contraindicated in animals with tuberculosis. Cushingoid syndrome, and peptic ulcer. Existence of congestive heart failure, diabetes, chronic nephritis, and osteoporosis are relative contraindications. In the presence of infection, appropriate antibacterial agents should also be administered and should be continued for at least 3 days after discontinuance of the hormone and disappearance of all signs of infection. Do not use in viral infections.
Warning: Clinical and experimental data have demonstrated that corticosteroids administered orally or parenterally to animals may induce the first stage of parturition when administered during the last trimester of pregnancy and may precipitate premature parturition followed by dystocia, fetal death, retained placenta, and metritis. Additionally, corticosteroids administered to dogs, rabbits, and rodents during pregnancy have resulted in cleft palate in offspring. Corticosteroids administered to dogs during pregnancy have also resulted in other congenital anomalies, including deformed forelegs, phocomelia, and anasarca.
Precautions: Solu-Delta-Cortef (prednisolone sodium succinate) may suppress systemic manifestations such as fever and also signs of toxemia. In some instances this alteration of the inflammatory reaction may be beneficial; however, it may also mask the signs of infection and tend to facilitate the spread of microorganisms. In infections characterized by overwhelming toxicity, prednisolone sodium succinate therapy in conjunction with indicated antibacterial therapy is effective in reducing mortality and morbidity. It is essential that the causative organism be known and an effective antibacterial agent be administered concurrently. The injudicious use of the adrenal hormones in animals with infections can be hazardous.
Side Effects: The therapeutic use of Solu-Delta-Cortef (prednisolone sodium succinate) is unlikely to cause undesired accentuation of metabolic effects. However, if continued corticosteroid therapy is anticipated, a high protein intake should be provided to keep the animal in positive nitrogen balance. A retardant effect on wound healing has not been encountered, but such a possibility should also be considered when it is used in conjunction with surgery. Euphoria, or an improvement of attitude, and increased appetite are usual manifestations.
Undesirable effects of adrenocorticoid administration are sodium and water retention, potassium loss, glycosuria, hyperglycemia, polyuria, and polydipsia.
Preparation of Solutions
1. Remove protective cap, give the plungerstopper a quarter-turn and press to force diluent into the lower compartment.
2. Gently agitate to effect solution.
3. Sterilize top of plunger-stopper with a suitable germicide.
4. Insert 18 gauge or smaller needle *squarely through center* of plunger-stopper until tip is just visible. Invert vial and withdraw dose.

No additional diluent should be added, and the solution should be injected directly into the vein or muscle. If desired, the solution may be incorporated into the following infusion solution: Dextrose 5% Injection, Dextrose 5% and Sodium Chloride Injection, Dextrose 10% Injection, Dextrose 10% and Sodium Chloride Injection, Ringer's Injection, Fructose 10%, and Lactated Potassic Saline Injection (Darrows Solution) *but must not be added to calcium infusion solutions.* If the solution should become cloudy after reconstituting, it should not be used intravenously.
Storage Conditions: 1. Store unreconstituted product at controlled room temperature 15°–30°C (59°–86°F).
Protect from light. Store in carton.
2. Do not store reconstituted product. Use immediately. Discard any unused reconstituted Solu-Delta-Cortef.

Dosage and Administration: Horses. The dosage for horses is 50 to 100 mg as an initial dose. This may be given intravenously over a period of ½ to 1 minute, or intramuscularly, and may be repeated in inflammatory, allergic, or other stress conditions, at intervals of 12, 24, or hours, depending upon the size of the animal, the severity of the condition, and the response to treatment. When steroid therapy is to be more prolonged, as in a chronic arthritic condition, Depo-Medrol® (methylprednisolone acetate) Sterile Aqueous Suspension or Predef 2X® (isoflupredone) Sterile Aqueous Suspension may be injected intramuscularly and continued daily, depending on the severity of the condition and response to treatment.

Dogs. The usual *intravenous* dose in shock and shocklike states ranges from 2.5 to 5 mg per lb of body weight as an initial dose, followed by equal maintenance doses at 1-, 3-, 6-, or 10-hour intervals as determined by the condition of the patient.

Dogs and Cats. The *intramuscular* dose in inflammatory, allergic, and less severe stress conditions, where immediate effect is not required, is usually 1 to 5 mg ranging upwards to 30 to 50 mg in large breeds of dogs. This may be repeated in 12 to 24 hours and continued for 3 to 5 days, if necessary. When steroid therapy is to be more prolonged, as in a chronic arthritic or dermal condition, Depo-Medrol Sterile Aqueous Suspenion may be used. If permanent corticosteroid effect is required, oral therapy with prednisolone tablets may be substituted as soon as possible. When therapy is to be withdrawn after prolonged corticosteroid administration, the daily dose should be reduced gradually over a number of days, in stepwise fashion.

Choice of appropriate concentration of Solu-Delta-Cortef (prednisolone sodium succinate) will help minimize discard of unused drug. It is suggested that the 10 mg/ml formulation be used to treat cats and horses of any size as well as dogs weighing less than 40 pounds. For intravenous treatment of shock in dogs weighing over 40 pounds use the 50 mg/ml formulation. Do not use 50 mg/ml formulation in dogs and cats for intramuscular use.

All intravenous injections should be administered slowly.

How Supplied: 10 ml (100 mg or 500 mg/10 ml) Sterile Mix-O-Vial®

SPECIAL FORMULA 17900–FORTE™

(penicillin procaine-novobiocin oil suspension)
Suspension
For udder instillation in lactating cattle only

Composition: Each 10 ml syringe contains:

Penicillin G Procaine 100,000 Int. Units
Novobiocin Sodium equiv. to
Albamycin® (novobiocin) 150mg
Chlorobutanol Anhydrous
(chloral derivative—used as a preservative) 50mg
in a special bland vehicle.

Store at controlled room temperature 15°–30°C (59°–86°F)

Shake Well Before Using.

Indications: Special Formula 17900-Forte (penicillin procaine-novobiocin oil suspension) is indicated for the treatment of bovine mastitis caused by susceptible strains of *Staphylococcus aureus, Streptococcus agalactiae, Streptococcus dysgalactiae,* or *Streptococcus uberis.* Use Special Formula 17900-Forte at the first signs of any alteration in the appearance of the milk, or if the teat or udder appear inflamed, or if other symptoms appear that indicate an infection of the mammary gland. Infections should be treated immediately after determining that the leukocyte count is elevated or that *Staphylococcus aureus, Streptococcus agalactiae, Streptococcus dysgalactiae,* or *Streptococcus uberis* has been isolated from the milk.

Warning:

1. Milk taken from treated animals within 72 hours (6 milkings) after latest treatment must not be used for food.
2. Treated animals must not be slaughtered for 15 days following last treatment.
3. Administration of this product in any manner other than shown under dosage may result in drug residues.
4. Not for human use.

Caution: For udder instillation in lactating dairy cattle only.

If redness, swelling, or abnormal milk persists, discontinue use and consult veterinarian.

Discard empty container; Do Not Reuse.

Dosage: Infuse one (1) syringe of Special Formula 17900-Forte (penicillin procaine-novobiocin oil suspension) into each infected quarter. Repeat this treatment once after a 24-hour interval.

Directions for Use: *Treatment.* Milk out udder completely, wash udder and teats thoroughly with warm water containing a suitable dairy antiseptic. Dry thoroughly. Using the alcohol pad provided, wipe off end of teat, using a separate pad for each teat to be treated. Warm Special Formula 17900-Forte (penicillin procaine-novobiocin oil suspension) to body temperature and shake thoroughly. Remove cap from tip of syringe and insert tip into teat canal; push plunger to dispense entire contents, massage the quarter to distribute the suspension up into the milk cistern.

Do not milk for at least six (6) hours after treatment; thereafter the animal should be milked at regular intervals. Mastitis should not be considered cured unless bacteriologic examination of the milk shows absence of causative microorganisms approximately three (3) weeks after treatment.

Reinfection. After successful treatment, reinfection may occur unless good herd management, sanitary and mechanical safety measures are practiced. Animals that have had repeated attacks of mastitis may have considerable scar tissue in the udder and are apt to be easily reinfected. These animals should be watched carefully to detect recurrence of infection and possible spread to other animals.

How Supplied: 10 ml Plastets®

TRITOP® Topical Ointment

(neomycin sulfate, isoflupredone acetate, tetracaine hydrochloride ointment)
For topical ear and skin use in dogs, cats and horses

Composition: Topical Tritop (neomycin sulfate, isoflupredone acetate, tetracaine hydrochloride ointment) contains in each gram the potent antiinflammatory agent Predef® (isoflupredone acetate) 1 mg (0.1%); the antibiotic neomycin sulfate, 5 mg (0.5%) (equivalent to 3.5 mg neomycin); and the topical anesthetic tetracaine hydrochloride, 5 mg (0.5%). This combination is well suited for the treatment or adjunctive therapy of many ear and skin conditions, as well as a dressing for superficial wounds occurring in dogs, cats and horses. Its action is specific as to anti-inflammatory, bactericidal, and anesthetic properties.

Isoflupredone Acetate

It has been reported by research workers that isoflupredone acetate (Predef) is 14 times as potent as hydrocortisone as an anti-inflammatory steroid as measured by the cotton pellet implantation assay. Isoflupredone acetate markedly inhibits inflammatory reaction through its controlling influence on connective tissue and vascular components. Topically applied isoflupredone acetate is rapidly effective. In otitis externa, wounds of the concha, ulcerations of the ear flaps, and irritated lesions of the skin, the inflammatory response may also be effectively inhibited by isoflupredone acetate. Chronic conditions respond more slowly and relapses are more frequent.

Neomycin

Neomycin is an antibiotic substance derived from cultures of the soil organism *Streptomyces fradiae.* Its antimicrobial range includes both gram-positive and gram-negative organisms commonly responsible for or associated with otic infections, such as staphylococci, streptococci, *Escherichia coli, Aerobacter aerogenes,* and many strains of Proteus and Pseudomonas organisms. It is not active against fungi. Neomycin is unusually nontoxic for epithelial cells in tissue culture and is nonirritating in therapeutic concentrations. The presence of neomycin in Topical Tritop (neomycin sulfate, isoflupredone acetate, tetracaine hydrochloride ointment) affords control of susceptible infection caused by neomycin-sensitive organisms.

Tetracaine

Tetracaine hydrochloride is a topical anesthetic agent that is more potent than either procaine or cocaine in comparable concentrations and has greater ability than procaine to penetrate mucous membranes. The duration of anesthetic action of tetracaine exceeds that produced by either butacaine or phenacaine.

Many investigators have demonstrated that local anesthesia plays a significant

Continued on next page

Upjohn—Cont.

part in the promotion of healing, especially where pain is a prominent factor. It is believed that trauma stimulates local pain receptors, which results in reflex vasodilation, edema, tenderness, and muscular spasm.
If the reflex is abolished through use of a local anesthetic such as tetracaine, amelioration of these tissue changes that interfere with healing is favored. The local anesthetic action of tetracaine has proved to be of great value in alleviating the pain reflex in painful skin and ear conditions.
Advantages of Topical Tritop
1. Potent anti-inflammatory effect of isoflupredone acetate.
2. Broad-spectrum bactericidal effect of neomycin.
3. Rapid anesthetic effect of tetracaine.
4. Prompt relief of symptoms.
5. Reduces further self-inflicted trauma.
6. Ease of application.

Clinical Indications: Topical Tritop (neomycin sulfate, isoflupredone acetate, tetracaine hydrochloride ointment) is indicated as treatment or adjunctive therapy of certain ear and skin conditions in dogs, cats and horses caused by or associated with neomycin susceptible organisms and/or allergy. In addition, it is indicated as superficial dressing applied to minor cuts, wounds, lacerations, abrasions, and for post surgical application where reduction of pain and inflammatory response is deemed desirable.
Topical Tritop is useful in treating such conditions as acute otitis externa in dogs and to a lesser degree, chronic otitis externa in dogs. It also is effective in treating anal gland infections and moist dermatitis in the dog and is a useful dressing for minor cuts, lacerations, abrasions, and post surgical therapy in the horse, cat, and dog.
Topical Tritop may also be used following amputation of dewclaws, tails and claws, following ear trimming and castrating operations.
Precautions and Warning: Not for human use.
Incomplete response or exacerbation of corticosteroid responsive lesions may be due to the presence of non-susceptible organisms or to prolonged use of antibiotic-containing preparations resulting in overgrowth of non-susceptible organisms, particularly Monilia. Thus, if improvement is not noted within two or three days, or if redness, irritation, or swelling persists or increases, the diagnosis should be redetermined and appropriate therapeutic measures initiated.
Tetracaine and neomycin have the potential to sensitize. Care should be taken to observe animals being treated for evidence of hypersensitivity or allergy to Topical Tritop (neomycin sulfate, isoflupredone acetate, tetracaine hydrochloride ointment). If such signs are noted, therapy with Topical Tritop should be stopped.
Dosage and Administration: In treatment of otitis externa and other inflammatory conditions of the external ear canal, a quantity of ointments sufficient to fill the external ear canal may be applied one to three times daily. When used on the skin or mucous membranes, cleanse the affected area, apply a small amount of the ointment and spread or rub in gently. The involved area may be treated one to three times a day, and these daily applications continued in accordance with the clinical response. Limit treatment to the period when local anesthesia is essential to control self-inflicted trauma.
How Supplied: 10 Gm Tubes with Special Applicator tip.
Caution: Federal (U.S.A.) law restricts this drug to use by or on the order of a licensed veterinarian.

Vet-A-Mix, Inc.
604 WEST THOMAS AVENUE
SHENANDOAH, IOWA 51601

AQUA–LITE
A Buffered Electrolyte Powder
For Use in Drinking Water of Pigs

Composition: Sodium chloride, calcium lactate, potassium phosphate dibasic, magnesium gluconate, glycine, potassium chloride, sodium acetate, citric acid, dextrose, fructose, lactose, sucrose, dextrin, flavoring and artificial coloring.
Indications: For use in swine of all ages for the correction of dehydration due to stress conditions associated with weaning, handling and diseases, especially associated with diarrhea.
Dosage and Administration: Aqua-Lite is intended for administration in drinking water. Dosage can either be calculated by body weight or water intake.
Automatic Medicator: Prepare a stock solution by dissolving the contents of one package into one gallon of warm water. Set proportioner to dispense one ounce of stock solution per gallon of drinking water. To assure freshness, prepare stock solutions daily. Do not store over 24 hours without refrigeration.
Stock Tank Administration: Dissolve one cup of Aqua-Lite per 25 gallons of drinking water or one pound (2.5 cups) in each 64 gallons of drinking water. One 2 pound package will treat 125–130 gallons of drinking water. For administration to litters, mix one ounce (3 tablespoons) in each 4 gallons of water.
Adminstration In The Feed: Mix 3 packages (6 pounds) in each ton of complete feed and feed for 5 to 7 days or until symptoms disappear.
Aqua-Lite is a concentrated water soluble electrolyte powder that has been buffered to maintain an acid pH. It is palatable to swine of any age, but specifically designed for excellent acceptance by young weaned pigs and feeder pigs.
Ambient temperature, humidity, ventilation and health conditions, such as dehydration and fever, will cause water intake to vary. As a generalization water consumption in pigs will be 8–12% of their body weight daily.

Dose Table For Swine

Number of Head	Body Weight Per Pig (lb)	Approximate Gal. Water Consumed Daily
100	15	10–30
100	30	40–60
100	60	80–100
100	90	100–130

Note: Store at room temperature and protect from light. Avoid excessive heat (104° F). Once an Aqua-Lite bag is opened, reseal and tape or place the unused portion in an airtight container.
How Supplied: 2 pound (907.2 g) packets

BLOAT-PAC®

Composition: Vegetable Oil, polyglycerol oleate, polyethylene glycol monooleate, butylated hydroxyanisole, butylated hydroxytoluene, citric acid, ethoxyquin, propylene glycol and propyl gallate.
Indications: For the treatment of acute bloat of cattle, sheep and goats, especially during forage or "frothy"bloat.
Dosage:

Mature Cattle	150-300 ml
Heifers	125-250 ml
Calves	100-200 ml
Lambs and Kids	50-100 ml

Note: *Bloat-Pac* may become cloudy by exposure to low temperatures. It will clear by gentle warming and remain clear at room temperatures. Method Number I —Intrarumenal Injection
Step 1. Insert long needle directly into the rumen through the left paralumbar space with a quick hard thrust. The paralumbar space corresponds to the point of highest distention in an acutely bloated animal. The hissing of escaping gas will indicate the needle is in the rumen.
Step 2. Place short needle on the tip of the plastic syringe, withdraw the proper dose of Bloat-Pac from the 500 ml bottle and inject through long needle into the rumen. More than one syringeful may be necessary in large animals.
Step 3. Allow long needle to remain in the rumen for a few minutes to relieve distention. Then remove needle. Method Number II —Oral
Bloat-Pac may be given as a drench, but administration via a stomach tube is preferable.
Caution: If administered to milking dairy cows, do not market milk for 24 hours after treatment.
How Supplied: 500 ml bottle and gallons.

BOVI-FORM K
Water Dispersible Oxytetracycline Hydrochloride with Potassium and Sodium

Composition:
Active Drug Ingredient *Per 400 g*
Oxytetracycline HCl ....25 grams (25,000 mg)
Electrolytes: Potassium 2400 mEq, Sodium 1200 mEq, Chloride 3600 mEq

Note: One level teaspoonful contains approximately 5 grams of Bovi-Form K or 312.5 mg of oxytetracycline hydrochloride. One level tablespoonful contains approximately 15 grams of Bovi-Form K or 937.5 mg of oxytetracycline hydrochloride.
Indications: An effective oral treatment for diseases when caused by organisms susceptible to oxytetracycline.
Dosage and Administration: Mix in milk, dry rations or drinking water.
Calves and Beef Cattle *—Bacterial enteritis* (scours). 400 grams per 5000 to 25,000 pounds body weight to furnish 1.0 to 5.0 mg oxytetracycline HCl per pound per day.
Bacterial pneumonia (shipping fever). 400 grams per 12,500 to 50,00 pounds body weight to furnish 0.5 to 2.0 mg oxytetracycline HCl per pound per day for 3 to 5 days preceding shipment and 3 to 5 days following arrival in feed lot.
Swine *—Bacterial enteritis (scours) vibrionic dysentery and necrotic enteritis due to salmonellosis.*
400 grams per 10,000 pounds body weight to furnish 2.5 mg oxytetracycline HCl per pound per day.
Sheep *—Bacterial enteritis (scours), lamb dysentery or white scours of lambs.*
Mix 1600 grams in each ton of feed. To increase rate of gain mix 200 to 400 grams in each ton of feed.
Drinking Water Treatment for all Species. Mix 400 grams per 100 to 150 gallons drinking water to furnish 165 to 250 mg oxytetracycine HCl per gallon.
How Supplied: 400 gram bottles, 10 kg pails

DIET-DERM
Polyunsaturated Fatty Acids with Vitamins A, D and E for Diet Supplementation

Composition: Each 5 ml contains: Linoleic acid 2080.0 mg.; Linolenic acid 317.5 mg.; other Unsaturated Fatty Acids —Arachidonic, oleic, palmitoleic, clupanodonic 1430.0 mg.; (all above as glycerides).
Lecithin 54.0 mg.; Vitamin A 1250 I.U.; Vitamin D_3 250 I.U.; Vitamin E 10 I.U.; Polyoxyethylene sorbitan monooleate 7.5 mg.; Sorbitan monooleate 92.5 mg.
With approved antioxidants and preservatives.
Indications: For the prevention and correction of dry skin (*xerodermia*) and dry hair (*xerasia*) when conditions are due to deficiencies of polyunsaturated fatty acids and/or vitamins A, D and E in the diet.
Dosage and Administration: ***For Dogs and Cats*** —Administer each directly as suggested below:
Under 5 kilograms (11 pounds) ¼ Teaspoonful.
5-10 kilograms (11-22 pounds) ½ Teaspoonful.
10-25 kilograms (22-55 pounds) 1 Teaspoonful.
Over 25 kilograms (55 pounds) 1½ Teaspoonful.
In severe cases give two to four times the above dosages.
One teaspoonful approximates 5 ml.
How Supplied: 8 oz. bottles and gallons.
For Veterinary Use Only.

DIRO-FORM
(brand of diethylcarbamazine citrate) Chewable Tablets

Composition: Each scored oval tablet contains Diethylcarbamazine citrate, 45 mg.
Each quarter-scored round tablet contains Diethylcarbamazine citrate, 60 mg, 150 mg or 180 mg.
Indications: Diro-Form Chewable Tablets are indicated for use in the prevention of infection with *Dirofilaria immitis* (heartworm disease) in dogs. Diro-Form Chewable Tablets may be given to dogs of all ages.
Precautions and Side Effects: Overdosage may cause emesis. The compound causes no cumulative toxic effects.
Dosage and Administration: Diro-Form Tablets are chewable tablets and are palatable to most dogs. Tablets may be fed free choice, from the hand or may be crumbled and placed on the food. Diro-Form Chewable Tablets, 45 mg, are scored and Diro-Form Chewable Tablets, 60 mg, 150 mg and 180 mg, are quarter scored for convenient adjustment of dosage.
For the Prevention of Heartworm Disease in Dogs. Diro-Form Chewable Tablets are given orally (once a day) at a dosage rate of 3 mg Diethylcarbamazine citrate per pound of body weight. Young dogs may be started on the preventive program at two months of age. Administration of Diro-Form Chewable Tablets in heartworm endemic areas should start 1 month before the beginning of mosquito activity and be continued daily throughout the mosquito season and for approximately 2 months thereafter. Continuous low level administration during the mosquito season effectively prevents maturation of recently inoculated heartworm larvae into adults (*Dirofilaria immitis*). A dog on prophylactic therapy should be examined for the presence of microfilaria every six months.
Recommended Dosage Schedule for Prevention of Heartworm:

Body Weight	45 mg Tablets
7½ lbs	½ tablet
15 lbs	1 tablet
Body Weight	**60 mg Tablets**
5 lbs	¼ tablet
10 lbs	½ tablet
20 lbs	1 tablet
Body Weight	**150 mg Tablets**
12½ lbs	¼ tablet
25 lbs	½ tablet
50 lbs	1 tablet
Body Weight	**180 mg Tablets**
15 lbs	¼ tablet
30 lbs	½ tablet
60 lbs	1 tablet

Warning: Dogs with established heartworm infections should not receive Diro-Form Chewable Tablets until they have been converted to a negative status by the use of adulticidal and microfilaricidal drugs. Inadvertent administration to heartworm infested dogs may cause adverse reactions due to pulmonary occlusion.
Caution: U.S. Federal law restricts this drug to use by or on the order of a licensed veterinarian. Do not use in dogs that may be harboring adult heartworms.
KEEP OUT OF REACH OF CHILDREN.
How Supplied:

45 mg scored tablets	
Bottle of 100	List No. 2603
Bottle of 200	List No. 2605
60 mg quarter-scored tablets	
Bottles of 100	List No. 2611
Bottle of 200	List No. 2612
150 mg quarter-scored tablets	
Bottle of 50	List No. 2604
Bottle of 100	List No. 2607
180 mg quarter-scored tablets	
Bottle of 50	List No. 2621
Bottle of 100	List No. 2622
Bottle of 200	List No. 2623

For Veterinary Use Only

EQU–LIN
Equine Liniment Gel

Composition: Isopropyl alcohol 70% v/v, methyl salicylate 8% v/v, menthol, 1.5% w/v, camphor 1.5% w/v.
Indications: For use in horses as an aid in the temporary relief of minor stiffness and soreness caused by overexertion.
Administration:
Massage: Apply full strength as needed.
Leg Brace: Mix 3 tablespoonfuls of Equ-Lin with 16 fl. oz. of witch hazel or water, and 6 fl. oz. of vinegar. Shake bottle vigorously, apply mixture freely and rub legs thoroughly.
Body Wash: Mix 4 tablespoonfuls of Equ-Lin with 32 fl. oz. of witch hazel or hot water. Apply mixture freely over horse's body.
Warning: Not to be used in horses intended for food.
Combustible mixture, do not use or store near heat or open flame. Do not use while smoking. For external use only. Use only as directed. Use otherwise may be dangerous. Keep out of reach of children to avoid accidental poisoning. Do not apply to irritated skin. If excessive irritations develop, discontinue use and consult a veterinarian. Avoid getting in eyes or on mucous membranes.
How Supplied: 12 fl. oz. Bottles

HYDRA–LYTE
Oral Electrolyte Replacement With Nutrients

Composition: Dextrose, glycine, potassium chloride, sodium acetate, sodium chloride and sodium citrate.
Indications: For use as a nutritional source of energy and as an aid in the replacement of normal body fluids and electrolytes to correct dehydration, acidosis and hypoglycemia in young calves, lambs and foals which are severely affected by infectious diarrhea.

Continued on next page

Vet-A-Mix—Cont.

Administration: Hydra-Lyte readily dissolves in water and is easily absorbed. Prepare solution by dissolving the contents of both compartments of this package in two quarts of warm water. Prepare the solution just prior to use and administer with an esophageal probe, nursing bottle or pail. Milk or milk replacer should be discontinued for the first two days of therapy.
Dosage: Administer two quarts of Hydra-Lyte solution to each calf or foal twice daily for the first two days. Important: milk or milk replacer should not be used during this period. On the third and fourth day administer one quart Hydra-Lyte solution mixed with either one quart of milk or milk replacer to each calf or foal two times each day. Lambs will require about one fourth of the above dosage.
Most treated animals can be returned to normal feeding on the fifth day, but treatment can be continued on the fifth through seventh day.
Note: In cases of severe dehydration or large neonatal animals, two quarts of Hydra-Lyte solution should be administered to each calf or foal four times each day for the first two days. One fourth this dosage is required for lambs. Use the same dosage regimen for the third and fourth days as recommended above.
How Supplied: 5.76 ounce (163.4 g) packets

ISOTONE-A

Composition: A balanced electrolyte-nutrient formula for oral use in the treatment of dehydration, acidosis and hypoglycemia in young animals severely affected with infectious diarrhea.
Formula: When contents of both compartments (in each 81.5 gram packet) are dissolved in water to a total volume of 3,000 ml, each 1,000 ml will contain; Potassium 28.5 mEq, Sodium 71.5 mEq, Bicarbonate 60.0 mEq, Chloride 40.0 mEq, Magnesium 5.0 mEq, Gluconate 5.0 mEq, Lactose 10.0 milliosmoles, Glucose 82.4 milliosmoles, Total Osmolarity 300.0 milliosmoles, Total metabolizable Energy 73.7 Kcal.
Product Rationale: Dehydration is one significant consequence of diarrhea caused by infectious enteritis in newborn animals. In severe cases metabolic acidosis exists with a marked depletion of electrolytes and water.
A clinician must possess knowledge of body fluids and electrolytes if therapy is to be successful. The three body fluid compartments, i.e., plasma, interstitial and cellular, normally possesses an osmolarity of approximately 300 milliosmoles (mosom) per liter and in dehydrated animals the osmolarity may be expected to be elevated. Water passively moves from compartment of lower to higher osmotic pressure until body fluid compartments become isotonic. Nutrients in the gastrointestinal tract are not absorbed through the epithelium until the contents become isotonic with blood. Obviously, oral administration of fluids with high osmolarity, i.e., greater than 300 to 400 mosm/liter, to dehydrated animals will cause further dehydration.
Electrolytes can be considered as either "fixed" or metabolizable. Fixed ions, when absorbed, must be excreted unchanged; metabolizable ions can be metabolized and excreted as CO_2, urea or water. Examples of fixed ions are Na^+, K^+, CA^{++}, Mg^{++}, Cl^-, So_{4-}, and $HPO4_-$, HCO_{3-}, acetate$_-$, lactate$_-$, and citrate$_-$. Of course, Ca^{++} and the phosphate anions can be either fixed in bone or excreted. The relative amounts of fixed and metabolizable ions are important because of the influence on osmolarity, the acid-base balance and kidney concentrating ability.
Salts of fixed cations and metabolizable anions are alkalinizing, i.e. $NaHCO_3$, $KHCO_3$ and magnesium citrate. Salts of fixed cations and fixed anions are netural, i.e. NaCl, KCl, and $MgSO_4$. Utilizing normal saline solution in diarrheic animals may correct the dehydration but obviously will not alleviate the acidosis. A combination of fixed and metabolizable anions is recommended in both parenteral and oral fluid therapy. This permits the gut epithelium and kidney tubules to establish acid-base homeostasis.
Therapy with oral and parenteral fluids should be designed to replace the total body deficit, and should not be based only on plasma electrolyte and acid-base analyses. Blood plasma is a transport medium and tends to remain homeostatic and constant. In diarrheic animals acidosis and hyperkalemia are common, despite the fact that cellular potassium may be subnormal. Potassium repletion should be restricted mainly to oral therapy, and intravenous infusions of solutions containing greater than 5 mEq of potassium per liter are contraindicated in hyperkalemic animals. Energy in a readily assimilable form, is secondary only to the establishment of hydration and initial acid-base balance. The presence of glucose in the gut enhances electrolyte absorption, as well as sparing protein utilization for energy purposes. Neonatal animals can utilize glucose and lactose; but they are not equipped to digest such sugars as sucrose and the di and trisaccharides in corn syrup.
Overfeeding is considered to be a predisposing or aggravating factor in neonatal infectious enteritis. The theory is supported by scientific evidence which has demonstrated that over feeding, or use of nutrients which are poorly digested, results in unassimilated foods appearing in the lower enteric tract and which serve as substrates to support the overgrowth of bacteria. Therapeutic nutrition should therefore be designed to supply frequent feeding of highly digestible and readily assimilable nutrients.
Parenteral Therapy: Comatose animals are best treated initially by intravenous infusions of isotonic alkalinizing solutions. The quantities recommended depend on the body size and the degree of dehydration. Calves may need 2 to 5 liters; lambs may require 0.25 to 0.50 liters. Infusions should be made slowly and may require several hours to establish near-normal hydration and kidney function. An ideal solution is half-strength (0.63%) $NaHCO_3$ and half-strength (0.425%) NaCl. Potassium should not exceed 5 mEq/liter; Ca^{++} and Mg^{++} are not critically needed at this stage. Other permissible solutions are Hartman's saline-lactate, Ringer's lactate, and salinebicarbonate with dextrose. Normal saline solution and 5% dextrose are not recommended; all hypertonic solutions are contraindicated.
Oral Therapy: Oral infusions of nutrient liquids are indicated in moribund animals that are not yet comatose and following parenteral therapy. Oral fluid therapy may normally continue from 24 to 72 hours, depending on the type of fluids used and the clinician's judgment. This time is used to complete homeostasis, and initiate chemotherapy and control of etiological infectious agents before resumption of feeding nutrients that are more slowly digested.
Certain general principles should be observed. The formulas should contain both chloride and metabolizable anions; sodium to potassium ratios should range from 1:1 to 3:1 Magnesium is desirable to reduce the possibility of tetany. Glucose or lactose enhances electrolyte assimilation and furnishes energy. High levels of magnesium, phosphates and sulfate should not be used due to their cathartic action. The inclusions of eggs, sucrose and corn syrup are *absolutely contraindicated.* Solutions should be isotonic, with an osmolarity of 300 to 350 milliosmoles/liter. Infusions should be frequent at intervals of 6 hours or less. Large feedings may overload the gut, and if fluids contain free amino acids from protein hydrolysates the animal may be subject to hyperaminoacidemia. When synthetic oral solutions are replaced with milk or milk replacer, feedings should be small and frequent. Vegetable protein supplements such as soybean oil meal, cottonseed meal, and linseed meal should be avoided during the first 3 to 4 weeks. Finally, fluid therapy is meant to rectify an acute pathological crisis. It is not designed to replace sanitation immunological procedures and chemotherapy.
Packaging for Isotone-A: The importance of including both fixed and metabolizable alkalinizing anions in the Isotone-A Formula has been previously emphasized. Some commercial preparations do not contain metabolizable anions because of physical and chemical incompatibility and instability when such mixtures are kept in storage. Powders which contain mixtures of citrate, carbonates and certain organic compounds will undergo chemical and physical changes harmful to such formulas.
Isotone-A was formulated with these vital metabolizable anions included. This was made possible by physical separation through the use of a double compartment packet, which insures optimum freshness at the time of re-constitution. Isotone-A provides a complete spectrum of

V

ingredients consistent with current scientific knowledge.
Directions for Use: Dissolve the contents of one 81.5 gram packet in clean, warm water (preferably distilled or deionized) and add to a total volume of 3 liters. This product contains no preservatives or antioxidants, so solutions should be mixed fresh before administration or kept refrigerated up to 24 hours. Solutions should be warmed to body temperature (37°C or 100°F) before administration. Solution should be infused into the stomach by use of a stomach hose or drenching tube.
Dosages: (1) If patients have been treated initially by intravenous infusions give 50 ml of solution for each kg body weight initially, followed by 25 ml/kg (55 ml/5 lb) every 6 hours for 24 hours. Thereafter, give 50 to 100 ml of solution for each kg of body weight (110 ml/5 lb to 225 ml/5 lb) for a total of 48 to 72 hours and gradually resume feeding milk or high quality milk replacers.
(2) Severely dehydrated animals which have not been treated by intravenous infusions should receive 50 ml/kg body weight initially and 25 to 50 ml/kg (55 to 110 ml/5 lb) 3 hours later. Thereafter, give 25 ml/kg (55 ml/5 lb) every six hours and continue as described above.
The average size baby calf may receive up to 3 liters initially and 1 to 2 liters every 6 hours.
The infectious etiological agents should be treated with appropriate chemotherapeutic agents or antibiotics.
Contraindications: There are no known contraindications to the use of Isotone-A. Since solutions prepared from Isotone-A contain high levels of potassium and lactose the product should not be used parenterally.
Glossary of Terms: Equivalent: One grammolecular weight of an atom (or radical) divided by its valence. A *milliequivalent* is one thousandth of an equivalent. *Milliosmole*—Equal to one thousandth of one gram mole of total dissolved substance. Used to measure the ability of solutes to cause osmosis and osmotic pressure. *Osmolarity*—A property of a solution which depends on the concentration of total solute per unit of total volume of solution.
How Supplied: 81.5 gram packets
For Veterinary Use Only

KAO-FORTE

Composition: Each fluid ounce contains: Kaolin 9000 mg; Pectin 200 mg, in a smooth stable liquid suspended with carboxy methyl cellulose.
Indications: For absorption of toxins and protection of the intestinal mucosa in simple diarrheas of dogs and cats, horses, cattle and swine.
Contraindications: There are no known contraindications to kaolin and pectin therapy. (See warning below).
Dosage: Dogs and Cats: 1 to 2 tablespoonfuls.
Horses and Cattle: 4 to 10 fl. oz.
Colts and Calves: 2 to 3 fl. oz.
Swine: ½ to 2 fl. oz.
Repeat every 2 to 4 hours or as indicated until condition improves. If improvement is not evident in 48 hours additional chemotherapy is indicated.
Warning: Do not use for more than two days or in the presence of a high fever. Do not use in very young animals unless treatment is supervised by a veterinarian.
Shake Well Before Each Use.
Protect from Freezing.
How Supplied: 1 gallon.

LIPO-FORM
Lipotropic Substances and Vitamins Chewable Tablets

Composition: Each tablet contains: Choline 125 mg; (Equivalent to Choline Dihydrogen Citrate 305 mg); dl-Methionine 100 mg; Inositol 25 mg; Vitamin E 10 I.U.; Vitamin B_{12} 3.50 mcg; Niacin 10.00 mg; Thiamine Mononitrate 0.10 mg; Riboflavin 0.22 mg; Pantothenic Acid 0.25 mg; Pyridoxine Hydrochloride 0.11 mg; Folic Acid 22.00 mcg. In a palatable protein base with desiccated liver.
Indications: For use as a supplementary dietary source of the lipotropic factors: choline, methionine and inositol in the canine.
Dosage and Administration: The usual daily dose is one to two tablets per 10 kilograms (22 pounds) of body weight. In severe cases increase the dosage level, preferably by giving twice daily.
Individualize the dosage according to the condition of the animal being treated.
Caution: Avoid prolonged excessive dosage administration. In rare cases animals may experience gastrointestinal irritation. In the event of stomach upset administer tablets during or after feeding.
How Supplied: 50 and 500 tablet bottles.

LIPOTINIC BOLUSES
Oral Niacin Supplement

Composition:
Nicotinic acid ....6000 mg (niacin)
Thiamine mononitrate.................250 mg
Riboflavin.....................................250 mg
Pyridoxine hydrochloride............100 mg
Vitamin B_{12}..................................100 mcg
Ingredients: Nicotinic acid, Thiamine mononitrate, Riboflavin, Pyridoxine hydrochloride, Vitamin B_{12} supplement, Dextrin, Starch, Lactose, Modified cellulose, Magnesium stearate, Artificial color.
Indications: For use as a niacin and B vitamin supplement in lactating cattle.
Dosage: Administer one bolus in the morning and one bolus in the evening for 10 consecutive days to high producing dairy cows when supplementation of nicotinic acid (niacin) is required. It is recommended that all high producing dairy cows receive Lipotinic Boluses either two weeks before or immediately following calving to lower blood ketone levels and increase serum glucose.
Administration: Lipotinic Boluses can be given with either a balling gun or broken and mixed into the feed.
How Supplied: 20 Bolus Bottles
For Veterinary Use Only

METHIO-FORM
DL-Methionine for Urinary Acidification of cats and dogs
Chewable Tablets

Composition: Each scored tablet contains:
DL-Methionine ....500 mg (6.7 mEq)
In a palatable protein base
Indications: For use in acidifying the urine of cats and dogs and as an aid in the prevention and treatment of feline urological syndrome (FUS), when lowering the pH and buffering the urine is of value. As an aid in controlling the odor from feline and canine urine residues.
Contraindications: Do not administer to animals with severe liver, kidney or pancreatic diseases, or those which are acidotic due to conditions such as uncontrolled diabetes mellitus or urinary obstruction.
Dosage:
Cats: The usual daily dose is 2.5 to 5.0 mEq/kg body weight or 1/2 to one tablet per 1 to 1.5 kg (2.5 to 3 lb) body weight. Average size adult cats normally should receive 1 1/2 to 3 tablets (10-20 mEq) daily.
Dogs: The usual daily dose is 2 to 4 mEq/kg body weight.
Small Breeds—7 kg (15 lb) or under, 1/2 to 4 tablets.
Medium Breeds—7-15 kg (15-33 lb), 2 to 7 tablets.
Large Breeds—15-30 kg (33-66 lb), 4 to 13 tablets.
Administration: Daily doses vary with diets and amount of acidification needed. After dosages have been determined, they may be used continuously. Methio-Form Chewable Tablets may be fed free choice, from the hand or may be crumbled and mixed into the food.
Note: In rare cases animals may experience gastrointestinal disturbance. In those cases administer during or after feeding or in 2 to 3 divided doses.
Caution: U.S. Federal Law restricts this drug to use by or on the order of a licensed veterinarian.
How Supplied: 50, 150, and 500 tablet bottles.
Patent Pending

METHIO-FORM
Brand of DL-Methionine for Urinary Acidification of Cats and Dogs
Palatable Granules

Composition: Each 3.08 grams contains:
DL-Methionine ....746 mg (10.0 mEq)
In a palatable protein base
Indications: For use in acidifying the urine of cats and dogs and as an aid in the prevention and treatment of feline urological syndrome (FUS), when lowering the pH and buffering the urine is of

Continued on next page

Vet-A-Mix—Cont.

value. As an aid in controlling the odor from feline and canine urine residues.
Contraindications: Do not administer to animals with severe liver, kidney or pancreatic diseases, or those which are acidotic due to conditions such as uncontrolled diabetes mellitus or urinary obstruction.
Dosage:
Cats: The usual daily dose is 2.5 to 5.0 mEq/kg body weight or 1/2 to one level teaspoon per 2 to 2.5 kg (4 to 5 lb) body weight. Average size adult domestic cats normally should receive one to 2 level teaspoons (10-20 mEq) daily.
Dogs: The usual daily dose is 2 to 4 mEq/kg body weight.
Small Breeds—7 kg (15 lb) or under, 1/2 to 3 level teaspoons.
Medium Breeds—7-15 kg (15-33 lb), 1 1/2 to 5 level teaspoons.
Large Breeds—15-30 kg (33-66 lb), 3 to 9 level teaspoons.
Note: One level teaspoonful contains 3.08 grams Methio-Form Palatable Granules.
Administration: Daily doses vary with diets and amount of acidification needed. After dosages have been determined, they may be used continuously. Methio-Form Palatable Granules may be sprinkled on top of or mixed into the food.
Note: In rare cases animals may experience gastrointestinal disturbance. In those cases administer during feeding in 2 to 3 divided doses.
Caution: U.S. Federal Law restricts this drug to use by or on the order of a licensed veterinarian.
How Supplied: 4 ounce and one pound bottles

Patent Pending

V

METHIO-TABS
DL-Methionine for urinary acidification of cats and dogs

Composition: Each scored tablet contains either
DL-Methionine .... 200 mg (2.68 mEq)
DL Methionine .... 500 mg (6.70 mEq)
Indications: For use as an aid in acidifying the urine of cats and dogs.
Dosage: Daily dosages vary with diets and amount of acidification needed. After dosages have been determined, they may be used continuously.
Cats: The usual daily dose is 2.5 to 5.0 mEq/kg body weight.
200 mg Tablets: One to two tablets per 1 to 1.5 kg (2.5 to 3 lb) body weight. Average size adult cats normally should receive 4 to 8 tablets (10–20 mEq) daily.
500 mg Tablets: One-half to one tablet per 1 to 1.5 kg (2.5 to 3 lb) body weight. Average size adult cats normally should receive 4 to 8 tablets (10–20 mEq) daily.
Dogs: The usual daily dose is 2 to 4 mEq/kg body weight.
200 mg Tablets: Small Breeds—7 kg (15 lb) or under, 1 to 10 tablets. Medium Breeds—7–15 kg (15–33 lb), 5 to 18 tablets. Large Breeds—15–30 kg (33–66 lb), 10 to 32 tablets.
500 mg Tablets: Small Breeds—7 kg (15 lb) or under, ½ to 4 tablets. Medium Breeds—7–15 kg (15–33 lb), 2 to 7 tablets. Large Breeds—15–30 kg (33–66 lb), 4 to 13 tablets.
Contraindications: Do not administer to animals with severe liver, kidney or pancreatic disease, or which are acidotic.
Caution: In rare cases, animals may experience gastrointestinal disturbance. In those cases, administer tablets during or after feeding or in 2 to 3 divided doses.
How Supplied: Methio-Tabs, 200 mg—1000 Tablet Bottles, Methio-Tabs, 500 mg—1000 Tablet Bottles

METHIO-VET PELLETS
DL-Methionine for Equine

Composition: Each pound contains 160 mg DL-Methionine.
Indications: For use as a nutritional supplement in horses when a methionine deficiency exists as evidenced by laminitis.
Dosage: The usual daily dose for a 1,000 to 1,200 pound horse is 10 grams of DL-methionine (2 level measures of Methio-Vet Pellets) for 7 days followed by 5 grams of DL-methionine (1 level measure of Methio-Vet Pellets) per day for 21 additional days.
Note: One level measure contains approximately ½ ounce of Methio-Vet Pellets equivalent to 5 grams of DL-methionine.
The enclosed measure is equivalent to 1 fluid ounce (29.6 mL).
Administration: Methio-Vet Pellets may be top dressed or mixed with the daily ration.
How Supplied: 5 pound jars

MEq-10
DL-Methionine and Ammonium Chloride
Chewable Tablets

Composition: Each scored tablet contains
DL-Methionine .... 560 mg (7.5 mEq)
Ammonium chloride .134 mg (2.5 mEq)
In a palatable protein base (10.0 mEq)
Indications: For use in acidifying and buffering the urine of cats and dogs and as an aid in the prevention and treatment of Feline Urological Syndrome (F.U.S.).
Contraindications: Do not administer to animals with severe liver, kidney or pancreatic diseases, or which are acidotic due to conditions such as uncontrolled diabetes mellitus or urinary obstruction.
Administration: Daily doses vary with diets and amount of acidification needed. After dosages have been determined, they may be used continuously. MEq-10 Chewable Tablets may be fed free choice, from the hand or may be crumbled and mixed into the food.
Dosage:
Cats: The usual daily dose is 2.5 to 5.0 mEq/kg body weight, or 1/2 to one tablet per 2 to 2.5 kg (4 to 5 lb) body weight. Average size adult domestic cats normally should receive one to 2 tablets (10-20 mEq) daily.
Dogs: The usual daily dose is 2 to 4 mEq/kg body weight.
Small Breeds —7 kg (15 lb) or under, 1/2 to 3 tablets.
Medium Breeds —7-15 kg (15-33 lb). 1 1/2 to 5 tablets.
Large Breeds —15-30 kg (33-66 lb), 3-9 tablets.
Note: In rare cases animals may experience gastrointestinal disturbance. In those cases administer chewable Tablets during or after feeding or in 2 to 3 divided doses.
Caution: U.S. Federal Law restricts this drug to use by or on the order of a licensed veterinarian.
How Supplied: 50 and 500 tablet bottles

Patent Pending

MEq-20
DL-Methionine and Ammonium Chloride
Palatable Granules

Composition: Each 4.5 grams contains
DL-Methionine .... 1120 mg (15.0 mEq)
Ammonium chloride .... 268 mg (5.0 mEq)
In a palatable protein base (20.0 mEq)
Indications: For use in acidifying and buffering the urine of cats and dogs and as an aid in the prevention and treatment of Feline Urological Syndrome (F.U.S.)
Contraindications: Do not administer to animals with severe liver, kidney or pancreatic diseases, or which are acidotic due to conditions such as uncontrolled diabetes mellitus or urinary obstruction.
Dosage:
Cats: The usual daily dose is 2.5 to 5.0 mEq/kg body weight or 1/4 to 1/2 teaspoonful per 2 to 2.5 kg (4 to 5 lb) body weight. Average size adult domestic cats normally should receive 1/2 to 1 teaspoonful (10-20 mEq) daily.
Dogs: The usual daily dose is 2 to 4 mEq/kg body weight.
Small Breeds—7 kg (15 lb) or under, 1/4 to 1 1/2 teaspoonful.
Medium Breeds—7-15 kg (15-33 lb) 3/4 to 2 1/2 teaspoonful.
Large Breeds—15-30 kg (33-66 lb, 1 1/2 to 4 1/2 teaspoonful.
Note: One rounded teaspoon contains 4.5 grams MEq-20 Palatable Granules
Administration: Daily doses vary with diets and amount of acidification needed. After dosages have been determined, they may be used continuously. MEq-20 Palatable Granules may be sprinkled on top of or mixed into the food.
Note: In rare cases animals may experience gastrointestinal disturbance. In those cases administer during feeding in 2 to 3 divided doses.
Caution: U.S. Federal Law restricts this drug to use by or on the order of a licensed veterinarian.
How Supplied: 4 ounce and one pound bottles

MEq-30®
DL-Methionine and Ammonium Chloride
Chewable Tables

Composition: Each scored tablet contains
DL-Methionine ...... 1680 mg (22.5 mEq)
Amonomium
Chloride .... 402 mg (7.5 mEq)
In a palatable protein base (30.0 mEq)
Indications: For use in acidifying and buffering the urine of dogs and cats. As an aid in the prevention and treatment of Feline Urological Syndrome (F.U.S.).
Contraindications: Do not administer to animals with severe liver, kidney or pancreatic disease, or which are acidotic.
Administration: MEq-30® Chewable Tablets may be fed free choice, from the hand or may be crumbled and mixed in the food. Daily dosages vary with diets and amount of acidification needed. After dosages have been determined, they may be used continuously.
Dosage:
Dogs: The usual daily dose is 2 to 4 mEq/kg body weight.
Small Breeds —7 kg (15 lb), 1/4 to 1 tablet.
Medium Breeds —7-15 kg (15-33 lb), 1/2 to 2 tablets.
Large Breeds —15-30 kg (33-66 lb), 1 to 3 tablets.
Cats: The usual daily dose is 2.5 to 5.0 mEq/kg body weight, or 1/4 tablet per 2 to 2.5 kg (4 to 5 lb) body weight. Average size adult domestic cats normally should receive 1/2 tablet (15 mEq) daily.
Note: In rare cases animals may experience gastrointestinal disturbance. In those cases administer tablets during or after feeding or in 2 to 3 divided doses.
Caution: Federal law restricts this drug to use by or on the order of a licensed veterinarian.
How Supplied: 50 tablet bottles
Patent Pending

PIPA-TABS, 50 mg
(Piperazine dihydrochloride)
Piperazine Wormer

Composition: Each scored tablet contains: piperazine dihydrochloride equivalent to 50 mg piperazine base.
Indications: For treatment and control of ascarids; *Toxocara canis* in dogs and *Toxacaris leonina* in cats.
Dosage and Administration: The recommended piperazine dosage for dogs and cats is 25 mg piperazine base per pound of body weight. The initial dose of Pipa-Tabs, 50 mg is 1 tablet per 2 pounds of body weight. A second dose should be administered after 10 days.
In heavily infested animals a third dose should be given after another 10 day rest period. In thin and undernourished animals the dosage should be reduced to one-third (8 to 10 mg per pound of body weight) and given over a three day period.
Dogs and cats may be wormed at 6 to 8 weeks of age.
Precautions: Although piperazine is a drug with a high degree of safety, an occasional animal may show nausea, vomiting or muscular tremors. Such side effects are usually associated with overdosage; therefore, the recommended dosage should be followed carefully. Animals with known kidney pathology should be treated only by a veterinarian.
Caution: Consult a veterinarian before using in severely debilitated animals.
How Supplied: 500 Tablet Bottles

PIPA-TABS, 250 mg
(Piperazine dihydrochloride)
Piperazine Wormer

Composition: Each scored oval tablet contains: piperazine dihydrochloride equivalent to 250 mg piperazine base.
Indications: For treatment and control of ascarids; *Toxocara canis* in dogs and *Toxacaris leonina* in cats.
Dosage and Administration: The recommended piperazine dosage for dogs and cats is 25 mg piperazine base per pound of body weight. The initial dose of Pipa-Tabs, 250 mg is 1 tablet per 10 pounds of body weight. A second dose should be administered after 10 days.
In heavily infested animals a third dose should be given after another 10 day rest period. In thin and undernourished animals the dosage should be reduced to one-third (8 to 10 mg per pound of body weight) and given over a three day period.
Dogs and cats may be wormed at 6 to 8 weeks of age.
Precautions: Although piperazine is a drug with a high degree of safety, an occasional animal may show nausea, vomiting or muscular tremors. Such side effects are usually associated with overdosage; therefore, the recommended dosage should be followed carefully. Animals with known kidney pathology should be treated only by a veterinarian.
Caution: Consult a veterinarian before using in severely debilitated animals.
How Supplied: 500 Tablet Bottles

PIP-POP 320
Flavored Piperazine Wormer
Water Soluble Powder

Composition: Each 620 gram package contains the equivalent of 320 grams anhydrous piperazine base (as piperazine dihydrochloride) with sodium benzoate, flavoring agents and artificial coloring.
Indications: Helminthiasis in swine, horses, sheep, dogs, cats, poultry, and calves as follows: ***Swine:*** *Ascaris lumbricoides.* ***Horses:*** Ascarids *(Parascaris equorum),* strongyles *(Strongylus vulgaris),* small strongyles and pinworms *(Oxyuris equi).* ***Sheep:*** *Oesophogostomum spp.* ***Dogs and Cats:*** *Toxocara canis* and *Toxascaris leonina.* ***Chickens and Turkeys:*** *Ascaridia spp.* ***Calves:*** *Neoascaris vitulorum* and *Oesophagostomum spp.*
Directions: Pip-Pop 320 may be mixed directly with the feed or dissolved and added to the drinking water.
Pip-Pop 320 Medicated Feeds—Thoroughly mix the contents of one can of Pip-Pop in 325-350 lbs of ground feed. This should be the only source of feed. Allow swine to eat feed until it is completely consumed. This quantity of feed will treat 6375 lb live weight of swine.
Pip-Pop 320 Medicated Drinking Water—The contents of one package dissolved in one-half gallon of water will produce a concentrate which contains 17% piperazine base. The contents of one package dissolved in one gallon of water will produce a concentrate which contains 8.5% piperazine base.
[See table above].
Caution: Consult veterinarian before using in severely debilitated animals.

Pip-Pop Medicated Drinking Water	8.5% solution		17% solution	
Swine, per 100 lbs.	2	fl oz	1	fl oz
Horses, per 100 lbs.	2	fl oz	1	fl oz
Sheep, per 100 lbs.	2	fl oz	1	fl oz
Dogs and Cats, per 10 lbs.	2½ ml-3½ ml		1¼ ml-1¾ ml	
Chickens under 6 weeks, per 100 birds	2	fl oz	1	fl oz
Chickens over 12 weeks, per 100 birds	4	fl oz	2	fl oz
Turkeys under 12 weeks, per 100 birds	4	fl oz	2	fl oz
Turkeys over 12 weeks, per 100 birds	4 to 8	fl oz	2 to 8	fl oz
Calves, per 100 lbs.	3	fl oz	1½	fl oz

RUMEN-EZE
Emulsified Treatment for Frothy Bloat

Composition: Rumen-Eze is an emulsion containing vegetable oil, emulsifiers and preservatives.
Indications: Rumen-Eze is intended for use as an aid in the treatment of frothy bloat in cattle and sheep.
Dosage and Administration: Administer the contents of the special dosing container orally as a drench to relieve bloat in average size mature cattle. Young cattle and sheep should receive 6 to 12 fluid ounces as the severity of the condition indicates.
Caution: If administered to milking dairy cows, do not market the milk for 96 hours after treatment.
How Supplied: 12 fluid ounce dosing bottle

SULECTRO-SOL ONE
Flavored Sulfathiazole Sodium, Electrolytes for Automatic Medicators

Composition: SulEctro-Sol One contains 325 grams (5016 grains) of sulfonamide per 500 grams. Sulfonamides are normally administered at the rate of 65 to 100 milligrams (1 to 1½ grains) per pound of body weight initially, or the first day. Daily maintenance dosage is about one-half of the initial dosage. Con-

Continued on next page

Vet-A-Mix—Cont.

tinuous administration of sulfonamides should normally not exceed a period of 96 hours.
SulEctro-Sol One is primarily intended for administration in drinking water, but may be administered individually or in feed if desired. Provide adequate water intake during treatment. Dosage may be calculated either by body weight or by water intake.
Indications: SulEctro-Sol One is intended for use as an antibacterial agent, and electrolyte replacer. It should be used in the treatment and prevention of infections responsive to sulfonamide drugs. It is also useful for the treatment of bacterial infections secondary to virus infections.
Swine: Pneumonia, enteritis, pyosepticemia (navel ill), and other bacterial infections.
Cattle & Horses: Shipping fever complex, pneumonia, enteritis, pyosepticemia (navel ill) and equine strangles. Mix stock solution by dissolving 500 grams in one gallon warm water. Allow no other available sources of water during treatment.
Swine, Cattle & Horses: First 24 hours —mix one pint of stock solution in each 5-7½ gallons drinking water. Next 48-72 hours —mix one pint in each 7½-10 gallons drinking water. Do not administer medicated water for more than five days.
Warning: This product contains sulfonamides and may cause toxic symptoms and irreparable kidney damage if blood levels become too high. Avoid overdosage and low water intake during treatment. Discontinue treatment if toxic symptoms appear. The use of this drug should be discontinued 10 days before slaughter, or sale of milk for human consumption. Do not administer to horses to be used for human food.
How Supplied: 500 gram packets and 12.5 kilogram pails

V

TANNI-GEL
Astringent and Antiseptic Gel

Composition: Isopropyl alcohol 70% v/v, Salicylic acid 4% w/v, Tannic acid 4% w/v and Benzocaine 1% w/v in a special gelatinous base.
Indications: For use as an aid in the management of moist dermatitis and to toughen the foot pads of dogs. Tanni-Gel can be used as an astringent and drying agent for weeping wounds in large animals.
Dosage and Administration: Apply directly to skin lesion every 6–8 hours until the lesion is dry. Continue one application daily until healing is complete. Apply undiluted to foot pads and between the toes.
Note: The benzocaine in Tanni-Gel minimizes the stinging sensation when applied to sensitive skin.
Warning: For external use only. Avoid getting into eyes or on mucous membranes.
How Supplied: 4 fluid ounce dispensing bottle

THIMER-LYTE
Flavored Sulfathiazole Sodium, Electrolytes for Stock Tank Application

Composition:
ACTIVE DRUG INGREDIENT:

	Per pound	
Sulfathiazole sodium ...	295 g ...	65%

ELECTROLYTES: Sodium chloride and potassium chloride in a water soluble base containing flavoring, coloring and stabilizing agents.
Indications: *SWINE*-Bacterial scours *(E. Coli)*, Bacterial pneumonia *(Pasteurella spp.)*
CATTLE—Shipping fever complex *(Pasteurella spp.)*, calf diphtheria *(Spherophorus necrophorus)*.
Dosage and Administration: *FOR SWINE AND CATTLE:* Prepare stock solution by dissolving one pound in one gallon of very warm water.
First 24 hours—mix one pint of stock solution in each 5–6 gallons of drinking water (approximately one gallon of stock solution to make 45 gallons of drinking water).
24–120 hours—mix one pint of stock solution in each 10–12 gallons of drinking water or approximately one gallon of stock solution to make 95 gallons of drinking water.
Analysis: ThiMer-Lyte contains 4550 grains of sulfonamide per pound. Sulfonamides are normally administered at the rate of 65–100 milligrams (1–1½ grains) per pound of body weight initially, or the first day. The daily maintenance dosage is about one-half of the initial dose. Continuous administration of sulfathiazole sodium should normally not exceed a period of 96 hours. Provide adequate water intake during treatment. Dosage may be calculated either by body weight or by water intake. Factors such as temperature, humidity and disease will cause water intake to vary. As a generalization cattle and swine will drink approximately 1 gallon per 100 pounds body weight per day.
Warning: To avoid drug residues in cattle and swine, withdraw medicated drinking water ten (10) days prior to slaughter for food.
Caution: For best advice in control and treatment of animal disease, consult a veterinarian. Only medicated water must be used. Check carefully to insure adequate sulfonamide dosage and water consumption. Treat for a maximum of 5 consecutive days only. If no improvement is observed after 2 to 3 days, discontinue treatment and redetermine diagnosis. Discontinue if sulfonamide toxicosis symptoms appear, such as loss of appetite, depression, rough hair coat, sunken eyeballs, crystals in the urine and reduced urine output.
Note: Do not use in cattle producing milk for human consumption.
How Supplied: One pound packets and 25 pound pails

THYRO-FORM
(brand of levothyroxine sodium) Chewable Tablets

Composition: Each scored oval tablet contains either:
1. Levothyroxine sodium U.S.P. 0.2 mg (200 mcg)
2. Levothyroxine sodium U.S.P. 0.8 mg (800 mcg)

Indications: For use in the canine for correction of conditions associated with low circulating thyroid hormone (hypothyroidism).
Dosage and Administration: The initial dose should be 10–20 mcg/kg body weight (approximately 5–10 mcg/lb). Response to the administration of Thyro-form Chewable Tablets (brand of levothyroxine sodium) should be evaluated every four weeks until an adequate maintenance dose is established. In most dogs, with the exception of the toy breeds, this is usually in the range of 0.2 mg (200 mcg) to 0.8 mg (800 mcg) total daily dose. Thyro-Form Chewable tablets may be fed free choice from the hand or crumbled and placed on the food.
Warning: Administer with caution to animals with clinically significant heart disease, hypertension or other complications for which a sharply increased metabolic rate might prove hazardous. Use in pregnant bitches has not been evaluated.
Caution: Federal law restricts this drug to use by or on the order of a licensed veterinarian.
Store at room temperature and protect from light. Avoid excessive heat (104°F).
Important: Read package insert carefully and completely before use.
KEEP OUT OF REACH OF CHILDREN.
How Supplied:
0.2 mg (200 mcg) tablets —Bottles of 100 tablets; bottles of 500 tablets.
0.8 mg (800 mcg) tablets —Bottles of 50 tablets; bottles of 500 tablets.
For Veterinary Use Only

THYRO-L
Levothyroxine Sodium Powder

Composition: Each Pound (453.6 g) Contains:
Levothyroxine Sodium, U.S.P. ......0.22% (1.0 g)
Indications: For use in horses for correction of conditions associated with low circulating thyroid hormone (hypothyroidism).
Dosage: Doses should be individualized and animals should be monitored daily for clinical signs of hyperthyroidism or hypersensitivity. Suggested initial doses are one to 10 mg levothyroxine sodium (T4) /100 lb body weight (2 to 20 mg/100 kg) once per day or in divided doses. Response to the administration of Thyro-L should be evaluated clinically every week until an adequate maintenance dose is established. In most horses, this is usually in the range of 35 to 100 mg total daily dose of T4 (one to 3 level tablespoonfuls Thyro-L).
Note: One level teaspoonful contains 12 mg of T4; one level tablespoonful contains 36 mg of T4.

Administration: Thyro-L may be top dressed or mixed with the daily ration.
Warning: Administer with caution to animals with clinically significant heart disease, hypertension or other complications for which a sharply increased metabolic rate might prove hazardous. Use in pregnant mares has not been evaluated.
Caution: Federal law restricts this drug to use by or on the order of a licensed veterinarian.
How Supplied: One pound bottles and 10 pound pails.

THYRO-TABS
(levothyroxine sodium tablets, USP)

Composition: Each Thyro-Tabs Tablet contains Synthetic Crystalline Levothyroxine (l-thyroxine) Sodium, USP.
Indications: For use for the correction of conditions associated with low circulating thyroid hormone (hypothyroidism) in dogs.
Dosage and Administration: The initial dose should be 10-20 mcg/kg body weight (approximately 5-10 mcg/lb.). Response to the administration of Thyro-Tabs should be evaluated every four weeks until an adequate maintenance dose is established. In most dogs, with the exception of the toy breeds, this is usually in the range of 0.2 mg (200 mcg) to 0.8 mg (800 mcg) total daily dose.
Warning: Administer with caution to animals with clinically significant heart disease, hypertension or other complications for which a sharply increased metabolic rate might prove hazardous. Use in pregnant bitches has not been evaluated.
Caution:
Store at room temperature and protect from light.
Avoid excessive heat (104°F).
Read package insert carefully and completely before use.
KEEP OUT OF REACH OF CHILDREN.
Caution: Federal law restricts this drug to use by or on the order of a licensed veterinarian.
How Supplied: Available as scored, color coded tablets in 5 concentrations:

Package	Potency	Color
1000's	0.1 mg	Yellow
1000's	0.2 mg	Pink
1000's	0.3 mg	Green
1000's	0.5 mg	White
1000's	0.8 mg	Purple

For Veterinary Use Only

TOXIBAN GRANULES
TOXIBAN SUSPENSION

Composition: ToxiBan Granules and ToxiBan Suspension contain a medicinal grade activated carbon (MedChar), and colloidal kaolin. They are intended for use as adsorbents of orally ingested toxicants.
ToxiBan Granules contain 47.5% MedChar (charcoal), 10% kaolin and 42.5% wetting and dispersing agents, and are free-flowing and wettable for rapid constitution in water. They may also be mixed in the dry form with food.
ToxiBan Suspension contains 10.4% charcoal and 6.25% kaolin in an aqueous base, and is a stable suspension which is intended for use as a convenient emergency treatment of small animals or small numbers of large animals.
MedChar, contained in both products, is a small particle size type of vegetable charcoal that possesses a relatively high activity as an adsorbent of organic chemicals. It has been processed by Vet-A-Mix to enhance its adsorptive power and reduce dustiness. The kaolin is a fine particle size N.F. grade.
Indications: ToxiBan is of value as a symptomatic treatment of poisoning by most organic chemical compounds. ToxiBan should be used in conjunction with other conventional treatments, such as atropine sulfate for organophosphates and carbamates or 2-PAM for organophosphates. ToxiBan is an effective adsorbent for most cyclical compounds; such as organochlorine, organophosphate, and carbamate insecticides, herbicides, rodenticides, parasiticides, alkaloids, depressants and analgesics.
Administration: Dilute suspensions of ToxiBan Granules and ToxiBan Suspension should be stirred or agitated frequently during administration to keep the liquid uniform and prevent equipment clogging. A stomach tube or rumen tube is preferred for administration in all animals, but an oral drench may be used in an emergency. The suspension can be poured through a funnel attached to a stomach tube in most animals. Alternate methods are use of a stomach pump or syringe to inject the suspension through a stomach tube.
Administration equipment should be flushed with a dose of cold water before removing the stomach tube. Equipment used to administer ToxiBan cleans easily with water and detergent or water alone.
Poisoned animals should be watched closely after treatment, since specific or systemic treatment may need be repeated. Repeat treatment with ToxiBan is not usually indicated in acute toxicosis *unless* the condition of the animal appears to worsen or remains static 12 hours after the initial treatment, when a second dose of ToxiBan should be administered.
Dosage Schedule: ToxiBan Granules —For individual administration it is most convenient to mix in water and give via a stomach or rumen tube as a thin suspension. To make a suspension mix one volume measure with 5 to 7 parts of cold water. (Ex: one level cup ToxiBan Granules to 6 cupfuls water) and shake or stir vigorously for 10 seconds.
Large Animals —0.75 to 2.0 grams per kg (0.35 to 0.9 g/lb) body weight; or one pound (453.6 grams) for an animal weighing 225 to 600 kg (500 to 1300 lb.)
Small Animals —1.0 to 2.0 grams per kg (0.5 to 1.0 g/lb) body weight.
[See table above].
2 g ToxiBan Granules = activity of 9 ml ToxiBan Suspension.
ToxiBan Suspension —Give as is or mixed with small amount of cold water, preferably by use of an stomach tube.
Small Animals —6.0 to 12.0 ml per kg (3.0 to 6.0 ml/lb.) body weight.
Large Animals —4.0 to 12.0 ml per kg (2.0 to 6.0 ml/lb. body weight.
Contraindications: There are no contraindications to the use of charcoal as such; however, ToxiBan is not generally considered effective against lead, mercury and inorganic arsenic or other heavy metals. ToxiBan should not be given in conjunction with oral chemotherapy as the charcoal may adsorb the therapeutic agent.
How Supplied: Granules, 5 kilogram pails. Suspension, 240 ml bottles.
For Veterinary Use Only.

Dosage:
Measure Equivalents

Measure	Equivalent Measures	MedChar	Kaolin
TOXIBAN GRANULES			
1 level teaspoon	2.0 g	1.0 g	0.2g
1 level tablespoon	5.0 g	2.4 g	0.5 g
1 level cup	120.0 g	57.0 g	12.0 g
one pound	453.6 g	215.5 g	45.4 g
TOXIBAN SUSPENSION			
1 level teaspoon	5 ml	0.5 g	0.3 g
1 level tablespoon	15 ml	1.5 g	0.9 g
1 cupful (8 fl oz)	240 ml	25.0 g	15.0 g
1 litre	1000 ml	104.0 g	62.5 g

VETA-METH
Solution, 12.5%

Composition: Oral solution (Not Sterilized)
Sulfamethazine Sodium ....12.5% w/v
15 ml (approximately 1 tablespoon) contains 1.880 mg (or 29 grains) of sulfamethazine sodium.
Indications: For the control and treatment of the following diseases when caused by one or more of the following pathogenic organisms sensitive to sulfamethazine.
Cattle —Bacterial Pneumonia and Shipping Fever Complex *(Pasteurella spp; Haemophilus spp; Klebsiella spp)* Bacterial Enteritis (Scours) *(E. coli)*, Foot Rot *(Spherophorus necrophorus)*, Diphtheria *(Spherophorus necrophorus)*, Acute Metritis *(Streptococcus spp)*
Swine —Bacterial Scours —Necro *(E. coli)*, Bacterial Pneumonia *(Salmonella spp)*
Sheep —Bacterial Pneumonia and Shipping Fever Complex *(Pasteurella spp, Haemophilus spp.), Diphtheria (Spherophorus necrophorus)*
Dosage: *Cattle, Calves, Sheep and Swine*

Continued on next page

V

Vet-A-Mix—Cont.

First Day: 90 ml (6 tablespoons or 3 fl oz.) for each 100 lbs. of body weight. 2nd, 3rd, 4th and 5th days: 45 ml. (3 tablespoons or 1½ fl. oz.) for each 100 lbs. body weight.
Dosage and Administration: *Cattle, Calves, Sheep and Swine*
Drinking Water: Add the dose listed to that amount of water that will be consumed in one day. Check consumption carefully. Factors such as temperature, humidity and disease will cause water intake to vary. As a generalization, the above animals will drink approximately 1 gallon per 100 lbs. body weight per day. Dairy cattle may drink up to 2 gallons per day.
Feed: Add the dose listed above to that amount of feed that will be consumed in 2 to 4 hours. Animals not eating or drinking should be dosed by drench or with Veta-Meth Boluses. For best results, separate the animals to be treated and treat sick animals individually.
Warning: To avoid drug residues —*Cattle, Calves and Sheep*—Withdraw medication ten (10) days prior to slaughter for food.
Swine—Withdraw medication fifteen (15) days prior to slaughter for food.
Note: Do not use in cattle producing milk for human consumption.
Caution: For best advice in control and treatment of animal disease, consult a veterinarian. Only medicated water must be used. Check carefully to insure adequate Veta-Meth dosage and water consumed. For best results treat sick animals individually by drench or with Veta-Meth Boluses. Treat for 5 consecutive days only. If no improvement is observed after 2 or 3 days, discontinue treatment and redetermine diagnosis. Discontinue treatment if sulfonamide toxicity symptoms, such as loss of appetite, depression, rough hair coat, and sunken eyeballs, appear.
How Supplied: Gallons.
Sale to Veterinarians Only

V

VETA-METH
Tablets, 5 gram

Composition: Each scored tablet contains:
Sulfamethazine, U.S.P. 5 grams
Indications: In cattle for the control and treatment of bacterial pneumonia and bovine respiratory disease complex (shipping fever complex) *(Pasteurella spp.), colibacillosis* (bacterial scours) *(E. Coli), necrotic pododermatitis* (foot rot) *(Spherophorus necrophorus)* calf diphtheria *(Spherophorus necrophorus),* acute metritis *(Streptococcus spp.).*
Dosage and Administration: Initial dose —give one 5 g tablet for each 50 pounds (22.5 kg) body weight. Follow within 12 to 24 hours with maintenance dose.
Daily maintenance dose —give one 5 g tablet for each 100 pounds (45 kg) body weight. Maintenance dose may be given once each 24 hour period. The maximum treatment period normally should not exceed five days.
Warning: Discontinue treatment if sulfonamide toxicity symptoms appear. Supply adequate water during treatment. The use of this drug should be discontinued 8 days before slaughter for human consumption. Do not use in cows producing milk for human consumption. Keep all medication out of the reach of children.
How Supplied: 50 Tablet Bottles
For Veterinary Use Only

VETA-METH
Tablets, 15 gram

Composition: Each scored tablet contains:
Sulfamethazine, U.S.P..............15 grams
Indications: In cattle for the control and treatment of bacterial pneumonia and bovine respiratory disease complex (shipping fever complex) *(Pasteurella spp.), colibacillosis* (bacterial scours) *(E. Coli), necrotic pododermatitis* (foot rot) *(Spherophorus necrophorus),* calf diphtheria *(Spherophorus necrophorus),* acute metritis *(Streptococcus spp..)*
Administration: *Initial dose*—give one 15 g tablet for each 150 pounds (78 kg) body weight. Follow within 12 to 24 hours with maintenance dose.
Daily maintenance dose—give one 15 g tablet for each 300 pounds (135 kg) body weight. Maintenance dose may be given once each 24 hour period. The maximum treatment period normally should not exceed five days.
Warning: Discontinue treatment if sulfonamide toxicity symptoms appear. Supply adequate water during treatment. The use of this drug should be discontinued 8 days before slaughter for human consumption. Do not use in cows producing milk for human consumption. Keep all medication out of the reach of children
How Supplied: 50 Tablet Bottles
For Veterinary Use Only

VETA-METH
Tablets, 25 grams

Composition: Each scored tablet contains:
Sulfamethazine, U.S.P. 25 grams
Indications: In cattle for the control and treatment of bacterial pneumonia and bovine respiratory disease complex (shipping fever complex) *(Pasteurella spp.), colibacillosis* (bacterial scours) *(E. coli), necrotic pododermatitis* (foot rot) *(Spherophorus necrophorus),* calf diphtheria *(Spherophorus necrophorus),* acute metritis *(Streptococcus spp.).*
Dosage and Administration: *Initial dose*—give one 25 g tablet for each 250 pounds (113 kg) body weight. Follow within 12 to 24 hours with maintenance dose.
Daily maintenance dose—give one 25 g tablet for each 500 pounds (225 kg) body weight. Maintenance dose may be given once each 24 hour period. The maximum treatment period normally should not exceed five days.
Warning:
Discontinue treatment if sulfonamide toxicity symptoms appear. Supply adequate water during treatment.
The use of this drug should be discontinued 8 days before slaughter for human consumption.
Do not use in cows producing milk for human consumption.
Keep all medication out of the reach of children.
How Supplied: 50 Tablet Bottles
For Veterinary Use Only

VILEC-SOL
Water Dispersible
Vitamin Complex-Electrolytes for Domestic Animals and Poultry

Composition: Guaranteed analysis:per 500 grams

Vitamin A, U.S.P. Units	500,000
Vitamin D_3, U.S.P. Units	100,000
Riboflavin	1,200 mg
Calcium dl-Pantothenate	8,700 mg
Equivalent to d-Pantothenic Acid	3,600 mg
Pyridoxine Hydrochloride	250 mg
Menadione Sodium Bisulfite (vitamin K analogue)	250 mg
dl-Alpha Tocopheryl Acetate (vitamin E)	100 mg
Nicotinic Acid	8,000 mg
Thiamine Mononitrate	500 mg
Vitamin B_{12}	1,000 mcg

Ingredients: Vitamin A acetate, irradiated ergosterol (source of vitamin D_3), calcium d-pantothenate, dl-alpha tocopheryl acetate, vitamin B_{12} supplement, riboflavin, nicotinic acid, thiamine mononitrate, pyridoxine hydrochloride, menadione sodium bisulfite, potassium chloride, sodium chloride, magnesium gluconate, calcium gluconate, sodium citrate, and BHT & BHA (antioxidants and preservatives).
Indications: For the replacement of electrolytes and vitamins, especially during dehydration due to diarrhea or vomiting or during periods of reduced feed intake. ViLec-Sol may be used for all domestic animals and poultry.
Directions: *Corrective level:* For use during severe dehydration and for correction of vitamin deficiencies. Mix 500 grams in each 100 gallons drinking water. Allow no other sources of water. Individual dosage is 5 grams (one level teaspoon) twice daily for each 100 lbs. body weight. Treat as long as indicated. As condition improves and food intake increases, decrease the level of medication to one-half or less.
Stress level: As an adjunctive corrective treatment of dehydration, such as mild cases of enteritis. Mix 500 grams in each 200 to 400 gallons drinking water depending upon severity of condition and water intake.
How Supplied: 500 gram packets and 12.5 kilogram pails.
Sales to Graduate Veterinarians Only

Products are cross-indexed by generic and chemical names in the
Active Ingredients Section

Vet-Kem
A Division of Zoecon Corporation
12200 DENTON DRIVE
DALLAS, TX 75234

BREAKAWAY™
Flea & Tick Collar for Cats
kills fleas & ticks up to 5 months
new stretch band
one-piece buckle

Composition:
ACTIVE INGREDIENT: *o*-Isopropoxyphenyl methylcarbamate† 9.4%.
INERT INGREDIENTS: 90.6%.

Directions For Use: Thread flat end of collar through buckle hole and tighten as necessary, so at least two ridges are covered by buckle. Collar must be worn loosely, but securely enough to prevent easy removal. Cut off any excess length and discard in trash.
Do not use on kittens under 6 weeks of age.

Unique Feature: The expandable section molded into collar will stretch under weight of average-size cat and allow cat to free itself if it becomes hooked or entangled by collar. Since both expandable section and plastic buckle are molded into collar, probability of neck irritation and buckle failure is reduced. To release collar, squeeze buckle between thumb and finger and pull sharply.

Results Expected: The flea and tick collar starts killing fleas and ticks when it is placed around the cat's neck. Fleas will be killed and new ones which may temporarily appear on the cat will also be killed during the 5 months collar is worn. Ticks are tough occasional pests of cats and will be killed within a few days.
For continuous protection, replace collar when effectiveness diminishes.

Caution: Do not open inner envelope until ready to use. Do not allow children to play with this collar. Dust will form on this collar during storage. Do not get dust or collar in mouth, harmful if swallowed. Do not get dust in eyes, will cause temporary pupillary constriction.* In case of contact, flush eyes with water. Wash hands thoroughly with soap and water after handling collar. The dust released by this collar is a cholinesterase inhibitor.

Note to Physician: Atropine and *homatropine are antidotal.
When collar is first worn, observe neck area every few days for irritation. Any collar, when fastened too tightly, may cause skin irritation. Remove collar at the first sign of irritation or adverse reaction. Collar is intended for use as an insecticide generator and is not to be taken internally by man or animal. Do not use on sick or convalescing animals. Do not use any other pesticide on cat while collar is worn.

Storage & Disposal: Store in original unopened container; away from children. Do not reuse container or used collar. Wrap and put in trash.
Seller makes no warranty, express or implied, concerning the use of this product other than indicated on the label. Buyer assumes all risk of use and handling of this material when such use and handling are contrary to label instructions.
EPA Reg. No. 2724-275-11785
Available Through Veterinarians
BREAKAWAY is a trademark of Zoecon Corporation.
For detailed directions for use, limitations, restrictions, exceptions, and precautions, carefully read product label.

DURSBAN*
Flea & Tick Collar for Dogs

Composition: Active Ingredient:
Chlorpyrifos [*0,0*-Diethyl *0*-(3,5,6-trichloro-2-pyridyl) phosphoro thioate] 8.0%
Inert Ingredients: 92.0%
Keep out of reach of children
* DURSBAN is a registered trademark of The Dow Chemical Company

Precautionary Statements: *Hazards to Humans and Domestic Animals–Caution:* Do not open protective pouch until ready to use. Do not allow children to handle collar. Wash hands thoroughly with soap and water after handling collar. Do not use on sick or convalescing dogs. Do not use other pesticides on dogs while collar is worn. Do not use on dogs under 12 weeks of age. This product contains a cholinesterase inhibitor. Some breeds or individuals may be sensitive. Remove collar if symptoms of cholinesterase inhibition (which may include salivation, vomiting, and/or diarrhea) occur. Atropine is antidotal only if symptoms of cholinesterase inhibition are present.

Directions for Use: It is a violation of Federal law to use this product in a manner inconsistent with its labeling.
Buckle collar around dog's neck. Collar should be worn loosely to prevent irration. Attach collar so two or three fingers may be inserted easily between collar and dog's neck. Cut off any excess length and dispose of it. When collar is first worn, observe neck area every few days for irritation.
Remove collar at first sign of irritation or adverse reaction.
This collar starts killing fleas and ticks as soon as it is placed around dog's neck. Fleas on the dog will be killed and new ones, which may temporarily appear on the dog, will also be killed while collar is worn.
Ticks are tough and are killed slowly. When the collar is first placed on dog, adult ticks will be killed over entire body in a few days and will fall off, or may then be easily removed. Ticks appear on dogs in three stages. In the first two stages, ticks are smaller than a match head and are difficult to see. The collar will also control these immature stages. Use in addition to regular collar. This collar has been shown to provide effective flea kill up to 11 months and tick kill up to 7 months plus aiding in tick control for an additional 2 months. Replace when effectiveness diminishes.
Kills ticks that may carry and transmit Rocky Mountain spotted fever and tularemia. This collar will also aid in the prevention of Sarcoptic Mange for up to 5 months.

Storage & Disposal: Store in original unopened container; away from children. Do not reuse container, pouch or used collar. Wrap and put in trash collection. Seller makes no warranty, express or implied, concerning the use of this product other than indicated on the label. Buyer assumes all risk of use and handling of this material when such use and handling are contrary to label instructions.
EPA Reg. No. 2724-282-11785
For detailed directions for use, limitations, restrictions, exceptions, and precautions, carefully read product label.

FLEA AND TICK DOG COLLAR

Composition:
Active Ingredient:
o-Isopropoxyphenyl methylcarbamate 9.4%
Inert Ingredients: 90.6%

Indications: Kills fleas up to 5 months. Kills ticks up to 5 months.

Directions: Buckle collar around dog's neck. Collar should be worn loosely to prevent irritation. Attach collar so two or three fingers may be inserted easily between collar and dog's neck. Cut off any excess length and dispose of it. The collar starts killing fleas as soon as it is placed around dog's neck. Fleas on the dog will be killed and new ones which may temporarily appear on the dog will also be killed while collar is worn. Use in addition to regular collar. This product has been shown to provide effective flea control for up to 21 weeks. *Replace collar when effectiveness diminishes.*
Ticks are tough and are killed slowly. When collar is first placed on dog, adult ticks will be killed over entire body in a few days and will fall off or may then be easily removed. Ticks appear on dogs in three stages. In the first two stages, ticks are smaller than a match head and are difficult to see. The collar will also control these immature stages. This product has been shown to provide effective tick control up to 5 months. If ticks are a problem, this collar should be worn continuously. Kills ticks that may carry and transmit Rocky Mountain spotted fever and tularemia. Temporary wetting will not reduce effectiveness. If your dog goes swimming or is out in the rain, it is not necessary to remove the collar. The continuous action collar will rapidly replace any flea and tick killing material removed. *Replace when effectiveness diminishes.*

Caution: Do not open protective pouch until ready to use. Do not allow children to handle this collar. Dust will form on this collar during storage. Do not get dust or collar in mouth, harmful if swallowed. Do not get dust in eyes, will cause temporary pupillary constriction*. In case of contact, flush eyes with water. Wash hands thoroughly with soap and water after handling collar. The dust released by this collar is a cholinesterase inhibitor.

Note to Physician: Atropine and *homatropine are antidotal.

Continued on next page

Vet-Kem—Cont.

When collar is first worn, observe neck area every few days for irritation. Remove collar at the first sign of irritation or adverse reaction. Collar is intended for use as an insecticide generator and is not to be taken internally by man or animals. Do not use on sick or convalescing dogs. Do not use other pesticides on dog while collar is worn.
Storage & Disposal: Store in original container; away from children. Do not reuse container or used collar. Wrap and put in trash.
How Supplied:
For Small and Medium dogs 20″
For Large dogs 26″
For detailed directions for use, limitations, restrictions, exceptions, and precautions, carefully read product label.
EPA Reg. No. 2724-254-11785
Seller makes no warranty, express or implied, concerning the use of this product other than indicated on the label. Buyer assumes all risk of use and handling of this material when such use and handling are contrary to label instructions.

FLEA® AND TICK POWDER

Composition:

Active Ingredient:	
Carbaryl (1-naphthyl *N*-methylcarbamate)	5.0%
Inert Ingredients:	95.0%

Directions for use: This product may be used as an aid in the control of Brown Dog Ticks on dogs and premises and is effective against fleas on dogs and cats.
Dosage and Administration: *For Control of Ticks and Fleas on Dogs and Cats:* Dust powder liberally over the animal and rub thoroughly into the skin. Be sure to apply also to the feet, between the toes and on the legs. Comb out dead ticks a few hours after treatment.
When dusting mother cats, remove the mother for treatment and return her to the kittens after one or two hours. Repeat at weekly intervals if needed.
In Kennels, Dog Houses: Dust in and around sleeping quarters and other areas where ticks and fleas occur.
Caution: Harmful if swallowed or inhaled. Avoid breathing dust and contact with skin; wash thoroughly after using. Keep out of reach of children. Avoid storage near feed and food products. Do not treat kittens or puppies under four weeks of age. Minimize treatment of eyes and face.
Storage & Disposal: Store in original closed container; away from children. Do not reuse empty container. Wrap and put in trash.
How Supplied: Available in 5 oz containers.
For detailed directions for use, limitations, restrictions, exceptions, and precautions, carefully read product label.
EPA Reg. No. 2724-75-11785
Seller makes no warranty, express or implied, concerning the use of this product other than indicated on the label. Buyer assumes all risk of use and handling of this material when such use and handling are contrary to label instructions.

FLEA & TICK PUMP SPRAY
For Dogs & Cats

Composition: Active Ingredients: Pyrethrins .150%; Technical Piperonyl Butoxide* 1.5%; N-Octyl Bicycloheptene Dicarboximide .333%; 2,3:4, 5-Bis(2-Butylene) Tetrahydro-2-Furaldehyde .200% Ingredients: 97.817%
*Equivalent to 1.2% (butylcarbityl) (6-propylpiperonyl) ether and .3% related compounds.
Precautionary Statements/Practical Treatments
Hazards to Humans & Domestic Animals—
Caution: Harmful if swallowed or inhaled. Avoid breathing mist. Avoid contact with eyes. In case of contact, immediately flush eyes with plenty of water. Get medical attention if irritation persists. Wash hands with soap and water after using.
Environmental Hazards: This product is toxic to fish. Keep out of lakes, ponds, streams, tidal marshes and estuaries. Do not contaminate water by cleaning of equipment or disposal of wastes.
Physical/Chemical Hazards: Flammable. Keep away from heat and open flame.
Directions for Use: It is a violation of Federal law to use this product in a manner inconsistent with its labeling.
Remove cap and insert trigger sprayer.
Dogs and Cats: To kill fleas, lice and ticks, cover animal's eyes with hand and with a firm, fast stroke to get a proper spray mist, spray head, ears and chest until damp. With fingertips, rub into face around mouth, nose and eyes. Then spray neck, middle and hindquarters, finishing legs last. For best penetration of spray to skin, direct spray against the natural lay of the hair. On long haired dogs, rub your hand against the lay of the hair, spraying the ruffled hair directly behind the hand. Make sure spray thoroughly wets ticks. Repeat treatment as needed.
Puppies and Kittens: Treat same as cats and dogs except nursing puppies and kittens, spray only along animal's back or on your fingertips and rub into animal's fur.
Pet Sleeping Quarters: Spray around baseboards, windows, door frames, wall cracks and local areas of floors. If mosquitoes, gnats or flies are present, spray lightly into the air. Repeat as needed. The bedding should be sprayed and then replaced with fresh bedding for best results. Con-current treatment of animals is recommended.
Horse: To repel gnats, flies and mosquitoes, apply a light mist sufficient to wet the surface of the hair. To control stable flies, horse flies, deer flies and face flies, apply at a rate of 2 oz. per adult horse, sufficient to wet the hair thoroughly. Repeat treatment as needed.
Storage and Disposal: Do not use or store near heat or open flame. Do not allow to freeze. Do not contaminate food or feed. Do not use empty container. Wrap container and put in trash collection.
SOLD BY VET-KEM
A Division of Zoecon Corporation
12200 Denton Drive - Dallas, Texas 75234
VET-KEM is a trademark of Zoecon Corporation
Seller makes no warranty, express or implied, concerning the use of this product other than indicated on the label. Buyer assumes all risk of use and handling of this material when such use and handling are contrary to label instructions.
EPA Reg. No. 43288-8-11785
For detailed directions for use, limitations, restrictions, exceptions, and precautions, carefully read product label.

FLEA & TICK SHAMPOO for dogs & cats
Kills fleas, lice, and ticks
Adds luster & groomability to pet's coat

Composition: Active ingredients: Piperonyl butoxide, technical* .50%; Pyrethrins, 0.5%; Petroleum distillate, .12%. (*Equivalent to .40% (butylcarbityl) (6-propylpiperonyl) ether and .10% related compounds.)
Inert ingredients: 99.33%
An insecticidal shampoo rich in coconut conditioners that aid in building body, luster, and groomability to the coats of dogs and cats. The insecticidal ingredients are highly and rapidly effective against fleas, ticks, and lice when used as directed.
Directions: It is a violation of Federal law to use this product in a manner inconsistent with its label.
Wet the dog or cat and apply a generous amount of shampoo, working it well into the coat. For best results, the dog or cat should be left in a lathered state for 4 to 5 minutes before rinsing with warm water.
Precautionary Statements: HAZARDS TO HUMANS & DOMESTIC ANIMALS—CAUTION: Harmful if swallowed. Do not inhale. Keep out of eyes and avoid contact with mucous membranes. In case this product should get in the eyes, flush immediately with water. In case of infection or skin irritation, discontinue use and consult a veterinarian. Avoid contamination of feed or foodstuffs.
Disposal: Do not reuse empty container. Wrap container and put in trash collection.
Seller makes no warranty, express or implied, concerning the use of this product other than indicated on the label. Buyer assumes all risk of use and handling of this material when such use and handling are contrary to label instructions.
How Supplied: 8 oz. and 1 gallon container
Available through veterinarians
EPA Reg. No. 29909-2-11785
For detailed directions for use, limitations, restrictions, exceptions, and precautions, carefully read product label.

V

4 MONTH FLEA COLLAR FOR CATS

Composition:
Active Ingredient:
Carbaryl (1-naphthyl *N*-methylcarbamate) 8.5%
Inert Ingredients: 91.5%

Directions: Remove the collar from package and place around cat's neck, adjust for proper fit and buckle in place. Collar must be worn loosely, but securely enough to prevent easy removal and loss of the collar. Cut off any excess length of collar, leaving ample length for expansion as the cat grows. Dispose of excess collar by discarding in trash. Check and adjust collar periodically to assure a proper fit. Do not use on kittens under six weeks of age.

Results Expected: The flea collar starts killing fleas when it is placed around the cat's neck. Fleas on the cat will be killed and new ones which may temporarily appear on the cat will also be killed during the 4 months (17 weeks) collar is worn. For continuous protection, replace collar when effectiveness diminishes.

Caution: Do not open inner envelope until ready to use. Do not allow children to play with this collar. Collar is intended for use as an insecticide generator and is not to be taken internally by man or animal. Not intended for use on humans.
Some animals may be sensitive to this collar. Any collar, when fastened too tightly, may cause skin irritation. If irritation persists after proper adjustment, remove the collar. Do not use any other pesticide on cat while collar is worn. Do not use on sick or convalescing animals.

Storage & Disposal: Store in original unopened container; away from children. Do not reuse container or used collar. Wrap and put in trash.

How Supplied: Individual packages.
For detailed directions for use, limitations, restrictions, exceptions, and precautions, carefully read product label.
EPA Reg. No. 2724-272-11785
Seller makes no warranty, express or implied, concerning the use of this product other than indicated on the label. Buyer assumes all risk of use and handling of this material when such use and handling are contrary to label instructions.

MEDICATED TAR & SULPHUR SHAMPOO for dogs
Deep cleansing

Composition: Coal Tar, 0.5%; Colloidal Sulphur, 5%; Salicylic Acid, 1%; P-Chloro-m-xylenol, 1%; in a therapeutic, penetrating shampoo base.

Indications: Dermatitis associated with flaking skin, crust, excessive skin oil, seborrhea and eczema, flea bite dermatitis.

Caution: KEEP OUT OF REACH OF CHILDREN. Do not use on cats. For external use only. KEEP OUT OF EYES.

Directions: Shake well before using. Wet dog thoroughly. Massage shampoo into skin and coat. Add more water during bath as necessary. Rinse. For best results, apply a second time and leave lather on for ten minutes before rinsing thoroughly. Persistent cases may require additional treatment. Use as directed by your veterinarian.
Seller makes no warranty, express or implied, concerning the use of this product other than indicated on the label. Buyer assumes all risk of use and handling of this material when such use and handling are contrary to label instructions.

How Supplied: 8 oz. container
Available through veterinarians
For detailed directions for use, limitations, restrictions, exceptions, and precautions, carefully read product label.

PARAMITE®
Insecticidal Collar
For Dogs

Composition:
Active Ingredient:
N-(Mercaptomethyl) phthalimide *S*-(*O,O*-dimethyl phosphorodithioate) 15.0%
Inert Ingredients: 85.0%

Indications: Kills ticks and fleas up to 7 months. Aids in prevention of Sarcoptic mange up to 7 months.

Directions: It is a violation of Federal law to use this product in a manner inconsistent with its labeling.
Buckle collar around dog's neck. Collar should be worn loosely to prevent irritation. Attach collar so two or three fingers may be inserted easily between collar and dog's neck. Cut off any excess length and dispose of it. When collar is first worn, observe neck area every few days for irritation. Remove collar at first sign of irritation or adverse reaction. Collar is intended for use only as an insecticide generator and is not to be taken internally by man or animals. Use in addition to regular collar. Do not use on sick or convalescing dogs. Do not use other pesticides on dogs while collar is worn. Product not to be used on puppies under 12 weeks of age. Remove collar when bathing.
The collar starts killing fleas as soon as it is placed around dog's neck. Fleas on the dog will be killed and new ones, which may temporarily appear on the dog, will also be killed while collar is worn. This product has been shown to provide effective flea kill up to 7 months plus aiding in kill for an additional 3 months. Replace collar when effectiveness diminishes.
Ticks are tough and are killed slowly. When the collar is first placed on dog, adult ticks will be killed over entire body in a few days and will fall off, or may then be easily removed. Ticks appear on dogs in three stages. In the first two stages, ticks are smaller than a match head and are difficult to see. The collar will also kill these immature stages. This product has been shown to provide effective tick kill up to 7 months plus aiding in kill for an additional 3 months. If ticks are a problem, this collar should be worn continuously. Kills ticks that may carry and transmit Rocky Mountain spotted fever and tularemia. Replace when effectiveness diminishes.
The collar will also aid in the prevention of Sarcoptic Mange for up to 7 months.

Hazards to humans and domestic animals.

Caution: Dust will form on this collar during storage. Do not get dust or collar in mouth, or allow dust in eyes. Do not open protective pouch until ready to use. Do not allow children to handle collar.
Statement of practical treatment: If dust is on skin—Wash promptly with soap and water. Rinse thoroughly. If dust is in eyes—Rinse eyes with plenty of water. Get medical attention if irritation persists.

Note to physician: The dust released by this collar is a cholinesterase inhibitor. If signs of cholinesterase inhibition appear, Atropine is antidotal.

Storage & Disposal: Store in original unopened container; away from children. Do not reuse container or used collar. Wrap and put in trash.
Seller makes no warranty, express or implied, concerning the use of this product other than indicated on the label. Buyer assumes all risk of use and handling of this material when such use and handling are contrary to label instructions.
EPA Reg. No. 2724-279-11785
Keep out of Reach of Children
Available through Veterinarians

How Supplied: For small and medium dogs 20"
For large dogs 26"
For detailed directions for use, limitations, restrictions, exceptions, and precautions, carefully read product label.
PARAMITE is a trademark of Zoecon Corporation.

PARAMITE®
Insecticidal Dust
For Dogs

Composition:
Active Ingredient:
N-(Mercaptomethyl) phthalimide
S-(*O,O*-dimethyl
phosphorodithioate) 5.0%
Inert Ingredients: 95.0%

Indications: Controls Sarcoptic Mange and fleas and ticks on dogs.

Directions: It is a violation of Federal law to use this product in a manner inconsistent with its labeling.
This product is effective in controlling Sarcoptic Mange on dogs. It controls fleas on dogs for up to 21 days. Brown Dog Ticks and American Dog Ticks on dogs will be controlled up to 14 days.
For Control of Sarcoptic Mange on Dogs: Treat dog using ¼ teaspoon (tsp) (0.5 g) of dust per pound of body weight weekly for 3 weeks. Treat entire dog paying particular attention to infected areas and rub thoroughly into hair to the skin. If no improvement is observed in 21 days, consult your veterinarian.
For Control of Ticks and Fleas on Dogs: Apply dust liberally over the animal at the rate of ¼ teaspoon (tsp) (0.5 g) per pound of body weight beginning at the head and rub thoroughly into hair to the skin. Be sure to treat the legs and feet. Minimize treatment of eyes and face. Do not treat puppies under 12 weeks of age.

Continued on next page

Vet-Kem—Cont.

Hazards to humans and domestic animals.

Caution: Harmful if swallowed or inhaled. Avoid breathing dust. Avoid contact with eyes. Avoid unnecessary contact with skin or clothing. Wash thoroughly after using.

Statement of practical treatment: If swallowed—Drink one or two glasses of water and induce vomiting by touching back of throat with finger. Do not induce vomiting or give anything by mouth to an unconscious person;. Get medical attention immediately. If inhaled—Remove victim to fresh air and apply respiration if indicated. If in eyes—Flush with plenty of water. Get medical attention if irritation persists.

Note to physician: This product contains an organophosphorous insecticide. Atropine is antidotal.

Storage & Disposal: Store in original closed container; away from children. Do not reuse empty container. Wrap and put in trash.

Seller makes no warranty, express or implied, concerning the use of this product other than indicated on the label. Buyer assumes all risk of use and handling of this material when such use and handling are contrary to label instruction.

EPA Reg. No. 2724-277-11785

Keep out of Reach of Children

Available Through Veterinarians

For detailed directions for use, limitations, restrictions, exceptions, and precautions, carefully read product label.

PARAMITE is a trademark of Zoecon Corporation.

PARAMITE®
Sponge-On or Dip for Dogs & Cats

Composition:

Active Ingredients:

N-(Mercaptomethyl) phthalimide *S* (*O, O*-Dimethyl phosphorodithioate)	11.60%
Aromatic petroleum solvent	72.90%
Inert Ingredients:	15.50%

Protect from temperatures below 20°F.

An insecticide for the control of sarcoptic mange on dogs, and for fleas and ticks on dogs and cats.

Directions: Sarcoptic mange on dogs is characterized by loss of hair, thickened skin and intense itching, caused by the mite *Sarcoptes scabiei varcanis.* Mix 1 oz (2 tbs) PARAMITE with 1 gal water. Dip dog until skin is wet and allow to shake dry. Do not rinse. If no improvement is seen within 14 days, consult your veterinarian. If mange mites reinfest your dog, retreatment may be necessary.

Fleas and ticks on dogs: Mix 1 oz (2 tbs) PARAMITE with 1 gal water. Dip or sponge on solution until skin is wet. For maximum residual control, allow to dry on animal.

Occasionally, cats get ticks.

Fleas and ticks on cats: Mix ½ oz (1 tbs) PARAMITE with 1 gal water. Dip or sponge on solution until skin is wet. For maximum residual control, allow to dry on animal.

Retreat as necessary but not more often than every 7 days. Do not treat dogs or cats under 8 weeks of age. The PARAMITE solution may be stored or used for 30 days.

Observe the following use precautions.

Warning: PARAMITE is a cholinesterase inhibitor. Do not use this product on animals simultaneously or within a few days before or after treatment with or exposure to cholinesterase inhibiting drugs, pesticides, or chemicals. Do not treat sick or debilitated animals.

May be harmful if swallowed, inhaled or absorbed through skin. If swallowed, do not induce vomiting. Immediately give large quantities of water or milk. If vomiting does occur, give fluids again. Never give anything by mouth to an unconscious person. Call a physician or Poison Control Center immediately.

Do not get in eyes, on skin or clothing. Do not breathe spray mist. Use only in well ventilated areas. Wear rubber gloves, goggles and protective clothing. In case of skin contact, wash immediately with soap and water; for eyes, flush with water. Wash all contaminated clothing with soap and hot water before re-use. Do not store near heat or open flame. Do not contaminate food or feed.

This product is toxic to fish and wildlife. Keep out of lakes, streams or ponds. Do not apply where runoff is likely to occur. Do not contaminate water by cleaning of equipment or disposal of wastes. Apply this product only as specified on this label.

Storage & Disposal: Store in original container; away from children. Do not reuse container. Wrap and put in trash.

Note to Physician and Veterinarian: PARAMITE is an organophosphorous insecticide. Atropine is antidotal. Usual symptoms of organophos phorous poisoning in man include: headache, blurred vision, weakness, nausea, discomfort in the chest, vomiting, abdominal cramps, diarrhea, salivation, sweating, and pinpoint pupils. Usual symptoms of organophosphorous poisoning in animals include salivation and labored breathing.

EPA Reg. No. 2724-169-11785

How Supplied: 4 oz bottles, gallon and 5 gallon cans.

For detailed directions for use, limitations, restrictions, exceptions, and precautions, carefully read product label.

Seller makes no warranty, express or implied, concerning the use of this product other than indicated on the label. Buyer assumes all risk of use and handling of this material when such use and handling are contrary to label instructions.

PARAMITE is a trademark of Zoecon Corporation.

PET SPRAY

Composition:

Active Ingredients:

Carbaryl (1-naphthyl *N*-methylcarbamate)	0.500%
Pyrethrins	0.050%
Technical piperonyl butoxide	0.100%
N-octyl bicycloheptene dicarboximide	0.166%
Inert Ingredients	99.184%

Dosage and Administration: Remove cap and press down plastic button with hole away from you. Hold at a convenient distance from the animal (approximately 6 inches) so that the spray penetrates to the skin. Work from the back of the animal toward the front of the animal; fluffing the hair may help permit the spray to penetrate. Keep the spray moving constantly. Spray only enough that the hair and skin are slightly damp. Wet ticks with spray. Do not allow spray to get in eyes or on scrotum.

For cats, spray on the basis of a 4 to 6 second application for a 5 pound cat, for dogs spray on the basis of a 20 to 30 second application for a 25 pound dog. Repeat treatment if necessary, but not more often than once weekly. Also treat bedding, interior of kennel and other places where ticks and fleas may be found. The cool sensation caused by the spray, as well as the hissing sound, may temporarily frighten nervous pets. Pets are expected to become accustomed to this treatment.

Caution: Harmful if swallowed or inhaled. Avoid contact with skin. Avoid breathing spray mist. Do not contaminate food or water. Wash hands after use. Keep out of reach of children. Do not allow spray to get in eyes. Avoid treatment of or exposure to kittens and puppies less than 4 weeks old.

Contents under pressure. Do not puncture. Do not use or store near heat or open flame. Exposure to temperatures above 130°F may cause bursting. Never throw container into fire or incinerator.

Storage & Disposal: Store in a cool area away from children. Do not reuse empty can. Wrap and put in trash.

How Supplied: 14 oz cans.

For detailed directions for use, limitations, restrictions, exceptions, and precautions, carefully read product label.

EPA Reg. No. 2724-90-11785

Seller makes no waranty, express or implied, concerning the use of this product other than indicated on the label. Buyer assumes all risk of use and handling of this material when such use and handling are contrary to label instructions.

SIPHOTROL™
Premise Spray
With Pyrethrins
For Use in the Home
Kills Adult and Pre-Adult Fleas

Composition: Active Ingredients: (Isopropyl (*E,E*)-11-methoxy-3,7,11-trimethyl-2,4 dodecadienoate) 0.03%

Pyrethrins 0.20%; Piperonyl butoxide, technical* 1.00%; *N*-octyl bicycloheptene dicarboximide 1.00%.

Inert Ingredients: 97.77%

*Equivalent to 0.80% (butylcarbityl) (6-propylpiperolyn) ether and 0.20% related compounds.

Keep Out of Reach of Children

Vet-Kem SIPHOTROL Premise Spray with PRECOR® insect growth regulator and Pyrethrins.

For Use Indoors: SIPHOTROL Premise Spray kills adult and pre-adult fleas. Prevents pre-adult fleas from hatching into adult biting fleas for 17 weeks. SIPHOTROL Premise Spray contains a unique combination of ingredients that kills adult and pre-adult fleas before they grow up to bite. It reaches fleas hidden in carpets, rugs, upholstery and pet bedding. Protects your home from reinfestation and flea buildup, your pets and family from bites. One treatment gives continuous protection against pre-adult fleas for 17 weeks.
SIPHOTROL Premise Spray kills fleas, ticks, roaches, waterbugs, silverfish, crickets, ants, centipedes, sowbugs and spiders. Leaves no bad smell, no sticky mess and will not stain furnishings.
For Use on Dogs
SIPHOTROL Premise Spray also kills fleas and ticks on dogs. To protect your pet against fleas outdoors, use a VET-KEM flea and tick collar, PARAMITE® dust or dip.
Precautionary Statements: *Hazards to Humans and Domestic Animals* —Caution: Harmful if swallowed or absorbed through skin. Avoid breathing spray mist. Avoid contact with skin. In case of contact, immediately flush skin with plenty of water. When used in commerical food processing, storage, preparation or serving areas, or in the house, all processing surfaces and utensils should be covered during treatment, or thoroughly washed before use. Cover exposed food. Do not apply while processing, preparation, or serving are underway. Remove pets, birds and cover fish aquarium before spraying.
Physical or Chemical Hazards: Contents under pressure. Do not use or store near heat or open flames. Exposure to temperature above 130°F may cause bursting. Do not puncture or incinerate. Shake well before using.
Directions for use: It is a violation of Federal law to use this product in a manner inconsistent with its labeling.
For Use Indoors
Fleas and Ticks: Hold can either right side up or upside down 2–3 feet from surfaces to be treated. Be sure to apply uniformly using a sweeping motion to carpets, rugs, drapes and all surfaces of upholstered furniture. One can will treat a surface area equivalent to approximately three 9′ x 12′ rooms. Avoid wetting furniture and carpeting. Do not spray wood surfaces as water spotting may occur. A fine mist or spray applied uniformly is all that is necessary to kill fleas. Re-treat as necessary.
To Kill Roaches, Waterbugs, Silverfish, Crickets, Ants, Centipedes, Sowbugs, and Spiders, apply directly to pests.
For Use in Pet Area
Be sure to treat pet bedding and other resting places as these are primary hiding places for fleas and ticks. No need to remove pet bedding after treatment. Follow directions as for indoor other areas.
For Use On Dogs
Fleas and Ticks: Spray at a distance of 6–12 inches until the entire coat is damp. Ruffle coat and spray against the lay of the hair for best coverage. Be sure spray wets ticks for best results. Re-treat as necessary.
Storage & Disposal: Store in a cool area away from children. Do not reuse empty container. Wrap and put in trash.
Seller makes no warranty, express or implied, concerning the use of this product other than indicated on the label. Buyer assumes all risk of use and handling of this material when such use and handling are contrary to label instructions.
EPA Reg. No. 2724-298-11785
For detailed directions for use, limitations, restrictions, exceptions, and precautions, carefully read product label.
SIPHOTROL and PARAMITE are trademarks of Zoecon Corporation.

SIPHOTROL® Plus with PRECOR®
Insect Growth Regulator
Kills both adult and pre-adult fleas
17 week continuous flea protection in the home.

Composition: ACTIVE INGREDIENTS:
Methoprene [Isopropyl *(E,E)*-11-methoxy-3,7,11-trimethyl-2,4-dodecadienoate] .15%
Permethrin (3-phenoxyphenyl)Methyl (±)*cis-trans*-3-(2,2-dichloroethenyl)-2,2-dimethylcyclopropanecarboxylate .50%
INERT INGREDIENTS: 99.35%
Indications: Siphotrol Plus contains a unique combination of ingredients that kills both adult and pre-adult fleas, plus kills cockroaches, flies and ticks. Even kills fleas before they grow up to bite. PRECOR, a unique ingredient in Siphotrol Plus, continues to kill fleas for 17 weeks by preventing their development into adult biting stage. Siphotrol Plus reaches fleas hidden in carpets, rugs, drapes, upholstery, pet bedding, floor cracks. Protects your home from reinfestation and flea buildup, your pets and family from bites. Siphotrol Plus leaves no bad smell or sticky mess and, used as directed, does not stain furnishings. To protect your pet against fleas outdoors, use a Vet-Kem flea or flea and tick collar.
Precautionary Statements:
Hazards to Humans and Domestic Animals—Warning: May cause eye irritation. Do not get in eyes. Avoid contact with skin and clothing. Harmful if inhaled. Avoid breathing vapors. Cover or remove fish bowls before use. Do not apply to animals or humans. Avoid contamination of food and foodstuffs. Do not use in edible product areas of food processing plants, restaurants, or other areas where food is commercially prepared, processed or stored. Do not use in serving areas while food is exposed.
Statement of Practical Treatment: If in eyes, flush with plenty of water. Get medical attention if irritation persists. If inhaled, remove victim to fresh air. Apply artificial respiration if indicated. If on skin, remove contaminated clothing and wash affected areas with soap and water.
Physical and Chemical Hazards: Contents under pressure. Do not use or store near heat or open flame. Do not puncture or incinerate container. Exposure to temperature above 130°F may cause bursting.
Directions for Use: It is a violation of Federal law to use this product in a manner inconsistent with its labeling.
For most effective results, entire dwelling should be treated. Use 1 fogger for each 12,000 cu. ft. (or 1,500 sq. ft.). 1. Close outside doors and windows and turn off fans and air conditioners. Open interior doors, cupboards and closets of areas to be treated. 2. Extinguish open flames except pilot lights. 3. Remove pets, but be sure to leave pet bedding as this is a primary hiding place for fleas and must be treated to get best results. No need to discard pet bedding after treatment. 4. Cover or remove fish tanks and bowls. Cover or remove exposed food, dishes, utensils, food handling equipment and plastic items such as eye glasses, stereo covers and notion boxes. Leave rugs, drapes, slip covers, upholstered furniture in place. Used as directed this product will not harm them, just the fleas hiding inside. 5. Place fogger on a raised area such as a table or chair with newspapers covering the area directly under the can. 6. Keeping at arm's length, point top of can away from face and press down actuator tab to lock in position and start fogging action. Set in an upright position and leave treated area for 2 hours. 7. After 2 hours, open all doors and windows, turn on air conditioners and fans and let treated area air for 30 minutes. 8. All food processing surfaces should be covered during treatment and thoroughly cleaned before using.
Storage & Disposal: Store in a cool area away from children. Do not reuse empty container. Wrap and put in trash.
How Supplied: 12 ounce (340g). EPA Reg. No. 2724-291-11785.
Available through veterinarians.
Seller makes no warranty, express or implied, concerning the use of this product other than indicated on label. Buyer assumes all risk of use and handling of this material when such use and handling are contrary to label instructions.
PRECOR and SIPHOTROL are trademarks of Zoecon Corporation.

SIPHOTROL® PLUS II HOUSE TREATMENT
with Pyrethrins, DURSBAN® & PRECOR® insect growth regulator
kills visible adult fleas
stops hatching eggs from developing into adult fleas for 17 weeks

Composition:
Active Ingredients: Methoprene [Isopropyl (E, E)-11-methoxy-3, 7, 11-trimethyl-2, 4-dodecadienoate] 0.014%; Chlorpyrifos [0,0-Diethyl 0-(3, 5, 6-trichloro-2-pyridyl) phosphorothioate] 0.225%; Pyrethrins 0.050%; Piperonyl Butoxide, technical* 0.100%; N-octyl bicycloheptene dicarboximide 0.165%.
Inert Ingredients: 99.446%.
*Equivalent to 0.08% (butylcarbityl) (6-propylpiperonyl) ether and 0.02% related compounds.

Continued on next page

Vet-Kem—Cont.

SIPHOTROL Plus II House Treatment contains a unique combination of ingredients that kills pre-adult fleas before they grow up to bite, and kills adult fleas. It reaches fleas hidden in carpets, rugs, upholstery and pet bedding. It protects your home from flea buildup; you, pets and family from bites. One treatment gives continuous protection against pre-adult fleas for 17 weeks. SIPHOTROL Plus II House Treatment kills fleas, ticks, roaches, ants, spiders, crickets, silverfish, earwigs, and pillbugs on contact. Leaves no bad smell, no sticky mess and will not stain furnishings. To protect your pet against fleas outdoors, use a Vet-Kem flea and tick collar, pet dust, pet spray, pet dip, or pet shampoo.
Precautionary Statements:
HAZARDS TO HUMANS AND DOMESTIC ANIMALS — CAUTION: Harmful if swallowed or absorbed through the skin. Avoid breathing spray. Avoid contact with skin, eyes, or clothing. Wash thoroughly after handling. Leave treated areas and do not return for at least one hour. Do not allow children or pets to walk on treated surfaces until they are completely dry. *Do not spray on pets or humans.* Avoid contamination of food and foodstuffs. Do not use in edible product areas of food processing plants, restaurants, or other areas where food is commercially prepared or processed. Do not use in serving areas while food is exposed.
Statement Of Practical Treatment: *If swallowed,* call physician or Poison Control Center. Drink 1 or 2 glasses of water and induce vomiting by touching finger to back of throat. Never give anything by mouth to an unconscious or convulsing person. Note to Physician: Chlorpyrifos is a cholinesterase inhibitor. Atropine sulfate by injection is antidotal only if symptoms of cholinesterase inhibition are present. *If on skin,* remove contaminated clothing and wash affected areas with soap and water. *If in eyes,* flush eyes with plenty of water. If irritation persists, call physician.
Directions for use — It is a violation of Federal law to use this product in a manner inconsistent with its labeling.
SHAKE WELL BEFORE USING.
Fleas: For maximum effectiveness, treat entire carpeted area. Adjust spray nozzle to create a fine spray. Treat carpets, rugs, drapes and all surfaces of upholstered furniture. Old bedding of pets should be removed and replaced with clean, fresh bedding after treatment of pet area. Retreat as necessary. Use in homes, garages, attics, apartments and hotels. One bottle will treat a surface area equivalent to approximately four 10′ × 10′ rooms. Avoid wetting furniture and carpeting. A fine spray applied uniformly is all that is necessary to kill fleas.
No need to remove plants from the home while applying product. Do not spray directly on plants. Remove birds, nursing puppies and cats, and cover fish bowls before spraying. To kill ticks, roaches, ants, spiders, crickets, silverfish, earwigs, and pillbugs, apply directly to pests.
STORAGE & DISPOSAL: Store in original container, away from children. Protect from freezing or high temperatures. Do not reuse empty container. Wrap and put in trash.
CAUTION — KEEP OUT OF REACH OF CHILDREN
How Supplied: 32 oz. & 64 oz. non-aerosol spray bottle.
EPA Reg. No. 2724-309-11785
Available through veterinarians
SIPHOTROL and PRECOR are trademarks of Zoecon Corporation.
DURSBAN is a registered trademark of the Dow Chemical Company
For detailed directions for use, limitations, restrictions, exceptions, and precautions, carefully read product label.

SIPHOTROL® 10
Fogger for fleas

Composition: Active Ingredient: Methoprene [Isopropyl (E,E)-11-methoxy-3,7,11-trimethyl 2,4 dodecadienoate] 0.15%
Inert Ingredients: 99.85%
Indications: SIPHOTROL 10 Fogger contains PRECOR®, a unique ingredient that kills pre-adult fleas. It reaches pre-adult fleas hidden in carpets, rugs, drapes, upholstery, pet bedding, floor cracks. Protects your home from reinfestation, and flea buildup, your pets and family from bites.
One treatment with SIPHOTROL 10 Fogger gives continuous protection for 10 weeks. No cleanup necessary. Does not leave a bad odor and, used as directed, does not stain furnishings.
Note: If a large number of adult fleas (the biting stage) are present, a flea killer effective against adults like VET-FOG® should be used, since SIPHOTROL 10 contains a unique ingredient that kills only pre-adult fleas. To protect your pet against fleas outdoors, use a Vet-Kem flea or tick collar.
Directions: It is a violation of Federal law to use this product in a manner inconsistent with its labeling.
1. Close outside doors and windows, turn off fans and air conditioners. 2. Extinguish open flames except pilot lights. 3. Remove pets, but be sure to leave pet bedding, as this is a primary hiding place for pre-adult fleas and must be treated to get best results. No need to discard pet bedding after treatment. Not necessary to cover or remove fish tanks or bowls. 4. Remove or cover exposed food, dishes and plastic items such as eye glasses, stereo covers, and notion boxes. Leave rugs, drapes, slip covers, upholstered furniture in place. Used as directed, this product will not harm them, just the pre-adult fleas hiding inside. 5. Place fogger on raised area such as a table or chair with newspapers covering area directly under the can. 6. Keeping at arm's length, point top of can away from face and press down actuator tab to lock in position and start fogging action. Set in upright position and leave treated area for 30 minutes. 7. After 30 minutes, open all doors and windows, turn on air conditioners and fans, and let treated area air for 30 minutes.
Caution: *Hazards to humans and domestic animals:* Harmful if swallowed, inhaled or absorbed through skin. Avoid breathing vapors. Causes eye irritation. Do not get in eyes. Avoid contact with skin or clothing. In case of eye contact, immediately flush eyes with plenty of water. Get medical attention. For skin, wash with plenty of water. Get medical attention if irritation persists.
Physical and Chemical Hazards: Contents under pressure. Do not use or store near heat or open flame. Do not puncture or incinerate container. Exposure to temperature above 130°F may cause bursting.
For detailed directions for use, limitations, restrictions, exceptions, and precautions, carefully read product label.
Storage and Disposal: Store in a cool area away from children. Do not reuse empty container. Wrap and put in trash.
EPA Reg. No.2724-287-11785
Keep out of Reach of Children
Available through Veterinarians
How Supplied: 6 oz can for 750 sq. ft. of floor space. 12 oz can for 1500 sq. ft. of floor space.
Seller makes no warranty, express or implied, concerning the use of this product other than indicated on the label. Buyer assumes all risk of use and handling of this material when such use and handling are contrary to label instructions.
SIPHOTROL, PRECOR and VET-FOG are trademarks of Zoecon Corporation.

TICK AND FLEA COLLAR FOR CATS

Composition:

Active Ingredient:	
o-Isopropoxyphenyl methylcarbamate	9.4%
Inert Ingredients:	90.6%

Indications: Kills ticks and fleas up to 5 months.
For cats of all sizes.
Directions: Remove collar from package and place around cat's neck. Adjust for proper fit and buckle in place. Collar must be worn loosely but securely enough to prevent easy removal and loss. Cut off any excess length of collar, leaving ample length for expansion as the cat grows, and dispose of by discarding in trash.
Check and adjust collar periodically to assure a proper fit.
Do not use on kittens under 6 weeks of age.
Results Expected: The tick and flea collar starts killing ticks and fleas when it is placed around the cat's neck. Fleas will be killed and new ones which may temporarily appear on the cat will also be killed during the 5 months collar is worn. Ticks are tough occasional pests of cats and will be killed within a few days. For continuous protection, replace collar when effectiveness diminishes.
Caution: Do not open inner envelope until ready to use. Do not allow children to play with this collar. Dust will form on this collar during storage. Do not get dust or collar in mouth, harmful if swallowed.

Do not get dust in eyes, will cause temporary pupillary constriction*. In case of contact, flush eyes with water. Wash hands thoroughly with soap and water after handling collar. The dust released by this collar is a cholinesterase inhibitor.

Note to Physician: Atropine and *homatropine are antidotal.

When collar is first worn, observe neck area every few days for irritation. Any collar, when fastened too tightly, may cause skin irritation. Remove collar at the first sign of irritation or adverse reaction. Collar is intended for use as an insecticide generator and is not to be taken internally by man or animal. Do not use on sick or convalescing animals. Do not use any other pesticide on cat while collar is worn.

Storage & Disposal: Store in original unopened container; away from children. Do not reuse container or used collar. Wrap and put in trash.

Seller makes no warranty, express or implied, concerning the use of this product other than indicated on the label. Buyer assumes all risk of use and handling of this material when such use and handling are contrary to label instructions. EPA Reg. No. 2724-275-11785

For detailed directions for use, limitations, restrictions, exceptions, and precautions, carefully read product label.

VET-FOG™

pressurized fogger

For apartments, houses, kennels, or buildings up to 12,000 cu. ft.

Entire contents released from one spot.

Fog penetrates throughout area.

Composition:

ACTIVE INGREDIENT: Permethrin (3-phenoxyphenyl) methyl (±)cis-trans-3-(2,2-dichloroethenyl)-2,2-dimethyl-cyclopropanecarboxylate .50%

INERT INGREDIENTS: 99.50%

Kills cockroaches. flies, ticks and fleas. Reaches fleas hidden in carpets, rugs, drapes, upholstery, pet bedding, floor cracks. Protects your home from flea buildup, your pets and family from bites. Leaves no bad smell or sticky mess and, used as directed, does not stain furnishings.

Precautionary Statements:

HAZARDS TO HUMANS AND DOMESTIC ANIMALS—WARNING: May cause eye irritation. Do not get in eyes. Avoid contact with skin and clothing. Harmful if inhaled. Avoid breathing vapors. Cover or remove fish bowls before use. Do not apply to animals or humans.

Statement of Practical Treatment: If in eyes, flush with plenty of water. Get medical attention if irritation persists.

Physical and Chemical Hazards: Contents under pressure. Do not use or store near heat or open flame. Do not puncture or incinerate container. Exposure to temperatures above 130°F may cause bursting.

Directions for Use: It is a violation of Federal law to use this product in a manner inconsistent with its labeling. For best results, entire dwelling should be treated (with particular attention to kitchens and bathrooms). Use one fogger for each 12,000 cubic feet (or 1,500 square feet). 1. Close outside doors and windows and turn off fans and air conditioners. Open interior doors, cupboards and closets of areas to be treated. 2. Extinguish open flames except pilot lights. 3. Remove pets, but be sure to leave pet bedding as this is a primary hiding place for fleas and must be treated to get best results. No need to discard pet bedding after treatment. 4. Cover or remove fish tanks and bowls. Cover or remove exposed food, dishes, utensils, food handling equipment and plastic items such as eye glasses, stereo covers, and notion boxes. Do not use in commercial food processing or food storage areas. Leave rugs, drapes, slip covers, upholstered furniture in place. Used as directed this product will not harm them, just the fleas hiding inside. 5. Place fogger on a raised area such as a table or chair with newspapers covering the area directly under the can. 6. Keeping at arm's length, point top of can away from face and press down actuator tab to lock in position and start fogging action. Set in an upright position and leave treated area for 2 hours. 7. After 2 hours, open all doors and windows, turn on air conditioners and fans, and let the treated area air for 30 minutes. 8. All food processing surfaces should be covered during treatment or thoroughly cleaned before using.

Storage and Disposal: Storage—Store in a cool area away from children. Disposal—Replace cap. Wrap container in layers of newspaper and discard in trash. Do not incinerate or puncture.

Seller makes no warranty, express or implied, concerning the use of this product other than indicated on the label. Buyer assumes all risks of the use and handling of this material when such use and handling are contrary to label instructions.

How Supplied: 6 oz. can and 12 oz. can.

EPA Reg No. 2724-292-11785

Available Through Veterinarians

For detailed directions for use, limitations, restrictions, exceptions, and precautions, carefully read product label.

VET-KEM and VET-FOG are trademarks of Zoecon Corporation

YARD & KENNEL SPRAY

Concentrate

Composition: Active Ingredients: Chlorpyrifos ([0, *0*-diethyl *0*-[3,5,6-trichloro-2-pyridyl]) phosphorothioate) 6.7%; Petroleum distillates 76.8%

Inert Ingredients: 16.5%

Directions: It is a violation of Federal law to use this product in a manner inconsistent with its labeling.

In Yards: Apply 1 pint (16 fl oz) of Yard & Kennel in 78 gallons of water as a coarse, low pressure spray to cover 2600 sq ft, 1¼ oz of Yard & Kennel Spray in 6 gallons of water covers 200 sq ft. Spray may be applied with a garden hose sprayer. Retreat as necessary. Thoroughly water immediately after treatment to wash the insecticide into the treated area. For best results, the lawn should be moist at time of treatment. See note below.

In kennels & dog houses: apply 10½fl oz of Yard & Kennel Spray in 1 gallon of water to buildings, resting areas, walls and floors. Old bedding of pets should be removed and replaced wth clean, fresh bedding after treatment. See note below.

Note: Remove pets before spraying. Do not treat pets with this product. Keep children and pets out of treated areas until spray has dried. Do not use on azaleas, camellias, poinsettias, rose bushes, or variegated ivy because of possible injury to these plants.

Caution: *Hazards to humans and domestic animals:* Harmful if swallowed or absorbed through the skin. Avoid contact with skin, eyes or clothing. Do not smoke while using. Wash thoroughly after handling. Wash contaminated clothing before reuse. In case of contact, immediately flush exposed eyes or skin with plenty of water. Get medical attention if irritation persists. Avoid breathing spray mist or vapors. Keep children and pets off treated areas until spray has dried.

Note to Physician: Active ingredient is a cholinesterase inhibitor. Treat symptomatically. *Antidote:* Atropine by injection only.

Environmental Hazards:

This product is toxic to fish, birds and other wildlife. Keep out of any body of water. Do not contaminate water by cleaning of equipment or disposal of wastes. Do not apply where runoff is likely to occur. Do not apply when weather conditions favor drift from areas treated.

Physical or Chemical Hazards: Do not use, pour, spill or store near heat or open flame.

Disposal: Do not reuse empty container. Wrap container and put in trash collection.

For detailed directions for use, limitations, restrictions, exceptions, and precautions, carefully read product label.

EPA Reg No. 7001-301-11785

Seller makes no warranty, express or implied, concerning the use of this product other than indicated on the label. Buyer assumes all risk of use and handling of this material when such use and handling are contrary to label instructions.

IDENTIFICATION PROBLEM?
Consult the
Product Identification Section
where you'll find
products pictured
in full color.

Vita Plus Industries Inc.
953 E. SAHARA AVE. #21B
LAS VEGAS, NV 89104

BENZALKONIUM WITH ZINC CREME
For dogs, cats and horses

Description: Benzalkonium with zinc creme combines a .20% concentrate of Benzalkonium chlorides. Other ingredients are water, Glyceryl Stearate, Propylene Glycol, Peg 9-Stearate, Isopropyl Palmitate, Cetyl Alcohol, Carbamide, Zinc Oxide, Peg 75 Lanolin, Methyl Paraben, Allantoin, Bittrex.
Indications: The preparation is intended for use topically for ringworm, and is also especially useful in disorders complicated or threatened by bacterial or fungal infection. The Zinc Oxide is helpful as an aid in the treatment of minor wounds, abrasions and inflammation of the outer epidermal layers.
Note: Efficiency is neutralized by soap or detergent residue.
Warning: Not for use on animals intended for food. For external use only. Keep out of reach of children. In case of contact with eyes or other mucous membrane, flush immediately with water. Obtain medical attention for eye irritation.
Precautions: Benzalkonium with zinc creme is not intended for the treatment of deep abscesses or deep-seated infections such as inflammed lymph vessels. If redness, irritation, or swelling persists, discontinue use.
Dosage and Administration: Apply a thin ribbon of creme directly to the lesion. Rub gently until Benzalkonium disappears into the skin. Apply daily until new hair growth occurs. Leave treated area uncovered. Fresh lesions usually show visible clinical results within 7–10 days.
How Supplied: Benzalkonium with Zinc Creme is supplied in 1 oz. (30 grm) tubes.
Storage: Store at room temperature. Avoid excessive heat.

V

Wayne Pet Food Division
See CONTINENTAL GRAIN COMPANY

Winthrop Veterinary
Sterling Animal Health Products
Division of Sterling Drug Inc.
90 PARK AVENUE
NEW YORK, NY 10016

CARBOCAINE®-V HYDROCHLORIDE
brand of mepivacaine hydrochloride injection, USP
Sterile Injection 2%
Potent Local Anesthetic with Rapid and Prolonged Effect for Use in Horses

Description: Mepivacaine hydrochloride, 1-methyl-2', 6'-pipecoloxylidide monohydrochloride, is a white, crystalline, odorless powder, readily soluble in water, and very stable in aqueous solution. It is available as a 2% sterile aqueous solution containing sodium chloride (for isotonicity) and 0.1% methylparaben (as preservative). The pH is adjusted with sodium hydroxide or hydrochloric acid.
Action and Advantages: Mepivacaine hydrochloride is a potent local anesthetic whose effectiveness and safety have been well established in human medicine and dentistry. Laboratory and clinical studies in animals have confirmed its value in veterinary medicine. Its anesthetic activity is two to two and a half times that of procaine, and it is equal to or better than that of lidocaine. The compound has shown excellent tissue compatibility in laboratory animals and in horses. Moderate transient edema at the site of injection may occur in rare instances.
CARBOCAINE-V hydrochloride produces rapid and marked local anesthesia lasting for several hours. This enables the veterinarian to proceed with intended manipulations without delay and to complete the work under desensitization which is adequate even for prolonged operations. The innate vasoconstrictive activity of CARBOCAINE-V hydrochloride may be enhanced by the addition of epinephrine at 1:100,000. The addition should be carried out aseptically for current use and any unused portion should be discarded.
Indications and Dosage:
CARBOCAINE-V hydrochloride is recommended for infiltration, nerve block, intraarticular and epidural anesthesia for horses. It has also been found useful for topical anesthesia of the laryngeal mucosa prior to ventriculectomy. As with other local anesthetics, the dosage varies considerably depending on the anesthetic technic, body area to be desensitized and the surgical procedure. Pharmacological studies in various species of animals, including horses, have shown that the drug produces complete and effective anesthesia at dosages that are no more than half those needed when procaine is used.
The following dosages have generally proved satisfactory in the horse and are therefore suggested as a guide:
For nerve block—(diagnosis of lameness, firing, pain relief in osteoarthritis, navicular disease)—3 to 15 mL
For epidural anesthesia—(animal standing)—5 to 20 mL
For intraarticular anesthesia—(removal of fracture chips, bone and bog spavin, arthritis)—10 to 15 mL
For Infiltration—(alone or in combination with nerve block or intraarticular anesthesia)—as required.
For anesthesia of the laryngeal mucosa prior to ventriculectomy
CARBOCAINE-V hydrochloride may be administered topically or by infiltration or by a combination of the two. For topical application, a total of 25 to 40 mL applied by spray (3 mL/application) is usually adequate. For infiltration, 20 to 50 mL will suffice.
Warning: Not for use in horses intended for food.
Precautions: When administered by skilled persons, CARBOCAINE-V hydrochloride may be employed safely for local infiltration, for common nerve blocking procedures, for intraarticular and epidural anesthesia. The following precautions, which are observed with respect to all local anesthetics, also apply to this anesthetic. (1) Injections should always be made aseptically and with frequent aspirations. If blood is aspirated, the needle should be relocated and the injections continued cautiously. (2) When used for epidural anesthesia, care should be taken to avoid injection into the subarachoid space. The skin should be shaved and sterilized, and the needles used must be sharp and of the proper length. (3) The depth of anesthesia should be checked by pricking the area before manipulations are begun.
How Supplied: CARBOCAINE-V hydrochloride, brand of mepivacaine hydrochloride injection, USP, Sterile 2% Injection is supplied in rubber-capped multiple-dose vials of 50 mL.
Caution: Federal law restricts this drug to use by or on the order of a licensed veterinarian.

CW-127D

INSTRACAL™
Cold Disinfectant for Veterinary Instruments and Equipment

Composition:
Active Ingredients—Ethyl alcohol 4.640%, soap 1.180%, o-Phenylphenol 0.518%, o-Benzyl-p-chlorophenol 0.250%, Isopropyl alcohol 0.083%, Tetrasodium ethylenediamine tetraacetate 0.072%.
Inert Ingredients—93.257%. Contains sodium nitrite.
EPA Reg. No. 675-15-7738.
Actions:
Tuberculocidal*
Bactericidal* for Staphylococcus and Pseudomonas
Fungicidal* for pathogenic fungi
Virucidal* for Influenza A_2 virus, Herpes simplex virus, Adenovirus Type 2, and Vaccinia virus
*On environmental surfaces
Indications: Cold disinfectant for veterinary instruments and equipment.
Contains Rust Inhibitor
Directions for use for Cold Disinfection:

Surgical and Dental Instruments: After thorough mechanical cleaning (with particular attention to removal of any contaminating matter from crevices, joints, and hollow spaces) immerse in INSTRACAL Cold Disinfectant for 15 minutes or until ready to use. To remove from the solution, grasp with sterile forceps. Rinse with sterile water.
Hypodermic Needles and Syringes: Flush with INSTRACAL Cold Disinfectant. Immerse in INSTRACAL Cold Disinfectant for 15 minutes and flush with sterile distilled water.
Rubber Gloves, Tubes, and Other Rubber Articles: Immerse in INSTRACAL Cold Disinfectant for no more than 15 minutes. Remove and immerse in 70% alcohol for one minute.
Optical Instruments: Rinse to remove mucus and exudate, and immerse in INSTRACAL Cold Disinfectant for 15 minutes but no longer. Assure thorough contact by flushing. On removal, flush and rinse with sterile water. For rapid drying, immerse for a few seconds in 70% alcohol. For future use, store in sterile wrap.
Storage and Disposal
Store in original container in areas inaccessible to small children.
Do not reuse empty container. Wrap and discard in trash.
Caution: Harmful if swallowed. Avoid contact with skin and eyes. In case of contact, flush immediately with water. If eye irritation persists, get medical attention. Avoid contamination of food.
Keep out of reach of children.
How Supplied: Plastic bottles of 1 gallon.

ROCCAL®-D
Virucide† •Disinfectant•Detergent• Deodorant

†Virucidal for *Canine Distemper virus, Canine Herpes virus,* and *Pseudorabies virus* at dilutions recommended for hard inanimate surfaces.
Composition:
Active Ingredients:

Alkyl* dimethyl benzyl ammonium chlorides	20.00%
*(67% C12, 25% C14, 7% C16, 1% C8, C10, and C18)	
Monoethanolamine ethylenediamine tetraacetate	1.75%
Essential oils	2.50%
Inert Ingredients	80.00%

EPA Reg. No. 7738-3
Directions: It is a violation of Federal Law to use this product in a manner inconsistent with its labeling. Dilute with water as directed.
FOR DISINFECTION OF ALL HARD INANIMATE SURFACES including floors, walls, examination tables, operating tables, diagnostic and therapeutic equipment and devices, furniture, cages, and carts.
Clean all surfaces with a suitable detergent and rinse thoroughly with water. Apply ROCCAL-D dilution by mop, sponge, or spray to thoroughly wet the surfaces for at least 10 minutes before allowing the surfaces to air dry.
For use in veterinary hospitals and premises, and where effectiveness against *Pseudomonas aeruginosa* is required, apply ROCCAL-D at 1:200 dilution.
For use as a general disinfectant in areas such as kennels, runs, vehicles, animal bathing areas, laboratory animal facilities, and nonfood areas in barns, apply ROCCAL-D at 1:400 dilution.
FOR DISINFECTION OF EATING AND DRINKING UTENSILS for animals not intended as food sources for human consumption. Scrape and prewash with warm water, soak in ROCCAL-D 1:400 dilution for at least 10 minutes, and rinse with potable water. Prepare fresh solution daily or sooner if it becomes soiled or diluted.
For use by professional and paraprofessional personnel in veterinary hospitals and other animal facilities.
Preparation of Use Dilutions:
Dilution 1:400: Add 10 mL (2 teaspoons) of ROCCAL-D disinfectant to 1 gallon of water.
Dilution 1:200: Add 20 mL (4 teaspoons) of ROCCAL-D disinfectant to 1 gallon of water.
Do not mix ROCCAL-D disinfectant with soap or anionic detergents.
Danger: Keep out of reach of children. Corrosive to tissues. Causes eye damage and skin irritation. Do not get in eyes, on skin, or on clothing. Wear goggles or face shield and rubber gloves when handling the concentrate. Harmful or fatal if swallowed. Avoid contamination of food.
First Aid: In case of contact, immediately flush eyes or skin with plenty of water for at least 15 minutes. For eyes, call a physician. Remove and wash contaminated clothing before reuse.
If swallowed, drink promptly a large quantity of milk, egg whites, gelatin solution or if these are not available, drink large quantities of water. Avoid alcohol. Call a physician immediately.
Note to Physician: Probable mucosal damage may contraindicate the use of gastric lavage. Measures against circulatory shock, respiratory depression, and convulsion may be needed.
Storage and Disposal
STORAGE: Store in original container in areas inaccessible to small children. Keep securely closed. Do not contaminate food or feed.
DISPOSAL: Do not reuse empty containers. Rinse thoroughly with water and detergent. Discard in trash.
Bactericidal by AOAC Use-Dilution Test for:
Pseudomonas aeruginosa
Staphylococcus aureus
Streptococcus faecalis
Salmonella choleraesuis
Salmonella typhimurium
Escherichia coli
Klebsiella pneumoniae
Enterobacter aerogenes
Proteus mirabilis
Corynebacterium diphtheriae
†Virucidal for:
Canine Distemper virus
Canine Herpes virus
Pseudorabies virus
at dilutions recommended for hard inanimate surfaces.
How Supplied: Plastic bottles of 1 gallon.

SEBBAFON®
Dermatologic Shampoo

Composition: Each 100 mL contains precipitated sulfur 5 g, sodium salicylate 0.5 g in a pleasantly scented emollient base of entsufon sodium, lanolin cholesterols, and petrolatum.
Actions: SEBBAFON dermatologic shampoo provides detergent, keratolytic and keratoplastic activity combined with the fungicidal and acaricidal actions of a specially prepared sulfur. Because of its emollient properties and pH equal to normal skin, the shampoo restores normal skin texture and the skin's natural acid mantle. The detergent and lipid components are responsible for the restoration of natural luster to the hair coat.
Indications: For external use as a cleansing shampoo and as an aid in the treatment of fungal, parasitic, and nonspecific dermatoses of dogs and cats.
Dosage and Administration:
1. Shake before using.
2. Wet animal thoroughly with warm water.
3. Apply 1 to 2 ounces of shampoo and work into a lather for several minutes.
4. If inadequate lathering results, rinse hair coat with warm water and repeat application of shampoo.
5. Avoid getting shampoo into the eyes and mouth. As a precaution, a bland ophthalmic ointment may be placed in the eyes before bathing.
6. Rinse well with warm water.
7. Dry animal thoroughly.

Caution: For external use only on dogs and cats. Not for routine bathing. Proper care should be taken to rinse the treated area thoroughly after each application, especially areas exhibiting skin lesions. Keep out of the reach of children. In case of accidental ingestion, seek professional assistance or contact a poison control center immediately.
How Supplied: Plastic bottles of 5 fl oz and 1 gallon.

W

SEBBATIX®
Insecticidal Shampoo for Dogs and Cats

Composition: Three agents blended in a lathering shampoo base provide broad-spectrum insecticidal activity.
Active Ingredients:

Pyrethrins	0.05%
Piperonyl butoxide, technical*	0.12%
N-octyl bicycloheptene dicarboximide	0.20%
Essential Oils	0.50%
Petroleum distillate	0.28%
Inert Ingredients:	98.85%

*Equivalent to 0.096% (butylcarbityl)-(6-propylpiperonyl)-ether and 0.024% related compounds.

Continued on next page

Winthrop—Cont.

EPA Reg. No. 7738-7.
Indications: SEBBATIX insecticidal shampoo is indicated for use on dogs and cats. SEBBATIX insecticidal shampoo kills fleas, lice, and ticks and cleans and conditions the hair coat.
Warnings: Do not treat puppies or kittens under 4 weeks of age. This product is toxic to fish. Keep out of lakes, streams, or ponds. Apply this product only as specified on the label. Keep out of the reach of children.
Harmful if swallowed.
Administration: Rinse the entire hair coat thoroughly with warm water to remove water-soluble deposits and loose soil. Massage the hair coat and skin thoroughly with sufficient SEBBATIX insecticidal shampoo to produce an adequate cover of lather over the entire body surface. Allow lather to stand undisturbed for 5 minutes. Rinse the hair coat and skin thoroughly with warm water and dry.
How Supplied: Plastic bottles of 5 fl oz and 1 gallon.
Storage and Disposal
Store in original container in areas inaccessible to small children. Keep securely closed. Do not contaminate food or feed. Do not reuse empty container. Rinse thoroughly with water and detergent. Discard in trash.

TALWIN®-V Ⓒ
brand of pentazocine lactate injection, USP

Analgesic for Veterinary Use

Description: TALWIN-V is a clear, sterile solution of pentazocine lactate in water for injection, prepared from pentazocine, USP, with the aid of lactic acid. Each 1 mL contains an equivalent of 30 mg pentazocine base.
Actions: TALWIN-V is an analgesic drug for veterinary use. Its activity has been demonstrated in controlled laboratory studies in experimental animals, including horses and dogs. Analgesic efficacy and safety of TALWIN-V for both species have been demonstrated under clinical conditions as well.
Horse—In the horse, TALWIN-V manifests strong analgesic properties in acute abdominal pain arising in the digestive organs. In most cases, a single parenteral injection brings about prompt relief of colicky signs, alleviation of stress and anxiety, and a generally calm attitude. This enables the veterinarian to safely examine the animal, establish a diagnosis, and administer appropriate treatment. TALWIN-V administered intravenously produces excellent analgesia within minutes after injection. Unlike other narcotic analgesics, it produces little or no sedation and it does not depress respiration and cardiac function at the recommended therapeutic dose. The duration of pain relief following intravenous injection is usually short (20 to 30 minutes), but adequate in many cases of acute colic. A more prolonged control of pain (2 to 4 hours) is attained following intramuscular injection. Quick onset and extended duration of analgesia have been demonstrated upon an initial dose of TALWIN-V injected intravenously, followed by one or more intramuscular injections.
Dog—In the dog, TALWIN-V proved to be a safe analgesic agent for the amelioration of pain of diverse etiology including fractures, trauma, and postoperative. TALWIN-V was administered intramuscularly as the sole analgesic in 119 clinical cases. Among these cases, pain was categorized as severe in approximately 44 percent and moderate in approximately 53 percent. Onset of analgesia was rapid and of significant duration. Analgesic effects were significant in 61 percent of trial patients evaluated three hours postmedication.
In the dog, TALWIN-V does not exhibit undesirable pharmacologic activity characteristic of other strong analgesics. In clinical trials as well as in laboratory studies, no sedation or respiratory depression was noted, Minimal bradycardia was noted in one laboratory study, whereas heart rate remained unchanged in another.
Indications: *Horse*—TALWIN-V is recommended for the symptomatic relief of pain of colic in horses. A colicky horse is usually unapproachable, and reacts to severe abdominal distress with extreme behavior which is spontaneous, unpredictable, and frequently violent. The untreated animal resents examination, whereas control of pain makes the animal manageable. TALWIN-V is indicated to relieve pain and thus facilitate handling and examination to determine the underlying cause of colic. The drug is also indicated to minimize the threat of self-inflicted injury to the colicky horse. TALWIN-V has been shown to provide satisfactory relief of pain in different breeds of horses, including ponies, and in various types of colic (flatulent, spasmodic, impaction, torsion, etc).
Dog—In the dog, TALWIN-V is indicated primarily for the amelioration of pain accompanying postoperative recovery from fractures, trauma, and spinal disorders. Amelioration of pain reduces the threat of aggravating the existing pathologic condition and allows for rest which is important for healing and repair of damaged tissues. Additionally, alleviation of pain facilitates physical and x-ray examination and permits application of proper treatment.
Contraindication: Reproduction studies have not been conducted in the target species. Therefore, this product cannot be recommended for administration to pregnant bitches or dogs and bitches intended for breeding.
Warnings: Not for use in horses intended for food.
Not for human use.
Precautions: *Horse*—TALWIN-V, brand of pentazocine lactate injection is indicated only for the control of pain due to various types of colic in horses. Relief of colicky signs results from the analgesic effect of TALWIN-V. Appropriate measures for the treatment of colic should be instituted as soon thereafter as possible.
Dog—In the dog TALWIN-V is indicated to provide analgesia only at recommended dose levels.
Adverse Reactions: *Horse*—Clinical investigations in horses demonstrated that TALWIN-V is a safe and effective drug for the symptomatic control of pain due to colic. Adverse reactions were not observed among horses medicated at the recommended dose level. Horses receiving larger doses, especially by the intravenous route, exhibited mild to moderate transient reactions proportionate to the dose. For example, during clinical investigations, 31 of a group of 75 horses received intravenous doses which exceeded the recommended dose by at least 50 percent. Adverse reactions consisting of transient incoordination were reported for only 10 of these animals.
In controlled laboratory studies, 11 TALWIN-V injections were given to horses in four days at the recommended dose level and at levels which exceeded this by three- and six-fold, respectively. Adverse reactions were noted only among horses medicated at three or six times the recommended dose level. Following intravenous administration, transient slight to moderate ataxia and nervousness were noted at both excessive dose levels; at the higher level, unsteady gait, excitability, localized muscular twitching, and slight perspiration were also noted. At the lower dose level, a slight elevation of pulse and respiratory rates was recorded following the initial intravenous injection only. Drowsiness and sedation, common reactions of narcotic analgesics, were not observed following intravenous or intramuscular administration of TALWIN-V.
Dog—In open clinical trials among dogs, mild to moderate salivation was the only significant adverse reaction noted. Frequency was limited to approximately 3 percent of the animals medicated at the recommended dose level.
In a laboratory study, 8 dogs received TALWIN-V within the recommended dose range twice daily for three successive days. The two doses were administered about 6 hours apart. Six of the animals remained normal throughout the study. The other two animals manifested occasional and transient salivation; there was one instance of emesis. In this same study, 4 dogs similarly medicated received slightly more than 2 mg/lb twice daily for three days. Two dogs remained normal, and the other 2 manifested occasional, transient salivation. In one, this was accompanied on one occasion by fine tremors. In the other dog, slight, transient swelling at the injection site was noted following only one injection. Four other dogs were similarly medicated with TALWIN-V for three days at 2.72 mg/lb twice daily. Adverse reactions noted among these animals included tonic convulsions (one instance), slight, transient ataxia (2 dogs), swelling at the injection site (2 dogs) and fine tremors (3 dogs). All dogs medicated at this high

dose level survived and returned to a normal state.

Dosage and Administration: *Horse*—Many cases of acute equine colic pain respond well to a single intravenous injection of TALWIN-V at 0.15 mg of active drug per lb of body weight (equivalent to 5 mL per 1000 lb of body weight). Injections are best made slowly into the jugular vein. In cases of severe pain, it is recommended that a second dose at the same level (0.15 mg per lb) be injected intramuscularly 10 to 15 minutes following the initial dose. Horses with stubborn impaction colic pain have been maintained on TALWIN-V for as long as four days without untoward reactions. It is important that a careful physical examination of the animal be made as early as possible and that appropriate therapeutic or surgical measures be instituted soon afterwards.

Dog—TALWIN-V, brand of pentazocine lactate injection, is recommended for administration to dogs by intramuscular administration only. An initial dose of 0.75 mg/lb of body weight (equivalent to 0.25 mL for each 10 lb of body weight) usually produces adequate analgesia. As much as 1.50 mg/lb of body weight (equivalent to 0.5 mL for each 10 lb of body weight) may be administered. In clinical trials, dogs with moderate to severe pain received TALWIN-V within the recommended dose range. Analgesic effects were evaluated periodically during 3 hours postmedication. The percentage of animals showing good to excellent analgesia during the observation period may be summarized as follows.

[See table above].

15 minutes	30 minutes	1 hour	2 hours	3 hours
64%	69%	77%	67%	61%

In laboratory studies, dogs received TALWIN-V, brand of pentazocine hydrochloride injection, within the recommended dose range twice daily for three successive days. The two doses were administered about six hours apart. When medication is repeated, it is advisable to vary the injection site.

How Supplied: Multiple-dose vials of 10 mL, each 1 mL containing pentazocine lactate equivalent to 30 mg base, 2 mg acetone sodium bisulfite, 1.5 mg sodium chloride, and 1 mg methylparaben as preservative, in water for injection. Box of 1 (NDC 0959-0019-01).

The pH of TALWIN-V solution is adjusted between 4 and 5 with lactic acid or sodium hydroxide.

Caution: Federal law restricts this drug to use by or on the order of a licensed veterinarian.

TW 240-I

WINSTROL® -V
Brand of stanozolol
Potent Anabolic Therapy for Dogs, Cats, and Horses

Description: WINSTROL-V is 17-methyl-2′ *H*-5α-androst-2-eno [3, 2-c] pyrazol-17 β-ol. It is a member of a unique series of heterocyclic steroids synthesized at the Sterling-Winthrop Research Institute. The unique endocrinologic activity of this compound was produced by the fusion of a pyrazole ring to a steroid nucleus. When administered to animals, WINSTROL-V was found to have an unusual pattern of biologic activity in that its anabolic (tissue-building) effect far outweighed its weak androgenic (masculinizing) influence.

Indications: Anabolic therapy with WINSTROL-V is indicated whenever excessive tissue breakdown or extensive repair processes are proceeding. Such processes usually diminish protein reserves in the tissues, thus leading to negative nitrogen balance. WINSTROL-V is indicated to reverse tissue-depleting processes and restore constructive metabolism. Anabolic therapy is intended primarily as an adjunct to other specific and supportive therapy, including nutritional therapy. Optimal results can be expected only when dietary intake is adequate and well balanced.

Dogs and Cats

WINSTROL-V is indicated when the therapeutic objective is to improve appetite, promote weight gain, and increase strength and vitality. For these reasons it is recommended for anorexia, unthriftiness, weight loss, debility, cachexia, inanition and poor haircoat when these accompany disease, trauma, or old age. Since certain skin conditions occurring in older dogs (alopecia and some types of eczema, for example) are caused by metabolic disorders based on negative nitrogen balance, WINSTROL- V may help to control such conditions.

Horses

WINSTROL-V is recommended as an aid for treating debilitated horses when the therapeutic objective is to improve appetite, promote weight gain, improve general physical conditions, and accelerate recovery. Clinical conditions most amenable to treatment are debilitated states resulting from illness, surgery, traumatic injuries, or plain overwork. In clinical investigations, administration of WINSTROL-V frequently had a marked effect on horses exhibiting diminished vitality and vigor due to overexertion.

Contraindications: Because the data regarding use during pregnancy are insufficient, WINSTROL-V should not be administered to pregnant dogs and cats. In the absence of data on the effects of WINSTROL-V on stallions and pregnant mares or the teratogenicity on offspring, WINSTROL-V should not be used in these animals.

Warning: For use in dogs, cats, and horses. Not for use in horses intended for food.

Precautions: Animals with impaired cardiac and renal function should be watched closely when receiving anabolic therapy because of the possibility of sodium and water retention. Special caution should be exercised in aged dogs suffering from chronic interstitial nephritis. In such cases, the progress of the disorder should be checked by means of laboratory tests and treatment discontinued if the drug appears to aggravate the disease.

Adverse Reactions: Mild androgenic effects may be noted after prolonged therapy with excessively high doses.

Dosage and Administration: Whenever indicated, anabolic therapy should be prescribed in conjunction with or as a follow-up to other therapeutic measures.

Dogs and Cats

The suggested oral dose for cats and small breeds of dogs is ½ to 1 tablet twice daily and for large breeds of dogs, 1 to 2 tablets twice daily, depending on body weight. If preferred, the tablets can be crushed and administered in feed. Treatment should be continued for at least several weeks, depending on the condition and response of the animal. In certain chronic conditions, especially in aged dogs, treatment can be continued for several months without untoward reactions.

Because the injectable form is absorbed slowly, injections may be given at weekly intervals. The suspension is best administered by deep intramuscular injection into the thigh. The recommended dose for cats and small breeds of dogs is 0.5 mL (25 mg) and for larger dogs 1 mL (50 mg). If desired, the two dosage forms of WINSTROL-V can be combined in a regimen of therapy. Many investigating clinicians gave an initial dose of the injectable form and then dispensed tablets for daily administration at home.

Horses

Only the sterile suspension is recommended for administration to horses. The recommended dose is 25 mg per 100 pounds of body weight intramuscularly, equivalent to 5 mL (250 mg) for a 1000 pound animal. Deep intramuscular injection in the gluteal region is recommended. Medication may be repeated at weekly intervals up to and including four weeks. In clinical trials, many animals required no more than one or two doses to achieve desirable therapeutic results.

How Supplied: WINSTROL-V, brand of stanozolol, is available as scored tablets of 2 mg, bottles of 50 and 500, and as a sterile suspension, containing 50 mg per mL, multiple-dose vials of 10 and 30 mL.

Caution: Federal law restricts this drug to use by or on the order of a licensed veterinarian.

Pharmacology: WINSTROL-V is classified as an "anabolic steroid" because of its pronounced stimulatory effects on constructive metabolism. The drug increases the retention of nitrogen and minerals, reverses tissue-depleting processes, and promotes better utilization of dietary protein. Its anabolic effects lead to improvement in appetite, increased vigor, and notable gains in weight. In this respect, it differs greatly from other steroids, such as the androgens, estrogens, and the corticosteroids. Methyltestosterone also possesses anabolic action, but its predominant androgenic activity makes

Continued on next page

Winthrop—Cont.

in unsuitable for long-term anabolic therapy. Although the frequently undesirable virilizing effects of the male sex hormones may be overcome by androgen-estrogen combinations, this does not improve their anabolic function. The corticosteroids (cortisone, prednisone, prednisolone, dexamethasone) comprise an entirely different group of steroids, which are well known for their antiinflammatory and antirheumatic activities. As a rule, prolonged use of the corticosteroids results in a catabolic (tissue-wasting) effect which may be relieved by anabolic therapy.
In a wide variety of tests on animals, WINSTROL-V, brand of stanozolol, was shown to possess high anabolic potency, whereas its androgenic effect was very low. The drug has been available to the medical profession since 1961, and over 60 publications describing its safety and efficacy in man have appeared. Extensive clinical investigations by veterinary practitioners have confirmed its anabolic action and therapeutic usefulness in dogs, cats, and horses.

WW 17 K

WINSTROL®-V
Brand of stanozolol
Chewable Tablets
Potent Anabolic Therapy for Dogs

Description: WINSTROL-V is 17-Methyl-2′*H*-5α-androst-2-eno[3, 2-c] pyrazol-17β-ol. It is a member of a unique series of heterocyclic steroids synthesized at the Sterling-Winthrop Research Institute. The unique endocrinologic activity of this compound was produced by the fusion of a pyrazole ring to a steroid nucleus. When administered to animals, WINSTROL-V was found to have an unusual pattern of biologic activity in that its anabolic (tissue-building) effect far outweighed its weak androgenic (masculinizing) influence.
Clinical Pharmacology: The male sex hormone, testosterone, exerts two principal pharmacologic effects. One is the masculinization or androgenic effect, the other, an anabolic or tissue-building effect. Efforts to clinically exploit anabolic effects apart from androgenic effects led to development of synthetic anabolic steroids. WINSTROL-V is one of them. These efforts at synthesis centered around modification of the testosterone molecule to retain maximum anabolic effect while minimizing androgenic effect. WINSTROL-V represents significant separation of the two effects. Its anabolic activity far exceeds its androgenic activity. This spectrum of activity is clinically applicable to geriatric dogs suffering from wasting disease of old age as well as to adult or young dogs recovering from debilitating disease.
Negative nitrogen and calcium balances in wasting disease of old age lead to loss of both soft and hard tissue. WINSTROL-V is indicated in such cases. WINSTROL-V is indicated also to reverse tissue-depleting processes that accompany diseases such as canine distemper, malnutrition, or heavy parasitism or result from corticosteroid overdosage in dogs of any age. Similarly, WINSTROL-V is indicated to hasten and assist tissue repair following surgery or trauma or whenever healing is delayed in soft or hard tissue.
Anabolic steroids also manifest nonspecific stimulation of erythropoiesis. They have proven useful in acquired aplastic anemia, myeloproliferative disorders, and lymphoma with associated nonregenerative anemia in dogs and cats. Approximately one-third of these animals so afflicted respond favorably to anabolic steroids.
Clinical effects of WINSTROL-V therapy are manifold and include among them: stimulation of appetite; promotion of body weight gain; improvement of hair coat; increase of vigor, and increase of strength.
Since therapeutic activity of WINSTROL-V is a function of its tissue-building activity, its administration should always be accompanied by an adequate diet that includes protein and calcium in quantities over and above those ordinarily fed.
Indications: Anabolic therapy with WINSTROL-V is indicated whenever excessive tissue breakdown or extensive repair processes are proceeding. Such processes usually diminish protein reserves in the tissues, thus leading to negative nitrogen balance. WINSTROL-V is indicated to reverse tissue-depleting processes and restore constructive metabolism. Anabolic therapy is intended primarily as an adjunct to other specific and supportive therapy, including nutritional therapy. Optimal results can be expected only when dietary intake is adequate and well balanced.
WINSTROL-V is indicated when the therapeutic objective is to improve appetite, promote weight gain, and increase strength and vitality. For these reasons it is recommended for anorexia, unthriftiness, weight loss, debility, cachexia, inanition and poor haircoat when these accompany disease, trauma, or old age. Since certain skin conditions occurring in older dogs (alopecia and some types of eczema, for example) are caused by metabolic disorders based on negative nitrogen balance, WINSTROL-V may help to control such conditions.
Contraindications: Because the data regarding use during pregnancy are insufficient, WINSTROL-V should not be administered to pregnant dogs.
Warning: For use in dogs.
Precautions: Animals with impaired cardiac and renal function should be watched closely when receiving anabolic therapy because of the possibility of sodium and water retention. Special caution should be exercised in aged dogs suffering from chronic interstitial nephritis. In such cases, the progress of the disorder should be checked by means of laboratory tests and treatment discontinued if the drug appears to aggravate the disease.
Adverse Reactions: Mild androgenic effects may be noted after prolonged therapy with excessively high doses.
Dosage and Administration: Whenever indicated, anabolic therapy should be prescribed in conjunction with or as a follow-up to other therapeutic measures.
The suggested dose for small breeds of dogs is ½ to 1 tablet twice daily and for large breeds of dogs, 1 to 2 tablets twice daily, depending on body weight. Treatment should be continued for at least several weeks, depending on the condition and response of the animal. In certain chronic conditions, especially in aged dogs, treatment can be continued for several months without untoward reactions.
How Supplied: Chewable tablets of 2 mg, bottles of 50 and 250
Caution: Federal law restricts this drug to use by or on the order of a licensed veterinarian.

WV-97

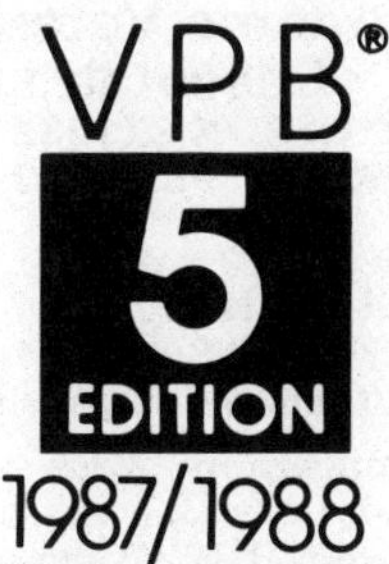

SECTION 7

Diets and Nutritional Supplements

The information provided in this section was supplied through the direct cooperation of the manufacturer and is designed to provide a convenient reference on diets and nutritional supplements employed in the practice of veterinary medicine. Products are arranged alphabetically under the name of the manufacturer.

A

Adams Veterinary Research Labs., Inc.

P.O. BOX 971039
MIAMI, FL 33197

FELI-TINIC

Nutritional Supplement for FUS Cats. Contains no magnesium.

Composition: Each 30 cc Contains: Ferric Glycerophosphate (soluble) 60 mg, Vitamin B-12 (Cyanocobalamin) 25 mg, Vitamin B-1 (Thiamin) 50 mg, Vitamin B-2 (Riboflavin) 5 mg, Vitamin B-6 (Pyrodoxine) 5 mg, Niacinamide 200 mg, Pantothenol 10 mg, Inositol 10 mg, Choline di-hydrogen Citrate 50 mg, 1-Lysine Monohydrochloride 100 mg, Methionine 6.25 mg, Paba (para-aminobenzoic Acid) 6 mg, Plus Beef Peptone, Trace Minerals, Copper Manganese, Zinc, Potassium and Cobalt in a sweet Sorbitol base, with Methyl Paraben 0.1%, Propyl Paraben 0.5% as preservatives.
Indications: Nutritional supplement with iron, B-complex, liptotropic factors, amino acids, trace minerals and sorbitol. Hematinic for FUS cats, containing no magnesium.
Dosage and Administration: Cats—1 to 2 teaspoonful (5 to 10 ml) daily depending on size. Kittens, ½ teaspoonful (1 to 2 ml) twice daily.
Caution: Keep out of reach of children.
How Supplied: 6 oz. plastic bottle with dropper and 1 gallon bottles. Sold only through licensed veterinarians.

NUTRI-TINIC

Nutritional Supplement

Composition: Each 30 cc Contains: Ferric Glycerophosphate (soluble) 60 mg, Vitamin B-2 (Cyanocobalamin) 25 mcgm, Vitamin B-1 (Thiamin) 50 mg, Vitamin B-2 (Riboflavin) 5 mg, Vitamin B-6 (Pyridoxine) 5 mg, Niacinamide 200 mg, Pantothenol 10 mg, Inositol 10 mg, Choline di-hydrogen Citrate 50 mg, 1-Lysine Monohydrochloride 100 mg, Methionine 6.25 mg, Paba (para-aminobenzoic Acid) 6 mg, Plus Beef Peptone, Trace Minerals, Copper Manganese, Zinc, Potassium, Cobalt and Magnesium in a sweet Sorbitol base, with Methyl Paraben 0.1%, Propyl Paraben 0.5% as preservatives.
Indications: Nutritional supplement with iron, B-complex, liptotropic factors, amino acids, trace minerals and sorbitol. Hematinic for dogs, cats, horses, cattle, kittens, puppies, foals and calves.
Dosage and Administration: Shake well before using.
Dogs and cats: 1 to 2 teaspoonsful daily depending on size. Puppies and Kittens: ½ teaspoonful daily.
Calves and Foals up to Yearlings: ½ to 1 oz. daily.
Yearlings and Adult Horses: 1 to 3 oz. daily.
Caution: Keep out of reach of children.
How Supplied: 6 oz. plastic bottles with droppers and 1 gallon bottles. Sold only through licensed veterinarians.

Beecham Laboratories

501 FIFTH STREET
BRISTOL, TN 37620

LIXOTINIC®

Composition: Each 60 ml (2 fluid ounces) contains: Peptonized Iron, 1,000 mg; Copper, 2.64 mg; Cyanocobalamin (B_{12}), 25 mcg; Thiamine Hydrochloride (B_1), 25 mg; Riboflavin (B_2), 15 mg; Niacinamide, 120 mg; Liver Fraction 1, 2.0 Gm.
Indications: Lixotinic is a premium quality supplement which provides nutrients essential for the production of hemoglobin in red blood cells and also those nutrients which help correct stress-induced deficiencies (debilitating illness, heavy training, pregnancy, endurance racing, convalescence).
All nutrients are provided in a highly available form for maximum results.
Dosage and Administration: Horses, 1 to 2 ounces; Calves and foals, ½ to 1 ounce; Cats and dogs, 1 teaspoonful (5 ml) per 25 lbs. body weight. Administer orally or pour over feed daily.
How Supplied: Gallons; amber glass.

PET-CAL™

Composition: Each tablet contains: calcium 600 mg; phosphorus 464 mg; vitamin D, 400 I.U. in a highly palatable base.
Indications: Pet-Cal is intended as a dietary supplement, particularly for fast growing large breeds of puppies, pregnant and lactating bitches, or whenever aid is required in the control of calcium deficiencies. Pet-Cal may also be used when a negative calcium balance occurs.
Dosage and Administration: For diet supplement, administer 1 tablet per 20 pounds of body weight daily. Pet-Cal may be given by hand just prior to feeding or may be crumbled and mixed with food if desired.
How Supplied: Bottles of 60 and 180 tablets.

PET-F.A. LIQUID®

A Liquid Fatty Acid Supplement with Zinc

Composition: Each teaspoon contains: Polyunsaturated fatty acids (as glycerides) 3900 mg; Zinc, 10 mg; Vitamin A, 1000 units; Vitamin D, 100 units; Vitamin E, 10 units; Lecithin, 50 mg.
Indications: Supplementation of diet to aid in prophylaxis and treatment of fatty acid, Vitamins A, D, E and Zinc deficiencies.
Dosage and Administration: Shake well before using. For dogs and cats. Administer once daily according to the following schedule:

Body Weight	*Dose*
Under 10 lbs	¼ teaspoonful
10 to 20 lbs	½ teaspoonful
20 to 50 lbs	1 teaspoonful
50 lbs or over	1½ teaspoonful

Quantity should be adjusted according to condition and size of the pet. Mix or pour over food.
How Supplied: 8 oz squeeze bottle for easy teaspoon measurements.

PET-TABS®

Composition: Each Pet-Tabs tablet contains: Vitamin A, 1000 I.U.; Vitamin D, 100 I.U.; Niacinamide, 10 mg; Thiamine, 810 mcg; Riboflavin, 1 mg; Pyridoxine, 82 mcg; Vitamin B_{12}, 0.2 mcg; Vitamin E, 2 I.U.; Iron, Peptonized, 6 mg; Zinc, 1.5 mg; Cobalt, 14 mcg; Potassium, 16 mcg; Iodine, 52 mcg; Copper, 50 mcg; Magnesium, 230 mcg; Manganese, 60 mcg; Linoleic acid, 30 mg; Calcium, 100 mg; Phosphorous, 77 mg; palatable protein base.
Indications: Pet-Tabs are recommended as a dietary supplement for dogs and cats of all sizes and ages to aid in the prevention of vitamin and mineral deficiencies.
Dosage and Administration: ***Dogs:*** under 10 lbs, ½ Pet-Tab daily; over 10 lbs, 1 Pet-Tab daily; growing pups, 1 to 2 Pet-Tabs daily; sick, convalescing, pregnant or nursing dogs, 2 Pet-Tabs daily. ***Cats:*** ½ to 1 Pet-Tab daily depending on size and condition.
Pet-Tabs are made with a special taste appeal to dogs and cats. Administer by hand just prior to feeding, or crumble and mix with food.
How Supplied: Bottles of 60 and 180 tablets, 12 per case, and bottles of 500.

PET-TABS® /F. A. GRANULES

Composition: Each 10 gm, or 1 packette (approximately 1 tbsp) contains Vitamin A, 1000 I.U.; Vitamin D, 100 I.U.; Niacinamide, 10 mg; Thiamine, 810 mcg; Riboflavin, 1 mg; Pyridoxine, 82 mcg; Vitamin B_{12}, 0.2 mcg; Vitamin E, 2 I.U.; Zinc (as gluconate) 10 mg; Iron Peptonized, 6 mg; Cobalt, 14 mcg; Potassium, 16 mcg; Iodine, 52 mcg; Copper, 50 mcg; Magnesium, 230 mcg; Calcium, 100 mg; Phosphorus, 77 mg; Manganese, 60 mcg; TBHQ, as preservative, 0.2 mg; total unsaturated fatty acids (as glycerides), 598 mg; palatable protein base.
Indications: Supplementation of diet to aid in prophylaxis and treatment of fatty acid, multiple vitamin, and mineral deficienceis. As such, Pet-Tabs/F.A. Granules should prove beneficial in the improvement and maintenance of healthy skin and coats on cats and dogs.
Dosage and Administration: Dogs: ½ to 2 packettes or tablespoons daily. **Cats:** ½ to 1 packette or tablespoon daily. Quantity should be adjusted according to size and condition of the pet. Mix with or sprinkle on food.
How Supplied: Pet-Tabs/F.A. Granules are supplied in convenient 10 gm packettes 30 per carton, and economical bulk canisters containing 650 gm; both in cases of 12.

PET-TABS® FELINE

Composition: Each Pet-Tabs Feline tablet contains: Vitamin A, 1500 I.U.; Vitamin D, 150 I.U.; Vitamin E, 4 I.U.;

Thiamine 810 mcg; Riboflavin, 1 mg; Niacinamide, 4 mg; Calcium Pantothenate, 1 mg; Pyridoxine 410 mcg; Inositol, 10 mg; Zinc, 0.3 mg; Manganese, 0.2 mg; Magnesium, 3 mg; Calcium, 40 mg; Phosphorus, 31 mg; Iron (peptonized), 5 mg; Copper, 0.2 mg; Cobalt, 100 mcg; Iodine, 100 mcg; Choline, 50 mg. Linoleic Acid, 20 mg; in a palatable protein base with flavoring agent.
Indications: For supplementation of diet to aid in prophylaxis and treatment of multiple vitamin and mineral deficiencies.
Dosage and Administration: For diet supplement: 1 tablet daily. For sick, convalescing, pregnant or nursing cats—2 tablets daily.
Pet-Tabs Feline are made with a special taste appeal to cats. Administer from the hand just prior to feeding, or crumble and mix with food. Should the animal at first refuse Pet-Tabs Feline, moisten the tablet very slightly to release the flavor.
How Supplied: Bottles of 60.

PET-TABS®, JR.

Composition: Each Pet-Tabs, Jr. tablet contains: Vitamin A, 500 I.U.; Vitamin D, 50 I.U.: Niacinamide, 5 mg; Thiamine, 405 mcg; Riboflavin, 0.5 mg; Pyridoxine, 41 mcg; Vitamin B_{12}, 0.1 mcg; Vitamin E, 1 I.U.; Iron Peptonized, 3 mg; Zinc, .75 mg; Cobalt, 7 mcg; Potassium, 8 mcg; Iodine, 26 mcg; Calcium, 50 mg; Phosphorus, 38 mg; Copper, 25 mcg; Magnesium, 115 mcg; Manganese, 30 mcg; Linoleic Acid, 15 mg; Palatable Protein Base.
Indications: For supplementation of diet to aid in prophylaxis and treatment of multiple vitamin and mineral deficiencies.
Dosage and Administrations: For Diet Supplement—Dogs and cats under 10 lbs—1 PetTabs, Jr. daily. Dogs and cats over 10 lbs—2 PetTabs, Jr. daily. Growing pups—2 to 4 PetTabs, Jr. daily. For sick, convalescing, pregnant or nursing dogs and cats—4 Pet-Tabs, Jr. daily. Pet-Tabs, Jr. are made with a special taste appeal to dogs and cats. Administer free choice just prior to feeding, or crumble and mix with food. Should the animal at first refuse Pet-Tabs, Jr. moisten the tablet very slightly to release the flavor.
How Supplied: Bottle of 50.

PET-TABS® PLUS
A Palatable Vitamin-Mineral Supplement For Special Nutritional Needs

Composition: Each Pet-Tabs Plus tablet contains Vitamin A, 1500 I.U.; Vitamin D, 150 I.U.; Pyridoxine 247 mcg; Pantothenic Acid, 684 mcg; Vitamin C, 10 mg; Niacinamide, 3.4 mg; Thiamine 243 mcg; Riboflavin, 655 mcg; Vitamin B_{12}, 7 mcg; Vitamin E, 15 units; Folic Acid, 55 mcg; Biotin, 30 mcg; Vitamin K, 300 mcg; Linoleic Acid, 30 mg; Choline, 50 mg; Calcium, 100 mg; Phosphorus, 77 mg; Iron Peptonized 6 mg; Cobalt, 14 mcg; Iodine, 52 mcg; Magnesium, 189 mcg; Copper, 50 mcg; Manganese, 60 mcg; Zinc, 1.5 mg; in a palatable protein base with flavoring agents.
Indications: For dietary supplementation in dogs with special nutritional needs due to sickness, debilitation or convalescence.
Advantages: Highly palatable; easily chewed; added vitamins for debilitated and older dogs; no mixing or measuring; helps maintain health and vigor in older, or convalescing animals.
Dosage and Administration: For diet supplementation dogs under 20 lbs should receive ½ tablet daily; dogs over 20 lbs 1 tablet.
Pet-Tabs Plus tablets are made with special taste appeal, and may be administered by hand prior to feeding, or crumbled and mixed with food.
How Supplied: Bottles of 60, 180, and 365 tablets.

PET-TINIC® WITH COPPER
Liquid Vitamin-Mineral Supplement for Small Animals

Composition: Each ml (one dropperful) contains:
Peptonized iron ....16.7 mg
Copper ....44.0 mcg
Cyanocobalamin (B_{12})................0.42 mcg
Thiamine Hydrochloride (B_1)..........418.0 mcg
Riboflavin (B_2)...........................200.0 mcg
Niacinamide......................................2.0 mg
Pyridoxine Hydrochloride (B_6)........250.0 mcg
Liver Fraction 1 ....33.3 mg
Indications: Supplementation of diet to aid in prophylaxis and treatment of iron, copper, amino acid and B-Vitamin deficiencies in young or orphaned animals and convalescent or debilitated animals.
Dosage and Administration: Puppies and kittens: ½ ml (½ dropper) per 5 pounds of body weight twice a day. Palatable drops may be placed directly in pet's mouth or over food.
Pet-Tinic does not require refrigeration.
How Supplied: One ounce (30 ml) amber glass bottles with dropper in dispensing boxes; four ounce amber glass bottles.

Products are cross-indexed by generic and chemical names in the **Active Ingredients Section**

DAILY FEEDING GUIDE

Weight of Dog	9	20	45	65	90*
8 oz. Volume Cups	½–1	1½–2	3½–4	5½–6	7½–8

The amount of food needed by adult dogs will vary according to breed, size, age, temperament, climate and amount of activity. In climates with temperatures above 80°F, intake may be reduced by as much as 25%. Hard working dogs may require more food. As a guide, start with the amounts shown in the Daily Feeding Guide and vary the amount to keep your dog in the proper body condition.
*For dogs over 90 lbs., feed 1 cup per 13 lbs. body weight.

Continental Grain Company
Wayne Pet Food Division
10 SOUTH RIVERSIDE PLAZA
CHICAGO, IL 60606

WAYNE® DOG FOOD

Wayne Dog Food guarantees pets of all ages complete and balanced nutrition to keep them healthy and in top condition and has been recommended by breeders, trainers and veterinarians for over fifty years. Beginning with research conducted at the Wayne Research Kennels near Libertyville, IL, Wayne Dog Food is produced to meet the standards of professional dog owners worldwide. You can guarantee dogs the benefits of professional quality nutrition when you recommend Wayne Dog Food.
Here's why Wayne Dog Food is recommended:

- Complete and balanced nutrition from multiple protein sources. The blend of animal, plant and dairy proteins helps insure top nutrition to keep dogs healthier.
- Dogs love the natural taste of Wayne Dog Food, because each bite is packed with protein-rich meat and bone meal.
- Linoleic acid for a rich, shiny hair coat and healthy skin.
- Firm stools for easier clean-up.
- No added artificial colors eliminate unsightly stains or whisker coloring.
- Two convenient shapes to suit every dog's needs. Bite size and chunk size provide you with a choice for every dog-large or small.

[See table above].
Feeding Puppies. For owners preferring a special puppy diet, Wayne PuppyOs® is recommended. If you should choose to feed Wayne Dog Food, puppies should start eating BITE SIZE (dry or moistened) at about 4 weeks of age. Feed the moistened food 3 times a day at the start. Gradually reduce the added moisture. Puppies like to chew on dry food. Change to twice-a-day feeding at six months.

WAYNE DOG FOOD GUARANTEED ANALYSIS

Crude Protein ....(Min.) 25.0%
Crude Fat ....(Min.) 8.0%
Crude Fiber ....(Max.) 4.5%
Moisture................................(Max.) 12.0%

Ingredients
Meat and bone meal, kibbled corn, kibbled wheat, ground soy grits, wheat middlings, corn gluten feed, dried bakery

Continued on next page

Continental—Cont.

product, dried beet pulp, corn gluten meal, soybean oil, animal fat preserved with BHA, dried whey product, cheese meal, brewers dried yeast, salt, vitamin A supplement, D-activated animal sterol (source of Vitamin D_3), vitamin B_{12} supplement, vitamin E supplement, menadione sodium bisulfite (source of vitamin K activity), riboflaven supplement, niacin, calcium pantothenate, choline chloride, thiamine, pyridoxine hydrochloride, folic acid, cobalt carbonate, iron carbonate, copper oxide, manganous oxide, ethylenediamine dihydriodide, zinc oxide and propylene glycol, propyl gallate, citric acid (preservatives).

C

WAYNE® PUPPYOS® Puppy Food
Complete and balanced for growing puppies.

Every bite of Wayne PuppyOs is packed with a high protein formula, fortified with extra vitamins and minerals known to be essential to growing puppies. Puppies love the easy to chew, unique O-shaped, milky coated PuppyOs. As a result of testing over 140 different formulas for taste, shape and nutritional balance, Wayne PuppyOs is the choice of professional breeders, veterinarians and pet owners who want to provide the best in puppy nutrition. Wayne PuppyOs provides puppies the complete nutrition necessary during this fast-growing first year of life.

Why PuppyOs are recommended:

- Puppies get off to a fast start because of the increased palatibility from real milk ingredients.
- Sound bone development and body growth from a complete and balanced diet.
- Unique blend of extra nutrients that all growing puppies need.
- Unique and convenient milk-coated "O" shape is easy for puppies to chew.
- Can be fed dry or moistened—you and your puppy decide.
- Linoleic acid added for healthy skin condition and shiny hair coat.
- Convenient package sizes of 5, 25 and 40 lbs. for one puppy or a litter.

DAILY FEEDING GUIDE

Weight of Puppy	Cups* of Wayne PuppyOs
5 lbs.	½ to 1 cup
10 lbs.	1½ to 2 cups
15 lbs.	2½ to 3 cups
20 lbs.	3 to 3½ cups
25 lbs.	4 to 4½ cups

*Use a standard 8 oz. measuring cup.

Remember, this is a feeding guide.—Some puppies may require more while others require less. This will depend on the adult size, age, breed, temperament and amount of exercise.

Easy to serve.—Feed it dry, straight from the bag, or just add warm water and stir it to bring out Wayne PuppyOs milky sauce.

For a fast start—Let nursing puppies begin eating Wayne PuppyOs 3 to 4 weeks of age. Combine 1 cup of water with 1 cup of PuppyOs. The milky coating in PuppyOs will become a rich and nutritious sauce that you should feed twice daily until weaning at 5 to 6 weeks of age.

Keep puppies growing after 6 weeks of age—If you prefer to continue to moisten their food, mix at the rate of 1 cup of warm water with 2 or 3 cups of PuppyOs until the milky sauce forms. Feed this mixture 3 times a day until 6 months of age and 2 times a day from 6 months to 1 year of age. Use the DAILY FEEDING GUIDE as an estimate of the daily feeding level.

If fed dry, keep the bowl filled all the time. This method (self-feeding) is ideal for puppies as they can regulate food consumption to meet their nutritional needs. Always provide plenty of fresh water.

When fully grown—At about 1 year old, begin to serve Wayne® Dog Food or Wayne Gold Label®. At each feeding, gradually decrease the amount of PuppyOs as you increase the serving of Wayne or Gold Label. Allow 1 week to complete this change in diet.

WAYNE PUPPY OS PUPPY FOOD GUARANTEED ANALYSIS

Crude Protein	(Min.)	28.0%
Crude Fat	(Min.)	9.0%
Crude Fiber	(Max.)	5.0%
Moisture	(Max.)	12.0%

Ingredients

Meat and bone meal, soybean meal, ground corn, wheat middlings, ground wheat, corn gluten meal, dried skimmed milk, corn gluten feed, dried beet pulp, dried bakery product, soybean oil, animal fat preserved with BHA, dried whey, cheese meal, brewers dried yeast, salt, vitamin A supplement, D-activated animal sterol (source of Vitamin D_3), vitamin B_{12} supplement, vitamin E supplement, menadione sodium bisulfite complex (source of Vitamin K activity), riboflavin supplement, niacin, calcium pantothenate, choline chloride, thiamine, pyridoxine hydrochloride, folic acid, copper oxide, cobalt carbonate, iron carbonate, manganous oxide, ethylenediamine dihydriodide, zinc oxide and chemical preservatives consisting of BHA, propylene glycol, propyl gallate and citric acid.

GOLD LABEL® Dog Food
The High Density Food for Special Dogs

The high nutrient density of Wayne® Gold Label® dog food allows feeding at reduced levels compared with most other dry dog foods, and still meet total nutritional requirements. Here's what Wayne Gold Label dog food provides for special dogs:

- Perfect balance of animal and vegetable protein for strength, stamina and energy.
- Unique package of vitamins and minerals to keep dogs healthier.
- Linoleic acid for a rich, shiny hair coat and healthy skin.
- Complete and balanced nutrition means Gold Label will meet your dog's nutritional requirements from puppyhood through old age.
- More taste appeal—taste tests have proven that special dogs prefer the beef, poultry, fish and dairy flavors of Wayne Gold Label.
- High density nutriton means less stool volume and easier clean-ups.
- No added artificial colors unlike other leading dog foods-eliminates unsightly stains.

FEEDING GUIDELINES

ADULT DOGS

Because of the high nutrient density of Wayne Gold Label dog food, you can recommend that dogs be fed about one half the serving size you would with most other dry dog foods.

A food scoop is enclosed in every bag of Gold Label dog food. It holds sufficient food for one feeding for the average size dog.

However, the amount needed by your dog may vary. You know your dog best. Hard working dogs, lactating bitches, and dogs engaged in demanding activities will require larger portions or more frequent feedings. Adjust serving size according to your dog's particular needs. Always provide plenty of clean, fresh water.

PUPPIES

Puppies require more food than an adult dog of the same weight. They should be fed three times per day until 6 months of age, and twice a day to one year of age. Always provide plenty of clean, fresh water.

Wayne "Good As Gold" Money-Back Guarantee

With a heritage of over 50 golden years of professional quality pet foods, Wayne is proud to stand behind this product with an unconditional "good as gold" money-back guarantee.

If customers are not 100% satisfied, they should send unused portion along with their receipt to Wayne Pet Food, P. O. Box 459, Libertyville, IL 60048 for a full refund.

Guaranteed Analysis

Crude Protein	(Min.)	30.0%
Crude Fat	(Min.)	20.0%
Crude Fiber	(Max.)	3.0%
Moisture	(Max.)	12.0%

Ingredients:

Beef meal, ground corn, corn gluten meal, animal fat (preserved with BHA), wheat middlings, poultry by-product meal, soybean oil (source of linoleic acid), ground wheat, brewers dried yeast, fish meal, digest (containing poultry by-products, beef and brewers yeast), dehydrated cheese, dried whey product, dried beet pulp, salt, L-lysine, dried egg, L-tryptophan, vitamin A supplement, D-activated animal sterol (source of vitamin D_3), vitamin B_{12} supplement, vitamin E supplement, menadione sodium bisulfite complex (source of vitamin K activity), riboflavin supplement, niacin, calcium pantothenate, choline chloride, thiamine, biotin, cobalt carbonate, iron carbonate, copper oxide, manganous oxide, ethylenediamine dihydriodide, zinc oxide, sodium selenite and BHA, propylene glycol, propyl gallate, citric acid (preservatives).

TAIL WAGGER® Flavored Gravy Dog Food

Like each of us, dogs have taste buds, too! And like humans, dogs appreciate variety in their diets. That's why Tail Wagger® Dog Foods have been formulated to provide a choice of a dog's four favorite flavors—Beef, Cheese, Chicken and Liver—in a thick juicy gravy. But, Tail Wagger Dog Foods offer more than just great taste.

IDEAL NUTRITION WITH GREAT TASTE

Every bag of Tail Wagger Dog Food meets or exceeds the nutrient requirements established by the National Research Council for all stages of a dog's life. With Tail Wagger Dog Foods you can be certain your favorite pet is getting the nutrition necessary for growth and energy plus the proper balance of protein, vitamins and minerals for a good hair coat and strong bones and teeth. And remember, the great taste of Tail Wagger Dog Foods means your dog will get the nutrition it needs regardless of which Tail Wagger flavor you choose to feed on any given day.

VARIETY FOR THE DOG THAT DESERVES A BREAK

The four flavors of Tail Wagger Dog Foods—Beef, Cheese, Chicken and Liver—give you the opportunity to provide your best friend with a break from having to face the same flavor day in and day out. The advantage of Tail Wagger Dog Foods is that they're so palatable your dog will switch from one flavor to another without batting an eye.

BACKED BY 50 YEARS OF QUALITY, EXPERIENCE

Tail Wagger Dog Foods are the result of 50 years experience in the research, development and production of quality products by Wayne Pet Foods. Each of the four flavors of Tail Wagger Dog Food has been extensively tested for its nutritional value and taste preference at our Research Kennels. The Beef, Cheese, Chicken and Liver flavors that make up Tail Wagger Dog Foods are those which dogs like yours prefer.

FEEDING DIRECTIONS

For a THICK, FLAVORED GRAVY DINNER that your dog will love, add one part warm water to 4–5 parts of Wayne Tail Wagger Flavored Gravy Dog Food and stir to make the gravy.

[See table above].

DAILY FEEDING GUIDE

	Weight of Dog	8 oz. Volume Cup[1]/Day	Cups of Warm Water[2]
Toy or miniature (Poodle,	5 lbs.	1	1/4
Chihuahua, Pekingese, etc.)	15 lbs.	2	1/2
Small (Scottie, Cocker,	25 lbs.	3	3/4
Fox Terrier, etc.)	36 lbs.	4	1
Medium (Springer Spaniel,	45 lbs.	5	1 1/4
Dalmation, Bulldog, etc.)	54 lbs.	6	1 1/2
Large (Irish Setter,	63 lbs.	7	1 3/4
Collie, Labrador, etc.)	72 lbs.	8	2
Giant (Great Dane,	81 lbs.	9	2 1/4
St. Bernard, Wolfhound, etc.)	90 lbs.[3]	10	2 1/2

[1]The amount of food needed by adult dogs will vary according to breed, size, age, temperament, climate and amount of activity. In climates with temperatures above 80°F, intake may be reduced as much as 25%. Hard working dogs may require more food. As a guide, start with the amounts shown in the Daily Feeding Guide and vary the amount to keep your dog in the proper body condition.

[2]In addition, always provide plenty of fresh water for drinking.

[3]For dogs over 90 lbs. feed approximately 1 cup per 12 lbs. body weight.

GUARANTEED ANALYSIS

Crude Protein	(Min.)	22.0%
Crude Fat	(Min.)	6.0%
Crude Fiber	(Max.)	5.0%
Moisture	(Max.)	12.0%

WAYNE® CAT FOOD

The new and improved tuna taste with reduced ash formula is a complete and balanced diet which meets or exceeds the nutritional requirements for the growing kitten and the maintenance of the adult cat as established by the National Research Council.

Guaranteed Analysis

Crude Protein	(Min.)	30.0%
Crude Fat	(Min.)	9.0%
Crude Fiber	(Min.)	4.5%

A complete and balanced diet, with poultry, fish and dairy flavors, Wayne Cat Food is the result of testing over 450 different formulations for taste, shape and nutritional preference.

Here's why you should feed your special cat Wayne Cat Food:

- Improved taste—Cats prefer our new tuna flavor.
- 25% lower ash—New ash content is only 7%.
- New and improved balance of animal, vegetable and milk protein for palatability and overall performance.
- Complete and balanced nutrition for growth in kittens or maintenance of adult cats.
- Wayne Cat Food is pressure cooked to enhance flavor, while also breaking down starches to improve digestibility.
- Fortified with the proper balance of minerals and vitamins.
- 9% fat for flavor, and energy for lactating females.

How to Feed

Adult Feeding

Feeding Wayne Cat Food straight from the bag makes feeding simple and easy. Wayne Cat Food is nutritious and its flavor is appealing to the cat. The average adult cat will eat daily approximately one full 8 oz. cup of Wayne Cat Food. When fed dry, feed enough so the cat can go to the food a number of times a day. Some cats prefer their food to be moistened. Add a small amount of warm liquid to slightly moisten Wayne Cat Food. Should your cat refuse to eat for a brief period (a number of hours or a day or so), do not become alarmed. The normal temperament of the cat is to occasionally refuse to eat for a short time. Also when changing from a canned wet product to a dry food, the cat may be reluctant to eat for a short interval and this is normal behavior.

Kitten Feeding

Wayne Cat Food is also well suited for kitten feeding. From 3 to 6 weeks of age start feeding well moistened Wayne Cat Food several times a day. Cut down gradually on the moisture until the cat is completely on dry food at from 3 to 6 months of age. After 6 months of age, follow the adult cat feeding information given above.

Remember: always provide plenty of fresh water.

Ingredients:

Ground corn, poultry by-product meal, soybean meal, wheat middlings, animal fat preserved with BHA, ground wheat, corn gluten meal, condensed fish solubles, cheese meal, corn fermentation solubles, dried skimmed milk, digest (containing poultry by-products, tuna and brewers yeast—source of tuna taste), brewers dried yeast, cheddar cheese, dried whey, salt, vitamin A supplement, D-activated animal sterol (source of vitamin D_3), vitamin B_{12} supplement, vitamin E supplement, menadione sodium bisulfite complex (source of vitamin K activity), riboflavin supplement, niacin, calcium pantothenate, choline chloride, thiamine, cobalt carbonate, iron carbonate, copper oxide, manganous oxide, ethylenediamine dihydriodide, zinc oxide and BHA, propylene glycol, propyl gallate and citric acid (preservatives).

WAYNE® GUINEA PIG DIET 8602-00

A complete and balanced diet for free choice feeding in self-feeders.

Guaranteed Analysis

Crude Protein	(Min.)	17.0%
Crude Fat	(Min.)	4.0%
Crude Fiber	(Max.)	12.0%

Protein from plant and milk sources provides the amino acid balance necessary for efficient reproduction and growth. Fat, from soybean oil, provides the extra energy needed during lactation and

Continued on next page

Continental—Cont.

growth, and helps provide a shiny hair coat.

Vitamin and mineral fortification maintains top condition, promotes growth and reproduction, regulates body functions. Vitamin C is added to prevent scurvy.

Soybean oil adds essential fatty acids needed for good hair coat, it also acts as a natural preservative so no chemical preservatives are added.

Constant formula will not mask or alter research results.

Code dated to assure freshness.

How to Feed

Feed Wayne Guinea Pig Diet in a self-feeder which may be attached to either the side or the front of the cage. Feeding bowls should not be used, since guinea pigs housed in wire cages will sit in the bowls and contaminate the feed. A constant supply of fresh water should be provided. If desired, feed greens or add Vitamin C to the drinking water several times a week.

Ingredients:

Ground corn, dehydrated alfalfa meal preserved with ethoxyquin, soybean meal, wheat middlings, dried whey, cane molasses, soybean oil, ascorbic acid, vitamin A supplement, D-activated animal sterol (source of vitamin D_3), vitamin B_{12} supplement, vitamin E supplement, menadione sodium bisulfite complex (source of vitamin K activity), riboflavin supplement, niacin supplement, calcium pantothenate, choline chloride, ground limestone, calcium phosphate, salt, copper oxide, iron sulfate, manganous oxide, ethylenediamine dihydriodide and zinc oxide.

WAYNE® RODENT BLOX®
8604-00

Complete and balanced, constant formula diet for mice, rats and hamsters.

Guaranteed Analaysis

Crude Protein	(Min.) 24.0%
Crude Fat	(Min.) 4.0%
Crude Fiber	(Max.) 4.5%

Blox available in two lengths, hardness-tested to prevent waste.

Meal will mix efficiently and uniformly with various ingredients for testing purposes.

Constant formula will not mask or alter research results.

Amino acid balance from fish, plant and milk protein sources and fat from soybean oil assures top performance of animals during maintenance, gestation and lactation. Soybean oil acts as a natural preservative, so no chemical preservatives are added.

Vitamin and mineral fortification helps animals stay in top condition without supplementation.

Quality assured by chemical and biological testing. Rodent Blox are produced only at a special plant with no antibiotics or estrogens in inventory, thus eliminating the possibility of mix up.

Code dated to assure freshness.

How to Feed

This complete diet is to be fed free choice in a self-feeder. Keep a constant supply of fresh water available.

Ingredients:

Corn and wheat flakes, ground corn, soybean meal, fish meal, wheat middlings, wheat red dog, dried whey, brewers dried yeast, soybean oil, animal liver meal, cane molasses, vitamin A supplement, D-activated animal sterol (source of vitamin D_3), vitamin E supplement, menadione sodium bisulfite complex (source of vitamin K activity) riboflavin supplement, niacin supplement, calcium pantothenate, choline chloride, thiamine, ground limestone, calcium phosphate, salt, manganous oxide, copper oxide, iron carbonate, ethylenediamine dihydriodide, cobalt carbonate and zinc oxide.

WAYNE® MOUSE BREEDER BLOX®
8626-00

A complete and balanced diet to meet energy and protein needs of mice during maximum reproduction and experimental stress.

Guaranteed Analysis

Crude Protein	(Min.) 20.0%
Crude Fat	(Min.) 10.0%
Crude Fiber	(Max.) 2.0%

Oval cross section blox move down in feeders without excessive waste; assures top production performance at least cost.

Protein and fat combine to meet energy and protein needs of mice during maximum reproduction and experimental stress, also meets the needs of certain strains of inbred mice. Assures top reproduction and growth; breeder can produce more mice on less feed.

Constant formula with only natural preservatives will not alter or mask research results.

Fortified with vitamins and minerals so animals stay in top condition without additional supplementation. Fortification is sufficient so that product can be pasteurized.

Quality assured by chemical and biological testing. Mouse Breeder Blox are produced only at a special plant with no antibiotics or estrogen in inventory, thus eliminating the possibility of mix up.

Code dated to assure freshness.

How to Feed

Mouse Breeder Blox is a complete diet to be fed free choice in a self-feeder. A constant supply of fresh water should always be available.

Ingredients:

Ground wheat, fish meal, dried skim milk, dried whey, animal fat preserved with BHA, soybean oil, brewers dried yeast, wheat middlings, casein, vitamin A supplement, D-activated animal sterol (source of vitamin D_3), vitamin B_{12} supplement, vitamin E supplement, menadione sodium bisulfite complex (source of vitamin K activity), riboflavin supplement, niacin supplement, calcium pantothenate, choline chloride, folic acid, pyridoxine hydrochloride, thiamine, calcium phosphate, salt, magnesium oxide, copper oxide, iron sulfate, iron carbonate, ethylenediamine dihydriodide, cobalt carbonate and zinc oxide.

WAYNE® MRH 22/5 RODENT BLOX®
8640-00

Free choice diet for mice, rats and hamsters. Vitamin fortification is sufficient so that product can be pasteurized.

Guaranteed Analysis

Crude Protein	(Min.) 22.0%
Crude Fat	(Min.) 5.0%
Crude Fiber	(Max.) 4.5%

Protein from animal and plant sources and fat from soybean oil are balanced to provide the protein-energy levels required for top performance by random bred and certain inbred strains of mice, rats and hamsters during maintenance, gestation and lactation. Soybean oil also acts as a natural preservative, so no chemical preservatives are added.

Vitamin and mineral fortified so animals stay in top condition without additional supplementation.

Quality assured by chemical and biological testing. MRH 22/5 Rodent Blox is produced at a special plant, where no antibiotics or estrogens are carried in inventory, thus eliminating the possibility of mixup.

Oval cross section blox can be fed in self-feeders.

Constant nutrition assures uniform production and testing results.

Code dated to assure freshness.

How to Feed

This is a complete diet, to be fed free choice in a self-feeder. Keep a constant supply of fresh water available.

Ingredients:

Soybean meal, ground corn, corn and wheat flakes, wheat middlings, fish meal, dried whey, brewers dried yeast, soybean oil, cane molasses, vitamin A supplement, D-activated animal sterol (source of vitamin D_3), vitamin B_{12} supplement, vitamin E supplement, menadione sodium bisulfite complex (source of vitamin K activity), riboflavin supplement, niacin supplement, calcium pantothenate, choline chloride, folic acid, thiamine, ground limestone, calcium phosphate, salt, manganous oxide, copper oxide, iron carbonate, ethylenediamine dihydriodide, cobalt carbonate and zinc oxide.

WAYNE® STERILIZABLE RODENT BLOX®
8656-00

Can be autoclaved; provides complete and balanced nutrition and maximum feeding efficiency whether sterilized or pasteurized for mice, rats, and hamsters.

Guaranteed Analysis

Crude Protein	(Min.) 24.0%
Crude Fat	(Min.) 4.0%
Crude Fiber	(Max.) 4.5%

Protein from animal and plant sources and fat from soybean oil supply the balance of protein and energy required by most random bred and certain inbred strains of mice, rats and hamsters for top performance. Soybean oil acts as a natu-

ral preservative, so no chemical preservatives are added.
Fortified with 9 vitamins and 9 minerals. Extra amounts of Vitamin A, Pantothenic Acid, Thiamine, and Menadione Sodium Bisulfite Complex (Vitamin K) are added because these vitamins are partially destroyed during autoclaving.
Special formulation prevents the product from sticking together or browning during autoclaving so that anti-caking agents are not needed. Specially constructed paper bag with offset pin holes allow autoclaving the entire bag at once.
Quality assured by chemical and biological testing. Sterilizable Rodent Blox are produced at a special plant, where no antibiotics or estrogens are carried in inventory, eliminating the possibility of mix up.
Oval cross section blox will feed efficiently in self feeder and minimize waste.
Code dated to assure freshness.

How to Feed

The free-flowing characteristic of autoclaved Wayne Sterilizable Rodent Blox allows them to be self-fed. A constant source of fresh water should be supplied in addition to the feed.

Ingredients:

Corn and wheat flakes, soybean meal, wheat red dog, ground corn, wheat middlings, fish meal, brewers dried yeast, soybean oil, animal liver meal, vitamin A supplement, D-activiated animal sterol (source of vitamin D_3), vitamin E supplement, menadione sodium bisulfite complex (source of vitamin K activity), riboflavin supplement, niacin supplement, calcium pantothenate, choline chloride, thiamine, ground limestone, calcium phosphate, salt, manganous oxide, copper oxide, iron sulfate, ethylenediamine dihydriodide, cobalt carbonate and zinc oxide.

WAYNE® F6 RODENT BLOX® 8664-00

Constant formula diet for free choice feeding to mice, rats and hamsters.

Guaranteed Analysis

Crude Protein	(Min.)	24.0%
Crude Fat	(Min.)	6.0%
Crude Fiber	(Max.)	4.5%

Protein from fish, plant and milk sources and fat from soybean oil provide the level of protein plus the extra energy needed by certain strains of mice, rats and hamsters. Some inbred strains require more energy. Soybean oil provides essential fatty acids and acts as a natural preservative, so no chemical preservatives are added.
Vitamin and mineral fortified so no supplementation is needed.
Quality assured by chemical and biological testing. F6 Rodent Blox are produced only in a special plant, where no antibiotics or estrogens are carried in inventory, eliminating the possibility of mix up.
Constant formula will not alter or mask research results.
Code dated to assure freshness.

How to Feed

A complete diet to be fed free choice in a self-feeder. Keep a constant supply of fresh water available.

Ingredients:

Soybean meal, corn and wheat flakes, ground corn, wheat red dog, fish meal, wheat middlings, cane molasses, soybean oil, dried whey, brewers dried yeast, animal liver meal, vitamin A supplement, D-activated animal sterol (source of vitamin D_3), vitamin E supplement, menadione sodium bisulfite complex (source of vitamin K activity), riboflavin supplement, niacin supplement, calcium pantothenate, choline chloride, thiamine, ground limestone, calcium phosphate, salt, manganous oxide, copper oxide, iron carbonate, ethylenediamine dihydriodide, cobalt carbonate and zinc oxide.

WAYNE® LAB DOG DIET 8653-00

Constant formula, complete and balanced dog diet for use in research investigations.

Guaranteed Analysis

Crude Protein	(Min.)	25.0%
Crude Fat	(Min.)	9.0%
Crude Fiber	(Max.)	5.0%

Protein selected for balance of amino acids for fast economical growth in puppies; for adult dogs to maintain body weight during hard work or during lactation.
Fat provides extra palatability and energy to keep research dogs and lactating bitches in top condition.
Vitamin and mineral fortification meets or exceeds dog's needs as established by the National Research Council; required for regulation of body fluids, strong bones and teeth, growth and maintenance, good blood, skin and coat condition.
Constant formula will not mask or alter research results.
Contains no antibiotics: Wayne Lab Dog Diet is produced only in Peoria, Illinois, and Everson, Pennsylvania. These plants produce only pet and research animal feeds; therefore, no antibiotics or estrogens are present in inventory, which eliminates the possibility of mix-up.

How to Feed

Wayne Lab Dog Diet may be fed dry as it comes from the bag, or moistened. Follow the recommended Daily Feeding or use the self-feeding program.

Daily Feeding Guide

Weight of Dog	*Cups of Dog Food
11–22 pounds	1–2
33–44 pounds	3–4
55–66 pounds	5–6
77–88 pounds**	7–8

*Use a standard 8 oz. size measuring cup.

**For dogs 90 pounds and over, feed approximately one cup of dog food per 12 pounds of body weight.

Feeding the Research Dog: Wayne Lab Dog Diet is designed to be fed to dogs under research conditions. Select the feeding method that keeps the research dog in proper body condition. For very active dogs, use the self-feeding program, or feed a controlled amount of Wayne Lab Dog Diet dry or moistened. The amount of food the research dog needs will depend on size, age, breed, temperament, and the amount of exercise the dog receives.
Feeding the Expectant Mother: It is very important that the expectant mother receives a nutritionally balanced dog food during pregnancy and nursing. Wayne Lab Dog Diet provides complete nutrition to keep her in the proper body condition. During pregnancy, feed her twice a day or use the self-feeding program. For the first few feedings of the mother after the puppies are born, moisten Wayne Lab Dog Diet. From this point on, use the self-feeding program plus feeding her moistened food once a day. Always provide plenty of fresh water.
Feeding the Puppies: Puppies will start eating Wayne Lab Dog Diet, moistened or dry, when they are about four weeks old. To start them eating, add one cup of liquid to one cup of dog food. At first, feed the moistened food three times each day. As puppies grow, gradually reduce the number of feedings to twice daily. The self-feeding program is ideal for puppies as they like to chew on dry food. The puppies can also eat when they are hungry, assuring proper nutrition. Puppies require twice as many nutrients per unit of body weight as do adult dogs.
Those preferring a special puppy diet should use Wayne PuppyOs Puppy Food—a complete and balanced diet, fed either dry or by adding warm water.

Feeding Methods

Self-Feeding the Dog: An easy solution to the actual feeding of your dog is to use the simple self-feeding program. This proven and accepted plan places Wayne Lab Dog Diet before your dog all the time. Use a feeding bowl or self-feeder. Self-feeding dry dog food will save labor and your dog will eat when he is hungry. Always provide plenty of fresh water. There are some dogs that may not adjust to the self-feeding program and will have to be fed a controlled amount of food.
To Moisten Wayne Lab Dog Diet: Add one cup of liquid to four cups of dog food. Feed this flavorful mixture once or twice daily as desired. Discard unused moistened food.

Ingredients:

Soybean meal, ground corn, wheat middlings, meat and bone meal, corn gluten feed, animal fat preserved with BHA, ground wheat, dried beet pulp, dried whey product, cheese rind, salt, vitamin A supplement, D-activated animal sterol (source of Vitamin D_3), vitamin B_{12} supplement, vitamin E supplement, menadione sodium bisulfite (source of vitamin K activity), riboflavin supplement, niacin, calcium pantothenate, choline chloride, thiamine, cobalt carbonate, iron carbonate, copper oxide, manganous oxide, ethylenediamine dihydriodide, zinc oxide and chemical preservatives consisting of BHA, propylene glycol, propyl gallate and citric acid.

Continued on next page

Continental—Cont.

WAYNE® 25% MONKEY DIET 8663-00

Once a day feed that meets known nutrient requirements for monkeys of all breeds and ages.

Guaranteed Analysis

Crude Protein	(Min.) 25.0%
Crude Fat	(Min.) 5.0%
Crude Fiber	(Max.) 5.0%

Protein from milk, plant and fish sources and fat from animal fat and soybean oil are combined to meet the nutrient needs of monkeys during maintenance, gestation, lactation and growth. Contains optimum balance of essential fatty acids necessary for growth and a good hair coat.

Fortified with 13 vitamins and 9 minerals: contains Vitamin D_3, because research has shown that New World monkeys cannot utilize Vitamin D_2. Extra fortification of folic acid, pyridoxine, Vitamin B_{12}, iron and copper helps prevent anemia, especially when conditioning primates for use in laboratories. Only one diet is needed for either New or Old World monkeys.

Pressure cooking breaks down starches which improves palatability, results in firm stools and helps prevent digestive disturbances. Special ingredients are added to satisfy the monkey's taste.

Convenient oblong blox are easily eaten by primates of all sizes.

Constant nutrition in every batch helps provide uniform production and testing results.

Code dated to assure freshness.

How to Feed

Feed Wayne Monkey Diet at approximately 4% of body weight once a day, preferably in the morning. If desired, supplement with one-fourth of an orange three times a week during breeding or illness.

Ingredients:

Ground corn, soybean meal, corn gluten meal, ground wheat, corn gluten feed, sugar (sucrose), dried whey product, fish meal, dried beet pulp, dehydrated alfalfa meal preserved with ethoxyquin, brewers dried yeast, animal fat preserved with BHA, soybean oil, vitamin A supplement, D-activated animal sterol (source of vitamin D_3), vitamin B_{12} supplement, vitamin E supplement, menadione sodium bisulfite complex (source of vitamin K activity), riboflavin supplement, niacin, calcium, pantothenate, choline chloride, thiamine hydrochloride, pyridoxine hydrochloride, ascorbic acid, folic acid, ground limestone, dicalcium phosphate, salt, manganous oxide, copper oxide, iron carbonate, ethylenediamine dihydriodide, cobalt carbonate, zinc oxide and calcium propionate, propylene glycol, propyl galate and citric acid (preservatives).

WAYNE® RABBIT RATION 8600-00

Complete and balanced, pelleted diet to meet the nutritional needs of the rabbit during growth, reproduction and maintenance.

Guaranteed Analysis

Crude Protein	(Min.) 17.0%
Crude Fat	(Min.) 2.0%
Crude Fiber	(Max.) 15.0%

Protein level meets requirements of rabbits during all stages of production; helps doe provide sufficient quantities of milk during lactation.

Fiber from alfalfa meal is provided to help digestive disturbances and aids in improving palatability, resulting in uniform production.

Fortified with 10 vitamins and 9 minerals, assuring the producer that the rabbits will be maintained in top condition and utilize feed efficiently.

Pellet form helps prevent food waste.

May be medicated with sulfaquinoxaline at 0.025% as an aid in prevention of coccidiosis. Medicated Rabbit Ration can be fed without changing the diet, reducing stress and taking care of disease problems at the same time.

How to Feed

If rabbits are hand-fed, the number of feedings per day is largely a matter of personal preference and convenience. However, regularity is more important than the number of feedings. In warm weather, rabbits generally consume more feed at night than during the day.

The most economical and efficient growth of rabbits for meat, the self-feeding plan is strongly recommended for does and litters up to weaning time. Self-feeding is also recommended for developing rabbits to heavier weights after weaning.

For good breeding results, avoid getting rabbits too fat. Feeding requirements for rabbits will vary with the breed, age, size, and weather conditions. Through observation and controlled feeding, the proper body condition can be maintained for maximum performance.

WAYNE FEEDING PROGRAM

Stage	Daily Feed Allowance
Maintenance	
Does or Bucks	
6– 8 lbs.	3 to 4 oz.
8–10 lbs.	4 to 5 oz.
10–12 lbs.	5 to 6 oz.
Pregnant Does	
6– 8 lbs.	5 to 6 oz.
8–10 lbs.	6 to 7 oz.
10–12 lbs.	7 to 8 oz.
Lactation	Self-feed
Growing Rabbits	Self-feed

Water: Rabbits should have access to fresh, clean water at all times. A good supply of water is needed by the rabbits to fully utilize the nutrients for growth and reproduction.

Salt: Mineral needs are supplied by Wayne Rabbit Ration, if fed as directed. Some rabbits may require extra salt. Attach an iodized or trace mineralized salt spool to the wall of each hutch to insure adequate salt for all rabbits.

Warning: Rabbit Ration with Sulfaquinoxaline must be withdrawn 10 days before rabbits are slaughtered for food.

Ingredients:

Grain products, plant protein products, processed grain by-products, forage product, cane molasses, vitamin A supplement, D-activated animal sterol (source of vitamin D_3), vitamin B_{12} supplement, vitamin E supplement, menadione sodium bisulfite complex (source of vitamin K activity), riboflavin supplement, niacin supplement, calcium pantothenate, choline chloride, folic acid, ground limestone, calcium phosphate, salt, copper oxide, iron sulfate, manganous oxide, ethylenediamine dihydriodide and zinc oxide.

WAYNE® 15% RABBIT RATION 8630-00

Complete and balanced diet to meet the nutritional requirements of the rabbit during various stages of production.

Guaranteed Analysis

Crude Protein	(Min.) 15.0%
Crude Fat	(Min.) 2.5%
Crude Fiber	(Max.) 18.0%

Protein, fat and fiber levels assure good performance and palatability, help minimize digestive disturbances and excessive weight gains during maintenance and growth.

Fortified with 10 vitamins and 9 minerals, so rabbits will stay in good condition and utilize feed efficiently.

Pelleted to prevent waste, thus reducing feed cost.

May be medicated with sulfaquinoxaline at 0.025% as an aid in prevention of coccidiosis; no stress from diet change while caring for disease problems.

How to Feed

Feed continuously as the sole ration to rabbits.

Stage of Production	Daily Feed Allowance
Maintenance	
Does or Bucks	
6– 8 lbs.	3 to 4 oz.
8–10 lbs.	4 to 5 oz.
10–12 lbs.	5 to 6 oz.
Pregnant Does	
6– 8 lbs.	5 to 6 oz.
8–10 lbs.	6 to 7 oz.
10–12 lbs.	7 to 8 oz.
Lactation	Self-Feed
Growing Rabbits	Self-Feed

Feeding Tips—If rabbits are hand-fed, the number of feedings per day is largely a matter of personal preference and convenience. Regularity is more important than the number of feedings. In warm weather, rabbits generally consume more feed at night than during the day.

For most economical and efficient growth of rabbits for meat, the self-feeding plan is strongly recommended for does and litters up to weaning time. Self-feeding is also recommended for developing rabbits to heavier weights.

For good breeding results, avoid getting rabbits too fat. Feeding requirements for rabbits will vary with the breed, age, size, and weather condition. Through observation and controlled feeding, the proper

body condition can be maintained for maximum performance.
Rabbits should have access to fresh, clean water at all times. A good supply of water is needed by the rabbit to fully utilize the nutrients present in Wayne 15% Rabbit Ration.
Warning: Wayne 15% Rabbit Ration with Sulfaquinoxaline must be withdrawn 10 days before rabbits are slaughtered for food.
Ingredients:
Grain products, plant protein products, processed grain by-products, forage product, 15% roughage product, cane molasses, vitamin A supplement, D-activated animal sterol (source of vitamin D_3), vitamin B_{12} supplement, vitamin E supplement, menadione sodium bisulfite complex (source of vitamin K activity), riboflavin supplement, niacin supplement, calcium pantothenate, choline chloride, folic acid, ground limestone, calcium phosphate, salt, copper oxide, iron sulfate, manganous oxide, ethylenediamine dihydriodide and zinc oxide.

WAYNE® CERTIFIED 25% MONKEY DIET 8726-00

WAYNE® CERTIFIED LAB DOG DIET 8727-00

WAYNE® CERTIFIED RODENT BLOX® 8728-00

Minimizing variables in laboratory studies is a prime concern of researchers. Good Laboratory Practices Regulations from the FDA require periodic analysis of feed for substances that might be capable of interfering with the study. The products listed above will be analyzed and certified to contain not more than certain levels of specified environmental contaminants. To help laboratories comply with the regulations, analysis will be completed before the products are shipped from Peoria. Specifications for maximum levels of environmental contaminants are listed below.
[See table above].
If other analyses are needed they can be provided by requesting analysis prior to manufacture. Charges for additional analysis will be based on current rates at the time. Normally, delivery of products will be within 6 weeks from the time an order is placed.
These products are identical in formulation to the present Rodent Blox, Lab Dog Diet, and 25% Monkey Diet. Additional testing and quality assurance monitoring is used to insure minimal levels of certain environmental contaminants. Key ingredients and certain nutrients are analyzed before and after manufacture by Wayne and by independent laboratories.

Products are cross-indexed by generic and chemical names in the **Active Ingredients Section**

CONTAMINANT CERTIFICATION PROFILE

	Rodent Blox	Lab Dog Diet	25% Monkey Diet
Arsenic, ppm	1.00	1.00	1.00
Cadmium, ppm	0.50	0.50	0.50
Lead, ppm	1.50	3.00	1.50
Mercury, ppm	0.20	0.20	0.20
Aflatoxin, ppb	10.00	10.00	10.00
Aldrin, ppm	0.03	0.03	0.03
Dieldrin, ppm	0.03	0.03	0.03
Endrin, ppm	0.03	0.03	0.03
Heptachlor, ppm	0.03	0.03	0.03
Heptachlor Epoxide, ppm	0.03	0.03	0.03
Lindane, ppm	0.05	0.05	0.05
Chlordane, ppm	0.05	0.05	0.05
DDT Related Substances, ppm	0.15	0.15	0.15
PCB, ppm	0.15	0.15	0.15
Thimet, ppm	0.50	0.50	0.50
Diazanon, ppm	0.50	0.50	0.50
Disulfaton, ppm	0.50	0.50	0.50
Methyl Parathion, ppm	0.50	0.50	0.50
Malathion, ppm	0.50	0.50	0.50
Parathion, ppm	0.50	0.50	0.50
Thiodan, ppm	0.50	0.50	0.50
Ethion, ppm	0.50	0.50	0.50
Trithion, ppm	0.50	0.50	0.50

Coopers Animal Health Inc.

520 WEST 21ST ST.
P.O. BOX 419167
KANSAS CITY, MO 64141-0167

EQUIFORM™
Vitamin and Mineral Supplement for Horses

Ingredients: Dried Cane Molasses, Dicalcium Phosphate, Dried Extracted Streptomyces Meal and Fermentation Solubles, Corn Distillers Dried Solubles, Condensed Whey Fermentation Solubles, Condensed Corn Fermentation Solubles, Corn Distillers Dried Grains, Heat Processed Walnut Meal, Dried Whey, Animal Fat (preserved with BHA), Dried Whey Fermentation Solubles, Cheese Rind, Dried Buttermilk, Dried Skim Milk, Yeast Culture, Vitamin A Supplement, D-Activated Animal Sterol (source of Vitamin D-3). Alpha Tocopherol Acetate (source of Vitamin E), Menadione Sodium Bisulfite Complex (source of Vitamin K Activity), Vitamin B-12 Supplement, Riboflavin Supplement, Calcium Pantothenate, Niacin Supplement, Choline Chloride, Folic Acid, Thiamine Mononitrate, Ascorbic Acid (source of Vitamin C), Natural and Artificial Flavors Added, dl-Methionine, Iron Ammonium Citrate, Iron Choline Citrate, Ferrous Fumarate, Iron Gluconate, Zinc Methionine, Extracted Yucca Meal, L-lysine Hydrochloride, Beta-Carotene, Copper Sulfate, Magnesium Oxide, Cobalt Carbonate, Potassium Chloride, Zinc Sulfate, Manganese Sulfate, Ethylene Diamine Dihydriodide, Dried Lactobacillus acidolphilus Fermentation Product, Dried Lactobacillus lactis Fermentation Product, Dried Lactobacillus plantarum Fermentation Product, Dried Streptococcus cremoris Fermentation Product, Dried Streptococcus Diacetilactis Fermentation Product, Dried B-Subtillis Fermentation Product, Dried Aspergillus oryzae Fermentation Product, Dried Brewers Yeast, Calcium Carbonate, Salt, Corn Oil, Pyridoxine Hydrochloride (source of Vitamin B-6), Smectite Vermiculite, Lecithin, Ethoxyquin (a preservative), Biotin, and Sodium Selenite.
Feeding Directions: Feed at the rate of one ounce per 250 pounds of body weight per day to Horses. Feed as the sole source of selenium. Do Not Exceed 5 ounces per head per day so as not to exceed the maximum permitted intake of Selenium per head per day. (Each measure holds one ounce)

Guaranteed Analysis Per Pound:

Calcium (Ca), minimum %	8.5
Calcium (Ca), maximum %	9.5
Phosphorus (P), minimum %	6.0
Salt (NaCl), minimum %	.75
Salt (NaCl), maximum %	1.75
Magnesium (Mg), minimum %	.80
Manganese (Mn), minimum %	.22
Iron (Fe), minimum %	.66
Copper (Cu), minimum %	.036
Zinc (Zn), minimum %	.23
Cobalt (Co), minimum %	.006
Iodine (I), minimum %	.007
Selenium (Se), minimum %	.0007
Vitamin A, USP Units minimum	250,000.00
Vitamin D-3, USP Units minimum	45,000.0
Vitamin E. Int. Units minimum	2,240.0
Vitamin B-12, mgs. minimum	1.0
Menadione (Vitamin K), mgs. minimum	10.0
Riboflavin, mgs. minimum	120.0
d-Pantothenic Acid, mgs. minimum	120.0
Niacin, mgs. minimum	610.0
Choline, mgs. minimum	3,770.0
Folic Acid, mgs. minimum	80.0
Biotin, mgs. minimum	6.0
Thiamine, mgs. minimum	78.0
Vitamin B-6, mgs. minimum	74.0

Continued on next page

Coopers—Cont.

dl Methionine, minimum %	.1

How Supplied: 7.5 and 30 pound pails.

MULTI-PRIME®
B-Complex Vitamin/Iron Supplement For Dogs and Cats

Composition: Each fluid ounce contains:

Ferrous sulfate (Fe 0.414%)	334.0 mg
Choline dihydrogen citrate	100.0 mg
Inositol	100.0 mg
Niacinamide	100.0 mg
Thiamine mononitrate (vitamin B_1)	50.0 mg
d-Panthenol	10.0 mg
Riboflavin (vitamin B_2)	8.0 mg
Pyridoxine HCl (vitamin B_6)	5.0 mg
Cyanocobalamin (vitamin B_{12})	10.0 mcg
Alcohol	5% by volume

Ingredients: Sucrose, Water, Honey, Sorbitol, Alcohol, Ferrous Sulfate, Niacinamide, Choline Dihydrogen Citrate, Inositol, Citric Acid, Propylene, Glycol, Thiamine Mononitrate, Benzoic Acid, True Apple Flavor, d-Panthenol, Riboflavin, Pyridoxine Hydrochloride, Synthetic Apple Flavor, Cyanocobalamin.
Actions and Uses: An aromatic, palatable vitamin/iron liquid supplement flavored with pure honey and apple flavor, particularly for dogs and cats on poor rations or for run-down, debilitated individuals and for the very young.
Dosage and Administration: Administer orally, may be mixed with food.
PUPPIES and CATS: ½ to 1 teaspoonful daily.
ADULT DOGS: 1 tablespoonful daily for 30 days, then 1 to 2 teaspoonfuls daily.
How Supplied: 8 oz and 1 gallon bottles.

VI-NATURA®
Vitamin/Iron Nutritional Supplement For Horses
Compounded with pure honey

Composition: Each fluid ounce contains:

Ferrous sulfate (Fe 0.414%)	334.0 mg
Niacinamide	100.0 mg
Thiamine mononitrate (vitamin B_1)	50.0 mg
d-Panthenol	10.0 mg
Riboflavin (vitamin B_2)	8.0 mg
Pyridoxine HCl (vitamin B_6)	5.0 mg
Cyanocobalamin (vitamin B_{12})	10.0 mcg
Alcohol	5% by volume

Flavored with pure honey and apple flavor.
Action and Uses: An aromatic, palatable equine vitamin/iron liquid supplement flavored with pure honey and apple flavor, particularly for horses on poor quality rations or for rundown, debilitated individuals and for the very young. Contains iron, vitamin B_{12} and other B-complex vitamins.
Dosage and Administration: Add to feed at recommended amounts:
FOALS: ½ oz daily.
ORPHAN FOALS, COLTS and YEARLINGS: 1 oz daily.
MATURE HORSES: 3 oz daily for 15 days, then 1 oz daily.
For Veterinary Use Only
How Supplied: 1 qt and 1 gal plastic containers.

Evsco Pharmaceuticals
Affiliate of Immunogenetics, Inc.
P.O. BOX 209, HARDING HIGHWAY
BUENA, NJ 08310

HI-VITE™ DROPS
With Liver and Iron

Composition: Each fluid ounce contains: Vitamin A 150,000 I.U.; Vitamin D_2 24,000 I.U.; Vitamin E 50 I.U.; Vitamin B_1 (Thiamine HC1) 60 mg; Riboflavin (B_2) 16 mg; Pyridoxine HCI (B_6) 32 mg; Nicotinamide 240 mg; D-Panthenol 100 mg; Liver Fraction 13 g; Liver Extract 3 g; Iron (as Ferric Ammonium Citrate) 52 mg. Also contains sugar, sorbitol, Polysorbate 80, propylene glycol, peptone, citric acid, sodium saccharin, BHA (an antioxidant), water, Methyl Paraben (a preservative), Sodium Benzoate (a preservative).
Indications: A vitamin supplement with liver and iron added.
Dosage and Administration: *For puppies and kittens,* ½ dropperful twice daily. *Dogs and cats,* one dropperful 2-3 times daily. This water dispersible vitamin mixture may be mixed in milk or food; or may be given by dropping directly on the tongue if desired.
How Supplied: 1 oz (29.57 ml) bottles

LINOPLEX™

Composition: Each fluid oz (29.6 ml) contains:

Linoleic Acid	13.9 g
Oleic Acid	7.0 g
Linolenic Acid	1.3 g

(all as the glycerides and other fatty acids derived from soy bean oil and wheat germ oil)

Vitamin A	6000 I.U.
Vitamin D_2	600 I.U.
Vitamin E	15 I.U.

Also contains lecithin, polysorbate 80, sorbitan monooleate and Tenox 6.
Indications: An aid in the treatment and prevention of skin and coat disorders caused by vitamin and/or unsaturated fatty acids deficiencies.
Dosage: For dogs and cats administer once daily by adding to food.

Under 10 lbs	¼ teaspoonful
10-20 lbs	½ teaspoonful
20-30 lbs	¾ teaspoonful
30-50 lbs	1 teaspoonful

Over 50 lbs according to weight.
How Supplied: One gallon (128 fl ozs) (3.785 liters)

NUTRI-CAL®

Description: Each ounce contains: Vitamin A 5000 I.U.; Vitamin D 250 I.U.; Vitamin E 30 I.U.; Thiamine HCL (B_1) 10 mg; Riboflavin (B_2) 1 mg; Pyridoxine HCL (B_6) 5 mg; Vitamin B_{12} (Cyanocobalamin) 10 mcg; Nicotinamide 10 mg; Calcium Pantothenate 10 mg; Folic Acid 1 mg; Iron (from Iron peptonized) 2.5 mg; Manganese (from Manganese Sulfate) 5.0 mg; Magnesium (from Magnesium Sulfate) 2.0 mg; Iodine (from Potassium Iodide) 2.5 mg. Also contains fats [vegetable (soya bean oil) and animal (cod liver oil)]; carbohydrates (malt syrup, corn syrup, molasses), protein (peptone); Methyl Cellulose; with Sodium Benzoate as a preservative.
Product Use: Provides supplemental caloric and nutritional intake in dogs and cats. Will not burden the digestive tract. Also provides an additional source of energy for hunting and working dogs.
Directions for Use: Place a small amount in animal's mouth to acquaint the animal with its palatability and flavor. When used as a supplement, give 1½ teaspoons per 10 pounds of body weight daily. When used as a main source of nutrition, give 3 teaspoonsful (1 tablespoon) per 10 pounds of body weight daily.
How Supplied: 4¼ (120.5 grams) ounce tubes.

ORALGIENE™

Composition: Each Oralgiene tablet contains 500 mgs of available Amino Acids derived from vegetable and animal sources.
Indications: A palatable, chewable tablet for the control of objectionable breath odors due to digestive problems in dogs and cats.
Dosage and Administration: Oralgiene may be hand fed, or may be crumbled and placed in the animal's food.
Initial Dosage for Dogs and Cats: 5 to 20 lbs. 1–2 tablets daily 20–50 lbs. 2–3 tablets daily 50 lbs. and over 3 tablets daily.
Maintenance Dosage (after first week of therapy): 5 to 20 lbs. 1 tablet daily, 20 to 50 lbs. 1–2 tablets daily. Over 50 lbs. 2 tablets daily.
Daily dosage schedule should be administered in divided dosage and may be adjusted according to animal's response to therapy.
How Supplied: 60 tablet bottles.

IDENTIFICATION PROBLEM?
Consult the
Product Identification Section
where you'll find
products pictured
in full color.

Fort Dodge Laboratories, Inc.

800 FIFTH STREET
FORT DODGE, IA 50501

B-SOL® ℞
Sterile Solution

Indications: For prevention of Vitamin B Complex deficiencies in non-ruminating calves, nursing lambs, swine and horses. Symptoms of deficiency can include one or more of the following: inappetence, poor condition, enteritis, scours, anorexia and hypersensitivity.
Each ml. contains:

Thiamine Hydrochloride	10 mg
Riboflavin	2 mg
Pantheno	50 mg
Nicotinamide	100 mg
Pyridoxine Hydrochloride	2 mg
with benzyl alcohol 1.5% as preservative	0.1%

EDTA disodium salt, 0.55% chloride, 0.35% sodium, distilled water q.s.
Dosage and Administration:
Horses and non-ruminating calves: 1 ml. per 100 lb. bodyweight.
Nursing Lambs and Swine: 1 to 1.5 ml. per 100 lb. bodyweight.
Inject intramuscularly or subcutaneously using aseptic technique. Repeat as indicated.
Caution: Federal law restricts this drug to use by or on the order of a licensed veterinarian.
Keep out of reach of children.
How Supplied: 100 ml.

CAL-DEXTRO® NO. 2 ℞
Sterile Solution

Indications: A source of sterile injectable calcium, phosphorus, magnesium and dextrose for use in the treatment of milk fever (parturient paresis), grass tetany and other conditions in cattle, swine and sheep where calcium, phosphorous and magnesium deficiencies may occur.
Composition: Each ml. contains:

Calcium (as gluconate salt)	16.84 mg (8.42 g/500 ml)
Phosphorus	9.6 mg (4.8g/500 ml)
Magnesium	3.76 mg (1.88g/500 ml)
Dextrose	165.0 mg (82.5 g/500 ml)

With boric acid not more than 21.14 mg; bromine (as bromide) not more than 7.0 mg; sodium 2.0 mg; distilled water q.s.
Dosage and Administration: Administer intravenously, intramuscularly, subcutaneously or intraperitoneally. Warm to body temperature before administration to reduce any likelihood of shock reaction.
Cattle: 500 ml. to 750 ml.
Swine and Sheep: 50 ml. to 125 ml.
Precautions: This product should be administered using aseptic technique. Administration should be made slowly and to effect, with monitoring of the animal during administration. In cases where accelerated respiration rate or heart rate is observed during treatment, the administration should be stopped until these vital signs return to an acceptable rate at which time injection can be continued. If part or all dosage is given by subcutaneous or intramuscular administration, it is advised that a maximum of 25 ml. per injection site be used. Any unused portion should be discarded. Do not use if material has precipitated. Keep out of reach of children.
To Open Container: Wipe cap, top and neck of bottle with 70% alcohol. Screw down cap until a snap is heard indicating bottle top seal is broken. Carefully unscrew cap removing top of bottle. Attach sterile IV administration unit.
Caution: Federal law restricts this drug to use by or on the order of a licensed veterinarian.
How Supplied: Pkg. 12-500 ml.

CAL-DEXTRO® C ℞
Sterile Solution

Indications: A source of sterile injectable calcium for use in treatment of milk fever (parturient paresis) in cattle or in treatment of hypocalcemia in cattle, sheep, swine and horses.
Composition: Each ml. contains:

Calcium (as gluconate salt)	22.00 mg (11.0 g/500 ml)

With dextrose not more than 44.9 mg; boric acid not more than 25.2 mg; bromine (as bromide) not more than 7.0 mg; sodium 2.0 mg; distilled water q.s.
Dosage and Administration: Administer intravenously, intramuscularly, subcutaneously or intraperitoneally. Warm to body temperature before administration to reduce any likelihood of shock reaction.
Cattle and horses: 500 ml. to 750 ml.
Swine and sheep: 50 ml. to 125 ml.
Precautions: This product should be administered using aseptic technique. Administration should be made slowly and to effect, with monitoring of the animal during administration. In cases where accelerated respiration rate or heart rate is observed during treatment, the administration should be stopped until these vital signs return to an acceptable rate at which time injection can be continued. If part or all dosage is given by subcutaneous or intramuscular administration, it is advised that a maximum of 25 ml. per injection site be used. Any unused portion should be discarded. Do not use if material has precipitated.
Keep out of reach of children.
To Open Container: Wipe cap, top and neck of bottle with 70% alcohol. Screw down cap until a snap is heard indicating bottle top seal is broken. Carefully unscrew cap removing top of bottle. Attach sterile IV administration unit.
Caution: Federal law restricts this drug to use by or on the order of a licensed veterinarian.
How Supplied: Pkg. 12—500 ml.

CAL-DEXTRO® K ℞
Sterile Solution

Indications: A source of sterile injectable calcium, potassium and dextrose for treatment of milk fever (parturient paresis) in cattle.
Composition: Each ml. contains:

Calcium (as gluconate salt)	16.84 mg (8.42g/500 ml)
Potassium	1.04 mg (0.52 g/500 ml)
Dextrose	165.0 mg (82.5g/500 ml)

With boric acid not more than 21.14 mg; bromine (as bromide) not more than 7.0 mg; sodium 2.0 mg; chloride 0.9 mg; distilled water q.s.
Dosage and Administration: Administer intravenously, intramuscularly, subcutaneously or intraperitoneally. Warm to body temperature before administration to reduce any likelihood of shock reaction. ***Cattle***—500 ml. to 750 ml.
Precautions: This product should be administered using aseptic technique. Administration should be made slowly and to effect, with monitoring of the animal during administration. In cases where accelerated respiration rate or heart rate is observed during treatment, the administration should be stopped until these vital signs return to an acceptable rate at which time injection can be continued. If part or all dosage is given by subcutaneous or intramuscular administration, it is advised that a maximum of 25 ml. per injection site be used. Any unused portion should be discarded. Do not use if material has precipitated.
Keep out of reach of children.
To Open Container: Wipe cap, top and neck of bottle with 70% alcohol. Screw down cap until a snap is heard indicating bottle top seal is broken. Carefully unscrew cap removing top of bottle. Attach sterile IV administration unit.
Caution: Federal law restricts this drug to use by or on the order of a licensed veterinarian.
How Supplied: Pkg. 12-500 ml

CAL-DEXTRO® SPECIAL ℞
Sterile Solution

Indications: Use in cattle as an aid in the treatment of calcium, phosphorus, magnesium and glucose deficiencies.
Composition:
Each ml. contains:

Calcium (as gluconate salt)	22.00 mg. (11.0 g./500 ml)
Phosphorus	1.022 mg. (511 mg./500 ml)
Magnesium	0.402 mg. (201 mg./500 ml)
Dextrose	150.00 mg. (75.0 g./500 ml)

With boric acid not more than 25.17 mg; bromine (as bromide) not more than 7.0 mg; sodium 2.0 mg; distilled water q.s.
Dosage and Administration: Administer intravenously, intramuscularly, subcutaneously or intraperitoneally. Warm to body temperature before administration to reduce any likelihood of shock reaction.
Cattle: 500 ml. to 750 ml.
Precautions: This product should be administered using aseptic technique. Administration should be made slowly and to effect, with monitoring of the animal during administration. In cases where accelerated respiration rate or

Continued on next page

F

Fort Dodge—Cont.

heart rate is observed during treatment, the administration should be stopped until these vital signs return to an acceptable rate at which time injection can be continued. If part or all dosage is given by subcutaneous or intramuscular administration, it is advised that a maximum of 25 ml. per injection site be used. Any unused portion should be discarded. Do not use if material has precipitated. Keep out of reach of children.
To Open Container: Wipe cap, top and neck of bottle with 70% alcohol. Screw down cap until a snap is heard indicating bottle top seal is broken. Carefully unscrew cap removing top of bottle. Attach sterile IV administration unit.
Caution: Federal law restricts this drug to use by or on the order of a licensed veterinarian.
How Supplied: Pkg. 12-500 ml.

CLOVITE®
Conditioner For All Species of Animals

Composition:
Minimum Vitamin Guarantee (each pound contains):

Vitamin A	110,000 U.S.P. Units (242 u/gm)
Vitamin D	50,000 U.S.P. Units (110 u/gm)
Vitamin B_{12}	136 mcg (0.3 mcg/gm)

Ingredients: Soybean meal, Soy flour, Vitamin A and D oil, dicalcium phosphate, Vitamin B_{12} supplement, Vitamin D_3 supplement, Choline chloride, Vitamin E supplement, Calcium pantothenate, Niacin, Pyridoxine hydrochloride, Thiamine hydrochloride, Riboflavin, Biotin.
Dosage and Administration:
All Farm Animals: 1 to 3 lb. to each 100 lb. feed.
Mature Cattle (milking or on full feed): 1 to 3 lb. to each 100 lb. feed. Many dairymen prefer adding a handful to each feeding. Feedlot operators simply top off feed with the prescribed amount of Clovite.
Calves (bucket fed): 1 to 2 tablespoonfuls daily in milk or ground feed.
Range Cattle: Supplemental feeding is simplified by mixing with salt—1 part to 10 parts salt, or 2½ lb. to 25 lb. salt. (These calculations are based on normal consumption of ¼ lb. salt per day by a 1,000 lb. cow and ⅛ lb. per day by a 400 lb. steer.) To prevent the oxidation that tends to destroy all vitamin A compounds on prolonged exposure, mix only the amount normally consumed in a 3-week period.
Young Foals and Weanlings: 1 to 2 tablespoonfuls daily.
Brood Mares (latter half of pregnancy and lactation): 2 tablespoonfuls twice a day.
Ponies: 1 tablespoonful daily.
Colts, Stallions and Horses in training: 1 tablespoonful per 400 lb. daily.
Poultry: 1 lb. to each 100 lb. feed.
Baby Pigs: 3% of the creep-feed.
Mink: 1 level teaspoonful daily.
How Supplied: 5 lb. pail, 25 lb. bag, 100 lb. drum.

CLOVITE® + IRON
Conditioner
Vitamin Supplement
for All Species of Animals

Composition:
Minimum Vitamin Guarantee (each pound contains):

Vitamin A	110,000 U.S.P. Units (242 u/gm)
Vitamin D	50,000 U.S.P. Units 110 u/gm)
Vitamin B_{12}	136 mcg (0.3 mcg/gm)
Iron	1.6 gm (3.5 mg/gm)

Ingredients: Soybean meal, Soy flour, Vitamin A and D oil, Iron proteinate, Dicalcium phosphate, Butylated hydroxytoluene, Butylated hydroxyanisole (preservatives), Vitamin B_{12} supplement, Vitamin D_3 supplement, Choline chloride, Vitamin E supplement, Calcium pantothenate, Niacin, Pyridoxine hydrochloride, Thiamine hydrochloride, Riboflavin, Biotin.
Dosage and Administration:
Young Foals and Weanlings: 1 to 2 tablespoonfuls daily.
Brood Mares (latter half of pregnancy and lactation): 2 tablespoonfuls twice a day.
Colts, Stallions and Horses in Training: 1 tablespoonful per 400 lb. daily.
Ponies: 1 tablespoonful daily.
All Farm Animals: 1 to 3 lb. to each 100 lb. feed.
Mature Cattle (milking or on full feed): 1 to 3 lb. to each 100 lb. feed. Many dairymen prefer adding a handful to each feeding. Feedlot operators simply top off feed with the prescribed amount of Clovite®.
Calves (bucket fed): 1 to 2 tablespoonfuls daily in milk or ground feed.
Range Cattle: Supplemental feeding is simplified by mixing with salt—1 part to 10 parts salt, or 2½ lb. to 25 lb. salt. (These calculations are based on normal consumption of ¼ lb. of salt per day by a 1,000 lb. cow and ⅛ lb. per day by a 400 lb. steer.) To prevent the oxidation that tends to destroy all vitamin A compounds on prolonged exposure, mix only the amount normally consumed in a 3-week period.
Baby Pigs: 3% of the creep-feed.
Dogs and Cats: 1 to 4 teaspoonfuls daily.
Poultry: 1 lb. to each 100 lb. feed.
Mink: 1 level teaspoonful daily.
How Supplied: 5 lb. pail

CLOVITE® PET CONDITIONER
Vitamin Supplement

Composition: Minimum Vitamin Guarantee (each pound contains):

Vitamin A	110,000 U.S.P. Units (242 u./gm)
Vitamin D	50,000 U.S.P. Units (110 u./gm)
Vitamin B_{12}	136 mcg. (0.3 mcg./gm)

Ingredients: Soybean meal, Soy flour, Vitamin A and D oil, Dicalcium phosphate, Vitamin B_{12} supplement, Vitamin D_3 concentrate, Choline chloride, Vitamin E supplement, Calcium pantothenate, Niacin, Pyridoxine hydrochloride, Thiamine hydrochloride, Riboflavin, Biotin.
Dosage and Administration: ***Dogs and Cats***—1 level standard measuring teaspoonful per each 10 pounds of bodyweight daily. This dosage should be doubled for growing pups and kittens, lactating animals and animals in the last half of pregnancy. Dosage may be varied as prescribed by the veterinarian.
How Supplied: Pkg. 12—1 pound.

D-CA-FOS®
A Natural Bone Ash With Vitamin D_3 Supplement

Indications: A supplemental source of Vitamin D, calcium and phosphorus for animals which have rations known to be deficient in these nutrients.
Composition: Calcium (Ca) not less than 31.0%; Calcium (Ca) not more than 36.0%; Phosphorus (P) not less than 15.0%; Vitamin D_3 62,500 U.S.P. units per pound with starch and silicon dioxide.
Dosage and Administration:
Horses: 2 to 4 rounded tablespoonfuls per 500 lb. bodyweight.
Cattle: 3 to 5 rounded tablespoonfuls per 500 lb. bodyweight.
Sows: 4 to 8 rounded tablespoonfuls.
Dogs: 1 to 2 rounded teaspoonfuls per 10 lb. bodyweight.
May be mixed with the normal feed ration or thoroughly mixed with water and administered as a drench.
Will provide the recognized daily minimum requirements for these nutrients.
Caution: *Keep out of reach of children.*
How Supplied: Pkg. 12—1 pound. 25 lb. drum.

FERREXTRAN® 100
(iron dextran injection)

Description: Ferrextran 100 is a sterile solution containing the equivalent of 100mg of elemental iron per ml. with 0.5% phenol as preservative.
Action: Ferrextran 100 contains iron dextran complex which provides a rapidly absorbed and readily utilizable form of iron for the prevention and treatment of baby pig anemia.
Pig anemia retards growth and can cause death.
Iron deficiency is the main cause of baby pig anemia. Pigs are born with only small amounts of iron (approximately 50mg) in their bodies. In order to maintain health and realize maximum growth, a baby pig must receive from outside sources, 7 mg of iron per day for the first three weeks of life. The sow's milk, regardless of the feed she eats, can supply only about 1 mg of additional iron per pig per day. Thus, the need for a readily available outside iron source is apparent. Without this additional iron, over 90% of

F

the newborn pigs may develop anemia within the first few days of life. It has been shown by many investigators that pig anemia retards growth. Anemia lowers the body defense against disease, allowing for scours, pneumonia and other conditions to develop. Pig anemia can cause death and is capable of destroying entire litters.
Route of Administration: Ferrextran 100 is for intramuscular injection only.
Dosage:
Prevention—For the prevention of iron deficiency anemia, administer intramuscularly an amount of drug containing 100 to 150mg of elemental iron (1 to 1½ ml. of Ferrextran 100) to pigs from 1 to 3 days of age.
Treatment—For the treatment of iron deficiency anemia, administer intramuscularly an amount of drug containing 100 to 200mg of elemental iron (1 to 2 ml. of Ferrextran 100) per pig. Dosage may be repeated in 10 days to 2 weeks.
General Information: Ferrextran 100 is quickly absorbed, completely utilized and non-toxic. Ferrextran 100 provides high hemoglobin levels for the critical three week period and when used in proper dosages, "booster" doses are seldom necessary.
Years of experience have proven that usually baby pig losses are concentrated in the first three weeks of life. Overlaying and such diseases as joint ill, scours and hypoglycemia are most damaging during this period. Anemia may increase the susceptibility of the baby pig to these conditions.
Side Effects: Acute poisoning which may result in fatalities in extreme cases is characterized clinically by prostration with muscular weakness.
NOTICE: Organic iron preparations injected intramuscularly into pigs beyond 4 weeks of age may cause staining of the muscle tissue.
How Supplied: Ferrextran 100 is supplied in 100 ml. multiple dose vials containing the equivalent of 100mg of elemental iron per ml.

FERRISOL® SOLUTION

Indications: Use in animals as a dietary supplement for animals which have rations deficient in these trace minerals.
Composition: Each fluid ounce contains: Green Iron and Ammonium Citrate 1.3 gram; Copper Acetate 8.1 mg; Cobalt Sulfate 0.23 gram with corn sugar, sodium benzoate, water.
Dosage and Administration: Administer orally.
Horses: one (1) fluid ounce.
Cattle: two (2) fluid ounces.
Swine: ¼ to ½ teaspoonful per pig (diluted with equal amount of water if desired).
For suckling pigs: paint udder and teats of sow once or twice daily.
For older pigs: two (2) ounces per 100 pigs daily in drinking water.
Caution: Keep out of the reach of children.
How Supplied: 1 gallon.

V.A.L.® SYRUP
Alcohol 4.75% by Volume

Indications: Highly palatable source of B-vitamins; amino acids and liver fraction 1. Use in animals as a dietary B-complex supplement.
Composition: Each fluid ounce contains: Thiamine Hydrochloride 2 mg; Riboflavin 2 mg; Calcium Pantothenate 12 mg; Nicotinamide 15 mg; Pyridoxine Hydrochloride 2 mg; Protein Hydrolysates (as source of amino acids) 3.5 g; Liver Fraction 1.5 g; Aromatic Syrup base with Sodium Benzoate as a preservative q.s.
Dosage and Administration:
Dogs and cats weighing under 12 lbs. - 1 teaspooonful per day; 12 to 30 lbs. - 2 teaspoonfuls per day; 30 to 50 lbs. - 3 teaspoonfuls per day; over 50 lbs. - 4 teaspoonfuls per day.
For growing puppies and kittens double the dosage.
Horses and Cattle: 1 to 2 tablespoonfuls twice daily.
Caution:
Keep out of the reach of children.
How Supplied: Pkg. 12-5.5 oz.
1 gallon.

VITATONE®

Indications: Use in dogs and cats as a vitamin and mineral dietary supplement.
Composition: Minimum Guarantee (each pound contains):

Vitamins	
A	120,000 U.S.P. Units
D	10,000 U.S.P. Units
B_1 (Thiamine hydrochloride)	19 mg
B_2 (Riboflavin)	41 mg
Niacin	212 mg
d-Pantothenic Acid	177 mg
Choline	1,280 mg
Vitamin E	192 Units
Pyridixine Hydrochloride	22 mg
B_{12}	59 mcg
Folic acid	48 mg
Minerals	
Iodine (I)	.003%
Manganese (Mn)	.005%
Copper (Cu)	.007%
Cobalt (Co)	.004%
Iron (Fe)	.130%
Zinc (Zn)	.003%
Potassium (K)	.002%
Calcium (Ca)	2.0% min.—3.0% max.
Phosphorus (P)	1.6% min.—2.6% max.
Salt (NaCl)	1.3% min.—2.3% max.
Linoleic Acid	1.200%

Ingredients: Yeast culture, dried whey, dicalcium phosphate, soybean meal, wheat germ oil, vitamin A supplement, iron sulfate, vitamin B_{12} supplement, choline chloride, nicotinic acid, calcium pantothenate, vitamin E acetate, copper sulfate, zinc chelate, manganese sulfate, cobalt carbonate, riboflavin, vitamin D_3 supplement, thiamine hydrochloride, potassium iodide, pyridoxine hydrochloride.
Dosage: Orally per day. Growing puppies and kittens—2 level standard measuring teaspoons for each 10 pounds of bodyweight. Adult dogs and cats—1 level teaspoon for each 10 pounds bodyweight. Pregnant dogs and cats—increase the regular dosage by 50%. Lactating dogs and cats—the regular adult dosage should be doubled.
Caution: Keep out of the reach of children.
How Supplied: Pkg. 12—1 lb.

Gaines Pet Foods
General Foods Corporation
250 NORTH STREET
WHITE PLAINS, NY 10625

GAINES CYCLE® DOG FOODS

Cycle products are specifically formulated for the dog's stage of life—puppy, adult, older adult.
Dogs, like people, have changing nutritional needs. All dogs require the same basic nutrients with only the amounts varying depending on physiology and age.

GAINES CYCLE 1 FOR PUPPIES —Dry

Indications: Cycle 1 is a palatable product formulated for the nutritional needs of the growing puppy. It supplies more nutrients per unit of product than the leading full feeding products. Growth studies at the Gaines Nutrition Center demonstrate that Cycle 1 provides nutrients in the amounts needed for optimal growth. Cycle 1 is also indicated for hard working dogs, during pregnancy and lactation, and dogs under stressful conditions.
Ingredients: Ground Wheat, Soybean Meal, Meat and Bone Meal, Ground Corn, Animal Fat Preserved with BHA, Salt, Beef Digest, Iron Oxide, Zinc Oxide, Vitamin E Supplement, Vitamin A Supplement, Calcium Pantothenate, Vitamin B_{12} Supplement, Vitamin D Supplement, Riboflavin Supplement, Copper Oxide, Ethylenediamine Dihydriodide, Pyridoxine Hydrochloride, Thiamin Mononitrate.
Analyses:

Average Product Analyses

Protein	27.6%	Ash	7.7%
Fat	11.9%	Carbohydrate	40.2%
Fiber	3.7%	Moisture	8.9%
		Salt	1.4%

Ca:P 1.25:1

Contains 290 KCal Metabolizable Energy per 8 oz. cupful.
Digestibility:

Dry Matter	76%
Protein	81%

Vitamins and minerals are supplied at the following minimums:

Vitamins		
Vitamin A	2283	IU/lb
Vitamin D	228.3	IU/lb
Vitamin E	22.8	IU/lb
Thiamin	0.45	mg/lb
Riboflavin	1.0	mg/lb
Pantothenic Acid	4.57	mg/lb
Niacin	5.21	mg/lb
Pyridoxine	0.45	mg/lb
Folic Acid	0.08	mg/lb
Biotin	0.05	mg/lb
Vitamin B_{12}	0.01	mg/lb
Choline	548.4	mg/lb

Continued on next page

G

Gaines—Cont.

Minerals		
Calcium	1.1	%
Phosphorus	0.9	%
Potassium	0.6	%
Sodium Chloride	1.0	%
Magnesium	0.04	%
Iron	27.27	mg/lb
Copper	3.3	mg/lb
Manganese	2.3	mg/lb
Zinc	137.3	mg/lb
Iodine	0.70	mg/lb
Selenium	0.05	mg/lb

Feeding Instructions:

Body Weight	*Cups Per Day for Puppies*
Up to 5 lbs.	1–2
10	3
20	5
30	6½
40	8
50	9½
Over 50	Add 1 cup per 8 lbs. body weight.

Feedings per day should be adjusted according to the age of the puppy. We suggest the following:

Feedings Per Day	4	3	2	1
Age in Months	0–3	3–6	6–12	12–18 (giant breeds)

Adjust suggested feeding amounts depending upon size, age, exercise, environment, etc. Pregnant, lactating or hard working dogs may require one and one half times more food per pound of body weight as puppies of the same weight.

For maximum results use no supplements and should canned food be used, mix only Cycle 1 canned.

How Supplied: Available in 5, 10, and 25 pound bags.

GAINES CYCLE 2 FOR NORMALLY ACTIVE ADULTS—Dry

Indications: Cycle 2 provides good taste and superior nutrition for the normally active adult dog. It supplies all the nutrients known to be needed for maintenance of the adult dog. One of the key elements to the Cycle feeding concept is that to maximize adult response, longevity, and reduce the problems of overfeeding generally associated with full feeding or all purpose dog foods, an adult food should deliver maintenance nutrition.

Maintenance and life span studies continually in progress at the Gaines Nutrition Center demonstrate that Cycle 2 provides everything known to be needed for maintenance of the adult dog. Cycle 2 should not be used for puppies or for pregnant or lactating bitches since they will not be able to eat sufficient amounts for maximum performance.

Ingredients: Ground Corn, Ground Wheat, Meat and Bone Meal, Soybean Meal, Animal Fat Preserved with BHA, Salt, Calcium Carbonate, Beef Digest, Iron Oxide, Zinc Oxide, Vitamin E Supplement, Vitamin A Supplement, Calcium Pantothenate, Vitamin B_{12} Supplement, Vitamin D Supplement, Riboflavin Supplement, Copper Oxide, Ethylenediamine Dihydriodide, Pyridoxine Hydrochloride, Thiamin Mononitrate.

Analyses:

Average Product Analyses

Protein	20.2%	Ash	6.8%
Fat	10.9%	Carbohydrate	49.6%
Fiber	3.4%	Moisture	9.1%
		Salt	1.4%

Ca:P 1.25:1

Contains 272 KCal Metabolizable Energy per 8 oz. cupful.

Digestibility:

Dry Matter	78%
Protein	78%

Vitamins and minerals are supplied at the following minimums:

Vitamins		
Vitamin A	2077.00	IU/lb
Vitamin D	207.70	IU/lb
Vitamin E	20.80	IU/lb
Thiamin	0.42	mg/lb
Riboflavin	0.91	mg/lb
Pantothenic Acid	4.18	mg/lb
Niacin	4.73	mg/lb
Pyridoxine	0.42	mg/lb
Folic Acid	0.07	mg/lb
Biotin	0.04	mg/lb
Vitamin B_{12}	0.009	mg/lb
Choline	498.5	mg/lb
Minerals		
Calcium	1.00	%
Phosphorus	0.80	%
Potassium	0.55	%
Sodium Chloride	1.00	%
Magnesium	0.04	%
Iron	24.90	mg/lb
Copper	3.00	mg/lb
Manganese	2.10	mg/lb
Zinc	124.80	mg/lb
Iodine	0.64	mg/lb
Selenium	0.05	mg/lb

Feeding Instructions:

Body Weight	*Cups Per Day for Adults*
Up to 5 lbs.	1–2
10	3
20	5
30	6½
40	8
50	9½
Over 50	Add 1 cup per 8 lbs. body weight.

Adjust suggested feeding amounts depending upon size, age, exercise, environment, etc. Cycle 2 should not be used for growing, pregnant, lactating or hard working dogs.

For maximum results add no supplements and mix only canned Cycle 2 should canned food be used.

How Supplied: Available in 5, 10, and 25 lb. bags.

GAINES CYCLE 3 FOR THE LESS ACTIVE ADULT DOG—Dry

Indications: Many household pets are very inactive and, therefore, receive far too many calories and excessive protein when fed full feeding or all purpose dog foods. Cycle 3 has less protein and fewer calories than most dog foods. Studies at the Gaines Nutrition Center have demonstrated complete maintenance nutrition along with good taste.

Cycle 3 may also be conveniently used as a weight reduction diet. Because it has a higher fiber content, weight reduction programs are easier to stay with since the dog's appetite is fulfilled. Studies at the Gaines Nutrition Center have shown that weight reduction goals can be met in 4 to 6 weeks with proper feeding.

Cycle 3 should not be used for growth, pregnant or lactating bitches, or hard working dogs.

Ingredients: Wheat Middlings, Ground Corn, Soybean Meal, Meat and Bone Meal, Ground Wheat, Soybean Hulls, Animal Fat Preserved with BHA, Salt, Calcium Carbonate, Beef Digest, Iron Oxide, Zinc Oxide, Vitamin E Supplement, Vitamin A Supplement, Calcium Pantothenate, Vitamin B_{12} Supplement, Vitamin D Supplement, Riboflavin Supplement, Copper Oxide, Ethylenediamine Dihydriodide, Pyridoxine Hydrochloride, Thiamin Mononitrate.

Analyses:

Average Product Analyses

Protein	20.6%	Ash	5.7%
Fat	9.8%	Carbohydrate	47.2%
Fiber	7.0%	Moisture	9.7%
		Salt	1.0%

Ca:P 1.2:1

Contains 244 KCal Metabolizable Energy per 8 oz. cupful.

Digestibility:

Dry Matter	66%
Protein	76%

Vitamins and minerals are supplied at the following minimums:

Vitamins		
Vitamin A	2077.00	IU/lb
Vitamin D	207.70	IU/lb
Vitamin E	20.80	IU/lb
Thiamin	0.42	mg/lb
Riboflavin	0.91	mg/lb
Pantothenic Acid	4.18	mg/lb
Niacin	4.13	mg/lb
Pyridoxine	0.42	mg/lb
Folic Acid	0.07	mg/lb
Biotin	0.04	mg/lb
Vitamin B_{12}	0.009	mg/lb
Choline	498.50	mg/lb
Minerals		
Calcium	1.00	%
Phosphorus	0.80	%
Potassium	0.55	%
Sodium Chloride	1.00	%
Magnesum	0.04	%
Iron	24.90	mg/lb
Copper	3.00	mg/lb
Manganese	2.10	mg/lb
Zinc	124.80	mg/lb
Iodine	0.64	mg/lb
Selenium	0.05	mg/lb

Feeding Instructions:

Body Weight	*Cups Per Day for Adults*
Up to 5 lbs.	1–2
10	3
20	5
30	6½
40	8
50	9½
Over 50	Add 1 cup per 8 lbs. body weight.

For best results follow the feeding instructions. For weight reduction reduce the recommended quantities slightly. Weight reductions should be made over a four to eight week period.

For client aid booklets on obesity and weight reduction, write Gaines Cycle 3, Rt. 3 Hieland Rd., St. Anne, Ill. 60964

How Supplied: Available in 5, and 10, pound bags.

GAINES CYCLE 4 FOR THE OLDER (OVER 7 YEARS) ADULT DOG—Dry

Indications: Cycle 4 provides a unique formula for maintenance of older dogs. Full Feeding (general purpose) dog foods over-deliver protein and calories for the older dog. Cycle 4 provides a lower quantity of a higher quality (better amino acid balance) protein along with fewer calories and lower quantities of calcium, phosphorus, and salt for more appropriate nutritional maintenance of the dog over 7 years of age.

Ingredients: Ground Corn, Ground Wheat, Soybean Meal, Animal Fat Preserved with BHA, Meat and Bone Meal, Heat Processed Soybeans, Dried Whey Product, Calcium Carbonate, Dried Whey, Dried Skim Milk, dl-Methionine, Beef Digest, Cereals Distillers Dried Solubles, Salt, Iron Oxide, Choline Chloride, Zinc Oxide, Vitamin E Supplement, Calcium Pantothenate, Vitamin B_{12} Supplement, Vitamin A Supplement, Riboflavin Supplement, Niacin, Pyridoxine Hydrochloride, Vitamin D Supplement, Copper Oxide, Ethylenediamine Dihydriodide, Biotin, Thiamin Mononitrate.

Analyses:

Average Product Analyses

Protein	19.2%	Ash	6.0%
Fat	9.7%	Carbohydrate	52.3%
Fiber	3.4%	Moisture	9.4%
Calcium	0.5%	Salt	0.3%
Phosphorus	0.4%		

Ca:P 1.2:1

Contains 263 KCal Metabolizable Energy per 8 oz. cupful.

Digestibility:

Dry Matter	79%
Protein	79%

Vitamins and minerals are supplied at the following levels:

Vitamins		
Vitamin A	NLT	3115.60 IU/lb
Vitamin D	NLT	311.60 IU/lb
Vitamin E	NLT	31.20 IU/lb
Thiamin	NLT	0.82 mg/lb
Riboflavin	NLT	1.82 mg/lb
Pantothenic Acid	NLT	8.30 mg/lb
Niacin	NLT	9.50 mg/lb
Pyridoxine	NLT	0.82 mg/lb
Folic Acid	NLT	0.07 mg/lb
Biotin	NLT	0.08 mg/lb
Vitamin B_{12}	NLT	0.02 mg/lb
Choline	NLT	996.98 mg/lb
Minerals		
Calcium	NLT	0.5 %
Phosphorus	NLT	0.4 %
Potassium	NLT	0.50 %
Sodium Chloride	NMT	0.3 %
Magnesium	NLT	0.04 %
Iron	NLT	24.90 mg/lb
Copper	NLT	3.00 mg/lb
Manganese	NLT	2.10 mg/lb
Zinc	NLT	124.80 mg/lb
Iodine	NLT	0.64 mg/lb
Selenium	NLT	0.05 mg/lb

NLT = not less than
NMT = not more than

Feeding Instructions:

Body Weight	*Cups Per Day for Adults*
Up to 25 lbs.	1–3
25–50	3–5
50–90	5–8
Over 90	1 cup per 12 lbs. of body weight.

For best results, adjust feeding amounts depending upon size, age, exercise, environment, etc. Do not use for growth, pregnant or lactating bitches, or hard working dogs. Use no supplements. Should canned dog food be used, mix only with Cycle 4 canned.

How Supplied: Supplied in 5 and 10 pound bags.

GAINES CYCLE 1 FOR PUPPIES—Canned

Indications: Cycle 1 is a palatable product formulated for the nutritional needs of the growing puppy. it supplies more nutrients per unit of product than the leading full feeding products. Growth studies at the Gaines Nutrition Center demonstrate that Cycle 1 provides nutrients in the amounts needed for optimal growth. Cycle 1 is also indicated for hard working dogs, during pregnancy and lactation, and dogs under stressful conditions.

Ingredients (beef flavor): Water, Soybean Grits, Beef By-Products, Chicken, Wheat Flour, Animal Fat Preserved with BHA, Soybean Flour, Dicalcium Phosphate, Salt, Caramel Color, Soybean Oil, Choline Chloride, Iron Oxide, Xanthan Gum, Artificial Flavor, Magnesium Oxide, Ferrous Sulfate, Zinc Oxide, Vitamin E Supplement, Ethoxyquin (a preservative), Calcium Pantothenate, Vitamin A Supplement, Copper Oxide, Vitamin B_{12} Supplement, Niacin, Manganous Oxide, Biotin, Vitamin D Supplement, Riboflavin Supplement, Pyridoxine Hydrochloride, Ethylenediamine Dihydriodide, Thiamin Mononitrate, Folic Acid.

Analyses:

Average Product Analyses

Protein	11.0%	Ash	2.5%
Fat	6.7%	Carbohydrate	8.4%
Fiber	0.8%	Moisture	70.6%
		Salt	0.44%

Ca:P 1.22:1

Contains 497 KCal Metabolizable Energy per 14 oz. can.

Digestibility:

Dry Matter	81%
Protein	83%

Vitamins and minerals are supplied at the following minimums (% or per pound):

Vitamins		
Vitamin A	723.5	IU
Vitamin D	72.3	IU
Vitamin E	7.20	IU
Thiamin	0.15	mg
Riboflavin	0.32	mg
Pantothenic Acid	1.45	mg
Niacin	1.65	mg
Pyridoxine	0.15	mg
Folic Acid	0.02	mg
Biotin	0.01	mg
Vitamin B_{12}	0.003	mg
Choline	174.00	mg
Minerals		
Calcium	0.35	%
Phosphorus	0.29	%
Potassium	0.19	%
Sodium Chloride	0.32	%
Magnesium	0.013	%
Iron	8.7	mg
Copper	1.04	mg
Manganese	0.73	mg
Zinc	15.90	mg
Iodine	0.22	mg
Selenium	0.016	mg

Feeding Instructions:

Body Weight (lbs.)	*Cans/Day for Puppies*
5 & Under	½–1
5–10	1–2
10–20	2–3
20–30	3–4
30–40	4–5
Over 40	1 can per 10 lbs. of body weight

Feeding per day should be adjusted according to the age of the puppy. We suggest the following:

Feedings Per Day	4	3	2	1
Age in Months	0–3	3–6	6–12	12–18 (giant breeds)

Adjust suggested feeding amounts depending upon size, age, exercise, environment, etc. Pregnant, lactating or hard working dogs may require one and one half times more food per pound of body weight as puppies of the same weight. For maximum results, use no supplements. Cycle 1 canned may be mixed with Cycle 1 dry for variety.

How Supplied: Available in 14 oz. cans. Also in liver, chicken, and beef and cheese flavors.

G

GAINES CYCLE 2 FOR NORMALLY ACTIVE ADULTS—Canned

Indications: Cycle 2 provides good taste and superior nutrition for the normally active adult dog. It supplies all the nutrients known to be needed for maintenance of the adult dog. One of the key elements to the Cycle feeding concept is that to maximize adult response, longevity, and reduce the problems of overfeeding generally associated with full feeding or all purpose dog foods, an adult food should deliver maintenance nutrition. Maintenance and life span studies continually in progress at the Gaines Nutrition Center demonstrate that Cycle 2 provides everything known to be needed for maintenance of the adult dog. Cycle 2 should not be used for puppies or for pregnant or lactating bitches since they will not be able to eat sufficient amounts for maximum performance.

Ingredients (beef flavor): Water, Beef By-Products, Chicken, Wheat Flour, Soybean Grits, Dicalcium Phosphate, Salt, Caramel Color, Soybean Oil, Potassium Chloride, Choline Chloride, Iron Oxide, Xanthan Gum, Artificial Flavor, Magnesium Oxide, Ferrous Sulfate, Zinc Oxide, Vitamin E Supplement, Ethoxyquin (a preservative), Calcium Pantothenate, Vitamin A Supplement, Copper Oxide, Vitamin B_{12} Supplement, Manganese Oxide, Niacin, Biotin, Vitamin D Supplement, Riboflavin Supplement, Pyridox-

Continued on next page

Gaines—Cont.

ine Hydrochloride, Ethylenediamine Dihydriodide, Thiamin Mononitrate, Folic Acid.

Analyses

Average Product Analyses

Protein	8.3%	Ash	2.5%
Fat	6.3%	Carbohydrate	8.8%
Fiber	0.6%	Moisture	73.5%
		Salt	0.39%

Ca:P 1.27:1

Contains 456 KCal Metabolizable Energy per 14 oz. can.

Digestibility:

Dry Matter	85%
Protein	84%

Vitamins and minerals are supplied at the following minimums (per pound):

Vitamins		
Vitamin A	590.0	IU
Vitamin D	59.0	IU
Vitamin E	5.9	IU
Thiamin	0.12	mg
Riboflavin	0.26	mg
Pantothenic Acid	1.18	mg
Niacin	0.34	mg
Pyridoxine	0.12	mg
Folic Acid	0.02	mg
Biotin	0.01	mg
Vitamin B_{12}	0.003	mg
Choline	142.0	mg
Minerals		
Calcium	0.29	%
Phosphorus	0.23	%
Potassium	0.16	%
Sodium Chloride	0.29	%
Magnesium	0.01	%
Iron	7.1	mg
Copper	0.86	mg
Manganese	0.59	mg
Zinc	15.9	mg
Iodine	0.18	mg
Selenium	0.01	mg

Feeding Instructions

Body Weight (lbs.)	*Cans/Day*
Up to 12	½–1
12–25	1–2
25–50	2–3
50–90	3–5
Over 90	1 can/20 lbs. of body weight

Adjust suggested feeding amounts depending upon size, age, exercise, environment, etc. Cycle 2 should not be used for growing, pregnant, lactating or hard working dogs.

For maximum results, add no supplements and mix only with Cycle 2 dry.

How Supplied: Available in 14 oz. cans. Also in liver, chicken, and beef and cheese flavors.

GAINES CYCLE 3 FOR THE LESS ACTIVE ADULT DOG—Canned

Indications: Many household pets are very inactive and, therefore, receive far too many calories and excessive protein when fed full feeding or all purpose dog foods. Cycle 3 has less protein and fewer calories than most dog foods. Studies at the Gaines Nutrition Center have demonstrated complete maintenance nutrition along with good taste.

Ingredients (beef flavor): Water, Chicken, Soybean Grits, Wheat Flour, Beef By-Products, Soybean Hulls, Dicalcium Phosphate, Salt, Beef Digest, Caramel Color, Soybean Oil, Potassium Chloride, Choline Chloride, Iron Oxide, Xanthan Gum, Artificial Flavor, Vitamin E Supplement, Ethoxyquin (a preservative), Magnesium Oxide, Ferrous Sulfate, Zinc Oxide, Calcium Pantothenate, Vitamin A Supplement, Vitamin B_{12} Supplement, Niacin, Biotin, Vitamin D Supplement, Riboflavin Supplement, Pyridoxine Hydrochloride, Copper Oxide, Thiamin Mononitrate, Manganous Oxide, Ethylenediamine Dihydriodide, Folic Acid.

Analyses:

Average Product Analyses

Protein	8.0%	Ash	2.4%
Fat	3.6%	Carbohydrate	9.8%
Fiber	2.0%	Moisture	74.2%
		Salt	0.39%

Ca:P 1.20:1

Contains 372 KCal Metabolizable Energy per 14 oz. can.

Digestibility:

Dry Matter	72%
Protein	79%

Vitamins and minerals are supplied at the following minimums (per pound):

Vitamins		
Vitamin A	590.0	IU
Vitamin D	59.0	IU
Vitamin E	5.9	IU
Thiamin	0.12	mg
Riboflavin	0.26	mg
Pantothenic Acid	1.18	mg
Niacin	1.35	mg
Pyridoxine	0.12	mg
Folic Acid	0.02	mg
Biotin	0.01	mg
Vitamin B_{12}	0.002	mg
Choline	141.6	mg
Minerals		
Calcium	0.30	%
Phosphorus	0.23	%
Potassium	0.16	%
Sodium Chloride	0.29	%
Magnesium	0.01	%
Iron	7.1	mg
Copper	0.86	mg
Manganese	0.59	mg
Zinc	15.90	mg
Iodine	0.18	mg
Selenium	0.01	mg

Feeding Instructions:

Body Weight (lbs.)	*Cans/Day*
Up to 12	½–1
12–25	1–2
25–50	2–3
50–90	3–5
Over 90	1 can/20 lbs. of body weight

For best results, follow the feeding instructions. Mix only with Cycle 3 dry.

For weight reduction reduce the recommended quantities slightly. Weight reductions should be made over a four to eight week period.

For client aid booklets on obesity and weight reduction write Gaines Cycle 3, Rt. 3 Hieland Rd., St. Anne, Ill. 60946

How Supplied: Available in 14 oz. cans. Also in liver, chicken, and beef and cheese flavors.

GAINES CYCLE 4 FOR THE OLDER DOG (OVER 7 YEARS) ADULT DOG —Canned

Indications: Cycle 4 provides a unique formula for maintenance of older dogs. Full Feeding (general purpose) dog foods over-deliver protein and calories for the older dog. Cycle 4 provides a lower quantity of a higher quality (better amino acid balance) protein along with fewer calories and lower quantities of calcium, phosphorus, and salt for more appropriate nutritional maintenance of the dog over 7 years of age.

Ingredients (beef flavor): Water, Chicken, Wheat Flour, Beef By-Products, Soybean Hulls, Soybean Meal, Dicalcium Phosphate, Animal Fat Preserved with BHA, Heat Processed Soybeans, Dried Whey Product, Beef Digest, Caramel Color, Choline Chloride, Soybean Oil, Dried Whey, Salt, Dried Skim Milk, Iron Oxide, Cereals Distillers Dried Solubles, dl-Methionine, Xanthan Gum, Magnesium Oxide, Artificial Flavor, Ferrous Sulfate, Zinc Oxide, Vitamin E Supplement, Ethoxyquin (A Preservative), Calcium Pantothenate, Vitamin A Supplement, Copper Oxide, Manganous Oxide, Vitamin B_{12} Supplement, Niacin, Biotin, Vitamin D Supplement, Riboflavin Supplement, Ethylenediamine Dihydriodide, Pyridoxine Hydrochloride, Thiamin Mononitrate, Folic Acid.

Analyses:

Average Product Analyses

Protein	6.3%	Ash	2.7%
Fat	4.6%	Carbohydrate	9.3%
Fiber	2.5%	Moisture	74.6%
Calcium	0.52%	Essential Fatty Acids	0.89%
Phosphorus	0.39%	Salt	0.10%

Ca:P 1.3:1

Contains 387 KCal Metabolizable Energy per 14 oz. can.

Digestibility:

Dry Matter	71%
Protein	78%

Vitamins and minerals are supplied at the following levels (per pound):

Vitamins			
Vitamin A	NLT	884.5	IU
Vitamin D	NLT	88.5	IU
Vitamin E	NLT	8.8	IU
Thiamin	NLT	0.24	mg
Riboflavin	NLT	0.52	mg
Pantothenic Acid	NLT	2.36	mg
Niacin	NLT	2.69	mg
Pyridoxine	NLT	0.24	mg
Folic Acid	NLT	0.02	mg
Biotin	NLT	0.024	mg
Vitamin B_{12}	NLT	0.005	mg
Choline	NLT	283.0	mg
Minerals			
Calcium	NLT	0.15	%
Phosphorus	NLT	0.11	%
Potassium	NLT	0.16	%
Sodium Chloride	NMT	0.15	%
Magnesium	NLT	0.01	%
Iron	NLT	7.1	mg
Copper	NLT	0.86	mg
Manganese	NLT	0.59	mg
Zinc	NLT	15.9	mg
Iodine	NLT	0.18	mg
Selenium	NLT	0.01	mg

NLT = not less than

NMT = not more than

Feeding Instructions:

Body Weight (lbs.)	*Cans/Day*
Up to 12	½–1
12–25	1–2
25–50	2–3
50–90	3–5
Over 90	1 can/20 lbs. of body weight

For best results, adjust feeding amounts depending upon size, age, exercise, environment, etc. Do not use for growth, pregnant or lactating bitches, or hard working dogs. Use no supplements. Mix only with Cycle 4 dry.
How Supplied: Available in 14 oz. cans. Also in liver, chicken, and beef and cheese flavors.

Glenwood Inc.

83 N. SUMMIT STREET
TENAFLY, NJ 07670

CALPHOSAN® SOLUTION
(Veterinary)
intramuscular/subcutaneous calcium solution

Composition: CALPHOSAN solution, each 10 ml. contains 50 mg. calcium glycerophosphate, 50 mg. calcium lactate and 0.25% phenol (as preservative), in a physiological solution of sodium chloride.
Advantages: Intramuscular or subcutaneous injections of CALPHOSAN raise blood serum calcium levels, without pain, inflammatory reactions or sloughing.
Indications: For use as an aid in the treatment of canine eclampsia.
Administration: SMALL DOGS—5 to 10 ml. subcutaneously (back of neck) or intramuscularly. LARGE DOGS—10 ml. for each 100 lbs. of body weight, or as indicated.
Contraindications: As there is a similarity in the actions of calcium and digitalis on the contractility and excitability of the heart muscle, CALPHOSAN is contraindicated in fully digitalized animals.
Availability: CALPHOSAN SOLUTION (Veterinary) 60 ml—NDC 0516-0060-66 and 250 ml. vials—NDC 0516-0060-44.
CALPHOSAN SUSPENSION (Veterinary) . . . ten times the concentration of CALPHOSAN SOLUTION (Veterinary) . . . is available for use as an aid in the supportive treatment of milk fever in cattle.

CALPHOSAN® SUSPENSION
(Veterinary)
intramuscular calcium suspension

Composition: Ten times the concentration of Calphosan Solution . . . for use in large animals. Calphosan is a specially processed suspension of calcium glycerophosphate and calcium lactate in a physiological solution of sodium chloride. Each 1 ml. of CALPHOSAN SUSPENSION contains 50 mg. calcium glycerophosphate, 50 mg. calcium lactate, and 0.25% phenol (as preservative).
Advantages: Deep intramuscular injections of CALPHOSAN SUSPENSION raise blood serum calcium levels, without pain, inflammatory reactions or sloughing.
Indications: For use as an aid in the supportive treatment of milk fever in cattle.
Administration: DAIRY CATTLE—30 to 60 ml. by **deep** intramuscular injection . . . alone or in combination with intravenous calcium. In more severe cases, an additional administration may be required the following day.
Contraindications: As there is a similarity in the actions of calcium and digitalis on the contractility and excitability of the heart muscle, CALPHOSAN is contraindicated in fully digitalized animals. **Any** suspension may cause the development of an aseptic abscess when injected. This event has been reported very rarely with use of Calphosan Suspension, and the probability is negligible.
Availability: CALPHOSAN SUSPENSION (Veterinary) in 30 ml.—NDC 0516-0080-33 and 240 ml. vials—NDC 0516-0080-44.
CALPHOSAN SOLUTION (Veterinary) . . . one-tenth the concentration of CALPHOSAN SUSPENSION (Veterinary) . . . is available for use as an aid in the treatment of canine eclampsia.

Haver

Mobay Corporation
Animal Health Division
SHAWNEE, KS 66201

HAVOLAC™ FOOD SUPPLEMENT

Composition: Non-fat milk solids; Soya Bean oil; Lactose; Vitamin A concentrate; Vitamin D concentrate; Moisture, Protein, 7.31%; Fat, 6.5%; Carbohydrates, 10.23%; Mineral content, 1.46%; Moisture, 74.5%; and Calories, 40, per fluid ounce. Analysis: Protein, 30.00 gm; Fat, 26.72 gm; Carbohydrate 42.10 gm; Calcium, 1026 mg; Phosphorus, 796 mg; Potassium, 1179 mg; Magnesium, 99 mg; Chlorine, 995 mg; Sodium, 490 mg; Copper, 0.108 mg; Iron, 0.383 mg; Thiamine, 0.245 mg; Riboflavin, 1.69 mg; Niacin, 0.88 mg; Ascorbic acid, 4.75 mg; Vitamin A, 2170 USP; Vitamin D, 566, Fatty acid composition: Saturated, 17.3%; Total Oleic, 58.5% Linoleic, 22.8%; Linolenic, 1.3%; and Arachidoni O.
Indications: Animal milk replacer and food supplement for dogs, cats and other pets.
Dosage and Administration: ***Puppies and kittens***—½ ounce (1 tablespoon per pound) of body weight in addition to normal diet. Increase slightly for small breeds and decrease for larger breeds. ***Adult cats***—3 ounces per day; ***Adult dogs***—1 ounce for each 5 lbs of body weight.
How Supplied:
Code: 0627—12 oz cans

Hill's Pet Products, Inc.

P.O. BOX 148
TOPEKA, KANSAS 66601

SCIENCE DIET® CANINE GROWTH®

Description: Science Diet Canine Growth is a nutrionally balanced diet specifically designed to be fed during the vital growth period of puppyhood (from weaning until maturity). It supplies the high protein, high energy, and balanced vitamins and minerals that puppies need, in a portion size they can easily eat. With Canine Growth, puppies receive the sound healthy foundation necessary for an optimum adult life.
Major Ingredients: *Dry:* Ground Corn, Poultry By-Product Meal, Soy Grits, Animal Fat (Preserved with BHA, Propyl Gallate, Citric Acid), Dried Whole Egg, Meat Meal, Brewers Rice, Vegetable Oil.
Canned:
Water, Meat By-Products, Ground Barley, Chicken, Ground Corn, Liver, Soy Grits, Animal Fat, Wheat Germ Meal, Vegetable Oil.
Average Analysis: (as fed)

Dry	
Moisture	9.0%
Dry Matter	91.0%
Protein	27.0%
Fat	18.5%
NFE	34.5%
Ash	7.5%
Fiber	3.5%
Calcium	1.5%
Phosphorus	1.2%
Sodium	0.42%
Potassium	0.87%
ME (kcal/lb.)	1843
ME (kcal/cup)	384
Canned:	
Moisture	69.4%
Dry Matter	30.6%
Protein	8.9%
Fat	6.6%
NFE	12.2%
Ash	2.3%
Fiber	0.6%
Calcium	0.40%
Phosphorus	0.31%
Sodium	0.12%
Potassium	0.25%
ME (kcal/can)	615

Dry Weight Analysis:

Dry:	
Protein	29.6%
Fat	20.3%
NFE	37.9%
Ash	8.2%
Fiber	3.8%
Calcium	1.6%
Phosphorus	1.3%
Sodium	0.46%
Potassium	0.96%
Canned:	
Protein	29.1%
Fat	21.6%
NFE	39.9%
Ash	7.5%
Fiber	2.0%
Calcium	1.3%

Continued on next page

Hill's—Cont.

Phosphorus 1.0%
Sodium 0.39%
Potassium 0.82%

Recommended Feeding

Dry:

Canine Growth can be offered to your puppy 2 or 3 times a day for 20 minutes. Allow him to eat whatever amount he wants and remove the remaining Growth. This method of feeding is recommended from the time the puppy is weaned until it reaches most of its adult size. Usually 6 months for small breeds to as much as 14 months for large dogs. Very young puppies (4–5 weeks) may be fed Canine Growth dampened slightly with water, if necessary. Supplemenation is not necessary. Feed dry as soon as the puppy is able to chew. When the puppy has attained adult size, switch to Canine Maintenance.

Canned:

Feed puppies 2 or 3 times a day, as much food as they will eat in a 20 to 30 minute period. The unused portion should be refrigerated, but returned to room temperature before the remainder is fed. This method can be used from weaning through the period of maximum growth. When mature, they should be changed to Canine Maintenance, either canned or dry.

Packaging

Canine Growth is available in 10 lb., 20 lb., and 40 lb. bags, and 15½ oz. cans, 24 cans per case.

SCIENCE DIET® CANINE MAINTENANCE®

Description: Science Diet Canine Maintenance is formulated to meet the requirements of adult dogs. Because of its high digestibility and caloric density, Canine Maintenance is biologically efficient and therefore requires minimum food intake. In addition, stool volume is greatly reduced. Canine Maintenance is a nutritionally complete diet which requires no supplementation.

Major Ingredients: *Dry:* Ground Corn, Meat Meal, Soy Grits, Brewers Rice, Animal Fat (preserved with BHA, Propyl Gallate, Citric Acid), Wheat Bran, Dried Whole Egg, Brewers Dried Yeast, Vegetable Oil.

Canned:

Water, Meat By-Products, Chicken, Ground Barley, Ground Corn, Liver, Soy Grits, Wheat Germ Meal, Vegetable Oil.

Average Analysis (as fed)

Dry:

Moisture 9.0%
Dry Matter 91.0%
Protein 23.0%
Fat 14.5%
NFE 45.9%
Ash 4.3%
Fiber 3.3%
Calcium 0.6%
Phosphorus 0.6%
Sodium 0.33%
Potassium 0.65%
ME (kcal/lb.) 1752
ME (kcal/cup) 336

Canned:

Moisture 71.7%
Dry Matter 28.3%
Protein 7.8%
Fat 5.5%
NFE 12.9%
Ash 1.7%
Fiber 0.4%
Calcium 0.24%
Phosphorus 0.17%
Sodium 0.13%
Potassium 0.26%
ME (kcal/can) 570

Dry Weight Analysis:

Dry:

Protein 25.3%
Fat 15.9%
NFE 50.4%
Ash 4.7%
Fiber 3.6%
Calcium 0.66%
Phosphorus 0.66%
Sodium 0.36%
Potassium 0.71%

Canned:

Protein 27.5%
Fat 19.4%
NFE 45.6%
Ash 6.0%
Fiber 1.4%
Calcium 0.85%
Phosphorus 0.60%
Sodium 0.50%
Potassium 0.92%

Recommended Feeding:

A guide to daily feeding for Canine Maintenance is as follows:

Weight of dog	Suggested Feeding
10 lbs.	1 cup or ⅔ can
20 lbs.	2 cups or 1¼ can
40 lbs.	3½ cups or 2 cans
60 lbs.	4¾ cups or 2½ cans
80 lbs.	5¾ cups or 3¼ cans
100 lbs.	7 cups or 3¾ cans

Food requirements may vary depending on breed, environment, exercise, temperament and stress factors. Adjustments of intake may be necessary for individual animals.

Packaging

Canine Maintenance is available in 10 lb., 20 lb., 40 lb. bags, and 15½ oz. cans, 24 cans per case.

SCIENCE DIET® CANINE PERFORMANCE®

Description: Active dogs require increased energy to match their increased physical activity. Activities such as field trials, dog shows, obedience trials, hunting, guard duty, etc. produce the need for a high energy, nutritionally balanced food that gives the dog the capability to perform to his optimum potential and the added conditioning he needs. Science Diet Canine Performance is scientifically formulated to meet this specific need.

Major Ingredients: *Dry:* Ground Corn, Poultry By-Product Meal, Animal Fat (preserved with BHA, Propyl Gallate, Citric Acid), Dried Whole Egg, Peanut Hulls (a source of fiber), Brewers Dried Yeast.

Canned:

Water, Chicken, Liver, Meat By-Products, Ground Corn, Brewers Rice.

Average Analysis (as fed)

Moisture 9.0%
Dry Matter 91.0%
Protein 28.0%
Fat 23.8%
NFE 31.2%
Ash 4.9%
Fiber 3.1%
Calcium 1.0%
Phosphorus 0.7%
Sodium 0.37%
Potassium 0.58%
ME (kcal/lb.) 2016
ME (kcal/cup) 568

Canned:

Moisture 72.1%
Dry Matter 27.9%
Protein 8.2%
Fat 8.9%
NFE 9.0%
Ash 1.6%
Fiber 0.2%
Calcium 0.25%
Phosphorous 0.20%
Sodium 0.12%
Potassium 0.19%
ME (K cal/can) 664

Dry Weight Analysis:

Dry:

Protein 30.76%
Fat 26.2%
NFE 34.2%
Ash 5.4%
Fiber 3.4%
Calcium 1.1%
Phosphorus 0.77%
Sodium 0.41%
Potassium 0.64%

Canned:

Protein 29.4%
Fat 31.9%
NFE 32.3%
Ash 5.7%
Fiber 0.7%
Calcium 0.9%
Phosphorous 0.7%
Sodium 0.43%
Potassium 0.61%

Recommended Feeding:

Weight of dog	Suggested Feeding
10 lbs.	⅔ cup or ½ can
20 lbs.	1¼ cups or 1 can
40 lbs.	2 cups or 1¾ cans
60 lbs.	2¾ cups or 2 cans
80 lbs.	3½ cups or 2¾ cans
100 lbs.	4 cups or 3¼ cans

Food requirements will vary depending on breed, evironment, temperament and stress factors. Food intake should be adjusted to maintain optimum body weight.

Packaging

Canine Performance is available in 20 lb. bags and 15½ oz cans, 24 cans per case.

SCIENCE DIET® CANINE SENIOR®

Description: Science Diet Canine Senior is formulated to supply the different nutritional needs required by older dogs because of subtle changes which alter the physiological functions of the dog's system. The aging animal is progressively deficient in its ability to capably digest, absorb, and assimilate all nutritional elements. Canine Senior is formulated to help the older dog's digestion, allowing for maintenance and continuing health and activity.

Major Ingredients: *Dry:* Ground Corn, Poultry By-Product Meal, Brewers Rice, Animal Fat (preserved with BHA, Propyl Gallate, Citric Acid), Peanut Hulls (a source of fiber), Dried Skimmed Milk, Vegetable Oil, Wheat Germ Meal, Dried Whole Egg, Cellulose Flour, Brewers Dried Yeast.

Canned: Water, Chicken, Brewers Rice, Meat By-Products, Ground Barley, Ground Corn, Liver, Vegetable Oil, Wheat Germ Meal, Whole Egg, Cellulose Flour, Brewers Dried Yeast.

Average Analysis (as fed):

Dry:

Moisture	9.0%
Dry Matter	91.0%
Protein	17.0%
Fat	9.8%
NFE	57.2%
Ash	3.6%
Fiber	3.4%
Calcium	0.63%
Phosphorus	0.55%
Sodium	0.23%
Potassium	0.32%
ME (kcal/lb.)	1675
ME (kcal/cup)	293

Canned:

Moisture	72.8%
Dry Matter	27.2%
Protein	5.3%
Fat	4.3%
NFE	15.7%
Ash	1.2%
Fiber	0.7%
Calcium	0.23%
Phosphorus	0.13%
Sodium	0.08%
Potassium	0.1%
ME (kcal/can)	528

Dry Weight Analysis:

Dry:

Protein	18.7%
Fat	10.8%
NFE	62.9%
Ash	4.0%
Fiber	3.7%
Calcium	0.69%
Phosphorus	0.60%
Sodium	0.25%
Potassium	0.35%

Canned:

Protein	19.5%
Fat	15.8%
NFE	57.7%
Ash	4.4%
Fiber	2.6%
Calcium	0.84%
Phosphorus	0.48%
Sodium	0.29%
Potassium	0.37%

Recommended Feeding:

Feed an amount of Canine Senior to maintain body weight. Avoid overfeeding which leads to obesity. The following amounts may be used as a guide.

Weight of dog	Suggested Feeding
10 lbs.	1½ cups or ⅔ can
20 lbs.	2 cups or 1¼ can
40 lbs.	3½ cups or 2 cans
60 lbs.	5 cups of 2¾ cans
80 lbs.	6 cups or 3½ cans
100 lbs.	7¼ cups or 4 cans

Consumption may vary depending on factors such as environment (including temperature), exercise, temperament and stress. Because this is a highly concentrated, highly digestible food, less food will be required than with ordinary commercial dog foods.

Packaging:

Canine Senior is available in 10 lb., 20 lb. and 40 lb. bags, and 15½ oz. cans, 24 cans per case.

SCIENCE DIET® FELINE GROWTH®

Feline Growth is formulated especially for kittens from weaning to maturity, and contains the extra nutrients needed by kittens and pregnant/nursing cats. Feline Growth is properly balanced with the extra calories, protein, vitamins and minerals kittens need for optimum growth, until they mature at approximately one year of age.

It is also the ideal diet for pregnant/nursing cats since it provides the optimum balance of extra calories, protein, calcium and phosphorus needed for fetal development and milk production. Feline Growth is also *extremely* effective in maintaining the pregnant/nursing cat's proper weight.

Major Ingredients:

Dry:

Ground Corn, Poultry By-Product Meal, Animal Fat (preserved with BHA, Propyl Gallate, Citric Acid), Meat Meal, Dried Whole Egg, Soy Mill Run, Brewers Dried Yeast.

Canned:

Water, Liver, Chicken, Whole Egg, Poultry By-Product Meal, Soybean Meal, Brewers Rice, Meat Meal, Brewers Dried Yeast.

Average Analysis: (as fed)

Dry:

Moisture	9.0%
Dry Matter	91.0%
Protein	34.32%
Fat	26.76%
NFE	22.42%
Fiber	1.0%
Ash	6.5%
Caclium	1.25%
Phosphorus	1.14%
Sodium	0.39%
Magnesium	0.09%
ME (kcal/lb.)	2029
ME (kcal/cup)	541

Canned:

Moisture	69.8%
Dry Matter	30.2%
Protein	14.8%
Fat	9.6%
NFE	3.27%
Fiber	0.33%
Ash	2.2%
Calcium	0.33%
Phosphorus	0.3%
Sodium	0.16%
Magnesium	0.033%
ME (kcal/can)	658

Dry Weight Analysis:

Dry:

Protein	37.71%
Fat	29.4%
NFE	24.64%
Fiber	1.1%
Ash	7.14%
Calcium	1.37%
Phosphorus	1.25%
Sodium	0.43%
Magnesium	0.1%

Canned:

Protein	49.0%
Fat	31.79%
NFE	10.83%
Fiber	1.1%
Ash	7.28%
Calcium	1.1%
Phosphorus	0.99%
Sodium	0.53%
Magnesium	0.11%

Recommended Feeding:

Feed kittens and pregnant/nursing cats free-choice, a bowl of food available at all times. This method is recommended for kittens from weaning to maturity and for reproducing females from breeding or detection of pregnancy to weaning.

Packaging:

Science Diet Feline Growth is available in 4 lb. and 10 lb. bags, and 15 oz. cans, 24 cans per case.

SCIENCE DIET® FELINE MAINTENANCE®

Description of Use: Feline Maintenance is a highly concentrated food, containing the optimum balance of high quality protein and calories non-reproducing cats need to maintain health and proper weight control throughout their adult years. It also incorporates the findings of recent scientific breakthroughs in the study of lower urinary tract diseases—known as the feline urologic syndrome (F.U.S.). As a result, it is restricted in minerals, *especially magnesium*, and supports maintenance of an acid urine pH to help prevent F.U.S. Because Feline Maintenance is high in calories and contains readily digestible nutrients, cats eat less. Therefore, they consume 50% less magnesium than they would if fed the average supermarket brands.

Major Ingredients: *Dry:* Ground Corn, Poultry By-Product Meal, Brewers Rice, Animal Fat (preserved with BHA, Propyl Gallate, Citric Acid), Meat Meal, Dried Whole Egg, Brewers Dried Yeast, Calcium Carbonate, Iodized Salt, DL-Methionine.

Canned: Meat By-Products, Water, Liver, Ground Corn, Animal Fat, Brewers Rice, Calcium Carbonate, Iodized Salt, DL-Methionine.

Average Analysis: (as fed)

Dry:

Moisture	9.0%
Dry Matter	91.0%
Protein	31.7%
Fat	21.8%
NFE	31.63%
Fiber	1.0%
Ash	4.87%
Calcium	0.87%
Phosphorus	0.55%
Sodium	0.29%
Magnesium	0.07%
ME (kcal/lb.)	1879

Continued on next page

H

Hill's—Cont.

ME (kcal/cup) 470
Canned:
Moisture 70.5%
Dry Matter 29.5%
Protein 12.2%
Fat 7.6%
NFE 7.8%
Fiber 0.2%
Ash 1.7%
Calcium 0.26%
Phosphorus 0.23%
Sodium 0.16%
Magnesium 0.022%
ME (kcal/can) 594
Dry Weight Analysis:
Dry:
Protein 34.84%
Fat 23.96%
NFE 34.76%
Fiber 1.1%
Ash 5.35%
Calcium 0.96%
Phosphorus 0.6%
Sodium 0.32%
Magnesium 0.08%
Canned:
Protein 41.36%
Fat 25.76%
NFE 26.44%
Fiber 0.68%
Ash 5.76%
Calcium 0.88%
Phosphorus 0.73%
Sodium 0.54%
Magnesium 0.075%
Recommended Feeding:
Feed cats free-choice, a bowl of dry food available at all times, or the dry or canned food in one or more meals of 20–30 minutes each. The average 8 lb. cat will maintain proper weight when fed about one-third to one-half cup of dry food or one-third to one-half can of food per day. This amount will vary with individual cats. Feed an amount to maintain *optimum weight.*
Packaging:
Feline Maintenance is available in 4 lb., 10 lb. and 20 lb. bags and 15 oz. cans, 24 cans per case.

SCIENCE DIET® MIXIT®

Description of Use: Science Diet Mixit is a special, highly palatable formula which provides the answer to problem eaters. It is a balanced meat product for owners who feel they must add meat to dry food. (Mixit will not upset the nutritional balance of dry dog food.) For owners wishing to break their dogs of the "canned food habit," Mixit may be added in decreasing portions until the dog accepts straight dry ration.
Major Ingredients: Liver, Meat By-Products, Water, Sucrose, Corn Flour, Vegetable Oil.
Average Analysis (as fed):
Moisture 76.9%
Dry Matter 23.1%
Protein 12.0%
Fat 5.3%
NFE 4.0%
Ash 1.8%
Fiber 0.1%
Calcium 0.27%
Phosphorus 6.23%
Sodium 0.24%
Potassium 0.35%
ME (kcal/can 462
Dry Weight Analysis:
Protein 51.9%
Fat 22.9%
NFE 17.3%
Ash 7.8%
Fiber 0.43%
Calcium 1.2%
Phosphorus 1.0%
Sodium 1.0%
Potassium 1.5%
Recommended Feeding:
For problem eaters, add to dry food. To break dogs of the "canned food habit," add in decreasing portions until the dog accepts straight dry ration.
Packaging:
Mixit is available in 14½ oz. cans, 24 cans per case.

PRESCRIPTION DIET® CANINE k/d®
Dietary Animal Food

Prescription Diet k/d is a dietary animal food containing a restricted but adequate level of protein and phosphorus, and a moderate level of salt. It is capable of supporting long-term maintenance of adult dogs.
Nutritional Characteristics:
Protein—moderately restricted, high quality
Fat and Carbohydrate—increased
Minerals—restricted
Vitamins—increased
Sodium—moderately restricted
Indications: k/d is recommended as a nutritional aid in the dietary management of mature dogs with:
1. Acute or chronic renal failure
2. Hepatic disease (high dietary fat tolerated)
3. Congestive heart failure
4. Endocrine imbalances (diabetes mellitus, hypothyroidism, etc.)

Contraindications: Cats, puppies and reproducing bitches due to restricted protein and minerals.
Metabolizable Energy (Kcal):
Canned—612/can
Dry—352/cup* (1943/lb)
*An 8 oz. cup of k/d contains 2.9 oz. by weight.
Feeding Guide: The following intakes are intended as a starting point only and should be adjusted to maintain optimum body weight.

BODY WEIGHT (LB.)	AMOUNT OF k/d CAN	AMOUNT OF k/d DRY (CUPS)
5	⅓	⅔
10	⅔	1
20	1	2
40	1¾	3¼
60	2½	4¼
80	3	5¼
100	3⅔	6¼

Ingredients: *Canned*—Water, Ground Corn, Chicken, Brewers Rice, Liver, Animal Fat, Whole Egg, Iodized Salt, Minerals and Vitamins.
Dry—Ground Corn, Brewers Rice, Dried Whole Egg, Animal Fat, Sucrose, Iodized Salt, Minerals and Vitamins.
Packaging: *Canned:* Cases of 24 • 15¾ oz. cans
Dry: 10 and 20 lb. bags

PRESCRIPTION DIET® CANINE u/d®
Dietary Animal Food

Prescription Diet u/d is a dietary animal food containing a severely restricted level of protein and phosphorus, and a moderately restricted level of salt, and promotes a basic urine. It is capable of supporting long-term maintenance of adult dogs.
Nutritional Characteristics:
Protein—severely restricted, high quality
Fat and Carbohydrate—increased
Minerals—severely restricted
Vitamins—increased
Sodium—moderately restricted
Indications: u/d is recommended as a nutritional aid in the dietary management of mature dogs with:
1. Advanced renal failure or end stage kidneys
2. Recurrent urolithiasis—cystine and urate
3. Advanced hepatic disease

Contraindications: Cats, puppies and reproducing bitches due to restricted protein and minerals.
Metabolizable Energy (Kcal):
Canned—662/can
Dry—295/cup* (2061/lb.)
*An 8 oz. cup of u/d contains 2.3 oz. by weight.
Feeding Guide: Prescription Diet u/d in either form will support long-term adult maintenance. In most cases supplementation is contraindicated. Individual requirements will vary depending upon breed, environment, season, exercise, temperament, and stress factors, including disease. The following intakes are intended as a starting point only and should be adjusted to maintain optimum body weight.

BODY WEIGHT (LB.)	AMOUNT OF u/d CAN	AMOUNT OF u/d DRY (CUPS)
5	⅓	¾
10	⅔	1⅓
20	1	2⅓
40	1¾	4
60	2⅓	5⅓
80	3	6¾
100	3½	8

INGREDIENTS: *Canned*—Water, Cornstarch, Brewers Rice, Animal Fat, Sucrose, Whole Egg, Liver, Cellulose Flour, Vegetable Oil, Potassium Chloride, Iodized Salt, Minerals and Vitamins.
Dry—Ground Corn, Brewers Rice, Sucrose, Dried Whole Egg, Animal Fat, Cellulose Flour, Iodized Salt, Potassium Chloride, Minerals and Vitamins.

Packaging: *Canned:* Cases of 24 • 15¾ oz. cans
Dry: 10 and 20 lb. bags.

PRESCRIPTION DIET® CANINE s/d®
Dietary Animal Food

Prescription Diet s/d is a dietary animal food containing severely restricted levels of protein, phosphorus and magnesium, and an increased level of salt.
Nutritional Characteristics:
Protein—severely restricted, high quality
Fat and Carbohydrate—increased
Magnesium, Phosphorus and Calcium—severely restricted
Sodium—increased
Indication: s/d is recommended as a nutritional aid in the dietary management of mature dogs with struvite uroliths.
Contraindications: Cats, puppies and reproducing bitches due to restricted protein and minerals. Dogs with congestive heart failure due to increased sodium.
Metabolizable Energy (Kcal): 670/can
Feeding Guide: Prescription Diet s/d will support adult maintenance, but because of its high sodium and restricted protein and mineral contents, long-term maintenance is not recommended. In most cases supplementation is contraindicated. Vitamin-mineral supplements should not be given when feeding s/d. The following intakes are intended as a starting point only and should be adjusted to maintain optimum body weight.

BODY WEIGHT (LB.)	AMOUNT OF s/d CAN
5	⅓
10	½
20	1
40	1⅔
60	2¼
80	2¾
100	3¼

Ingredients: Water, Cornstarch, Animal Fat, Sucrose, Whole Egg, Liver, Cellulose Flour, Iodized Salt, Vegetable Oil, Potassium Chloride, Vitamins and Minerals.
Packaging: Canned: Cases of 24 • 15¾ oz. cans.

PRESCRIPTION DIET® CANINE c/d™
Dietary Animal Food

Prescription Diet Canine c/d is a dietary animal food containing restricted but adequate levels of protein, phosphorus and magnesium, and promotes an acid urine. It is useful in the prevention of struvite calculi, and is nutritionally adequate for the long-term maintenance of adult dogs.
Nutritional Characteristics:
Protein—reduced
Minerals—mildly restricted
Indications: Canine c/d is recommended as a nutritional aid in the dietary management of adult dogs to prevent struvite uroliths. It is also an ideal maintenance diet for adult dogs.
Contraindications: Cats, puppies and reproducing bitches due to restricted protein and minerals.
Metabolizable Energy (Kcal):
Canned: 600/can
Dry: 365/cup* (1947/lb.)
*An 8 oz. cup of c/d contains 3.0 oz. by weight.
Feeding Guide: The following intakes are intended as a starting point only and should be adjusted to maintain optimum body weight.

BODY WEIGHT (LB.)	AMOUNT OF c/d CAN	DRY (CUPS)
5	⅓	⅔
10	⅔	1
20	1	2
40	2	3¼
60	2⅔	4⅓
80	3⅓	5½
100	4	6½

Ingredients: *Canned*—Water, Brewers Rice, Liver, Meat By-Products, Chicken, Ground Corn, Animal Fat, Iodized Salt, Minerals and Vitamins.
Dry—Ground Corn, Poultry By-Product Meal, Animal Fat, Soy Grits, Whole Dried Egg, Soybean Mill Run, Vegetable Oil, Brewers Dried Yeast, Iodized Salt, DL-Methionine, Minerals and Vitamins.
Packaging: *Canned:* Cases of 24 • 15¾ oz. cans
Dry: 10 and 20 lb. bags.

PRESCRIPTION DIET® CANINE g/d®
Dietary Animal Food

Prescription Diet g/d is a dietary animal food with mild restriction of energy, protein, phosphorus and sodium. Other nutrients are present at levels which take into consideration the structural and metabolic changes associated with aging. It is capable of supporting long-term maintenance of adult dogs.
Nutritional Characteristics:
Protein—mildly restricted
Fat and Carbohydrate—mildly restricted
Fiber—increased
Vitamins—increased
Minerals—mildly restricted
Unsaturated fatty acids—increased
Salt—mildly restricted
Indications: g/d is recommended as a nutritional aid in the dietary management of:
1. The geriatric dog
2. Congestive heart failure
3. Endocrine imbalances (diabetes mellitus, hypothyroidism, etc.)

Contraindications: Cats, puppies and reproducing bitches due to restricted protein and minerals.
Metabolizable Energy (Kcal):
Canned—463/can
Dry—268/cup* (1592/lb.)
*An 8 oz. cup of g/d contains 2.7 oz. by weight.
Feeding Guide: Prescription Diet g/d in either form will support long-term adult maintenance. In most cases supplementation is contraindicated. Individual requirements will vary depending upon breed, environment, season, exercise, temperament, and stress factors, including disease. The following intakes are intended as a starting point only and should be adjusted to maintain optimum body weight.

BODY WEIGHT (LB.)	AMOUNT OF g/d CAN	DRY (CUPS)
5	½	¾
10	¾	1½
20	1½	2½
40	2½	4½
60	3½	6
80	4⅓	7½
100	5	9

Ingredients: *Canned*—Water, Brewers Rice, Chicken, Ground Corn, Liver, Cellulose Flour, Whole Egg, Vegetable Oil, Dried Skim Milk, Brewers Dried Yeast, Iodized Salt, Minerals and Vitamins.
Dry—Ground Corn, Peanut Hulls, Poultry By-Product Meal, Brewers Rice, Animal Fat, Dried Whole Egg, Dried Skimmed Milk, Wheat Germ Meal, Vegetable Oil, Brewers Dried Yeast, Iodized Salt, Minerals and Vitamins.
Packaging: *Canned:* Cases of 24 • 15¾ oz. cans
Dry: 10 & 20 lb. bags

PRESCRIPTION DIET® CANINE p/d®
Dietary Animal Food

Prescription Diet p/d is a high energy, high quality protein dietary animal food in a form highly utilizable by the dog. It is capable of supporting all phases of the normal canine life cycle.
Nutritional Characteristics:
Protein—increased
Fat—increased
Carbohydrate—decreased
Minerals and Vitamins—increased
Indications: p/d is recommended as a nutritional aid in the dietary management of:
1. Nutritional deficiency diseases, i.e. anemias, dermatoses of dietary origin, eclampsia, malnutrition, protein depletion and skeletal diseases
2. Weaning and growing puppies
3. Gestating and lactating bitches
4. Malnourished dogs prior to, and/or following surgery

Metabolizable Energy (Kcal):
Canned: 663/can.
Dry: 395/cup* (1900/lb.)
*An 8 oz. cup of p/d contains 3.3 oz. by weight.
Feeding Guide: Prescription Diet p/d will support growth and reproduction. In most cases supplementation of p/d with other foods or supplements is contraindicated.

1. For Adults
Feed the same amounts of p/d as recommended for k/d. Please note that the

Continued on next page

Hill's—Cont.

amounts recommended are starting points only and should be adjusted to maintain optimum body weight.

2. For Puppies

Feed as much p/d as the pups will eat in 20–30 minutes, but no more than twice the amount recommended in the feeding chart, 2–3 times per day, and remove any remaining food.

Feed approximately the following amounts:

[See table below].

3. For Lactation—Feed lactating bitches ad lib (as much as they want). Limit food intake only if necessary to control obesity.

Ingredients: *Canned*—Water, Chicken, Liver, Whole Egg, Ground Corn, Ground Barley, Meat By-Products, Soy Grits, Brewers Dried Yeast, Iodized Salt, Minerals and Vitamins.

Dry—Ground Corn, Poultry By-Product Meal, Soy Grits, Animal Fat, Brewers Rice, Dried Whole Egg, Vegetable Oil, Brewers Dried Yeast, Minerals and Vitamins.

Packaging: Canned: Cases of 24 • 15¾ oz. cans

Dry: 10 and 20 lb. bags

PRESCRIPTION DIET® CANINE i/d®

Dietary Animal Food

Prescription Diet i/d is a bland, low-residue, dietary animal food, having restricted levels of fat and fiber. It is made from ingredients that are highly digestible and nonirritating. It is capable of suporting all phases of the normal canine life cycle.

Nutritional Characteristics:

Protein—high quality

Fat—restricted

Carbohydrate—highly digestible

Fiber—restricted

Electrolytes and Vitamins—increased

Indications: i/d is recommended as a nutritional aid in the dietary management of:

1. Gastrointestinal conditions, i.e. enteritis, gastritis, intestinal parasitism and gastrointestinal surgical patients
2. Early weaning
3. Hepatic disease
4. Pancreatic insufficiency
5. Bloat

Metabolizable Energy (Kcal):

Canned—581/can

Dry—325/cup* (1735 lb.)

*An 8 oz. cup of i/d contains 3.0 oz. by weight.

Feeding Guide: The following intakes are intended as a starting point only and should be adjusted to maintain optimum body weight.

1. For Maintenance

BODY WEIGHT (LB.)	AMOUNT OF i/d CAN	DRY (CUPS)
5	⅓	⅔
10	⅔	1
20	1	2
40	2	3½
60	2½	4⅔
80	3¼	5⅔
100	3¾	6¾

2. For Growth

See feeding guide for Canine p/d. Feed approximately 15% more Canine i/d than Canine p/d.

Ingredients: *Canned*—Water, Whole Egg, Liver, Chicken, Brewers Rice, Ground Corn, Dextrose, Brewers Dried Yeast, Potassium Chloride, Minerals and Vitamins.

Dry—Ground Corn, Dried Whole Egg, Ground Rice, Meat Meal, Casein, Animal Fat, Vegetable Oil, Brewers Dried Yeast, Iodized Salt, Potassium Chloride, Minerals and Vitamins.

Packaging: *Canned:* Cases of 24 • 15¾ oz. cans

Dry: 10 and 20 lb. bags

PRESCRIPTION DIET® CANINE h/d®

Dietary Animal Food

Prescription Diet h/d is a dietary animal food containing a severely restricted but adequate level of sodium. It is capable of supporting long-term maintenance of adult dogs.

Nutritional Characteristics:

Sodium—severely restricted

Potassium—increased

Protein—mildly restricted

Fat and Carbohydrate—increased

Vitamins—increased

Indications: h/d is recommended as a nutritional aid in the dietary management of:

1. Congestive heart failure
2. Hepatic and renal diseases accompanied by sodium retention

Contraindications: Dehydration, diarrhea and reproduction in the bitch due to severely restricted sodium level.

Metabolizable Energy (Kcal):

Canned—648/can

Dry—336/cup* (1920/lb.)

*An 8 oz. cup of h/d contains 2.8 oz. by weight.

Feeding Guide: Prescription Diet h/d in either form will support long-term adult maintenance. In most cases supplementation is contraindicated. Individual requirements will vary depending upon breed, environment, season, exercise, temperament, and stress factors, including disease. The following intakes are intended as a starting point only and should be adjusted to maintain optimum body weight.

BODY WEIGHT (LB.)	AMOUNT OF h/d CAN	DRY (CUPS)
5	⅓	⅔
10	⅔	1
20	1	2
40	1¾	3⅓
60	2⅓	4⅓
80	2¾	5½
100	3⅓	6½

Ingredients: *Canned*—Water, Chicken, Ground Corn, Liver, Brewers Rice, Vegetable Oil, Potassium Chloride, Minerals and Vitamins

Dry—Ground Corn, Brewers Rice, Meat Meal, Dried Whole Egg, Animal Fat, Soybean Meal, Vegetable Oil, Potassium Chloride, Minerals and Vitamins.

Packaging: *Canned:* Cases of 24 • 15¾ oz. cans

Dry: 10 and 20 lb. bags

PRESCRIPTION DIET® CANINE r/d®

Dietary Animal Food

Prescription Diet r/d is a low calorie dietary animal food which has a portion of its fat and digestible carbohydrates replaced by indigestible fiber. This simultaneously reduces the digestible caloric density while maintaining bulk. The diet is capable of supporting long-term maintenance of adult dogs.

Nutritional Characteristics:

Fat—severely restricted

Carbohydrate (digestible)—restricted

Fiber—greatly increased

Indications: r/d is recommended as a nutritional aid in the dietary management of:

1. Obesity and predisposition to obesity
2. Constipation
3. Hypothyroidism in obese patients
4. Hyperlipoproteinemia
5. Diabetes mellitus (patients at or above normal weight with no other disease problem).

Contraindications:

1. Puppies and reproducing bitches due to restricted caloric content.
2. Renal failure due to protein and sodium contents.
3. Cardiac failure due to sodium content.

Metabolizable Energy (Kcal):

Canned—300/can

Dry—186/cup* (1000/lb.)

*An 8 oz. cup of r/d contains 3.0 oz. by weight.

Feeding Guide: For active weight reduction DETERMINE THE AMOUNT TO BE FED BASED ON THE DESIRED WEIGHT RATHER THAN THE OBESE WEIGHT. The following intakes are intended to be a starting point only and should be adjusted to produce desired weight loss. Full client cooperation must

Amount of p/d for 24 hrs. (cans or cup of dry)

MATURE WT. (LB.)	6 WKS CANS	6 WKS CUPS	9 WKS CANS	9 WKS CUPS	12 WKS CANS	12 WKS CUPS	6 MOS. CANS	6 MOS. CUPS
10	⅓	½	⅖	⅔	½	1	¾	1¼
20	¾	1¼	1	1⅔	1¼	2	1½	2½
50	1⅛	1¾	1⅓	2¼	1¾	3⅛	2⅓	4
70	1⅔	2½	2¼	3¾	3	5¼	3⅓	5½
130	1¾	3⅓	2⅔	4⅓	3½	6	4⅓	7⅓

be obtained and all food intake rigidly controlled.

NORMAL WEIGHT (LB.)	AMOUNT OF r/d (REDUCING) CAN	DRY (CUPS)
5	1/3	2/3
10	2/3	1
20	1	1 3/4
40	1 3/4	3
60	2 1/3	4
80	2 3/4	5
100	3 1/3	6

Ingredients: *Canned*—Water, Liver, Soybean Mill Run, Meat By-Products, Brewers Rice, Powdered Cellulose, Vegetable Oil, Brewers Dried Yeast, Iodized Salt, Minerals and Vitamins.
Dry—Peanut Hulls, Ground Corn, Poultry By-Product Meal, Soybean Meal, Soybean Mill Run, Iodized Salt, Vegetable Oil, Minerals and Vitamins.
Packaging: *Canned:* cases of 24 • 15½ oz. cans
Dry: 10 and 20 lb. bags.

PRESCRIPTION DIET® CANINE d/d®

Dietary Animal Food

Prescription Diet d/d is a dietary animal food having a reduced likelihood of eliciting an allergic response because it contains ingredients that are uncommonly eaten by dogs. It is capable of supporting all phases of the normal canine life cycle.
Nutritional Characteristics:
Protein and Fat—derived solely from ovine tissues and rice
Carbohydrate—derived solely from rice
Unsaturated fatty acids—increased
Indications:
1. d/d is recommended as a nutritional aid in the dietary management of allergic dermatitis and/or gastroenteritis of dietary origin.
2. d/d is also clinically useful as a test diet for the differential diagnosis of food allergies.

Alternative Hypoallergenic Diets:
Prescription Diet k/d dry:
Protein sources—Corn, rice, egg, milk
Prescription Diet u/d dry:
Protein sources—Corn, rice, egg
Metabolizable Energy (Kcal): 585/can
Feeding Guide: Prescription Diet d/d will support all phases of the canine life cycle. In most cases supplementation is contraindicated. Individual requirements will vary depending upon breed, environment, season, exercise, temperament, and stress factors, including disease. The following intakes are intended as a starting point only and should be adjusted to maintain optimum body weight.

BODY WEIGHT (LB.)	AMOUNT OF d/d CAN
5	1/3
10	2/3
20	1
40	2
60	2½
80	3
100	3 3/4

Ingredients: Water, Mutton By-Products, Brewers Rice, Mutton Liver, Rice Oil, Iodized Salt, Potassium Chloride, Minerals and Vitamins.
Packaging: *Canned:* Cases of 24 • 15 3/4 oz. cans

CONTROL DIET® HRH®

Dietary Animal Food

Control Diet HRH is a medicated, high energy diet containing two anthelmintic drugs. It is capable of supporting long-term maintenance of adult dogs.
Nutritional Characteristics:
Fat — increased
Carbohydrate — highly digestible
Drug additives — diethylcarbamazine (Caricide®) and styrylpyridinium (Styrid®)
Indications: Control Diet HRH is recommended as a nutritional aid in the dietary management of:
1. Working dogs
2. Heartworms
3. Hookworms and roundworms

Contraindications: Heartworm positive dogs (dog should be converted to a negative status before initiating feeding of HRH).
Metabolizable Energy (Kcal):
586/cup* 2134/lb.
*An 8 oz cup of HRH contains 4.4 oz. by weight.
Feeding Guide: Control Diet HRH will support long-term adult maintenance. In most cases supplementation is contraindicated. Individual requirements will vary depending upon breed, environment, season, exercise, temperament, and stress factors, including disease. The following intakes are intended as a starting point only and should be adjusted to maintain optimum body weight.

BODY WEIGHT (LB.)	AMOUNT OF HRH CUPS
5	1/3
10	2/3
20	1¼
40	2
60	2½
80	3 1/8
100	3 3/4

Ingredients: Animal Fat, Soy Flour, Meat Meal, Dextrose, Dried Whole Egg, Dried Skimmed Milk, Vegetable Oil, Brewers Dried Yeast, Minerals and Vitamins.
Packaging: Dry: 25 lb. pails

PRESCRIPTION DIET® FELINE c/d®

Dietary Animal Food

Prescription Diet Feline c/d is a dietary animal food containing restricted, but adequate, levels of minerals thereby minimizing their urinary excretion. It is capable of supporting long-term maintenance of adult cats.
Nutritional Characteristics: Magnesium, Phosphorus and Calcium—restricted
Calories (fat)—increased
Indications: Feline c/d is recommended as a nutritional aid in the dietary management of:
1. Feline urologic syndrome (prevention of recurrence)
2. Anorexia—feline or canine

Contraindications: Reproducing queens due to mineral restriction.
Metabolizable Energy (Kcal):
Canned—604/can
Dry—519/cup* (1934/lb.)
*An 8 oz. cup of Feline c/d contains 4.3 oz. by weight.
Feeding Guide: Prescription Diet Feline c/d in any form will support long-term adult maintenance. In most cases supplementation is contraindicated. Individual requirements will vary depending upon breed, environment, season, exercise, temperament, and stress factors, including disease. The following intakes are intended as a starting point only and should be adjusted to maintain optimum body weight.

BODY WEIGHT (LB.)	AMOUNT OF FELINE c/d CAN OR CUP
5	1/4
7–8	1/3
10	2/5
15	3/5

Ingredients: *Canned*—Liver, Meat By-Products, Water, Ground Corn, Animal Fat, Dried Skimmed Milk, Brewers Dried Yeast, Iodized Salt, DL-Methionine, Minerals and Vitamins.
Dry—Poultry By-Product Meal, Ground Corn, Brewers Rice, Animal Fat, Meat Meal, Dried Whole Egg, Soybean Mill Run, Iodized Salt, Brewers Dried Yeast, DL-Methionine, Minerals and Vitamins.
Packaging: *Canned:* Cases of 24 • 15 oz. cans
Dry: 4 and 10 lb. bags

PRESCRIPTION DIET® FELINE s/d®

Dietary Animal Food

Prescription Diet Feline s/d: Prescription Diet Feline s/d is a dietary animal food containing restricted levels of magnesium, phosphorus and calcium, and an increased level of salt to increase urine volume and reduce urinary mineral concentration. Metabolism of Feline s/d results in the maintenance of an acid urine.

Continued on next page

Hill's—Cont.

Nutritional Characteristics:
Fat—increased
Magnesium, Phosphorus and Calcium—severely restricted
Sodium—increased
Indications: Feline s/d is recommended as a nutritional aid in the dietary management of mature cats with:
1. Struvite uroliths
2. Feline urologic syndrome (initial management)
Contraindications: Kittens and reproducing queens because of restricted minerals.
Metabolizable Energy (Kcal): 645/can
Feeding Guide: Prescription Diet Feline s/d will support long-term adult maintenance but, because of its high sodium content, it is not recommended for long-term feeding unless urolithiasis and/or F.U.S. recurs when Feline c/d is being fed. Supplementation, including use of urinary acidifiers, is contraindicated. The following intakes are intended as a starting point only and should be adjusted to maintain optimum body weight.

BODY WEIGHT (LB.)	AMOUNT OF FELINE s/d CAN
5	1/4
7–8	1/3
10	2/5
15	3/5

Ingredients: Liver, Meat By-Products, Water, Animal Fat, Ground Corn, Brewers Rice, Powdered Cellulose, Iodized Salt, DL-Methionine, Minerals and Vitamins.
PACKAGING: *Canned:* Cases of 24 • 15 oz. cans

PRESCRIPTION DIET® FELINE k/d®
Dietary Animal Food

Prescription Diet Feline k/d is a dietary animal food containing a restricted but adequate level of protein and phosphorus. It is capable of supporting long-term maintenance of adult cats.
Nutritional Characteristics:
Protein—restricted
Fat and Carbohydrate—increased
Magnesium, Phosphorus and Calcium—restricted
Vitamins—increased
Sodium—moderately restricted
Indications: Feline k/d is recommended as a nutritional aid in the dietary management of mature cats with:
1. Acute or chronic renal failure
2. Hepatic disease
Contraindications: Kittens or reproducing queens because of restricted protein and minerals.
Metabolizable Energy (Kcal):
Canned —722/15 oz. can
Feeding Guide: Prescription Diet Feline k/d will support long-term adult maintenance. In most cases supplementation is contraindicated. Individual requirements will vary depending upon environment, season, exercise, temperament, and stress factors, including disease. The following intakes are intended as a starting point only and should be adjusted to maintain optimum body weight.

BODY WEIGHT (LB.)	AMOUNT OF FELINE k/d CAN (15 oz.)
5	1/5
7–8	1/3
10	2/5
15	1/2

Ingredients: Water, Liver, Meat By-Products, Ground Corn, Animal Fat, Brewers Rice, Whole Egg, Iodized Salt, Minerals and Vitamins.
Packaging: *Canned:* Cases of 24 • 15 oz. cans

PRESCRIPTION DIET® FELINE p/d®
Dietary Animal Food

Prescription Diet Feline p/d is a high energy, high quality protein dietary animal food balanced to meet the nutrient requirements of the cat. It is capable of supporting all phases of the feline life cycle.
Nutritional Characteristics:
Calories (fat)—increased
Vitamins—increased
Magnesium—restricted
Indications: Feline p/d is a dietary animal food recommended as a nutritional aid in the dietary management of:
1. Nutritional deficiency diseases, i.e. anemias, dermatoses of dietary origin, malnutrition, protein depletion and skeletal diseases
2. Weaning and growing kittens
3. Gestating and lactating queens
4. Malnourished cats prior to and/or following surgery
Metabolizable Energy (Kcal):
Canned —610/can
Feeding Guide: Prescription Diet Feline p/d will support growth, reproduction and long-term adult maintenance. In most cases supplementation is contraindicated. Individual requirements will vary depending upon the environment, season, exercise, temperament and phase of the life cycle. Growing kittens and lactating queens can be fed ad lib. The following intakes are intended to be a starting point only and should be adjusted to maintain optimum body weight. Lactating queens will require 2 to 2.5 times their maintenance intake by the fifth week depending upon the number of kittens nursing.
1. **For Maintenance:** Feed the same amount of Feline p/d as recommended for Feline c/d.
2. **For Growth:**

AGE OF KITTEN	AMOUNT OF FELINE p/d CAN
6 weeks	1/8
2 months	1/8
3 months	1/5
4 months	1/4
5 months	1/3

3. **For Lactation**
[See table below].

BODY WEIGHT (LB.)	CANS OF FELINE p/d FOR 24 HOURS 1 WK	2 WKS	3 WKS	4 WKS	5 WKS	6 WKS	7 WKS
5	1/4	1/4	1/3	2/5	1/2	2/5	1/4
8	1/3	1/3	2/5	1/2	2/3	1/2	1/3
10	2/5	2/5	1/2	2/3	4/5	2/3	2/5

Ingredients: Liver, Meat By-Products, Water, Ground Corn, Whole Egg, Animal Fat, Dried Skimmed Milk, Brewers Dried Yeast, Iodized Salt, DL—Methionine, Minerals and Vitamins.
Packaging: *Canned:* Cases of 24 • 15 oz. cans.

PRESCRIPTION DIET® FELINE r/d®
Dietary Animal Food

Prescription Diet Feline r/d is a low calorie dietary animal food which has a portion of its fat and digestible carbohydrates replaced by indigestible fiber. This simultaneously reduces the digestible caloric density while maintaining bulk. The diet is capable of supporting long-term maintenance of adult cats.
Nutritional Characteristics:
Fat—restricted
Carbohydrate (digestible)—restricted
Fiber—increased
Minerals—restricted
Indications: Feline r/d is recommended as a nutritional aid in the dietary management of:
1. Obesity and predisposition to obesity in mature cats
2. Constipation
3. Hairballs
Contraindications: Kittens and reproducing queens because of restricted caloric content.
Metabolizable Energy (Kcal):
Canned —350/can
Feeding Guide: Prescription Diet Feline r/d will support long-term adult maintenance. In most cases supplementation is contraindicated. For active weight reduction DETERMINE THE AMOUNT TO BE FED BASED ON THE DESIRED WEIGHT RATHER THAN THE OBESE WEIGHT. The following are intended to be a starting point only and should be adjusted to produce desired weight loss. Full client cooperation must be obtained and all food intake rigidly controlled. Following weight loss increase amount fed sufficiently to maintain weight and prevent weight gain.

NORMAL WEIGHT (LB.)	AMOUNT OF FELINE r/d (REDUCING) CAN
5	1/3
7–8	1/2
10	3/5
15	3/4

Ingredients: Water, Meat By-Products, Liver, Cellulose Flour, Corn Flour, Iodized Salt, DL-Methionine, Minerals and Vitamins.
Packaging: *Canned:* Cases of 24 • 15 oz. cans

PRESCRIPTION DIET® FELINE h/d®
Dietary Animal Food

Prescription Diet Feline h/d is a dietary animal food containing a restricted but adequate level of sodium. It is capable of supporting long-term maintenance of adult cats.
Nutritional Characteristics:
Sodium—restricted
Potassium—increased
Vitamins—increased
Minerals—restricted
Indications: Feline h/d is recommended as a nutritional aid in the dietary management of:
1. Congestive heart failure
2. Hepatic disease accompanied by sodium retention

Contraindications: Dehydration and diarrhea due to restricted sodium level.
Metabolizable Energy (Kcal):
Canned —594/can
Feeding Guide: Prescription Diet Feline h/d will support long-term adult maintenance. In most cases supplementation is contraindicated. Individual requirements will vary depending upon breed, environment, season, exercise, temperament, and stress factors, including disease. The following intakes are intended as a starting point only and should be adjusted to maintain optimum body weight.

BODY WEIGHT (LB.)	AMOUNT OF FELINE h/d CAN
5	1/4
7–8	1/3
10	2/5
15	3/5

Ingredients: Liver, Meat By-Products, Water, Ground Corn, Animal Fat, Brewers Dried Yeast, Potassium Chloride, DL-Methionine, Minerals and Vitamins.
Packaging: *Canned:* Cases of 24 • 15 oz. cans

Body Weight	Dose	Strokes of pump
Under 10 lb	1/4 teaspoonful	1
10 to 20 lb	1/2 teaspoonful	2
20 to 50 lb	1 teaspoonful	4
50 lb & over	1 1/2 teaspoonfuls	6

Norden Laboratories, Inc.
601 W. CORNHUSKER
P.O. BOX 80809
LINCOLN, NE 68521

FELOBITS®
A Palatable Vitamin, Mineral and Fatty Acid Supplement for Cats and Kittens

Composition: Each tablet contains: D-Sorbitol 145.0 mg; Vitamin A 1500 IU; Vitamin D_3 150 IU; Vitamin E 2 IU; Thiamine mononitrate 1.0 mg; Riboflavin 1.0 mg; Niacinamide 4.0 mg; Calcium pantothenate 0.5 mg; Pyridoxine HC1 (B_6) 0.5 mg; Inositol 10.0 mg; Zinc 0.145 mg; Manganese 0.11 mg; Magnesium 3.0 mg: Linoleic Acid 20.0 mg; Choline (as the bitartrate) 50.0 mg; Calcium (as calcium phosphate) 46.0 mg; Phosphorus (as calcium phosphate) 35.6 mg; Iron (as ferrous fumerate) 5.0 mg; Cobalt (as cobalt sulfate) 0.1 mg; Iodine (as potassium iodide) 0.1 mg.
Suggested Daily Dosage: One tablet per day, or as directed by your veterinarian, given whole or crumbled on food. Daily use of Felobits provides broad supplementation of vitamins and minerals, linoleic acid to support feline high fat requirements, and important fat metabolizing agents.
Felobits have special flavor appeal for cats. Each tablet is scored by quarters for easy dosing in kittens.
Regularly scheduled examinations by your veterinarian help assure a healthy, happy pet.
How Supplied: Bottles of 50, 200 tablets.

GERIBITS®
A Palatable Vitamin and Mineral Supplement For Older Dogs

Composition: Each tablet contains: Vitamin A, 1800 IU; Vitamin D_3, 180 I.U.; Vitamin E, 20 I.U.; Thiamine mononitrate (B_1), 2.0 mg; Riboflavin, 2.0 mg; Pyridoxine HC1 (B_6), 2.0 mg; Folic acid, 0.2 mg; Calcium pantothenate, 1.0 mg; Niacinamide, 10.0 mg; Choline (as the bitartrate) 50.0 mg; Inositol, 10.0 mg; Vitamin B_{12} crystalline, 50.0 mcg; Linoleic acid, 30.0 mg; D-Sorbitol, 145.0 mg; Elemental iron (as ferrous fumarate) 9.5 mg; Copper (as copper acetate) 0.5 mg; Cobalt (as cobalt sulfate) 0.5 mg; Calcium (as dicalcium phosphate) 46.0 mg; Phosphorus (as dicalcium phosphate) 35.6 mg; Zinc (as zinc sulfate) 1.0 mg; Manganese (as manganese sulfate) 0.5 mg; Magnesium 3.0 mg; Iodine (as potassium iodide) 0.6 mg.
Suggested Daily Dosage: One tablet per day, or as directed by your veterinarian, given whole or crumbled on food.
Geribits are specially formulated to provide supplemental vitamins and essential minerals to aging pets. Essential amino acids are obtained from the ingredients which make up the palatable base of the tablet. Geribits have special flavor appeal for dogs.
Regularly scheduled examinations by your veterinarian help assure a healthy, happy dog.
How Supplied: Bottles of 50, 200 tablets.

NUTRIDERM®
Special Dietary Supplement

Composition: Each ml contains:

Vitamin A	230 I.U.
Vitamin D_2	54 I.U.
Vitamin E	1.8 I.U.

Indications: A palatable formulation containing vitamins A, D_2 and E with supportive essential fatty acids and sorbitan derivatives.
Directions: For dogs or cats. Administer orally once daily according to following schedule:
[See table above].
How Supplied: 4 1/2 oz plastic bottle, 4 1/2 oz. with pump, 12 oz with pump, gallon.

VI-SORBIN*
Vitamin-Iron Preparation with Sorbitol

Composition: Each 5 ml (1 teaspoonful) contains: Vitamin B_{12} (cyanocobalamin), 8.34 mcg; Vitamin B_6, (pyridoxine hydrochloride) 2.0 mg; Ferric pyrophosphate (soluble) 100.0 mg; Folic acid 0.5 mg; Sorbitol solution U.S.P. 4.4 ml; (equiv. to not less than 73% w/v of D-Sorbitol); Aromatic base q.s.
Indications: Useful as a nutritional vitamin and mineral supplement for both young and very old animals and for horses on the racing circuit.
Dosage: *Dogs:* 1 to 3 teaspoonfuls daily, depending upon size. Administer directly or mix with feed when possible. *Cats:* 1/2 teaspoonful daily (mix in milk if desired). *Puppies and kittens:* 1/4 teaspoonful daily. *Calves, and foals* up to yearlings: 1/2 fl oz daily. *Yearlings and adult horses:* 1 fl oz daily.
Important: Protect from light. Dispense only in amber bottles. Do not refrigerate.
*Reg. TM of SmithKline Beckman Corporation.
For Veterinary Use Only.
How Supplied: 4 1/2 oz, 900 ml, 1 gal.

Continued on next page

Norden—Cont.

VI-SORBITS®
A Palatable Vitamin-Iron Supplement for Dogs.

Composition: Each tablet contains:

Elemental iron	9.5 mg
Vitamin B_{12} crystalline	8.0 mcg
Folic Acid	0.2 mg
Riboflavin (B_2)	1.0 mg
Niacinamide	10.0 mg
D-Sorbitol	145.0 mg
Vitamin A	1250 I.U.
Vitamin D_3	125 I.U.
Vitamin E	2 I.U.
Pyridoxine hydrocholoride (B_6)	1.0 mg
Thiamine mononitrate (B_1)	1.0 mg
Calcium pantothenate	0.5 mg
Calcium (as calcium phosphate)	100.0 mg
Phosphorus (as calcium phosphate)	77.3 mg
Magnesium	1.0 mg
Copper (as cupric acetate)	0.5 mg
Linoleic Acid	20.0 mg

Dosage and Administration: One tablet per day, or as directed by your veterinarian, given whole or crumbled on food.

Vi-Sorbits are a source of supplemental vitamins and iron when used as recommended.

Vi-Sorbits have special flavor appeal for dogs. Each tablet is scored for easy dosing in small puppies.

Regularly scheduled examinations by your veterinarian help assure a healthy, happy dog.

Caution: Keep container in a cool, dry place. Keep out of the reach of children. For Veterinary Use Only.

Osborn
AN ESSAR CORPORATION
P. O. BOX 1590
FORT DODGE, IOWA 50501

CAL-PHOS PALATABS®
Calcium, Phosphorus & Vitamin D

Composition: Each tablet contains: Calcium 580 mg, Phosphorus 450 mg., Vitamin D3 400 I.U. in a protein chewable base.

Indications: For preventing calcium and phosphorus deficiences during rapid growth, pregnancy and lactation.

Dosage and Administration: One tablet per 20 pounds body weight daily. Cal-Phos Palatabs® may be given free choice or crumbled and mixed with food.

How Supplied: 50's

CONVAL™
Composition:
Each Pound Contains:
Vitamins:—Vitamin A, 4480 I.U., Vitamin D_3 3,000 I.U., Vitamin E 56 I.U., Thiamin HCl 0.060 mg., Riboflavin 2.240 mg., Pantothenic Acid 6.670 mg., Niacin 11.280 mg., Pyridoxine HCl 0.060 mg., Folic Acid 0.112 mg., Biotin 0.006 mg., Vitamin B_{12} 0.056 mg., Choline Chloride 0.720 mg., Menadione SBC 1.125 mg., *Amino Acids:*—Lysine 7,450 mg., Methionine 1,950 mg., Cystine 1,095 mg., Threonine 4,975 mg., Valine 6,325 mg., Isoleucine 5,525 mg., Leucine 9,195 mg., Phenylalanine 5,145 mg., Tyrosine 3,625 mg., Histidine 2,740 mg., Arginine 6,070 mg., Aspartic Acid 11,220 mg., Serine 6,325 mg., Glutamic Acid 21,640 mg., Proline 8,605 mg., Glycine 4,595 mg., Alanine 4,680 mg.

In an especially prepared essential fatty acid base containing arachidonic, linoleic and linolenic acids and natural flavors.

Guaranteed Analysis: Protein (Min) . . . 24.00%; Fat (Min) . . . 9.00%; Fiber (Max) . . . 0.75%.

Indications: Conval is indicated particularly during the postsurgical convalescent period and during periods of general hospitalization and confinement. Conval is also indicated for general geriatric debilitation and may be used following periods of chronic disease conditions such as chronic gastritis or enteritis in the dog.

Dosage: *Slight Negative Nitrogen Balance* . . . One tablespoon* for each 30 pounds body weight twice daily mixed in dog food.

Moderate Negative Nitrogen Balance . . . Two tablespoonfuls* for each 15 pounds of body weight twice daily mixed in dog food.

Severe Negative Nitrogen Balance . . . Four tablespoonfuls for each 15 pounds of body weight twice daily mixed in dog food.*

Conval may be used as an adjunct to parenteral therapy.

*NOTE: A special dosage tablespoon is provided which will deliver approximately one ounce.

How Supplied: 2 lb.

GERIATRIC VITAMIN PALATABS®
Palatable Chewable Supplement for Mature Dogs and Cats

Composition: Each tablet contains Thiamine Mononitrate 2 mg., Riboflavin 1.5 mg., Pyridoxine Hydrochloride 2 mg., Niacinamide 10 mg., Calcium Pantothenate 2 mg., Cyanocobalamin (Vitamin B12) 10 mcg., Folic Acid 0.2 mg., Vitamin A 1850 I.U., Vitamin C 10 mg., Vitamin D_3 185 I.U., Vitamin E Acetate 10 I.U., DiCalcium Phosphate 300 mg., Iron Amino Acid Chelate 15 mg., Copper Amino Acid Chelate 1.5 mg., Magnesium Amino Acid Chelate 0.3 mg., Zinc Amino Acid Chelate 2 mg., Potassium Iodide 0.6 mg., Cobalt Gluconate 0.03 mg., Biotin 0.03 mg., Inositol 2 mg., Selenium 25 mcg., in a protein chewable base.

Indications: Vitamin and Mineral supplement specially formulated for mature dogs and cats.

Dosage and Administration: One-half tablet per 20 pounds body weight per day. Geriatric Vitamin Palatabs may be given freely by hand or crumbled and mixed with food.

How Supplied: 150's

HEMA-GLO™
Iron Nutritional Supplement

Composition: Elemental Iron (Fe) 1.9%.

Indications: A source of oral iron with trace elements and methionine. Aids in the control and treatment of iron deficiency anemia and following those conditions which may tend to induce anemia.

Dosage and Administration: *For growing and adult swine, cattle and poultry:* mix 5 lbs. Hema-Glo per ton of complete feed.

Nursing Pigs: When pigs are 3 days of age, place on creep feed in a pan by itself at the rate of ½ oz. daily or 1½ oz. every 3rd day and continue feeding until pigs reach 4 to 5 weeks of age.

Dogs: Feed ½ oz. daily per 10 lbs body weight.

How Supplied: 5-lb. bags.

METHIONINE PALATABS®

Composition: Each chewable tablet contains, 500 mg D-L Methionine in a protein chewable base.

Indications: For use as an aid to acidify the urine of dogs and cats and to control the ammoniacal odor of urine.

Contraindications: Not for use in animals with severe liver or kidney damage.

Dosage and Administration: Give ½ tablet per 20 pounds of body weight, 2 to 3 times a day.

Methionine Palatabs may be given freely by hand or crumbled and mixed with food.

For optimal results, Methionine Palatabs should be given after food to lessen the chance of stomach upsets.

How Supplied: Bottle of 50's

VITA-GLO™
Conditioner Vitamin Supplement. For all Species of Animals.

Composition: plant protein products, processed grain by-products, vitamin A & D supplement, fish oil, dicalcium phosphate, vitamin B_{12} supplement, choline chloride, vitamin E supplement, calcium pantothenate, niacin, pyridoxine hydrochloride, thiamine, riboflavin, biotin.

Minimum vitamin guarantee (each pound contains)

Vitamin A	160,000 U.S.P. units (352 u/gm)
Vitamin D	64,000 I.C. units (141 u/gm)
Vitamin B_{12}	160 mcg (0.35 mcg/gm)

Suggested Dosage:
All Farm Animals: 1–3 lb. to each 100 lb. feed.
Poultry: 1 lb. to each 100 lb. feed.
Young Foals and Weanlings: 1–2 tablespoonfuls daily.
Brood Mares: (latter half of pregnancy and lactation) 2 tablespoonfuls twice a day.
Ponies: 1 tablespoonful daily.
Colts, Stallions & Horses in Training: 1 tablespoonful per 400 lb. daily.
Mature Cattle: (milking or on full feed) 1–3 lb. to each 100 lb. of feed. Many dairymen prefer a handful to each feeding.

Feedlot operators simply top off feed with the prescribed amount of Vita-Glo.
Calves: (bucket fed) 1–2 tablespoonfuls daily in milk or ground feed.
Range Cattle: supplemental feeding is simplified by mixing with salt—1 part to 10 parts salt, or 2½ lb. to 25 lb. salt. (These calculations are based on normal consumption of ¼ salt per day by a 1,000 lb. cow and ⅛ by a 400 lb. steer.) To prevent the oxidation that tends to destroy all vitamin A compounds on prolonged exposure, mix only the amount normally consumed in a 3-week period.
Baby Pigs: 3% of the creep-feed.
Mink: 1 level teaspoonful daily.
How Supplied: 25 lb. Bags

VITA-MIN PALATABS®

Composition: Each Vita-Min Palatab contains Vitamin A 1500 I.U., Vitamin D3 150 I.U., Vitamin E2 I.U., Thiamin Mononitrate 1,000 mcg, Riboflavin 1,000 mcg, Pyridoxine 1,000 mcg, Niacinamide 10 mg., Vitamin B_{12} 8 mcg, Calcium Pantothenate 500 mcg, Iron Amino Acid Chelate 10 mg., Copper Amino Acid Chelate 50 mcg, Potassium Iodide 60 mcg, Manganese Amino Acid Chelate 200 mcg, Zinc Amino Acid Chelate 1.5 mg., Choline Bitartrate 2 mg. with polyunsaturated fatty acid ingredients composed of Linoleic, Linoleic and Achrodonic Acids combined with Calcium 125 mg., and Phosphorus 75 mg., in a protein chewable base.
Indications: Vita-Min Palatabs provide supplemental essential dietary vitamins and minerals with essential fatty acids in a highly palatable chewable tablet. Vita-Min Palatabs are designed for dogs of all ages and are especially useful in aiding in providing dietary needs of young growing dogs. Dogs which have special dietary needs following dehibilitation or convalescence may also be given Vita-Min Palatabs at increased dosages.
Dosage and Administration: Vita-Min Palatabs may be given freely by hand or crumbled and offered over the food.
Dogs up to 20 lbs.: ½ tablet daily.
Dogs 20-40 lbs.: 1 tablet daily.
Dogs 40 lbs & over: 1½ tablets daily.
Dogs with special nutritional requirements may be given double dosage for a period of 2 weeks.
How Supplied: 50's, 100's.

Pfizer Inc.

Agricultural Division
235 EAST 42ND STREET
NEW YORK, NY 10017

VITAMIN A & D
Injectable Emulsifiable Nutrient
A source of Vitamins A & D

Composition: Pfizer Vitamin A & D Injectable Emulsifiable is a solution of vitamins A & D for use in cattle, sheep, and swine.
Each ml contains: 500,000 I.U. of vitamin A and 75,000 I.U. of vitamin D; compounded with 5% polysorbate 80, 2% benzyl alcohol, 10% ethanol w/v; (5 I.U. of vitamin E; 0.75% BHT, and 0.75% BHA as preservatives); in an emulsifiable base.
Administration: Pfizer Vitamin A & D Injectable Emulsifiable may be administered by intramuscular injection. Intramuscular injection should be made with a 14 or 16 gauge needle, 1 or 2 inches long. The preferred route of administration is deep injection into heavy musculature. Dosage levels in all species should be related to weight as well as age. Care should be taken not to inject the product into the blood stream.
Suggested Dosages:

Calves	¼ to 1 ml
Yearlings and Feedlot Cattle	1 to 2 ml
Beef and Dairy Cows	1 to 2 ml
Breeding Cattle	1 to 2 ml
Adult or Breeding Sheep	½ to 1 ml
Adult or Breeding Swine	½ to 1 ml

For breeding animals dosage may be repeated in two or three months as needed. For market animals administer at least two months before marketing.
Caution: Handle aseptically. Use entire contents when first opened.
Storage Conditions: Keep from freezing. Store in a dark, cool place—not above 50°F (10°C).
Caution: KEEP OUT OF THE REACH OF CHILDREN. LIVESTOCK DRUG, NOT FOR HUMAN USE. RESTRICTED DRUG, USE ONLY AS DIRECTED.
For Veterinary Use Only.

Pitman-Moore, Inc.

P.O. BOX 344
WASHINGTON CROSSING, NJ 08560

VITAMYCIN*
Powder
Vitamin-Mineral Supplement
This Product Does Not Have Antibiotic Activity

Composition: Each pound contains:

Cyanocobalamin as cobalamin concentrate	2.5 mg
Niacin	8 g
Racemic calcium pantothenate	5 g
Thiamine mononitrate	1 g
Riboflavin (Feed Grade)	2 g
Vitamin A as palmitate (USP Units)	1,000,000 units
Cholecalciferol (International Chick Units)	1,000,000 units
Choline chloride	5 g
Ferrous sulfate	5 g
Dibasic calcium phosphate hydrous	2.5 g
Calcium gluconate	2.5 g
Cupric sulfate	100 mg
Cobalt sulfate monohydrate	500 mg
Wheat germ oil	2 g
Menadione (Vit. K_3)	200 mg
Soya lecithin	5 g
Zinc sulfate	454 mg

Indications: Recommended for conditions caused by deficiencies of only those vitamins and minerals listed.
Dosage and Administration: Individual dose: swine, sheep, calves, ¼ to 1 teaspoonful twice daily; cattle and horses, 2 to 8 teaspoonsful twice daily. Feed mixes: livestock, 1 lb per 100 lbs feed; poultry, 1 lb per 1000 lbs feed. Dogs, 1 teaspoonful daily in feed. Puppies, ¼ to ½ teaspoonful.
How Supplied: Pound and 25 lb carton.
*Trademark

S

Specialty Pet Products, Inc.

P.O. BOX 58
NASHVILLE, TN 37202

ANF 30

Specifically formulated for the working or show animal where the highest level of nutritional performance is required, ANF 30 has been created to produce the results professionals demand. Despite its preference by professionals, this carefully balanced formulation is ideal for the highly active family pet as well, particularly in high-stress situations such as pregnancy and lactation. Formulated with the highest-quality chicken protein and fats, ANF 30 is noted for its palatability and nutritional density. ANF 30 is the perfect dry diet for dogs of all ages with high energy requirements.
ANF 30 is available in 8 lb., 20 lb. and 40 lb. bags, and 26 oz. cartons.
Feeding Guidelines: Daily intakes of ANF 30 should correspond to body weights of mature healthy dogs according to the following guidelines.

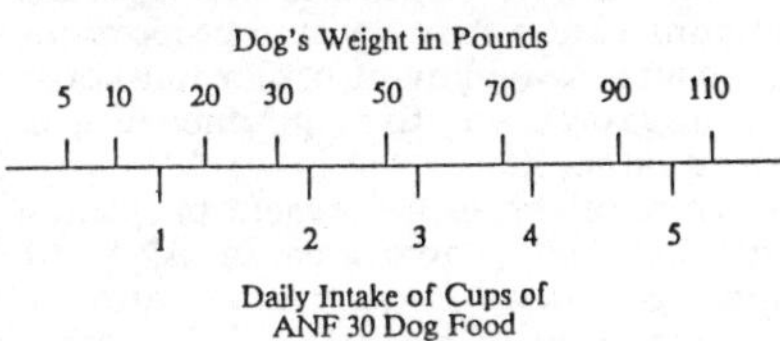

Variation in nutrient requirements between individual dogs is large. One dog in seven needs 20% more or less than the average values in these guidelines.
Food requirements may decrease slightly in hot weather, and increase in the cold. They are also increased by hard work and stress.

Continued on next page

Specialty—Cont.

The daily intake should be gradually increased during the last month of pregnancy, even more during lactation. Feeding should be divided into two or three meals if greatly exceeding the amounts indicated above for maintenance.

After weaning, puppies should receive about twice the amounts of ANF Dog Food in the feeding guidelines for corresponding body weight. After the pups are about one-half their expected mature weight, daily intakes should be reduced gradually to equal the amounts for corresponding desired mature body weights.

Alternatively, if feeding ANF 30 or ANF Puppy Food after weaning, puppies should start to receive small amounts of dry food, moistened with water, about two weeks before weaning. After weaning we suggest that your puppy be allowed to free feed. In larger breeds controlled feeding may be desirable. Always have plenty of fresh water available.

One standard measuring cup will hold 4 oz. of ANF 30.

Main Ingredients: ANF 30 contains chicken by-products, chicken, chicken fat and corn, plus minerals and vitamins, including vitamin C.

Calories: ANF 30 typically contains 2200 gross calories per pound or 1900 available calories per pound. Typically a cupful (4 oz.) of ANF 30 contains 550 gross calories or 500 available calories.

Nutritional Features: A significant amount of available calories in ANF 30 are in the form of high quality protein. This protein level is optimal for even the most demanding conditions encountered by healthy dogs.

An optimal balance among amino acids is built into ANF 30 by the main ingredients. Methionine, the amino acid most susceptible to damage during processing, is supplemented in the formulas. Oxidation of methionine also yields acid that tends to lower the pH of the urine and prevent crystal formation.

The fat contents of ANF 30 are in optimal balance with proteins and other essential nutrients.

Calcium, phosphorus and vitamin D are present in ANF 30, not only in optimal amounts, but also in optimal proportions to ensure development of normal bones during growth and to help remodeling of bones in adults.

All trace minerals are present in optimal amounts and proportions in ANF 30. There is no need for supplementation of any kind (unless prescribed by a veterinarian). All vitamins known to be required by dogs are present in concentrations that meet or exceed currently accented standards. In addition, ANF 30 contains vitamin C, which may be beneficial to some dogs subjected to demanding situations and stress.

Guaranteed Analysis

Crude protein minimum 30.0%
Crude fat minimum 18.0%
Crude fiber maximum 3.5%
Moisture maximum 10.0%
Ash maximum 9.0%

Ingredients: Chicken-by-products, chicken, corn, poultry fat, poultry meal, beet pulp, cane molasses, dried eggs, mono-calcium phosphate, di-calcium phosphate, brewer's dried yeast, calcium carbonate, salt, DL-methionine, sodium propionate, ethoxyguin, vitamin A supplement, vitamin D_3 supplement, DL-alpha tocopheryl acetate, menadione sodium bisulphite complex (source of vitamin K activity), riboflavin supplement, calcium pantothenate, niacin choline chloride, vitamin B_{12} supplement, pyridoxine hydrochloride, thiamine hydrochloride, biotin, folic acid, ascorbic acid, manganous oxide, iron sulfate, iron carbonate, zinc oxide, copper oxide, cobalt carbonate, calcium iodate, sodium selenite.

ANF PUPPY FOOD

ANF Puppy Food has been specifically formulated to meet the critical nutritional needs of the growing puppy from weaning until 12 to 18 months of age. The growing puppy's special needs demand a puppy food high in protein and digestible fats, and rich in balanced vitamins and minerals. ANF Puppy Food contains the natural protein and fat of chicken to meet the important nutritional requirements of every growing puppy.

ANF Puppy Food should be fed dry with plenty of water available at all times.

Natural Palatability: ANF Puppy Food is so palatable that weaning is seldom a problem. Puppies love the natural taste and aroma of ANF Puppy Food right from the start. Chicken and egg proteins, carefully blended, properly proportioned and prepared under exacting conditions, make ANF Puppy Food appealing to even the most finicky eaters. We recommend feeding ANF Puppy Food dry with plenty of water available at all times.

Feeding Instructions: ANF Puppy Food has been specifically formulated to meet the critical nutritional needs of the growing puppy from weaning until 12 to 18 months of age. Puppies should start to receive small amounts of dry food moistened with water about 2 weeks before weaning. After weaning we suggest your puppy be allowed to free feed. In large breeds controlled feeding may be desirable. Always have plenty of fresh water available.

Ingredients: Chicken by-products, chicken, corn, chicken fat (preserved with ethoxyguin), beet pulp fish meal, cane molasses, dried eggs, dried whey, mono & di-calcium phosphate, brewer's dried yeast, calcium carbonate, salt, potassium chloride, DL-methionine, sodium propionate (a preservative), vitamin A acetate, d-activated animal sterol (source of vitamin D_3), DL-alpha tocopheryl acetate (source of vitamin E), menadione sodium bisulphite complex (source of vitamin K activity), riboflavin supplement, calcium pantothenate, niacin supplement, chloine chloride, vitamin B_{12} supplement, pyridoxine hydrochloride, thiamine hydrochloride, biotin, folic acid, ascorbic acid (source of vitamin C), manganous oxide, iron sulfate, iron carbonate, zinc oxide, copper oxide, cobalt carbonate, calcium iodate, sodium selenite.

TAMIAMI

Tamiami's superiority stems from ingredients that cats adapted to throughout their evolution. Cats remain true to their nutritional heritage and have several specific nutrient requirements in addition to those of dogs and humans.

Cats find animal proteins extremely palatable and assimilable. Animal proteins have a high biologic value and an optimal profile of amino acids. Chicken fat has an ideal balance between saturated and polyunsaturated fatty acids.

Sufficient corn and rice are added to allow optimal balancing of protein, minerals and vitamins and to provide readily digestible carbohydrates. These carbohydrates faclitate digestion during dietary transitions or times of stress.

Feeding Guidelines: We recommend free feeding of dry Tamiami. Make dry Tamiami available at all times so that your cat can satisfy its nutritional needs at will. Most mature cats will require about one-half cupful (2 oz.) of dry Tamiami per day.

Variation in nutrient requirements between individual cats is large. One cat in seven needs 20% more or less than average. That is why many cat fanciers prefer to make dry food available at all times.

For best reproductive performance, the daily intake should be gradually increased about two to three weeks after a queen has been bred. Feeding should be further increased early in lactation. The food should be divided into two or three meals when the daily intake greatly exceeds the above amounts.

Kittens should start to receive a small amount of moistened Tamiami about two weeks before weaning. This relaxes the demand for milk production by the queen and accustoms the kitten to digestion of solid food.

Following weaning, dry Tamiami should be made available free choice to growing kittens.

Clean water should be available at all times in a separate dish.

Calories: Dry Tamiami typically contains 2300 gross calories or 2000 available calories per pound. One-half cupful typically contains 290 gross calories or 250 available calories.

Nutritional Features: Approximately 30% of the available calories in Tamiami is in the form of high quality protein. This protein level is optimal for even the most demanding conditions encountered by healthy cats. More protein is unnecessary for healthy cats during any stage of the life cycle.

An optimal balance among amino acids is built into Tamiami by the main ingredients. The amino acid most susceptible to damage during processing, methionine, is supplemented in both formulas. Methionine also helps acidify the urine,

an important factor in managing the Feline Urologic Syndrome.
The fat content of Tamiami is balanced optimally against protein and other essential nutrients. Adding more fat will tend progressively to create imbalances with these nutrients.
Calcium, phosphorus and vitamin D are present in Tamiami in optimal amounts and proportions to ensure development of normal bones during growth and to help remodeling of bones in adults.
Special attention has been given to phosphorus and magnesium in Tamiami. The levels reflect recommended minimums for healthy cats. These two minerals contribute to struvite crystals in the urine.
All trace minerals are present in optimal amounts and proportions in Tamiami.
All vitamins known to be required by cats are present in concentrations that meet or exceed currently accepted standards. In addition, Tamiami contains vitamin C, which may be beneficial in cats subjected to demanding situations and stress.

THE FELINE UROLOGIC SYNDROME (FUS)

A crucial feature in FUS is the formation of struvite crystals in the urine. The chances of such crystalization are diminished by several features of Tamiami.
This special cat food contains an optimal level of salt which promotes thirst and water intake. Tamiami's fiber content is lower than in most cat foods leaving more water available for urine formation. Dilution helps to prevent crystals.
Tamiami's high level of sulfur-containing amino acids, including added methionine, as well as the addition of ascorbic acid, helps to acidify the urine and prevent the formation of crystals. Nearly minimal contents of magnesium and phosphorus further help to prevent crystal formation.

Guaranteed Analysis

Crude protein minimum	32.00%
Crude fat minimum	20.00%
Crude fiber maximum	3.75%
Moisture maximum	10.00%
Ash maximum	6.50%

Ingredients: Chicken by-products, corn, poultry fat, beef pulp, fish meal, poultry meal, dried eggs, brewer's yeast, mono-calcium carbonate, phosphoric acid, salt, DL-methionine, sodium propionate, ethoxyguin, vitamin A supplement, vitamin D_3 supplement, DL-alpha tocopheryl acetate, menadione sodium bisulphite complex (source of vitamin K activity), riboflavin supplement, calcium pantothenate, niacin, choline chloride, vitamin B_{12} supplement, pyridoxine hydrochloride, thiamine hydrochloride biotin folic acid, ascorbic acid, manganous oxide, iron sulfate, iron carbonate, zinc oxide, copper oxide, cobalt carbonate, calcium iodate sodium selenite.
Tamiami Cat Food is available in 8 lb. and 20 lb. bags and in 26 oz. cartons.

	Prevention of Deficiencies	Nutritional Adjunct
Cattle and Horses	1 or 2 boluses, per day; 3 to 5 days, preceding shipment or parturition.	2 or 3 boluses, per day for 3 to 5 days, following parenteral therapy.
Sheep and Swine	½ or 1 bolus, per day; 3 to 5 days, preceding shipment or parturition.	1 or 2 boluses, per day for 3 to 5 days, following parenteral therapy.

Syntex Animal Health, Inc.
4800 WESTOWN PARKWAY, SUITE 200
WEST DES MOINES, IA 50265
Subsidiary of Syntex Agribusiness, Inc.
PALO ALTO, CA

AMCAL BOLUS

Composition: Each Bolus contains:

Calcium Metalosate® (equiv. to 4.37 g calcium)	12.0 g
Phosphorus Complex (equiv. to 3.7 g phosphorus)	10.0 g
Magnesium Metalosate® (equiv. to 1.36 g magnesium)	4.0 g
Potassium	1.44 g
Vitamin D_3	50,000 I.U.

with Ground Licorice Root, Condensed Beet Solubles Product, Condensed Whey Solubles, Dried Extracted Torula Yeast Fermentation Solubles, Dextrose, Squalene, Hydrolyzed Corn Protein, Anethol and Condensed Fermented Corn Extractives.
Indications: A Bolus for use as nutritional support and to prevent nutritional deficiencies of the minerals calcium, phosphorus, and magnesium.
Dosage and Administration: The Bolus dosage should be adjusted and administered depending upon the condition of the animal, or as directed by the veterinarian.
[See table above].
The boluses may be administered orally with a balling gun, or crushed and suspended in milk or water and given as a drench or sprinkled on the daily feed ration. A balanced ration and access to ample water supply should be provided.
Store in a Cool, Dry Place at Room Temperature. Avoid Exposure to Moisture.
Keep out of the Reach of Children
How Supplied: 50 boluses
For Veterinary Use Only.

DIA-GLO L A®
Nutritional Supplement for Skin and Hair Coat Maintenance
For veterinary use only

Description: DIA-GLO L A (Large Animal) is a nutritional additive containing a combination of vitamins, iron, copper, cobalt and polyunsaturated fatty acids. This combination of nutriments has been designed to aid skin and hair condition plus low blood iron levels resulting from dietary inadequacies of these nutriments.
The keen competition between the highly developed animals of today stresses the need for close supervision of complete condition both internal and external. The condition of the skin and a high luster of the hair coat are of prime importance to all show animals. It has often been said, "To be a champion, an animal must look like a champion."
It has been well established that inadequate nutritional requirements, insufficient fatty acids in the diet, and/or vitamin deficiencies result in dryness of the skin and hair coat, desquamation, loss of hair, and increased susceptibility to infection.
DIA-GLO L A has been carefully formulated into a combination of nutritious ingredients which play an important role in developing and keeping the skin of animals soft, smooth and pliable and the hair coat sleek and lustrous and which assist in obtaining proper blood iron levels when these conditions exist due to dietary deficiencies.
How Supplied: DIA-GLO L A is available as follows:
4 lb. containers
10 lb. containers

S

DIA-GLO S.A.®
Veterinary Use Only.

A nutritional supplement especially designed for maintenance of healthy skin and hair coat of dogs, cats, hamsters, chinchillas, parakeets, canaries and other pets.
The Analysis Guaranteed for Dia-Glo S.A.® is as follows:

Vitamin A, (110.2 I.U./g) units/lb	50,000
Vitamin B_6 (50 mcg/g) mg/lb	22.7
Vitamin E, (0.441 I.U./g) I.U./lb	200
Calcium Pantothenate, (8.81 mcg/g)	4
Zinc* (100 mcg/g) (Zn) Minimum	0.01%
Polyunsaturated Fatty Acids, g/lb	62.2

Ingredients: Soy Flour with Soybean Oil Added, Vegetable Oils (Safflower, Soybean, and Corn), Sugar, Silicon Dioxide, Natural and Artificial Flavors Added, Vitamin E Supplement, Zinc Proteinate, Vitamin A Supplement, Ethoxyquin (a preservative), Pyridoxine Hydrochloride, Calcium Pantothenate.
*As Zinc Proteinate, Mfd. under U.S. Patent 3775132, other patents pending.
Directions: Dia-Glo S.A.® should be mixed in or sprinkled over the pet's food daily according to the recommendations below.

Continued on next page

Syntex—Cont.

Weight of Pet	Daily Requirements
10 lbs or less	1 rounded teaspoonful
10 lbs to 20 lbs	2 rounded teaspoonsful
20 lbs to 50 lbs	1 rounded tablespoonful
50 lbs or more	2 rounded tablespoonsful

Note: Dia-Glo S.A.® has exceptional palatability and taste appeal for all pets. Dia-Glo S.A.® is also available in 10 lb plastic pails.

DIAMINO 4X
Pediatric Drops for Small Animals

Composition: Each fluid ounce of Diamino 4X contains:

Nicotinamide ....80 mg
Riboflavin ....8 mg
Thiamine Hydrochloride ....32 mg
Pyridoxine Hydrochloride ....16 mg
Calcium Pantothenate ....48 mg
Liver Fraction 1 ....3 gm
Amino Acids (Protein Hydrolysates) ....4.5 gm
Iron Sulfate....240 mg
Aromatic Syrup Base, q.s.

Indications: Diamino 4X is designed as an oral iron, B vitamin, liver and amino acid supplement for young and orphaned small animals.

Dosage and Administration: For pets weighing up to 3 pounds: ½ ml, 2 or 3 times daily. For pets weighing over 3 pounds: 1 ml, 2 or 3 times daily.
Shake well before using.
Store in a cool place.
For animal use only.

EQUINE PROLEEN® 775
Dia-Quin Brand

Ingredients: Soybean Meal, Wheat Middlings, Concentrated Steffen Filtrate, Ground Licorice Root, Choline Chloride, Hydrolyzed Corn Protein, Condensed Extracted Glutamic Acid Fermentation Product, Dried Whey-Product, Corn Distillers, Dried Grains with Solubles, Ferrous Carbonate, Condensed Fermented Corn Extractives with Germ Meal and Bran Dehydrated, Lignin Sulfonate, Dried Whey, Manganous Oxide, Animal Fat Preserved with BHA, BHT, Propyl Gallate and Citric Acid, Riboflavin Supplement, Vitamin E Supplement, Shark Liver Oil Preserved with BHA and BHT, Vitamin A Supplement, Vitamin B_{12} Supplement, Sodium Sulfate, Vitamin D_3 Supplement, Copper Oxide, Calcium Pantothenate, Niacin Supplement, Thiamine Hydrochloride, Natural and Artificial Flavors Added, Calcium Iodate, Menadione Sodium Bisulfite Complex, Cobalt Carbonate, Zinc Oxide.
[See table below].

Indications: The requirements of all horses are not the same. They vary with the individual according to age, size and usage. Equine Proleen® 775 Dia-Quin Brand added to the diet according to directions, will help provide the necessary fortification to meet the known daily requirements for (1) Suckling foals; (2) Growing colts; (3) Broodmares; (4) Stallions: (5) Horses in training, and racing; and (6) During stress (in all cases of increased body demand such as during and following illness, shipping, surgery, and like conditions).

Note: It may be advisable on certain individuals to feed a minimum amount of the supplement until the animal adjusts to the taste. Acceptablility of Proleen® by the equine approaches 100%.

EQUINE PROLEEN® 775

Weight	Amount to Feed Daily	Units Vitamin A Supplied Daily	Grams Proleen® Supplied Daily
100–200 lbs.	2 Teaspoonsful	8,750 I.U.	7
200–400 lbs.	1 Tablespoonful	13,250 I.U.	10
400–700 lbs.	1½ Tablespoonsful	19,875 I.U.	15
700–1000 lbs.	2 Tablespoonsful	26,500 I.U.	20
Broodmares (Gestation & Lactation) Stallions (In Service)			
400–700 lbs.	1½ Tablespoonsful	19,875 I.U.	15
700–1000 lbs.	2 Tablespoonsful	26,500 I.U.	20
1000–1200 lbs.	2½ Tablespoonsful	33,125 I.U.	25
1200–or more	3 Tablespoonsful	39,750 I.U.	30 (1 oz.)
Maintenance—Adult Horses & Ponies			
400–600 lbs.	2 Teaspoonsful	8,750 I.U.	7
600–800 lbs.	1 Tablespoonful	13,250 I.U.	10
800–1000 lbs.	1½ Tablespoonsful	19,875 I.U.	15
1000–or more	2 Tablespoonsful	26,500 I.U.	20
Racing—Heavy Training—Stress			
400–600 lbs.	1½ Tablespoonsful	19,875 I.U.	15
600–800 lbs.	2 Tablespoonsful	26,500 I.U.	20
800–1000 lbs.	3 Tablespoonsful	39,750 I.U.	30
1000–1200 lbs.	3½ Tablespoonsful	46,375 I.U.	35
1200–or more	4 Tablespoonsful	53,000 I.U.	40

How Supplied: 10 and 25 lb containers.

PROLEEN® T20 BOLUS

Composition: Guaranteed Analysis: Each Bolus Contains:

Protein*, gm	9.0
Nitrogen Free Extract, gm	12.5
Vitamin A, I.U.	Not less than 30,000
Vitamin D_3, I. U.	Not less than 10,000
Choline chloride, mg	Not less than 50
Riboflavin, mg	Not less than 15
Niacin, mg	Not less than 10
d-Pantothenic Acid, mg	Not less than 15
Vitamin B_{12}, mcg	Not less than 20
Potassium (K), mg	500
Sodium (Na), mg	250
Phosphorous (P), mg	1,400
Magnesium (Mg), mg	100
Iron (Fe), mg	10
Zinc (Zn), mg	25
Copper (Cu), mg	3
Manganese (Mn), mg	5
Iodine (I), mg	7
Sulfur (S), mg	50

*Consists of amino acids, peptides and polypeptides readily available to the rumen metabolic processes.

Ingredients: Hydrolyzed Starch, Marine Protein Concentrate, Ground Licorice Root, Condensed Beet Solubles Product, Condensed Whey Solubles, Dried Extracted Torula Yeast Fermentation Solubles, Hydrolyzed Corn Protein, Condensed Fermented Corn Extractives, Shark Liver Oil, Artificial Flavoring, Sodium Chloride, Potassium Iodide, Sulfur, Magnesium Proteinate, Iron Proteinate, Copper Proteinate, Manganese Proteinate and Cobalt Proteinate in an Amino Acid-phosphorylated complex with isolated Fish Solubles, Isolated Soy Protein Concentrate, Vitamin A Acetate (stability improved), Vitamin D_3 (stability improved), Alpha Tocopherol Acetate (a preservative), Riboflavin Supplement, Niacinamide, Calcium Pantothenate, and Vitamin B_{12} Supplement, Calcium Phosphate Monobasic.

Indications: Proleen® T^{20} Boluses are indicated for use in ruminants of all ages whenever supplemental amounts of protein, energy, vitamins, trace elements, electrolytes or micro-nutrients are required.

Dosage and Administration: Administer 1 bolus for each 200–300 pound of body weight once or twice daily depending upon the nutrient intake of the animal. The boluses can be given with a balling gun, broken, crushed and sprinkled on daily feed ration, crushed, suspended in milk or water and given as a drench or by stomach pump and tube.
In cases of severe nutrient depletion the number of boluses used can be doubled.

How Supplied: Boxes of 50 Boluses.
For Veterinary Use Only.

Products are cross-indexed by generic and chemical names in the **Active Ingredients Section**

S

The Upjohn Company
7000 PORTAGE ROAD
KALAMAZOO, MICHIGAN 49001

BRYTIN™
Pellets

Composition: Each ounce contains:

Vitamin A (40,000 Int. Units)	12 mg
Vitamin D (8,000 Int. Units)	200 mcg
Thiamine Mononitrate	24 mg
Riboflavin	40 mg
Niacin	120 mg
Pyridoxine Hydrochloride	12 mg
Calcium Pantothenate	48 mg
Cyanocobalamin	120 mcg
Vitamin E	80 Int. Units
Folic Acid	12 mg
Choline (as choline chloride)	600 mg
Iron (from ferrous gluconate)	60 mg
Iodine (from copper iodate)	3 mg
Copper (as copper oxide)	12 mg
Manganese (as manganese oxide)	60 mg
Zinc (as zinc oxide)	270 mg
Cobalt (as cobalt carbonate)	0.27 mg
Diabasic Calcium Phosphate equiv. to Calcium	1,800 mg
Phosphorus	1,391 mg

Using the plastic scoop provided, one level scoop will deliver approximately one ounce.
Suggested Daily Dosage as a Vitamin-Mineral Supplement: Mature Horses, 1 ounce (1 scoop).
Foals, ⅛ to ½ ounce.
Warning: Keep out of reach of children.
Not for human use.

PETDROPS®
Multiple Viatamin Drops

Composition: Each 0.6 ml contains:

Vitamin A	5000 Int Units
Vitamin D_3	1000 Int Units
Thiamine Hydrochloride	1 mg
Riboflavin (as 5 phosphate sodium)	1 mg
Ascorbic Acid	30 mg
Niacinamide	10 mg
Pyridoxine Hydrochloride	1 mg
dl-alpha-Tocopheryl Acetate	5 mg
Dexpanthenol	3 mg

A nutritional tonic and dietary supplemental for dogs and cats—particularly the young and old in each species.
Indications: Pediatric and geriatric nutritional tonic or dietary supplement, listlessness, dietary imbalance or deficiency, lack of appetite, rapid tiring, convalescence, animals being wormed, and general conditioning for breeding, showing or working.
Dosage and Administration:
Dogs and Cats—As a reconstructive tonic and dietary supplement—0.3 to 0.6 ml (indicated by graduations on the dropper) one or two times daily.
Petdrops may be administered by dropping directly into the mouth or on the food.
Warning:
Not for human use.
Store at room temperature.
How Supplied: ½ fl oz (15 ml).
For Veterinary Use Only

UNILACT®
Liquid or Powder
Replacement for bitch's milk
Feed Supplement for Dogs and Pets

Composition: Ingredients: Skimmed Milk, Water, Vegetable Oils, Casein, Egg Yolk, Calcium Carbonate (Precipitated), Potassium Phosphate Monobasic, Lecithin, Calcium Hydroxide, Choline Chloride, Sodium Bicarbonate, Potassium Chloride, Carrageenan, Salt, Potassium Phosphate Dibasic, Magnesium Carbonate, Magnesium Sulfate, Vitamin E Supplement, Vitamin A Supplement, Iron Sulfate, Zinc Sulfate, Niacin Supplement, Calcium Pantothenate, Copper Sulfate, Vitamin B_{12} Supplement, Vitamin D_3 Supplement, Manganese Sulfate, Riboflavin, Thiamin Hydrochloride, Pyridoxine Hydrochloride, Potassium Iodide, Folic acid.
Guaranteed Analysis: Crude Protein, Min., 4.5%; Crude Fat, Min., 6.0%; Crude Fiber, none; Moisture, Max., 85.0%; Ash, Max., 1.0%.
How to Feed: Feeding newborn mammals a replacement formula always entails some risk, and your veterinarian should be consulted for advice on feeding Unilact and on sound management practices.
For growing puppies, household pets, field and working dogs, show dogs, old and convalescent pets and all furbearing animals: Feed one tablespoon of Unilact Liquid for every 5 pounds of body weight by mixing into daily ration.
For brood matrons: Feed Unilact as above until two weeks after whelping, one-half this amount during the third week, one-fourth during the fourth week, and then discontinue until the puppies are weaned and the bitch has dried up. Normal supplementation with Unilact can then be resumed.
From birth through the second week: All puppies should receive their dam's milk for at least two days if possible. The colostrum milk gives extra nutrition and temporary immunity against some diseases. The table below shows the amount of Unilact to be fed each pup for one day: Divide the amount of Unilact to be fed each pup into equal portions per feeding. For example, three feedings daily, ⅓ of the preceding amount at each feeding; four feedings daily, ¼ of the preceding amount at each feeding, etc.
Puppies' needs will vary and the amounts suggested in the table are a guide but may have to be increased or decreased depending on the individual. Large breeds do well when fed every 8 hours, medium size breeds every 6 hours and toy breeds or weak pups of any size every 3 or 4 hours. Feed at body temperature.
For very small and weak puppies an eye dropper or doll bottle with nipple can be used for nursing. A regular baby bottle and nipple or spoon feeding can be used for average or large size puppies. When pups are old enough to lap Unilact, they may be switched to bowl feeding.
Weaning the pups: During the third or fourth week, mix Unilact Liquid with dog meal to produce a gruel-like mixture. Start the pup off with small amounts of the mix and increase gradually so that the pups are on solid food by the end of the weaning period. Weaned pups should continue to receive Unilact at the rate of one tablespoon per 4 lbs of body weight.
After Unilact has been opened, it should be refrigerated. Discard any opened, unused Unilact Liquid after 72 hours. Caution: Prevent from freezing.
Total Daily ration Per Pup

Weight of pups	*Tablespoons of Unilact powder or Liquid Formula Each Pup Daily*
2 oz	1½
4 oz	2
6 oz	3
8 oz	4
12 oz	5
1 lb	6
2 lbs	12
3 lbs	20

Note: Weigh the pup at least once a week to assure adequate feeding.
Available in 12 oz cans of powder and 14 oz cans of liquid.

UNIPET®
Tablets

Composition: Each tablet supplies: Animal Protein, 500 mg; Brewer's Feed Yeast, 400 mg; Dibasic Calcium Phosphate, Hydrous, 275 mg; Ferrous Gluconate (equiv. to 1.87 mg iron), 16.2 mg; Wheat Germ Oil, 30 mg; Lecithin, 15 mg; Cephalin, 15 mg; Inositol-Phosphatides, 15 mg; Soy Bean Oil, 25 mg; Choline, 2.5 mg; Vitamin A (1,500 International units), 0.45 mg; Vitamin D (150 International units), 3.75 mcg; Thiamine Mononitrate (B_1), 1 mg; Riboflavin (B_2), 1 mg; Pyridoxine Hydrochloride (B_6), 0.1 mg; Niacinamide, 10 mg; Folic Acid, 0.05 mg; Cyanocobalamin (B_{12}), 0.2 mcg.
A palatable vitamin-mineral-protein nutritional supplement for dogs and cats.
Daily Dosage and Administration: Dogs—1 to 4 tablets. Puppies—½ to 1 tablet.
Cats—½ to 1 tablet.
(Tablets may be fed directly to the animal or crumbled and mixed with the food.)

UNIPET–C®
Tablets

Composition: Each tablet supplies: Animal Protein, 250 mg; Brewer's Feed Yeast, 200 mg; Dibasic Calcium Phosphate, Hydrous, 125 mg; Ferrous Gluconate (equiv. to 0.93 mg iron) 8.1 mg; Wheat Germ Oil, 15 mg; Lecithin, 7.5 mg; Cephalin, 7.5 mg; Inositol Phosphatides, 7.5 mg; Soy Bean Oil, 12.5 mg; Choline, 1.25 mg; Vitamin A, 0.225 mg (750 11 units); Vitamin D, 1.875 mcg (75 Interna-

Continued on next page

U

Upjohn—Cont.

tional units); Thiamine Mononitrate (B_1), 0.5 mg; Riboflavin (B_2), 0.5 mg; Pyridoxine Hydrochloride (B_6), 0.05 mg; Niacinamide, 5 mg; Folic Acid, 0.025 mg; Cyanocobalamin (B_{12}), 0.1 mcg.
Vitamin-Mineral-Protein nutritional supplement for cats, kittens and puppies.
Daily Dosage and Administration: Cats: 1 to 2 tablets. Kittens: ½ to 1 tablet. Puppies: 1 to 2 tablets.
(Tablets may be fed directly to the animal or crumbled and mixed with the food).

UNIPET® SENIOR
Tablets

Composition: Each tablet supplies: Animal Protein, 500 mg; Brewer's Feed Yeast, 450 mg; Dibasic Calcium Phosphate Hydrous, 250 mg; Ferrous Gluconate (equiv. to 12 mg iron), 105 mg; Wheat Germ Oil, 30 mg; Lecithin, 15 mg; Cephalin, 15 mg; Inositol Phosphatides, 15 mg; Soy Bean Oil, 25 mg; Choline, 2.5 mg; Vitamin A (1500 International units), 0.45 mg; Vitamin D (150 International units), 3.75 mcg; Vitamin E 10 International units; Thiamine Mononitrate (B_1), 1 mg; Riboflavin (B_2), 1 mg; Pyridoxine Hydrochloride (B_6), 0.2 mg; Niacinamide, 10 mg; Folic Acid, 0.05 mg; Calcium Pantothenate, 0.55 mg; Cyanocobalamin (B_{12}), 2 mcg; Copper (as sulfate), 1.5 mg; Cobalt (as carbonate), 0.5 mg; Magnesium (as oxide), 20 mg; Manganese (as sulfate), 1 mg; Iodine (as potassium iodide), 0.05 mg; Zinc (as oxide), 1 mg.
A palatable vitamin-mineral-protein supplement for older dogs and cats or those with special needs.
Dosage: Dogs—1 tablet daily per 20 pounds body weight.
Cats—½ tablet daily.
(Tablet may be fed directly to the animal or crumbled and mixed with the food.)
Warning: Hazardous for human use.

U

Vet-A-Mix, Inc.
604 WEST THOMAS AVENUE
SHENANDOAH, IOWA 51601

ADD-PLEX
A Conditioner For All Species Of Animals

Composition:

Guaranteed Analysis:	***per pound***
Vitamin A	400,000 IU
Vitamin D_3	100,000 IU
Cobalt sulfate monohydrate	150 mg
Equivalent to elemental Cobalt	30 mg

Also contains 2% dicalcium phosphate and supplemental amounts of riboflavin, pantothenic acid, niacin, vitamin B_{12}, vitamin E, thiamine and vitamin K_3.
Ingredients: Vitamin A acetate, vitamin D_3 supplement, riboflavin supplement, calcium pantothenate, niacin supplement, vitamin B_{12} supplement, vitamin E supplement, thiamine mononitrate, menadione sodium bisulfite, cobalt sulfate monohydrate, BHT (butylated hydroxytoluene, a preservative), dicalcium phosphate, vegetable oil, and soybean meal.
Indications: A vitamin supplement with minerals for use in domestic animals and poultry.
Dosage and Administration: Supplementation level for all domestic animals. Mix in the feed at the rate of 1/2 to 1 pound in each 100 pounds of feed.
Mature Cattle: 1/2 to 1 pound to each 100 pounds of feed.
Dairy: Individual dose may be fed on grain at the rate of 1-2 ounces (2-4 rounded teaspoons) per day for each 1,000 pounds body weight.
Feedlot: Top dress the prescribed amount on the grain.
Range Cattle: Mix with salt at the rate of 1 pound to 25 pounds salt. Normal consumption is 1/4 pound salt per day per 1,000 pound cow and 1/8 pound salt per 400 pound steer per day. Mix only the amount of salt consumed in a 2-3 week period.
Horses: Top dress the prescribed amount on the grain.
Foals and Ponies: 1 to 2 tablespoons daily.
Colts, Stallions, Brood Mares and Horses in training: 1 tablespoon per 400 pounds body weight.
Sheep and Swine: 1 pound per 100 lb feed.
Poultry: 1/2 pound per 100 lb feed.
How Supplied: 25 pound pails, 50 pound bags

ADE-SOL
Water Dispersible
A Concentrated Vitamin A, D & E Supplement for All Species of Livestock and Poultry

Composition: Guaranteed Analysis:

	Per lb	Per Gram
Vitamin A (as Palmitate) U.S.P. Units	4,800,000	10,582
Vitamin D_3, I.C. Units	960,000	2,116
Equivalent to U.S.P. Units	960,000	2,116
Vitamin E (a-alpha tocopheral acetate)	I.U.-5,600	12.3

In a base composed of dextrose, lactose, sucrose, gelatin, gum arabic, and butylated hydroxytoluene (a preservative).
One level teaspoon contains 4 to 5 grams.
The dosages indicated are nutritional and will provide the approximate recommended daily allowance of vitamin A, excess vitamin D, and minimum requirements of vitamin E (suggested levels for poultry—levels for other animals unknown).
May be administered in water, milk or rations. When administering in cold drinking water, the rate of dispersion will be improved by dissolving the required amount in a small quantity of warm water first. When administering in rations, it is recommended that the required dosage be premixed into a small amount of ground grain or supplement.
If daily administration is impractical, Ade-Sol may be given less frequently, but in large doses (Example: 7 times the daily dosage may be given once each week).
During deficiency symptoms, double the dosage levels indicated below.
Cattle, Horses & Sheep: To furnish RDA (recommended daily allowance) give ¼ teaspoon per 1,000 lbs or one oz (2 tablespoons) per 25,000 lbs body weight per day. Mix in drinking water, grain ration or protein supplement. This dosage can be approximated by administering in drinking water at the rate of one teaspoon per 40 gallons water, one tablespoon per 120 gallons or 4 oz per 1,000 gallons. For growing animals double the above RDA levels. During reproduction and lactation give 3 to 4 times the RDA levels.
Feeder Calves: Use 2 teaspoons per 1,000 lbs or 8 oz per 25,000 lbs body weight per day for 3 to 5 days. The calculated dosage may be mixed in drinking water, grain ration or protein supplement This dosage can be approximated by administering in drinking water at the rate of 1 teaspoon per 5 gallons water, one tablespoon per 15 gallons or 8 oz per 250 gallons. After treatment reduce the level to match body requirements and intake of vitamins from other sources.
Small Calves: Administer thoroughly mixed in milk or on the tongue as dry powder. Give ½ teaspoon per calf at birth; thereafter give ½ to one teaspoon per calf once each week. An alternate method is to mix 1/8 to ¼ teaspoon in each 2 gallons milk fed each day. Mix in calf meals at the rate of ½ to one pound per ton of ration. Lambs should receive proportionate amounts.
Swine & Poultry: To furnish RDA mix in drinking water at the rate of ½ teaspoon per 5 gallons water, one tablespoon per 30 gallons water, or 4 oz per 250 gallons water. Mix in rations at the rate of 8 oz per ton of complete ration or of total feed intake. Breeder flocks and turkeys should receive twice these amounts.
Note: Keep container sealed when not in use. When administering in drinking water, avoid mixing more than the amount normally consumed in a 24 hour period.
How Supplied: 1 lb bottles and 15 lb pails.

AVI-CON
Concentrated water soluble vitamins for birds

Composition: Each 200 mg dose supplies:

Vitamin A acetate	200 IU
Vitamin D_3	25 IU
Vitamin E	1 IU
Thiamine mononitrate	100 mcg
Riboflavin	300 mcg
Pyridoxine hydrochloride	100 mcg
Vitamin B_{12}	1 mcg
Biotin	4 mcg
Choline	4000 mcg
Folic acid	60 mcg
Niacin	1000 mcg

Pantothenic acid .... 300 mcg
Menadione (K_3) .... 200 mcg

Indications: A dietary and supportive supplement designed to provide the vitamins necessary for normal health and feathering.

Dosage and Administration: To assure freshness, prepare a water/vitamin mixture every day. For dietary supplementation, mix two (2) measures in each fluid ounce of drinking water each day. For young, ailing or aged birds, mix four measures in each fluid ounce of drinking water each day.

Note: Because of the special water soluble base, Avi-Con will remain a fresh, free flowing powder as long as the container is kept tightly closed when not in use. Accelerated tests show optimum vitamin stability when compared to other vitamin preparations for birds. Avi-Con, like all other bird vitamins, will remain potent for a limited period when mixed with drinking water. Do not mix more than the amount of drinking water that will be consumed in one day.

How Supplied: 50 gram and 250 gram bottles

BIO–METH
Biotin and DL-Methionine Supplement

Composition: Each pound contains not less than 96 milligrams d-Biotin and 32,000 milligrams DL-Methionine in a base composed of roughage products, calcium carbonate and mineral oil.

Indications: For use as a nutritional supplement in horses when a deficiency of DL-Methionine and biotin exists.

Dosage: Feed 70 grams (2 level measures) per head per day. Each 70 grams contains 15 mg d-Biotin and 5 grams DL-Methionine.

Administration: Top dress or mix with the daily ration. To facilitate proper adhesion slightly moisten the grain with water or liquid supplement.

How Supplied: 4 pound jars, 20 pound pails

BIOTIN–100
d-Biotin for Horses

Composition: Each pound contains 100 mg of d-Biotin in a base of rice hulls and mineral oil.

Indications: For use as a nutritional supplement in horses when a biotin deficiency exists.

Dosage: Feed 68 grams (2 heaping measures) per head per day. Each 68 grams contains 15 mg d-Biotin.

Administration: Top dress or mix with the daily ration. To facilitate proper adhesion slightly moisten the grain with water or liquid supplement.

How Supplied: 5 pound bags and 20 pound pails

EQU-AID PLUS
Vitamin-Mineral Supplement for Horses and Ponies

Composition:

Guaranteed Analysis:	*Per 2 ounce*
Vitamin A	40,000 IU
Vitamin D_3	5,000 IU
Vitamin E	100 IU
Riboflavin	40 mg
Niacin	80 mg
Thiamine mononitrate	20 mg
d-Pantothenic acid	100 mg
Pyridoxine hydrochloride	5 mg
Vitamin B_{12}	40 mcg
Iodine	2 mg
Iron	100 mg
Copper	20 mg
Cobalt	1 mg
Magnesium	100 mg
Manganese	100 mg
Selenium	1 mg
Zinc	280 mg
Phosphorus	1,200 mg
Calcium, not less than	4,200 mg
Calcium, not more than	5,000 mg
Salt, not more than	1,418 mg
DL-methionine	1,000 mg
L-Lysine monohydrate	1,000 mg
Vegetable oils, not less than	5,670 mg

(containing not less than 85% unsaturated fatty acids)

The dose cup enclosed with every container will provide approximately 2 ounces when level full.

Directions: Feed 2 ounces (one level measure) per day to colts and adult horses. Shetland ponies and very small breeds should receive proportionate amounts.

Note: Consider selenium concentrations in the total daily feed intake. The total added level should not exceed 0.10 ppm of selenium.

How Supplied: 5 lb Jars, 40 lb Pails, 100 lb Drums

EQU-SeE
Vitamin E and Selenium Supplement for Horses

Composition:

Guaranteed Analysis	Per lb	Per g
Selenium, mg	90.7	0.20
Vitamin E, IU	20,000	44.09

Ingredients: Sodium selenite, Vitamin E (as dl-alpha tocopheryl acetate), roughage products, calcium carbonate, mineral oil.

Indication: For use as a dietary source of selenium and vitamin E for horses.

Dosage and Administration: Equ-SeE can be administered by mixing the daily dose in the concentrate or by top dressing on some grain, preferably rolled or ground. The normal recommended dosage is one to 2 teaspoons per 1,000 lb (450 kg) body weight or ½ to 1 teaspoon per 10 lb (4.5 kg) total daily feed.

Recommended Daily Dosage

Body Weight	Dose
250 lb (115 kg)	¼-½ Teaspoon
500 lb (225 kg)	½-1 Teaspoon
750 lb (340 kg)	¾-1½ Teaspoon
1000 lb (450 kg)	1-2 Teaspoon

Note: One teaspoonful contains approximately 5 grams of Equ-SeE.

Caution: Follow label directions. The addition to feed of higher levels of the premix is not permitted. DO NOT EXCEED RECOMMENDED DOSAGE.

Warning: Consider selenium concentrations in the total daily feed intake. The total added level should not exceed 0.10 ppm of selenium.

ETHYODIDE
A Ten Percent Organic Iodine Compound to be Mixed in Rations, Salt or Water of Domestic Animals and Poultry

Composition: Each pound contains: Ethylenediamine Dihydriodide 45,360 mg (700 gr).

In a free flowing base of dextrose, sodium chloride, coloring, flavoring and stabilizers.

Indications: *Cattle*—Aid in the treatment of foot rot caused by *Spheropherous necrophorus* and lumpy jaw caused by *Actinobacillus lignierisi*. Aid in the treatment of respiratory infections by action as an expectorant.

And in the prevention of foot rot and soft tissue lumpy jaw and as nutritional source of iodine.

Swine—Aid in the control of respiratory difficulties by loosening mucus in the upper respiratory tract.

Chickens & Turkeys—Aid in the removal of mucus from the upper respiratory tract following treatment of CRD.

Dosage and Administration:

Cattle: Therapeutic Level—1 lb per 100 head per day for 2 to 3 weeks in water, feed or salt. For free choice administration in salt, mix 1 lb Ethyodide in 6 lbs salt and feed to provide 1 oz of mixture per head per day.

Preventive Level—1 lb per 900 head (500 mg Ethyodide per head) per day continuously in feed, salt or water. For salt administration mix 1 lb with 50 to 100 lb salt.

Swine: Give 1 lb per 100 to 200 head per day in water or feed for 5 to 7 days.

Chickens & Turkeys: Mix 2½ lb in each ton of ration for 5 to 7 days.

Warning: Treat animals and birds with caution until tolerance is determined because of the variation in susceptibility to iodides.

How Supplied: 1 lb jars and 25 lb pails.

FELO-FORM
Chewable Tablets

A Vitamin-Trace Mineral Supplement with Proven Palatability for cats Especially Formulated Without Struvite Forming Compounds

Composition: Each chewable tablet contains:

Taurine	10 mg
Methionine	100 mg
Vitamin A Acetate . . . 0.450 mg	1500 IU
Vitamin D_3 . . . 0.004 mg	50 IU
Vitamin E . . . 4.000 mg	4 IU
Thiamine mononitrate	1 mg
Riboflavin	1 mg
Niacin	4 mg
d-Pantothenic Acid	1 mg
Pyridoxine hydrochloride	0.2 mg
Inositol	10 mg
Choline bitartrate	50 mg
Biotin	10 mcg
Folic acid	2 mcg
Zinc	0.3 mg

(as zinc oxide)

Continued on next page

Vet-A-Mix—Cont.

Manganese ....0.2 mg
(as manganese sulfate)
Iron ....5.0 mg
(as ferrous gluconate)
Copper ....0.2 mg
(as copper sulfate)
Cobalt ....0.1 mg
(as cobalt sulfate)
Iodine ....0.2 mg
(as ethylenediamine dihydriodide)
In a palatable protein base with unsaturated fatty acids.
Indications: For use as a dietary supplement for cats and kittens. Because of the lack of struvite-forming elements, may be especially useful for feline prone to Feline Urological Syndrome.
Dosage and Administration: Felo-Form Chewable Tablets may be fed free choice, from the hand or crumbled and mixed into the food. For additional flavor release, moisten the tablets before offering to the cat.
Recommended Daily Dosage
Kittens: One-half tablet
Adult cats: One tablet for diet supplementation, two tablets for convalescing, pregnant or nursing cats.
Note: Use Osteo-Form 181 Chewable Tablets when calcium, phosphorus and magnesium are needed for an increase in dietary supplementation or intake.
How Supplied: 100 and 500 tablet bottles.

K-SOL
Water Soluble

Composition: Vitamin K_3, a vitamin K analogue.

Guaranteed Analysis	Per Pound
Menadione Sodium Bisulfite	8,000 mg

In a base composed of dextrose, lactose, sucrose and butylated hydroxytoluene (a preservative).
Each gram of K-Sol contains 17.6 mg; one ounce contains 500 mg menadione sodium bisulfite. One level teaspoonful contains approximately 5 grams of K-Sol representing 88 mg menadione sodium bisulfite.
Indications: For use as a source of vitamin K_3 (a vitamin K analogue) for all species of livestock and poultry.
Dosage and Administration: K-Sol contains the water soluble analogue of the fat-soluble vitamin K.
Poultry: To furnish the RDA (recommended daily allowance) of vitamin K, mix in the drinking water at the rate of one teaspoonful per 40 gallons of drinking water or 2 ounces per ton of complete ration. Breeder flocks should receive four times the above level. For treatment of vitamin K deficiencies, mix in the drinking water at a rate of one to two teaspoonfuls per 10 gallons water or one ounce per 30 gallons water. Treat for as long as indicated.
Swine: To aid in the treatment of vitamin K deficiencies, mix in the drinking water at the rate of one to two teaspoonfuls per 10 gallons water or 8 to 16 ounces per 500 gallon water. Mix 8 to 16 ounces per ton of complete ration. Treat for 3 to 5 days or as long as indicated.
Cattle, Sheep and Horses: To aid in the treatment of vitamin K deficiency, administer one teaspoonful per each 500 pounds orally or one ounce per 2500 pounds body weight. Mix one pound per 500 gallons of drinking water. Treat for 3 to 5 days or as long as indicated.
Note: Keep container sealed when not in use.
Store at room temperature and protect from light.
Avoid excessive heat (104°F).
KEEP OUT OF REACH OF CHILDREN
How Supplied: One pound bottle.

METHIO-VET POWDER
DL-Methionine For Equine

Composition: Each pound contains DL-methionine 99%.
Indications: For use as a nutritional supplement in horses when a methionine deficiency exists as evidenced by laminitis.
Dosage: The usual dose for a 1000 to 1200 pound horse is 10 grams (4 slightly rounded teaspoonsful) per day for 7 days followed by 5 grams (2 slightly rounded teaspoonsful) per day for 21 additional days.
Administration: Methio-Vet Powder may be top dressed or mixed into the daily ration. To facilitate proper adhesion of Methio-Vet Powder, slightly moisten the grain with water or liquid supplement before mixing.
Note: One slightly rounded teaspoonful contains approximately 2.5 grams of DL-methionine powder.
How Supplied: 1 pound bottles, 5 pound jars, 10 pound pails and 25 pound pails

NUTRI-FORM G CHEWABLE TABLETS
A High Potency Vitamin-Mineral Geriatric and Stress Formula

Composition: Each chewable tablet contains:
Vitamin A ....1100 IU
Vitamin D_3 ....110 IU
Vitamin E ....22 IU
Thiamine mononitrate ....2.2 mg
Riboflavin ....4.8 mg
Niacin ....25 mg
Pyridoxine HCl ....2.2 mg
Vitamin B_{12} ....50 mcg
Pantothenic acid ....11 mg
Folic acid ....200 mcg
Biotin ....22 mcg
Zinc
(as zinc oxide) ....11 mg
Iodine
(as EDDI) ....120 mcg
Selenium
(as sodium selenite) ....24 mcg
Choline
(as choline chloride) ....26 mg
Inositol ....5 mg
Methionine ....200 mg
Lysine HCl ....25 mg
Brewer's Yeast ....650 mg
Unsaturated fatty acids ....15 mg
In a palatable base composed of liver, meat and yeast
Indications: For use as a nutritional supplement in mature or stressed dogs and cats.
Dosage and Administration: Nutri-Form G Chewable Tables may be fed free choice, from the hand or may be crumbled and mixed into the food. For additional flavor release, moisten the tablets before offering to the pet.
Recommended Daily Dosage

Dogs -	
Small breeds	One-half tablet
Medium breeds	One tablet
Large breeds	Two tablets
Extra large breeds	3-4 tablets
Cats -	
All breeds and sizes	One tablet

How Supplied: 50 and 150 Tablet Bottles

OSTEOFORM IMPROVED

Composition: A palatable, readily assimilable supplement for the correction of dietary deficiencies of calcium and phosphorus in dogs, cats, horses, swine and cattle.

Contents per 425 grams:	
Calcium, not more than	32.4%
Calcium, not less than	27.0%
Phosphorus, not less than	16.5%
Vitamin A	153,000 I.U.
Vitamin D_3	15,300 I.U.
Vitamin C	1,000 mg

Indications: For use as an aid in the prevention and correction of dietary deficiencies of calcium phosphorus and vitamins A, D_3 and ascorbic acid in swine, cattle, horses, dogs and cats.
Dosage and Administration: OsteoForm Improved may be added to the daily ration or mixed with milk or water.
Dogs and Cats: To aid in the correction of dietary deficiencies, give 1 to 2 heaping teaspoonfuls (1–12 grams) for each 10 pounds body weight per day for as long as indicated. For the prevention of dietary deficiencies and during healing of fractures, give ½ the above dose.
Horses: To aid in the correction of dietary deficiencies, give 1 to 3 slightly rounded tablespoonfuls (12–36 grams) to foals and 3 to 5 tablespoonfuls to yearlings and adults each day for as long as indicated. As a dietary supplement give ½ the above dose.
Cattle: As a dietary supplement, give 2 to 4 tablespoonfuls per day.
Swine: As a dietary supplement, especially for brood sows, give 1 to 2 tablespoonfuls per day.
When using OsteoForm Improved as a maintenance dietary supplement, calcium and phosphorus from other food sources should be considered.
KEEP OUT OF REACH OF CHILDREN.
How Supplied: 425 gram bottles; 12.5 kilogram pail.
For Veterinary Use Only

OSTEO-FORM 181
(brand of calcium-phosphorous with vitamins)
Chewable Tablets

Composition: Each Scored Tablet Contains:

Calcium	600 mg
Phosphorus	335 mg
Vitamin A	750 I.U.
Vitamin D	75 I.U.
Ascorbic Acid (Vitamin C)	10 mg

In a palatable protein base

Ingredients: Bone ash, Vitamin A acetate, activated animal sterol (source of Vitamin D), calcium carbonate, calcium phosphate dibasic, ascorbic acid, bone meal, meat byproducts and dried yeast.

Indications: For use as an aid in the prevention and correction of dietary deficiencies of calcium, phosphorus and vitamins A, D_3, and ascorbic acid in dogs and cats.

Dosage and Administration: OsteoForm 181 Tablets may be fed free choice, from the hand or may be crumbled and mixed into the food.

For an aid in the correction of rickets and eclampsia give 2 to 4 OsteoForm 181 Tablets per 5 kilograms (11 pounds) of body weight daily as necessary.

For the prevention of dietary deficiencies and during healing of fractures give 1 to 2 OsteoForm 181 Tablets for each 5 kilograms (11 pounds) of body weight per day.

Note: Two OsteoForm 181 Tablets are equivalent to one slightly rounded teaspoonful of OsteoForm Improved Powder.

Caution: When using OsteoForm 181 Tablets as a maintenance dietary supplement, calcium and phosphorus from other food sources should be considered.

KEEP OUT OF REACH OF CHILDREN

How Supplied: 50, 150 and 500 tablet bottles

For Veterinary Use Only

PET–FORM®

(brand of vitamin-mineral dietary supplement with Essential Unsaturated Fatty Acids) Chewable Tablets

Composition: Each Tablet Contains:

Vitamin A Acetate	0.450 mg (1,500 I.U.)
Vitamin D_3	0.004 mg (150 I.U.)
Vitamin E (dl-alpha tocopheryl acetate)	2.0 mg (2.0 I.U.)
Thiamine mononitrate	1.0 mg
Riboflavin	1.0 mg
Niacin	10.0 mg
Pyridoxine hydrochloride	0.1 mg
Vitamin B_{12}	3.0 mcg
d-Pantothenic acid	0.5 mg
Folic acid	0.05 mg
Choline chloride	20.0 mg
Calcium (from calcium phosphate dibasic and calcium carbonate)	200 mg
Phosphorus (from calcium phosphate dibasic)	100 mg
Iron (as ferrous gluconate)	6.0 mg
Copper (as copper sulfate)	0.375 mg
Cobalt (as cobalt sulfate)	0.125 mg
Iodine (as ethylenediamine dihydriodide)	0.5 mg
Zinc (as zinc oxide)	1.0 mg
Manganese (as manganese sulfate)	1.0 mg
Protein (from liver, meat and yeast)	500 mg
dl-Methionine	27 mg
Unsaturated fatty acids	25 mg

Indications: Use as a dietary supplement for dogs and cats.

Dosage and Administration: Pet-Form Tablets may be fed free choice, from the hand or may be crumbled and mixed into the food.

As an aid in dietary supplementation, Pet-Form Tablets provide eleven vitamins and eight minerals plus supplemental amounts of protein and essential unsaturated fatty acids in a palatable base.

Recommended Daily Dosage:

Dogs:

Small Breeds—One half to one Pet-Form Tablet.

Medium Breeds—One Pet-Form Tablet.

Large Breeds—Two to four Pet-Form Tablets.

Cats:

All Breeds and Sizes—One Pet-Form Tablet.

KEEP OUT OF REACH OF CHILDREN

How Supplied: 50, 150 and 500 tablet bottles

For Veterinary Use Only

PLEX-SOL C

Water Dispersible

Composition: A concentrated high potency vitamin complex for domestic animals, pet birds, poultry and laboratory animals, i.e. rats, guinea pigs, hamsters and monkeys.

Guaranteed Analysis	Per Kilogram
Vitamin A	2,000,000 I.U.
Vitamin D_3	250,000 I.U.
Vitamin E	5,000 I.U.
Vitamin C (Ascorbic Acid)	40,000 mg
Menadione (K3 from Menadione sodium bisulfate)	2,000 mg
Niacin	10,000 mg
d-Pantothenic Acid	2,484 mg
Riboflavin	2,500 mg
Thiamine Mononitrate	1,000 mg
Pyridoxine Hydrochloride	1,000 mg
Vitamin B_{12}	10 mg
Folic Acid	500 mg

Ingredients: Vitamin A supplement (improved stability), vitamin D_3 supplement; vitamin E supplement, ascorbic acid, menadione sodium bisulfite complex, niacin supplement, calcium pantothenate, riboflavin supplement, thiamine mononitrate, pyridoxine hydrochloride, vitamin B_{12} supplement, folic acid, in a water soluble base of dextrose, sucrose, magnesium sulfate, sodium sulfate and BHT (a preservative.)

Indications: For use as a dietary and supportive supplement in cattle, swine, poultry, pet birds and laboratory animals such as rats, guinea pigs, hamsters and monkeys.

Directions for Use: *For mixing in the daily ration:* For prevention, thoroughly and evenly mix 5 grams in each kilogram (2.2 pounds) of diet; 1 kilogram in each 200 kilograms of ration; 4.5 kilograms in each 2000 pounds of ration.

For mixing in the drinking water: For prevention, mix 5 grams in each liter of water; 1 kilogram in each 200 liters of water, or 950 grams in each 50 gallons of water. For therapeusis, double the above dosages.

Keep container closed when not in use. Do not store at temperatures exceeding 80°F (27°C).

KEEP OUT OF REACH OF CHILDREN

How Supplied: 500 gram bottles and 10 kilogram pails.

For Veterinary Use Only

SUPER SeE

Composition: Guaranteed Analysis Per Pound

Selenium	90.7 mg
Vitamin E	20,000 I.U.

Ingredients: Sodium selenite, vitamin E (as dl alpha tocopheryl acetate), roughage products, calcium carbonate and mineral oil.

Indications: For the control or correction of vitamin E and selenium deficiencies in beef cattle, dairy cattle, sheep, swine, chickens, ducks and turkeys.

Dosage and Administration: *Beef cattle, dairy cattle, sheep, swine, chickens, ducks:* Thoroughly and evenly mix 1 pound of Super SeE per ton of complete ration. This will furnish a level of 0.1 p.p.m. of selenium.

Turkeys: Thoroughly and evenly mix 2 pounds of Super SeE per ton of complete ration. This will furnish a level of 0.2 p.p.m. of selenium.

Caution: Follow label directions. The addition to feed of higher levels of this premix is not permitted.

Warning: This product must be evenly and thoroughly mixed in rations to avoid toxicoses. When used in feeds mixed with vertical and on-the-farm mixers, thoroughly premix one pound of Super SeE with approximately 50 pounds of ground grain or supplement before mixing in a one ton batch.

How Supplied: 1 lb packets, 25 lb pails, 50 lb bags

VETA-LAC®

Fortified Dry Milk with Vitamins, Minerals, and Methionine

Composition: Guaranteed Analysis

Protein, not less than	26.0%
Fat, not less than	20.0%
Fiber, not more than	1.0%
Ash, not more than	8.0%
Calories, per kilogram	4500.0
Calories, per 400 grams	1800.0
Calories, per 100 grams	450.0
Calories, per measure	67.5

Ingredients: Dried skim milk, vegetable oils, edible animal fats, lecithin, vitamin A, vitamin D_3, vitamin E, vitamin B_{12}, thiamine mononitrate, riboflavin, folic acid, pyridoxine hydrochloride, pantothenic acid, niacin, choline bitartrate, ascorbic acid, inositol, dl methionine, di-calcium phosphate, ferrous sulfate, cobalt sulfate , copper sulfate, manganese sulfate, magnesium oxide, zinc oxide, ethylenediamine dihydriodide,

Continued on next page

Vet-A-Mix—Cont.

sodium phosphate, sodium citrate, flavorings, emulsifiers and preservatives.
Indications: For orphan puppies and kittens. For young animals whose mothers are furnishing inadequate or unsatisfactory milk. During convalescence from illness or during vomiting, when low roughage diets are required. For overweight dogs.
Dosage and Administration: *Orphan puppies and kittens* —place 3 level measures of Veta-Lac into a clean, dry container. Add clean, very warm water to eight fluid ounces (½ pint or 1 cup). *Strong puppies and kittens* should normally be fed six times during each 24 hours (weak or very small animals should be fed every 2 hours) for the first few days. The number of feedings may be reduced to four times every 24 hours by the end of the first week.

Liquid (Re-Constituted) Veta-Lac Feeding Guide

Weight of Animal	Amount of Liquid To Be Fed Daily
2 ounces (57 grams)	½–1 measure*
4 ounces (113 grams)	1 measure
8 ounces (227 grams)	2 measures
1 pound (454 grams)	3 measures
2 pounds (907 grams)	6 measures

*1 measure =1 fl oz =approx. 2 tablespoonfuls

Dry Feeding Veta-Lac
(Dietary Supplementation)
Sprinkle Dry Veta-Lac over regular or canned feeds in amounts shown below:

Dogs:

Small Breeds	1 Measure
Medium Breeds	3 Measures
Large Breeds	6 Measures
Cats:	1 Measure

How Supplied: 400 grams and 5 kg pails.
For Veterinary Use Only

VITA-PLEX SeE

Composition: For the correction or prevention of vitamin and selenium deficiencies of swine and turkeys.

Guaranteed Analysis:	Per Pound
Selenium	18 mg
Vitamin E	2,000 I.U.
Vitamin A	200,000 I.U.
Vitamin D_3	50,000 I.U.
Riboflavin	500 mg
d-Pantothenic Acid	1,650 mg
Niacin	2,000 mg
Thiamine Mononitrate	100 mg
Vitamin B_{12}	2 mg

Ingredients: Sodium selenite, vitamin E supplement, vitamin A supplement (with improved stability), D-activated animal sterol (source of vitamin D_3), riboflavin supplement, calcium pantothenate, niacin supplement, thiamine mononitrate, vitamin B_{12} supplement, corn distillers dried grains with solubles, soybean meal and ethoxyquin (a preservative).
Indications: For the control or correction of vitamin and selenium deficiencies in beef cattle, dairy cattle, sheep, swine, chickens, ducks and turkeys.
Caution: Follow label directions. The addition to feed of higher levels of this premix is not permitted.
Dosage and Administration: *Beef Cattle, Dairy Cattle, Sheep, Swine, Chickens, Ducks:* Thoroughly and evenly mix 5 pounds of *Vita-Plex SeE* per ton of complete ration. This will furnish a level of 0.1 p.p.m. of selenium.
Turkeys: Thoroughly and evenly mix 10 pounds of *Vita-Plex SeE* per ton of complete ration. This will furnish a level of 0.2 p.p.m. of selenium.
Caution: Use only in selenium deficient rations. A determination of selenium content in the complete ration is recommended.
How Supplied: 5 pound and 50 pound bags.
For Veterinary Use Only

Vita Plus Industries Inc.
953 E. SAHARA AVE. #21B
LAS VEGAS, NV 89104

GERI-VITE With Selenium
A palatable vitamin and mineral supplement for older cats and dogs.

Composition: Each tablet contains:

Vitamin B_1 (Thiamin HCl)	100 mcg.
Vitamin B_2 (Riboflavin)	200 mcg.
Vitamin B_6 (Pyridoxine HCl)	100 mcg.
Vitamin B_{12} (Cobalamin Concentrate)	2 mcg.
Calcium (Oyster Shell)	150 mg.
Zinc (Zinc Oxide)	5 mg.
Vitamin E (dl Alpha Tocopheryl Acetate)	10 IU
Selenium (Yeast)	10 mcg.

In a base of Liver, Malt, Ascorbic Acid, and Wheat Germ.
Suggested Daily Dosage:
1 tablet a day per 10 pounds of body weight. 6 tablets per day maximum for large breeds. Geri-Vite may be given by hand or crumbled on food. Geri-Vite is specially formulated to provide nutritional anti-oxidants essential to aging pets. A supplement for healthy skin, hair, bones and muscle tone. Special base gives flavor appeal to cats and dogs. Dosage may be given in half the regular amounts for use as a preventive supplement.
How Supplied: Bottle of 90 tablets.

SUPER-TABS
A palatable Vitamin/Mineral supplement for cats and dogs also containing nutritional anti-oxidants.

Composition:
Each tablet provides:

Calcium (Dicalcium Phosphate)	150	mg.
Phosphorus (Dicalcium Phosphate)	33	mg.
Iron (Ferrous Fumerate)	3	mg.
Copper (Cupric Acetate)	0.8	mg.
Magnesium (Magnesium Oxide)	3	mg.
Manganese (Manganese Sulfate)	0.5	mg.
Zinc (Zinc Oxide)	5	mg.
Iodine (Kelp)	150	mg.
Vitamin A (Fish Liver Oil)	500	IU
Vitamin D (Fish Liver Oil)	50	IU
Vitamin E (Mixed d-alpha Tocopherol)	5	IU
Vitamin B_1 (Thiamin HCl)	100	mcg.
Vitamin B_2 (Riboflavin)	200	mcg.
Vitamin B_6 (Pyridoxine HCl)	100	mcg.
Vitamin B_{12} (Cobalamine Concentrate)	2	mcg.
Biotin	10	mcg.
Folic Acid	25	mcg.
Pantothenic Acid (d-Calcium Pantothenate)	1	mg.
Niacin	1	mg.
Choline Bitartrate	100	mg.
Selenium (Yeast)	10	mcg.

In a base containing Sodium, Potassium, Liver, Honey and Carob.
Indications: Super-Tabs provide essential vitamins and minerals with nutritional antioxidants useful for supplementation in the general care of cats and dogs of all ages. Super-Tabs may also be given at increased dosages for convalescence or debilitation.
Dosage and Administration: Super-Tabs may be given in tablet-form or crumbled on food.

Small Dogs— (Up to 10 lbs.)	1 tablet per day
Medium Dogs— (20 lbs.)	2 tablets per day
Large Breeds (60–100 lbs.)	6 tablets per day

Cats—1 tablet per day
(Or as directed by veterinarian)
How Supplied: Bottles of 50 or 150 tablets.

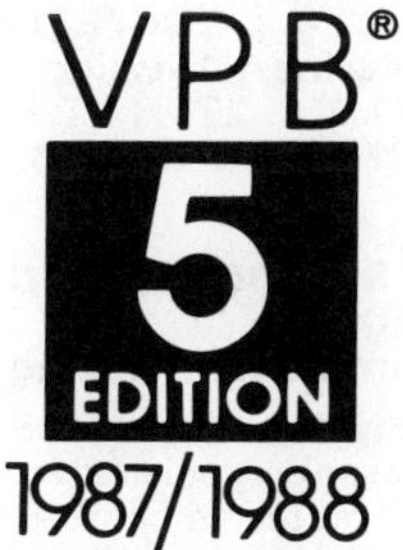

SECTION 8

Diagnostic Aids and Supplies

The information provided in this section was supplied through the direct cooperation of the manufacturer and is designed to provide a convenient reference on diagnostic aids and supplies employed in the practice of veterinary medicine. Products are arranged alphabetically under the name of manufacturer.

Barry Laboratories, Inc.
Veterinary Division
461 N.E. 27TH ST.
POMPANO BEACH, FL 33064

B

ALLERGENIC EXTRACT, FLEA ANTIGEN
for Intradermal Testing

Description: The vial contains an aqueous allergenic extract of fleas commonly found on canines (Ctenocephalides spp.). It is a dilution of allergen as labelled in a buffered saline menstruum pH 7.4 containing 0.5% Sodium Chloride; 0.8% Dibasic Sodium Phosphate; 0.145% Monobasic Potassium Phosphate; and 0.4% Phenol as preservative.

Actions: The mechanism of allergenic extract (Flea Antigen) is under investigation at this time. However, in sensitive canines, intradermal injection of antigen causes the release of histamine and other chemical mediators from mast cells as a result of its interaction with lgE skin sensitizing antibody.

Indications: Allergenic extract, Flea Antigen (intradermal strength), is indicated in the diagnosis of flea bite allergic dermatitis.

How Supplied: Flea Antigen for intradermal testing is supplied in 5.0 ml vials at a concentration of 1:600 dilution W/V.

ALLERGENIC EXTRACT INTRADERMAL TEST KIT

Description: The intradermal test kit contains the following:

1. 26 one ml vials of concentrated allergenic extract 1:20 dil. w/v. Each vial is a dilution of allergen as labelled in a glycerol-saline solution pH 7.4 containing: 0.5% Sodium Chloride; 0.8% Dibasic Sodium Phosphate; 0.145% Monobasic Potassium Phosphate; 50% Glycerine and 0.4% Phenol as preservative.
2. 52 vials of diluent for preparation of intradermal testing strength. Each vial contains 2.9 ml of sterile buffered saline solution pH 7.4 with the same inactive ingredients as above, excluding Glycerine.
3. One 5 ml vial of Diagnostic Control pH 7.4 containing the same inactive ingredients as the allergenic extracts except that the concentration of Glycerine is 1.7%

Actions: The mechanism of allergenic extracts is under investigation at this time. However, in sensitive canines, intradermal injection of antigen causes the release of histamine and other chemical mediators from mast cells as a result of its interaction with lgE skin sensitizing antibody.

Indications: Allergenic extracts, when properly diluted, are indicated in the diagnosis of canine inhalant dermatitis.

Products are cross-indexed by generic and chemical names in the **Active Ingredients Section**

Coopers Animal Health Inc.
520 WEST 21ST ST.
P.O. BOX 419167
KANSAS CITY, MO 64141-0167

EAS™ ALKALINE PHOSPHATASE TEST KIT
Two-minute test for Alkaline Phosphatase in Heparinized Plasma or Serum.
For use with Coopers EAS (Electronic Animal Sensor)

Product Description: EAS Alkaline Phosphatase Test Kit consists of one pipette, one reagent bottle, disposable vials and enzyme strips for the determination of alkaline phosphatase in heparinized plasma or serum.

EAS Alkaline Phosphatase Test Kit is used with strip carrier that is designated with a yellow arrow.

Test Principle: EAS Alkaline Phosphatase Test Kit is for exclusive use in determination of alkaline phosphatase in heparinized plasma or serum (for concentrations 0–600 IU/l).

Three drops of heparinized plasma or serum are added to an unused vial (provided). Then three drops of alkaline phosphatase reagent are added to the same vial, swirled gently and allowed to react for 1 minute. The test strip is immersed into the solution after 60 seconds countdown on the sensor (buzzer will sound 3 seconds prior to 60-second mark). After an additional 60 seconds, the buzzer sounds and the screen flashes zero, the strip is removed from the vial and excess moisture is removed by *side blotting* as described in WIPE TECHNIQUE. The strip is then inserted into the sensor, the door closed and a value readout appears on the screen. The reflected light intensity is measured as the density of developed color to obtain the alkaline phosphatase concentration in the sample.

REAGENT COMPOSITION FOR EAS ALKALINE PHOSPHATASE
Composition and properties

Phenolphthalein Monophosphate	0.09 mg
Buffer	10%
Non-reactive Ingredients	90%

Warnings and Precautions: EAS Alkaline Phosphatase Kit is for *in-vitro* diagnostic use. The Test Kit should be stored in a secure area away from small children.

Storage and Handling: Kit should be stored under 30°C (86°F) in a dark, dry, cool place. After opening, Test Kit should be kept at 4°C (39°F). Mark the date on the vial when first opened.

Specimen Collection and Preparation: EAS Alkaline Phosphatase Kit is intended for use with heparinized plasma or serum. Citrate and EDTA inhibit alkaline phosphatase and should **NOT** be used. Whole blood should not be used.

Limitations of Procedure: Increases in alkaline phosphatase occur when the specimen is stored at room temperature. Do not use severely hemolyzed specimens.

Performance Characteristics: EAS Alkaline Phosphatase Kit is specific for Serum Alkaline Phosphatase. When used with EAS (Electronic Animal Sensor), readings are comparable to other quantitative methods for Serum Alkaline Phosphatase.

Wipe Technique:

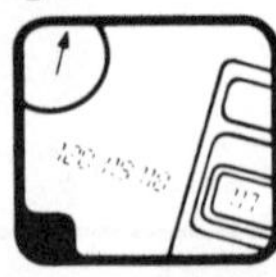

1. Proper timing is critical for this technique. Add strip to reagent and sample mixture at 60 seconds. Begin *side blot* as soon as sensor has completed 120-second count.

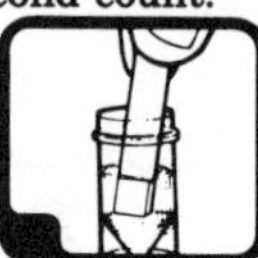

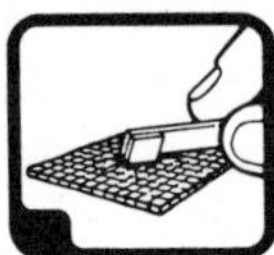

2. Using a piece of cotton gauze as a blotter, remove strip from vial and place side edge of strip gently on gauze. Excess liquid will be removed from pad surface. **DO NOT PLACE PAD FACE DOWN ON GAUZE.**

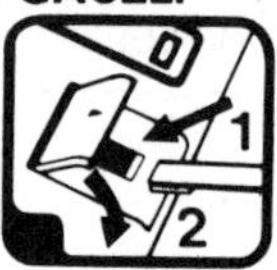

3. Immediately insert the strip into the sensor as directed in the operating manual.

Specifications

1. Range :0–660 IU/l
2. Specimen :Heparinized plasma or serum
3. Required Sample Volume :150–200 μl
4. Reaction Time :120 seconds
5. Storage :At room temperatures below 30°C (86°F) in closed container

Caution

1. To prevent the deterioration of sensitivity of EAS Alkaline Phosphatase Test Kit, store in a dark, dry, cool place. Avoid excessive humidity, temperature extremes and direct sunlight.
2. When Test Kit is stored under refrigeration, allow it to return to room temperature before using.
3. Do not touch the test pad area, also avoid contamination with volatile chemicals.
4. Do not remove the desiccant packed in the container.
5. If stored properly, the Test Kit is usable up to the expiration date indicated on the label. Do not use any discolored or mutilated test strips.

Precautions for Specimens

1. Use only heparinized plasma or serum.
2. Use specified amount of sample for testing.
3. The reaction of color development progresses slowly under low temperatures and may result in low measurement values. If frozen serum is used, allow it to return to room temperature before proceeding with the test. It is recommended to conduct measurements at

room temperatures between 15°C–30°C (59°F–86°F).

Availability: EAS Alkaline Phosphatase Kit is available in test kits of 25 tests.

EAS™ B.U.N. REAGENT STRIPS
One minute Test for Blood Urea Nitrogen in Whole Blood, Heparinized Plasma or Serum
For use with the COOPERS EAS (Electronic Animal Sensor)

Product Description: EAS B.U.N. Reagent Strips are disposable plastic reagent strips for the determination of blood urea nitrogen in whole blood, heparinized plasma or serum. A semi-permeable membrane is employed to serve as a barrier to prevent blood cells from entering into the reagent test pad area.

EAS B.U.N. Reagent Strips are packaged in a vial with a tight-fitting cap. Each strip is stable and ready for use when removed from the vial. At the beginning of a 60-second time period, one drop of whole blood, heparinized plasma or serum is applied to the reagent test pad area, which changes color in response to the concentration of blood urea nitrogen in the blood.

EAS B.U.N. Reagent Strips are used with strip carrier designated with a green arrow.

Test Principle: EAS B.U.N. Reagent Strip is for exclusive use in determination of blood urea nitrogen (for concentration 5–100 mg/dl).

The reagent pad area of the strip is prepared for optical measuring of the degree of color development which is proportional to the urea nitrogen concentration in the blood sample.

A small amount of whole blood, heparinized plasma or serum is used as the sample, for rapid and accurate measurement of blood urea nitrogen.

The reagent pad area is composed of urease and a pH indicator. It is coated with a substance impermeable to blood cells.

When whole blood, heparinized plasma or serum is applied on the reagent pad area, only low molecule weight components such as urea permeate underneath the surface of the test pad membrane. The area is then enzymatically decomposed by urease to ammonia and carbon dioxide. This ammonia changes to an ammonium hydroxide, and as the pH increases, the color of pH indicator changes. The degree of the color development corresponds to the concentration of urea nitrogen in blood. The blood cell components remaining on the surface of the reagent pad area are removed by wiping with lint-free tissue. A monochromatic light corresponding to the hue of developed color illuminates the reagent area. The reflected light intensity is measured as the density of developed color to obtain the urea nitrogen concentration in blood.

REAGENT COMPOSITION FOR EAS B.U.N. STRIP

Composition and properties

Urease	37.5μg
Bromothymol Blue	22.0μg
Non-Reactive Ingredients	15.0μg

Configuration of EAS B.U.N. Reagent Strip

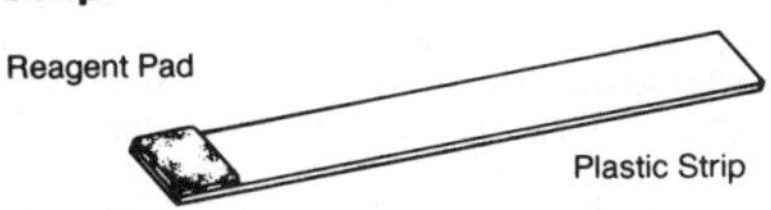

Warnings and Precautions: EAS B.U.N. Reagent Strips are for *in vitro* diagnostic use. EAS B.U.N. Reagent Strip should be stored in a secure area away from small children.

Storage and Handling: Store strips at temperatures under 30°C (86°F) in a dark, dry, cool place. Avoid exposing reagent strips to moisture, light and heat to prevent deterioration of reagents. Do not remove the desiccant from the bottle and keep the bottle tightly capped. Do not touch test pad area of the reagent strip. Do not transfer the strips to any other containers. Mark the date the vial was first opened in the space allotted on the label.

Specimen Collection and Preparation: EAS B.U.N. Reagent Strips are intended for use with whole blood, heparinized plasma or serum. If desired, venous whole blood samples with common anticoagulants (citrate, heparin or EDTA) may be used.

Limitation of Procedure: This procedure is free from interference if fresh whole blood, heparinized plasma or serum is used. Whole blood with fluoride as preservative should be avoided. Uric acid and ascorbic acid (when occurring in physiological blood concentrations) do not affect the reaction. Hematocrits greater than 55% can cause lower results.

Performance Characteristics: EAS B.U.N. Reagent Strips are specific for blood urea nitrogen determination. When used with EAS (Electronic Animal Sensor), readings are comparable to other quantitative methods for blood urea nitrogen.

Wipe Technique:

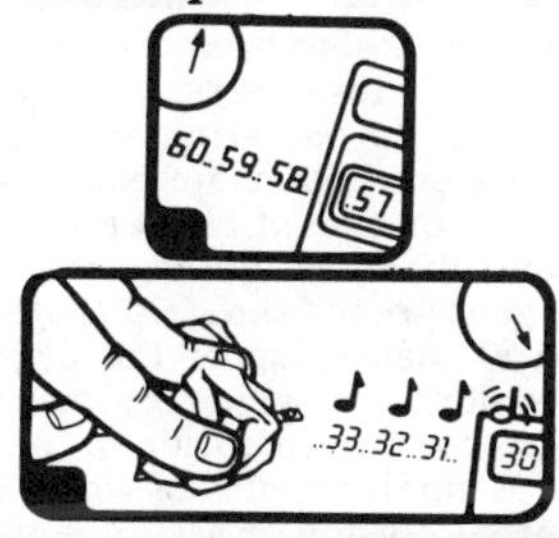

1. Proper timing is critical for this technique. Begin to wipe as soon as the sensor has completed 30 seconds of the 60 second countdown. Improper timing will result in erroneous readings.

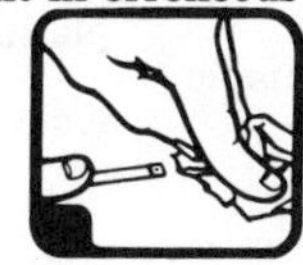

2. Wipe off blood from reagent pad in one forward motion using a lint-free tissue. DO NOT APPLY PRESSURE DIRECTLY ON REAGENT PAD.

3. When buzzer sounds and zero flashes, immediately insert strip into sensor as directed in the operating manual. B.U.N. Reagent Strip is for exclusive use in determination of blood urea nitrogen (for concentrations 5–100 mg/dl).

The reagent area of the strip is prepared for optical measuring of the degree of color development, which is proportional to the urea nitrogen concentration in the blood sample. A small amount of whole blood, heparinized plasma or serum is used as the sample for rapid, and accurate measurement of blood urea nitrogen.

Specifications

1. Range :5–100 mg/dl
2. Specimen :Whole blood, heparinized plasma or serum
3. Required Sample Volume :about 50μl–100μl
4. Reaction Time :60 seconds
5. Storage :At room temperatures below 30°C (86°F)

Caution

1. To prevent the deterioration of sensitivity of reagent strips, store in a dark, dry, cool place. Avoid excessive humidity, temperature extremes and direct sunlight.
2. If reeagent strips are stored under refrigeration, allow them to return to room temperature before opening the container and remove only required number of strips and re-cap container immediately.
3. Do not touch the reagent area, also avoid contamination with volatile chemicals.
4. Do not remove the desiccant packed in the container.
5. If stored properly, the reagent strips are usable up to the expiration date indicated on the label. Do not use any discolored or mutilated reagent strips.

Precautions for Specimens

1. Use only whole blood, heparinized plasma or serum.
2. For determination use a sufficient amount of whole blood, heparinized plasma or serum.
3. The reaction of color development progresses slowly under low temperatures and may result in low measurement value. If frozen heparinized plasma or serum is used, allow it to return to room temperature before measurement. It is recommended to conduct measurements at room temperatures between 15°–30°C (59°–86°F).

Availability: EAS B.U.N. Reagent Strips are available in a vial of 25 strips.

Continued on next page

C

Coopers—Cont.

EAS™ GLUCOSE REAGENT STRIPS
One minute Test for Glucose in Whole Blood, Heparinized Plasma or Serum For use with the COOPERS EAS (Electronic Animal Sensor)

Product Description: EAS Glucose Reagent Strips are disposable plastic reagent strips for the determination of glucose in whole blood, heparinized plasma or serum. A semi-permeable membrane is employed to serve as a barrier to prevent blood cells from entering into the reagent test pad area.

EAS Glucose Reagent Strips are packaged in a vial with a tight-fitting cap. Each strip is stable and ready for use when removed from the vial. At the beginning of a 60-second time period, one drop of whole blood, heparinized plasma or serum is applied to the reagent test pad area, which changes color in response to the concentration of glucose in the blood.

EAS Glucose Reagent Strips are used with strip carrier designated with a green arrow.

Test Principle: EAS Glucose Reagent Strip chemistry is based on the glucose oxidase/peroxidase reaction. D-glucose is oxidized to gluconic acid and hydrogen peroxide in the presence of atmospheric oxygen and glucose oxidase as a catalyst. In the presence of peroxidase indicators the reagent strip is oxidized to produce various shades of green color.

REAGENT COMPOSITION FOR EAS GLUCOSE STRIP

Composition and properties

ABTS	0.5%
Glucose Oxidase	0.2%
Peroxidase	0.6%
Non-Reactive Ingredients	98.7%

Configuration of EAS Glucose Reagent Strip

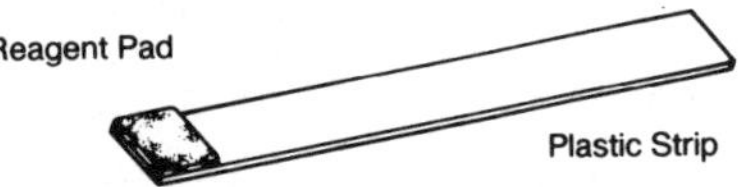

Warnings and Precautions: EAS Glucose Reagent Strips are for *in vitro* diagnostic use. EAS Glucose Reagent Strips should be stored in a secure area away from small children.

Storage and Handling: Store strips at temperatures under 30°C (86°F) in a dark, dry, cool place. Avoid exposing reagent strips to moisture, light and heat to prevent deterioration of reagents. Do not remove the desiccant from the bottle and keep the bottle tightly capped. Do not touch test pad area of the reagent strip. Do not transfer the strips to any other containers. Mark the date the vial was first opened in the space allotted on the label.

Specimen Collection and Preparation: EAS Glucose Reagent Strips are intended for use with whole blood, heparinized plasma or serum. If desired, venous whole blood samples with common anticoagulants (oxalate, citrate, heparin and EDTA) may be used. Blood glucose undergoes glycolysis rapidly after drawing. To prevent glycolysis, use blood samples immediately.

Limitation of Procedure: This procedure is free from interference if fresh whole blood, heparinized plasma or serum is used. Whole blood with fluoride as preservative should be avoided. Uric acid and ascorbic acid (when occurring in physiological blood concentrations) do not affect the reaction. Hematocrits greater than 55% can cause lower results.

Performance Characteristics: EAS Glucose Reagent Strips are specific for glucose determination. When used with EAS (Electronic Animal Sensor), readings are comparable to other quantitative methods for blood glucose.

Wipe Technique: Please follow exactly:

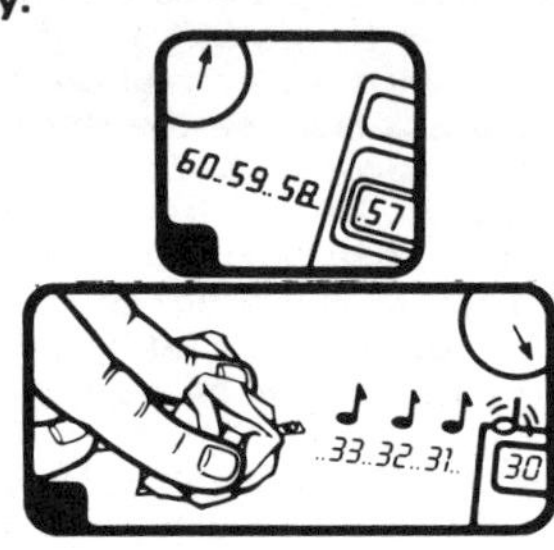

1. Proper timing is critical for this technique. Begin to wipe as soon as the sensor has completed 30 seconds of the 60 second countdown. Improper timing will result in erroneous readings.

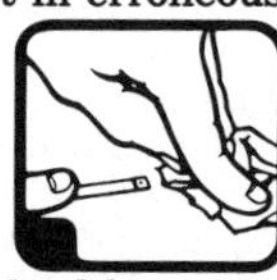

2. Wipe off blood from reagent pad in one forward motion using a lint-free tissue. DO NOT APPLY PRESSURE DIRECTLY ON REAGENT PAD. Countdown continues an additional 30 seconds.

3. When buzzer sounds and zero flashes, immediately insert strip into sensor as directed in the operating manual. Glucose Reagent Strip is for exclusive use in determination of blood glucose (for concentrations 25–250 mg/dl).

The reagent area of the strip is prepared for optical measuring of the degree of color development, which is proportional to the glucose concentration in the blood sample. A small amount of whole blood, heparinized plasma or serum is used as the sample for rapid, and accurate measurement of glucose.

Specifications

1. Range :25–250 mg/dl
2. Specimen :Whole blood, heparinized plasma or serum
3. Required Sample Volume :about 50µl–100µl
4. Reaction Time :60 seconds
5. Storage :At room temperature below 30°C (86°F)

Caution

1. To prevent the deterioration of sensitivity of reagent strips, store in a dark, dry, cool place. Avoid excessive humidity, temperature extremes and direct sunlight.
2. If reagent strips are stored under refrigeration, allow them to return to room temperature before opening the container and remove only required number of strips and re-cap container immediately.
3. Do not touch the reagent area, also avoid contamination with volatile chemicals.
4. Do not remove the desiccant packed in the container.
5. If stored properly, the reagent strips are usable up to the expiration date indicated on the label. Do not use any discolored or mutilated reagent strips.

Precautions for Specimens

1. Use only whole blood, heparinized plasma or serum.
2. For determination use a sufficient amount of whole blood, heparinized plasma or serum.
3. The reaction of color development progresses slowly under low temperatures and may result in low measurement value. If frozen heparinized plasma or serum is used, allow it to return to room temperature before measurement. It is recommended that measurements be conducted at room temperatures between 15°–30°C (59°–86°F).

Availability: EAS Glucose Reagent Strips are available in a vial of 25 strips.

EAS™ SGPT TEST KIT
Six minute test for Serum Glutamic Pyruvic Transaminase in heparinized plasma or serum.
For use with COOPERS EAS (Electronic Animal Sensor)

Product Description: EAS SGPT Reagent Test Kit consists of one pipette, two reagent bottles, disposable vials and enzyme strips for the detemination of SGPT in heparinized plasma or serum. The test consists of a wet phase and a test strip for final reading.

EAS SGPT Reagent Test Kit is used with strip carrier that is designated with a yellow arrow.

Test Principle: EAS SGPT Test Kit is exclusive for determination of SGPT in heparinized plasma or serum (for concentrations 0–400 IU/l).

Five drops of heparinized plasma or serum are added to the freeze-dried reagents in the provided vial, swirled gently and allowed to react for five minutes. Following the reaction interval, 4 drops of Solution A are added to the mixture in the vial. Immediately add 9 drops of Solution B and swirl to obtain uniform color. The reagent pad is then immersed into the solution for the final 60-second countdown. The pad area will change color in response to the concentration of SGPT in the sample. When the buzzer sounds and the screen flashes zero, the strip is removed from the vial and the excess moisture is removed by *side blotting* as described in WIPE TECHNIQUE. The strip is then inserted into the sensor, the door closed and a value readout appears on the screen. The reflected light intensity is measured as the density of developed color to obtain the SGPT concentration in the sample.

FREEZE-DRIED REAGENT COMPOSITION

L-alanine, α-ketoglutaric acid 2.28%
Nitrophenylhydrazine .... .02%
Buffer 97.70%

Warnings and Precautions: EAS SGPT Kit is for *in vitro* diagnostic use. The Test Kit should be stored in a secured area away from small children.

Storage and Handling: Kit should be stored under 30°C (86°F) in a dark, dry, cool place. After opening, Test Kit should be kept at 4°C (39°F). Mark the date on the vial when first opened.

Specimen Collection and Preparation: EAS SGPT Kit is intended for use with heparinized plasma or serum. Whole blood should not be used.

Limitations of Procedure: Freezing and thawing of sample impair SGPT stability. Prolonged storage should be at −40°C, short term storage, 0°C–4°C (32°F–39°F).

Performance Characteristics: EAS SGPT Kit is specific for Serum SGPT. When used with EAS (Electronic Animal Sensor), readings are comparable to other quantitative methods for Serum SGPT.

Wipe Technique:

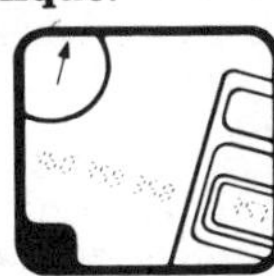

1. Proper timing is critical for this technique. Improper timing will result in erroneous readings.

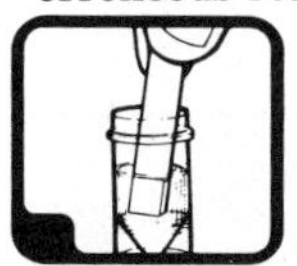

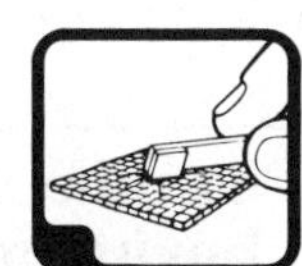

2. Using a piece of cotton gauze as a blotter, remove strip from vial and place side edge of strip gently on gauze. Excess liquid will be removed from pad surface. **DO NOT PLACE PAD FACE DOWN ON GAUZE.**

3. Immediately insert the strip into the sensor as directed in the operating manual.

Specifications

1. Range :0–400 IU/l
2. Specimen :Heparinized plasma or serum
3. Required Sample Volume :300 μl
4. Reaction Time :6 minutes
5. Storage :At room temperatures below 30°C (86°F) in closed container provided in kit.

Caution

1. To prevent the deterioration of sensitivity of EAS SGPT Test Kit, store in a dark, dry, cool place. Avoid excessive humidity, temperature extremes and direct sunlight.
2. When Test Kit is stored under refrigeration, allow it to return to room temperature before using.
3. Do not touch the test pad area, also avoid contamination with volatile chemicals.
4. Do not remove the desiccant packed in the container.
5. If stored properly, the Test Kit is usable up to the expiration date indicated on the label. Do not use any discolored or mutilated test strips.

Precautions for Specimens

1. Use heparinized plasma or serum.
2. Use a specified amount of sample for testing.
3. The reaction of color development progresses slowly under low temperatures and may result in low measurement value. If frozen serum is used, allow it to return to room temperature before proceeding with the test. It is recommended to conduct measurements at room temperaturės between 15°–30°C (59°F–86°F).

Availability: EAS SGPT Reagent Kit is available in test kits of 25 tests.

TUBERCULIN
Mammalian, Human Isolates, Intradermic

Description: Tuberculin, Mammalian, Human Isolates, Intradermic is prepared from culture filtrates of *Mycobacterium tuberculosis* (strains Pn, C, and Dt) which are heat-inactivated and concentrated 40% of their original volume by evaporation. The cultures are grown on a synthetic media and tested in accordance with U.S.D.A. requirements.

Indications: For intradermal testing of cattle, goats, swine and non-human primates for mammalian tuberculosis.

Equipment: Intradermic tuberculin syringes graduated in hundredths of a ml and equipped with a 26 gauge needle, 3/8-inch in length. The needle should be cleaned with alcohol and dried before each use.

Directions:

Intradermic Test: For cattle and goats, inject 0.1 ml between the superficial layers of the caudal fold skin; cattle—2 ½ inches, goats—1 inch distal to the base of the tail. For swine, inject 0.1 ml into the skin on the upper surface of the ear. Care should be exercised to ensure that the point of the needle does not penetrate through the skin. For non-human primates, follow the procedures recommended in the current 'Guide for Laboratory Animal Facilities and Care' as promulgated by the Committee on the Guide for Laboratory Animal Resources, National Academy of Sciences—National Research Council, or equivalent.

If the skin is clean, it is not necessary to disinfect or otherwise clean the surface. Soiled skin should be cleaned with cotton, either dry or moistened with 50% alcohol. Strong disinfectants must not be applied near the injection site. Care must be taken to ensure that all traces of alcohol are removed from both the injection site and needle prior to each injection. This is necessary to avoid any inflammation from the disinfectant which might be mistaken for a reaction.

A positive reaction is indicated by an induration (swelling) of the skin at the site of injection. The test should be interpreted at 72 ± 6 hours by palpation and observation (additional observations may be made at 48, 96 and 120 hours).

Precautions:

Store in dark at not over 45°F. or 7°C. Protect from freezing.

This test should not be repeated at less than 60 day intervals.

Veterinarians interested in the use of this product should contact regulatory officials within their state or county for specific directions and legal requirements pertaining to its use.

Restricted to use by or under the direction of a veterinarian.

How Supplied: 10 ml vials

TUBERCULIN
PPD Bovis, Intradermic

General Information: Tuberculin, PPD Bovis, Intradermic was developed by the United States Department of Agriculture and is to be used for the official Tuberculin test in cattle. This purified protein derivative (PPD) of *Mycobacterium bovis* Strain AN-5 is considered more specific than the Mammalian O.T. for bovine tuberculosis and has been adopted for official use under the Cooperative United States, Federal and State Bovine Tuberculosis Eradication Program.

Tuberculin, PPD Bovis, Intradermic contains 1.0 ± 0.1 mg per ml of tuberculoprotein derived from cultures of *M. bovis* concentrated by ultrafiltration and purified by ammonium sulfate precipitation and dialysis. Each serial is produced and tested in accordance with current United States Department of Agriculture, (USDA) regulations and must meet the requirements set forth for purity, safety, potency and special chemical characteristics prior to release for marketing.

This PPD reagent must be used in accordance with the Uniform Methods and Rules adopted by the United States Animal Health Association and approved by USDA. Under this agreement, accredited veterinarians are restricted to the use of the single caudal fold test procedure for official testing. Other procedures concerning retesting of suspected animals by comparative cervical test (C-C test) or for cleanup testing of infected herds in the United States (0.2 ml intradermal dose, caudal fold or cervical site) can only be conducted as approved by State or Federal Regulatory Veterinarians.

Indications: For intradermal testing of cattle for bovine tuberculosis.

Equipment: Intradermic tuberculin syringes graduated in hundredths of a ml

Continued on next page

C

Coopers—Cont.

and equipped with a 26 gauge needle, 3/8 inch in length. The needle should be cleaned with alcohol and dried before each use.
Directions: Intradermic Test: Inject 0.1 ml of Tuberculin PPD Bovis, Intradermic between the superficial layers of the caudal fold skin approximately 2½ inches distal to the base of the tail. Care should be exercised to ensure that the point of the needle does not penetrate through the skin.
If the skin is clean, it is not necessary to disinfect or otherwise clean the surface. Soiled skin should be cleaned with cotton, either dry or moistened with 50% alchohol. Strong disinfectants must not be applied near the injection site. Care must be taken to ensure that all traces of alcohol are removed from both the injection site and needle prior to each injection. This is necessary to avoid any inflammation from the disinfectant which might be mistaken for a reaction.
A positive reaction is indicated by an induration (swelling) of the skin at the site of injection. The test should be interpreted at 72 ± 6 hours by palpation and observation.
Caution: Store in dark at not over 45°F or 7°C. Protect from freezing.
This test should not be repeated at less than 60 day intervals.
Veterinarians interested in the use of this product should contact regulatory officials within their state or country for specific directions and legal requirements pertaining to its use.
RESTRICTED TO USE BY OR UNDER THE DIRECTION OF A VETERINARIAN.
How Supplied: 10 ml vials

Daniels Pharmaceuticals, Inc.
2527 25TH AVENUE NORTH
ST. PETERSBURG, FL 33713

FECAL FLOT DRY

Composition: Sodium Nitrate
Indications: For use in fecal flotation analysis.
Directions: Fill container with distilled water up to the brim. As the contents go into solution, the water level will drop. **Do not** add additional water. This procedure will produce a specific gravity of 1.25 to 1.30.
Warning: Keep out of reach of children.
How Supplied: 1 Gallon & 5 lb. containers.

Products are cross-indexed by generic and chemical names in the **Active Ingredients Section**

Evsco Pharmaceuticals
Affiliate of Immunogenetics, Inc.
P.O. BOX 209, HARDING HIGHWAY
BUENA, NJ 08310

CLIPPER-AID™

Composition: Special lubricating oil, silicones, and isopropyl alcohol.
Indications: Helps lubricate and cool clipper blades.
Directions: Spray CLIPPER-AID through teeth of clipper blades after each use, allowing spray to remain on blade for at least one minute before using blade again. Older blades may need extra oiling.
Caution: Avoid spraying into eyes.
Warning: Flammable. Contents under pressure. Do not puncture or incinerate container. Do not expose to heat or flame. Do not store above 130°F. Keep Out of Reach of Children.
How Supplied: 12 oz. Spray Can.

DIFIL-TEST®

Description: Contains a reusable filter membrane holder, lysing solution dispenser and plastic tray plus microfilariae stain, lysing solution and filter membranes for 50 canine heartworm tests.
Indications: For the detection of canine heartworm microfilariae.
How Supplied: Difil Test Kit contains reusable membrane holder, lysing, solution, dispenser and plastic tray plus microfilariae stain, lysing solution and filter membranes for 50 canine heartworm tests.

FECALYZER®

Description: The Fecalyzer disposable diagnostic system is designed so that the odorfree sample collecting device is also the complete apparatus for assaying the fecal sample. The attached cap closes tightly for transporting the sample and for disposal after assay. Cross-contamination is avoided by using a new Fecalyzer for each sample.
Directions: The client is instructed to remove insert, press small end of insert into sample, return insert to holder, close lid and return to veterinarian. To assay sample, lid is opened and flotation solution (Fecasol) is added to level of holes in insert. The insert is rotated back and forth. Blades at bottom of insert and container mix the sample and separate ova from fecal matter. Insert is seated firmly and flotation solution added to form meniscus. Debris is trapped in lower section while ova float to surface where slide or coverslip has been placed on meniscus. After 15–20 minutes, slide is placed on microscope for examination, Fecalyzer is capped and discarded.
How Supplied: Each box contains 100 individual Fecalyzer test units, clipboard/worktray, instruction card, pad of 100 client instruction sheets, and 100 pressure-sensitive identification labels.

FECASOL®

Description: Sodium nitrate solution having a specific gravity of 1.200.
Indications: May be used for all flotation techniques in performing fecal analyses. Gives optimum results when used with the Fecalyzer system.
How Supplied: Gallon Bottle (13.785 liters).

Fort Dodge Laboratories, Inc.
800 FIFTH STREET
FORT DODGE, IA 50501

LEPTOSPIRA ANTIGENS

Indications: For use in a simple, macroscopic agglutination test for serodiagnosis of leptospirosis. The antigen is a chemically killed, refined, concentrated, standardized suspension of *Leptospira* organisms of the serotype indicated on label.
Advantages of this type of antigen are: the simplicity of the test; ability to read the test without aid of a microscope; and no necessity for maintenance of living cultures of Leptospira organisms for use in the test.
The antigen can be used in a rapid platescreen test to differentiate positive serum from negative, and, in a rapid plate test to determine the titer of positive serum.
Care should be exercised in the collection and handling of the blood samples in order to keep hemolysis to a minimum.
Complete detailed directions are given in each package insert.
How Supplied:
Bio. 306 *L. pomona,* 5 ml
Bio. 307 *L. canicola,* 5 ml
Bio. 308 *L. icterohaemorrhagiae,* 5 ml
Bio. 309 *L. grippotyphosa,* 5 ml
Bio. 310 *L. hardjo,* 5 ml.
These products are not returnable for credit or exchange.

Granite Division, Environmental Diagnostics, Inc.
P. O. BOX 908
2990 ANTHONY ROAD
BURLINGTON, NC 27215

EZ-SCREEN TEST SYSTEM

The EZ-SCREEN test kits consist of Quik-Cards® and dropper bottles of reagent. EZ-SCREEN is a colorimetric indicator test for the presence of a minute amount of a specific substance in a liquid or liquid extract. The test can be qualitative or semiquantitative. Results are available within five minutes of collecting the sample. In its simplest configuration, it consists of two or more areas of solid-phase antibody on a filter-like material sandwiched between two thin plastic sheets.
Some characteristics of EZ-SCREEN are:
*High Concentration Kinetics — the

speed of the antigen/antibody reactions and substrate development are vastly increased, requiring seconds rather than minutes or hours.

- *Low Rate of Antigen/Antibody Dissociation—the displacement of test antigen by labeled antigen is virtually eliminated, thereby increasing sensitivity, reducing background, and increasing contrast for clearer semiquantitative determinations.
- *Inherent Separation—the lack of mixing of solutions which are sequentially added to the filter-like material results in inherent separation of reaction steps, thereby eliminating the need for centrifugation, decanting or homogeneous chemistries.
- *Multicomponent Packaging—the short shelf-life of many enzyme substrates in solution requires that the liquid and dry components be separately packaged and mixed just prior to use. The EZ-SCREEN test reagents are lyophilized and separated in a single package which includes premeasured quantities of both the liquid and dry components. The user squeezes the ampule to combine the reagents into a drop dispenser.

EZ-SCREEN tests are available for the detection of antibiotics, insecticides, pesticides, drugs, and diseases. Presented herein are seven selected EZ-SCREEN tests. EZ-SCREEN: SULFAMETHAZINE is described in detail, the specifics of the other EZ-SCREEN tests are comparable.

EZ-SCREEN: AFLATOXIN

Description: The EZ-SCREEN: AFLATOXIN test is specific for the qualitative detection of Aflatoxin in feed, grain, milk (B_1), and cereal samples. This test will detect Aflatoxin levels of 5 ppb or greater.
How Supplied: 2, 5, 10, 25, 50, or 100 Test kits.
Test configuration, reagents supplied, test procedure, interpretation of results, quality assurance, limitations, and storage are the same as those for EZ-SCREEN: SULFAMETHAZINE.
PATENTED AND PATENTS PENDING

EZ-SCREEN: CHLORAMPHENICOL

Description: The EZ-SCREEN: CHLORAMPHENICOL test is specific for the qualitative detection of Chloramphenicol in urine, serum, and tissue samples. This test will detect levels of Chloramphenicol residues of 50 ppb or greater.
How Supplied: 2, 5, 10, 25, 50, or 100 Test kits.
Test configuration, reagents supplied, test procedure, interpretation of results, quality assurance, limitations, and storage are the same as those for EZ-SCREEN: SULFAMETHAZINE.
PATENTED AND PATENTS PENDING

EZ-SCREEN: GENTAMICIN

Description: The EZ-SCREEN: GENTAMICIN test is specific for the qualitative detection of Gentamicin in urine, serum, tissue, and feed samples. This test will detect levels of Gentamicin residues of 100 ppb or greater.
How Supplied: 2, 5, 10, 25, 50, or 100 Test kits.
Test configuration, reagents supplied, test procedure, interpretation of results, quality assurance, limitations, and storage are the same as those for EZ-SCREEN: SULFAMETHAZINE.
PATENTED AND PATENTS PENDING

EZ-SCREEN: NEOMYCIN

Description: The EZ-SCREEN: NEOMYCIN test is specific for the qualitative detection of Neomycin in urine, serum, tissue, and feed samples. This test will detect levels of Neomycin residues of 100 ppb or greater.
How Supplied: 2, 5, 10, 25, 50, or 100 Test kits.
Test configuration, reagents supplied, test procedure, interpretation of results, quality assurance, limitations, and storage are the same as those for EZ-SCREEN: SULFAMETHAZINE.
PATENTED AND PATENTS PENDING

EZ-SCREEN: PENICILLIN (Beta-Lactams)

Description: The EZ-SCREEN: PENICILLIN test is specific for the qualitative detection of Penicillin in milk, urine, serum, plasma, and feed samples. This test will detect levels of Penicillin residues of 2 ppb (nanograms/ml) or greater.
How Supplied: 2, 5, 25, 50 or 100 Test kits.
Test configuration, reagents supplied, test procedure, interpretation of results, quality assurance, limitations, and storage are the same as those for EZ-SCREEN: SULFAMETHAZINE.
PATENTED AND PATENTS PENDING

EZ-SCREEN: SULFADIMETHOXINE

Description: The EZ-SCREEN: SULFADIMETHOXINE test specific for the qualitative detection of Sulfadimethoxine in serum and feed samples. This test will detect levels of Sulfadimethoxine residues of 0.1 ppm or greater.
How Supplied: 2, 5, 10, 25, 50, or 100 Test kits.
Test configuration, reagents supplied, test procedure, interpretation of results, quality assurance, limitations, and storage are the same as those for EZ-SCREEN: SULFAMETHAZINE.
PATENTED AND PATENTS PENDING

EZ-SCREEN: SULFAMETHAZINE

Description: The EZ-SCREEN: SULFAMETHAZINE test is specific for the qualitative detection of Sulfamethazine in urine, serum, and feed samples. EZ-SCREEN: SULFAMETHAZINE is available in two sensitivities: 0.1 ppm or greater.
How Supplied: 2, 5, 10, 25, 50, or 100 Test Kits.
Reagents Supplied:

A. QUIK-CARD®
B. SULFAMETHAZINE ENZYME (Red Cap)
C. CONTROL REAGENT (Green Cap)
D. STANDARD REAGENT (0.1 ppm) SULFAMETHAZINE—(White Cap)
E. SUBSTRATE TUBES (Blue Cap)
F. SAMPLE PIPETTES

Test Procedure: PERFORM TEST SLOWLY AND CAREFULLY. Allow all reagents to come to room temperature (23°–29° C.; 73°–84° F.) before starting the test.
When reagents are added to the QUIK-CARD®, allow the drops to fall freely onto the card. DO NOT TOUCH the drops off the tips of the bottles or pipettes. The drop size will be uniform by following this procedure, and the bottles of reagents will not become contaminated.

1. The samples have been collected and prepared according to directions.
2. Crush one blue-capped Substrate ampule for each sample to be tested. Shake vigorously for 20 seconds. CAUTION: Do not squeeze the ampule so hard as to force the pieces of broken glass through the walls of the ampule.
3. Crush the green-capped Control ampule and apply one drop of the liquid to the control port (C).
4. Using the small plastic pipettes provided, apply two drops of the sample to the sample port (S).
5. Allow these drops to totally absorb into the card.
6. Crush the red-capped Enzyme ampule and apply one drop of liquid from the ampule to both the spots and allow drops to totally absorb into the card.
7. Wipe carefully around the outside of the ports to remove any excess liquid which has remained. DO NOT BLOT THE PORT DIRECTLY.
8. Crush the blue-capped Substrate ampule and apply one drop of liquid from the ampule to all ports and allow these to totally absorb.
9. Apply one to two more drops of liquid from the blue-capped Substrate ampule to all the ports.
10. Interpret the results of each test on the card after two minutes.

Interpretation of Results:

1. The interpretation of the results for the QUIK-CARD® test should be done in approximately 2 minutes after the addition of the last drop of Substrate Reagent.
2. The C port should always turn a purplish-blue color. If this does not occur, the card test is invalid. Recheck the procedure or contact Granite Division, Environmental Diagnostics Inc. for assistance.
3. NEGATIVE—If sample port (S) is approximately the same color (purplish-blue) as the control port (C), the sample contains less than 0.1 ppm of SULFAMETHAZINE.
POSITIVE—If sample port (S) is colorless or noticeably lighter than the control spot (C), the sample contains at least 0.1 ppm SULFAMETHAZINE.

Continued on next page

Granite—Cont.

Quality Assurance: Although each lot of EZ-SCREEN: SULFAMETHAZINE has been quality controlled prior to shipment, the customer should confirm the performance of the test.
The Standard Reagent (white cap), supplied with the EZ-SCREEN Kit, can be used as a check for positive results. Apply two drops of liquid from the white capped vial to the sample port, in place of a urine or feed sample. Perform the rest of the test as described in the test procedure section. If the card and test reagents are working properly, the sample port should remain colorless.
Limitations: EZ-SCREEN: SULFAMETHAZINE is specific for the detection of SULFAMETHAZINE. This test is only a qualitative screen for Sulfamethazine. Quantification must be done with an alternative method.
Storage: Store the kits for the EZ-SCREEN: SULFAMETHAZINE at 2°–8° C (36°–48°F). DO NOT FREEZE any of the reagents. Do not expose reagents to elevated temperatures [greater than 35° C (95° F)] for prolonged periods.
PATENTED AND PATENTS PENDING

EZ-SCREEN: TYLOSIN

Description: The EZ-SCREEN: TYLOSIN test is specific for the qualitative detection of Tylosin in urine, serum, tissue, and feed samples. This test will detect levels of Tylosin residues of 100 ppb or greater.
How Supplied: 2, 5, 10, 25, 50, or 100 Test kits.
Test configuration, reagents supplied, test procedure, interpretation of results, quality assurance, limitations, and storage are the same as those for EZ-SCREEN: SULFAMETHAZINE.
PATENTED AND PATENTS PENDING

Haver
Mobay Corporation
Animal Health Division
SHAWNEE, KS 66201

FOALCHEK®
Diagnostic Equine Immunoglobulin G Test Kit

Description: FOALCHEK® is a latex agglutination test for IgG in foals.
Indications: The FOALCHECK® test evaluates passive transfer of colostral immunoglobulins. The recommended time to test is 12 to 15 hours after the first nursing. FOALCHEK® indentifies neonates with inadequate IgG levels at a time when treatment can be carried out by the most efficient means.
Kit Contents:
10 glass bottles of diluent
1 plastic squeeze bottle of Polystyrene Latex Particles
1 vial containing twenty 5-microliter heparinized capillary pipettes
1 vial containing wood mixing sticks
10 disposable plastic Pasteur pipettes
1 agglutination slide (block with three test rings)
Test Procedure:
1) Collect sample—either whole block or serum may be used.
2) File one 5-microliter capillary pipette with serum or two 5-microliter capillary pipettes with blood. The pipette must be filled from tip to tip.
3) Drop filled capillary pipette(s) into diluent vial.
4) Allow 5 minutes for the specimen to disperse throughout the diluent.
5) Shake vial to insure mixing.
6) Place two drops of specimen diluent in the first ring of the glass slide, three drops in the second ring and four drops in the third ring, using the plastic Pasteur pipette (hold vertically). Work from left to right.
7) Add two drops of Polystyrene Latex Particles to each ring. Hold dropper bottle vertically. Work from left to right.
8) Stir with wood mixing sticks. Work from left to right.
9) Rotate slide and look for agglutination.

Interpretation: Specimens with high IgG levels will agglutinate in all three rings within 15 seconds, indicating adequate passive transfer. If the rings do not agglutinate, the slide should be rotated an additional 45 seconds, then read. Questionable or weak agglutinations should be considered negative. Hemolysis does not interfere with the test. The following table should be used to interpret the results. Timing is important. [See table below].
Serum provides a more precise assessment of the foal's immune status. Therefore, when whole blood indicates PFPT or FPT, serum can also be tested for a more exact measurement.
Precautions:
1) The accuracy of the test is dependent upon delivery of consistent-size drops of both Polystyrene Latex Particles and serum diluent. Therefore, hold the dropper bottle and pipettes vertically when dispensing drops.
2) Avoid air bubbles in the drops of liquid.
3) Wipe excess blood or serum from the outside of the pipettes.
4) Rinse and dry the glass slide between tests.
5) Store latex between 35° and 45°F (2° - 7°C). High temperatures can degrade particles.
6) Do not open diluent until ready to use. If diluent has a cloudy appearance, do not use.
7) If the Polystyrene Latex Particles are difficult to squeeze from the vial, or if they have a stringy appearance, or if separation has occurred, do not use.

Packaging: Code 0119 FOALCHEK® Test Kit
Code 3938 FOALCHEK® Latex
Code 3939 00 FOALCHEK® Glass Plate

Agglutination	IgG mg/dl	Interpretation
all three rings +	>400	Adequate passive transfer
– + +	200 - 400	Partial failure of passive transfer (PFPT)
– – +	<200	Failure of passive transfer (FPT)

PARA BAN™-S
Insecticide Fogger

Composition: methylcarbamate 1.00%; 2,2-dichlorovinyl dimethyl phosphate 0.47%; Related compounds 0.03%.
Inert ingredients: 98.50%
Indications: Kills exposed roaches, ants, ticks, fleas, spiders, flying moths and scorpions.
For use only when building is vacated by humans and pets.
Directions: It is a violation of Federal Law to use this product in a manner inconsistent with its labeling. Use at least one canister for each 5,000 cubic feet of unobstructed area. Use additional units for remote rooms or where free flow of mist is not assured.
Important: Locate fogger in center of room or area being treated. Place newspapers under fogger unit and for three or four feet around the can to prevent staining or marring surfaces. Close doors and windows. Remove pets and cover or remove fish bowls. Cover or remove exposed foods and dishes. Open cabinets and doors to areas to be treated. Shut off fans and air conditioners. Put out all open flames except pilot light. Place at least 6 feet away from pilot light. Keep at arm's length when releasing. Point top of can away from face and eyes. Refer to the product label for more detailed information.
Warning:
Contents under pressure.
Do not puncture or incinerate container or throw into fire.
Exposure to temperatures above 130F. may cause bursting.
Disposal: Do not reuse empty container. Wrap container and put in trash collection.
How Supplied:
Code: 2013—12 oz

IDENTIFICATION PROBLEM?
Consult the
Product Identification Section
where you'll find
products pictured
in full color.

Molecular Genetics Inc.

10320 BREN ROAD EAST
MINNETONKA, MINNESOTA
55343

COLI-TECT® 99

Coli-Tect® 99: An Aid To Diagnosis
When interpreting the results of the Coli-Tect® 99 kit, a positive test result indicates the presence of K-99 bearing *E. coli* in the sample tested. The stronger the color development, the greater the concentration of pilus antigen in the sample and the greater the probability of the *E. coli* being directly involved. Color developments of lesser intensity may indicate one of the following:

1. The organism is the primary etiological agent, but it has not yet reached its peak level or has passed its peak level.
2. The K-99 organism is present, but is not the primary etiological agent.

It is strongly recommended that at least two animals in early stages of diarrhea be tested in each herd or group of affected animals before firm conclusions are reached relative to the etiology of infectious diarrhea.

The possibility of other etiological agents such as rotavirus, coronavirus, clostridia, coccidia, cryptosporidia and others should not be ignored. A thorough review of nutritional, environmental and other management practices, as well as necropsy and herd involvement observations, need to be considered in making a diagnosis.

Escherichia coli
Enterotoxigenic *Escherichia coli* (ETEC) bearing the K-99 pilus is a major cause of diarrhea in newborn calves, lambs and piglets (1). Pili (also known as fimbriae) are hair-like projections on the surface of the bacteria. The K-99 pilus plays a major role in facilitating adherence and colonization in the small intestine (2,3).

Description of Colibacillosis
Neonatal pigs, calves and lambs are very susceptible to diarrheal disease caused by ETEC, but clinical infections caused by ETEC have not been reported in adult animals. Calves and lambs become resistant to experimental challenge with K-99 ETEC by two days of age (4).

E. coli scours is characterized by diarrhea and progressive dehydration. Death may occur in a few hours and perhaps even before severe diarrhea develops. The color and consistency of the feces are of little value in making a diagnosis of any type of diarrhea (5).

The haircoat of an infected animal becomes rough as dehydration develops, and an emaciated appearance often occurs before death. Upon necropsy, food is usually found in the stomach. The intestine may contain varying amounts of yellowish to grayish ingesta with mucus. Pathological changes of the gastrointestinal tract include hyperemia, dilation of a flaccid small and large intestine, increased fluid contents, possible villar atrophy and some hemorrhage and edema.

Diagnosis of Colibacillosis
Definitive diagnosis of K-99 colibacillosis requires that the following criteria be met:

1. High number of K-99 *E. coli* are present (e.g. $\geq 10^8$ organisms/gm) in the posterior small intestine. (2)
2. Clinical symptoms consistent with colibacillosis are present. As previously mentioned, these clinical symptoms include:
   a. watery diarrhea;
   b. animal is less than 1 week old (1–5 days in calves);
   c. dehydrated.

References

1. Orskov, I., and Orskov, F. 1983. Serology of *Escherichia coli* Fimbriae. Prog. Allergy, 33:80-105.
2. Smith, H.W., and Huggins, M.B. 1977. The influence of plasmid determined and other characteristics of enteropathogenic *Escherichia coli* or their ability to proliferate in the alimentary tracts of piglets, calves and lambs. J. Med. Microbiology 11:471-492.
3. Moon, H.W. 1981. Protection against enteric colibacillosis in pigs suckling orally vaccinated dams: evidence for pili as protective antigens. AM. J.Vet. Res. 42:173-177.
4. Runnels, P.L., Moon, H.W., Schneider, R.A.: Development of Resistance with Host Age to Adhesion of K99 *Escherichia coli* to Isolated Intestinal Epithelial Cells. Infection and Immunity, April 1980, p.: 298–300.
5. Hudson, D., White, R.G. Calf Scours, Causes, Prevention and Treatment. University of Nebraska, Extension Service Publication G75-269.

Coli-Tect® 99 is a Registered Trademark of Molecular Genetics, Inc.
U.S. Veterinary License No. 284

Manufactured by
Molecular Genetics, Inc.
10320 Bren Road East
Minnetonka, MN 55343

Norden Laboratories, Inc.

601 W. CORNHUSKER
P.O. BOX 80809
LINCOLN, NE 68521

ClinEase™-FeLV
Feline Leukemia Virus Antigen Test Kit

Feline Leukemia Virus (FeLV): FeLV is a retrovirus which is transmitted between cats primarily via saliva and urine. As a consequence of viral replication, FeLV and viral antigens appear in the blood; the predominant viral antigen is p27. Cats which persistently express p27 have a much higher incidence of lymphoid and myeloid malignancies and degenerative conditions such as anemia and thymic atrophy. Persistent infection can also be immunosuppressive, which predisposes cats to numerous secondary infections. In some cats there is only a transient appearance of p27, and these animals generally remain healthy.

All FeLV-infected cats are potentially contagious when they have p27 in their blood, whether the p27 expression is transient or not. 'ClinEase-FeLV' is designed to identify whether unhealthy animals are infected with FeLV or whether apparently healthy cats may be contagious carriers.

Assay Principles: Monoclonal antibodies specific to FeLV p27 antigen are adsorbed to the plastic wells in the kit. Other anti-p27 monoclonal antibodies conjugated with the enzyme are contained in the diluent. When p27 in serum or plasma is incubated in the wells with diluent, immune complexes form; antigen molecules are bound by both enzyme-conjugated antibodies and antibodies adsorbed to the well. Free antibodies are then removed by a brief wash. With addition of the chromogen/substrate mixture, a green color will develop in the sample if antigen is present, bound by enzyme-conjugated antibodies. Intensity of color is proportional to the antigen-antibody concentration, and no color will develop in the absence of p27 antigen. 'ClinEase-FeLV' is highly specific and sensitive. Accurate scoring of the results can be made visually, without instrumentation. Alternatively, results can be scored by means of a microtiter plate reading instrument.

Reagents and Materials Included in the Kit:

1. 48 wells coated with monoclonal antibodies against FeLV p27.
2. Black-labeled bottle: 0.8 ml Negative Assay Control Solution. Contains preservative.
3. Red-labeled bottle: 0.8 ml Positive Assay Control Solution (FeLV p27 antigen, feline origin). Contains preservative.
4. Orange-labeled bottle: 2.6 ml Diluent containing Peroxidase-Conjugated Monoclonal Antibodies against FeLV p27. Contains preservative.
5. Green-labeled bottle: 2.6 ml Substrate A/Chromogen Solution (ABTS).
6. Blue-labeled bottle: 2.6 ml Substrate B Solution (peroxide).
7. Reusable plastic microwell holder.

Additional Materials Required But Not Provided:

1. Pipettes for delivery of approximately 0.05 ml test serum to the test wells.
2. Deionized or distilled water.
3. Paper towels or other absorbent material.

Precautions:

1. Remove foil only from those wells to be used immediately.
2. Do not freeze. Store kit at 2°C.–8°C. Do not allow reagents to stand at room temperature for longer than necessary to run the test.
3. Always include positive and negative assay controls for each group of samples tested.
4. Use a separate pipette for each sample.

Continued on next page

N

Norden—Cont.

5. Handle serum samples as if capable of transmitting FeLV. Sterilize or burn positive samples and materials they contact.
6. Use only distilled or deionized water.
7. Do not use reagents from other kits.
8. Do not use expired reagents.
9. Do not reuse wells or reagents.
10. For veterinary use only.

Storage and Stability: Do not freeze. Store kit at 2°C.–8°C. Date of expiration is stamped on kit box.

Specimens: Use serum or plasma. Hemolysis does not interfere with the assay. Fresh, refrigerated or frozen samples may be used. Bacterial contamination may interfere with the accuracy of the test.

Procedures:

1. Place wells in the holder (1 per sample plus 2 for assay controls). Write sample identification and well location in the record log. In subsequent steps, hold dropper bottles in vertical position to minimize variation in amount of substance delivered.
2. Place one drop of Negative Assay Control (black-labeled bottle) into the first well, one drop of Positive Assay Control (red-labeled bottle) into the second well, and one drop (0.05 ml) of the serum sample into the third well. Use additional wells for additional samples.
3. Add **1 drop** of Diluent/Conjugate (orange-labeled bottle) to every well. Allow each sample to incubate **at least 15 and no more than 30 minutes** at room temperature.
4. Invert and drain wells onto 3 or 4 stacked paper towels or other absorbent material. Fill wells with distilled or deionized water. Make sure each well is filled with water and no air bubbles are trapped. Invert onto paper towels or flick into sink. Be sure the wells are empty before starting next wash cycle. Repeat 4 more times, for a total of 5 washes.
5. Add **1 drop** of Substrate A/Chromogen (green-labeled bottle) and **1 drop** of Substrate B (blue-labeled bottle) to every well. Incubate at room temperature for 10 minutes and look for development of green color. If the results are not clear, incubate an additional 10 minutes.

Interpretation of Results:

1. ANY SAMPLE GIVING COLOR DEVELOPMENT GREATER THAN THE NEGATIVE ASSAY CONTROL indicates an FeLV infection.
2. The Negative Assay Control should remain nearly colorless for up to 20 minutes if the washes have been done thoroughly. Some positive samples will cause intense color to develop as soon as 1 minute after addition of Substrate. If color development in the negative control well approaches that of the positive control well, repeat the assay, being sure to wash thoroughly as described above.
3. The **Positive Assay Control** only indicates that the kit is properly functioning and it is **not for comparison with cat serum samples.** If the positive control well does not develop intense color after 20 minutes of incubation, repeat the assay. Be sure to follow the instructions carefully.
4. Animals giving test results that are weakly positive or ambiguous should be retested in 2–3 months to determine if the infection is "transient". Any questionable samples should be retested with a fresh serum sample.

Retesting:

1. *Negatives:* Most free-roaming cats which have tested negative should be retested yearly. Cats in frequent contact with other cats should be tested every 6 months. Isolated cats should be retested once (from 2 months to 1 year after the first test). Isolated animals testing negative twice need not be retested.
2. *Positives:* To determine if the infection is persistent or transient, a second test is necessary 2 months to 1 year after the first test. All positive cats should be isolated from other cats.

Quality Control: If the Positive Assay Control fails to yield the expected color development after 2 attempts, the kit should not be used and the Veterinary Services department of Norden Laboratories should be contacted.

'ClinEase-FeLV' was developed and is manufactured by Cambridge BioScience Corp.

FLEAVOL®
Beautifying-Cleansing Shampoo

Composition:

Active Ingredients:	
Pyrethrins	0.05%
Piperonyl butoxide, tech.*	0.50%
Diisopropyl cresols	0.10%
Inert Ingredients	99.35%
Total	100.00%

*Equivalent to 0.40% butylcarbityl (6-propylpiperonyl) ether and 0.10% of related compounds.

Indications: A fine detergent shampoo that cleans and beautifies without heavy sudsing. Grooms perfectly, rinses thoroughly, leaves coat soft, lustrous and clean smelling. Rids pets of fleas and lice.

Directions: *Small animals*—Place dog or other small animal in tub and thoroughly soak with warm water, taking two or three minutes to wet the hair. Apply "Fleavol" on head and ears and lather head, then repeat procedure with neck, chest, middle and hind quarters, finishing legs last. Let animal stand 5 minutes (10 minutes is even better)—this is an important part of both flea-killing and grooming procedure. Rinse thoroughly. "Fleavol" washes away quickly and easily.

Show livestock—For grooming large animals for show purposes, wet coat thoroughly. Dilute one part "Fleavol" with four parts warm water and apply with brush or low pressure spray gun. Rub to lather, then rinse.

Store in original container in a cool area away from heat or open flame. Do not reuse container. Rinse thoroughly before discarding in trash.

Caution: Keep Out of Reach of Children. Harmful if swallowed.

How Supplied: 12-6 oz plastic bottles, 1 gal, 5 gal.

Pitman-Moore, Inc.
P.O. BOX 344
WASHINGTON CROSSING, NJ 08560

BACTASSAY*
Bacterial Test Media
For *in vitro* diagnostic use.

Indications: For the identification and antibiotic susceptibility testing of aerobic pathogenic bacteria.

Directions: Refer to Pitman-Moore Veterinary Manual for full use directions.

Caution: Do not use these plates if contaminated, or if media appears dry and opaque. Destroy after use. Keep out of the reach of children. Store under refrigeration below 40°F. Do not freeze.

How Supplied: 10 sterile disposable test plates. Packages of cotton swabs.

*Trademark

DERMASSAY*
Dermatophyte Diagnostic System

Reagent Composition: Dermassay Clearing Solution contains dimethyl sulfoxide and potassium hydroxide.

Dermassay Staining Solution contains lactic acid, phenol, poirrier's blue, and inert ingredients.

Warning: Caustic—Avoid skin contact. If solution comes in contact with skin, flush with large amounts of water. Do not take internally. Avoid inhalation.

Principle: Fungal infections are caused by a variety of agents. Suspect lesions should be examined grossly, microscopically and culturally. The reagents in Dermassay Dermatophyte Diagnostic System along with Fungassay* Dermatophyte Test Medium facilitate the microscopic examination of the suspicious material and of the cultural growth.

Gross examination is helpful to select suspicious hairs which are then examined microscopically for arthrospores, hyphae and hair damage using the Dermassay Clearing Solution.

Suspicious specimens should also be cultured on Fungassay to determine the presence of pathogenic fungi.

Definitive identification of dermatophyte organisms from cultures can be made by microscopic examination of the growth mat produced in culture by using the Dermassay Staining Solution.

Store at controlled room temperature (59°–86°F). See accompanying literature for full directions.

How Supplied: Dermassay Clearing Solution, two 7 ml vials. Dermassay Staining Solution, one 7 ml vial. Forceps and Scraper.

*Trademark

D-TEC*CB
CANINE BRUCELLOSIS AGGLUTINATION ANTIGEN and REAGENT SERUM.
Canine Origin
Canine Brucellosis Diagnostic Test

Plate Test for Brucella Canis Antibodies
Store at 2–7°C (35–45°F)
Diagnostic Reagent—For Veterinary Use Only

Description: Thc rapid slide agglutination test (RSAT) for the diagnosis of *Brucella canis* was described by George and Carmichael (Proc. Council Res. Workers in Animal Disease, November 1973). The basis of the test is direct agglutination of the killed stained antigen by *Brucella canis* antibodies.
Indications: The reagents are used to presumptively diagnose infection with *Brucella canis.*
General Information: Canine brucellosis is a chronic infection with *Brucella canis* that causes generalized lymphadenitis and mild to severe reproductive symptoms. Prostatitis, epididymitis, scrotal dermatitis, testicular atrophy, and impotence can be present in the male; abortion typically in the final two weeks of gestation, resorption, infertility, and vaginal discharge can be present in the female. Its incidence in the continental United States is approximated by current surveys to be between 1% and 10%. *Brucella canis can infect man, and caution should be exercised when handling serums to be tested.*
The test has been shown to presumptively diagnose infection with *Brucella canis* by detecting specific antibody that is formed 1 to 4 weeks after infection.
The basis for serodiagnosis of canine brucellosis is the 2-Mercaptoethanol Tube Agglutination Test (2ME-TAT) and the Rapid Slide Agglutination Test (RSAT). The 2ME-TAT and RSAT have demonstrated excellent correlation in experimentally infected dogs.
In field situations, it has been recognized that an occasional healthy dog, culturally negative for *Brucella canis* will react positively in the RSAT, but not in the 2ME-TAT. The 2-Mercapto ethanol-Rapid Slide Agglutination Test (2ME-RSAT) has been developed in an attempt to eliminate discrepancies between the RSAT and the 2ME-TAT.
Certain non-specific agglutinins, reported to occur in the sera of normal dogs, are removed from canine sera when 2-mercaptoethanol is employed in the 2ME-TAT. Because of this occurrence 2-mercaptoethanol is employed in the modified Rapid Slide Agglutination Test procedure.
Procedure for Rapid Slide Agglutination Test (RSAT)

1. Bring reagents to room temperature 21°C (70°F) and shake well before use.
2. Divide a clean 1″ × 3″ slide in half by drawing a line with a wax pencil across the width.
3. Place one drop of antiserum (white label) (positive control) on one side.
4. Use one disposable plastic pipette and a rubber bulb to place one drop of test serum on the other side of the slide. Each test kit contains 25 disposable pipettes to prevent serum cross-contamination. Do not dispose of pipette until 2ME-RSAT is completed.
5. Add one drop of the *B. canis* agglutination antigen close to each serum drop, being careful not to touch serum with dropper.
6. Mix each antigen-serum with a separate end of an applicator stick, spreading to a circular area 2 cm in diameter. Do not allow the positive control test to touch the suspect serum test.
7. Rock slide very slowly and gently, and observe for agglutination for no longer than 2 minutes. A white background facilitates reading. If the serum is negative (absence of agglutination), no further testing is required; the animal is considered not to be infected with *B. canis.* If the slide test is positive perform the 2ME-RSAT.

Procedure for 2-Mercaptoethanol-Rapid Slide Agglutination Test (2ME-RSAT)

1. Add 2 drops of 2-mercaptoethanol, 0.2M solution to a tube containing 2 drops of the serum to be tested and mix well.
2. Place 1 drop of mixture on a clean dry slide.
3. Add 1 drop of *B. canis* agglutination antigen to the serum solution and mix well.
4. Observe for agglutination for no longer than 2 minutes.

When the RSAT-positive sample also tests positive by 2ME-KSAT, the animal is presumptively diagnosed as being infected with *B. canis.* Blood should be subjected to cultural examination for *B. canis.*
When the RSAT-positive sample tests negative by 2ME-RSAT, the animal may be in the early stage of *B. canis* infection, or alternatively, its serum may contain non-specific agglutinins to *B. canis.* To distinquish between these two conditions, a second serum sample should be collected in approximately thirty days and retested by the 2ME-RSAT procedure. Only if this sample tests positive should the animal be presumptively diagnosed as having *B. canis* infection.
Definitive diagnosis of canine brucellosis is based upon isolation of *B. canis* from the animal.

NEGATIVE TEST
No agglutination within two minutes

POSITIVE TEST
Agglutination within two minutes

Precaution: Antigen and accompanying antiserum have been standardized and should be used together. Store components at 2–7°C (35–45°F). Do not allow reagents to stand at room temperature for excessive periods of time. Do Not Freeze.
How Supplied: One kit supplies 2.5 ml antigen, 2.5 ml 2-mercaptoethanol, 0.2M solution, and 1.3 ml anti-serum sufficient to perform a minimum of 25 tests (Procedure one and/or Procedure two).
Reference:

1. A Plate Agglutination Test for the Rapid Diagnosis of Canine Brucellosis. Lisle W. George and L. E. Carmichael, presented November, 1973. Proceedings of the Council of Research Workers in Animal Diseases.

D-TEC* DF
Canine Heartworm Antibody Test Kit

General Information
Heartworm *(Dirofilaria immitis)* infection is a clinical diagnostic problem for the veterinarian with endemic areas existing in the U.S. and many other countries throughout the world. Reported incidences of infection in dogs range anywhere from 3–52 percent.[1] Though not recognized as the natural host animal, increased reported incidences of infection in cats has made this animal an acceptable alternate host.[2,3]
The onset of infection begins with mosquitoes passing infective third stage larvae through punctures in the skin of the animal. Third and fourth stage larvae remain in the connective tissues for about four months, after which the immature adults migrate to the right ventricle and pulmonary artery by way of the venous circulation. Further maturation of the parasites in the heart takes two to three months, where the young adults become sexually mature and mate, producing microfilariae. The time from initial infection through the maturation of the worm but before the production of microfilariae is called the prepatent period. Infection with the production of microfilariae is termed patent infection. The presence of adult worms can produce misleading signs of lung disease (chronic cough), congestive heart disease (ascites and lung edema), and possibly liver disease (weakness and jaundice).
The most common method of diagnosis is detection of circulating microfilariae in blood samples. However, it is not unusual to have adult worm infection without the presence of microfilariae, a condition termed occult infection. Examination of blood samples fails to detect occult infections as well as prepatent infections. Anywhere from 10 to 67 per cent of dogs with adult worms in the heart do not have demonstrable circulating microfilariae.[4] In cats, diagnosis of infection is even more difficult, with lower numbers of adult worms and circulating microfilariae than with dogs.[5]
The D-TEC* DF enzyme-linked immunosorbent assay (ELISA) diagnostic test kit detects the presence of *D. immitis* specific IgG antibodies in the blood of infected dogs and cats. This ELISA test correctly identifies prepatent infections (approximately two months after exposure), patent infections (with low to moderate numbers of circulating microfilariae) and occult infections, allowing the veterinarian to make a thorough examination

Continued on next page

P

Pitman-Moore—Cont.

of the animal before prescribing any treatment.
Since some animals with a high number of microfilariae may not have detectable free specific antibodies circulating, it is recommended that the blood first be screened for microfilariae before using this kit.

Preparation and Test Procedure
Carefully read and observe the following directions:

1 Prepare Washing Fluid by putting 100 ml distilled water in a wash bottle. Dissolve one PBS tablet, add two drops of Tween 20, and mix by inverting the bottle several times. (It will take approximately 20 minutes for the tablet to dissolve). This may be used for one week if stored at room temperature, or two months if refrigerated.
2 Add 20 microliters from each test serum to a test tube.
3 Add one drop of Positive Reference to a test tube.
4 Add one drop of Negative Reference to a test tube.
5 Add one drop of Absorbing Solution to each tube. Let stand at room temperature, while proceeding with Steps 6–10.
6 Cut a 3-well section from the plate when only one sample is to be tested. (Cut a larger section of wells if multiple samples are to be tested.) Keep the unused portion of the plate sealed and stored under refrigeration.
7 Remove cover and empty fluid from wells.
8 Wash plates as follows:
a. Fill the wells with Washing Fluid and empty quickly.
b. Fill with Washing Fluid, wait 1 minute and empty. Repeat this procedure 2 more times.
c. Quickly rinse twice with distilled water.
d. Shake off all the fluid and then tap the plate hard, twice, to remove the last traces of fluid.
9 Add three drops of Diluent to each well.
10 Incubate at room temperature for approximately 10 min.
11 Add washing fluid to the samples as follows using the plastic calibrated Transfer Pipet.
1) If the test sera is from a dog: Add 0.25 ml
2) If the test sera is from a cat: Add 0.50 ml
3) To the Reference sera: Add 0.25 ml to each
Mix all samples well.
12 Transfer 50 microliters of diluted Negative Reference to the upper well and 50 microliters of diluted Positive Reference to the bottom well. If several tests are run simultaneously, only one set of references is needed.
13 Transfer 50 microliters (0.05 ml) from each test sample to one of the remaining wells. To avoid contamination of samples, use a clean pipet tip or capillary tube for each.
14 Incubate wells at room temperature for 15 minutes.
15 While the samples are incubating, prepare the Substrate Solution as follows: In the empty dropper bottle provided, place one OPD tablet in 6 ml of distilled water. To prevent contamination of this reagent, avoid touching the tablet with the bare hand or metal. Dissolve tablet with occasional shaking, then add one drop of hydrogen peroxide, replace the dropper tip and mix. Substrate Solution is unstable and must be used within 2 hours. After use, the remaining fluid should be discarded and the bottle rinsed with distilled water.
16 After the incubation period, empty the fluid from the wells and wash the plate by repeating Step 8 a–d.
17 Add three drops of Diluent to each well.
18 Add one drop of Conjugate to each well.
19 Incubate at room temperature for 15 minutes.
20 After the incubation period, empty the wells and wash the plate by repeating Step 8 a–d.
21 Add four drops of Substrate Solution to each well.
22 Incubate at room temperature until fluid in the positive control well is distinctly yellow-green in color; fluid in the negative control well should remain colorless (or slightly colored).
23 Add two drops of Developer to each well in order to terminate the reaction and produce an amber color in the positive wells.
24 Score results.

Caution: DEVELOPER CONTAINS STRONG ACID. AVOID CONTACT WITH SKIN AND EYES.

Scoring Results
For the test to be valid, the fluid in the Positive Reference well must be distinctly amber colored, while that in the Negative Reference well must be either colorless or slightly amber. When the color of the test sample is distinctly more intense than that of the Negative Reference well, the sample is scored as positive; otherwise, it is scored as a negative. If the result is unclear, retest the animal in thirty days, using a fresh sample.

Interpretation of the Results
A negative test result shows that the animal has no detectable antibodies to *D. immitis*, indicating either no exposure or a recent (less than 2 months) infection. If a recent exposure is suspected, the animal should be retested 6–8 weeks later. A positive test shows that the animal has developed antibodies against *D. immitis* and indicates either a prepatent or occult infection. Antibodies may persist for several weeks, or even months, after successful treatment for heartworm.

Principle of the D-TEC* DF Test
To perform the assay, the sample (plasma or serum) and absorbing reagent are mixed to eliminate any non-specific, cross-reacting antibodies. After dilution, a portion is incubated in one of the wells in the test plate that has been precoated with heartworm antigen. Antibodies against the heartworm parasite, if present in the sample, will immunologically bind to the antigen coated well. The presence of IgG antibodies is detected by the addition of an anti-cat and anti-dog IgG peroxidase conjugate, followed by an enzyme substrate. Development of a distinctly colored product will indicate the presence of heartworm parasite antibodies.

Description of the D-TEC* DF Test
D-TEC* DF is a highly sensitive, specific and rapid ELISA test for *Dirofilaria immitis* antibodies in dogs and cats. Neither special training nor elaborate laboratory equipment is needed. The result of one or more tests can be determined within 1 hour (approximately 25 minutes working time) from the start of the assay. The diagnostic test kit contains both positive and negative references that are to be included each time the assay is performed.

Materials Needed but not Provided in the Kit
1. Distilled water —500 to 600 ml.
2. A system for delivery of 20 microliters (0.02 ml) and 50 microliters (0.05 ml).
3. Test tubes for preincubation of test serum.
4. Two wash bottles.

Specimen Information
Since some animals with a high number of circulating microfilariae may not have detectable free specific antibodies, it is recommended that the blood be screened for microfilariae before using this kit. Twenty microliters of plasma or serum is required for this ELISA assay. Fresh, refrigerated, or frozen samples may be tested. Hemolysis does not significantly interfere with the test.

Precautions
1. Store the kit at 2–7°C (35–45°F). Do not allow reagents to stand at room temperature for extended periods of time. Protect from direct light.
2. Conduct the test using freshly prepared Substrate Solution.
3. Use only distilled water for preparation of the reagents.
4. Avoid contamination of the OPD tablet, Hydrogen peroxide, and the prepared Substrate Solution with organic or metallic materials.
5. Use a separate pipet tip for each sample.
6. Follow the instruction exactly. Improper washing or contamination of the Substrate Solution may produce non-specific color development.
7. Include the Positive and Negative References each time the test is performed.
8. Reagents provided are intended for use with test wells in this kit. Do not use reagents from kits of other serials.
9. For Veterinary Use Only.

Contents of Test Kit
Three *D. immitis* antigen coated plates (5 × 3 well/plate—45 wells). Contains preservative.
One vial Diluent—17.0 ml. Contains preservative.

One vial Heartworm Ab. Negative Reference—1.0 ml. Contains preservative.
One vial Heartworm Ab. Positive Reference—1.0 ml. Contains preservative.
One vial Anti Feline and Canine IgG Peroxidase Conjugate—2.5 ml. Contains preservative.
One empty bottle for preparation of Substrate Solution.
One vial Developer—5.0 ml.
One vial Phosphate-Buffered Saline (PBS) Tables—(6).
One vial Polyoxyethylene Sorbitan Monolaurate (Tween 20)—1.0 ml.
One vial Ortho-Phenylenediamine Tablets—(15).
One vial Hydrogen Peroxide, 3% Aqueous Solution—1.0 ml.
One vial Absorbing Solution—2.5 ml.
One calibrated plastic Transfer Pipet.

References

1. Grieve, Robert B., Lok, James B., and Glickman, Lawrence T., *Epidemiologic Reviews, 5;* (1983), pgs. 220–245.
2. Calvert, Clay A. and Mandell, Carol P., *JAVMA, 180 (5);* (1980), pgs. 550–552.
3. Otto, G.F., *Proceedings Heartworm Symposium '74;* pgs. 6–13.
4. Otto, G.F., *Proceedings of the Heartworm Symposium '77;* pgs. 22–30.
5. Donahue, Joyce M.R., *Proceedings Heartworm Symposium '74;* pgs. 59–65.

U.S. Veterinary License No. 264
PITMAN-MOORE, INC.
Washington Crossing, N.J. 08560

*Trademark
Made in U.S.A.
9050049 PM2

D–TEC* FOAL IGG
Coagglutination Test Kit

General Information: The D-TEC* Foal IgG Test Kit is a rapid coagglutination test for detection of IgG antibodies in foal serum. The neonate depends on maternal antibodies for immune defense against infection. The newborn foal is born with little or no circulating immunoglobulins. Failure of passive transfer occurs if there is: premature lactation, delayed or deficient suckling, malabsorption or stress. Failure of passive transfer can occur in as high as 24% of foals.[1] To adequately determine failure of passive transfer of maternal antibodies, foals should be bled 18 to 72 hours after birth. Foals with IgG values less than 400 mg/dl are considered deficient in passive transfer of colostral anitbodies.[2,3]
Early diagnosis provides the clinician opportunity to implement effective treatment.

Principle Of The Test: Rabbit Anti-Horse IgG antibody has been coated to inactivated methylene-blue stained Protein A producing *Staphylococcus aureus* cells. Diluted samples are mixed with coated cells. Samples containing Horse IgG will produce agglutination of the cells by immunologically binding with the antibody coated on the cells.

Description Of The Test: D-TEC Foal IgG is designed to give the veterinarian a rapid, definitive screening of the IgG levels in foal serum 18 to 72 hours after birth. The controls in the kit are used to differentiate failure, partial failure and adequate transfer of colostral antibody. The test can be performed within five minutes. Neither special training nor elaborate equipment is required. The screening test contains positive and negative references that are to be included each time the assay is performed.

Use Of D-TEC Foal IgG Test: The kit is recommended for the semi-quantitative determination of IgG in new born foal serum or plasma.

Specimen Information: Ten microliters (0.010 ml) of serum or plasma (collected with heparin or EDTA) is required. Fresh, refrigerated or frozen samples may be tested. Enough serum can be obtained from 3–5 ml of blood.

Preparation And Test Procedure

1. a. Allow contents of kit to come to room temperature 21°C (70°F) before use.
   b. Thoroughly mix Staph A reagent by gentle shaking before use.
   c. Do not handle surface of slide card.
2. Use capillary pipet and black rubber bulb provided to pipet 10 μl (0.010 ml) of serum or plasma. Carefully wipe outside of pipette with tissue. DO NOT TOUCH TIP OF PIPET. Check volume of sera in capillary. Expel the serum or plasma into one of the prefilled buffered diluent vials. (Pipet is graduated 10 μl).
3. Recap the vial and mix well by swirling. DO NOT SHAKE.
4. Place one drop of Staph A reagent (mix well before use) into each of the four circles on the disposable agglutination card.
5. Place one drop of the High (600 mg/dl) Positive Control into the first circle (not into the Staph A Reagent).
6. Using plastic tubing with amber bulb provided, transfer one drop of the diluted sample into the second circle. (not into the Staph A Reagent).
7. Place one drop of the Low (300 mg/dl) Positive Control into the third circle (not into the Staph A Reagent).
8. Place one drop of the Negative Control into the fourth circle (not into the Staph A Reagent).
9. Using a wooden stirrer, quickly mix the drops on each circle together with a circular motion, filling almost the entire circled area, starting with circle No. 1 (600 mg/dl) control).
10. Rock the card with a circular motion and observe for approximately 15 seconds. Place on flat surface. DO NOT ROCK.
11. Observe the rate of agglutination by comparing the sample with the 600 mg/dl control, then with the 300 mg/dl control. No significance is given to reactions that occur after 2 minutes.

Interpretation Of Results:
If the sample agglutinates first or at the same time as the 600 mg/dl control, then the sample is ≥600 mg/dl, or adequate transfer.
If the sample agglutinates after the 600 mg/dl control, but faster than the 300 mg/dl control, then the sample is between 300–600 mg/dl, or partial failure of passive transfer.
If the sample agglutinates slower than the 300 mg/dl control, then the sample is less than 300 mg/dl or failure of passive transfer.
The negative control should be smooth with no agglutination.

Contents Of D-TEC Foal IgG Test Kit:

One vial Staph A coated cells contains Preservative	1.0 ml
Five vials PBS Buffer Diluent contains Preservative	10.0 ml ea.
One vial Negative Control contains Preservative	1.0 ml
One vial 300 mg/dl Control contains Preservative	1.0 ml
One vial 600 mg/dl Control contains Preservative	1.0 ml
Disposabe slide cards	5
Capillary pipettes	10
Pipette tubing	6
Wooden stirrers	25
Capillary pipette bulb (black)	2
Pipette tubing bulb (amber)	2

Precautions: 1. Store the kit under refrigeration 2–7°C (35–45°F).
2. Include the 300 mg, 600 mg and negative controls each time the test is performed.
3. Reagents provided are intended for use in this kit. Do not use reagents from kits of other serials.
4. For veterinary use only.

References

1. Crawford TB, McGuire TC, Hallowell AL and Mac Comber LE: Failure of Colostral Antibody Transfer in Foals: Its Effect, Diagnosis and Treatment. Proceedings of the 23rd Annual Convention, American Association of Equine Practitioners p 265–274, 1977.
2. McGuire TC and Crawford TB: Passive Immunity in the Foal: Measurement of Immunoglobulin Classes and Specific Antibody. Am. J. Vet. Res. 34: 1299–1303, 1973.
3. Rumbaugh GE, Ardans AA, Ginno D and Trommershausen-Smith A: Identification and Treatment of Colostrum Deficient Foals. JAVMA 174: 273–276, 1979.

*Trademark

D–TEC* MP
Mare Pregnancy Test Kit

General Information: D-TEC MP Mare Pregnancy Test Kit is a rapid micro enzyme-linked immunosorbent assay (ELISA) test for detection of pregnant mare serum gonadotropin (PMSG).
In pregnant mares, PMSG is reported to appear in plasma 37 to 42 days after conception, reaching peak concentration between 55 to 65 days and disappearing after 120 to 150 days of pregnancy.[1] The presence of PMSG in plasma forms the basis of the biological or immunological tests for pregnancy in mares. Unlike human chorionic gonadotropin, PMSG is not excreted by the kidneys therefore

Continued on next page

Pitman-Moore—Cont.

urine cannot be used for pregnancy tests in mares.

Plasma concentrations of PMSG in pregnant mares are known to reach 50 to 100 IU/ml during peak periods. D-TEC MP Mare Pregnancy Test Kit can detect as little as 0.4 IU/ml of PMSG. This kit has been found to correctly identify all pregnant mares, most of them being detected within 35 to 45 days after the last breeding[2]. The use of monoclonal antibody has eliminated the possibility of false positive reactions.

Principle of the D-TEC MP Test

To perform the D-TEC MP test, serum or plasma (with heparin or EDTA) is added to one of the wells in the test plate. The wells have been precoated with anti-PMSG 1gG. PMSG, if present in the sample, will immunologically bind to the antibody coated well. The presence of the bound PMSG is detected by the addition of specific antibody enzyme-conjugate, followed by enzyme substrate.

Development of a distinct color resulting from the reaction between substrate and immunologically immobilized enzyme indicates the presence of PMSG in the sample, confirming pregnancy of the mare.

Description of the D-TEC MP Test Kit

D-TEC MP is a highly sensitive, specific and rapid ELISA test for the detection of PMSG. Neither special training nor elaborate laboratory equipment is needed to perform the test. The results can be determined within approximately 1 hour with 15 minutes working time. The kit contains both positive and negative references that are to be included each time the assay is performed. There are sufficient reagents to test from 15 to 39 samples.

Materials Needed But Not Provided in the Kit

1. Distilled water.
2. Two wash bottles.

Use of D-TEC MP Test Kit

The kit is recommended for laboratory diagnosis and monitoring of pregnancy in mares.

Specimen Information

Fifty microliters (0.05 ml) of serum or plasma (collected with heparin or EDTA) is required. Fresh, refrigerated or frozen samples may be tested. Hemolysis does not significantly interfere with the test. Enough serum or plasma can be obtained from 5 ml of blood without centrifugation.

Preparation and Test Procedure: Carefully read and observe the following directions.

1. Prepare washing fluid as follows: Dissolve 1 PBS tablet per 100 ml distilled water, add 2 drops or 0.08 ml of Tween 20 for each 100 ml of solution and mix thoroughly, but, gently. At least 20 minutes are needed for the tablets to dissolve. This solution may be used for 1 week if stored at room temperature or 2 months if stored under refrigeration.
2. Cut a 3-well section from the plate when only one sample is run. Cut a larger section of two or more rows of 3 wells if multiple samples are tested. Use entire plate when testing 11 to 13 samples. Keep the unused portion of the plate sealed and stored under refrigeration.
3. Remove cover and empty fluid from wells.
4. Wash the plates as follows:
   a. Fill the wells with washing fluid and empty quickly.
   b. Fill with washing fluid, wait 3 minutes and empty. Repeat this procedure 2 more times.
   c. Quickly rinse twice with **distilled water.**
   d. Shake off all the fluid and then tap the tray hard, twice, to remove the last traces of fluid.
5. Add three drops of Diluent to each well.
6. Add one drop of Negative Reference to the upper well and add one drop of Positive Reference to the bottom well. If several tests are run simultaneously, only one set of references is needed.
7. Use 50 μl (0.05 ml) of sample to the remaining well or wells. To avoid contamination of samples, use a clean pipet tip or capillary tube for each.
8. Add one drop of Antibody-Peroxidase conjugate to each well.
9. Incubate for 45 minutes at room temperature.
10. Approximately 20 minutes before the end of incubation, prepare the Substrate Solution. In the empty dropper bottle provided, place one OPD tablet in 6 ml of distilled water. To prevent contamination of the reagent, avoid touching the tablet with the bare hand. Dissolve tablet with occasional gentle shaking, **then add one drop of hydrogen peroxide,** replace the dropper tip and mix. Substrate Solution is unstable and must be used within 2 hours. After use, the remaining fluid should be discarded and the bottle rinsed with distilled water.
11. After the 45 min. incubation period, empty the fluid from the wells and **wash the plate by repeating Step 4 (a through d).**
12. Add four drops of Substrate Solution to each well.
13. Incubate at room temperature until fluid in the positive reference well is distinctly yellow-green in color; fluid in the negative reference well should remain colorless (or slightly colored).
14. Add two drops of Developer to each well in order to terminate reaction and produce an amber color in the positive wells.
15. Score results.

Caution: The developer contains 5N sulfuric acid. Avoid contact with skin and eyes.

Scoring of Test Results

For the test to be valid, the fluid in the positive reference well must be distinctly amber colored, while that in the negative reference well must be either colorless or slightly amber. When the color of the test sample is distinctly more intense than that of the negative reference well, the sample is scored as positive: otherwise, it is scored negative.

Interpretation of the Results

In the majority of pregnant mares, PMSG appears in serum before 45 days after breeding. The levels of PMSG peak at 55 to 65 days of pregnancy and then decrease gradually to low levels or disappear altogether by 120 to 150 days after conception.

A positive test result indicates the presence of PMSG in the sample, confirming pregnancy in the mare. Mares with negative test results during 60 to 90 days after breeding are most likely not pregnant. A negative test result before 60 days or after 90 days does not rule out pregnancy as undetectable levels of hormone may be present during these stages of pregnancy. For early detection, it is recommended that testing be started approximately 35 days after breeding and animals with negative results be retested at 7 to 10 day intervals.

Precautions

1. Store the kit under refrigeration 2–7°C (35–45°F). Do not allow reagents to stand at room temperature for extended periods of time. Protect from direct light.
2. Conduct the test using freshly prepared Substrate Solution.
3. Use only distilled water for preparation of reagents.
4. Avoid contamination of the OPD tablet, hydrogen peroxide, and the prepared Substrate Solution with organic or metallic materials.
5. Follow the instructions exactly. Improper washing or contamination of the Substrate Solution may produce non-specific color development.
6. Include the positive and negative references each time the test is performed.

Contents of D-TEC MP Test Kit

Three anti-PMSG-IgG Coated Plates (5 × 3 wells/plate—Total 45 wells). Contains preservative.

One vial Diluent—17.0 ml. Contains preservative.

One vial Mare Pregnancy Negative Reference—1.0 ml. Contains preservative.

One vial Mare Pregnancy Positive Reference—1.0 ml. Contains preservative.

One vial anti-PMSG-1gG Peroxidase Conjugate—2.5 ml. Contains preservative.

One vial Phosphate Buffered Saline (PBS) Tablets—(6)

One vial Tween 20—1.0 ml.

One vial Ortho-Phenylenediamine (OPD) Tablets—(15)

One vial Hydrogen Peroxide, 3% Aqueous Solution—1.0 ml.

One vial Developer—5.0 ml.

One empty vial for preparation of Substrate Solution.

For Veterinary Use Only

References:

1. Ginter, O.J.: "Endocrinology of Pregnancy" (Chapter 10), *Reproductive Biology of the Mare,* pp. 321–324, McNaughton and Gunn, Inc., Ann Arbor, MI, 1979.
2. Mia, A.S., M. Tierney, and M.W. Rohovsky: A Rapid Micro-Elisa Test for Detection of Equine Pregnancy. *Proceedings of the 62nd Annual Meeting of the Conference of Research Workers in Animal Disease, Chicago, IL,* p, 18, November, 1981.

*Trademark

EQUINE INFECTIOUS ANEMIA
Immunodiffusion Antigen

Sale and use in the U.S. restricted to Laboratories or Individuals approved by State and Federal (USDA) Animal Health Officials.

FILARASSAY*F
Heartworm Microfilariae Diagnostic System
Filtration

Indications: For the determination of the presence of circulating microfilariae.

Summary and History: Filtration has long been used to prepare blood for examination to determine the presence or absence of circulating microfilariae. This procedure has been adapted for use in this kit.

Principle: The Filarassay F kit provides the practitioner with a rapid procedure for blood examination to determine the presence or absence of circulating microfilariae. The system is based on the lysis of red blood cells followed by concentration of microfilariae through filtration. If present, the microfilariae on the membrane remain alive and active. This kit also provides a stain solution so that a detailed study of the morphological characteristics of the microfilariae may be conducted to differentiate between species.

Reagent Information: Filarassay* Lysing Solution, Filarassay* Stain Solution and Filarassay* Anticoagulant (ethylenediaminetetraacetic acid—EDTA) are provided in quantities sufficient to perform 50 tests.

Caution: Do not take internally. For *in vitro* diagnostic use.

Storage: Store at controlled room temperature (59°–86°F).

Specimen Information:

1. One ml of blood obtained by venipuncture is required.
2. Prompt processing of the specimen will aid in accurate determination of the presence or absence of microfilariae.

General Information

Materials Provided:

1. Filarassay Lysing Solution—One 55 ml bottle
2. Filarassay Stain Solution—One 7 ml bottle
3. Filarassay Anticoagulant (EDTA)—One 10 ml vial
4. Phosphate Buffered Saline Tablets (PBS)—5 tablets
5. 50 filters
6. One filter holder
7. One mixing vial
8. One disposable 20 ml syringe
9. One calibrated 1 ml dropper
10. Detailed instructions

Materials Required But Not Provided:

1. Sterile disposable syringes—3 ml
2. Sterile disposable syringes—20 ml
3. Microscope slides and cover slips
4. Microscope capable of low and medium (1OX and 40X) magnification

Test procedure

Caution: Sodium fluoride-potassium oxalate must not be used as an anticoagulant since it kills the microfilariae, thereby precluding observation of movement. The use of heparin will cause difficulty in filtration. Use materials provided with this kit for best results.

Note: Discard all filters and syringes after use to avoid any possibility of contamination or cases of false positives.

1. Obtain 1 ml of blood by venipuncture using a 3 ml syringe containing 0.1 ml of EDTA,
2. Prepare Phosphate Buffered Saline Solution by dissolving one PBS tablet in 100 ml of distilled or clean tap water.
3. Assemble the filter holder as described below.
   a. Unscrew and remove the syringe attachment top, being careful not to misplace or damage the silicone "0" ring.
   b. Hold the top section of the filter holder and turn upside down.
   c. Place the silicone "0" ring in the inverted top section of the filter holder. Make sure that the ring is seated properly.
   d. Remove the filtering membrane from the package with colored separator paper: discard paper.
   e. Grasp the filter membrane by the edge with forceps and gently slide the filter membrane over the lip of the filter top and down on top of the "0" ring. Make sure that the "0" ring is completely covered by the filter membrane.
   f. Replace the base of the filter holder in the inverted top.
4. Place the 1 ml of blood into the provided vial or the disposable 20 ml syringe and add 1 ml of Filarassay Lysing Solution. Mix well to hemolyze the red blood cells.
5. Add sufficient Phosphate Buffered Saline Solution (prepared in Step 2 above) to the vial or syringe to make 10 ml of solution; mix thoroughly.
6. If the vial was used to make the solution, put the lysed blood in the syringe attached with the filter holder containing a 3 μm membrane. Otherwise, attach the syringe to the prepared filter holder.
7. Filter the lysed blood.
8. Unscrew the filter holder. Grasp the filter with forceps and gently slide it down to a microscope slide.
9. Cover with a cover slip and examine under a microscope with the condenser down. Observe for moving microfilariae.
10. If microfilariae are found, use Filarassay Stain Solution to aid in positive identification of species. Add three drops of stain per filter to be observed. Cover with a cover slip and examine under the microscope with the condenser up. The microfilariae are rapidly killed, stained and clarified.

Identification of Microfilariae

Microfilariae can be identified by their differences in size and morphological characteristics. The microfilariae of *Dirofilaria immitis* have a tapered head and straight tail. The microfiliariae of *Dipetalonema reconditum* have a blunt head and button-hooked tail and are smaller than those of *D. immitis.* [1–4].

Limitation of Procedure

When used according to directions, there are no known limitations to the Filarassay F Heartworm Microfilariae Diagnostic System—Filtration.

Reference:

1. Jackson, R. F. and Otto, G. F. Detection and Differentiation of Microfilariae. In: Proceedings of the Heartworm Symposium 1974. H. C. Morgan, Ed., V. M. Publishing, Inc., Bonner Springs, Kansas, 21–22, 1975.
2. Jackson, R. F., *et al.* Procedure for the Treatment and Prevention of Canine Heartworm Disease. J.A.V.M.A. 162(8):660–661, 1973.
3. Morgan, H. C..Canine Blood Parasites: Filariasis. Veterinary Medicine/Small Animal Clinician 61 (9):829–841, 1966.
4. Sawyer, Thomas, *et al.* The Cephalic Hook in Microfilariae of *Dipetalonema reconditum* in the Differentiation of Canine Microfilariae. In: Proceedings of the Helminthological Society of Washington 32(1): 15–20, 1965.

*Trademark

FUNGASSAY*
Dermatophyte Test Medium

Indications: Fungassay Dermatophyte Test Medium is a culture medium that provides a simple, rapid and practical method for confirming dermatophyte infections. The test is based on a color change within the medium caused by the growth of pathogenic fungi. Nearly all dermatomycoses seen in veterinary practice are due to Microsporum and Trichophyton infections. When hair or scales infected with these fungi are placed on Fungassay Dermatophyte Test Medium, growth of the organisms will cause the medium to change from amber to red.

Common Dermatophytes in Veterinary Practice:

Animal Species	*Dermatophytes*
Cats	M. + Canis
Dogs	M. canis
	M. gypseum
	T. ++ mentagrophytes
Cattle	T. verruco sum
Swine	M. nanum
Horses	M. gypseum
Monkeys	M. canis

Continued on next page

Pitman-Moore—Cont.

	T. mentagrophytes
Laboratory Rodents	M. gypseum
	T. mentagrophytes

Evaluation of Test Results: Evaluation of the test results can begin as early as 48 hours after innoculation. A pinkish color will appear in the amber medium under the specimen and developing colony. The color will intensify as growth proceeds and is due to alkaline metabolites produced by the dermatophytes. When a positive dermatophyte infection is present, the entire medium will turn red by the seventh to fourteenth day. If there is no growth within 10 days, redistribute the sample on the medium. Occasionally growth does not occur because of improper innoculation. A color change may occasionally be produced by a specimen heavily contaminated with saprophytic fungi or bacteria. However, this is not a problem because differentiation from dermatophytes can be made as follows:

Dermatophyte: A color change appears in the medium with colony growth —colony pigments are usually light colored.

Saprophyte Fungi: Colony growth is well established before any color change appears in the medium—colony pigments are usually dark colored.

Bacteria: The morphology of bacterial colonies differs from the morphology of fungal colonies.

Precautions: Refrigerate Fungassay Dermatophyte Test Medium for optimum storage. Warming to room temperature before using is not necessary.

Destroy the used Fungassay Dermatophyte Test Medium bottle by incineration to eliminate spread of all organisms.

How Supplied: Fungassay Dermatophyte Test Medium is supplied in a package containing 12 individual bottles.

*Trademark

LEUKASSAY*-B BOVINE LEUKEMIA GLYCOPROTEIN IMMUNODIFFUSION ANTIGEN, Ovine Cell Line Origin REAGENT SERUM and REFERENCE SERUMS, Bovine Origin

Description: The immunodiffusion test using a glycoprotein antigen of the virus for the diagnosis of bovine leukemia virus infection was described by Miller and Van Der Maaten. The Bovine Leukemia Glycoprotein Immunodiffusion (BL-GID) kit contains the following: glycoprotein antigen, antigen diluent, reagent serum, negative, weak positive and positive reference serums.

Indications: The BL-GID test is used to determine if animals are infected with bovine leukemia virus by detecting the presence of serum antibody against a specific bovine leukemia virus glycoprotein antigen.

Precautions: Store all reagents frozen after rehydration or first use. Antigen and accompanying reagent serum have been standardized and should be used together. Use a negative, positive and weak positive reference serum in one pattern on each plate where these would replace the test serum to assure proper sensitivity of the test. Fill all wells properly as described under 3 of preparation tion and use. Do not allow reagents to stand at room temperature for excessive periods of time while performing tests. Handle all reagents and their equipment as if capable of transmitting bovine leukemia. Contains sodium azide, gentamicin and amphotericin B as preservatives. Burn all containers and all unused contents. Autoclave all disposable test components and test specimens after use.

How Supplied: Each kit contains enough antigen, reagent serum and reference serum to perform 90 tests and 30 control tests as follows:

One vial BL-GID Antigen

Rehydrates to 3 cc (90 tests and 30 control tests)

One vial Sterile Diluent—3 cc

One vial Reagent Serum—9 cc (90 tests and 30 control tests)

One vial Negative Reference Serum—1 cc (10 control tests)

One vial Weak Positive Reference Serum—1 cc (10 control tests)

One vial Positive Reference Serum—1 cc (10 control tests)

*Trademark

LEUKASSAY* F
Feline Leukemia Virus Test Kit

General Information: The feline leukemia (FeLV) enzyme-linked immunosorbent assay (ELISA) diagnostic test kit detects the presence of FeLV group-specific (gs) antigens in the blood of infected cats. Feline Leukemia Virus is a cause of lymphosarcoma, the most commonly occurring feline neoplasm. It also induces non-regenerative anemia; a "panleukopenia-like" syndrome of dysentery and leukopenia; and a "fading kitten" syndrome resulting from atrophy of the thymus. Myeloid disorders, fetal resorptions and abortions are thought to be attributable to FeLV infection. However, all cats with these conditions may not be infected with FeLV. Sixty to 90% of cats with lymphosarcoma and 40–70% of cats with non-regenerative anemia have been found to be infected with FeLV (1,2). Because it is immunosuppressive, FeLV predisposes infected cats to a variety of secondary diseases. A great majority of cats suffering from hemobartonellosis, septicemia, feline infectious peritonitis, toxoplasmosis, glomerulonephritis, chronic oral ulcers and chronic skin conditions also have been found to be infected with FeLV. It has been observed that the incidence of leukemia was approximately 900% greater in FeLV-infected cats than in non-infected cats in the same households. The incidence of diseases other than leukemia was reported to be 400% greater in the FeLV-infected cats (3). Kittens may acquire FeLV *in utero*, but more commonly infection results from prolonged contact of susceptible cats with those having FeLV.

Principle of the Leukassay* F Test: During FeLV infection gs antigens are detectable in infected tissues, such as blood cells, and in plasma (1). To perform the Leukassay* F Test, the sample (whole blood with heparin or EDTA, plasma or serum) and the specific antibody-enzyme conjugate are added to one of the wells in the test plate. The wells have been precoated with antibody specific for FeLV gs antigens. When the sample is from an infected cat, gs antigens having multiple binding sites will be bound immunologically to both the coated antibody and the enzyme conjugated antibody. After addition of the substrate, a distinctly colored reaction product will be formed only if the well contains immunologically immobilized enzyme.

Description of the Leukassay* F Test Kit: Leukassay* F is a highly sensitive, specific and rapid ELISA test for FeLV gs antigens in kit form. Neither special training nor elaborate laboratory equipment is needed. The results of one or more tests can be determined within 25 minutes (approximately 10 minutes working time) from the start of the assay. The diagnostic test kit contains both positive and negative references that are to be included each time the assay is performed. Using Monoclonal Antibody, the test has been simplified and made highly specific.

Indications: The Leukassay* F Test is used to determine if cats are infected with FeLV. The testing of healthy cats is recommended as a routine part of a comprehensive health program. Because FeLV has a variety of manifestations and predisposes infected cats to other infectious diseases, the test has diagnostic value in the following conditions: neoplastic disease; non-regenerative anemia; leukopenia and enteritis (especially in cats immunized previously against feline panleukopenia); neo-natal death; abortion; fetal resorption and infertility; chronic skin disease or ulceration of the oral cavity; general unthriftiness; any condition unresponsive to specific therapy.

Leukemia virus-negative cats should be retested after they have been in contact with other cats for extended periods of time. A routine quarantine and testing program is rcommended to establish and maintain FeLV-free catteries(1).

Contents of Leukassay* F Test Kit: Three Anti-Feline Leukemia Virus gsa Immune Globulin G-Coated Plates, (5 × 3 Wells/Plate). Contains preservative.

One vial Feline Leukemia Virus Test Diluent (Reagent 1)—17.0 ml. Contains preservative.

One vial Feline Leukemia Negative Reference, Feline Origin (Reagent 2)—1.0 ml. Contains preservative.

One vial Feline Leukemia Positive Reference, Killed Virus, Feline Origin (Reagent 3)—1.0 ml. Contains preservative.

One vial Anti-Feline Leukemia Virus gsa Peroxidase-Conjugated Immune Globulin G (Reagent 4)—2.5 ml. Contains preservative.

One empty bottle for preparation of Substrate Solution (Reagent 5).
One vial Feline Leukemia Virus Test Developer (Reagent 6)—5.0 ml.
One vial Phosphate-Buffered Saline Tablets (Reagent A)—6 tablets.
One vial Polyoxyethylene Sorbitan Monolaurate, Tween 20, (Reagent B)—1.0 ml.
One vial Ortho-Phenylenediamine Tablets (Reagent C)—15 tablets.
One vial Hydrogen Peroxide, 3 percent Aqueous Solution (Reagent D)—1.0 ml.

Precautions: 1. Store the kit at 2–7° C (35–45°F) Do not allow reagents to stand at room temperature for extended periods of time. Protect from direct light.
2. Conduct the test using freshly prepared Substrate Solution.
3. Use only distilled water for preparation of reagents.
4. Avoid contamination of the OPD tablet, hydrogen peroxide, and the prepared Substrate Solution with organic or metallic materials.
5. Use a separate pipet tip for each sample.
6. Follow the instructions exactly. Improper washing or contamination of the Substrate Solution may produce non-specific color development.
7. Include the positive and negative references each time the test is performed.
8. Handle all samples as if capable of transmitting FeLV. Burn all unused biological components.
9. Reagents provided are intended for use with test wells in this kit. Do not use reagents from kits of other serials.
10. For Veterinary Use Only.

Materials Needed But Not Provided In The Kit Are: 1. *Distilled water* —400 to 500 ml.
2. A system for delivery of 50 µl (0.05 ml) sample to the test well. A micropipet with disposable tip, bulb dropper, or capillary tube capable of delivering 50 µl may be used. (If a bulb dropper is used, one drop is equivalent to 50 µl).
3. Two wash bottles.

Specimen Information: Fifty microliters of serum or plasma is required. Whole blood with heparin or EDTA may be used but requires stringent post incubation washing (see step 11). Fresh, refrigerated, or frozen samples may be tested. Hemolysis does not significantly interfere with the test.

Preparation And Test Procedure: *Carefully read and observe the following directions:*

1. Prepare Washing Fluid by putting 100 ml *distilled water* in a wash bottle. Dissolve one PBS tablet (Reagent A), add two drops of Tween 20 (Reagent B), and mix by inverting the bottle several times. (It will take approximately 20 minutes to dissolve the tablet). This may be used for two months if refrigerated.
2. Cut a 3-well section from the plate when only one sample is run. (Cut a larger section of two or more rows of 3 wells if multiple samples are tested.) Keep the unused portion of the plate sealed and stored under refrigeration.
3. Remove cover and empty fluid from wells.
4. Wash the plates as follows:
   a. Fill the wells with Washing Fluid and empty quickly.
   b. Repeat this procedure 2 more times.
   c. Quickly rinse twice with *distilled water.*
   d. Shake off all the fluid and then tap the tray hard, twice, to remove the last traces of fluid.
5. Add two drops of Diluent (Reagent 1) to each well.
6. Add one drop of Negative Reference (Reagent 2) to the upper well and add one drop of Positive Reference (Reagent 3) to the bottom well. If several tests are run simultaneously, only one set of references is needed.
7. Add 50 µl (0.05 ml) of sample to the remaining well or wells. To avoid contamination of samples, use a clean pipet tip or capillary tube for each.
8. Add one drop of Antibody-Peroxidase Conjugate (Reagent 4) to each well.
9. Incubate for 20 min. at room temperature.
10. Soon after the start of incubation, prepare the Substrate Solution (Reagent 5): In the empty dropper bottle provided, place one OPD tablet (Reagent C) in 6 ml of distilled water. To prevent contamination of the reagent, avoid touching the tablet with the bare hand. Dissolve tablet with occasional gentle shaking, *then add one drop of hydrogen peroxide* (Reagent D), replace the dropper tip and mix. Substrate Solution is unstable and must be used within 2 hours. After use, the remaining fluid should be discarded and the bottle rinsed with *distilled water.*
11. After the incubation period, empty the fluid from the wells and wash the plates as follows:
    a. Fill the wells with Washing Fluid, and empty quickly. If whole blood was used, flush wells thoroughly to remove excess red cell debris.
    b. Fill with Washing Fluid and empty. Repeat this procedure 2 more times.
    c. Quickly rinse twice with *distilled water.*
    d. Shake off all the fluid and then tap the tray hard, twice, to remove the last traces of fluid.
12. Add four drops of Substrate Solution (Reagent 5) to each well.
13. Incubate at room temperature until fluid in the positive reference well is distinctly yellow-green in color; fluid in the negative reference well should remain colorless (or slightly colored).
14. Add two drops of Developer (Reagent 6) to each well in order to terminate reaction and produce an amber color in the positive wells.
15. Score results.

CAUTION: THE DEVELOPER IS A STRONG ACID. AVOID CONTACT WITH SKIN AND EYES.

Scoring Of Test Results: For the test to be valid, the fluid in the positive reference well must be distinctly amber colored, while that in the negative reference well must be either colorless or slightly amber. When the color of the test sample is distinctly more intense than that of the negative reference well, the sample is scored as positive; otherwise it is scored negative. If the result is unclear, retest the animal in thirty days, using a fresh sample.

P

Interpretation of the Results: A positive test result indicates active FeLV infection. Because infection is transient in cats that develop immunity, FeLV (gs) antigen-positive animals should be retested in three or four weeks. A negative second sample would indicate immune clearance of FeLV. A positive second sample would indicate persistent infection. Persistence of FeLV infection is accompanied by a high risk that the cat will develop lymphosarcoma, non-regenerative anemia, or one of the other FeLV associated diseases. A persistently infected cat is likely to shed FeLV and is a potential source of infection. A negative test indicates the animal has little likelihood of having active FeLV infection at the time of assay. This cat may be susceptible to FeLV infection and should be retested periodically. Animals added to FeLV negative catteries should be tested at the time of purchase and again after they have been isolated from other cats for three weeks. A test and removal program has been proposed as a method of eliminating FeLV infection in breeding facilities and multiple cat households (1).

References:
1. Hardy, W.D. Jr. and McClelland, A. J. Veterinary Clinic North Am. 7:93 (1977).
2. Hardy, W.D. Jr., DVM, 10:20 (1979)
3. Essex, M., Hardy, W.D. Jr., Cotter, S.M., Lakowski, R.M. and Sliski, A. Infection and Immunity 11, 470 (1975)

Sold to Veterinarians Only
U.S. Veterinary License No. 264
*Trademark

OVASSAY*
Fecal Diagnostic System

Summary and History: Salts and sugars have long been used to produce high specific gravity media to aid in the separation of common parasite ova from the debris in fecal matter. The fecal flotation method has been adapted for use in this kit.

Principle: When a fecal specimen is homogenized in a solution with specific gravity of approximately 1.2, the common ova float at the top of the liquid while most of the fecal debris settles to the bottom. The top portion of the liquid is then collected on a coverslip and examined microscopically.

Continued on next page

Pitman-Moore—Cont.

Specimen Information:
1. Approximately two grams of feces are required.
2. Prompt processing of specimen will aid in the accurate diagnosis of parasitic infection.

Procedure:
Materials Provided:
1. Ovassay Collection Vials with Caps and Label/Scoops-55
2. Stirring Rods-50
3. Ovassay Fecal Diagnostic Devices-50
4. Ovassay Sodium Nitrate Crystals-40 fl oz (when reconstituted with water)
5. Instructions

Materials Required but Not Provided:
1. Microscope slides and coverslips ($22mm^2$)
2. Microscope capable of low and 100x magnification

Time Required for the Test:
Total Time: 20–25 minutes
Working Time: Approximately 5 minutes
Set Up Time: 30–45 seconds
Reading Time: 3–4 minutes

Test Procedure: Examine the specimen for any visible adult parasites or tapeworm segments.
1. Prepare Sodium Nitrate Solution according to the directions on the bottle of Ovassay Sodium Nitrate Crystals.
2. Fill the collection vial half full with the Ovassay Sodium Nitrate Solution prepared in Step 1.
3. Thoroughly mix the fecal specimen and solution with the stirring rod.
4. Gently place the Ovassay Fecal Diagnostic Device covered with the cap into the vial. Snap the device into place. Remove cap.
5. Add additional Ovassay Sodium Nitrate Solution until a convex meniscus is formed in the device.
6. Float a $22mm^2$ coverslip on the meniscus. Let stand for *at least 15 minutes* to allow the ova to float through the device and cling to the coverslip. (Overflow will be collected in the well on the device.)
7. Lift the coverslip straight up in a smooth, nonstop motion to avoid loss of ova and place on a microscope slide. Examine under low power and 100x for ova.
8. Place the cap onto the assembled vial-device and discard.

Examination of the Slide: Moving the slide systematically, scan the entire preparation. Identify all parasite eggs and grade the quantity of eggs to relate to light, medium or heavy infections. Do not confuse epithelial cells, air bubbles, etc. with the ova.

Limitation of Procedure: Generally, the ova of common nematode parasites are readily detected by this technique. Tapeworm eggs would be detected if gravid proglotids are found in the samples or if they burst and dessiminate eggs into the feces.

Specific Performance Characteristics: The Ovassay Fecal Diagnostic System has been found to compare favorably with standard flotation techniques for identifying parasitic infections. It requires a minimum of manipulative procedures, and the materaials and remaining debris are disposable in a manner that minimizes chances of contamination of the technician's hands or laboratory area.
*Trademark

PROGESTASSAY*
Milk Progesterone Test Kit

General Information
Progesterone is a steroidal hormone produced by the corpus luteum during the estrous cycle and pregnancy. Plasma progesterone levels accurately reflect the different stages of the estrous cycle as well as the pregnancy status. Since progesterone levels in milk correlate well with those of plasma, determination of milk progesterone levels is the most common test that has been used to predict pregnancy status and to detect estrus in cows. The test has also been used to diagnose various reproductive disorders and to monitor the effectiveness of treatment for infertility.

Principle of the Milk Progesterone Test
The enzyme linked immunosorbent assay (ELISA) for milk progesterone is based on the principle of competitive binding. Endogenous progesterone in milk competes with exogenous horseradish peroxidase-labeled (HRP) progesterone in the test reagent for binding sites on a limited quantity of a specific antibody. The amount of HRP-labeled progesterone bound to the antibody is inversely proportional to the amount of endogenous progesterone present; e.g. the higher the level of progesterone present in the milk, the fewer binding sites available for the HRP-labeled progesterone. The bound labeled progesterone is measured by allowing the HRP label to act on its substrate, hydrogen peroxide, in the presence of a chromogen which turns from colorless to a blue colored product. The comparison between the color produced by the control and the test may be made visually or spectrophotometrically.

Description of the Kit
PROGESTASSAY* Milk Progesterone Test Kit is a sensitive and rapid Dip-Stick ELISA test, using **highly specific monoclonal antibody,** for evaluation of the reproductive status of cows by comparative determination of milk progesterone. Neither special training nor elaborate laboratory equipment is needed. The results of one or more tests can be determined within 15 to 20 minutes (less than 5 minutes of working time) from the start of the assay. The kit contains two milk controls, one for estrus or follicular phase and the other for pregnancy or luteal phase. At least one milk control must be included each time the test is performed. Twenty to thirty-six samples may be tested in multiples of one to nine samples at a time.

Indications or Uses of the Test Kit
For *In-Vitro* use in the evaluation of the reproductive status of cows based on milk progesterone levels. This will assist in the following determinations:
a. Confirmation of non-estrus/estrus
b. Determination of non-pregnancy/pregnancy status
c. Detection of post parturient cyclicity and anestrus
d. Detection of silent estrus
e. Detection of embryonic or fetal death
f. Determination of luteal phase for effective use of luteolytic agents
g. Diagnosis of ovarian disorders
h. Monitoring of infertility treatments

Contents of the Kit
Monoclonal antibody coated dipstick—40 sticks
Progesterone-peroxidase conjugate concentrate—0.5 ml
Diluent for preparing progesterone-peroxidase conjugate (Reagent A)—45 ml
Washing Solution (Reagent B)—90 ml
Buffered Substrate (Reagent C)—45 ml
Substrate Chromogen (Reagent D)—10.5 ml
Estrus Milk Control (Control E)—5.5 ml
Pregnancy Milk Control (Control P)—5.5 ml
Pipeting syringe—1
Pipeting tips—61 tips
Rubber bulb droppers—3 droppers

Materials Needed but not Provided in the Kit†
1. 12 × 75 mm test tubes
2. Milk sample containers
3. PROGESTASSAY milk sample preservative
4. Test tube rack

†Available from Pitman-Moore

Storage and Stability
Store the kit at 2 to 7°C (35–45°F).
Do not freeze. Do not allow reagents to stand at room temperature for extended periods of time. Protect from direct light. Reagent D may develop a slight bluish color during storage which will not affect the test results.

Precautions
1. Do not run the test outdoors or in front of an open window. Ultraviolet light may interfere with the test.
2. Use only PROGESTASSAY* milk preservative. Lactab or other preservatives may interfere with the test.
3. Avoid contamination of the reagents with organic or metallic materials.
4. Use a separate tip for each sample.
5. Follow the instructions exactly. Contamination of the reagents may produce non-specific color development.
6. Do not interchange the droppers.
7. Do not touch the bulb end of the sticks.
8. Avoid bubbling air through the reagent during the use of a dropper.
9. Include the appropriate milk control each time the test is performed.
10. Reagents provided are intended for use as a unit combination. Do not use reagents from kits of other lots.
11. Reagents should be handled carefully, avoiding ingestion and contact with the skin.
12. For Veterinary Use Only.

Test Sample Information
The test kit has been standardized for testing fore milk or composite milk with PROGESTASSAY milk preservative.

The milk may be collected at regular milking time or any other time except within two hours following milking to avoid high-fat content strip milk. Milk may be collected from one or more healthy quarters after discarding first few squirts. The collection container should be filled approximately to a 10 ml volume. One drop of PROGESTASSAY milk preservative is added and mixed gently. (PROGESTASSAY milk preservative may be omitted if samples are refrigerated and tested within 24 hours). The sample should be properly identified and stored under refrigeration and **must not be frozen.** A milk sample with preservative is stable for 3 days at room temperature or 2 months under refrigeration provided no coagulation or curdling occurs. Several samples may be accumulated and tested at one time.

Milk Sampling Schedules:

a. **For confirmation of non-estrus/estrus:** A single sample on the day of suspected estrus.

b. **For determination of non-pregnancy/pregnancy:** One sample taken 20 to 23 days after insemination. Continuation of pregnancy may be confirmed with an additional sample taken on days 40 to 43 after breeding, or at the time of palpation.

c. **For determination of post-parturient cyclicity:** A minimum of three samples collected at 7 day intervals starting 25 to 30 days after parturition. Samples taken at 4 day intervals for 3 weeks may define the cycle more precisely.

d. **For detection of silent estrus:** Collect samples on alternate days starting from 7 days prior to the expected heat period estimated by testing for cyclicity.

e. **For detection of embryonic or fetal death:** Periodic samples following diagnosis of pregnancy, especially during the first 3 months of pregnancy.

f. **For determination of luteal phase for effective use of luteolytic agents:** Collect one sample within one day prior to administration of luteolytic agent followed by another sample 72–90 hours after treatment.

g. **For diagnosis of ovarian disorders:** One sample on the day of palpation. Two additional samples at 7 day intervals in doubtful cases.

h. **For monitoring infertility treatment:** Collect a minimum of three samples at 7 day intervals after therapy to detect the initiation of the estrous cycle. Samples taken at 4 day intervals for 3 weeks may define the cycle more precisely.

Patent Pending

PITMAN-MOORE, INC.
Washington Crossing, N.J.08560

Printed in U.S.A. 8-1-85 *Trademark
Made in U.S.A. 9050051 PM2

TOXOPLASMA GONDII ANTIBODY TEST KIT

General Information: Toxoplasmosis, a disease in cats caused by the intracellular parasite *Toxoplasma gondii,* is a diagnostic challenge to veterinarians. It is also one of the most widespread zoonotic diseases worldwide.[1] The sexual phase of T. gondii is known to occur only in cats and cats therefore serve as the definitive hosts; however, various mammalian and avian species may serve as intermediate hosts. In the cat, clinical disease may be dependent upon immunocompetence or age. Clinical signs vary from inapparent to more severe forms. Most cases are inapparent but the more severe signs are associated with lesions of the respiratory, gasrointestinal, CNS, myocardial, muscular, lymphatic and ophthalmic systems.

Serologic testing for T. gondii specific antibody in cats has utilized the Sabin-Feldman dye test, indirect hemagglutination, indirect flourescent antibody, or complement fixation.[2,4] Each method has inherent difficulties which make them difficult to routinely perform in the veterinary diagnostic laboratory. Diagnosis of infection has also included parasitologic examination. ELISA methodology, as described by Voller,[3] employs enzyme-labeled antiglobulin conjugates to detect specific antibody and has become a useful tool in veterinary serology. The test has been found to be a faster, simpler, and more economical alternative to standard tests where greater sensitivity, specificity and accuracy are desired.

Description Of The Test Kit: This test is designed to be a highly sensitive, specific and rapid test for the detection of Toxoplasma gondii specific IgG antibody in cat serum. The kit contains both negative and low positive reference control sera which are included each time the assay is performed. Visual or spectrophotometric evaluation of 16–46 test samples can be performed with this kit. Results can be obtained within 2½ hours.

Principle Of The Test: A test serum or plasma sample from a cat is added to one well of a test plate. Wells have been coated with *Toxoplasma gondii* antigen. T. gondii specific antibody, if present in the sample, will specifically bind to the attached antigen. Nonspecific antibody will not be bound and is therefore removed by washing. The amount of antibody bound to the antigen is detected by the addition of enzyme-conjugated anti-cat IgG and substrate.

When T. gondii specific IgG is present, the resulting enzymatic reaction upon the substrate will produce a colored product suitable for visual or spectrophotometric analysis. The intensity of color in the well is directly proportional to the amount of specifically bound antibody.

Specimen Information: Ten microliters (0.010 ml) of serum or plasma is required. Fresh, refrigerated or frozen samples may be tested.

Direction For Use: Read through the entire test procedure section prior to initiating the test.

Reagent Preparation Prior To Testing Procedure:

1. Prepare washing fluid as follows: Dissolve 1 PBS tablet per 100 ml distilled or deionized water, add 2 drops of 0.08 ml of Tween 20 for each 100 ml of solution. Mix thoroughly but gently. At least twenty minutes are needed for the tablets to dissolve. This solution may be used for 1 week if stored at room temperature or 2 months if refrigerated.
2. Allow all materials to come to room temperature before beginning the assay.
3. Record location of test samples on sides of wells or in carrier. Do not write on or touch the optically clear portion of the well bottom if the test is to be read spectrophotometrically at 550 nm.
4. Unused wells should be resealed in the plastic bag and stored with other unused components at 2–7°C. Keep dissicant pouch in bag with unused wells.

Testing Procedure: Remove appropriate number of strips from plastic bag and fasten them into the carrier plate. Reseal unused strips in plastic bag immediately. Begin wash procedure.

1. Washing Procedure.

a. Flood wells with the washing fluid and empty quickly.

b. Fill wells with washing fluid, wait 3 minutes and empty. Repeat this procedure twice.

c. Remove the last traces of fluid by tapping inverted carrier plate onto absorbent paper, being careful not to dislodge the strips from the carrier plate.

2. Serum or plasma addition.

a. Add 5 drops (or 0.200 ml) of diluent to each well.

b. Add 1 drop (0.04 ml) of negative reference to the upper well and add 1 drop (0.04 ml) of positive reference to the bottom well. If several tests are run simultaneously, only one set of references is needed.

c. Add 10 ul (0.010 ml) of test serum sample to the remaining well or wells. To avoid contamination of samples, use a clean pipette tip or capillary tube for each sample.

d. Incubate for 30 minutes at room temperature.

3. Enzyme-labeled conjugate addition.

a. Discard the fluid from the wells and wash the plate by repeating Step 1 (a through c).

b. Add 4 drops of diluent to each well.

c. Add 1 drop of conjugate to each well.

d. Incubate for 30 minutes at room temperature.

4. Substrate Addition.

a. Discard the fluid from the wells and wash the plate by repeating Step 1 (a through c).

b. Add 5 drops of substate solution to each well.

c. Incubate for 30 minutes at room temperature.

d. Add one drop of sodium hydroxide solution to each well to stop the reaction.

e. Shake slightly to insure proper mixing.

f. Score results.

CAUTION: SODIUM HYDROXIDE (1N) IS A STRONG ALKALI. AVOID CONTACT WITH SKIN OR EYES.

Continued on next page

Pitman-Moore—Cont.

Scoring Of Test Results: For a valid test, the fluid in the negative control reference well must be colorless or slightly pink, while the positive control reference well must be distinctly red-pink colored. When the test sample is the same as or distinctly more intensely colored than that of the positive reference control, the test well is positive. Otherwise, the test is scored negative.

Interpretation Of The Test Results: This kit is designed to detect antibody to T. gondii in cat serum.

A. If the test sample color intensity is less than the low positive reference control, the results indicate there is an absence of prior exposure to Toxoplasma gondii organisms or that antibody is not present in detectable quantities. Should clinical signs indicate otherwise, the cat should be tested again within a seven day interval.

B. If the test sample's color intensity is equivalent to or greater than that of the positive reference control, the results indicate there has been prior exposure to Toxoplasma gondii.

Precautions: 1. Refrigerate the kit at 2–7°C. Do Not Freeze Any Kit Components.

2. The product contains components preserved with sodium azide. Sodium azide may react with lead and copper plumbing to form explosive metal azides. In disposal, flush with a large volume of water to prevent azide build-up.
3. Sodium Hydroxide (1N) is a strong alkali. Avoid contact with skin and eyes.
4. Do not intermix reagents from different kits or serials.
5. Include controls each time the test is performed. Hyperlipemic or contaminated sera or plasma may give erroneous results.
6. Follow instructions exactly. The ELISA is a sensitive technique; care should be taken in dispensing reagents and timing incubation periods. Improper washing or contamination of test wells may produce nonspecific color development.
7. Temperatures above or below normal room temperature (20–25°C) may give erroneous results. All components should be at room temperature prior to use.
8. For Veterinary Use Only.

Contents Of The Kit: Six strips of eight T. gondii Antigen Coated Wells.
One vial Diluent—17.0 ml.
One vial T. gondii Negative Control Serum—1.5 ml
One vial T. gondii Positive Control Serum—1.5 ml
One vial Conjugate—2.5 ml
One vial Phosphate Buffered Saline Tablets—(PBS)—(6)
One vial Polyoxyethylene Sorbitan Monolaurate (Tween 20)—1.0 ml
One vial Sodium Hydroxide Solution—3.0 ml
Two vials Substrate Solution—12.0 ml
Fifty capillary tubes

Materials Needed But Not Supplied
1. Distilled water.
2. Wash bottle.
3. ELISA reader with 550 nm. filter needed for spectrophotometric reading if desired.
4. Well carrier plate.

References: 1. Burridge, M.J. 1980. Toxoplasmosis. Comp. Contin. Ed. 2(3):233–239.
2. Milatovic, D and I. Braveny. 1980. Enzyme-linked immunosorbent assay for the serodiagnosis of Toxoplasmosis. J. Clin. Pathol. 33.841–844.
3. Voller, A., D.E. Bidwell. (1975) Brit. J. Exp. Pathol. 56:338.
4. Walls, K.W., S.L. Bullock, and D.K. English. 1977. Use of the enzyme-linked immunosorbent assay (ELISA) and its microadaptation for the serodiagnosis of Toxoplasmosis. J. Clin. Microbiol. 5(3):273–277.

TechAmerica Group, Inc.

15TH & OAK
P.O. BOX 338
ELWOOD, KS 66024

DIASYSTEMS®–CANINE PARVO
Canine Parvovirus Test Kit
For use in dogs only

Indications: For IN VITRO use in the detection of Canine Parvovirus in feces by the Enzyme-linked Immunosorbent Assay (ELISA) Technique.

Summary and Explanation: Canine parvovirus is a member of the parvoviridae family, and is immunologically and biochemically similar to the feline panleukopenia virus and mink enteritis virus. Since 1978 canine parvovirus outbreaks have occurred simultaneously throughout widely separated areas of North America. In 1979 it was identified in outbreaks in Mexico, Central America, Asia, and South Africa. The disease is characterized in the acute stage by severe vomiting and diarrhea, leukopenia, rapid dehydration, myocarditis and hepatitis. The disease is often fatal. More than 10 viral particles can be shed per gram of feces in acute infections. Thus the feces have proven to be the main source for the transfer of infection to susceptible animals and can be used for the diagnosis of infection.

Diagnosis of parvovirus is presently based on clinical symptoms. Hemagglutination or hemagglutination inhibition tests can be run to confirm the presence of parvovirus in the feces of the dog. However, in many cases veterinarians may need to rapidly screen fecal samples of dogs that have parvo-like symptoms and to confirm the presence of the virus so that they may decide on a prompt and effective course of treatment.

Test Principles: DiaSystems®-Canine Parvovirus Test Kit is a two-site immunoassay utilizing two monoclonal antibodies specific to two different antigenic sites of canine parvovirus. The plastic wells precoated with one monoclonal antibody specific to canine parvovirus are incubated with the suspected sample (fetal extract) and a second monoclonal antibody is conjugated chemically to an enzyme horseradish peroxidase. Parvovirus particles are bound to wells and enzyme-linked antibody simultaneously. After washing away the unbound materials, a chromogenic enzyme substrate is added. Any change in color of the substrate to blue-green indicates the presence of canine parvovirus in the sample. There is no color change if parvovirus is not present in the sample. Visual comparison of color between the sample and the positive and negative references will accurately confirm the presence of parvovirus in dogs.

The canine parvovirus ELISA diagnostic test is highly specific, very sensitive and easy to perform. Results can be obtained in one hour and fifteen minutes. It is recommended that a positive and negative control be run each time. The use of monoclonal antibodies and ELISA technology provide a rapid and sensitive immunoassay to accurately diagnose the presence of parvovirus in fecal specimens.

Precautions:
1. Store the diagnostic kit at 2–8°C. Do not allow reagents to stand at room temperature for extended periods of time.
2. Include positive and negative references each time test is performed.
3. Use separate pipette for each fecal sample.
4. Be sure to fill the wells with Buffer Reagent and that no air is trapped in wells. Improper washing may produce nonspecific color development.
5. Handle all samples as if capable of transmitting parvovirus. Burn all unused biological components.
6. Do not use reagents from other kits.
7. Do not use expired reagents.
8. For veterinary use only.

Storage and Stability: Store the diagnostic kit at 2–8°C. Do not store below 2°C as a precaution against freezing. Reagents should be stable until expiration date, provided they have been stored properly.

Specimen Collection and Preparation For Testing: Use only canine fecal extract for test specimens. A swab of the suspected stool sample is resuspended in about 1 ml Buffer Reagent. Let sample settle for ten (10) minutes, the resultant supernatant is the fecal extract. Specimens may be stored at 2–8°C for one day. If longer storage is desired, store at −20°C. Visible indications of bacterial growth may interfere with performance and accuracy of the test.

Quality Control: Include positive and negative references each time test is performed.

In the event that the positive reference included in the kit does not react, the contents of the kit should not be used and the technical service department of TechAmerica Diagnostics should be contracted for information.

Results:
1. For the test to be valid, the references will appear as follows:
   a. Negative reference—no change to very little color change from initial substrate color.
   b. Positive control—substrate has turned blue-green.
2. A visual color change substantially higher than the negative reference indicates the presence of parvovirus in specimen.
3. Any test sample that is questionable should be repeated with fresh stool sample.

How Supplied: Kit of 12-46 tests.

DIASYSTEMS®-FeLV
Feline Leukemia Virus Test Kit

Indication: For the detection of FeLV group-specific antigens in cat serum by the Enzyme-linked Immunosorbent Assay (ELISA) Technique.

Summary and Explanation: The feline leukemia (FeLV) enzyme-linked immunosorbent assay (ELISA) diagnostic test kit detects the presence of FeLV group-specific (gs) antigens in the serum, plasma or blood of infected cats.

The feline leukemia viruses are infectiously transmitted feline oncornaviruses. FeLV is transmitted horizontally from most infected cats via saliva, urine, and milk.

FeLV causes five primary diseases in cats and is often fatal. These five (5) diseases include malignancies such as feline lymphosarcoma, myleogenous leukemia and degenerative diseases which include thymic atrophy, panleukopenia-like disease and nonregenerative anemia. Because it is immunosuppressive, FeLV predisposes infected cats to a variety of secondary diseases.

It is important that FeLV infected cats be identified and separated from non-infected cats. The group-specific antigen, p27, is found in high levels in the sera, plasma, or blood of infected cats and its presence is diagnostically significant for FeLV infection. The FeLV ELISA diagnostic kit utilizes two monoclonal antibodies that specifically recognize p27. The monoclonal antibodies provide sensitivity and easy use for the accurate diagnosis and identification of FeLV infected cats.

Test Principles: The plastic wells are precoated with a monoclonal antibody that specifically binds to the FeLV group-specific antigen, p27. The cat serum sample is incubated simultaneously with a second monoclonal antibody that is linked to an enzyme, horseradish peroxidase. Virus and free group-specific antigen are bound to the well and the enzyme-linked antibody at the same time. After binding, free antibody and unbound serum are washed away and a chromogenic enzyme substrate is added. A change in the color of the substrate to blue-green indicates FeLV is present.

The FeLV ELISA diagnostic test is highly specific, sensitive and easy to perform. Results can be obtained in twenty minutes. The diagnostic kit contains a high titer and a low titer positive reference as well as negative reference. Visual comparison of the color of samples and references will accurately determine the presence of FeLV in the sample.

Routine screening of FeLV should be included into a comprehensive health program. Testing of cats prior to vaccination for FeLV is highly recommended. This testing program is essential to establish FeLV free catteries.

Precautions:
1. Store the diagnostic kit at refrigerated temperature 2–8°C (35–46°F). **Use the kit cold directly from the refrigerator. Do not allow reagents to stand at room temperature continuously for more than thirty minutes.**
2. Use separate straw pipette for each sample.
3. Visible indications of bacterial growth in any of the reagents may interfere with the performance and accuracy of the test.
4. Be sure to fill the wells with distilled water and that no air is trapped in wells. Improper washing may produce nonspecific color development.
5. The use of tap water does not adversely affect the FeLV test results. However, the local variation in water supplies makes it difficult to recommend the use of tap water and to follow accepted scientific laboratory practices. TechAmerica feels the importance of accurate diagnosis compared with the low cost and ease of availability of distilled water makes it good laboratory practice to use distilled water with all diagnostic tests.
6. Handle all samples as if capable of transmitting FeLV. Burn all unused biological components.
7. Do not use reagents from other kits.
8. Do not use expired reagents.
9. For veterinary use only.

Storage and Stability: Store the diagnostic kit at refrigerated temperature 2-8°C (35-46°F). Do not store below 2°C (35°F) as a precaution against freezing. Reagents should be stable until expiration date, provided they have been stored properly.

Specimen Collection and Preparation For Testing: Use only feline serum, plasma or whole blood for test specimens. Specimens may be stored at refrigerated temperature 2–8°C (35–46°F) up to five days. If longer storage is desired, store frozen −20°C (−4°F). The presence of turbidity or visible indications of bacterial growth may interfere with the performance and accuracy of the test.

Quality Control: Include positive and negative references each time test is performed.

Results:
1. For test to be valid, the references must appear as follows:
   a. Negative reference—no color change from initial substrate color.
   b. Low positive reference—substrate has turned moderately blue-green.
   c. High positive reference—substrate has turned dark blue-green.
2. A color change in the test sample of equal or greater intensity than the low positive reference indicates the cat has a current FeLV infection. A color change less than the low positive inference but greater than the negative reference indicates a low level of FeLV present. If no chemical symptoms exist, the cat could be a possible carrier. Positive cats should be kept isolated and retested until they are no longer positive.
3. Cats that have been exposed for extended periods of time to a FeLV infected cat should be routinely screened for FeLV infection.
4. Any test sample that is questionable should be repeated with a fresh serum sample.

How Supplied: Kit 16 to 46 tests.

DIASYSTEMS®-OVUCARE™ COWSIDE
Bovine Milk Progesterone Kit

Introduction: DiaSystems-Ovucare is a simple and fast test which provides a reliable aid to the breeding status of lactating dairy and beef cows.

The test is used to measure the level of progesterone in a drop of cow's milk. The amount of progesterone is almost zero at estrus (heat) and then increases and remains at a high level during the remainder of the estrous cycle. At 17 to 20 days after the last heat the progesterone level falls suddenly indicating the onset of the next heat. This drop does not occur if the animal is pregnant. Although the test is not intended for pregnancy detection, continued high levels of progesterone at day 24 (with no drop at days 19, 20, 21) suggests pregnancy. This should be confirmed by rectal palpation at the appropriate time.

The test detects the amount of progesterone in the milk by means of a color change.

—pink for Estrus (low progesterone)

—virtually colorless for possible Pregnancy (high progesterone)

Two Controls (Estrus and Pregnancy) are provided. These are used with the test to enable comparisons to be made with the samples. When using the kit as a heat detection screen only, it is acceptable to omit the pregnancy control.

Sample Collection: Milk samples for testing should be taken from whole milk and must contain one potassium dichromate tablet per 20 ml. sample as preservative, if they are to be stored longer than 12 hours.

Results: If the sample is the same color or darker than the Estrus Control, then Estrus is indicated.

If the sample is the same color or lighter than the Pregnancy Control, then pregnancy is indicated or the cow is mid-way in a normal cycle.

If results are doubtful, take another sample the next day and retest.

Precautions: 1. Store the kit at 35–45°F (2–8°C). NEVER FREEZE.

2. The Controls contain a stabilizing agent which inparts a yellow color. This does not interfere with the performance of the test.

Continued on next page

TechAmerica—Cont.

3. For *in-vitro* diagnostic use only.
For professional advice contact your veterinarian.
[See table below].

DIASYSTEMS® OVUCARE™ 96 WELL PLASMA

Description: TechAmerica Group, Inc.'s progesterone EIA kit DiaSystems®-OVUCARE™ provides a simple, reliable and precise enzyme immunoassay for the measurement of progesterone in bovine plasma or serum.
Four standards 0.5, 1, 5 and 10 ng/ml are provided in the kit.
Each kit contains sufficient reagents for a total of 92 tests (samples and standards).
OVUCARE™ is used for estrus detetion and pregnancy testing in cows.
For *in-vitro* veterinary diagnostic use only.
Principle of the Assay: The DiaSystems®-OVUCARE™ test is based on the competitive binding of unlabelled progesterone present in the standard or plasma sample, and a fixed quantity of progesterone labelled with the enzyme alkaline phosphatase (AP), to binding sites on a limited amount of specific progesterone antibody.
The wells are pre-coated with antibody, providing a solid phase for the convenient separation of the bound progesterone from the free progesterone in the sample. After incubation, all components other than those bound to the plate wells are washed away.
The amount of AP-labelled progesterone remaining on the wells is inversely proportional to the concentration of the unlabelled progesterone present in the sample. The bound labelled progesterone is then measured by reacting the AP with its substrate during a second incubation.
The color produced is measured spectrophotometrically and the concentration of progesterone in the milk is determined from a standard curve. Alternatively, the color can be interpreted visually.
Recommended Equipment and Additional Materials:

DiaSysytems® Ovucare™
Instructions for Use
Place the kit in a refrigerator when not in use.
Bring kit to room temperature (65–80°F) before use.
To set up work station, separate the box into its three parts; the bottom section is your workstation.

Step 1 Gently shake both Controls and milk samples just before use. **ALWAYS USE A FRESH STRAW PIPETTE FOR EACH CONTROL AND EACH MILK SAMPLE.**

Step 2 Uncover the number of wells required by peeling back foil cover and discarding plastic inserts. Use ONE well for the Estrus Control, another for the Pregnancy Control and one for each sample. Empty well contents into sink. Tap dry on absorbent paper towels.

Step 3 To run the test add ONE drop Estrus Control, ONE drop Pregnancy Control and ONE drop of each milk sample to separate wells. To insure accurate measurement be sure to hold the pipettes vertically.

Step 4 TRACER
Add FOUR drops of TRACER into each exposed well. Cover the wells with the clear plastic kit lid to protect from contamination. Leave for 30 minutes at room temperature.

Step 5 After 30 minutes, empty wells and wash with cold running tap water for a few seconds and empty. Repeat twice and tap dry.

Step 6 DEVELOPER
Add FOUR drops of DEVELOPER to each well. Cover again. Leave at room temperature. After 15 minutes compare color intensities.

1. Shake

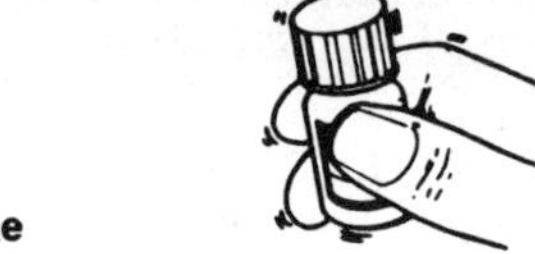

2. Strip

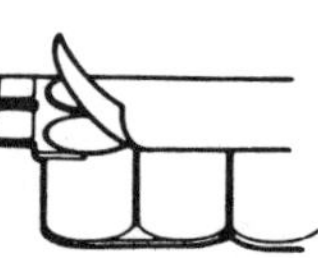

3. Empty

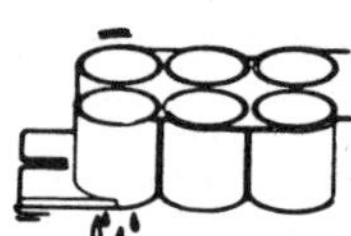

4. Add (left) 1 drop Estrus (right) 1 drop Pregnancy Control

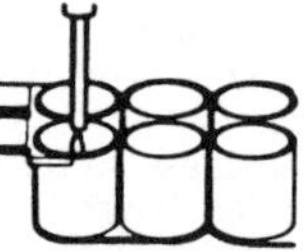

5. Add 1 drop of milk sample

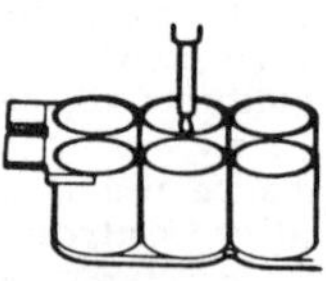

6. Add 4 drops of Tracer

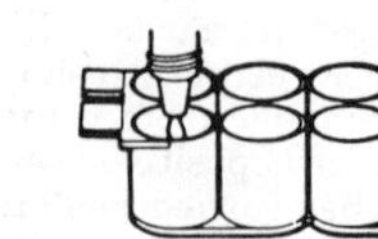

7. Wait 30 minutes.

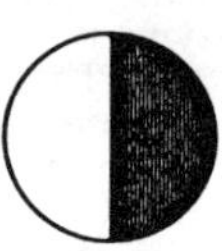

8. Empty wells and wash 3 times

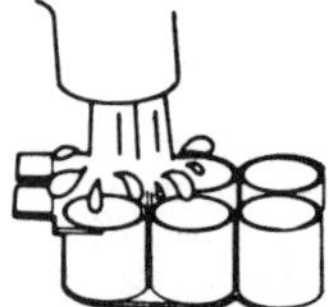

9. Add 4 drops Developer

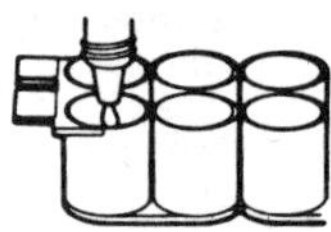

10. Wait 15 minutes

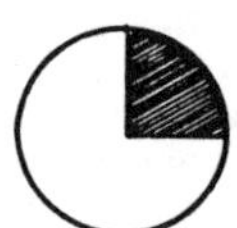

11. Assess results

200μL dispenser
100μL dispenser
10μL pipette
Elisa Plate/Strip reader

Reagents:

Conjugate
Progesterone-alkaline phosphatase conjugate 25mL.

Substrate Tablets
p-nitrophenyl phosphate 3 × 40mg.

Substrate Buffer
Diethanolamine 1M.
Magnesium chloride 0.5mM.
pH 9.8 25mL.

Stopping Solution
Di-potassium hydrogen orthophosphate 0.5M
EDTA 5mM pH 10.0 20mL.

Standards
Progesterone in plasma 0.5, 1, 5 and 10 ng/mL.
1mL.

Microtitre Wells
96 wells pre-coated with sheep anti-progesterone serum. The wells contain a stabilising buffer.

Substrate Reagent Preparation: Add 3 Substrate tablets to the Substrate Buffer and shake it to dissolve. If all the Substrate Reagent is not required immediately, it can be dispensed into clean plastic containers and stored at 2 to 8 degrees Centigrade for one week or 3 months at minus 20 degrees Centigrade. Repeated freezing and thawing does not effect its performance.

Sample Collection:

Plasma
Blood samples should be collected into heparinised collection vessels, eg Vacutainer (Becton Dickinson) or Monovette (Sarstedt).
For highest accuracy of progesterone measurement, centrifuge the blood sample within 30 minutes of collection and draw off the plasma into a clean container. The plasma sample will remain usable for up to 48 hours if kept cool, or will remain usable indefinitely if kept frozen.
If centrifugation is not immediately available, keep the blood sample as cool as possible and centrifuge within 24 hours of collection. Progesterone levels can fall by as much as 30% under these conditions.

Serum
Blood samples should be collected into a non-heparinised tube. Once the clot has formed the tube should be centrifuged and the serum drawn off into a clean container.
If a centrifuge is not available, the serum should be drawn off carefully after the clot has settled. In general progesterone values from serum samples will be lower than those for plasma samples by 20% to 30%. If kept cool serum samples will remain usable for up to 24 hours.

Mode of Use:
For the detection of estrus or pregnancy the OVUCARE™ assay may be used in one of two ways:
1. For a visual interpretation of the color development use Standard 1.
2. For a quantitative measurement of the sample progesterone level the color development of the samples and the four standards provided should be determined using an ELISA plate reader or spectrophotometer.

Test Procedure:
1. Shake samples and standards just before use.
2. Expose the number of wells required according to the following plan ie. one well for each standard and another well for each sample.

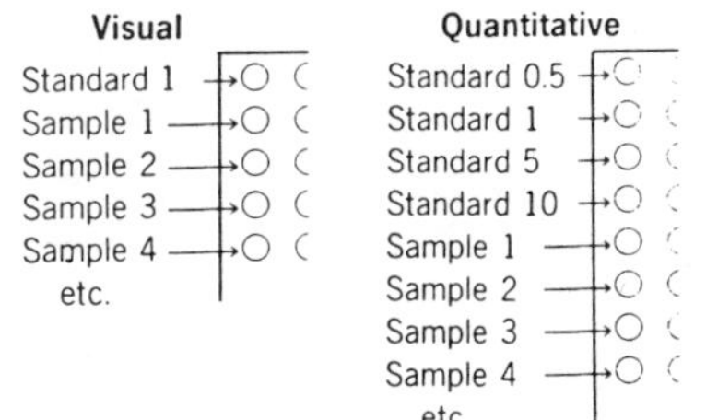

3. Empty the contents of the exposed wells and tap dry on absorbent paper.
4. Add 10μL of each standard to be used to the appropriate wells.
5. Add 10μL of each sample to be tested to the appropriate wells.
6. Add 200μL to conjugate to every exposed well.
7. Cover all wells and leave for about 30 minutes at room temperature (14 to 37 degrees C). Leave for about 40 minutes at 4 to 13 degrees C.
8. After covering wells prepare the substrate reagent as described in Section 4.
9. Empty wells and wash by filling with cold water and emptying. Repeat twice. Tap dry on absorbent paper.
10. Add 200μL of substrate reagent to all empty wells.
11. Cover wells and leave for about 30 minutes at room temperature (14 to 37 degrees C). At 4 to 13 degrees C leave for about 40 minutes.
12. Obtain results—see next section.

Results:

For Visual Method
Examine wells by eye after about 30 minutes.
Compare color intensity of each sample with Standard 1. A color the *same as*, or *more* intense than Standard 1 indicates a lower progesterone level, ie. estrus or non-pregnant. A color *paler* than Standard 1 indicates a higher progesterone level, ie. pregnant.

For Quantitative Method
When using a manual plate reader or spectrophotometer add 100μL of Stopping Solution to all wells.
Set spetrophotometer or plate reader to read absorbance at 405nm. Zero instrument on air. Draw a standard curve by plotting standard absorbance on the graph paper provided.
The progesterone concentration of the samples can then be read from the curve.

Performance:
A typical standard curve for the test is shown below:

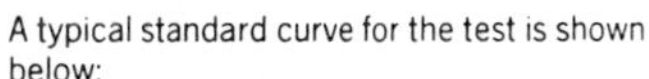

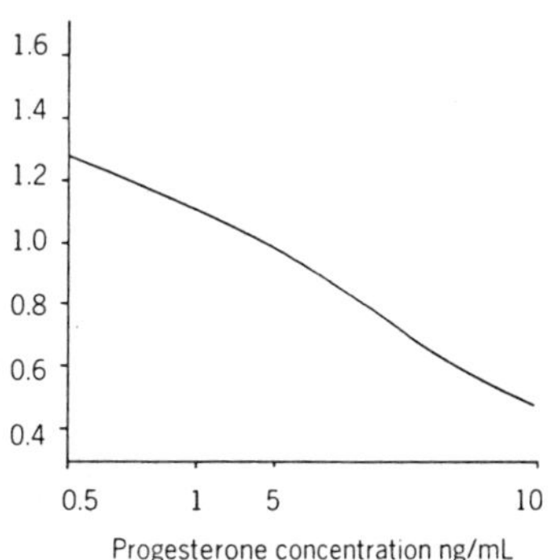

Progesterone concentration ng/mL
The absorbance value for Standard 0.5 (0.5ng/mL) should lie between 0.8 and 1.6 absorbance units and will vary according to incubation temperature.
A minimum difference of 0.3 absorbance units should be observed between the absorbance values for Standard 0.5 (0.5ng/mL) and Standard 10 (10ng/mL).
NOTE: Variations in color intensity and therefore the standard curve can be expected owing to daily changes in temperature. This does not affect the validity of the results.

Precision:
The intra-assay precision at 1 ng/mL progesterone in milk samples has been measured at 10% coefficient of variation.
The inter-assay precision at 1 ng/mL progesterone in milk samples has been measured at 25% coefficient of variation.

Precautions:
1. The stabilizing solution and the Conjugate contain sodium azide (0.05%) as a preservative. When emptying the well contents into a sink, thoroughly flush away with an excess volume of tap water.
2. Store the kit at 2 to 8 degrees Centigrade. DO NOT FREEZE.

Appendix 1

Antibiotic Therapy in Pet Birds and Reptiles

Thomas J. Burke, DVM, MS

Introduction

When compared to food producing and companion animals there is relatively little pharmacokinetic data available for birds and even less for reptiles. The author has attempted to incorporate existing studies into the following tables, but some of the material has been derived from the experience of many practitioners.

One fairly widely accepted "rule of thumb" for birds is to double the canine dose for large birds, and triple it for small ones. One adopting this policy must observe the patient closely for signs of toxicity (as well as idiosyncratic reactions), and also be prepared for some treatment failures. In general, the dosage interval for reptiles should be one-third that of dogs for most antibiotics with a low toxicity potential.

Culture and sensitivity results are of great importance, and appropriate samples should be obtained prior to the onset of any therapy.

Principles of Therapy

For birds, one must weight the benefits of accurate dosage for parenterally administered drugs versus the hazards of frequent handling. Antibiotics administered via the drinking water or food may be grossly misdosed because ill birds may drink or eat less (most common), or more than when they are in good health. Ailing birds are commonly placed in incubators to increase the environmental temperature. This alone can lead to increased water consumption.

Concomitant therapy with Gram-positive bacteria such as *Lactobacillus* is wise, especially when an antibiotic is administered per os. Such replacement therapy should be continued for 2 to 3 days beyond the cessation of antibiotic therapy.

For reptiles, the problem of medication administration is compounded by the fact that few regularly drink quantities of water on a daily basis; and many, especially snakes, do not eat daily. As poikilotherms their metabolism of any drug is dependent upon environmental temperature. For dose ranges listed in Table 2, the lower doses are suggested for patients kept at lower temperatures. Injection of a dose of drug into live prey usually results in erratic absorption by the patient, and the prey specimen may metabolize a fair amount of the compound if not immediately consumed. Thus this practice results in the least accurate dosage form of all.

All patients should be well hydrated prior to the administration of any drug as dehydration may potentiate toxicity via decreased renal and/or hepatic metabolism and excretion.

TABLE 1
Antibiotic Therapy for Pet Birds

Antibiotic	Species	Route	Dose	Frequency	Comments
Amikacin	All	IM	40 mg/kg	SID or BID	Potentially nephrotoxic. Stop therapy if polyuria occurs.
Ampicillin & Amoxicillin	All	IM	100 mg/kg	q 4 h	Dosage based on pharmacokinetic studies in Amazon parrots. Rapid renal clearance. Higher doses used in serious infections (e.g., septicemia). Many Gram negative pathogens resistant.
		IM	50 mg/kg	TID or QID	
		PO	150-200 mg/kg	BID or TID	
		PO-in drinking water	250 mg/8 oz	Change daily	
Carbenicillin	Psittacines	IM	100-200 mg/kg	SID or BID	Synergistic with aminoglycosides, but **must not** be mixed in the same syringe.
	Most	PO	200 mg/kg	BID	Crush tablets and mix with small amount of food or suspend in fruit juice with electric blender.
Cefotaxmine	Most	IM	50-100 mg/kg	TID	Apparent low toxicity, but may see nephrotoxicity when used in conjunction with an aminoglycoside.
Cephalexin	Most	PO	50 mg/kg	QID	
Cephalothin	Most	IM	100 mg/kg	QID	Not absorbed orally; must administer parenterally.

Antibiotic	Species	Route	Dose	Frequency	Comments
Chloramphenicol (propylene glycol base)	Most	IM	80 mg/kg	BID or TID	Pigeons excrete very rapidly; probably not satisfactory for use in this species.
	Macaws & Conures	IM	50 mg/kg	QID	Based on pharmacokinetic studies; note wide species vcariation in dose frequency necessary to maintain average therapeutic blood levels.
	Budgie	IM	50 mg/kg	BID	
	Bald eagle & Peackco	IM	50 mg/kg	SID	
Chloramphenicol (sodium succinate)	Most	IM	80 mg/kg	BID or TID	Can also be given IV - very rapid excretion.
Chloramphenicol	Most	PO	50-200 mg/kg	BID ro QID	Oral absorption very erratic; often poor. Solutions very bitter and should be given by gavage into crop; suspensions fairly well accepted. Can mix powder (capsule) form in soft foods or suspend in fruit juice.
Chlortetracycline	Large Psittacines	PO	5000 ppm in food 1% in pelleted feeds	Only source of food for 30-45 days	For treatment of psittacosis. Mash or nectar must be prepared daily—cool before adding drug. Oral absorption can be potentiated with citric acid.
	Lories & Lorikeets	PO	500 mg/L of nectar	Only source of food for 30-45 days	
	Small Psittacines	PO	0.5% impregnated in millet seed	Only source of food for 30-45 days	
	Most	PO	250 mg/pint of drinking water	Change TID	For general therapy. Candidial superinfection common following prolonged therapy.
Doxycycline	Psittacines	PO	18-26 mg/kg	BID	Less effect on GI flora than chloratetracycline
		IV	22-44 mg/kg	SID or BID	*Do not* give IM.
Erythromycin (soluble powder)	Most	PO	125 mg/L of water	Change daily	Useful in chronic respiratory diseases especially if mycoplasma infection is present.
Erythromycin (suspension)	Most	PO	44-88 mg/kg	BID	
Gentamicin	Most large	IM	5 mg/kg	BID or TID	Nephrotoxic dose has not been established in birds; the doses given here result in blood levels below the mammalian nephrotoxic dose when administered BID in most species tested. Serious infections may require initial dose frequency of TID or QID and polyuria may be seen; reduce dose frequency to BID as soon as possible or change to another antibiotic if sensitivity results indicate. SID dosing may be effective in mild infections.
	Most Small	IM	10 mg/kg	BID or TID	
	Raptors	IM	2.5 mg/kg	TID	
	Most	PO	40 mg/kg or 50-100 mg/L of water	SID or BID	For GI infections; not absorbed by intact mucosa; this may be altered by some enteric disease states.
	Most	Nebulizer	50 mg/10 ml of saline	TID	Clinically effective in treating respiratory infections. Nebulize for 15 minutes per treatment. Nebulizer should produce 3 μ droplets.
Kanamycin	Most	IM	10 mg/kg	BID	May be less nephrotoxic than gentamicin.
		PO	10-50 mg/L of water	Change daily	For GI infection and reducing potential pathogens in gut prior to stress (e.g., shipping); use for 2-3 days.
Lincomycin	Psittacines	PO	100-150 mg/kg	BID	Limited use because of spectrum of activity; may be useful in respiratory disease caused by mycoplasma and GI infections with campylobacter.
	Raptors	PO	100 mg/kg	SID	
Neomycin	Most	PO	10 mg/kg	BID or TID	For GI infections; not absorbed by intact mucosa. Do not use form containing methscopolamine bromide.
Nitrofurazone	Most	PO	⅛-¼ tsp of 9.3% soluble powder/L of water	Change daily for 7-10 days	Useful for GI infections and coccidia (except mynahs and toucans). Good for flock treatment of salmonellosis. Overdose may produce neurotoxicity and/or sudden death.
Oxytetracycline	Most	IM	200 mg/kg	SID	Long acting tetracycline. Not approved for treatment of psittacosis carriers.

Antibiotic	Species	Route	Dose	Frequency	Comments
Spectinomycin	Most	PO	5-8 mg/oz. of water	Change daily 5-10 days	Good for GI infections.
Streptomycin	Large birds	IM	10-15 mg/kg	BID	Appears to be quite toxic to small caged birds. Extensive use in poultry. Good for treatment of quail enteritis.
Sulfachloropyrida-zine	Most	PO	¼ tsp. of soluble powder/L of water	Change daily 7-10 days	Good for *E. coli* enteric infections.
Sulfadimethoxine	Most	PO	20 mg/kg	BID	May cause vomiting.
Sulfamethazine	Most	PO	30 mg/oz solution	Full strength instead of drinking water for 5-7 days	Good for coccidiosis. Watch for dehydration if patient refuses to drink.
Tetracycline HCl	Most	PO	¼ tsp. of soluble powder (10 g/6.4 oz)/L water	Change TID	Not approved for treatment of psittacosis carriers. Do not use in cachexic patients or those with enteritis.
			OR 250 mg/kg of oral suspension	BID	
Ticarcillin	Most	IM	200 mg/kg	BID to QID	Syngergistic with aminoglycosides. Low toxicity. Use QID in severe infections, especially *Pseudomonas*. May be given IV.
Tobramycin	Most	IM	See under gentamicin	See under gentamicin	Useful for gentamicin-resistant infection.
Trimethoprim and Sulfamethoxazole	Most	PO	100 mg/kg	BID	Use oral suspension rather than crushing tablets. Useful for coccidiosis in mynahs and toucans.
Tylosin	Most	PO	1 tsp. of soluble powder (250 g/8.81 oz.)/5 oz. of water	Change daily	Good in treatment of respiratory infections, especially sinusitis. Treat for up to 21 days if there is clinical response within 5 days. Dose may be tripled if necessary.
		IM	10-25 mg/kg	BID or TID	Good initial therapy for acute respiratory infections.

TABLE 2
Antibiotic Therapy for Reptiles

Antibiotic	Species	Route	Dose	Frequency	Comments
Ampicillin	All	IM or SQ	3-6 mg/kg	SID	Useful in mild mixed infections.
Carbenicillin	All	IM	75 mg/kg	SID	Useful in conjunction with aminoglycosides in severe systemic Gram-negative infections.
	All	IV	75 mg/kg	BID	
Cephaloridine	All	IM or SQ	10 mg/kg	BID	May be nephrotoxic.
Cephalothin	All	IM	20-40 mg/kg	BID	
Chloramphenicol	All	IM or SQ	40 mg/kg	SID	
		PO	100 mg/kg	SID	May not attain effective blood levels, especially in snakes.
Chlortetracycline	All	PO	200 mg/kg	SID	
Dihydrostrepto-mycin	All	IM	5 mg/kg	BID	Potentially toxic to kidneys, CNS and myocardium. Useful orally for GI infections including stomatitis.
Gentamicin	Snakes, Lizards	IM or SQ	2.5 mg/kg	q 72 h	Potential nephrotoxicity with long-term use and/or dehydration.
	Chelonians	IM	10 mg/kg	q 48 h	Do not use longer than 14 days.
Kanamycin	All	IM	10 mg/kg	SID	Potentially nephrotoxic.
Lincomycin	All	IM	6 mg/kg	SID	Limited use since most reptilian pathogens are Gram-negative.
Potassium Penicillin G	All	IM	10,000-80,000 u/kg	SID	Potassium ion may cause toxicity. Also limited use because of spectrum of activity.
Oxytetracycline	All	IM	6-10 mg/kg	SID	
Sulfadimethoxine	All	IM	30-90 mg/kg first day; 15-45 mg/kg subsequently	SID	
Sulfaquinoxaline	All	PO	0.04% in water	Change daily for 5 days	Useful as adjunctive therapy in treatment of superficial infections and stomatitis.
Tylosin	All	IM	25 mg/kg	SID	

Appendix 2

Drug Interactions

The interaction of two or more drugs may occur as a result of (1) mixing solutions outside the animal body, or (2) it may occur within the body after their administration by the same or different routes. The interactions that may occur include: (1) Direct chemical and physical interactions; (2) Altered absorption following administration by the oral or parenteral routes; (3) Effects on protein binding; (4) Changed rate of drug metabolism; (5) Increase or decrease in body clearance by renal, hepatic, and other routes; (6) Interaction of drugs at the receptor; (7) Interactions related to changes in acid base balance of body fluids. Any of the preceding can result in a variety of unexpected responses ranging from no response to a reduced response, to an increased response, of which may be associated with toxic reactions that may vary from minimal to severe (deaths).

Several solutions used for parenteral fluid therapy have been shown to inactivate certain antibiotics (for example, glucose solutions and potassium penicillin G). Combinations of antimicrobial agents may have altered activity against infectious agents that are termed (a) indifferent (b) additive (c) synergistic (d) and antagonistic.

For additional information, the reader is referred to *Hazards of Medication,* E. W. Martin, J. B. Lippincott Co., 1971 and *Clinical Pharmacology,* 2nd edition, H. F. Morelli and K. L. Melmon, "Drug Interactions," pp 982–1007, Macmillan, Inc., 1978.

Primary Drug(s)	Interacts Witn	Interaction
Acidifying Agents (Ex. ammonium chloride, methenamine, etc.)	Weak acid drugs	↑ response
	Weak base drugs	↓ response
Alkalizing Agents (sodium bicarbonate, Na_2HPO_4, etc.)	Weak acid drugs	↓ response
	Weak base drugs	↑ response
Aminoglycoside Antibiotics (Streptomycin, Dihydrostreptomycin, Neomycin, Kanamycin, Paromomycin, Gentamicin, Amikacin, Sisomicin, etc.)	Other aminoglycoside antobiotics &	↑ Neuromuscular blockade
		↑ Nephrotoxicity
	Ethacrynic Acid	↑ Ototoxicity
	Methoxyflurane	↑ Nephrotoxicity
	Tubocurarine	↑ Neuromuscular block
	General anesthetics	↑ Neuromuscular block
	Succinylcholine	↑ Neuromuscular block
	Polymixins	↑ Nephrotoxicity and neuromuscular blockade
Ammonium chloride	Sulfonamides	Crystalluria
Amphotericin B	0.9% NaCl	Precipitation of amphotericin
	Corticosteroids	↑ K+ depletion
	Digitalis	↑ Digitalis toxicity
	Tubocurarine	*Neuromuscular block
	Succinylcholine	↑ Neuromuscular block
Antacids (Aluminum hydroxide, Magnesium compounds, $NaHCO_3$, Calcium carbonate, etc.)	Nitrofurantoin	↓ Absorption of nitrofuratoin
	Oxacillin	↓ Absorption of oxacillin
	Penicillin	↓ Absorption of penicillin
	Sulfonamides	↓ Absorption of sulfonamides
	Tetracyclines	↓ Absorption of tetracyclines
	Iron	↓ Absorption of iron
Aspirin	Heparin	↑ Bleeding
Barbiturates	Acidifying agents	↑ Barbiturate potentiated
	CNS depressants	↑ Additive Effect
Calcium Salts	Digitalis glycosides	↑ Cardiac arrythmias
	Tetracyclines	↓ Absorption & Activity
	Aminoglycosides	↓ Neuromuscular blockade
Carbenicillin	Gentamicin	In vitro inactivation when mixed in same bottle or syringe

Carbonic Anhydrase Inhibitors (Acetazolamide)	Amphetamine	↑ Response to amphetamine
Cephalosporins	Gentamicin	↑ Nephrotoxicity
	Colistin	↑ Nephrotoxicity
	Lactated Ringers	↓ Cephalothin Na
Chloramphenicol	Iron	↓ Response to iron
	Cyanocobalamine	↓ Response to cyanocobalamine
	Dicumarol	↑ Clotting time
	Penicillins	Chloramphenicol may interfere with activity of penicillins
	Tolbutamide	Intense hypoglycemia
	Dipheylhydantoin	↓ Metabolism of diphenylhydantoin
	Barbiturate	Prolongs anesthesia (enzyme inhibition)
Clindamycin	Erythromycin	Possible Antagonism
Colistin	Cephalosporins	↑ Nephrotoxicity
	Anesthetics	Neuromuscular blockade
	Aminoglycosides	Neuromuscular blockade
Corticosteroids	Amphotericin B	↑ K+ depletion
Cyanocobalamine	Neomycin	↓ Absorption of cyanocobalamine
	Chloramphenicol	↓ Response to cyanocobalamine
Digitalis glycosides	Neomycin	↓ Absorption of digitalis
	Amphotericin B	↑ K+ depletions; digitalis toxicity
	Calcium products	↑ Cardiac arrythmias
	Furosemide	Digitalis toxicity
	Phenylbutazone	↑ Metabolism of digitalis
	Succinylcholine	Cardiac arrythmias
Diphenylhydantoin	Chloramphenicol	↓ Metabolism of diphenylhydantoin
	Phenothiazines	↓ Metabolism of diphenylhydantoin
	Halothane	Possible hepatotoxicity
Erythromycin	Clindamycin	Possible antagonism
	Lincomycin	Possible antagonism
	Penicillin	Possible antagonism
Estrogens	Phenobarbital	↑ Metabolism of estrogens
Furosemide	Digitalis glycosides	Digitalis toxicity
	Tubocurarine	↑ Effects of tubocurarine
Gentamicin	Carbenicillin	In vitro inactivation when mixed in same bottle or syringe
	Cephalosporins	↑ Nephrotoxicity
Griseofulvin	Phenobarbital	↓ Absorption of griseofulvin; barbiturate is potentiated
Halothane	Diphenylhydantoin	↑ Possible hepatotoxicity
Iron products	Chloramphenicol	↓ Response to iron
	Tetracycline	↓ Absorption of tetracycline
Kanamycin SO_4	Dextrose Soln pH 3.5-6.5	↓ Kanamycin
Kaolin-Pectin	Lincomycin	↓ Absorption of lincomycin and other drugs
	Tetracycline	↓ Absorption of tetracycline and other drugs
Lidocaine (i.v.)	Diphenylhydantoin	↑ Cardiac depression
Lincomycin	Erythromycin	Possible antagonism
Methenamine	Sulfonamides	↑ Crystalluria
Methicillin	Kanamycin, Tetracycline	Inactivate methicillin
	Normal sodium chloride injection or dextrose sol.	↓ Methicillin

Methoxyflurane	Tetracycline	↑ Nephrotoxicity
	Aminoglycosides	↑ Nephrotoxicity
Narcotics	Succinylcholine	↑ Neuromuscular block
	Tubocurarine	↑ Neuromuscular block
Neomycin	Digitalis glycosides	↓ Absorption of digitalis
	Peincillin-V	↓ Absorption of penicillin-V
	Cyanocobalamine	↓ Absorption of cyanocobalamine
	Alkalizers	↑ Activity
Nitrofurantoin	Antacids	↓ Absorption of nitrofuratoin
	Acidifiers	↑ Activity
Oxacillin	Antacids	↓ Absorption of oxacillin
Penicillins	Neomycin	↓ Absorption of penicillin
	Chloramphenicol	Chloramphenicol may interfere with activity of penicillin
	Dextrose solutions (pH 8.0 or greater)	Inactivate penicillin
	Erythromycin	Possible antagonism
	Tetracycline	Possible antagonism
	Antacids	↓ Absorption of penicillin
Phenobarbital	Estrogens	↑ Metabolism of estrogens
	Griseofulvin	↓ Absorption of griseofulvin
Phenothiazines	Diphenylhydantoin	↑ Metabolism of diphenylhydantoin
	Piperazine	↑ Phenothiazine toxicity
Phenylbutazone	Digitalis glycosides	↑ Metabolism of digitalis
Piperazine	Phenothiazines	↓ Phenothiazine toxicity
Polymyxin	Succinylcholine	↑ Neuromuscular block
	Tubocurarine	↑ Neuromuscular block
Procaine and related local anesthetics	Sulfonamides	Antagonism
Procainamide	Atropine	↑ Anticholinergic activity
Salicylates	Ammonium chloride	↑ Blood level of salicylates
	Ascorbic acid	↑ Blood level of salicylates
Sulfisoxazole	Thiopental	↑ Response to thiopental
Sulfonamides	Methanamine	↑ Crystalluria
	Antacids	↓ Absorption of sulfonamides
Succinylcholine	Narcotics	↑ Neuromuscular block
	Aminoglycosides	↑ Neuromuscular block
	Amphotericin B	↑ Neuromuscular block
	Polymyxin	↑ Neuromuscular block
	Digitalis glycosides	Cardiac arrythmias
Tetracyclines (Chlortetracycline, Oxytetracycline, Demethylchlortetracycline, Doxycline, Minocycline, etc.)	Antacids	↓ Absorption of tetracycline
	Penicillin	Possible antagonism
	Iron products	↓ Absorption of tetracycline
	Cations	↓ Absorption & Activity
	Methoxyflurane	↑ Nephrotoxicity
Thyroid hormone	Ketamine	Hypertension; tachycardia
Trimethoprim	Thiazides or furosemide	↑ Incidence of thrombocytopenia
Tubocurarine	Aminoglycosides	↑ Neuromuscular block
	Amphotericin B	↑ Neuromuscular block
	Furosemide	↑ Effects of tubocurarine
	Narcotics	↑ Neuromuscular block
	Polymyxin	↑ Neuromuscular block
Vitamin B Complex with Vitamin C	Chloramphenicol	↓ Antibiotic Activity
	Erythromycin	↓ Antibiotic Activity
	Nitrofurantoin	↓ Antib otic Activity
	Potassium Pen-G	↓ Antibiotic Activity

↑ = increased or enhanced

↓ = decreased or inhibited

Appendix 3

Toxicology

Emergency Treatment of Human Cases of Poisoning Caused by Veterinary Products.

GENERAL MANAGEMENT

Emetics. When someone has swallowed poison, giving an emetic is usually the quickest and most handy way of cleaning out the stomach. However, there are many patients who should *not* be given an emetic. Unconscious patients and those poisoned by petroleum distillates, strong acid or alkali should not be given emetics. Also, emetics may be ineffective in patients poisoned by antiemetics—for example, phenothiazine derivatives.

In treating a child, syrup of ipecac (15 to 20 ml followed by at least 20 ml of fluid) is preferable. However, ipecac should not be used if the child is in shock. Furthermore, if the child is given ipecac and does not vomit, gastric lavage is imperative.

Apomorphine, a good emetic for both adults and children, may be administered IM at a dose of 1 mg per 10 kg for adults and 1 or 2 mg for children. Nalorphine or levallorphan should be given later to counteract the emetic effect.

Do *not* administer hypertonic saline orally as a means of inducing emesis, especially in children, because severe hypernatremia may occur if the individual fails to vomit.

Gastric Lavage. Gastric lavage is useful if it is done within 3 or 4 hrs after the poison has been taken. It should *not* be done, however, on patients poisoned by a strong acid, alkali, or strychnine. Nor should it be done on patients poisoned by iron, if the iron has been taken more than 1 hr previously. (The danger is that since iron causes gastric necrosis, the lavage tube might perforate the stomach.)

Gastric lavage is also usually not performed on patients who have swallowed gasoline or other petroleum distillates, because of the risk of chemical pneumonitis.

These procedures should be followed in gastric lavage:

1. Aspirate as much of the stomach contents as possible before starting lavage.
2. Lavage the unconscious patient while he's lying on his side, his head lower than his body—for instance, over the edge of a table.
3. Use gastric tubes of ample caliber.
4. Use normal saline solution instead of tap water to lavage children—no more than 50 cc per lavage.
5. Repeat procedure until the return fluid is clear—usually about 10 times.

Certain antidotes can be administered through the gastric tube. Egg white and milk, for example, will help capture iron; sodium bicarbonate (1% solution) will convert iron to a less soluble form so that it will not be absorbed by the body. If the poison is unknown, administer activated charcoal—about 15 gm mixed with water to form a thin paste. If the poison is fat-soluble, do not administer milk or castor oil, since they will cause the poison to be more easily absorbed. Liquid paraffin or mineral oil, however, which are not absorbable, will help prevent further absorption of fat-soluble substances. Following lavage, replace lost fluids, lost blood or plasma, and correct any electrolyte imbalance.

A number of poisons are easily absorbed through the skin—for example, cholinesterase-inhibiting insecticides and halogenated hydrocarbons. To treat this type of poisoning, remove contaminated clothing and thoroughly wash the affected areas with soap and water. Do not use phenothiazine derivatives to treat emesis in these patients because phenothiazines may delay the recovery of enzyme activity.

If the patient has injected the poison into the arm or leg, tie off the extremity, apply ice locally, and inject a vasoconstrictor into the surrounding tissue.

Some inhalants may cause pulmonary edema. This condition calls for the administration of oxygen and a rapid-acting corticosteroid.

SPECIFIC ANTIDOTES

Atropine sulfate. For the treatment of cholinesterase-inhibiting insecticide poisoning—2 to 3 mg per injection repeated every few minutes as necessary. As much as 50 to 70 mg may be required.

Pralidoxime chloride. For the treatment of organic phosphate insecticide poisoning—500 mg IV as a 0.1* solution as the initial dose.

Levallorphan tartrate and nalorphine. For the treatment of poisoning due to morphine, codeine, other semisynthetic and synthetic narcotic analgesics as well as propoxyphene:

Levallorphan tartrate—1 mg IV followed by 1 or 2 doses of 0.5 mg at 10 to 15 minute intervals.

Nalorphine—5 to 10 mg IV repeated every few minutes as necessary.

Deferoxamine. For the treatment of iron poisoning. When a patient is in cardiovascular collapse, 1 gm IV at a rate not to exceed 15 mg per kg per hr. This may be followed with 0.5 gm every 4 hr for 2 doses. Depending on the response, subsequent doses of 0.5 gm may be given every 4 to 12 hr. Do not exceed 6 gm in 24 hr. As soon as the patient's condition improves, administer the drug IM. For less severely affected patients, administer the drug IM at the beginning, following the same schedule.

Sodium nitrite and sodium thiosulfate. For the treatment of cyanide poisoning—0.3 to 0.5 gm of sodium nitrite dissolved in 10 to 15 ml of water, given IV over a period of 3 or 4 minutes. Following this, 12.5 gm of sodium thiosulfate dissolved in 50 ml of water, given over a 10-minute period. If the drugs must be administered a second time, halve the dose.

Consult Appendix 9 for the telephone number of the poison control center nearest you. Additional management information is available from them.

(Reference: *Pocket Book of Medical Tables,* 19th edition, Smith, Kline and French Laboratories.)

Management & Treatment of Toxicological Emergencies in Animals

Without a complete accurate history, and physical and chemical evidence, it is often difficult to diagnose poisoning produced by many substances in animals. While there are relatively few true pathognomonic signs of toxicoses, the sequence of events and the nature and severity of clinical signs are very important aids to assist you in arriving at a diagnosis.

When treating cases of suspected poisoning, however, your objectives should include the following:

1. To maintain vital functions.
2. To identify the toxicant and eliminate the source of exposure.
3. To prevent or delay further absorption.
4. To administer specific antidotes, if available.
5. To promote the elimination of the absorbed toxicant.
6. To provide supportive therapy as required and good nursing care.

The tables which follow are presented as guides to help you differentiate between some of the more common types of poisoning encountered in both small and large animal practice. With the ever increasing and widespread use of plants for ornamental purposes in homes, the incidence of poisoning, especially in small animals, will probably increase, hence a selected guide to poisonous plants has also been included.

For specific treatment of individual poisons, the reader should consult a current text. Your local Poison Information/Control Center (Listed in Appendix 9) can tell you the chemical conmposition of most commercial products and also can provide antidotal information.

TABLE 1
A GUIDE TO COMMON TOXICANTS OF SMALL ANIMALS*

Toxicant	Source	Toxicity and Pathogenesis	Clinical Signs	Lesions	Diagnosis	Treatment
Heavy Metals						
Arsenic	Pesticides, herbicides, insecticides, paints, smelters, drugs, food additives.	Trivalent as most toxic (As_2O_3, arsenites). Toxicity varies greatly. Single toxic dose in dogs: As_2O_3-100-150 mg. Sodium arsenite 50-100 mg. General tissue poison. inactivates-SH groups, blocks cellular respiration, inhibits phosphonate groups.	**Acute**—1-2 days; extreme weakness, violent gastrointestinal upset, vomition purgation, black diarrhea. Fast weak pulse, normal temperature **Subacute**—2-7 days similar to acute but prolonged. Dehydration, thirst incoordination, coma.	Gastrointestinal inflammation, hemorrhages, ulcers and necrotic mucosa. Liver and kidney changes endocarditis, lung congestion, cardiac hemorrhages, skin dry and cracked (dermal exposure)	Clinical syndrome, chemical analysis of urine and feces. Tissue analysis; liver, spleen, kidney; 10-15 ppm.	British Anti-Lewisite (BAL) fluids. Sodium thiosulfate
Lead	Paints, puppy toys containing lead, putty, bathroom linoleum, golf balls, solder, and lotions containing lead acetate.	10-25 mg/Kg lead lethal to dogs. Repeated doses accumulate and are slowly eliminated in feces. Affects several areas of brain.	Signs: vomition, abdominal pain, hemoglobinuria, paralysis of masseter muscles of dogs. Anorexia, wasting, depression, weakened heart and respiration.	Mild gastroenteritis. May be no lesions. Petechial hemorrhages on heart. **Chronic:** liver and kidney degeneration.	Clinical signs and history Blood lead 35ug% or greater, Analysis of liver and kidney. 5ppm or greater. Basophilic stippling, Nucleated red blood cells without anemia Abdominal radiographs	Ca EDTA, Penicillamine Supportive care.
Insecticides						
Chlorinated hydrocarbon	Accidental or improper exposure of animals to sprays and/or dips	Toxicity depends on the compound. Action is hyperirritability of central nervous system. Cats are particularly susceptible.	Intermittent tonic clonic convulsive seizures, with intermittent periods of depression.	May be none. Agonal hemorrhages on visceral organs. Lung congestion, blanched intestines.	History and signs are important. Chemistry of little value. Differentiate from 1080, strychnine, garbage, lead, distemper.	No specific antidote. Control seizures with sedatives (eg phenobarbital)
Organo-phosphorus Carbamate	Accidental or improper exposure of animals to spray dips & collars Over medication with drugs containing organophosphate and/or carbamate compounds	Toxicity depends on compound. Cholinesterase inhibition causing over-stimulation of parasympathetic nervous system.	Salivation, vomition, diarrhea, miosis, severe dyspnea, stiffness followed by paralysis of skeletal muscles. Bradycardia.	May be none. Lung congestion and edema. Hemorrhages on heart, lungs and intestines.	History and clinical signs Chemical analysis of tissue of little value. Blood and tissue cholinesterase depression.	Atropine sulfate to effect (no salivation). 2-PAM (pralidoxime) for organophosphate compounds. Maintain respiration. Supportive care.
Rodenticides						
Alpha-napthyl thiourea (ANTU)	Rodenticide (gray powder) in bread and sausage containing baits, usually 1-3%.	Increases permeability of pulmonary capillaries. Pulmonary edema and/or pulmonary effusions.	**Initial:** Vomition, salivation, Gastric distress. **Later:** Dyspnea coughing, tachycardia, muted heart sounds, hypothermia.	Plural effusions and edema, hydrothorax Inflammation of trachea, bronchi and G.I. mucosa. Hyperemic kidneys and liver.	History and signs, hydrothorax and pulmonary changes.	No specific antidote available, Silicone aerosol, N-amylmercaptan, Emetics immediately after ingestion.
Sodium fluoro acetate (1080)	Rodenticide. Tasteless, water soluble; usually mixed with black dye. Dogs and cats may eat baits or rodents poisoned with 1080 and be poisoned.	0.05-0.5 mg/Kg MLD; Fluorocitrate formed which blocks cellular respiration. Inhibits aconitase	Dogs show signs in 15 min. to 2 hrs. Wild running and barking, defecation, intermittent tetanic convulsions terminating in death. Cats show both convulsions and cardiac depression. Animals not hyperirritable. Cyanosis.	May be no lesions. Gastrointestinal tract and bladder empty.	History of exposure signs displayed. Chemical analysis of liver, muscle. Differentiate from strychnine, chlorinated hydrocarbon, insecticides, and garbage.	No specific antidote available, Gastric lavage with milk or limewater, Glycerol monoacetate (Monacetin), Barbiturates to control seizures. Supportive care.

Strychnine	Rodenticide. Most common in dogs. Sometimes in cats. Used as toxic agent in many malicious poisonings.	0.75 mg/Kg lethal. Causes increased irritability to stimulation. Death from exhaustion or anoxia.	Nervous and restless 10 min. to 2 hrs. after exposure, followed by tetanic convulsions; all muscles tense. A period of relaxation is followed by seizures; cyanosis, dilated pupils, rapid weak pulse. Seizures may be initiated by touch or noise. Animals generally do not vomit.	No specific lesions. Stomach usually contains bait or rodent.	History and signs. Demonstration of strychnine in urine and stomach contents. Injection of urine into frog or mouse produces convulsions. Differentiate from 1080, garbage, and chlorinated hydrocarbon pesticides.	Control seizures, keep quiet. Potassium permanganate (to oxidize it) or tannic acid (to precipitate it) should be given orally.
Thallium	Dog or cat has access to rodent bait. Most often seen in dogs. Sale and manufacture of thallium containing rodenticides now illegal but cases still occur.	10-20 mg/Kg MLD; general cellular poison, distributed throughout body. Slowly excreted in urine. Cause vascular and hair follicle damages (Hair changes in dogs and sheep).	**Peracute**—1-4 days severe gastroenteritis dyspnea elevated temperature. Motor paralysis and dehydration. **Acute**—3-7 days mild gastroenteritis and motor paralysis; conjunctivitis injected sclera and oral mucous membranes. Bronchitis and pneumonia. Some alopecia in dogs. **Chronic**—7-10 days or longer. Mild signs of acute toxicity. Alopecia and scaling of skin of dogs.	**Peracute**—Hemorrhagic gastroenteritis and inflamed respiratory mucosa. **Acute**—milder gastroenteritis, congestion and hemorrhage in abdominal organs; fatty degeneration and necrosis of liver Petechia, perivascular cuffing and demyelination in brain. **Chronic**—skin hyperkeratosis parakeratosis, hypermia, and hyaline changes in dogs.	History of exposure. Urine test for thallium. Characteristic signs, lesions, course of disease. Liver and kidney analysis for thallium above 8 mg.%.	Dithizone, Prussian blue, and KCI orally. Supportive care and treatment. Antibiotics for secondary infections.
Vacor DLP-787	A new rodenticide, as a 10% tracking powder or as a 2% bait.	LD_{50} in dogs for technical material is 500-1000 mg/Kg. Values for cats vary from 62-500 mg/Kg. B vitamin antagonist	**Initial:** Nausea, abdominal pain, emesis, depression, constricted pupils **Intermediate** Anorexia general body pain, dilated pupils, dehydration, ataxia, deep breathing, reduced respiratory rate, Visual problems, lethargy tremors, slow pupilary, light response, hind limb weakness, decreased reflexes.	Dose Dependent **Gross:** Depressed foci in liver. Liver, adrenal and kidney weights increased. **Microscopic** Degenerative pigmentary and proliferative lessons of liver. Hyperplasia of gallbladder. Aspermatogenesis, casts, necrosis, degenerative and regenerative changes in kidneys. Pigment in spleen and bone marrow.	History of exposure & clinical signs. Identification of toxicant.	Induce emesis (early), nicotinanide. Supportive care.
Warfarin Pindone Dicoumarin	Rodenticide, moldy clover hay, "contaminated" rodents may poison cats and dogs.	Anticoagulants Single dose: 20-50mg/Kg **warfarin. 75-100mg/Kg** pindone. Multiple doses: 1-5mg/Kg for 5-15 days. Act by prolonging blood clotting time and and damaging blood vessels.	Signs generally reflect hemorrhage. Weakness, lameness, paralysis, anorexia, pale mucous membranes, vomition, blood in mouth and feces, progressive posterior paralysis, convulsions, death 1-10 days.	Multiple hemorrhage throughout muscles, viscera, body cavities, subdurally.	Lesions, prolonged clotting time. Chemical analysis of liver or other tissues.	Blood transfusion. Vitamin K_1 Keep warm and quiet.
Zinc phosphide	Rodenticide. 2.5 or 5% in sausage, bread, or cereal grains.	20-40mg/Kg. lethal dose. Toxicity due to phosphine gas(PH_3) liberated.	Loss of appetite, abdominal pain, lethargy, coma, death in 48-72 hours. Signs of asphyxia may be evident in terminal stages.	Venous congestion, capillary breakdown, lung edema, gastroenteritis. Carcass may have acetylene odor.	Detection of phosphine gas or zinc phosphide in stomach. Acetylene odor.	So specific antidote, Supportive care.
Miscellaneous						
Ethylene glycol	Permanent antifreeze and coolant, industrial solvent, rust remover, hydraulic fluid	6 ml/Kg and greater causes acute effects, CNS depression, Metabolized to oxalic acid which complexes with calcium.	**Initial** (1-6 hrs) Vomition, ataxia, rapid breathing, tachycardia. **Delayed** (24 hrs.) Vomition, anorexia, dehydration, weakness ataxia, convulsions, coma, death.	Gastritis, enteritis G.I. hemorrhage, pulmonary edema and hyperemia. Kidneys pale and streaked with grey or yellow. Birefringent oxalate crystals in convoluted renal tubules.	History of exposure, Clinical signs, Chemical and histochemical tests	Control convulsions, prevent or control pulmonary edema. Maintain fluid and electrolyte balance. Ethyl alcohol and $NaHCO_3$ IV. Supportive.

Garbage	Access to spoiled food or rodents, especially ham, chicken, milk, some vegetables.	*Staphylococcus* toxins-Lethal toxin, enterotoxin and others. *Clostridium botulinum* toxins—Motor paralysis, depression.	*Staph.* lethal toxin rapid; 5-15 min. to 24 hrs. Unsteadiness, difficult respiration, violent convulsions. *Staph.* enterotoxins-nausea, prostration abdominal pain, diarrhea within 4 hrs. Death rare. *Cl. botulinum*-motor paralysis, coma and death.	*Staph.*—lethal—usually stomach contains garbage. Hyperemia and hemorrhage of gastrointestinal tract. *Cl. botulinum*—may be no lesions. Some hemorrhages.	History, Clinical signs Isolate toxins and test in laboratory animals.	Supportive care and treatment. Alleviate shock, Maintain electrolyte balance, Antibiotics, Antitoxins for *Cl. Botulinum.*
Metaldehyde	Molluscicide, used in slug and snail killers in both liquid and solid form.	Dogs—approximately 400 mg/Kg cause toxicoses, geographical	Incoordination, rapid breathing, tachycardia, unconsciousness, cyanosis. Possibly hyperesthesia and muscle tremors leading to opisthotonus and convulsions. Nystagmus in cat.	Hyperemia of liver and kidneys. Degeneration of liver and ganglion cells in brain. Lungs hyperemic with interstitial hemorrhages. Odor of acetaldehyde Ecchymotic and petechial hemorrhages of G.I. mucosa	History and clinical signs, Chemical analysis for acetaldehyde	No specific antidote available; Supportive and symptomatic treatment for control of neurological signs and maintenance of electrolyte balance.
Neuro-toxins of toads or lizards.	Spray of toxin from the parotid salivary gland of *Bufo marinus (Bufo giganticus)* into mouth of dog or cat, or ingestion by animal. The blue Tail lizard and the Gila monster.	Apparently toxin absorbed through mucous membranes of oral cavity.	Onset within minutes, and may cause death within 15-20 minutes. Salivation, prostration convulsions.	None	History and clinical signs.	Irrigation of mouth. Injection of atropine sulfate and calcium gluconate. Tracheal intubation.

*Adapted from: Case, A. L. Norden News 47:23-25, 1972 after Ramsey, F. K., Buck, W. B. and Duncan, J. R., Anim. Hosp. 3:221-237, 1967.

References: 1. Buck, W. B., Osweiler, G. D. and Van Gelder, G. A., *Clinical & Diagnostic Veterinary Toxicology, 2nd Ed.*, Kendall/Hunt Publishing Co., Debuque, Iowa, 1976.
2. Clarke, E. G. C. and Clarke, M. L., *Veterinary Toxicology,* Lea & Febiger, Philadelphia, Pa., 1975.

TABLE 2
A GUIDE TO COMMON TOXICANTS OF LARGE ANIMALS, POULTRY & RELATED SPECIES

TOXICANT	SOURCE	TOXICITY AND PATHOGENESIS	CLINICAL SIGNS	LESIONS	DIAGNOSIS	TREATMENT
Heavy Metals						
Arsenic	Pesticides, herbicides, environmental industrial pollution, medications	Trivalent compounds, pesticides, etc. have greatest toxicity for all species. Phenylarsonic compounds, feed additives for swine and poultry, are considerably less toxic.	**Trivalents Acute:** G.I.-vomition, abdominal pain, watery and/or bloody diarrhea dehydration, circulatory collapse, depression death. **Phenylarsonic Acute:** Incoordination, some paralysis (still able to eat & drink) possible blindness. **Chronic: Swine:** slow partial paralysis of extremities, blindness, poor weight gain. **Poultry:** anorexia, ruffled feathers, depression, ataxia.	**Trivalents:** Reddening of gastric mucosa (abomasum), ulcerations, necrosis, liver and kidney lesions and necrosis, dry cracked skin. **Phenylarsonic Swine:** Skin erythema, muscle atrophy, Urinary bladder distension, peripheral nerve, optic tract and optic nerve lesions.	**Inorganic:** Rapid onset and sudden death, GI signs with CNS involvement, History and chemical evidence. **Phenylarsonic Swine & Poultry** - ataxia, paralysis of extremities without CNS involvement, high morbidity, low mortality.	Demulcents, lavage or emesis, B.A.L. (for trivalent form), fluids, Vitamin B complex, antibiotics, supportive therapy. **Phenylarsonic:** Swine and Poultry—withdraw medication, provide adequate drinking water, diuretics.

Lead	Paint and discarded containers, old crankcase oil and grease, batteries, trash piles, lead shot (wild fowl).	Cumulative, all species susceptable but swine relatively resistant. Combines with SH groups, interferes with hemoglobin synthesis and other enzymes, passes placental barrier.	**Cattle:** blindness, muscle twitching (head and neck region) teeth grinding and excessive salivation, hyperirritability, depression anorexia, bellowing **Horse:** Acute—colic and diarrhea. **Chronic:** laryngeal paralysis (roaring). **Sheep:** Primarily depression. **Wild fowl:** Weakness, anorexia and weight loss, paralysis (legs and wings).	**Cattle:** mild gastritis liver pale with centrilobular degeneration, kidneys hyperemic, some degeneration and presence of acid fast intramuscular inclusion bodies, brain edema and histological changes	History, rapid onset of clinical signs in acute cases, physical and chemical evidence - blood and urine analysis. Postmortem tissue analysis.	CaEDTA, supportive therapy, fluids (with care) magnesium sulfate as purge and to limit further absorption.
Mercury	Contaminated food sources Seed grains treated with mercury containing fungicides, Environmental pollution of air, soil and water. Antimildew and antifouling paints	Inhaled vapors, methyl and ethyl mercury most toxic. Sheep and cattle quite sensitive	**Cattle:** Stomatitis, salivation, gastroenteritis, skin changes, weakness, anorexia, nephritis, hemorrhage, expistaxis hematuria, bloody feces **Swine:** Severity and onset dose dependent with specific agent. Vomiting GI, CNS (stimulation and/or depression) weakness, cardiovascular, coma.	**Cattle:** Subacute interstitial nephritis and catarrhal bronchitis, enlargement and edema of lymph nodes. Enlarged splenic follicles. Subendocardial and subepicardial hemorrhage, G.I. hemorrhage, Focal necrosis in liver, CNS vascular lesions. **Swine:** GI inflammation and necrosis, liver and kidney changes. Degenerative vascular lesions in CNS.	History and clinical signs. Physical and chemical evidence of mercury.	BAL, Sodium thiosulfate, Prognosis poor, Meat from poisoned animals unfit for human consumption.
Insecticides and Pesticides						
Chlorinated Hydrocarbon	Accidental or improper exposure of animals to sprays and/or dips.	CNS stimulation, taken up by fat and other tissues—residue problems, excreted in milk	CNS stimulation, convulsive seizures with intermittent depression, muscle faciculation, abnormal posturing, continuous chewing, increased salivation.	Minimal and nonspecific Small generalized hemorrhages, pulmonary hemorrhage and congestion, brain congestion and edema.	History and clinical signs, convulsive seizures coupled with neuromuscular involvement, Chemical analysis. Detection in milk.	No specific antidote, sedation with long acting barbiturates, Phenobarbital may be useful to hasten metabolism, activated charcoal.
Organophosphate Carbamate	Accidental or improper exposure of animals to sprays and/or dips. Overmedication with drugs containing organophosphate and/or carbamate compounds.	Inhibition of acetylcholinesterase and pseudocholinesterase	Excessive parasympathetic stimulation. Muscle tremors followed by neuromuscular and respiratory paralysis. CNS stimulation but convulsive seizures are rare in food producing animals.	Minimal and nonspecific Pulmonary edema, excessive fluids in respiratory and GI tracts.	History and clinical signs, depression of tissue and blood cholinesterase. Analysis for toxicant of little value in tissues and fluids.	Atropine sulfate to effect (no salivation). 2-PAM (pralidoxime) only for organophosphate compounds. Maintain respiration, Supportive care.
Feed Related Toxicants						
Urea and Non protein nitrogen	Urea, biuret, ammonium salts, fertilizers, Errors in mixing and contamination of feeds.	Excessive production and absorption of NH_3 by ruminants. Alteration of acid-base balance.	Frothy salivation, teeth grinding, abdominal pain, polyurea, muscle tremors, weakness, incoordination, forced respiration, bloat, bellowing, tetanic spasms, terminal hyperthermia and anuria. Vomiting in sheep.	Nonspecific, pulmonary hemorrhage, and congestion, bloating, rapid decomposition, rumen pH less than 7.5	History and clinical signs, analysis of food. Rumen NH_3 greater than 80 mg/100 ml, elevated blood and/or serum ammonia nitrogen.	**Cattle:** Cold water orally, vinegar to lower rumen pH. Supportive and symptomatic treatment.

Water Deprivation/ Na^+ Toxicity	Limited water intake, Na^+ in feed coupled with diminished water intake.	Most common in swine and poultry, less frequent in cattle and sheep. Production of cerebral edema.	**Swine:** Increased thirst, pruritis, constipation, intermittent convulsive seizures, circling, blindness and deafness. **Poultry:** Similar, excessive thirst, respiratory difficulty, fluid discharge from beak, wet feces, limb paralysis. **Cattle:** Vomiting, diarrhea, abdominal pain, polyurea, blindness, convulsive seizures, partial paralysis, knuckling of fetlock joints, drag rear feet.	Gastric inflammation and ulceration, pinpoint ulcers (blood filled). **Swine:** eosinophilic meningoencephalitis, perivascular cuffing	History and clinical signs. Characteristic histopathology of CNS in swine. Elevated Na^+ in serum and CSF.	No specific antidote, limit and regulate water intake, diuretics and anticonvulsants but prognosis grave and mortality high.
Miscellaneous						
Fluoride	Environmental pollution, water, feed.	Accumulates in calcified tissues and alters the normal processes of mineralization	**Acute:** Excitement, seizures, incontinence, weight loss, stiffness, diminished milk production, salivation, nausea, vomiting, depression, cardiac failure, death. **Chronic:** Lesions in those teeth exposed during their developmental phases. Hyperostosis, intermittent lameness, altered hair coat.	Mottling and erosion of tooth enamel, roughened periosteal surface of bones, periosteal hyperostosis, uneven mineralization, areas of inmature bone, reabsorption on endosteal surface, excessive osteoid tissue. Gastroenteritis in acute cases.	History and clinical signs, skeletal fluorosis and intermittent lameness, Chemical analysis, radiographic examination.	No specific antidote, reduce intake levels, Aluminum sulfate, aluminum chloride, Calcium aluminate, calcium carbonate and defluorinated phosphate used as antagonists. Symptomatic and supportive treatment as indicated.

References: 1. Buck, W. B. Osweiler, G. D., and Van Gelder, G. A. **Clinical and Diagnostic Veterinary Toxicology, Second Edition,** Kendall/Hunt Publishing Co., Dubuque, Iowa, 1976.
2. Clarke, E. G. C. and Clarke, M. L., **Veterinary Toxicology,** Lea and Febiger, Philadelphia, Pa. 1975.

TABLE 3
A GUIDE TO SOME COMMON POISONOUS PLANTS*

Common name	Scientific name	Toxic part	Poisonous principles	Clinical signs and treatment
A. House Plants				
Hyacinth	*Hyacinthus orientalis*	Bulb		Intense digestive upset, gastric lavage or emesis, Symptomatic indication
Narcissus or daffodil	*Narcissus* sps.	Bulb	Toxic alkaloids (?)	Severe gastroentertis, vomition, purging, trembling, convulsions. Gastric lavage or emesis, Symptomatic medication
Oleander	*Nerium oleander*	All parts, green or dry. Food skewered on oleander branches becomes poisonous. Single leaf is lethal.	Cardiac glycosides: oleandroside, oleandrin, nerioside	Nausea, depression, lowered and irregular pulse, mydriasis, bloody diarrhea, paralysis, death. Atropine, emetics, gastric lavage, potassium, procaimamide, quinidine sulfate or disodium salt of EDTA. Symptomatic medication. This plant also can cause dermatitis.
Poinsettia	*Euphorbia pulcherrima*	Juice of leaves, stems, flowers, or fruit; green or dry	Various poisons in the acrid milky sap	Intense emesis, abdominal pains, diarrhea, delirium. Sap causes dermatitis externally and temporary blindness if rubbed in eyes. Use demulcents, intestinal astringents, gastric sedatives, nervous and circulatory stimulants
Dieffenbachia, Dumbcane	*Dieffenbachia seguine* or *picta*	All parts including sap	Calcium oxalate crystals, toxic protein	Ingestion produces rapid irritation, burning of surface of mouth, tongue, and lips, copious salivation and edematous swelling. May cause death if swelling blocks air passages of throat. Juice may cause intense irritation on skin. Treatment symptomatic, pain relieved with meperidine HCl; aluminum-magnesium hydroxide useful as demulcent and neutralizing agent.
Rosary pea, Crabs-eye, precatory bean, jequirity bean	*Abrus precatorius*	Seeds	The phytotoxin abrin and the tetanic glycoside abric acid	Extremely toxic. Less than one seed, if chewed, is fatal. Symptoms resemble tetanus or typhoid. Nausea, vomiting, severe diarrhea, weakness, cold perspiration, colic, weak and accelerated iulse and trembling of hands. Drowsiness coma, circulatory collapse, hemolytic anemia, oligouria, fatal uremia. Gastric lavage or emesis, maintain circulation, blood transfusion for anemia, sodium bicarbonate to alkalinize urine.
Castor bean	*Ricinus communis*	All parts, mainly seeds	The phytotoxin ricin	Produces burning sensation in mouth and throat. Two to four seeds may produce serious poisoning, about eight seeds considered lethal. Symptoms include nausea, vomiting, violent purging, bloody diarrhea, and dullness of vision. Gastric lavage, administration of saline cathartics, maintenance of fluid and electrolyte equilibrium and symptomatic measures recommended.
Mistletoe	*Phoradendron flavescens* (American) and *Viscum album* (European)	Berries	beta-phenylethylamine and tyramine	Several deaths among children have been attributed to eating the berries. Tea brewed from berries has caused fatality. Death occurred about 10 hours after symptoms of acute gastroenteritis and cardiovascular collapse. Gastric lavage or emesis supportive, potassium, procainamide, quinidine sulfate or disodium salt of EDTA.

Common name	Scientific name	Toxic part	Poisonous principles	Clinical signs and treatment
B. Flower Garden Plants				
Larkspur	*Delphinium ajacis* and *other species*	Young plant, seeds	Poisonous alkaloids, mainly delphinine which is a polycyclic diterpene	Ingestion produces digestive upset and symptoms of nervous excitement or depression. May be fatal. Perform gastric lavage and treat for alkaloid poisoning and CNS excitation using short-acting barbiturates because of subsequent depression.
Monkshood	*Aconitum napellus* and other species	Roots, seeds, leaves	Poisonous alkaloids, mainly aconitine which is a polycyclic diterpene	Poisonous alkaloids affect vagus nerve from brain causing a slowing of the heart. Other effects include tingling and numbing sensation of the lips and tongue, irregular pulse, dimness of vision and respiratory failure. Keep victim warm, horizontal. Treat for alkaloid poisoning. Use gastric lavage and circulatory stimulants if necessary.
Autumn crocus or Meadow saffron	*Colchicum autumnale*	All parts, bulbs, seeds	Colchicine alkaloid	Cerebral depression; circulatory collapse, diarrhea, nausea. Treat symptomatically with zinc sulfate, apomorphine, Lugol's solution, activated charcoal, saline cathartics, paregoric.
Star of Bethlehem	*Ornithogalum umbellatum*	All parts, bulbs, leaves fresh or dry	Alkaloids	Nausea, nervous symptoms and general disturbance of the intestinal tract. Treatment symptomatic.
Lily-of-the valley	*Convallaria majalis*	Leaves, flowers, roots	The cardiac glycosides convallarin and convallamarin	Heart stimulations similar to digitalis glycosides. Dizziness and vomiting may occur in 1-2 hours, if large quantities are eaten. Gastric lavage or emesis, symptomatic & supportive, potassium, procainamide, quinidine sulfate or disodium salt of EDTA.
Iris or Blue Flag	*Iris versicolor*	Leaves and root stalks	Acrid resinous substance irisin	Produces severe but not usually serious digestive upset. Acts on G.I. tract, liver, and pancreas, causing purging and congestion of the intestinal tract. Can also cause dermatitis. Antidote materials include Lugol's solution, antihistaminics, barbiturates, and paregoric.
Foxglove	*Digitalis purpurea*	Leaves and seeds	Several glycosides, mainly digitoxin, digitalin, and digitonin	One of the sources of the drug digitalis, used to stimulate the heart. In large amounts the active principles cause dangerously irregular heartbeat and pulse, usually digestive upset, and mental confusion. May be fatal. Have patient vomit and perform gastric lavage. Sedative drugs of value to control restlessness. Potassium chloride orally or I.V. if renal function not impaired; atropine sulfate (2 mg. in adults) blocks influence of exaggerated vagal tone. Use procaineamide HCl or quinidine sulfate for ventricular tachycardia. Disodium salt of EDTA.
Bleeding heart (Dutchman's breeches)	*Dicentra cucullaria*	Foliage, roots	Several isoquinoline-type alkaloids including apomorphine, protoberberine, and protopine	Symptoms include trembling, staggering, convulsions, and labored breathing. Has proved fatal to livestock. Treatment includes use of heart and respiratory stimulants and nerve sedatives.
Christmas rose	*Helleborus niger*	Rootstocks and leaves	Two very toxic glycosides, helleborin and helleborein	Causes purgation, gastric distress, and nervous effects. Juice produces skin inflammation and numbing sensations in mouth. Wash skin with soap. Have person vomit and treat for digitalis or aconite poisoning, depending upon symptoms.

Common name	Scientific name	Toxic part	Poisonous principles	Clinical signs and treatment
Four o'clock	*Mirabilis jalapa*	Root, seed	The alkaloid trigonelline	Irritant to skin and mucosa. The alkaloid has a laxative effect. Treatment symptomatic.
Sweet pea	*Larthyrus*	Seeds or peas	beta (gamma-L-glutamyl)-amino-propionitrile	Large quantities in diet produce paralytic syndrome in man called lathyrism. Remove from diet. Casein given to animals has protected against paralytic effect.
Morning glory, (Heavenly Blue, Pearly Gates, Flying Saucers, varieties)	*Ipomoea violacea*	Seeds	The clavine alkaloids ergine, isoergine, elymoclavine, and others; all chemically related to LSD	From 50-200 powdered seeds ingested are capable of inducing psychotomimetic effects for several hours. Used by thrill-seekers because of LSD-like effects. Produces nausea, uterine stimulation, euphoria. Has produced death by suicide presumably due to mental effects. Chlorpromazine effective as antidote.
C. Vegetable Garden Plants				
Rhubarb	*Rheum rhaponticum*	Leaf *blade* (not the petiole which is edible)	Oxalic acid	Severe intermittent abdominal pains, vomiting, and weakness. Muscular cramps and tetany due to hypocalcemia may occur. Large amounts of raw or cooked leaves can cause convulsions, coma, followed rapidly by death. Give milk or lime water and induce emesis or gastric lavage with lime water. Give calcium gluconate 10% I.V. injection if tetany or hypocalcemia appears. Supportive therapy.
Potato	*Solanum*	Green "sunburned" spots and sprouts of potato tubers, green stems and leaves	Solanine alkaloids	Cold, clammy skin; nausea; mental confusion; respiratory and cardiac depression. Has caused deaths. Symptomatic treatment.
D. Ornamental Plants				
Daphne	*Daphne mezereum* and other species	Berries, bark, leaves	Bitter glycoside daphnin and an acid resinous mixture	Plant intensely acrid, producing vesication when rubbed on skin. Ingestion produces burning sensation in mouth. Vomition, diarrhea with blood and mucus, stupor, weakness, convulsions, and death. Perform gastric lavage, treat for irritation of G.I. tract. For severe pain use meperidine (demerol) Symptomatic treatment.
	Wisteria *floribunda* (Japanese) and *W. Sinensis* (Chinese)	Seeds or pods	Poisonous resin and a glucoside wisterin	Mild to severe gastroenteritis with repeated vomiting, abdominal pain, and diarrhea. Induce emesis. Once toxic symptoms begun, treatment symptomatic, using antiemetics (chlorpromazine) and fluid replacement therapy. Flowers may be eaten.
Golden chain	*Laburnum anagyroides*	Bean-like capsules in which the seeds are suspended	The quinolizidine alkaloid cytisine	Excitement, incoordination, vomition, convulsions, coma, and death through asphyxiation. Considered very poisonous shrub or tree in Britain. Action similar to nicotine. Treat for alkaloid poisoning and symptomatically using lavage, glucose-saline solution 5%.
Mountain laurel	*Kalmia latifolia* and *augustifolia*	All parts	Andromedotoxin, a resinoid substance	Curare-like effect on skeletal muscle. Stimulation of striated muscle followed by depression. Inhibitory action on heart tissues. Slowing of pulse, hypotension, salivation lacrimation Rhinorrhea, vomiting Convulsions. Depresses the CNS, causing respiratory failure and ultimately death. Use diuretics, laxatives, nerve stimulants, and gastric sedatives or demulcents. Gastric lavage or emesis, activated charcoal, atropine

Common name	Scientific name	Toxic part	Poisonous principles	Clinical signs and treatment
Rhododendron, Western azalea	*Rhododendron albiflorum, macrophyllum, maximum, accidentale = (azalea occidentale)*	All parts	Ditto	Ditto
Yellow jessamine	*Gelsemium sempervirens*	Whole plant, berries	Toxic alkaloids gelsemine and gelseminine	These alkaloids chiefly depress and paralyze motor nerve endings. Depression of the motor neurons of the brain and spinal cord results in respiratory arrest. Profuse sweating, muscular weakness, convulsions. Gastric lavage or emesis atropine, support respiration. Morphine said to be a specific antidote.
Lantana	*Lantana camara*	Berries	A polycyclic triterpenoid named lantadene A	Extreme muscular weakness, gastrointestinal irritation, and circulatory collapse. Syndrome resembles, atropine poisoning in acute cases. Protosensitization. Gastric lavage or emesis Symptomatic and supportive treatment.
Yew	*Taxus baccata* and *T. canadensis*	All parts, especially *seed* if chewed; fleshy red pulp of fruit least harmful	Taxine, an alkaloid	Nausea, vomiting, diarrhea, abdominal pain, circulatory failure, and difficulty in breathing. The alkaloid depresses the heart function. Can cause dermatitis. Induce vomiting, perform gastric lavage. and treat for circulatory failure and alkaloid poisoning. Never feed clippings to horses!
E. Trees and Shrubs				
Wild and cultivated cherries	*Prunus serotina* (Wild black cherry), *virginiana* (Choke cherry), *pennsylvanica* (Pin cherry)	Twigs, leaves, bark, and fruit stones	Cyanogenitic glycosides including amygdalin, prunasin, etc. which release cyanide when eaten	Difficult breathing, vertigo, spasms, coma, and sickness of short duration. A rapid reaction and little outward signs of poisoning; death usually less than one hour after eating. Treat for cyanide poisoning. Use sodium thiosulfate and sodium nitrite injections; oxygen. Oxidizing substances such as potassium permanganate or H_2O_2 given as a drench may be of some help. Also vigorous respiratory, heart, and nerve stimulants would be of aid.
Oaks	*Quercus* sps.	acorns, young shoots, leaves when eaten in large quantities	Tannic acid and a volatile oil	Causes constipation, bloody stools, and gradual kidney damage. Takes a large amount for poisoning. Children should not be allowed to chew on acorns. Saline purgatives followed by emollients.
Elderberry, Black elder	*Sambucus canadensis* and other sps.	Shoots, leaves, bark, roots	Alkaloid and glycoside. Small amounts of hydrocyanic acid are produced under certain conditions	Children have been poisoned by using pieces of the pithy stems for blowguns. Fresh berries essentially harmless. These may produce nausea if too many are eaten. Symptoms include nausea and digestive upset. Treat for alkaloid and/or HCN poisoning.
Black locust	*Robinia pseudoacacia*	Bark, sprouts, foliage, seeds	The phytotoxin robin and a glycoside robitin	Anorexia, lassitude, weakness, nausea, vomition, coldness of extremities, and marked dilation of pupils. Pulse weak and irregular. Death occurs within 2-3 days. Treatment symptomatic. Use antispasmodics, digitalis to help heart action, demulcents.
Bloodroot	*Sanguinaria canadensis*	The underground stems, roots, and their red contents	The alkaloid sanguinarine	Causes irritation of the mucous membranes of the mouth, throat, and stomach causing intense burning, nausea, and vomiting. If absorbed, alkaloids affect the nervous system, depress the heart, cause coma, and produce temporary paralysis. Induce vomiting, then give warm milk. Perform gastric lavage and treat irritated G.I. tract. Prevent circulatory collapse.

Common name	Scientific name	Toxic part	Poisonous principles	Clinical signs and treatment
Poison ivy (Erroneously called poison oak)	*Toxicodendron radicans* or *Rhus toxicodendron*	All parts, even the smoke from burning it	An oil-resin called urushiol which is made up of phenolic substances like 3-n-pentadecylcatechol	Produces a severe allergenic response causing dermatitis upon contact resulting in inflammation, blistering, and vesicles. As skin breaks, a liquid exudes and scabs or crusts form. Combination of poison with skin proteins is immediate and yellow soap only washes off excess poison. Treatment topical with lotions and creams for symptomatic relief Oral and injectable products of limited value. Do not use alcohol or organic solvents on the skin as this will spread the urushiol.
Poison sumac	*Toxicodendron vernix*	Ditto	Ditto	Ditto
F. Plants in Wooded Areas				
Jack-in-the-pulpit	*Arisaema triphyllum* and other sps.	All Parts, especially the rhizome	Needle-like crystals of calcium oxalate	Calcium oxalate crystals become embedded in the mucous membranes of mouth provoking intense irritation and a burning sensation. In large doses may cause gastroenteritis. Seldom fatal. Treatment symptomatic, pain relieved with meperidine HCl; aluminum-magnesium hydroxide useful as demulcent and neutralizing agent.
Moonseed	*Menispermum canadense*	Roots and fruit	Bitter alkaloids	Fruits and leaves resemble those of grape vine and thus mistaken for this plant. Contains a single seed. (True grapes contain several small seeds.) The rough sharp ridges of the fruit pits may also cause mechanical injury to the intestines. Has caused loss of life in children. Treatment symptomatic.
Mayapple	*Podophyllum peltatum*	Green fruit, foliage, roots	A crude resinous material podophyllin	Ripe fruit (yellow) edible. Green fruit and other parts cause severe purging; gastroenteritis accompanied with vomition. May also cause dermatitis. Young plant eaten as pot herb has caused human death. Treatment symptomatic.
Baneberry, Snake berry	*Actaea rubra*, *A. alba*, and *A. spicata*	Berries, rootstock, sap	An essential oil	As few as six berries can cause gastroenteritis, diarrhea, vomiting, and delirium. If absorbed the acid principles can cause tachycardia and dizziness. Fatalities have been reported. Have person vomit. Perform gastric lavage. Support circulation and treat for gastric inflammation.
Fly agaric mushroom	*Amanita muscaria*	All parts	Muscarine	Intense sweating, salivation, wheezing, irregular breathing and heart beat, mental confusion, muscular twitching, possible vomiting, diarrhea, and abdominal pain. Can be fatal within an hour. Induce vomiting, gastric lavage. Treat for CNS stimulation and dehydration. Atropine is antidote for any poisoning by mushrooms containing muscarine.
Destroying angel, death cup	*Amanita phalloides*	All parts	Five related cyclopeptides, phalloidin, phallion, a, B, V, amanitin	No symptoms for 6-15 hours, then sudden severe seizure of extreme abdominal pain, vomition, and diarrhea. Hepatic and renal involvement in 3-4 days. CNS signs are usually terminal. There is no specific antidote, treatment being symptomatic and supportive. Mortality rate from 50 to 90 per cent. Corticosteroids, broad spectrum antibiotics, vitamins, C, K, B complex, and dextrose and sodium chloride injection are all recommended. Thioctic acid used as an investigational agent. Contact National Institutes of Health Clinical Center, 24 hours a day concerning use and availability of thioctic acid.

Common name	Scientific name	Toxic part	Poisonous principles	Clinical signs and treatment
Panter mushroom	*Amanita pantherina*	All parts	Muscarine	Same as with *Amanita muscaria*
Jack-o'-lantern fungus	*Clitocybe illudens* and related *species, C. sudorifica* and *C. morbifera*	All parts	Muscarine	Similar to *Amanita muscaria*, but in reported cases no fatalities have occurred. Common symptoms include vomition, perspiration, and salivation. Treat for muscarine poisoning.
False morels	*Helvela exculenta, H. gigas,* and *H. underwoodii*	All parts	An unknown protoplasmic poison	Activity essentially hepatotoxic, with additional effects on the hematopoietic system and CNS. Has latent period of 6-10 hours between ingestion and symptoms. Fatal poisonings rare in the U.S. Treatment same as with *Amanita phalloides*.
Inky cap	*Coprinus atramentarius*	All parts	Unknown	Ingestion of these followed by ingestion of alcohol yields symptoms (in certain individuals) which resemble those of the alcohol-disulfiram (Antabuse) syndrome. Symptoms occur from ½-2 hours after ingestion and include flushing, palpitations, dyspnea, hyperventilation, and tachycardia. Recovery usually spontaneous and complete; however, severe cases may require gastric lavage and symptomatic treatment.
G. Plants in Swamp or Moist Areas				
Water hemlock (Cowbane)	*Cicuta maculata* and other species	All parts, mostly the roots	Resin-like substance called cicutoxin	Symptoms appear in 15 minutes and include severe stomach pain, great mental excitation and frenzy, vomiting, salivation, violent spasmodic convulsions alternating with periods of relaxation. Pupils dilate and delirium common. Death may occur within 15 minutes after ingestion of a lethal amount. Perform stomach lavage, treat for picrotoxin poisoning because cicutoxin is related to it. Control convulsions with parenteral short-acting barbiturates. Use morphine if necessary.
Marsh marigold	*Caltha palustris*	Top leaves and stems	Protoanemonin, a volatile oil	Irritant sap may cause salivation, inflamed oral tissues, G.I. irritation, and diarrhea. May cause convulsions if ingested in large quantity. Oily purgatives, demulcents, and heart stimulants may be of value. When cooked, the "greens" can be eaten without ill effects.
Skunk cabbage	*Symplocarpus foetidus*	Leaves, rhizomes	Calcium oxalate crystals	Needles of calcium oxalate become embedded in the mucous membranes and produce intense irritation and a burning sensation. Mortality in human beings unknown. Treat with demulcents. Leaves can be eaten if cooked in several waters to which has been added sodium bicarbonate.
H. Plants in Fields, Meadows, Pastures, and Roadsides				
Green or false hellebore, Indian poke	*Veratrum viride*	Roots, leaves, and seeds	Mixture of veratrum alkaloids	Salivation, vomiting, sweating, hypotension, muscular weakness, shallow respiration, bradycardia. Shallow breathing, slow pulse, low temperature, convulsions, and death from asphyxia. Pulse rapid and irregular. Induce emesis, gastric lavage, saline cathartics, support respiration. Use atropine to block reflex bradycardia. Levarterenol or ephedrine used for hypotension. Epinephrine is contraindicated and remaining treatment is symptomatic and supportive.
Buttercups	*Ranunculus abortivus, R. acris,* and other sps.	All parts, especially the juice	Ranunculin and protoanemonin	Have vesicant properties. Orally cause salivation, inflamed tissues, G.I. irritation, and diarrhea. May cause convulsions if ingested in large quantity. Oily purgatives, demulcents, and heart stimulants may be of value.

Common name	Scientific name	Toxic part	Poisonous principles	Clinical signs and treatment
European bittersweet, climbing nightshade	*Solanum dulcamara*	Leaves and unripe green fruits	A glycoalkaloid solanine	Ingestion results in burning in the throat, nausea, dizziness, dilation of pupils, convulsions, and general muscular weakness. Other symptoms include G.I. irritation, anorexia, vomition, constipation, or diarrhea. Death is result of paralysis, although not all ingestions are fatal. Has poisoned children. Induce vomiting, treat for alkaloidal poisoning, give heart and nerve stimulants.
Black, deadly, or common night shade	*Solanum nigrum*	Ditto	Ditto	Ditto (Ripe berries and young stems and leaves, when cooked, may be edible.)
Horse or bull nettle	*Solanum carolinense*	Ditto	Ditto	Ditto (Caused death of 6-yr.-old child in Delaware County, Pennsylvania, in January of 1963.)
Poison hemlock	*Conium maculatum*	Leaves, stem, and fruit	Coniine and other related alkaloids	Cause nervousness, trembling, ataxia (lower limbs), dilation of pupils, weakened and slowed heartbeat, coldness of extremities or whole body, coma, and eventual death through respiratory failure. Perform gastric lavage. Treat for alkaloid poisoning and maintain respiration.
Jimson weed or thornapple	*Datura strammonium, D. mietel D. metaloides, D. suaveolens,* and other sps.	All parts, especially seeds	The solanaceous alkaloids atropine, hyoscyamine, and scopolamine	Symptoms include intense thirst, dilated pupils, vomiting, vertigo, dryness of mouth, rapid and weak pulse, partial blindness, excessive thirst, delirium, incoherence; later, slow respiration, low temperature, rapid and weak pulse, convulsions or coma preceding death. Handling leaves followed by rubbing eyes can cause dilation of pupils. Wash hands after handling. Use tannic acid, cholinergic drugs (pilocarpine, physostigmine), respiratory stimulants.
Pokeweed, pigeonberry, inkberry	*Phytolacca americana, P. decandra*	Roots and leaves; fruit is least toxic	A resinous material and a water-soluble saponin	Produces burning sensation in mouth, G.I. cramps, vomition, diarrhea. Later, visual disturbance, perspiration, salivation, lassitude, prostration, weakened respiration and pulse may be seen. If recovery does not occur in 24 hours, may be fatal. Treat by inducing vomiting. Perform gastric lavage and treat for circulatory and respiratory depression. References to poisoning of children by berries are not conclusive. Some persons make pies with berries. Young shoots edible after boiling in two changes of water.
Dogbane	*Apocynum cannabinum* (Indian hemp, dogbane), *A. androsaemifolium* (spreading dogbane)	Green or dry leaves and tops	The resinoid apocynin and glucosides apocynein and cymarin	Increase in temperature, pulse and blood pressure, cold sweating, dilation of pupils, discoloration of mouth, refusal to eat and drink, G.I. disturbance, finally death. Use emetic, then use gallic or tannic acid as an antidote.
Hemp, marihuana	*Cannabis sativa*	Leaves and flowering tops	A resinous mixture of tetrahydrocannabinols	Individual reaction extremely variable. Generally have period of euphoria and elation followed by a heightened sensitivity to stimulation. This is followed by hallucinations and mental confusion. With heavier doses, depression and comatose sleep follow. Little or no withdrawal symptoms on long use. Effects can be produced by smoking resin-containing parts or ingesting crude resin. Death may occur on overdose due to its effect on heartbeat. Federal law prohibits (without license) the possession of living or dried cannabis or parts of the plant. Treatment symptomatic. Gastric lavage, CNS stimulants.

*Adapted from: Der Marderosian A., Am. J. Pharmaceut. Ed. 30:55-79, 1966; and Arena, J.M., Clinical Symposia 30:1-47, 1978.
Reference: Kingsbury, J.M. *Poisonous Plants of the United States and Canada* Prentice-Hall, Inc. Englewood Cliffs, N.J., 1964.

Appendix 4

Principles of Fluid Therapy

Each cell of the body is bathed in tissue fluid containing electrolytes—sodium, potassium, calcium, magnesium, ammonium, chloride, bicarbonate, and hydrogen ions. The amount and composition of tissue fluids are maintained within remarkably narrow limits through the continuous activity of several homeostatic mechanisms. Profound physiologic derangements can be caused by alterations of the tissue fluids. These often occur as major or minor features of illness, trauma, or surgical procedures. Under such circumstances, it frequently becomes necessary to anticipate or correct deficits and imbalances by the administration of appropriate fluids. Successful treatment of fluid and electrolyte disturbances need not be complicated. The approaches outlined here should provide a sound physiologic basis for correct fluid and electrolyte therapy.

The principles of fluid therapy are based largely on animals studies, including dogs, but the practice of fluid therapy depends greatly on experience with human patients. Fortunately, the physiologic principles involved vary little from species to species. Thus, conditions such as water depletion, sodium depletion, acidosis, etc., are treated similarly irrespective of species.

The general principles of fluid therapy are few and simple: maintain the body in balance—replace any losses. Fluids lost should be replaced (replacement therapy) in terms of pre-existing loss and current loss. Water and electrolytes needed day by day must be provided to balance normal daily loss (maintenance therapy).

Allow the Body to Naturally Aid the Selection of Its Needs

Balanced electrolyte solutions are designed to be versatile, i.e., each fulfills its own general purpose despite variations in the exact requirements for replacement or maintenance from case to case. The designs take into account the ability of the body's homeostatic mechanisms to make final adjustments after the solution is administered.

The Body Balance Shifts to Compensate for Fluid Electrolyte Loss

When fluid is lost, the body usually reacts in ways which lead to a deficit of the extracellular fluid. Thus, the replacement solution should have an electrolyte content like that of extracellular fluid.

Acidosis Often Develops When Body Water is Lost

The loss of body water is usually accompanied by the loss of sodium and bicarbonate ions and the retention of chloride and hydrogen ions, with the development of acidosis. This may be corrected by the administration of sodium bicarbonate or its equivalents (organic acid anions which are metabolized to bicarbonate). Standard replacement solutions contain a little less chloride and nearly twice the bicarbonate equivalents of extracellular water, so they tend to correct acidosis. Further power to combat acidosis is obtained by the addition of sodium bicarbonate to the replacement solution.

Alkalosis Occasionally Develops with Vomiting

Less commonly, alkalosis may develop, usually in association with vomiting, gastric juice loss or sequestration. Water, hydrogen ions and chloride are lost. Some sodium is usually lost in partial compensation. Moreover, bicarbonate tends to be retained in order to compensate for hypochloremia. Under these circumstances, replacement is achieved by the administration of balanced electrolyte solutions.

Administer Potassium Cautiously if Urination Has Stopped

In nearly all conditions requiring fluid therapy, some potassium is lost from the body. So some potassium should be present in solutions designed for routine use. Potassium should not be given to animals with severely impaired renal tubule function manifested by anuria and acute uremia.

Oliguria is usually due to extrarenal factors which deplete the extracellular fluid, e.g., diarrhea, vomiting, blood loss (injury or surgery) and intestinal obstruction. The kidney has a strong reserve capacity to excrete potassium. Under these circumstances, the extracellular fluid volume should be restored by the administration of a solution containing a small amount of potassium which is usually needed to correct the potassium depletion which commonly accompanies both acidosis and alkalosis.

Fluid Volumes

Maintenance (to balance normal daily loss):
Canine 20—30 ml per lb daily
Feline 30—40 ml per lb daily
Replacement, Pre-existing loss (dehydration)
Mild —4% of body weight (none to slight signs of dehydration, but history of thirst, vomiting, diarrhea, or other fluid loss) replace 18 ml per lb body weight.
Moderate —6% of body weight (ocular and oral mucous membranes dry, hair coat dull, loss of skin resiliency) replace 27 ml per lb body weight.
Severe —8% of body weight (skin leathery and inelastic, conjunctiva congested and dry, oral mucosa dry and sticky, eyeballs may be sunken and soft, slow refilling capillary bed, urine slow or stopped) replace 37 ml per lb body weight.
Replacement, concurrent loss: This continuing loss must be replaced volume for volume.

This requires an on the spot estimation of loss from vomiting, diarrhea, or hemorrhage. If a liter is lost, a liter must be replaced.

Fluid volumes needed are the sum total of maintenance and replacement volumes: maintenance need, pre-existing replacement need, or concurrent replacement need. The sum of fluid volumes required can be a combination of any of these or a total of all three.

Dose requirements of each electrolyte will vary from case to case. The volume and composition of fluid given only approximates that which might be optimal, and the homeostatic mechanisms of the body are depended on to make further adjustments. In general, the fluid volume required for maintenance varies with age and body size. It is a volume equivalent to 7 to 10% body weight in young animals. This decreases progressively to 3 to 6% body weight in mature animals. The fluid volume required for replacement varies with the degree of loss, but it usually lies within the range of 3 to 10% body weight. The rate at which replacement fluid should be given depends on the degree of depletion, the animal's condition and the composition of the fluid. Under most circumstances, a replacement volume no greater than 3% of the body weight is given per hour and no more than 10% of body weight is administered per day. There are exceptions to this general rule, e.g., acute hemorrhage may call for rapid administration of large amounts of fluids. The total daily volume needed will include the maintenance requirement in addition to the replacement requirement, so it may reach a total equal to 20% body weight.

The Young Patient

A few special considerations should be kept in mind when treating the young. The body size is smaller, but the proportion of body water is larger, about 80% of the body weight in newborn animals. Moreover the metabolic rate and water turnover are 1.5 to 2 times higher than in mature animals. Thus a puppy weighing 250 g (0.5 lb) requires a fluid volume equal to 7% of its body weight, i.e., 15 to 20 ml for its daily maintenance.

Depletion develops more rapidly in young animals when intakes of water and electrolytes are impaired due to vomiting or when losses occur due to diarrhea. A very young animal may loss 5% of its body weight in a day. A severe situation usually takes longer to develop in an adult.

Routes of Administration

The **intravenous (IV) route** is used when a serious disturbance of water, electrolytes and protein balance has occurred. To meet the needs of the animal that requires large volume fluid therapy, continuous slow drip administration gives the best response. Fluids are well tolerated and efficiently absorbed, when given IV.

The **intraperitoneal (IP) route** may be used to correct major fluid imbalances. Fluids are well tolerated and even whole blood is absorbed fairly rapidly when given IP. However, adhesions and infections may occur with this route of administration. Aseptic technique should be carefully employed.

The **subcutaneous (SC) route** can be used for maintenance fluid therapy. Large volume replacement of fluids needed to correct serious dehydration cannot be absorbed from SC administration. Hypertonic solutions are not well absorbed from the site since the solution hyperosmolarity attracts water from the body and more dehydration may result before the fluid is redistributed. SC diffusion is said to be increased by the incorporation of hyaluronidase in the administered solution. This method is used with some success in the very young, and for cats.

Techniques of Administration

Administration of fluids by continuous slow drip gives far superior results for two major reasons: 1) The body has a chance to adjust and utilize fully the ingredients retained, and 2) The kidney is able to adjust its selectivity to retain only those things and in the correct amounts that the body needs.

IV administration by slow drip over long periods through the extremities is difficult in animals. Tubing and administration site exposure are vulnerable to the animal's reach, sometimes resulting in expensive equipment damage. Almost constant monitoring is necessary, a waste of manpower.

Variations of IV administration technique can overcome some of the problems mentioned above. Choose a venopuncture site (e.g., the jugular route) that is more difficult for the animal to reach and not conttantly in his sight. Allow lead-in tubing to approach animal from behind the head. Use plastic IV catheters for less site damage and easier administration. Utilization of IV catheters gives better site attachment for safer and surer administration.

They are adaptable to most uses, most depth settings, and for use on all animal sizes.

Types of Fluids

Fluids can be categorized in three basic groups: balanced polyelectrolyte solutions, simple hyerating solutions, and special solutions.

Balanced polyelectrolyte solutions will best satisfy the majority of fluid replacement and maintenance therapy uses because their electrolyte content closely emulates that of extracellular fluids. They are designed to offer, in physiologic proportions, all the electrolytes and buffers the body utilizes. The body's homeostatic mechanisms will select that part it has need of at the time in correct proportions and will eliminate the balance in the urine. Balanced polyelectrolyte solutions supply water, sodium, potassium, calcium, magnesium, ammonium, chloride, and bicarbonate ions. Potassium is present in small amounts. Potassium depletion has been found to develop rapidly in most conditions calling for fluid therapy. A clinical sign of potassium depletion is muscular weakness (e.g., skeletal muscle, the smooth muscle of the gastrointestinal tract and the heart). The animal's physicial strength improves with the restoration of potassium. Therefore, small amounts of potassium are now included in polyelectrolyte solutions designed for routine maintenance and replacement therapy.

Simple hydrating solutions contain varying amounts of only water, sodium, chloride, and dextrose. Most authorities agree that the usefulness of simple hydrating solutions for extensive hydration is limited. However, these fluids are excellent hydration solutions for use during renal shutdown. It is imperative that potassium-containing fluids be avoided if shutdown is due to acute renal failure or severe chronic renal impairment. Fluids in this group are indicated to supply the required amount of a specific deficit of water, sodium, chloride, or dextrose. Simple hydrating solutions can be useful as a vehicle to supply the needs of a specific additive, e.g., potassium. These solutions were formerly used for routine maintenance but are rapidly being replaced by the balanced polyelectrolyte solutions because of their superior ionic content and buffering systems.

Special solutions are designed to assist the veterinarian by doing a specialized task. For example, acidosis is corrected by the administration of bicarbonate or its equivalents; dextrose 50% is used to correct hypoglycemia.

(Modified from literature provided by Abbott Laboratories.)

Appendix 5

Drug Therapy in Laboratory Animals*

TABLE 1. ANTIBIOTIC THERAPY IN LABORATORY ANIMALS

Anitibiotic therapy is often a compromise between theoretical and practical treatment. Theorectically, antibiotic sensitivity tests should be performed before treatment is initiated, however, this is not always possible. Although sensitivity testing is *highly* recommended, one must keep in mind several factors:

1. *In vitro* results don't always apply in *in vivo*.
2. Laboratories may differ in antibiotic sensitivity results.
3. A nonpathogenic organism may have been tested.
4. There may be a mixed infection.
5. The antibiotic the organism is sensitive to may be toxic to the animal.
6. Antibiotic sensitivities may differ between strains, serotypes, and species of the same genus of bacteria, as well as with the passage of time.

A helpful "guide" to antibiotic therapy in laboratory animals based on an etiological agent is Antibiograms of Pathogenic Bacteria Isolated from Laboratory Animals by D. Owens, J. Wagner, and J. Addison in JAVMA 167(7):605–609, 1975.

Very little research has been done on either the minimum effective dose or the actual blood levels of antibiotics used for the treatment of laboratory animal diseases. For the most part, dosages, route of administration, and duration of treatment appear to be a combination of clinical experience and extrapolation of therapy for dogs and cats.

The following tables are limited to treatable diseases or conditions of rabbits and rodents. The antibiotics are not listed in any particular order and their incidental positioning opposite an etiologic agent does not imply that the antibiotic is specific for that organism.

Abbreviations used in this section are as follows:

ABBREVIATIONS

IM–intramuscular	**SC**–subcutaneously
IV–intravenous	**P/O**–per os
SID–once a day	**QID**–four times a day
BID–twice a day	**EOD**–every other day
TID–three times a day	
IU–international unit	**L**–liter
kg–kilogram	**ml**–milliliter
mg–milligram	**BW**–body weight

*Prepared by T.A. Bowman and C.M. Lang, Department of Comparative Medicine, The Milton S. Hershey Medical Center, The Pennsylvania State University, Hershey, PA 17033

A. Rabbits

Disease/condition	Possible Etiology	Treatment	Dosage[a]	Frequency	Route	Ref
BACTERIAL DISEASES:						
Rhinitis and/or Pneumonia	*Bordetella bronchiseptica*	Procaine penicillin	40,000-60,000 IU/kg	SID	IM	3,8
	Pasteurella multocida	Benzathine penicillin and procaine penicillin	12,000 IU/kg	EOD	IM	7
		Tetracycline or Oxytetracycline	300-100 mg/kg or 400-1,000 mg/L (Prepare fresh 3 times a week)	in divided dose of drinking water	P/O	4,7,8
		Oxytetracycline	10 mg/kg	SID	IM	5
		Ampicillin	10-25 mg/kg or 22-44 mg/kg	SID 5 to 7 days in divided doses	IM P/O	4 7
		Cephaloridine	10-25 mg/kg	SID 5 days	IM, SC	4
		Cephalothin sodium	13 mg/kg	QID for 6 days	IM	7,8
		Sulfamethazine or Sulfamerazine	80-100 mg/kg or 0.2% in drinking water for 7-10 days	SID	P/O	5,7 4
		Furazolidone	5 mg/kg or 5 mg/100 gm feed	SID	P/O	5

Disease/condition	Possible Etiology	Treatment	Dosage[a]	Frequency	Route	Ref
Diarrhea	*Bacillus piliformis*	Procaine penicillin	40,000-60,000 IU/kg	SID	IM	3,8
	Clostridium perfringens	Benzathine penicillin and procaine penicillin	120,000 IU/kg	EOD	IM	7
	Escherichia coli	Tetracycline or Oxytetracycline	30-100 mg/kg or 400-1,000 mg/L (prepare fresh 3 times a week)	in divided doses of drinking water	P/O	5,7,8
		Oxytetracycline	10 mg/kg	SID	IM	5
		Chloramphenicol succinate	50 mg/kg	BID-TID	IV, IM, SC	7,8
		± Fluids poor prognosis				
Mastitis	*Staphylococcus sp*	Procaine penicillin	40,000-60,000 IU/kg	SID	IM	3,8
	Streptococcus sp	Benzathine and procaine penicillin	120,000 IU/kg	EOD	IM	7
		Plus moist hot packs				
Moist Dermatitis and/or Cutaneous Abscesses	*Staphylococcus aureus*	Local application of hydrogen peroxide and iodine		BID	Topical	7
	Fusobacterium necrophorum	Zinc oxide or antibiotic ointment		SID-BID	Topical	9
		OPTIONAL PARENTERAL ANTIBIOTICS:				
		Tetracycline[b] or Oxytetracycline[c]	30-100 mg/kg	Divided doses of drinking water	P/O	5,7,8
			or 400-1,000 mg/L (make up fresh 3 times a week)			
	Pseudomonas aeruginosa	Procaine penicillin	40,000-60,000 IU/kg	SID	IM	3,8
	(Blue-green discoloration of the fur)	Benzathine penicillin and procaine penicillin	120,000 IU/kg	EOD	Im	7
		Chloramphenicol succinate	50 mg/kg	BID-TID	IM, IV, SC	7,8
		Gentamicin[b,c]	4 mg/kg	SID	IM, SC	5,7,8
Genital sores ± secondary lesions on hock, lips, nares, feet, ears, and eyelids. (Rabbit syphilis)	*Treponema cuniculi*	Procaine penicillin	40,000-60,000 IU/kg	SID for 3-5 days	IM	3,7
		Benzathine penicillin and procaine penicillin	120,000 IU/kg	EOD for 2-3 treatments	IM	7
MYCOTIC DISEASE:						
Ringworn	Usually *Trichophyton mentagrophytes*	Griseofulvin	25 mg/kg	SID for 2 wks.	P/O	2,7,9
		Antifungal ointment		BID for a minimum of 4 weeks	Topically	2

a - per kg of body weight unless states otherwise
b - Especially for *Pseudomonas sp*
c - Use with care—quite nephrotoxic in rabbits

B. Guinea pigs

NOTE: Antibiotics such as penicillin, lincomycin, erythromycin, and tylosin are *contraindicated* for guinea pigs as they may lead to fatal toxicity from overgrowth of intestinal gram negative organisms.[6,8]

Disease/condition	Possible Etiology	Treatment	Dosage	Frequency	Route	Ref
BACTERIAL DISEASES:						
Pneumonia	*Streptococcus pneumoniae*	Tetracycline HCl or Oxytetracycline	30-100 mg/kg	In divided doses of drinking water	P/O	5,7,8
			400-1,000 mg/L (Make up fresh 3 times a week)			
	Klebsiella pneumoniae	Oxytetracycline	10 mg/kg	SID	IM	5
	Pseudomonas aeruginosa	Cephaloridine	20-25 mg/kg or 11 mg/kg	SID for 5-10 days BID	IM SC or IM	1,2,7 8

Disease/condition	Possible Etiology	Treatment	Dosage	Frequency	Route	Ref
	Streptococcus pyogenes	Sulfamethazine	4 ml of 12.5% solution/500 ml drinking water for	1-2 weeks		8,9
			or 80-100 mg/kg	SID	P/O	5,7
	Bordetella bronchiseptica	Chloramphenicol sodium succinate	10-50 mg/kg	BID for 5 days	IM	3,8,9
		Gentamicin	5 mg/kg	SID for 5 days	IM or SC	4
Cervical Lymphadenitis	*Streptococcus zooepidemicus*	Chloramphenicol palmitate	50 mg/kg	SID-TID	P/O	2,5,7,9
		Oxytetracycline or Tetracycline HCl	30-100 mg/kg or 400-1,000 mg/L (Make up fresh 3 times a week)	in divided doses of drinking water	P/O	5,7,8
	Streptobacillus moniliformis	Oxytetracycline	10 mg/kg	SID	IM	5
		Cephaloridine	20-25 mg/kg	SID for 5-10 days	IM	1,2,7
			or 11 mg/kg	BID	SC or IM	8
		Local drainage plus flushing with hydrogen peroxide and iodine		BID 5-7 days		
Diarrhea	*Bacillus piliformis*	Oxytetracycline or Tetracycline HCl	30-100 mg/kg or 400-1,000 mg/L (Make up fresh 3 times a week)	in divided doses of drinking water	P/O	5,7,8
		Oxytetracycline	10 mg/kg	SID	IM	5
		Chloramphenicol palmitate	50 mg/kg	SID-TID	P/O	2,5,7,9
MYCOTIC DISEASES:						
Ringworm	Primarily *Trichophyton mentagrophytes*	Griseofulvin[d]	2.5 mg/100 gm	SID for 14 days	P/O	7,8
MISCELLANEOUS:						
Bleeding gums	Ascorbic acid (Vitamin C) deficiency	Ascorbic acid or green leafy vegetables such as kale, parsley, and spinach; lettuce is *not* adequate.	10-30 mg/kg	SID	P/O	3,8
Swollen joints			10 mg/kg BW in drinking water[e]		P/O	2

[d]-Derived from penicillin cultures so use with caution

[e]-May refuse to drink; metal or hard water will inactivate solutions of ascorbic acid

C. Hamsters

NOTE: Penicillins, Tylosin, Lincomycin, and Erythromycin will produce antibiotic toxicity in Hamsters.[7]

Disease/condition	Possible Etiology	Treatment	Dosage	Frequency	Route	Ref
Bacterial Diseases:						
Pneumonia	*Streptococcus sp*	Oxytetracycline or Tetracycline HCl	30-100 mg/kg or 400-1,000 mg/L (Make up fresh 3 times a week)	in divided doses of drinking water	P/O	5,7,8
	Pasteurella sp	Sulfamethazine or Sulfamerazine	100 mg/kg or 40 ml of 12.5% solution/gal drinking water	SID	P/O	7
		Gentamicin	0.5 mg/100 gm	SID for 5 days	IM or SC	2,4,5,7
Infected cheek Pouches	Bacterial	Evert the pouch and treat locally with hydrogen peroxide				7

Disease/condition	Possible Etiology	Treatment	Dosage	Frequency	Route	Ref
Diarrhea	Viral, bacterial, protozoal, and/or	Oxytetracycline or Tetracycline	30-100 mg/kg or 400-1,000 mg/L (Make up fresh 3 times a week)	divided doses of drinking water	P/O	5,7,8
		Gentamicin[f]	0.5 mg/100 gm BW	SID for 5 days	IM or SC	2,4,5,7
		Neomycin sulfate	100 mg/kg or 2-10 g/gal	SID for 5 days of drinking water	P/O	4,9 7,9
		Chloramphenicol succinate or	30-50 mg/kg	TID for 5-7 days	IM, IP	4
		Chloramphenicol palmitate	50 mg/kg	TID for 5-7 days		4
		Support Therapy: Fluids: Lactated Ringers	5-15% BW	SID	SC	2
		Kaolin with pectin[g]	1-2 ml	SID	P/O	2
		Liquid vitamin supplement		SID	P/O	2
		Better sanitation Poor prognosis				

[f]-Has had good results
[g]-If used in conjunction with oral antibiotics, these products may nullify the antibiotic activity.

D. Rats

Disease/condition	Possible Etiology	Treatment	Dosage	Frequency	Route	Ref
Bacterial Diseases:						
Rhinitis/pneumonia[h]	*Mycoplasma pulmonis*	Tetracycline or Oxytetra-cycline	400-1,000 mg/L (make fresh 3 times a week)	of drinking water		5,7,8
	Pasteurella sp	Chloramphenicol palmitate	20 mg/100 gm	TID	P/O	7
	Bordetella sp	Chloramphenicol succinate	30 mg/kg	SID for 5 days	IM	3
	Streptococcus pneumoniae	Procaine penicillin	40,000 IU/kg	SID	IM	3,8
		Sulfamerazine or Sulfamethazine	100 mg/kg or 40 ml of 12.5% solution/gal of drinking water	SID	P/O	7
		Ampicillin	2-10 mg/100 gm	BID	P/O	7
		Gentamicin	5 mg/100 gm BW	SID for 14 days	SC	7
			or 0.5 mg/100 gm	SID	IM	5,7
		Tylosin	0.2-0.8 mg/100 g BW	SID-BID for 5 days	IM	2,5,7
			or 2.5 g/gal	in drinking water for 21 days	P/O	7
		Cephaloridine	10-25 mg/kg	SID 5-7 days	IM or SC	4
Ulcerative Dermatitis	*Staphylococcus aureus*	Clip toenails				
		Systemic antibiotics previously listed for *S. aureus*				
Mycotic Diseases:						
Ringworm	*Trichophyton sp* *Microsporum sp*	Griseofulvin	2.5 mg/100 gm BW	SID for 14 days	P/O	7,8

[h]-In many cases antibiotic treatment controls but doesn't cure the disease or eliminate the carrier state

E. Mice

Disease/condition	Possible Etiology	Treatment	Dosage	Frequency	Route	Ref
Bacterial Diseases:						
Rhinitis/ Pneumonia	*Mycoplasma sp*	Oxytetracycline or Tetracycline	400-1,000 mg/L (Make up fresh 3 times a week)	of drinking water		5,7,8
	Pasteurella pneumotropica	Chloramphenicol palmitate	20 mg/100 gm	TID	P/O	7
	Bordetella bronchiseptica	Ampicillin	2-10 mg/100 gm	BID	P/O	7
		Penicillin[i]	100,000 IU/kg	BID	IM	7
	Klebsiella pneumoniae	Gentamicin	5 mg/100 gm	SID for 14 days	SC	7
		Cephaloridine	10-25 mg/kg	SID 5-7 days	IM or SC	4
	Pseudomonas aeruginosa	Sulfamethazine or Sulfamerazine	100 mg/kg or 4 ml of 12.5% solution/gal of drinking water	SID	P/O	7
Necrotic Dermatitis	*Streptococcus* Group G *Staphylococcus aureus*	Systemic antibiotics previously listed for these organisms				
Swollen Joints and Toes	*Streptobacillus moniliformis*	Penicillin[i]	100,000 IU/kg	BID	IM	7
Ringworm	*Trichophyton* sp *Microsporum* sp	Griseofulvin	2.5 mg/100 gm	SID for 14 days	P/O	7,8

[i]-Do not use procaine penicillin

REFERENCES:

1. Diaz, J. and Soave, O. Cephaloridine Treatment of Cervical Lymphadenitis in Guinea Pigs. Lab. Anim. Dig. 8:60-62. 1973.
2. Harkness, J. and Wagner, J. The Biology and Medicine of Rabbits and rodents. Lea and Febiger. Philadelphia. 1977.
3. IBID. 1983
4. Jacobson, E., Kollias, G., Peters, L. Dosages for Antibiotics and Parasiticides Used in Exotic Animals. The Compendium on Continuing Education for Veterinarians 5(4):315-324, 1983.
5. Kirk, R. (ed). Current Veterinary Therapy VI. W.B. Saunders Co., Philadelphia. 1977.
6. Owens, D., Wagner, J., and Addison, J. Antibiograms of Pathogenic Bacteria Isolated From Laboratory Animals. JAVMA 167(7):605-609. 1975.
7. Russell, R., Johnson, D., and Stunkard, J. A Guide to Diagnosis, Treatment, and Husbandry of Pet Rabbits and rodents. Veterinary Medical Publishing Co., Edwardsville, KS, 1981.
8. Siegmund, O. (ed). The Merck Veterinary Manual. Fifth edition. Merck and Co., Inc., Rahway. 1979.
9. Williams, C. Practical Guide to Laboratory Animals. C.N. Mosby Co., St. Louis. 1976.

TABLE 2
PARASITE CONTROL IN LABORATORY ANIMALS*

A. Internal Parasites

The control of internal parasites of laboratory animals is as much dependent on sanitation and good husbandry as it is on drugs. Some drugs suggested for parasite control in laboratory animals are only partially effective or are not parasiticidal but rather partially inhibit or delay the development of the parasites. In such instances, knowledge of the life cycle of the parasite and the action of the anthelmintic as well as good sanitation are equally important in parasite control.

Many naturally occurring parasites of feral animals used as laboratory subjects lack the appropriate intermediate hosts for transmission in a well controlled laboratory environment. Infestation with these parasites is often limited to a few individuals and is not a problem in laboratory propagated animals.

The following table represents a compilation of common internal parasites of laboratory animals for which anthelmintic therapy has been used successfully. A certain latitude in dosage exists for most of the agents especially those administered in the feed or water. Not included in the table are the avermectins. These broad spectrum parasiticides including Ivermectin are probably effective against many internal and external parasites of laboratory animals in single or multiple oral dosages of 200 μ gm/kg/day. Unfortunately, sufficient clinical trials are not yet available to justify their routine use in laboratory animals.

SPECIES	PARASITE	DRUG
Mice	Hymenolepis sp.	Niclosamide—50 to 100 mg/kg per day in feed; two weeks of treatment separated by one week without treatment
	Syphacia sp. & Heterakis sp.	Piperazine—160 to 200 mg/kg per day in H_2O (4 to 7 mg/ml) or feed for 3 to 10 days
		Pyrvinium pamoate[1]—0.0008% in H_2O or 0.0016% in feed for 30 days (intended dosage 1.6 mg/kg/day)
		Dichlorovos[2,3]—in food at 250 to 500 mg/kg of food for 1 day
		Trichlorfon[3] with Atropine (180:1)—1.75 in water over 7 to 14 days
		Dithiazanine iodide[4]—0.1 mg/gm food fed for 7 days
		Stilbazium iodide—0.1 mg/gm food for 2 days
	Giardia sp.	Metronidazole—15 mg/kg IP (1 dose) or 0.5% in H_2O for 11 days
		Quinacrine—0.25 mg/gm oral (1 dose)
Rat	Hymenolepsis sp.	Niclosamide—50 to 100 mg/kg per day in feed; two weeks of treatment separated by one week without treatment
	Syphacia sp[5] & Heterakis sp.	Piperazine—160 to 200 mg/kg per day in H_2O (4 to 7 mg/ml) or feed for 3 to 10 days
		Pyrvinium pamoate[1]—0.003% in H_2O or 0.012% in feed for 30 days
	Trichosomoides sp.	Methyridine 125 mg/kg (1 dose) IP or 65 mg/kg SQ (1 dose)
		Nitrofurantoin[6]—0.2% in Feed for 6 to 8 weeks
Hamster	Hymenolepis sp.	Niclosamide—50 to 100 mg/kg per day in feed; two weeks of treatment separated by one week without treatment
Rabbit	Eimeria sp.	Succinylsulfathiazole, Sulfamerazine or Sulfamethazine[7]—0.5 to 1.0% in feed
		Sulfaquinoxaline or Sulfamerazine[7]—0.02 to 0.10% in drinking water
		Sulfadiazine or Sulfaquinoxaline[7]—0.1 g/kg SQ of a 20% aqueous solution single dose followed by oral therapy (see above compounds)
	Passalurus sp.	Piperazine—200 mg/kg single oral dose
Guinea Pig	Eimeria sp.	Succinylsulfathiazole[7]—1.0% in drinking water
Nonhuman Primate	Hymenolepis sp.	Niclosamide—100 to 200 mg/kg single oral dose
	Oesophagostomum sp. & Trichostrongylus sp.	Thiabendazole—100 mg/kg single oral dose
	Stronygloides sp.	Thiabendazole—100 mg/kg single oral dose, repeat in 14 days
		Dithiazanine iodide[4]—20 mg/kg sid orally for 10 to 14 days
	Trichuris sp.[8]	Dithiazanine iodide[4]—20 mg/kg sid orally for 10 to 14 days
		Dichlorovos[2,3]—10 mg/kg sid for 2 days
		Thiabendazole—60 mg/day sid orally for 9 to 10 days or 100 mg/kg single oral dose, repeat in 14 days
		Methyridine—200 mg/kg SQ (1 dose)
	Enterobius sp.	Dithiazanine iodide[4]—20 mg/kg bid orally for 14 days
		Dichlorvos[2,3]—8 to 9 mg/kg sid orally for 2 days
		Pyrvinium pamoate[1]—5 mg/kg orally (1 dose), repeat in 14 days
	Anyclostoma sp. & Necator sp.	Dithiazanine iodide[4]—20 mg/kg bid orally for 14 days
		Dichlorvos[2,3]—8 to 9 mg/kg sid orally for 2 days
	Balantidium sp.	Carbarsone[9]—150 to 200 mg bid orally for 10 days
		5,7 Diiodo-8-hydroxyquin[10]—0.65 to 1.3 gm orally for 21 days
		Paromomycin—25 mg/kg/day tid orally for 10 days
	Entamoeba sp.	Fumagillin—20 mg bid orally for 14 days
		Carbarsone[9]—150 to 200 mg bid orally for 10 days
		5,7 Diiodo-8-Hydroxyquin[10]—0.65 to 1.3 gm orally for 21 days

*Prepared by W.J. White and C.M. Lang, Department of Comparative Medicine, The Milton S. Hershey Medical Center, The Pennsylvania State University, Hershey, PA 17033

[1]May color feces red

[2]Must be prepared immediately before use and as close as possible to the time of consumption

[3]Cholinesterase inhibitor; effects may last for 21 days following administration

[4]Will stain animals and surroundings, may cause diarrhea

[5]Dichlorovos or trichlorofon with atropine *may* also be effective at mouse dosage in this species

[6]High oral dosage produces serious neuropathy in this species

[7]These drugs are coccidostats and are not therapy for an active infection; continual administration is necessary for control

[8]Oral anthelmintics are relatively ineffective in eliminating this parasite

[9]Contains arsenic; contraindicated in hepatic or renal disease

[10]Often given with antibiotics; may cause yellow-brown staining of hair and may alter serum PBI

B. External Parasites

The drugs and procedures for treating external parasites in laboratory animals are similar for most species. In small rodents, dipping in a tepid insecticidal solution at weekly intervals for 2 to 3 weeks coupled with concomittant environmental sanitation procedures is usually effective. Room and cage cleaning and premisses insecticide application along with topical application of insecticides to the animals are the important aspects of the control program. All animals in the housing area should be treated but care should be exercised in treating pregnant animals and newborns. The cumulative and long lasting effects of organophosphates must be appreciated and steps taken to prevent overdose when multiple agents are used.

The following table summarizes some of the more commonly used agents. It does not include avermectins. Oral administration of these compounds may be effective in external parasite control of laboratory animals but sufficient clinical data is not yet available to justify their use.

AGENT	TYPE[1]	FORM	CONC.	APPLICATION	REMARKS
Carbaryl[2]	OP	Dust	5%	Apply to pelage at 1 to 3 week intervals	Commonly used & reasonably safe
		Sol.	1%	Place in ears at 10 day intervals	Treatment of earmites
Diazinon	OP	Sol.	0.03 to 0.06%	Apply as dip; repeat in 2 to 3 weeks	More commonly used for larger lab animals
Dichlorovos	OP	Plastic impregnated strip	—	Place over cage for 1 to 3 days; single application	Use restricted to small rodents; reasonably effective
		Plastic Impregnated pellets	—	Mix in bedding; single application	Use restricted to small rodents; reasonably effective
Malathion	OP	Sol.	2%	Dip once a week for 2 or 3 weeks	Safe & effective for most lab animals
		Dust	2 to 4%	Apply once a week for 2 to 3 weeks	Safe & effective for most lab animals
Methoxychlor	CH	Dust[3]	2 to 10%	Apply to pelage at 7 to 10 day intervals	Analogue of DDT; not very toxic
		Sol.	0.5%	Apply as dip at 10 to 14 day intervals	Analogue of DDT; not very toxic
Monosulfiram	S	Sol. in Alcohol	2.5 to 5.0%	Apply 2 to 3 times a week for 2 to 3 weeks	Not as effective as other preps. listed
Pyrethrins	BI	Sol.	0.05 to 0.02%	Apply as spray of dip	Safe "knock down" agent with little residual action
Rotenone	BI	Sol. in oil	0.12 to 1.0%	Place in ears 2 to 3 times/wk for 2 to 3 weeks	Treatment of ear mites

[1] OP—Organophosphate; BI—Botanical Insecticide; S—Sulfur Containing Agent; CH—Chlorinated Hydrocarbon
[2] Passed in milk of lactating animals; Teratogenic to hamsters at 300 mg/kg
[3] Dusts up to 2% are used in rats, mice, and hamsters

TABLE 3
ANESTHETIC, ANALGESIC AND SEDATIVE DRUG DOSAGES IN LABORATORY ANIMALS*

		Sedation/Analgesics			Anesthesia		
Drug	Species	I.V.	I.P.	I.M.	I.V.	I.P.	I.M.
Droperidol-fentanyl (ml/kg)	Mice			0.2-0.3			0.5
	Rats			0.13-.16			0.3
	Hamsters	Undesirable-CNS Stimulation					
	Guinea Pig			0.08-0.66			0.66-0.88
	Rabbits			0.15-0.17			
	NHP			0.06			0.11
Ketamine (mg/kg)[1]	Mice	25	25-50	22	50	100-200	400
	Rats		20	22	50	40-160	44
	Hamsters		100	40		200	100
	Guinea pigs			22-64			44-256
	Rabbits			22-35	15-20		44
	NHP	7-14		5-15	28-45		7-40
Meperidine (mg/kg)	Mice		40	60			
	Rats	25	50	44			
	Guinea pigs		1	2			
	Rabbits	10					
	NHP			2-10			
Pentobarbital (mg/kg)	Mice				40-70	40-80	
	Rats				25-40	35-40	
	Hamsters				30	50-90	
	Guinea pigs				30	15-30	
	Rabbits				25-40	40	
	NHP				25-33	30	
Thiopental (mg/kg)	Mice				25-50		
	Rats				25-48	40	
	Hamsters				20		
	Guinea pigs				20	55	
	Rabbits				25-50		
	NHP				22-25		
Xylazine (mg/kg)[2]	Rabbit					5	
	NHP					6	

1—Minimal analgesia properties 2—Used in conjunction with Ketamine at sedative level
*Prepared by H.C. Hughes and C.M. Lang, Dept. of Comparative Medicine, The Milton S. Hershey Medical Center, The Pennsylvania State University, Hershey, PA 17033

Appendix 6

Normal Values*

NORMAL VALUES—HEMATOLOGY

	Dog	Cat	Horse	Cow	Pig	Sheep
Erythrocytes:						
RBC $\times 10^6$/ul	6–9(6.8)	5–10(7.5)	7–13(9.5)	5–8(7.0)	5–8(6.5)	8–15(12)
Hemoglobin (g/dl)[1]	12–18(15)	8–15(12)	11–18(15)	8–14(11)	10–16(13)	8–16(12)
PCV (%)[2]	37–54(45)	24–45(37)	32–52(42)	26–42(34)	33–50(45)	24–49(38)
MCV (fl)	60–77(70)	39–55(45)	34–58(46)	40–60(52)	50–67(63)	23–48(33)
MCHC (g/dl)[1]	31–34(33)	31–34(33)	31–37(35)	26–34(31)	30–34(32)	29–35(32)
Leukocytes:†						
Total WBC	6.0–15	5.5–19	6.0–12.5	4.0–12	10–22	4.0–12
Neutrophils	3.0–11.8	2.5–12.5	2.7–6.7	1.5–4.0	3.2–10	1.0–5.6
Lymphocytes	1.5–5.0	2.0–7.0	2.0–5.0	3.0–7.5	4.5–13	2.0–9.0
Monocytes	0.1–0.8	0.1–0.6	0.2–1.0	0.1–.85	0.1–2.0	0.1–0.75
Eosinophils	0.1–0.75	0.1–0.75	0.2–1.5	0.2–1.0	0.2–2.0	0.1–1.0
Basophils	Rare	Rare	Rare	Rare	Rare	Rare
† All values $\times 10^3$						
Platelets $\times 10^5$/ul	2–5	2–7	1–4	2–8	2–5	2–8
Fibrinogen (mg/dl)[3]	100–500	100–300	100–500	300–700	100–300	300–600

[1] These values may be artificially increased by the presence of lipemia, hemolysis, or the presence of large numbers of Heinz bodie.
[2] Packed cell volume may be reduced in samples with excess EDTA.
[3] May be artificially increased with lipemia and hemolysis if plasma protein and fibrinogen are determined using a refractometer.

Prepared by E.H. Coles, Department of Laboratory Medicine, College of Veterinary Medicine, Kansas State University, Manhattan, Kansas 66506.

Serum chemistry (other than enzymes)

Some values were established in the clinical pathology laboratory at Kansas State University and others were taken from the current literature. They are should be used as a guideline. Normals vary from laboratory to laboratory according to the technique used. Veterinarians should obtain normal values for the clinical laboratory assaying their samples.

	Dog	Cat	Horse	Cow	Pig	Sheep
Ammonia (ug/dl)	19–120		13–108			
Bicarbonate (mEq/l)	17–23	17–23	22–34	21–35	17–25	20–27
Bilirubin, Total (mg/dl)	0.1–0.4	0.1–0.4	0.2–0.6	0.0–0.7	0.0–0.2	0.0–0.4
Bilirubin, Direct (mg/dl)	0.0–0.2	0.0–0.2	0.0–0.4	0.0–0.4	0.0–0.1	0.0–0.3
Calcium (mg/dl)	8.4–11.2	8.0–10.4	10.5–12.9	8.0–10.9	11.0–11.3	11.5–13.0
CO_2 Total (mm/l)	18–24	18–24	23–35	22–36	18–26	21–28
CO_2 Pressure (mmHg)	29–42	29–42	38–46	35–44	32–51	32–51
Chloride (mEq/l)	105–115	115–125	98–106	97–111	100–105	98–115
Cholesterol (mg/dl)	130–290	90–105	78–120	71–130	116–119	31–67
Creatinine (mg/sl)	0.5–1.2	0.5–1.2	1.2–1.9	1.0–2.4	1.0–2.7	1.2–1.9
Glucose (mg/dl)[2]	60–100	60–120	70–110	55–110	65–95	50–80
Iron (ug/dl)	94–122	68–215	73–140	57–162	91–199	166–222
Magnesium (mg/dl)	1.7–2.8	1.8–2.7	2.0–3.0	1.7–3.1	1.9–3.9	1.0–2.5
Phosphorus (mg/dl)[1,3]	2.8–5.5	2.5–6.5	2.0–3.9	4.0–7.0	4.0–11.0	4.0–7.0
Potassium (mEq/l)	3.7–5.5	3.5–5.0	2.7–4.4	3.5–5.5	4.9–7.1	4.0–6.0
Protein, Total (g/dl)[1]	6.0–7.7	5.5–8.5	6.1–8.4	6.0–8.9	3.5–6.1	6.0–7.9
Protein, Albumin (g/dl)	2.5–3.7	2.5–3.8	2.7–4.2	2.5–4.0	1.9–2.4	2.4–3.0
Sodium (mEq/l)	139–152	145–160	130–150	130–156	140–160	136–154
Urea Nitrogen (mg/dl)	10–25	10–30	8–24	5–25	8–24	18–31
Uric acid (mg/dl)	0–2	0–1	0.9–1.1	0–2		0–2

Serum Enzymes: (NORMAL VALUES FOR SERUM ENZYMES VARY FROM ONE LABORATORY TO THE NEXT. NORMALS MUST BE ESTABLISHED FOR EACH LABORATORY ACCORDING TO THE TECHNIQUE USED.)

	Dog	Cat	Horse	Cow	Pig	Sheep
Alkaline phosphatase (IU/l)[3]	14–84	10–44	60–320	25–220	80–269	98–278
ALT(GPT) (IU/l)[1]	14–70	10–70	10–30	10–40	22–68	60–84
AST(GOT) (IU/l)[1]	15–50	15–45	100–500	30–110	5–87	22–50
CK (IU/l)	1.2–28.4	7.2–28.2	2.4–23.4	4.8–12.1	2.4–22.5	8.1–12.9
GGT (IU/l)	1.2–6.4	1.3–5.1	4.3–13.4			
LDH (IU/l)[1]	45–233	63–273	162–412	692–1445	380–643	238–440
SDH (IU/l)	2.9–8.2	3.9–7.7	0.5–3.4	8–12	1.0–5.8	5.8–27.9

Abbreviations: ALT = alanine amino transferase (glutamic pyruvic transaminase); AST = alanine aspartate transferase (glutamic oxalacetic transaminase); CK = Creatinine kinase; GGT = gamma glutamyltransferase; LDH = Lactate dehydrogenase; SDH = Sorbitol dehydrogenase (more properly iditol dehydrogenase)

[1] Normals will be altered (most are increased) if hemolysis is present.

[2] Values may be greatly reduced if serum is not separated from RBC as soon as possible after collection. May be avoided if sample is collected in anticoagulant that preserves glucose (sodium fluoride).

[3] Values in young growing animals may be higher than in adults.

CONVERSION OF CONVENTIONAL UNITS TO SI UNITS—BLOOD AND SERUM

Component	*Conventional Units*	× *Factor*	= *Recommended SI Units*
Albumin	g/dl	10	g/L
Ammonia	μg/dl	0.554	μmol/L
Amylase	Somogyi units	1.85	U/L
Base excess	mEq/L	1	mmol/L
Bicarbonate	mmol or mEq/l	1	mmol/L
Bilirubin	mg/dl	17.1	μmol/L
BSP (dog and cat)	Percent retention	0.01	Fraction retention
Calcium	mg/dl	0.25	mmol/L
Carbon dioxide	mM	1	mmol/L
Chloride	mEq/L	1	mmol/L
Cholesterol	mg/dl	0.026	mmol/L
Cholinesterase	IU/L	1	U/L
Cortisol	μg/dl	27.6	mmol/L
Creatine kinase	U/L	1	U/L
Creatinine	mg/dl	88.4	μmol/l
Cr. clearance	ml/min	0.0167	ml/sec
Electrophoresis protein	gm/dl	10	g/L
Fibrinogen	mg/dl	0.01	g/L
Gamma GT	IU/L	1	U/L
Globulins	g/dl	10	g/L
Glucose	mg/dl	0.055	mmol/L
Haptoglobin	mg/dl	0.01	g/L
Hemoglobin	g/dl	10	g/L
Iron binding	μg/dl	0.179	μmol/L
Iron, total	μg/dl	0.179	μmol/L
Lipase	mIU/ml	1	U/L
Lipase	Cherry-Crandall units	278	u/L
Magnesium	mEq/L	0.5	mmol/L
Magnesium	mg/dl	0.41	mmol/L
Osmolality	Osm/Kg	1	mmol/L
Phosphatase, alkaline	IU/L	1	U/L
Phosphorus (inorganic)	mg/dl	0.01	g/L
Potassium	mEq/L	1	mmol/L
Protein, total	g/dl	10	g/L
Sodium	mEq/L	1	mmol/L
T_4 (RIA)	μg/dl	13	mmol/L
Transferases	IU/L	1	U/L
Urea nitrogen	mg/dl	0.357	mmol/L
Uric acid	mg/dl	0.059	mmol/L
Xylose absorption	mg/dl	0.067	mmol/L

Appendix 7

Fundamentals of Prescription Writing

A prescription is an order to a pharmacist written by a licensed medical practitioner to prepare the prescribed medication, to affix the directions, and to sell the preparation to the client or patient. The prescription is a legally recognized document and the writer is held responsible for its accuracy.

To be able to accurately and speedily write prescriptions requires considerable knowledge and practice. The prescription should be written legibly. If a practitioner has poor handwriting, the prescription should be printed or typewritten. The standard prescription blank should have printed on it the name, address, telephone number, and office hours of the doctor prescribing the medication. Space should also be provided for the practitioner to in write his/her DEA registration number. Many doctors avoid printing this number on their prescription blanks in advance, as a safeguard, in the event their forms become lost or stolen. It is also recommended that the statement "Please Label" be printed on the bottom of the form along with directions to the pharmacist concerning refilling the prescription. The former instructs the pharamcist to indicate the name and strength of the drug being prescribed on the container label. In an emergency situation, for example, accidental ingestion of a drug by a small child, such information can be lifesaving. The latter, on the other hand, clearly establishes the practitioners intent regarding subsequent refills, if any. Prescription order blanks bearing the name of a particular pharmacy, drug company or other advertising should be avoided.

At any time a prescription may become a medicolegal document. Therefore, it should be written in ink. It is also a good practice to keep an exact or carbon copy of the prescription for the files. This copy protects the doctor and serves to complete the record of treatment.

Components of Prescriptions. Prescriptions consist of the following:

1. The *date* the prescription was written.
2. The name and address of the owner and patient.
3. The *superscription* Rx is an abbreviation of the Latin word recipe ("take thou"). The stroke after the "R" is believed by some to be an abbreviation, others consider it the ancient invocation of Chaldean physicians to the Roman god Jupiter.
4. The *inscription* lists the names and amounts of drugs to be incorporated in the prescription.
5. The *subscription* gives instructions to the pharmacist. These may be entirely in English or with Latin abbreviations.
6. The *signa* (sig.), also called the transcription, consists of instructions for administration of the medication which the pharmacists is to write on the label.
7. The *signature* of the practitioner.
8. Prescriptions which contain controlled substances must also list the *DEA number* of the veterinarian. (See Appendix 10 for additional information pertaining to DEA numbers).

Language of Prescriptions. Years ago prescriptions were written exclusively in Latin. Today, with the exception of some conventional Latin abbreviations, the use of Latin in such orders has become practically obselete. It is strongly recommended that all prescriptions be written entirely in English. Some frequently used Latin abbreviations and their meanings are:

Latin Derivation	*Abbreviation*	*Meaning*
ad libitum	ad lib.	at pleasure; freely; as much as is wanted
ana	aa	of each
ante cibum	a.c.	before meals
aqua	aqua	water
aqua distillata	aqua distillata	distilled water
bis in die	b.i.d.	twice daily
capsula	caps	capsule
chartula	chart.	powder
cum	c	with
dentur tales doses	d.t.d.	give such doses
gutta, guttae	gtt.	a drop, drops
hora	h.	hour
hora sommi	h.s.	hour of sleep; at bedtime
misce	M	mix
non repetatur	non. rep.	do not repeat
numerus	No.	number
omni die	o.d.	every day
omni hora	o.h.	every hour
oculus dexter	o.d.	right eye
oculus sinistes	o.s.	left eye
os	os.	mouth
pilula	pil.	a pill
post	p	after
post cibum	p.c.	after meals
pro re nata	p.r.n.	according to circumstances; occasionally
quantum sufficit	q.s.	a sufficient amount
quarter in die	q.i.d.	four times a day

semis	ss	one-half
signa	sig.	write on label
sine	s	without
statim	stat	immediately
tabella	tab.	tablet
ter in die	t.i.d.	three times a day
tinctura	Tr.	tincture
unguentum	Ung.	ointment
ut dictum	ut dict.	as directed

Choice of Drug Name. Most drugs can be prescribed by their official names (USP or NF), by their generic names or by the manufacturers' proproprietary (trade) names.

Choice of system of Weights and Measures. Although some drugs are still available in the apothecaries system of weights and measures, the metric system offers a number of advantages and it is greatly preferred by most veterinarians. Consult Appendix 8 for conversion factors and additional information about both systems.

Classes of Prescription Orders. On the basis of the availability of the prescribed medication, prescription orders may be divided into two large classes: extemporaneous (compounded) and precompounded. An extemporaneous prescription is the type in which the veterinarian elects the drugs, doses, and the pharmaceutical forms that he desires and the pharmacist prepares the medication according to his art. The precompounded prescription order is one that calls for a drug or mixture of drugs supplied by a pharmaceutical company by its official or proprietary name in a form that the pharmacist dispenses without pharmaceutical alteration.

Dispensing and Safety Practices. When dispensing drugs, it is important that the veterinarian package the medication in properly labeled containers, preferably those equipped with safety-type closures. The use of such containers is strongly recommended to minimize the risk of accidental ingestion of the medication by young children. Proper labeling should include the name of the patient, name, address & phone number of the veterinarian, name & quantity of the drug dispensed, and specific directions for use of the drug. Stickers *warning* the person administering the drug to "Shake Well Before Using", "Keep Refrigerated" "Keep Away From Children" etc., for example, are readily available and are also recommended when appropriate.

Under no circumstances should drugs be dispensed in plain envelopes or in any other type of unlabeled container!

Appendix 8

Metric System, Apothecary System and Other Convenient Conversion Aids

THE METRIC SYSTEM

Linear Measure

1 millimeter (mm) = 0.04 inch (in)
1 centimeter (cm) = 0.4 in
1 decimeter = 4 in

---

1 inch (in) = 2.54 cm
1 foot (ft) = 30.48 cm
1 yard (yd) = 91.44 cm

To convert inches (in) to millimeters (mm) and centimeters (cm):

⅛ in = 3 mm
¼ in = 6 mm
½ in = 12.5 mm
¾ in = 18 mm
1 in = 2.5 cm
2 in = 5 cm
3 in = 7.5 cm
4 in = 10 cm
5 in = 12.5 cm
6 in = 15 cm
7 in = 17.5 cm
8 in = 20 cm
9 in = 22.5 cm
10 in = 25 cm
11 in = 27.5 cm
12 in = 30 cm

---

10 mm = 1 cm
100 cm = 1 meter (m)
1000 m = 1 kilometer (km)

Volume

1 milliliter (ml) = 1000 microliters
1 liter (l) = 100 ml

To convert liters (l) to ounces (oz), pints (pt), quarts (qt) and gallons (gal):

¼ l = 8½ oz
½ l = 1 pt 1 oz
1 l = 1 qt 2 oz
4 l = 1 gal 7 oz
10 l = 2¾ gal
25 l = 6¾ gal
50 l = 13¼ gal
100 l = 26½ gal

To convert ounces (oz), pints (pt), quarts (qt), and gallons (gal) to milliliters and liters (l):

1 oz = 29.6 ml
2 oz = 59.2 ml
3 oz = 88.8 ml
4 oz = 118.4 ml
5 oz = 148 ml
6 oz = 177.5 ml
7 oz = 207.2 ml
8 oz = 236.8 ml
1 pt = 473.2 ml
1 qt = 946 ml (or 0.946 l)
2 qt = 1.893 l
3 qt = 2.839 l
4 qt = 3.785 l

Weights

1 gamma = 1 microgram (mcg)
1,000 mcg = 1 milligram (mg)
1,000 mg = 1 gram (gm)
1,000 gm = 1 kilogram (kg)
1,000 gm = 1 kg = 2.2 lb

To convert ounces (oz) and pounds (lb) to grams (gm) and kilograms (kg):

1 oz = 28.3 gm
2 oz = 56.7 gm
3 oz = 85 gm
4 oz = 113.3 gm

5 oz	=	141.6 gm
6 oz	=	170 gm
7 oz	=	198.3 gm
8 oz	=	226.6 gm
9 oz	=	254.7 gm
10 oz	=	283.5 gm
11 oz	=	311.8 gm
12 oz	=	340 gm
13 oz	=	367.9 gm
14 oz	=	396.2 gm
15 oz	=	425 gm
(1 lb) 16 oz	=	453.6 gm
1 lb	=	453.6 gm
2 lb	=	907.2 gm
3 lb	=	1.4 kg
4 lb	=	1.8 kg
5 lb	=	2.3 kg
10 lb	=	4.5 kg
50 lb	=	22.7 kg
100 lb	=	45.4 kg
1,000 lb	=	453.6 kg
2,000 lb	=	907.2 kg

Temperature

To convert Centigrade (C) to Fahrenheit (F)

C	= *F*
36	96.8
36.5	97.7
37	98.6
37.5	99.5
38	100.4
38.2	100.8
38.4	101.1
38.6	101.5
38.8	101.8
39	102.2
39.2	102.6
39.4	102.9
39.6	103.3
39.8	103.6
40	104
40.2	104.4
40.4	104.7
40.6	105.1
40.8	105.4
41	105.8
41.2	106.2
41.4	106.6
41.6	106.8
41.8	107.2
42	107.6

Note: To convert degrees F to degrees C, subtract 32, then multiply by 5/9. To convert degrees C to degrees F, multiply by 9/5 then add 32.

Weight

20 grains (gr)	=	1 scruple
3 scruples	=	1 dram
8 drams	=	1 ounce

3 scruples	=	60 gr
1 ounce	=	480 gr
1 lb	=	5,760 gr (=16 oz Avoir.)

Volume

1 fluid dram	=	60 minims (m)
8 fluid dram	=	1 fluid ounce (fl oz)
1 fluid ounce	=	480 m = 8 fl drams
1 pint (pt)	=	7,680 m = 16 fl oz
1 quart (qt)	=	2 pt
1 gallon (gal)	=	4 qt

Approximate equivalents of milligrams (mg) and grains (gr):

0.2 mg	=	1/300 gr
0.3 mg	=	1/200 gr
0.4 mg	=	1/150 gr
0.5 mg	=	1/120 gr
0.6 mg	=	1/100 gr
1 mg	=	1/60 gr
3 mg	=	1/20 gr
6 mg	=	1/10 gr
10 mg	=	1/6 gr
15 mg	=	1/4 gr
25 mg	=	3/8 gr
30 mg	=	1/2 gr
60 mg	=	1 gr
120 mg	=	2 gr
200 mg	=	3 gr
300 mg	=	5 gr
500 mg	=	7½ gr
600 mg	=	10 gr
1,000 mg	=	15 gr

Approximate equivalents of grams (gm) and grains (gr):

0.0002 gm	=	1/300 gr
0.0003 gm	=	1/200 gr
0.0004 gm	=	1/150 gr
0.0005 gm	=	1/120 gr
0.0006 gm	=	1/100 gr
0.001 gm	=	1/60 gr
0.01 gm	=	1/6 gr
0.015 gm	=	1/4 gr
0.025 gm	=	3/8 gr
0.03 gm	=	1/2 gr
0.06 gm	=	1 gr
0.12 gm	=	2 gr
0.2 gm	=	3 gr
0.3 gm	=	5 gr
0.5 gm	=	7½ gr
0.6 gm	=	10 gr
1 gm	=	15 gr

Approximate equivalents of grams (gm), grains (gr) and drams.

4 gm	=	60 gr	=	1 dram
6 gm	=	90 gr	=	1½ drams
10 gm	=	150 gr	=	2½ drams
15 gm	=	240 gr	=	4 drams
30 gm	=	480 gr	=	8 drams (1 oz)

Approximate equivalents of milliliters (ml), minims (m), drams and ounces (oz.)

0.06 ml	=	1 m
0.5 ml	=	8 m
1 ml	=	15 m
4 ml	=	1 fluid dram
30 ml	=	1 fluid oz
250 ml	=	8 fluid oz
500 ml	=	16 fluid oz (pt)
1,000 ml	=	32 fluid oz (qt)

APPROXIMATE HOUSEHOLD MEASURES

1 teaspoonful	=	5 ml (cc)
3 teaspoonfuls	=	1 tablespoonful
1 tablespoonful	=	½ fl oz = 15 ml
1 jigger	=	1½ fl oz = 45 ml
1 cup	=	8 fl oz = 240 ml

CONVENIENT CONVERSION FACTORS

Dosage Forms
To convert dosage forms according to body weight, the following conversion table will provide *approximate* equivalents:

From		*To*
gr/lb × 65	=	mg/lb
gr/lb × 143	=	mg/kg
mg/lb × 0.015	=	gr/lb
mg/lb × 2.2	=	mg/kg
mg/kg × 0.007	=	gr/lb
mg/kg × 0.454	=	mg/lb

Example: A dosage form expressed as 1 gr/5 lb of body weight would be converted to mg/5 as follows: 1 × 65 = 65 mg/5 lb; 65 ÷ 5 = 13 mg/lb of body weight.
To convert lb to gm, multiply number of lb by 453.6.
Example: 5 lb × 453.6 = 2,268 gm.

Percentage & Parts Per Million (PPM)

To convert gm per ton %, multiply number of gm by 11 and move decimal point 5 places to the left.
Example: 100 gm of tetracycline × 11 = 1,100 or 0.011%.
To convert % to gm per ton, divide % by 11 and move decimal 5 places to the right.
Example: 0.011% tetracycline ÷ 11 = 0.001 or 100 gm.
To convert % to parts per million (ppm) move decimal point 4 places to the right.
Example: 0.011% tetracycline = 110 ppm.

Other relationships commonly used are:

10^{-3} gm/kg = 1 milligram/kilogram = 1 ppm

10^{-6} gm/gm = 1 microgram/gram = 1 ppb
10^{-9} gm/gm = 1 nanogram/gram = 1 ppb
10^{-12} gm/gm = picogram/gram = 1 ppt

Weights & Volume

To convert from one unit of measure to another, the following conversion table will provide *approximate* equivalents:

Weights

From		*To*
Grams × 0.03527	=	Ounces (av dp.)
Ounces × 28.349	=	Grams
Pounds × 0.4536	=	Kilograms

Volume

Liters × 1,000	=	Cubic centimeters
Ounces × 0.02957	=	Liters
Quarts × 0.9463	=	Liters
Gallons × 3.785	=	Liters

Electrolytes

To convert mg% (mg per 100 ml) to milliequivalents (mEq) per liter:

$$\frac{\text{mg\%} \times \text{valence} \times 10}{\text{atomic weight}} = \text{mEq per liter}$$

Many electrolytes are now expressed as mEq/liter of fluid. However, some products may still be expressed as gr or mg per 100 ml or 1,000 ml. To obtain mEq/liter, convert values given for product to mg% and use the above formula.

GUIDE TO METRIC PREFIXES

Prefix	*Meaning*
tera	one trillion times
giga	one billion times
mega	one million times
kilo	one thousand times
hecto	one hundred times
deca	ten times
deci	one tenth of
centi	one hundredth of
milli	one thousandth of
micro	one millionth of
nano	one billionth of
pico	one trillionth of

Appendix 9

Certified Regional Poison Control Centers

Information furnished by the American Association of Poison Control Centers. For information on animal poisonings contact:

National Animal Poison Control Center
University of Illinois
College of Veterinary Medicine
Department of Veterinary Sciences
2001 South Lincoln Avenue
Urbana, Illinois 61801
(217) 333-3611

ALABAMA

Tuscaloosa
Alabama Poison Center
809 University Boulevard, East
Tuscaloosa, AL 35401
(205) 345-0600 (Administrative)
(800) 462-0800 (Alabama only)

ARIZONA

Tucson
Arizona Poison and Drug Information Center
Arizona Health Sciences Center
Room 3204K
University of Arizona
Tucson, AR 85724
(602) 626-6016
(800) 362-0101 (Arizona only)

CALIFORNIA

Los Angeles
Los Angeles County Medical Association
Regional Poison Information Center
1925 Wilshire Boulevard
Los Angeles, CA 90057
(213) 484-5151
Sacramento
University of California Davis Medical Center
Regional Poison Control Center
2315 Stockton Boulevard
Sacramento, CA 95817
(916) 453-3414
San Diego
San Diego Regional Poison Center
University of California Medical Center
225 Dickinson Street, H925
San Diego, CA 92103
(619) 294-6000 (Emergency)
(619) 294-3666 (Administrative)
San Francisco
San Francisco Bay Area
Regional Poison Center
1E86, San Francisco General Hospital
1001 Potrero Avenue
San Francisco, CA 94110
(415) 666-2845
(800) 233-3360

COLORADO

Denver
Rocky Mountain Poison Center
645 Bannock Street
Denver, CO 80204-4507
(303) 893-7774

DISTRICT OF COLUMBIA

Washington, D.C.
National Capital Poison Center
3800 Reservoir Road, NW
Washington, D.C. 20007
(202) 625-3333

FLORIDA

Tampa
Tampa Bay Regional Poison Control Center
P.O. Box 18582
Tampa, FL 33679
(813) 251-6995
(800) 282-3171

GEORGIA

Atlanta
Georgia Poison Control Center
Grady Memorial Hospital
Box 26066
80 Butler Street, SE
Atlanta, GA 30335
(404) 589-4400

ILLINOIS

Springfield
Central and Southern Illinois
Poison Resource Center
St. John's Hospital
800 East Carpenter Street
Springfield, IL 62769
(217) 753-3330
(800) 252-2022

INDIANA

Indianapolis
Indiana Poison Center
1001 West Tenth Street
Indianapolis, IN 46202
(317) 630-7351
(800) 382-9097
(317) 630-6382 (Administrative)

IOWA

Iowa City
University of Iowa Hospitals and Clinics
Poison Control Center
Pharmacy Department
Iowa City, IA 52242
(319) 356-2922

KENTUCKY

Louisville
Kentucky Regional Poison Center of Kosair Children's Hospital
P.O. Box 35070
Louisville, KY 40232
(502) 562-7270
(800) 722-5725

LOUISIANA

Shreveport
Louisiana Regional Poison Control Center
1501 Kings Highway
P.O. Box 33932
Shreveport, LA 71130
(318) 425-1524
(800) 535-0525

MARYLAND

Baltimore
Maryland Poison Center
20 North Pine Street
Baltimore, MD 21201
(301) 528-7701

MICHIGAN

Detroit
Poison Control Center
Children's Hospital of Michigan
3901 Beaubien Boulevard
Detroit, MI 48201
(313) 494-5711
Grand Rapids
Blodgett Regional Poison Center
Blodgett Memorial Medical Center
1840 Wealthy Street, SE
Grand Rapids, MI 49506
(800) 442-4571 (AC 616 only)
(800) 632-2727 (Michigan only)

MINNESOTA

Minneapolis
Hennepin Poison Center
701 Park
Minneapolis, MN 55415
(612) 347-3141
St. Paul
Minnesota Poison Control System
640 Jackson Street
St. Paul, MN 55101
(612) 221-2113
(800) 222-1222

MISSOURI

St. Louis
Cardinal Glennon Children's Hospital
Regional Poison Center
1465 South Grand Avenue
St. Louis, MO 63104
(314) 772-5200

NEBRASKA

Omaha
Mid Plains Poison Control Center
Children's Memorial Hospital
8301 Dodge Street
Omaha, NE 68114
(402) 390-5434
(800) 642-9999

NEW JERSEY

New Jersey Poison Information and Education System
201 Lyons Avenue
Newark, NY 07112
(201) 926-8005
(800) 962-1253 (New Jersey only)
(201) 926-8008 (TTY/TTD only)

NEW MEXICO

Albuquerque
New Mexico Poison and Drug Information Center
University of New Mexico
Albuquerque, NM 87131
(505) 843-2551
(800) 432-6866

NEW YORK

East Meadow
Nassau County Medical Center's Long Island
Regional Poison Control Center
2201 Hempstead Turnpike
East Meadow, NY 11554
(516) 542-2323
New York
New York City Poison Center
455 First Avenue, Room 123
New York, NY 10016
(212) 340-4494

NORTH CAROLINA

Durham
Duke Poison Control Center
Box 3007
Duke University Medical Center
Durham, NC 27710
(919) 684-8111
(800) 672-1697 (North Carolina only)

OHIO

Cincinnati
Southwest Ohio Regional Poison Control System
Drug and Poison Information Center
University of Cincinnati College of Medicine
231 Bethesda Avenue ML 144
Cincinnati, OH 45267-0144
(513) 872-5111

Columbus
Central Ohio Poison Control Center
700 Children's Drive
Columbus, OH 43205
(614) 461-2012
(614) 228-1323

PENNSYLVANIA

Pittsburgh
Pittsburgh Poison Center
125 DeSoto Street
Pittsburgh, PA 15213
(412) 647-5600

UTAH

Salt Lake City
Intermountain Regional Poison Control Center
50 North Medical Drive, Building 428
Salt Lake City, UT 84132
(801) 581-2151

WASHINGTON

Seattle
Seattle Poison Center
Children's Orthopedic Hospital and Medical Center
Box 5371
4800 Sand Point Way, NE
Seattle, WA 98105
(206) 526-2121

Appendix 10

Information Regarding Registration with the Drug Enforcement Administration

This information was obtained from the Drug Enforcement Administration of the U.S. Department of Justice. For additional information, the veterinarian is also directed to Public Law 91-513, 91st Congress, H.R. 18583, October 27, 1970.

REGISTRATION:

United States Department of Justice
Drug Enforcement Administration
P.O. Box 28083, Central Station
Washington, D.C. 20005

Persons Required to Register

Every person who (1) manufactures, imports, distributes, dispenses, prescribes or administers any controlled substance, or who proposes to engage in the manufacture, importation, distribution, dispensing, prescribing, or administering of any controlled substance, or who (2) exports or proposes to engage in the exportation of controlled substances listed in Schedules I through IV, shall obtain annually a registration unless exempted by law or 21 CFR 1301.24-1301.29. Only persons actually engaged in such activities are required to obtain a registration; related or affiliated persons who are not engaged in such activities are not required to be registered. (For example, a stockholder or parent corporation of a corporation manufacturing controlled substances is not required to obtain a registration.)

Separate Registration for Independent Activities

(a) The following ten groups of activities are deemed to be independent of each other:

(1) Manufacturing (including repackaging and relabeling) controlled substances;

(2) Distributing controlled substances;

(3) Dispensing controlled substances listed in schedules II through V;

(4) Conducting research (other than research described in subparagraph (6) of this paragraph) with controlled substances listed in schedules II through V;

(5) Conducting instructional activities with controlled substances listed in schedules II through V;

(6) Conducting a narcotic treatment program using any narcotic drug listed in Schedules II, III, IV or V, however, pursuant to § 1301.24, employees, agents, or affiliated practitioners, in programs, need not register separately. Each program site located away from the principal location and at which place narcotic drugs are stored or dispensed must be separately registered and obtain narcotic drugs by use of order forms pursuant to § 1305.03;

(7) Conducting research and instructional activities with controlled substances listed in schedule I;

(8) Conducting chemical analysis with controlled substances listed in any schedule;

(9) Importing controlled substances; and

(10) Exporting controlled substances listed in schedules I through IV.

(The term "exporter" includes every person who exports, or who acts as an export broker for exportation of, controlled substances listed in schedules I through IV. The term "importer" includes every person who imports, or who acts as an import broker for importation of, controlled substances listed in any schedule.)

(b) Every person who engages in more than one group of independent activities shall obtain a separate registration for each group of activities, except as provided in this paragraph. Any person, when registered to engage in the group of activities described in each subparagraph in this paragraph, shall be authorized to engage in the coincident activities described in that subparagraph without obtaining a registration to engage in such coincident activities, provided that, unless specifically exempted he complies with all requirements and duties prescribed by law for persons registered to engage in such coincident activities.

(1) A person registered to manufacture or import any controlled substance or basic class of controlled substance shall be authorized to distribute that substance or class, but no other substance or class which he is not registered to manufacture or import;

(2) A person registered to manufacture any controlled substance listed in schedules II through V shall be authorized to conduct chemical analysis and preclinical research (including quality control analysis) with narcotic and nonnarcotic controlled substances listed in those schedules in which he is authorized to manufacture;

(3) A person registered to conduct research with a basic class of controlled substance listed in schedule I shall be authorized to manufacture or import such class if and to the extent that such manufacture is set forth in the research protocol filed with the application for registration, and to distribute such class to other persons registered or authorized to conduct research with such class or registered or authorized to conduct chemical analysis with controlled substances;

(4) A person registered or authorized to conduct chemical analysis with controlled substances shall be authorized to manufacture and import such substances for analytical or instructional purposes, to distribute such substances to other persons registered or authorized to conduct chemical analysis or instructional activities or research with such substances and to persons exempted from registration pursuant to 1301.26, to export such substances to persons in other countries performing chemical analysis or enforcing laws relating to controlled substances or drugs in those countries, and to conduct instructional activities with controlled substances; and

(5) A person registered or authorized to conduct research (other than research described in paragraph (a)(6) above) with controlled substances listed in schedules II through V shall be authorized to conduct chemical analysis with controlled substances listed in those schedules in which he is authorized to conduct research, to manufacture such substances if and to the extent that such manufacture is set forth in a statement filed with the application for registration to import such substances for research purposes to distribute such substances to other persons registered or authorized to conduct chemical analysis, instructional activities, or research with, such substances and to persons exempted from registration pursuant to 1301.26 and to conduct instructional activities with controlled substances;

(6) A person registered to dispense controlled substances listed in schedules II through V shall be authorized to conduct research (other than research described in paragraph (a)(6) of this section) and to conduct instructional activities with those substances.

(c) A single registration to engage in any group of independent activities may include one or more controlled substances listed in the schedules authorized in that group of independent activities. A person registered to conduct research with controlled substances listed in schedule I may conduct research with any substance listed in schedule I for which he has filed and has approved a research protocol.

Separate Registrations for Separate Locations

(a) A separate registration is required for each principal place of business or professional practice at one general physical location where controlled substances are manufactured, distributed, or dispensed by a person.

(b) The following locations shall be deemed not to be places where controlled substances are manufactured, distributed, or dispensed:

(1) A warehouse where controlled substances are stored by or on behalf of a registered person, unless such substances are distributed directly from such warehouse to registered locations other than the registered location from which the substances were delivered or to persons not required to register by virtue of subsection 302(c)(2) of the CSA (21 U.S.C. 822(c)(2);

(2) An office used by agents of a registrant where sales of controlled substances are solicited, made, or supervised but which neither contains such substances (other than substances for display purposes or lawful distribution as samples only) nor serves as a distribution point for filling sales orders; and

(3) An office used by a practitioner (who is registered at another location) where controlled substances are prescribed but neither administered nor otherwise dispensed as a regular part of the professional practice of the practitioner at such office, and where no supplies of controlled substances are maintained.

Exemption of agents and employees; affiliated practitioners

(a) The requirement of registration is waived for any agent or employee of a person who is registered to engage in any group of independent activities, if such agent or employee is acting in the usual course of his business or employment.

(b) An individual practitioner, as defined in § 1304.02 of this chapter (other than an intern, resident, foreign-trained physician, or physician on the staff of a Veterans Administration facility or physician who is an agent or employee of the Health Bureau of the Canal Zone Government), who is an agent or employee of another practitioner registered to dispense controlled substances may, when acting in the usual course of his employment, administer and dispense (other than by issuance of prescription) controlled substances if and to the extent that such individual practitioner is authorized or permitted to do so by the jurisdiction in which he practices, under the registration of the employer or principal practitioner in lieu of being registered himself. (For example, a pharmacist employed by a pharmacy need not be registered individually to fill a prescription for controlled substances if a pharmacy is so registered.)

(c) An individual practitioner, as defined in § 1304.02 of this chapter, who is an intern, resident, or foreign-trained physician or physician on the staff of a Veterans Administration facility or physician who is an agent or employee of the Health Bureau of the Canal Zone Government, may dispense, administer and prescribe controlled substances under the registration of the hospital or other institution which is registered and by whom he is employed in lieu of being registered himself, provided that:

(1) Such dispensing, administering or prescribing is done in the usual course of his professional practice;

(2) Such individual practitioner is authorized or permitted to do so by the jurisdiction in which he is practicing:

(3) The hospital or other institution by whom he is employed has vertified that the individual practitioner is so permitted to dispense, administer, or prescribe drugs within the jurisdiction;

(4) Such individual practitioner is acting only within the scope of his employment in the hospital or institution;

(5) The hospital or other institution authorizes the intern, resident, or foreign-trained physician to dispense or prescribe under the hospital registration and designates a specific internal code number for each intern, resident, or foreign-trained physician so authorized. The code number shall consist of numbers, letters, or a combination thereof and shall be a suffix to the institution's DEA registration number, preceeded by a hyphen (e.g., APO 123456-10 or APO 123456-A12); and

(6) A current list of internal codes and the corresponding individual practitioners is kept by the hospital or other institution and is made available at all times to other registrants and law enforcement agencies upon request for the purpose of verifying the authority of the prescribing individual practitioner.

[36 FR 18728, Sept. 21, 1971, as amended at 37 FR 15918, Aug. 8, 1872]

Application forms; contents; signature

(a) If any person is required to be registered, and is not so registered and is applying for registration:

(1) To manufacture or distribute controlled substances, he shall apply on DEA Form 225;

(2) To dispense controlled substances listed in schedules II through V, he shall apply on DEA Form 224;

(3) To conduct instructional activities with controlled substances listed in schedules II through V, he shall apply on DEA Form 224;

(4) To conduct research with controlled substances listed in schedules II through V (other than research described in §§ 1301.22(a)(6), he shall apply on DEA Form 225;

(5) To conduct research with narcotic drugs listed in schedules II through V, as described in § 1301.22(a)(6), he shall apply on DEA (or BND) Form 225;

(6) To conduct research with controlled substances listed in schedule I, he shall apply on DEA (or BND) Form 225, with three copies of a research protocol as described in § 1301.33(a) attached to the form, or, in the case of a clinical investigation, with three copies of a certificate of submission of an IND as described in § 1301.33(b) attached to the form (the researcher also submitting to the Food and Drug Administration three copies of a Notice of Claimed Investigational Exemption for a New Drug as required in § 1301.33(b));

(7) To conduct instructional activities with controlled substances listed in schedule I, he shall apply as a researcher on BND Form 225 with two copies of a statement describing the nature, extent, and duration of such instructional activities attached to the form; and

(8) To conduct chemical analysis with controlled substances listed in any schedule, he shall apply on DEA (or BND) Form 225.

(9) To conduct a narcotic treatment program, including a compounder, shall apply on DEA Form 363.

Each application for registration to handle any basic class of controlled substance listed in schedule I (except to conduct chemical analysis with such classes), and each application for registration to manufacture a basic class of controlled substance listed to schedule II, or to conduct research with any narcotic controlled substance listed in schedule II, shall include the Bureau Controlled Substances Code Number for each basic class or substance to be covered by such registration.

Each application shall include all information called for in the form, unless the item is not applicable, in which case this fact shall be indicated.

Each application, attachment, or other document filed as part of an application, shall be signed by the applicant, if an individual; by a partner of the applicant, if a partnership; or by an officer of the applicant, if a corporation, corporate division, association, trust or other entity. An applicant may authorize one or more individuals, who would not otherwise be authorized to do so, to sign applications for the applicant by filing with the Registration Branch of the Bureau a power of attorney on DEA Form 231a for each such individual. The power of attorney shall be signed by a person who is authorized to sign application under this paragraph and shall contain the signature of the individual being authorized to sign applications. The power of attorney shall be valid until revoked by the applicant.

Acceptance for Filing; Defective Applications; Inspection

If found to be complete, the application will be accepted for filing. A defective application will be returned to the applicant within 10 days following its receipt with a statement of the reason for not accepting the application for filing. A defective application may be corrected and resubmitted for filing at any time. Accepting an application for filing has no bearing on whether the application will be granted. An application may be amended or withdrawn after filing. The Director may inspect, or cause to be inspected, the establishment of an applicant or registrant.

Certificate of Registration; Denial of Registration

The Administrator shall issue a Certificate of Registration (DEA Form 223) to an applicant if the issuance of registration is required under the applicable provisions of section 303 of the Act (21 USC 823). In the event that the issuance of registration or reregistration is not required, the Admin. shall deny the application. Before denying any application, the Admin. shall issue an order to show cause and, if requested by the applicant, shall hold a hearing on the application.

For each registration or re-registration to manufacture controlled substances, the registant shall pay a fee $250.

For each registration or re-registration to distribute controlled substances, the registrant shall pay a fee of $125.

For each registration or re-registration to dispense, or to conduct research or instructional activities with, controlled substances listed in schedules II through V, the registrant shall pay a fee of $20.

For each registration or re-registration to conduct research or instructional activities with a controlled substance listed in schedule I, the registrant shall pay a fee of $20.

For each registration or re-registration to conduct chemical analysis with controlled substances listed in any schedule, the registrant shall pay a fee of $20.

For each registration or re-registration import controlled substances, the registrant shall pay a fee of $125.

For each registration or re-registration to export controlled substances, the registrant shall pay a fee of $125.

Time and Method of Payment; Refund

Registration and re-registration fees shall be paid at the time when the application for registration or re-registration is submitted for filing. Payment should be made in the form of a personal, certified or cashier's check or money order made payable to "Drug Enforcement Administration (DEA)." Payments made in the form of stamps, foreign currency, or third party endorsed checks will not be accepted. In the event that the application is not accepted for filing or is denied, the payment shall be refunded to the applicant.

Persons Exempt from Fee

(a) The Administrator shall exempt from payment of a fee for registration or re-registration the following persons:

(1) Any official or agency of the U.S. Army, Navy, Marine Corps, Air Force, Coast Guard, Veterans' Administration, Public Health Service, or Bureau of Prisons who or which is authorized to procure or purchase controlled substances for official use; and

(2) Any official, employee or other civil officer or agency of the United States, of any State, or any political subdivision or agency thereof, who or which is authorized to purchase controlled substances, to obtain such substances from official stocks, to dispense or administer such substances, to conduct research, instructional activities, or chemical analysis with such substances, or any combination thereof, in the course of his or its official duties or employment.

(b) In order to claim exemption from payment of a registration or re-registration fee, the registrant shall have completed the certification on the appropriate application form, wherein the registrant's superior (if an individual) or officer (if an agency) certifies to the status and address of the registrant and to the authority of the registrant to acquire, possess, or handle controlled substances.

(c) Important: Exemption from payment of a registration or re-registration fee does not relieve the registrant of any other requirements of duties prescribed by law.

Modification in Registration

Any registrant may apply to modify his registration to authorize the handling of additional controlled substances by submitting a letter of request to the United States Department of Justice, Drug Enforcement Administration, P.O. Box 28083, Central Station, Washington, D.C. 20005. The letter shall contain the registrant's name, address, registration number, and the substances and/or schedules to be added to his registration, and shall be signed by the same person who signed the most recent application for registration or re-registration. If the registrant is seeking to handle additional controlled substances listed in schedule I for the purpose of research or instructional activities, he shall attach three copies of a research protocol describing each research project involving the additional substances, or two copies of a statement describing the nature, extent, and duration of such instructional activities, as appropriate. No fee shall be required to be paid for the modification. The request for modification shall be handled in the same manner as an application for registration.

Termination of Registration

The registration of any person shall terminate if and when such person dies, ceases legal existence, discontinues business or professional practice. Any registrant who ceases legal existence, discontinues business or professional practice, shall notify the Director promptly of such fact.

Transfer of Registration

No registration or any authority conferred thereby shall be assigned or otherwise transferred except upon such conditions as the Administrator may specifically designate and then only pursuant to his written consent.

INVENTORY REQUIREMENTS:

Every registrant, other than an "individual practitioner" (definition and further explanation is stated below), shall on the day he is first registered and every two years thereafter, make a complete and accurate record of all stocks of controlled substances, on hand. The record must:

a. Indicate the date on which the inventory was taken and whether taken at close or opening of business.

b. Be signed by the person responsible for taking the inventory.

c. Be maintained at the location appearing on the registration for at least two years.

A registered individual practitioner is not required to keep records with respect to narcotic controlled substances listed in schedules II through V which he prescribes or administers in the lawful course of his professional practice; he shall keep records, however, with respect to such substances that he dispenses other than by prescribing or administering. A registered individual practitioner is not required to keep records with respect to nonnarcotic controlled substances listed in schedules II through V which he dispenses in any manner unless he regularly charges his patients, either separately or together with charges for other professional services, for such substances so dispensed (e.g., when he substitutes his services for those of a pharmacist).

The term "individual practitioner" means a physician, dentist, veterinarian, or other individual licensed, registered, or otherwise permitted by the United States or the jurisdiction in which he practices, to dispense a controlled substance in the course of professional practice, but does not include a pharmacist; a pharmacy, or an institutional practitioner.

Records Required

Every registrant required to keep records pursuant to 21 CFR 1304.03 shall maintain on a current basis a complete and accurate record of every controlled substance which is manufactured, imported, received, sold, delivered, exported or otherwise disposed of by him. As a general rule these records must contain the following for each transaction:

a. Full name or "brand" name, strength and form of substance(s). (Example: Dextroamphetamine 15 mg plus Amobarbital 60 mg capsules or "RAINBOW #2" R.Tm. capsules.)

b. Actual date of distribution, dispensing, receipt, etc. (an invoice date is not sufficient if it is not the actual date of the receipt, distribution, etc.)

c. Quantity received, sold, dispensed, or otherwise disposed of. (Example: 3 × 50 capsule bottles).

d. Name and address, (registration number, if applicable) of the person to whom the substance was sold, dispensed, etc., or from whom received, etc.

For more specific details, see 21 CFR, Part 1304. Records and Reports of Registrants; 21 CFR, Part 1305—Order Forms; and 21 CFR 1306—Prescriptions.

Copies of the "Comprehensive Drug Abuse Prevention and Control Act of 1970" (P.L. 91-513) and the regulations promulgated under this law can be obtained from the Superintendent of Documents, U.S. Government Printing Office, Washington, D.C. 20402 at a nominal cost.

SCHEDULES OF CONTROLLED SUBSTANCES

(Public Law 91-513)

ESTABLISHMENT

Sec. 202 (A) There are established five schedules of controlled substances, to be known as schedules I, II, III, IV, and V. Such schedules shall initially consist of the substances listed in this section. The schedules established by this section shall be updated and republished on a semiannual basis during the two-year period beginning one year after the date of enactment of this title and shall be updated and republished on an annual basis thereafter.

Placement on Schedules, Findings Required

(b) Except where control is required by United States obligations under an international treaty, convention, or protocol, in effect on the effective date of this part, and except in the case of an immediate precursor, a drug or other substance may not be placed in any schedule unless the findings required for such schedule are made with respect to such drug or other substance. The findings required for each of the schedules are as follows:

(1) Schedule I

(A) The drug or other substance has a high potential for abuse.

(B) The drug or other substance has no currently accepted medical use in treatment in the United States.

(C) There is a lack of accepted safety for use of the drug or other substance under medical supervision.

(2) Schedule II

(A) The drug or other substance has a high potential for abuse.

(B) The drug or other substance has a currently accepted medical use in treatment in the United States or a currently accepted medical use with severe restrictions.

(C) Abuse of the drug or other substances may lead to severe psychological or physicial dependence.

(3) Schedule III

(A) The drug or other substance has a potential for abuse less than the drugs or other substances in schedules I and II.

(B) The drug or other substance has a currently accepted medical use in treatment in the United States.

(C) Abuse of the drug or other substance may lead to moderate or low physical dependence or high psychological dependence.

(4) Schedule IV

(A) The drug or other substance has a low potential for abuse relative to the drugs or other substances in schedule III.

(B) The drug or other substance has a currently accepted medical use in treatment in the United States.

(C) Abuse of the drug or other substance may lead to limited physical dependence or psychological dependence relative to the drugs or other substance in schedule III.

(5) Schedule V

(A) The drug or other substance has a low potential for abuse relative to the drugs or other substances in schedule IV.

(B) The drug or other substance has a currently accepted medical use in treatment in the United States.

(C) Abuse of the drug or other substance may lead to limited physical dependence or psychological dependence relative to the drugs or other substances in schedule IV.

(c) Schedules I, II, III, IV, and V shall, unless and until amended pursuant to section 201, consist of the following drugs or other substances, by whatever official name, common or usual name, chemical name, or brand name designated.

SCHEDULE I

Opiates

(a) Unless specifically excepted or unless listed in another schedule, any of the following opiates, including their isomers, esters, ethers, salts, and salts of isomers, esters, ethers, and salts is possible within the specific chemical designation:

(1) Acetylmethadol
(2) Alfentanil
(3) Allylprodine
(4) Alphacetylmethadol
(5) Alphameprodine
(6) Alphamethadol
(7) Alpha-methylfentanyl (N-[1-(alpha-methy-beta-phenyl) ethyl-4-piperidyl] propionanilide; 1-(1-methyl-2-phenylethyl)-4-(N-propanilido) piperidine)
(8) Benzethidine
(9) Betacetylmethadol
(10) Betameprodine
(11) Betamethadol
(12) Betaprodine
(13) Clonitazene
(14) Dextromoramide
(15) Diampromide
(16) Diethylthiambutene
(17) Difenoxin
(18) Dimenoxadol
(19) Dimepheptanol
(20) Dimethylthiambutene
(21) Dioxaphetyl butyrate
(22) Dipipanone
(23) Ethylmethylthiambutene
(24) Etonitazene
(25) Etoxeridine
(26) Furethidine
(27) Hydroxypethidine
(28) Ketobemidone
(29) Levomoramide
(30) Levophenacylmorphan
(31) Morpheridine
(32) Noracymethadol
(33) Norlevorphanol
(34) Normethadone
(35) Norpipanone
(36) Phenadoxone
(37) Phenampromide
(38) Phenomorphan
(39) Phenoperidine
(40) Piritramide
(41) Proheptazine
(42) Properidine
(43) Propiram
(44) Racemoramide
(45) Tilidine
(46) Trimeperidine

Opium Derivatives

(b) Unless specifically excepted or unless listed in another schedule, any of the following opium derivatives, their salts, isomers, and salts of isomers whenever the existence of such salts, isomers, and salts of isomers is possible within the specific chemical designation:

(1) Acetorphine
(2) Acetyldihydrocodeine
(3) Benzylmorphine
(4) Codeine methylbromide
(5) Codeine-N-Oxide
(6) Cyprenorphine
(7) Desomorphine
(8) Dihydromorphine
(9) Drotebanol
(10) Etorphine
(11) Heroin
(12) Hydromorphinol
(13) Methyldesorphine
(14) Methyldihydromorphine
(15) Morphine methylbromide
(16) Morphine methylsulfonate
(17) Morphine-N-Oxide
(18) Myrophine
(19) Nicocodeine
(20) Nicomorphine
(21) Normorphine
(22) Pholcodine
(23) Thebacon

Hallucinogenic Substances

(c) Unless specifically excepted or unless listed in another schedule, any material, compound, mixture, or preparation, which contains any quantity of the following hallucinogenic substances, or which contains any of their salts, isomers and salts of isomers whenever the existence of such salts, isomers, and salts of isomers is possible within the specific chemical designation.

(1) 4-bromo-2.5-dimethoxy-amphetamine
Some trade or other names 4-bromo-2.5-dimethoxy-a-methyphenethylamine; 4-bromo-2.5-DMA.
(2) 2.5-dimethoxyamphetamine
Some trade or other names: 2.5-dimethoxy-a-methylphenethylamine; 2.5-DMA.
(3) 4-methoxyamphetamine
Some trade or other names: 4-methoxy-a-methylphenethylamine; paramethoxyamphetamine, PMA.
(4) 5-methoxy-3,4-methylenedioxy-amphetamine.
(5) 4-methyl-2.5-dimethoxy-amphetamine
Some trade and other names: 4-methyl-2.5-dimethoxy-a-methylphenethylamine; "DOM"; and "STP"
(6) 3,4 methylenedioxy amphetamine
(7) 3,4,5-trimethoxy amtpetamine
(8) Bufotenine
Some trade and other names: 3-(B-Dimethylaminoethyl)-5-hydroxyindole; 3-(2-dimethylaminoethyl)-5-indolol; N,N-dimethylserotonin; 5-hydroxy-N,N-dimethyltryptamine; mappine.
(9) Diethyltryptamine
Some trade and other names: N,N-Diethyltryptamine; DET.
(10) Dimethyltryptamine
Some trade and other names: DMT.
(11) Ibogaine
Some trade and other names: 7-Ethyl-6,6B,7,8,9,10,12,13-octahydro-2-methoxy-6,9-methano-5H-pyrido [1', 2':1,2] azepino [5,4-b] indole; tabernanthe iboga.
(12) Lysergic acid diethylamide
(13) Marihuana
(14) Mescaline
(15) Parahexyl-7374; some trade and other names: 3-Hexyl-1-hydroxy, 7,8,9,10-tetrahydro-

6,6,9-trimethyl-6H-dibenzo [b,d] pyran; Synhexyl.

(16) Peyote

Meaning all parts of the plant presently classified botanically as *Lophophora Williamsii Lemaire*, whether growing or not, the seeds thereof, any extract from any part of such plant, and every compound, manufacture, salts, derivative, mixture, or preparation of such plant, its seeds or extracts.

(interprets 21 USC 812 (c), Schedule I(c)(12)

(17) N-ethyl-3-piperidyl benzilate

(18) N-methyl-3-piperidyl benzilate

(19) Psilocybin

(20) Psilocyn

(21) Tetrahydrocannabinols

Synthetic equivalents of the substances contained in the plant, or in the resinous extractives of Cannibis, sp. and/or synthetic substances, derivatives, and their isomers with similar chemical structure and phamacological activity such as the following:

◇1 cis or trans tetrahydrocannabinol, and their optical isomers.

◇6 cis or trans tetrahydrocannabinol, and their optical isomers.

◇3.4 cis or trans tetrahydrocannabinol, and its optical isomers.

(Since nomenclature of these substances is not internationally standardized, compounds of these structures, regardless of numerical designation of atomic positions covered.)

(22) Ethlamine analog of phencyclidine

Some trade or other names: N-ethyl-1-phenylcyclohexylamine, (1-phenycyclohexyl) ethylamine, N-(1-phenylcyclohexyl) ethylamine, cyclohexamine, PCE

(23) Pyrrolidine analog of phencyclidine

Some trade or other names: 1(1-phenylcyclohexyl)-pyrrolodine, PCPy, PHP

(24) Thiophene Analog of Phencyclidine

Some trade or other names: 1-[1-(2-thienyl) cyclohexyl] piperidine; 2-Thienylanalog of Phencyclidine; TPCP, TCP.

(d) *Depressants.* Unless specifically excepted or unless listed in another schedule, any material compound, mixture, or preparation which contains any quantity of the following substances having a depressant effect on the central nervous system, including it salts, isomers, and salts of isomers whenever the existence of such salts, isomers, and salts of isomers is possible within the specific chemical designation:

(1) mecloqualone

(2) methaqualone

(e) Stimulants. Unless specifically excepted or unless listed in another schedule, any material, compound, mixture, or preparation which contains any quantity of the following substances having a stimulant effect on the central nervous system, including its salts, isomers, and salts of isomers:

(1) Fenethylline

(2) N-ethylamphetamine

SCHEDULE II

Substances, Vegetable Origin or Chemical Synthesis

(a) Unless specifically excepted or unless listed in another schedule, any of the following substances whether produced directly or indirectly by extraction from substances of vegetable origin, or independently by means of chemical synthesis, or by a combination of extraction and chemical synthesis:

(1) Opium and opiate, and any salt, compound, derivative, or preparation of opium or opiate, excluding apomorphine, dextrophan, nalbuphine, nalaxone, and naltrexone, and their respective salts, but including the following:

Raw opium
Opium extracts
Opium fluid extracts
Powdered opium
Granulated opium
Tincture of opium
Codeine
Ethylmorphine
Etorphine Hydrochloride
Hydrocodone
Hydromorphone
Metopon
Morphine
Oxycodone
Oxymorphone
Thebaine

(2) Any salt, compound, derivative, or preparation thereof which is chemically equivalent or identical with any of the substances referred to in clause (1), except that these substances shall not include the isoquinoline alkaloids of opium.

(3) Opium poppy and poppy straw.

(4) Coca leaves and any salt, compound, derivative, or preparation of coca leaves, and any salt, compound, derivative, or preparation thereof which is chemically equivalent or identical with any of these substances, except that the substances shall not include decocainized coca leaves or extraction of coca leaves, which extractions do not contain cocaine or ecgonine.

Opiates

(b) Unless specifically excepted or unless in another schedule, any of the following opiates, including their isomers, esters, ethers, salts, and salts of iosomers, esters, and ethers, whenever the existence of such isomers, esters, ethers, and salts is possible within a specific chemical designation.

(1) Alphaprodine

(2) Anileridine

(3) Bezitramide

(4) Bulk dextropropoxyphene (non-dosage forms)

(5) Dihydrocodeine

(6) Diphenoxylate

(7) Fentanyl

(8) Isomethadone

(9) Levomethorphan

(10) Levorphanol

(11) Metazocine

(12) Methadone

(13) Methadone-Intermediate, 4-cyano-2-dimethylamino-4, 4-diphenyl butane
(14) Moramide-Intermediate, 2-methyl-3-morpholino-1,1-diphenylpropane-carboxylic acid
(15) Pethidine (Meperidine)
(16) Pethidine-Intermediate-A-4-cyano-1-methyl-4-phenylpiperidine
(17) Pethidine-Intermediate-B, ethyl-4-phenylpiperidine-4-carboxylate
(18) Pethidine-Intermediate-C, 1-methyl-4-phenylpiperidine-4-carboxylic acid
(19) Phenazocine
(20) Piminodine
(21) Racemethorphan
(22) Racemorphan
(23) Sufentanil

Stimulants

(c) Unless specifically excepted or unless listed in another schedule, any material, compound, mixture, or preparation which contains any quantity of the following substances having a stimulant effect on the central nervous system:
(1) Amphetamine, its salts, optical isomers, and salts of its optical isomers.
(2) Any substance which contains any quantity of methamphetamine, including its salts, isomers, and salts of isomers.
(3) Phenmetrazine and its salts.
(4) Methylphenidate.

(e) Depressants. Unless specifically excepted or unless listed in another schedule, any material, compound, mixture, or preparation which contains any quantity of the following substances having a depressant effect on the central nervous system, including its salts, isomers, and salts of isomers whenever the existence of such salts, isomers, and salts of isomers is possible within the specific chemical designation:
(1) Amobarbital
(2) Pentobarbital
(3) Phencyclidine
(4) Secobarbital

(f) Immediate precursors. Unless specifically excepted or unless listed in another schedule, any material, compound, mixture, or preparation which contains any quantity of the following substances:
(1) Immediate precursor to amphetamine and methamphetamine:
(i) Phenylacetone
Some trade or other names: phenyl-2-propanone; P2P; benzyl methyl ketone; methyl benzyl ketone
(2) Immediate precursors to phencyclidine (PCP):
(i) 1-phenylcyclohexylamine
(ii) 1-piperidinocyclohexanecarbonitrile (PCC)

SCHEDULE III

(a) *Stimulants.* Unless specifically excepted or unless listed in another schedule, any material, compound, mixture, or preparation which contains any quantity of the following substances having a stimulant effect on the central nervous system, including its salts, isomers (whether optical, position, or geometric), and salts of such isomers whenever the existence of such salts, isomers, and salts of isomers is possible within the specific chemical designation.
(1) Those compounds, mixtures, or preparations in dosage unit form containing any stimulant substances listed in schedule II which compounds, mixtures, or preparations were listed on August 25, 1971, as excepted compounds under § 308.32, and any other drug of the quantitive composition shown in that list for those drugs or which is the same except that it contains a lesser quantity of controlled substances.
(2) Benzphetamine
(3) Chlorphentermine
(4) Clortermine
(5) Phendimetrazine

(b) *Depressants.* Unless specifically excepted or unless listed in another schedule, any material, compound, mixture, or preparation which contains any quantity of the following substances having a depressant effect on the central nervous system:
(1) Any compound, mixture or preparation containing:
(i) Amobarbital
(ii) Secobarbital
(iii) Pentobarbital
or any salt thereof and one or more other active medicinal ingredients which are not listed in any schedule.
(2) Any suppository dosage form containing:
(i) Amobarbital
(ii) Secobarbital
(iii) Pentobarbital
or any salt of any of these drugs and approved by the Food and Drug Administration for marketing only as a suppository.
(3) Any substance which contains any quantity of a derivative of barbituric acid or any salt thereof:
(4) Chlorhexado
(5) Glutethimide
(6) Lysergic acid
(7) Lysergic acid amide
(8) Methypryion
(9) Sulfondiethylmethane
(10) Sulfonethylmethane
(11) Sulfonmethane

(c) Nalorphine 9400.

Narcotic Drugs

(d) Unless specifically excepted or unless listed in another schedule, any material, compound, mixture, or preparation containing limited quantities of any of the following narcotic drugs, or any salts thereof:
(1) Not more than 1.8 grams of codeine per 100 milliliters or not more than 90 milligrams per dosage unit, with an equal or greater quantity of an isoquinoline alkaloid of opium.
(2) Not more than 1.8 grams of codeine per 100 milliliters or not more than 90 milligrams. per dosage unit. With one or more active, non-narcotic ingredients in recognized therapeutic amounts
(3) Not more than 300 milligrams of dihydrocodeinone per 100 milliliters or not more than 15 milligrams per dosage unit, with a

fourfold or greater quantity of an isoquinoline alkaloid of opium
(4) Not more than 300 milligrams of dihydrocodeinone per 100 milliliters or not more than 15 milligrams per dosage unit, with one or more active, non-narcotic ingredients in recognized therapeutic amounts
(5) Not more than 1.8 grams of dihydrocodeine per 100 milliliters or not more than 90 milligrams per dosage unit, with one or more active, non-narcotic ingredients in recognized therapeutic amounts
(6) Not more than 300 milligrams of ethylmorphine per 100 milliliters or not more than 15 milligrams per dosage unit, with one or more active, non-narcotic ingredients in recognized therapeutic amounts
(7) Not more than 500 milligrams of opium per 100 milliliters or per 100 grams, or not more than 25 milligrams per dosage unit, with one or more active, non-narcotic ingredients in recognized therapeutic amounts
(8) Not more than 50 milligrams of morphine per 100 milliliters or per 100 grams with one or more active, non-narcotic ingredients in recognized therapeutic amounts

SCHEDULE IV

(b) *Narcotic drugs.* Unless specifically excepted or unless listed in another schedule, any material, compound, mixture, or preparation containing any of the following narcotic drugs, or their salts calculated as the free anhydrous base or alkaloid, in limited quantities as set forth below:

(1) Not more than 1 milligram of difenoxin (DEA Drug Code No. 9168) and not less than 25 micrograms of atropine sulfate per dosage unit.

(2) Dextropropoxphene (alpha-(+)-4-dimethylamino-1,2-diphenyl-3-methyl-2-propionoxybutane)

(c) *Depressants.* Unless specifically excepted or unless listed in another schedule, any material, compound, mixture, or preparation which contains any quantity of the following substances, including its salts, isomers, and salts of isomers whenever the existence of such salts, isomers, and salts of isomers is possible within the specific chemical designation:

(1) Alprazolam
(2) Barbital
(3) Bromazepam
(4) Camazepam
(5) Chloral betaine
(6) Chloral hydrate
(7) Chlordiazepoxide
(8) Clobazam
(9) Clonazepam
(10) Clorazepate
(11) Clotiazepam
(12) Cloxazolam
(13) Delorazepam
(14) Diazepam
(15) Estazolam
(16) Ethchlorvynol
(17) Ethinamate
(18) Ethyl loflazepate
(19) Fludiazepam
(20) Flunitrazepam
(21) Flurazepam
(22) Halazepam
(23) Haloxazolam
(24) Ketazolam
(25) Loprazolam
(26) Lorazepam
(27) Lormetazepam
(28) Mebutamate
(29) Medazepam
(30) Meprobamate
(31) Methohexital
(32) Methylphenobarbital (mephobarbital)
(33) Nimetazepam
(34) Nitrazepam
(35) Nordiazepam
(36) Oxazepam
(37) Oxazolam
(38) Paraldehyde
(39) Petrichloral
(40) Phenobarbital
(41) Pinazepam
(42) Prazepam
(43) Temazepam
(44) Tetrazepam
(45) Triazolam

(d) *Fenfluramine.* Any material, compound, mixture, or preparation which contains any quantity of the following substances, including its salts, isomers (whether optical, position, or geometric), and salts of such isomers, when the existence of such salts, isomers, and salts of isomers is possible:

(1) Fenfluramine

(e) *Stimulants.* Unless specifically excepted or unless listed in another schedule, any material, compound, mixture, or preparation which contains any quantity of the following substances having a stimulant effect on the central nervous system, including its salts, isomers, (whether optical, position, or geometric), and salts of such isomers whenever the existence of such salts, isomers, and salts of isomers is possible within the specific chemical designation:

(1) Diethylpropion
(2) Mazindol
(3) Pemoline (including organometallic comlexes and chelates thereof)
(4) Phentermine
(5) Pipradrol
(6) SPA ((-)-1-dimethylamino-1,2,-diphenylethane)

(f) *Other substances.* Unless specifically excepted or unless listed in another schedule, any material, compound, mixture or preparation which contains any quantity of the following substances, including its salts:

(1) Pentazocine

SCHEDULE V

(b) *Narcotic drugs.* Unless specifically excepted or unless listed in another schedule, any material, compound, mixture, or preparation containing any of the following narcotic drugs and their salts, as set forth below:

(c) Narcotic drugs containing non-narcotic active medicinal ingredients. Any compound, mixture, or preparation containing any of the following limited quantities of narcotic drugs or salts thereof, which shall include one or more non-narcotic active medicinal ingredients in sufficient proportion to confer upon the compound, mixture, or preparation valuable medicinal qualities other than those possessed by the narcotic drug alone:

(1) Not more than 200 milligrams of codeine per 100 milliliters or per 100 grams.

(2) Not more than 100 milligrams of dihydrocodeine per 100 milliliters or per 100 grams.

(3) Not more than 100 milligrams of ethylmorphine per 100 milliliters or per 100 grams.

(4) Not more than 2.5 milligrams of diphenoxylate and not less than 25 micrograms of atropine sulfate per dosage unit.

(5) Not more than 100 milligrams of opium per 100 milliliters or per 100 grams.

(6) Not more than 0.5 milligram of difenoxin (DEA Drug Code No. 9168) and not less than 25 micrograms of atropine sulfate per dosage unit.

[39 FR 22143, June 20, 1974]

For information on excluded non-narcotic substances, exempt chemical preparations, and excepted stimulant or depressant compounds see 21 CFR 1308.21-1308.24 and 21 CFR 1308.31-1308.32.

Appendix 11

Diagnostic Laboratories

Alabama
State of Alabama Veterinary Diagnostic Laboratory
P.O. Box 127
Albertville, 35950
205-878-2471

Charles S. Roberts Veterinary Diagnostic Laboratory
P.O. Box 2209
Auburn, 36830
205-887-3433 (FTS)
534-4551

Poultry Producers Diagnostic Laboratory
1724-A 2nd Ave.
Cullman, 35055
205-739-1414

Alaska
Alaska State Federal Laboratory
P.O. Box 1088
Palmer, 99645
907-745-3236

Arizona
Arizona State Department of Health
1520 West Adams St.
Phoenix, 85007
602-255-1188

Department of Veterinary Science,
University of Arizona
Tucson, 85721
602-626-2356

Arkansas
Federal Brucellosis Laboratory
1 Natural Resources Drive
Little Rock, 72205
501-224-0525 (FTS)
740-5253

Arkansas Livestock and Poultry Commission
Diagnostic Laboratory
Highway 71 N., 3405 N. Thompson
Springdale, 72764
501-751-4869

Fish Farming Experimental Station
Box 860
Stuttgart, 72160
501-673-8761

California
County of Los Angeles
Department of Health Services Division
Comparative Medical and
Veterinary Public Health Service
12824 Erickson Ave.
Downey, 90242
213-922-8801

State of California Department of
Food and Agriculture Laboratory Services
2789 South Orange Ave.
Fresno, 93725
209-266-9418

Wildlife Investigations Laboratory
1701 Nimbus Road Suite D,
Rancho Cordova, 95670
916-355-0124

California Department of Agriculture
Veterinary Laboratory Services
3290 Meadowview Road
Sacramento, 95823
916-428-3172

San Diego County Veterinary Laboratory
5555 Overland Avenue, Bldg. 4
San Diego, 92123
714-565-5400

California Department of Agriculture
Veterinary Laboratory Services
P.O. Box 5579
San Bernardino, 92412
714-383-4287

Colorado
Veterinary Diagnostic Laboratory
Colorado State University
Fort Collins, 80523
303-491-6128

Connecticut
Department of Pathobiology
Box U-89 University of Connecticut
Storrs, 06268
203-486-3736

Delaware
Division of Standards and Inspection
State Department of Agriculture, Poultry and
Animal Health Section
P.O. Drawer D
Dover, 19901
302-736-4811 (FTS) 302-487-5122

Florida
State of Florida Department of Agriculture
Bureau of Diagnostic Laboratories
P.O. Box 460
Kissimmee, 32741
302-847-3185

Bureau of Diagnostic Laboratories, Miami Branch
(Direct all correspondence to Kissimmee, Fla., branch)
8701 N.W. 58th Street
Miami, 33178
305-592-3059

Georgia
Diagnostic Assistance Laboratory
College of Veterinary Medicine
University of Georgia
Athens, 30602
404-542-5568

Diagnostic and Investigational Laboratories
Route 2 Brighton Road
Tifton, 31793
912-386-3340

Hawaii
Hawaii Department of Agriculture
Veterinary Laboratory Branch
99-762 Moanalua Road
Aiea, 96701
808-488-3640

Idaho
Idaho Bureau of Animal Health Laboratories
P.O. Box 7249
Boise, 83707
208-334-3111

Illinois
Laboratories of Veterinary Diagnostic Medicine
University of Illinois
Urbana, 61801
217-333-1620

Indiana
Animal Disease Diagnostic Laboratory
School of Veterinary Medicine
Purdue University
West Lafayette, 47907
317-494-7440

Iowa
Veterinary Diagnostic Laboratory
Iowa State University
Ames, 50011
515-294-1950 (FTS) 865-1950

Kansas
Veterinary Diagnostic Laboratory
College of Veterinary Medicine
Manhattan, 66506
913-532-5650

Kentucky
Murray State University Diagnostic
and Research Center
P.O. Box 2000, North Drive
Hopkinsville, 42240

Louisiana
Louisiana Veterinary Medical
Diagnostic Laboratory
Louisiana State University
Baton Rouge, 70803
504-346-3193

Central Louisiana Livestock Diagnostic
Laboratory
Route 2, Box 51-F
Lecompte, 71346
318-443-6993

Northwest Louisiana Livestock Diagnostic and
Research Laboratory
P.O. Box 2156
Natchitoches, 71457
318-352-6272

Maine
University of Maine Pathology Diagnostic and
Research Laboratory
Hitchner Hall
Orono, 04473
207-581-7521

Maryland
Maryland Department of Agriculture
Animal Health Department Laboratory
4901 Calvert Road
College Park, 20740
301-454-3631

Massachusetts
Large Animal Diagnostic Laboratory
Paige Laboratory
University of Massachusetts
Amherst, 01003
413-545-2427

Michigan
Wildlife Pathology Laboratory
Michigan Department of Natural Resources
8562 E. Stoll Road R1
East Lansing, 48823
517-373-9358

Michigan Department of Agriculture
Laboratory Division
1615 S. Harrison Road
East Lansing, 48823
517-373-6410

Minnesota
Veterinary Diagnostic Laboratories
E220 Diagnostic and Research Building
College of Veterinary Medicine
University of Minnesota
St. Paul, 55101
612-373-0774

Mississippi
Mississippi Veterinary Diagnostic Laboratory
P.O. Box 4389
Jackson, 39216
601-354-6091

Missouri
Veterinary Medical Diagnostic Laboratory
College of Veterinary Medicine
University of Missouri
Columbia, 65211
314-882-6811 (FTS 875-5278)

Ralston Purina Veterinary Laboratory,
Veterinary Service Department
Checkerboard Square
St. Louis, 63164
314-982-2611

Montana
State of Montana Department of Livestock
Animal Health Division, Diagnostic Laboratory
P.O. Box 997
Bozeman, 59715
406-586-8558 (FTS) 585-4339

Nebraska
Diagnostic Laboratory
Department of Veterinary Science
University of Nebraska
Lincoln, 68583
402-472-1434 (FTS) 472-3818

Nevada
Animal Disease Laboratory,
Nevada Department of Agriculture
P.O. Box 11100
350 Capitol Hill Avenue
Reno, 89510
702-784-6229

New Hampshire
Veterinary Diagnostic Laboratory
University of New Hampshire
Durham, 03824
603-862-2726

New Jersey
Rutgers Poultry Health Laboratory
2569 Landis Ave.
Vineland, 08360
609-691-0360

New Mexico
State Federal Cooperative Laboratory
P.O. Box 464
Albuquerque, 87103
505-766-2573 (FTS)
474-2573

New York
Cornell University Duck Research Laboratory
Box 217 Old Country Road
Eastport, 11941
516-325-0600

Diagnostic Laboratory
New York State Veterinary College
at Cornell University
Box 786
Ithaca, 14850
607-256-6541

North Carolina
Rollins Animal Disease Diagnostic Laboratory
P.O. Box 12223
Cameron Village Station
Raleigh, 27605
919-733-3986

North Dakota
North Dakota State Veterinary Diagnostic Lab
North Dakota State University
Fargo, 58102
701-237-7511

Ohio
Ohio State University
Department of Veterinary Clinical Sciences
Clinical Path Lab
1935 Coffey Road
Columbus, 43210
614-422-1202

Oklahoma
Oklahoma Animal Disease Diagnostic Laboratory
College of Veterinary Medicine
Oklahoma State University
Stillwater, 74074
405-624-6623

Oregon
Oregon State Veterinary Diagnostic Laboratory
Oregon State University
Corvallis, 97339
503-754-3261

Pennsylvania
Division of Clinical Laboratory Medicine
School of Veterinary Medicine
Department of Clinical Studies
University of Pennsylvania
3800 Spruce Street
Philadelphia, 19174
215-243-7891

Laboratory of Pathology, School of Veterinary
Medicine, University of Pennsylvania
3800 Spruce St.
Philadelphia, 19104
215-898-8859

Pennsylvania Department of Agriculture
Bureau of Animal Industry Laboratory
Summerdale, 17093
717-787-8808 (FTS) 637-8808

Puerto Rico
Institute of Health Laboratories
Box 10427
Caparra Heights Station
Rio Piedras, 00922
809-764-8585

Rhode Island
Diagnostic Laboratory Department of Animal
Pathology
University of Rhode Island
Kingston, 02881
401-792-2487

South Carolina
Clemson University
Livestock-Poultry Health Department
P.O. Box 218
Elgin, 29045
803-788-2260 (FTS) 779-6760

South Dakota
Animal Disease Research and Diagnostic
Laboratory
South Dakota State University
Brookings, 57007
605-688-5171

Tennessee
C.E. Kord Animal Disease Laboratory
P.O. Box 40627 Mel. Sta.
Nashville, 37204
615-741-1506 (FTS) 853-1506

Texas
Texas Veterinary Medical Diagnostic Laboratory
Drawer 3040

College Station, 77841
713-845-3414

Utah
Utah State University Veterinary Diagnostic Laboratory
Utah State University
Logan, 84321
801-750-1880

State Chemist Office and State Federal Cooperative Laboratory
360 North Redwood Road
Salt Lake City, 84116
801-533-5421

Vermont
Animal Health Laboratory
Hills Science Building
University of Vermont
Burlington, 05405
802-656-2650

Virginia
Division of Animal Health and Dairies Regulatory Laboratory
116 Reservoir Street
Harrisonburg, 22801
703-434-3897

Washington
Washington Animal Disease Diagnostic Laboratory
Washington State University
P.O. Box 2037, College Station
Pullman, 99163
509-335-9696

Poultry Diagnostic Laboratory
Western Washington Research and Extension Center
Washington State University
Puyallup, 98371
206-593-8536

West Virginia
State Federal Cooperative Animal Health Laboratory
4720 Brenda Lane
Charleston, 25312
304-348-3418, 304-348-2231, and 304-348-2214 (FTS) 885-3418

Wisconsin
National Wildlife Health Laboratory
6006 Schroeder Road
Madison, 53711
608-252-5411 (FTS) 364-5411

Wyoming
Wyoming State Veterinary Laboratory
Box 950
Laramie, 82070
307-742-6638

Appendix 12

Food-Animal Withdrawal Times

BABY PIG DRUG LIST

Active Ingredients	Withdrawal Days
INJECTABLE	
Lincomycin	2
Erythromycin	2
ORAL	
Chlortetracycline hydrochloride	1
Spectinomycin dihydrochloride pentahydrate	21
Thiabendazole paste	30

BEEF CALF DRUG LIST

Active Ingredients	Withdrawal Days
INJECTABLE	
Sodium sulfachlorpyridazine	5
Sulfadimethoxine	7
Dihydrostreptomycin	30
Erythromycin	14
Levamisole	7
Oxytetracycline	15–22
Procaine penicillin G (*varies with brand name)	5–30*
Procaine penicillin G and dihydrostreptomycin	30
Sulfamethazine	10
Tylosin	21
ORAL	
Chlorhexidine dihydrochloride and dihydrostreptomycin sulfate	3
Chlortetracycline hydrochloride	1–3
Chlortetracycline bisulfate	3
Dihydrostreptomyin	30
Streptomycin	2
Sulfachlorpyridazine	7
Sulfamethazine, streptomycin, phthalysulfathiazole, and Kaolin	10
Tetracycline hydrochloride	12

Beef Calf Drug List (Cont.)

Active Ingredients	Withdrawal Days
Amprolium	Withdrawal Times for these drugs are listed in the Beef Cattle Section.
Chlortetracycline	
Chlortetracycline and sulfamethazine	
Famphur	
Haloxon	
Levamisole	
Ronnel	
Sulfabromomethazine	
Sulfadimethoxine	
Sulfamethazine	
Tetracycline	
IMPLANT	
Zeranol	65

BEEF CATTLE DRUG LIST

Active Ingredients	Withdrawal Days
INJECTABLE	
Dihydrostreptomycin	30
Erythromycin	14
Levamisole phosphate	7
Oxytetracycline	15–22
Procaine penicillin G (*varies with brand name)	5–30*
Procaine penicillin G and dihydrostreptomycin sulfate	30
Sulfadimethoxine	5
Sulfamethazine	10
Tylosin	21
LA-200	28
ORAL	
Amprolium	1
Chlortetracycline hydrochloride	2–3 (350 mg/head)
Chlortetracycline sulfamethazine	7
Famphur	4
Haloxon	7
Levamisole	2
Melengestrol acetate	2
Ronnel	10
Sulfabromomethazine	10

Beef Cattle Drug List (Cont.)

Sulfadimethoxine (*varies with dosage form)	7–12*
Sulfamethazine (*varies with dosage form)	10–28*
Sulfaquinoxaline	10
Tetracycline hydrochloride	5
Thiabendazole	3
TOPICAL	
Famphur	35
Fenthion	35–45
N-(mercaptomethyl) phthalimide S-(0,0-dimethyl phosphorodithioate)	21
IMPLANT	
Estradiol benzoate and testosterone propionate	60
Progesterone and estradiol benzoate	60
Zeranol	65

DAIRY CALF DRUG LIST

Active Ingredients	Withdrawal Days
INJECTABLE	
Dihydrostreptomycin sulfate	30
Erythromycin	14
Levamisole	7
Oxytetracycline	15–22
Procaine penicillin G	5
Procaine penicillin G and dihydrostreptomycin sulfate	30
Sodium sulfachlorpyridazine	5
Sulfamethazine	10
Sulfadimethoxine	7
Tylosin	8
ORAL	
Amprolium	1
Chlortetracycline hydrochloride	1–3
Chlortetracycline bisulfate (water)	3
Chlortetracycline and neomycin	1
Haloxon	7
Levamisole hydrochloride	2
Streptomycin	30
Sulfabromomethazine	10
Sulfachlorpyridazine	7
Sulfadimethoxine	7
Sulfamethazine	10
Sulfamethazine, streptomycin, phythalylsulfathiazole and kaolin	10
Tetracycline hydrochloride (water)	5
Thiabendazole	3
TOPICAL	
Famphur	35
Fenthion (add 45 days if retreated)	35–45

SHEEP AND GOAT DRUG LIST

Active Ingredients	Withdrawal Days	Milk Discard Milking (Hours)
INJECTABLE		
Dihydrostreptomycin sulfate	30	—
Erythromycin (sheep only)	3	—
Procaine pencillin G	5	6 (72)
Procaine penicillin G and dihydrostreptomycin (sheep only)	30	4 (48)
Sulfamethazine (sheep only)	10	
ORAL		
4-tert-Butyl-2-chlorophenyl methyl methylphosphoramidate	7	—
Haloxon	7	—
Levamisole (sheep only)	3	—
Sulfaquinoxaline	10	
Sulfisoxazole (sheep only)	10	
Thiabendazole	30	8 (96)
IMPLANT		
Zeranol (feedlot lambs only)	40	
INTRAVAGINAL		
Flurogestone acetate (sheep only)	30	

SWINE DRUG LIST

Active Ingredients	Withdrawal Days
INJECTABLE	
Dihydrostreptomycin	30
Erythromycin	7
Lincomycin	2
Oxytetracycline	20–26
Procaine penicillin G	7
Procaine penicillin G and dihydrostreptomycin	30
Sulfamethazine	15
Tylosin	14
LA-200	28
ORAL	
Arsanilic acid	5
Carbadox	70 (10 weeks)

Swine Drug List (Cont.)

Chlortetracycline (water)	1–5
Chlortetracycline bisulfate and sulfamethazine (feed)	15
Chlortetracycline, sulfamethazine, and procaine penicillin (feed)	15
Chlortetracycline, sulfathiazole, and procaine penicillin (feed)	7
Furazolidone	5
Hygromycin B	2
Levamisole (feed or water)	3
Lincomycin (feed)	6
Nitrofurazone	5

Swine Drug List (Cont.)

Procaine penicillin G and streptomycin sulfate (water)	2
Pyrantel tartrate	1
Roxarsone	5
Sodium arsanilate	5
Sodium sulfachlorpyridazine	4
Sodium sulfathiazole	10
Sulfamethazine	15
Sulfaquinoxaline	10
Tetracycline hydrochloride (water)	4
Tylosin (with vitamins)	2
Tylosin and sulfamethazine	15

Memorandum

Memorandum

Memorandum

Memorandum

Memorandum

Memorandum